CLINICAL
NUTRITION
Volume 1

Enteral and Tube Feeding

JOHN L. ROMBEAU, M.D.

Assistant Professor of Surgery,
University of Pennsylvania School of Medicine
Director, Nutritional Support Service and
    Surgical Metabolic Unit
Veterans Administration Medical Center
Philadelphia, Pennsylvania

MICHAEL D. CALDWELL, M.D., Ph.D.

Associate Professor, Section of Surgery
Brown University
Director, Nutritional Support Service and
    Surgical Metabolism Laboratory
Rhode Island Hospital
Providence, Rhode Island

Illustrations by David Low, M.D.

W.B. SAUNDERS COMPANY
Philadelphia•London•Toronto•Mexico City•Rio de Janeiro•Sydney•Tokyo

W. B. Saunders Company: West Washington Square
Philadelphia, PA 19105

1 St. Anne's Road
Eastbourne, East Sussex BN21 3UN, England

1 Goldthorne Avenue
Toronto, Ontario M8Z 5T9, Canada

Apartado 26370—Cedro 512
Mexico 4, D.F., Mexico

Rua Coronel Cabrita, 8
Sao Cristovao Caixa Postal 21176
Rio de Janeiro, Brazil

9 Waltham Street
Artarmon, N.S.W. 2064, Australia

Ichibancho, Central Bldg., 22–1 Ichibancho
Chiyoda-Ku, Tokyo 102, Japan

Library of Congress Cataloging in Publication Data
Main entry under title:

Enteral and tube feeding.

    (Clinical nutrition ; v. 1)
    1. Enteral feeding.   2. Tube feeding.   I. Rombeau,
John L.   II. Caldwell, Michael D.   III. Title.
IV. Series. [DNLM: 1. Nutrition.   2. Enteral feeding.
WB 400 C641]
RM216.C5775   1984   vol. 1   615.8′323s   83-2864
[RM225]   [615.8′323]
ISBN 0-7216-7644-8

ENTERAL AND TUBE FEEDING
Volume 1 of Clinical Nutrition   ISBN   0-7216-7644-8

Last digit is the print number: 9   8   7   6   5   4   3   2

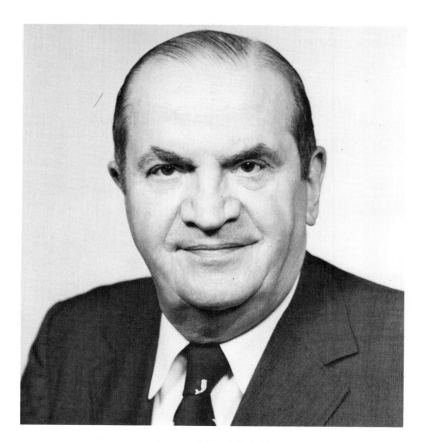

Henry T. Randall, M.D.

Contributors

CARL F. ANDERSON, M.D.

Professor of Medicine and Nephrology, Mayo Medical School; Consultant in Medicine and Nephrology, Mayo Clinic, Rochester, Minnesota

KEITH N. APELGREN, M.D.

Research Fellow, Brigham & Women's Hospital, Boston, Massachusetts

LENORA R. BAROT, M.D.

Instructor in Surgery, University of Pennsylvania School of Medicine, Philadelphia, Pennsylvania

CATHERINE H. BASTIAN, M.A., R.D.

Clinical Dietitian, Nutrition Service, Geisinger Medical Center, Danville, Pennsylvania

STACEY J. BELL, R.D.

Research Dietitian, Shriners Burns Institute, Boston, Massachusetts

MARIE BERNARD, M.D.

Assistant Professor of Medicine, Temple University School of Medicine; Co-director, Nutrition Support Service, Temple University Hospital, Philadelphia, Pennsylvania

JAMES BETZHOLD, M.D.

Assistant Director and Assistant Professor of Pediatrics, Albany Medical College, Albany, New York

PRESTON R. BLACK, M.D.

Clinical Fellow in Surgery, Harvard Medical School; Fellow in Pediatric Surgery, Children's Hospital Medical Center, Boston, Massachusetts

MARCIA C. BORAAS, M.D.

Instructor in Surgery, Department of Surgery, University of Pennsylvania School of Medicine, Philadelphia, Pennsylvania

JOHN F. BURKE, M.D.

Helen Andrus Benedict Professor of Surgery, Harvard Medical School; Chief of Trauma Services, Massachusetts General Hospital, Boston, Massachusetts

GORDON P. BUZBY, M.D.

Assistant Professor of Surgery, University of Pennsylvania School of Medicine; Attending Surgeon, Hospital of the University of Pennsylvania; Chief, General Surgery Section, Philadelphia Veterans Administration Medical Center, Philadelphia, Pennsylvania

MICHAEL D. CALDWELL, M.D., PH.D.

Associate Professor of Surgery, Division of Biology and Medicine, Section of Surgery, Brown University Program in Medicine; Director, Nutrition Support Service and Surgical Metabolism Laboratories, Rhode Island Hospital, Providence, Rhode Island

RONNI CHERNOFF

Associate Chief of CRECC for Education and Evaluation, Little Rock Veterans Administration Hospital, Little Rock, Arkansas

DANIEL DEBONIS, M.D.

Nutrition Research Fellow, Department of Clinical Nutrition, City of Hope National Medical Center, Duarte, California

SUSAN J. DEHOOG, R.D.

Director of Clinical Nutrition, University of Washington Hospital, Seattle, Washington

RICHARD H. DRISCOLL, JR., M.D.

Associate Clinical Professor of Medicine, Pennsylvania State University School of Medicine, Hershey, Pennsylvania; Associate, Department of Gastroenterology and Nutrition, Geisinger Medical Center, Danville, Pennsylvania

REBECCA MILLER ESVELT, R.D.

Consulting Dietitian, University of Washington Hospital, Seattle, Washington

LORETTA FORLAW, M.S.N., R.N., MAJOR A.N.C.

Nutritional Support Clinical Nurse Specialist, Department of Nursing, Walter Reed Army Medical Center, Washington, D.C.

RICHARD D. GOODENOUGH, M.D.

Resident and Instructor in Surgery, University of Rochester School of Medicine and Dentistry, Rochester, New York

GREGORY E. GRAY, PH.D.

Nutrition Fellow, Department of Clinical Nutrition, City of Hope National Medical Center, Duarte, California

HARRY L. GREENE, M.D.

Professor of Pediatrics, Vanderbilt University School of Medicine; Head, Division of Pediatric Gastroenterology, and Director, Clinical Nutrition Research Unit, Vanderbilt University Hospital, Nashville, Tennessee

BARBARA C. HANSEN, PH.D.

Associate Vice-President for Research and Dean of the Graduate School; Professor, Department of Physiology, School of Medicine; and Professor, Department of Psychology, College of Liberal Arts, Southern Illinois University, Carbondale, Illinois

LYN HOWARD, M.D.

Associate Professor of Medicine, Department of Pediatric Gastroenterology, Albany Medical College, Albany, New York

DANNY O. JACOBS, M.D.

Assistant Instructor in Surgery, University of Pennsylvania School of Medicine; Senior Resident in Surgery, Hospital of the University of Pennsylvania; Fellow in Nutrition and Metabolism, Philadelphia Veterans Administration Medical Center, Philadelphia, Pennsylvania

CHRISTINE KENNEDY-CALDWELL, M.S.N., R.N., C.S.

Pediatric Nutritionist and Clinical Nurse Specialist, Nutrition Support Service, Department of Surgery and Department of Nursing (Pediatric Division), Rhode Island Hospital, Providence, Rhode Island

P. P. KEOHANE, M.B., B.S., M.R.C.P.

Research Fellow in Clinical Nutrition, Department of Gastroenterology and Nutrition, Central Middlesex Hospital, London, England

G. M. LEVINE, M.D.

Associate Professor of Medicine, Temple University School of Medicine; Head, Division of Gastroenterology and Nutrition, Albert Einstein Northern Division, Philadelphia, Pennsylvania

DAVID A. LIPSCHITZ, M.D., PH.D.

Professor of Medicine, and Chief, Division of Hematology/Oncology, University of Arkansas Medical Sciences and Little Rock Veterans Administration Medical Center, Little Rock, Arkansas

DAVID W. LOW, M.D.

Clinical Instructor in Surgery, Hospital of the University of Pennsylvania, Philadelphia, Pennsylvania

MAUREEN M. MACBURNEY, R.D., M.S.

Assistant Director, Nutrition Support Service, Brigham & Women's Hospital, Boston, Massachusetts

GORDON K. McLEAN, M.D.

Associate Professor of Radiology, University of Pennsylvania School of Medicine; Chief, Angiography and Interventional Radiology Section, Department of Radiology, Hospital of the University of Pennsylvania, Philadelphia, Pennsylvania

MICHAEL M. MEGUID, M.D., PH.D.

Assistant Clinical Professor of Surgery, University of California, Los Angeles, School of Medicine; Associate Surgeon, Division of Surgery, and Director, Department of Clinical Nutrition, City of Hope National Medical Center, Duarte, California

GEORGE MELNIK, B.S. PHARMACY, R.PHARMACIST

Nutritional Support Pharmacist, Philadelphia Veterans Administration Medical Center, Philadelphia, Pennsylvania

THOMAS A. MILLER, M.D., F.A.C.S.

Associate Professor of Surgery and Director of Graduate Surgical Education, Department of Surgery, The University of Texas Medical School at Houston; Attending Surgeon, and Assistant Chief, "C" Surgical Service, Hermann Hospital, Houston, Texas

JOSEPH A. MOLNAR, M.D.

Research Fellow, Harvard Medical School, and Department of Surgery, Massachusetts General Hospital, Boston, Massachusetts

J. ROBERTO MORAN, M.D.

Assistant Professor of Pediatrics, Vanderbilt University School of Medicine; Attending Pediatric Gastroenterologist, Vanderbilt University Hospital, Nashville, Tennessee

JAMES L. MULLEN, M.D.

Associate Professor of Surgery, University of Pennsylvania School of Medicine; Attending Surgeon, Hospital of the University of Pennsylvania; Chief, Surgical Service, Philadelphia Veterans Administration Medical Center, Philadelphia, Pennsylvania

HENRY T. RANDALL, M.D., M.Sc.D. (SURGERY)

Professor Emeritus of Medical Science, Brown University Program in Medicine; Consulting Surgeon, Rhode Island Hospital, The Miriam Hospital, and Providence Veterans Administration Medical Center, Providence, Rhode Island

JOHN L. ROMBEAU, M.D.

Assistant Professor of Surgery, University of Pennsylvania School of Medicine, Hospital of the University of Pennsylvania and Philadelphia Veterans Administration Hospital, Philadelphia, Pennsylvania

BRIAN J. ROWLANDS, M.D., F.R.C.S.

Associate Professor of Surgery, The University of Texas Medical School at Houston; Attending Surgeon and Director of Nutritional Support Services, Hermann Hospital, Houston, Texas

VAL SELIVANOV, M.D.

N.I.H. Trauma & Burn Research Fellow, University of California, San Francisco, at San Francisco General Hospital

R. GREGG SETTLE, Ph.D.

Assistant Research Professor, Department of Otorhinolaryngology, University of Pennsylvania and the Philadelphia Veterans Administration Hospital Medical Center, Philadelphia, Pennsylvania

GEORGE F. SHELDON, M.D.

Professor of Surgery, University of California, San Francisco, School of Medicine; Chief, Trauma & Hyperalimentation Services, San Francisco General Hospital, San Francisco, California

D. B. A. SILK

Consultant Physician and Co-director, Department of Gastroenterology and Nutrition, Central Middlesex Hospital, London, England

WILLIAM P. STEFFEE, M.D., Ph.D.

Director, Department of Medicine, St. Vincent Charity Hospital & Health Center, Cleveland, Ohio

T. P. STEIN, Ph.D.

Associate Professor, University of Pennsylvania School of Medicine; Director, Nutritional Support Service, Graduate Hospital, Philadelphia, Pennsylvania

JAMES N. St. JOHN, M.D.

Assistant Professor of Neurological Surgery, University of California, Davis, School of Medicine; Chief, Neurological Surgery, Department of Surgery, Veterans Administration Medical Center, Martinez, California

PATRICK L. TWOMEY, M.D.

Assistant Professor of Surgery, University of California, Davis, School of Medicine; Chief, Gastrointestinal Surgery, Department of Surgery, Veterans Administration Medical Center, Martinez, California

DONALD M. WATKIN, M.D., M.P.H.

Manager, Occupational Health Division, Office of Aviation Medicine, Federal Aviation Administration, U.S. Department of Transportation; Research Professor of Medicine, George Washington University School of Medicine and Health Sciences, Washington, D.C.

ELLIOT WESER, M.D.

Professor and Deputy Chairman, Department of Medicine, Division of Gastroenterology and Nutrition, University of Texas Health Science Center at San Antonio; Staff Physician, Medical Center Hospital; Chief, Medicine Service, Audie L. Murphy Memorial Veterans Hospital, San Antonio, Texas

DOUGLAS W. WILMORE, M.D.

Director, Nutritional Support Service, and Surgeon, Brigham & Women's Hospital; Associate Professor of Surgery, Harvard Medical School, Boston, Massachusetts

KATHERINE WRIGHT, M.S.

Department of Pharmacy, Philadelphia Veterans Administration Medical Center, Philadelphia, Pennsylvania

ELEANOR A. YOUNG, Ph.D.

Associate Professor, Department of Medicine, Division of Gastroenterology and Nutrition, University of Texas Health Science Center at San Antonio; Consultant, Medical Center Hospital and Audie L. Murphy Memorial Veterans Hospital, San Antonio, Texas

LORRAINE SEE YOUNG, R.D., M.S.

Clinical Dietitian, Nutritional Support Service, Brigham & Women's Hospital, Boston, Massachusetts

Foreword

JONATHAN E. RHOADS

In previous studies of enteral nutrition at the Hospital of the University of Pennsylvania, both the rectal route and the jejunal route have been explored. The rectal route had broad appeal nearly a century ago, when a variety of nutrient enemas were used in medical practice. The original calorie-containing mixtures contained primarily milk and eggs with additives such as caffeine and whiskey. Their value was disputed in a study published by Edsal and Miller in 1902,[1] who analyzed the nitrogen in stools of patients who received these nutrient enemas. Their results showed that the majority of nitrogen contained in the protein of the enema was recovered in the stool.

The simplest large-bowel infusions were usually water or a 0.9 per cent sodium chloride solution. They were often given slowly by gravity drip, in a process called proctoclysis. Indeed the rectal route was widely used at the Hospital of the University of Pennsylvania when I began internship there in 1932. On one of the surgical services, the practice was to infuse a liter of water or physiologic saline solution while the patient was still under anesthesia. The other surgical service connected a rectal tube to an elevated bottle with the flow regulated by a screw clamp. The first service depended on anesthesia and opiates to prevent evacuation of the solution; the second service used a slow rate of administration to accomplish the same end.

Dr. Walter Ebeling, a surgical trainee with the late Dr. Eldridge Eliason, conducted laboratory studies on the effect of adding glucose to the proctoclysis. He showed that the net glucose absorption did not appear to increase beyond a 2 per cent concentration. More basic work was done in 1912 by Folin and Denis[2] at Harvard, who tested the absorption of alanine, glycine, and Witte's peptone in large bowel loops of cats. They were able to demonstrate absorption of amino acids and some larger protein moieties through an increase in non-protein nitrogen in the portal blood. In Germany, Abderhalden and associates achieved a brief period of nitrogen balance in a patient by infusing hydrolyzed protein into the rectum. In 1936 a group of workers at the University of Pennsylvania studied isolated loops of large bowel to exclude the possibility that small bowel enzymes enter the large bowel and further hydrolyze the introduced food. Again, absorption of amino acids, polypeptides, and some peptones appeared to take place. Such absorption was also demonstrated in isolated small bowel loops at an increased rate. At the suggestion of Dr. I. S. Ravdin, a two-lumen tube was designed by Dr. W. Osler Abbott and Mr. A. J. Rawson[5] to be used for jejunal feeding. One lumen was used for gastric drainage, while the other was connected to a small single-lumen tube that could be placed at operation through a gastroenterostomy for jejunal feedings. This tube was used mainly in patients undergoing a gastroenterostomy, with the small loop being placed in the efferent loop of jejunum with an opening about 12 in. below the stomach. While this tube was designed to be introduced through the nose, pharynx, and esophagus, it could also be introduced through a gastrostomy opening and we used it in this way for a considerable period of time. The gastrostomy avoided the considerable discomfort of an indwelling nasopharynx tube. However, it added slightly to the operative risk. In the early 1940s, Dr. Riegel[6, 7] and a group of collaborators compared patients using this form of jejunal feeding with those nourished by the intravenous route. An effort was made to provide an equal number of calories and grams of food nitrogen by the two routes. The obtained data showed that nitrogen balance was slightly better when the food was given into the jejunum, though statistical significance was not claimed for the difference. These experiments also compared the use of whole protein versus hydrolyzed protein for the jejunal feedings. While these studies were not pursued definitively, the group members concluded that there was no clear-cut advantage in hydrolyzing the protein before it was given. As a result, most of the later experiments used whole milk and milk powder as the principal source of protein.

My interest has been in both parenteral feeding and the development of intravenous hyperalimentation. However, the difficulties and dangers related to intravenous hyperalimentation make the enteral route preferable, assuming there are equivalent results and no significant contraindications. Indeed, the intravenous route was developed only for those patients in whom the enteral route could not be used. The main problem with enteral feedings has been that they sometimes produce cramps and diarrhea. Two investigations carried out by former colleagues have highlighted the mammalian bodies' control of osmolarity in the small bowel. In the first of these studies, Drs. Ravdin, Johnston, and Morrison[8] placed glucose in concentrations up to 50 per cent solution in the stomach of dogs, and then measured the concentration in the jejunum. The glucose concentration they found in the small intestine was 5.3 per cent. Thus, the pyloric mechanism, and gastric and duodenal secretions had, in effect, diluted the glucose by about ten times by the time it reached the sampling in the small intestine. Drs. Abbott, Karr, and Miller[9] repeated and substantially confirmed this work in humans by using a Miller-Abbott tube. Thus one of the difficulties with jejunal feedings may have been the use of small molecular nutrients, such as glucose, which reached too high a concentration. Another colleague, Dr. Thomas Machella,[10] showed that the symptoms of dumping syndrome could often be brought on by injecting concentrated glucose solutions through a tube in the jejunum. The glucose was believed to cause the influx of much water, distending the bowel locally. Somewhat later, however, Drs. Gerald Peskin and Leonard Miller[11] implicated serotonin as the agent mediating the symptoms of dumping syndrome. They postulated that this was released from the bowel wall, but whether this release was due to stretching the bowel wall by the influx of fluid or by direct action of the glucose remained uncertain. Other studies, and our own clinical experience, have shown successful use of jejunal feedings in some patients. In general, these feedings were made by placing food in a blender, grinding it to a smooth suspension, then injecting it through the jejunal tube. The feeding was usually chased with water or saline so that it would not become caked in the tube.

Following Russia's launching of Sputnik in 1957, plans were made to place a man in orbit around the earth and then to send a man to the moon. A concentrated form of food was necessary for these trips, one containing all essential nutriments yet having minimal bulk. Mixtures of amino acids were tried in this regard and, as the celestial market was small, it was conceived that these might be valuable for jejunal feedings. The dietary supplement Vivonex was developed in this way. One of the questions dealt with in this volume is whether there is an advantage to such expensive purified products as compared with appropriately blended regular food. This volume comprehensively presents the theory and the practice of enteral feeding. Each of the editors has an extensive background in the field of surgical nutrition, which, of course, overlaps into nutrition in general.

Dr. Rombeau joined the faculty at the University of Pennsylvania in 1978 after a distinguished career in California. Dr. Caldwell has served for three years as the original editor of the *Journal of Parenteral and Enteral Nutrition*, which is the official organ of the American Society for Parenteral and Enteral Nutrition. In this capacity he has seen and edited a tremendous range of reports on therapeutic nutrition. As editors, these two physicians have drawn upon many of the most talented clinical investigators in the field of enteral nutrition from the United States and Europe. Their coverage of the subject is presented in a logical, easy-to-find manner, and I believe this volume will prove very useful to both house officers and visiting staff so often confronted with serious nutritional deficits in their patients.

REFERENCES

1. Edsal, D. L., and Miller, C. W.: Study of two cases nourished exclusively per rectum; with a determination of absorption nitrogen metabolism and intestinal putrefaction. Trans. Stud. Coll. Physicians Philadelphia 24:255, 1902
2. Folin, O. and Denis, W.: The origin and significance of the ammonia in the portal blood. *J. Biol. Chem.* 11:116, 1912
3. Abderhalden, E., Frank, F. and Schittenhelm, A.: Rectal feeding of biuret-neg protein digest. *Z. Physiol. Chem.* 63:214, 1909
4. Rhoads, J. E., Stengel, A., Jr., Riegel, C., Cajori, F. A. and Frazier, W. D.: The absorption of protein split products from chronic isolated colon loops. *Am. J. Physiol.* 125:707–712, 1939
5. Abbott, W. O. and Rawson, A. J.: A tube for use in the postoperative care of gastroenterostomy cases. *J.A.M.A.* 108:1873, 1937
6. Riegel, C., Rhoads, J. E., Koop, C. E., et al.: Dietary requirements for nitrogen equilibrium in the period immediately following certain major surgical operations. *Am. J. Med. Sci.* 210:133–134, 1945
7. Riegel, C., Koop, C. E., Drew, J., Stevens, L. W. and Rhoads, J. E.: The nutritional requirements for nitrogen balance in surgical patients in the early postoperative period. *J. Clin. Invest.* 26:18, 1947
8. Ravdin, I. S., Johnston, C. G. and Morrison, P. J.: Comparison of concentration of glucose in the stomach and intestines after intragastric administration. *Proc. Soc. Exp. Biol. Med.* 30:955, 1933
9. Abbott, W. O., Karr, W. G. and Miller, T. G.: Intubation studies of the human small intestine: VII. Factors concerned in absorption of glucose from the jejunum and ileum. *Am. J. Digest. Dis. & Nutr.* 4:742, 1937
10. Machella, R. E.: The mechanism of the post-gastrectomy dumping syndrome. *Ann. Surg.* 130:145, 1949
11. Peskin, G. W. and Miller, L. D.: The role of serotonin in the "Dumping Syndrome." *Arch. Surg.* 85:701, 1962

Preface

In 1790 John Hunter published a monumental report entitled "A Case of Paralysis of the Muscles of Deglutition, Cured by an Artificial Mode of Conveying Food and Medicine into the Stomach" (Fig. 1). This report was significant for two reasons. First, it was one of the first reports of a patient being fed successfully via an enteric tube; and second, owing to Hunter's immense prestige coupled with the fact that the patient recovered, enteral feeding was given instant credibility. It was this report that probably heralded what is now known as tube feeding. Unfortunately, this method of feeding was not used extensively in the United States until the early twentieth century when it had a brief renaissance. Because of inadequate liquid diets and difficulties with formula delivery, tube feeding did not receive widespread acceptance and it was subsequently overshadowed by intravenous nutrition. It is ironic that the discovery of intravenous nutrition is probably most responsible for the renewed interest in enteral feeding. This is partly due to the increased awareness concerning all aspects of nutritional care that has been generated by the discovery of intravenous nutrition. The availability of therapeutic intravenous diets has necessitated that physicians learn about nutritional assessment, nutrient requirements, and (apropos of this text) how to feed a patient who is unable to eat yet still has a functional gastrointestinal tract. It is important that enteral nutrition not be viewed as a substitute for parenteral nutrition inasmuch as these two feeding methods are indicated in very different conditions. Enteral and parenteral nutrition are complementary rather than competitive.

Why is it necessary to compile a textbook on enteral nutrition? A major reason for this text is that the majority of hospitalized patients in need of specialized nutritional support have functioning gastrointestinal tracts and presumably should be fed enterally. However, we believe that this mode of therapy is greatly underutilized. What are the reasons for this underutilization? The explanation most frequently given is that "enteral feeding is too difficult to do and takes too long to advance the feedings to full nutrient requirements." Certainly there is marked variability in the tolerance of the gastrointestinal tract to enteral feeding. This variability requires that the clinician pay close attention to the details of feeding methods. It is often difficult to obtain good descriptions of enteral feeding methods and their respective rationale. The need to compile this information provides the raison d'être for this volume.

This book has been organized to answer four questions: What? Why? How? and When? It is our belief that prior to using these feeding techniques, the physician should have a basic understanding of the physiology of eating, digestion, absorption, substrate metabolism, and nutrient requirements. The current "state of the art" of new diets, enteral delivery systems, and methods is presented; however, we realize that much of this information may soon be outdated. The specific indications for enteral feeding are discussed in detail with an emphasis on the unique requirements and feeding techniques for different diseases. It is acknowledged that there are complications associated with enteral feeding and it is hoped that the appropriate preventive measures will be implemented by better identification of these problems. Finally, the future of any science lies in the quality of its research. Every attempt has been made to include data from the best available studies. It is to be emphasized, however, that there is a great need for well-controlled trials in most areas of enteral feeding.

The contributors have been chosen because of their proven clinical expertise and their objective documentation of this expertise. Those contributors selected work concurrently at the bedside and in the laboratory to provide the highest standard of enteral nutrition. Of necessity, one will find areas of conflict among the authors because of differences in interpretation, varying clinical experiences, and the unique aspects of many of these feeding methods.

Several administrative tasks have been implemented to provide a comprehensive and accurate reference source. All references have been checked for accuracy by an independent reviewer, and each reference includes all of the authors. To provide the most current references on each topic, most senior authors have submitted a list of additional references that have been published following the completion of their manuscripts and prior to the publication deadline.

We are indebted to our physician-illustrator, Dr. David W. Low, who came to the bedside, laboratory, and operating room to better communicate our information.

Our deepest gratitude goes to our mentors, Drs. Louella Kretschmar, C. J. Berne, Leonard Rosoff, Charles Frey, Robert Cargill, Curtis Artz, Biemann Othersen, John Exton, William Lacy, Charles Park, Ray Meng, James O'Neill, Ed Canham, Julius Mackie, and Jonathan Rhoads, who created and expanded the necessary academic environment that has nurtured our interest in clinical nutrition.

Our thanks go to Rosalind Corman and Sally Sepaga for their invaluable literary and grammatical help and to Linda Belfus from the W. B. Saunders Company for her cogent suggestions and editorial assistance. A special word of gratitude goes to Peggy Kless, whose indefatigable secretarial skills and equanimity were indispensable to the transcription of this text. Finally, our most grateful appreciation goes to our wives, Maureen and Christine, and children, Suzanne and Charlie, for their inordinate patience and understanding.

JOHN L. ROMBEAU, M.D.
MICHAEL D. CALDWELL, M.D., PH.D.

Contents

INTRODUCTION

The History of Enteral Nutrition

HENRY T. RANDALL

The history of enteral nutrition by means other than eating and drinking begins with rectal feeding. In a comprehensive review written 100 years ago, Bliss[1] quotes Herodotus, who wrote that the ancient Egyptians, many centuries before Christ, used nutrient enemas as a part of a custom of using emetics and enemas three days each month to preserve health.

Greek physicians made extensive use of clysters (a word for enemas derived from the Greek word for syringe) in the treatment of diarrhea, perferring this method to medication by mouth. They also used wine, milk, whey, and wheat and barley broths, which were intended to be nutritious as well as mildly laxative.

Probably the earliest form of rectal syringe was that used by the Egyptians, a piece of pipe with a bladder tied to one end. The form recommended by Hippocrates differed only in the placement of a number of small openings in the side of the pipe.

Other devices for rectal feeding were developed in the eighteenth and nineteenth centuries. A fountain syringe for continuous lavage of the lower bowel, and longer pipes, including the tube portion of a stomach pump, were employed to introduce food as high as the transverse colon.[1] Rubber tubing, as small as ⅛ inch in diameter, to which was attached a small funnel and a short segment of glass tubing to observe flow, was recommended as a simple method of rectal feeding. "Patients could be fed by inexperienced persons once instructed in use of the device."[2]

The type and variety of foods that were administered rectally are quite remarkable. In addition to milk, whey, and grain broths first used by the Egyptians and early Greek physicians, beef and chicken broths and raw eggs were commonly prescribed along with small amounts of brandy.[1] In a letter to *Lancet* in 1878, Brown-Séquard[3] commented on his personal use of a mixture of two thirds of a pound of beef and half as much fresh hog pancreas, finely ground together and pushed into the rectum with a wooden syringe. Three patients with esophageal spasm preventing the use of a stomach tube were fed twice a day by this means from five to eight days. He recommended the method as a useful alternative to forced feeding of patients who refused to eat.

Defibrinated blood was used in the United States for rectal feeding, including in the case of President Garfield. Rapid putrefaction of the blood and rectal irritation were described as limitations in its use. Peptonized beef broth and beef peptonoids together with whiskey were administered rectally every four hours for most of the President's 79 days of survival after he had been wounded by an assassin.[1]

Theories of reversal of peristaltic action, with perfusion of small bowel from the cecum, were used to sustain belief in the efficacy of rectal feeding. Case reports, including that of President Garfield and five others fed rectally, are included in the report by Bliss, despite his statement that "it is extremely improbable that assimilation takes place in the lower bowel, save as crystalline principles may dialyze through the mucous membrane."[1]

Use of the rectum to provide water, saline, glucose, and isotonic amino acid solutions by proctoclysis was advocated at least until the time of World War II, although tube feeding into the stomach or jejunum and peripheral parenteral infusions containing amino acids, glucose, minerals, and vitamins were considered preferable. Proctoclysis was given either in the form of a rectal tap of 300 ml every four hours, or continuously as a Murphy drip. Such drugs as paraldehyde, chloral hydrate, and suppositories containing opiates were also administered rectally.[4] Rectal irritation, even with isotonic solutions, limited the amount of nutrition that could be administered per day to about 400 calories and the duration of this form of treatment.

TUBE FEEDING INTO THE UPPER GUT

The first record of use of a tube for feeding into the esophagus is reported by His[5] to be by Capivacceus, who in 1598 introduced nutrient substances into the esophagus. He used a hollow tube with a bladder attached to one end, similar to tubes used for clysters. In 1617, Fabricius ab Aquapendente reported the use of a silver tube passed through the nostril into the nasopharynx for feeding patients with tetanus.[6] In 1646 Von Helmont fabricated flexible leather catheters, and subsequently Boerhaave recommended that such catheters be introduced into the stomach.[6, 7]

John Hunter appears to be the first to mention introduction of substances into the stomach by means of a hollow catheter and a syringe. Pareira[6] reported that Hunter used this method initially for the introduction of stimulating substances into the stomach of a patient being resuscitated from near drowning. Several years later, in 1790, Hunter successfully treated a patient with paralysis of the muscles of deglutition by using a tube made of a whale bone probe covered with an eelskin and attached to a bladder. The eelskin-covered probe was passed orogastrically for feeding. Hunter recommended that jellies, eggs beaten up with a little water, sugar, and milk or wine be used as food, and noted that medicines could be mixed with it.

The stomach pump, which subsequently became the first consistently used method of intragastric feeding, was initially used for gastric lavage and gastric decompression. Philip Syng Physick, Professor of Surgery at the University of Pennsylvania, is credited with the first use of a flexible orogastric tube for removal of poisonous substances from the stomach in about 1810.[6]

In 1823 Sir Astley Cooper observed a demonstration of removal of opium from the stomach of a dog, using a gum rubber tube inserted into the stomach and a complicated syringe invented by a Mr. Reed.[8] Three weeks later a Mr. Jukes demonstrated on himself the use of a gum rubber tube which he said he had invented to evacuate his own stomach of extract of licorice and water that he had drunk.[7] This demonstration prompted a letter to *Lancet* by a Mr. Alcock, who observed that a report on the identical apparatus had been published in France in 1814 and had even been proposed by Boerhaave a century before.[7]

Kussmaul, in 1867, used a flexible orogastric tube for gastric decompression, and Ewald and Oser introduced the soft rubber tube for gastric intubation in 1874.[5]

The stomach pump was in common use for feeding of refractory insane patients in England during the first half of the nineteenth century. In 1851 Reeve, in describing a new device he had invented for oral hypopharyngeal feeding of the insane, noted examples of laceration of the stomach and drowning with beef broth as complications of the use of the stomach pump for feeding.[9] He observed that "the circumstances of forcible injection of food or medicine into the stomach requires patience; it is always a troublesome task, and if confided to ignorant keepers is also a perilous one."

Nasopharyngeal feeding and rectal feeding both were used quite widely in the latter half of the nineteenth century. Clouston[10] in 1872 stated that "unquestionably the medical officers of asylums see far more of and therefore are much more experienced in overcoming attempted starvation than any other parts of the profession." He went on to state that at that time the best mode of feeding varied from case to case. It should be oral, if possible, using a common metal spoon or "a long small stiffish tube for passing well down into the esophagus by the nose." He stated that he used "an extremely simple arrangement within the reach of any medical man—a foot of ordinary India rubber tubing used for children's bottles with an ear speculum struck at one end of it. The other, well-oiled, is then passed into one nostril as far as the fauces and when the speculum is held up and liquid poured into it a small quantity at a time the patient gets (them) unmixed and must swallow them." He objected to the use of a syringe with the tubing on the ground that squirting materials forcibly through the tubing resulted in aspiration. Clouston stated that "when all other methods failed, as was true in many cases, a good stomach pump or, as some prefer, merely its esophageal tube with a funnel which can be attached to its end is our last resource and a never failing one." Two types of tubing were described: one apparently made entirely of an elastic rubber and the other consisting of a gum elastic containing spiral wire. Apparently, forcible restraint using four strong men was a standard part of the feeding procedure.

Advocates of nasal feeding commended the method for feeding of patients who were unable to swallow or unable to eat but who were conscious and to some degree cooperative. Dukes,[11] in 1876, described feeding a child at the time he was a resident medical officer at the Hospital for Sick Children in London by a method used for sane patients, those with diphtheria, severe stomatitis, and "for fasting girls and spoilt children." A yard of India rubber tubing of ⅛-inch bore, a bottle of any kind, and a piece of twine to tie the tube in the bottle formed a feeding system. The free end of the tube was passed just inside the nostril of the patient lying supine, then the fluid was allowed to run into the nose, with the flow controlled by compressing the tube with thumb and index finger. Dukes stated that this method was used instead of the stomach pump if it was not available or was unsuitable, as may have been the case with small children.

L. Emmett Holt, Professor of the Diseases of Children and Attending Physician at Babies Hospital in New York, advocated gavage feeding in acutely ill infants and children. In 1894[12] he described the technique as very simple: "a funnel, 18 inches of rubber tubing, a soft rubber catheter and a few inches of glass tubing for connections." A gag was recommended for older children. The catheter was introduced perorally with the child supine and restrained and the liquid food introduced in 10 to 30 seconds! A typical feeding in young children comprised 4 to 6 oz of milk and 1 oz of brandy with digitalis every six hours; in older children, 6 to 8 oz of milk was given. Pinching the catheter tightly on withdrawal prevented aspiration.

In 1895 Morrison[13] reported on the value of the stomach tube for feeding after intubation of the larynx of children with diphtheria. It was noted that following diphtheria children frequently had paralysis of the muscles of deglutition. Morrison wrote that many attempts were made to nourish children rectally but that rectal alimentation fell short of the desired effect because of the inability of the bowel to retain or absorb the proper amount of nourishment. A typical intragastric feeding was 6 oz of cream with 20 per cent fat content, 2 oz of brandy, 3 drops of tincture of nux vomica, and a digestive ferment; this was given three times a day. In his paper, Morrison reported the use of gastric intubation in 28 children, 12 of whom recovered. The method was to roll the child in a blanket using two assistants. A soft rubber catheter to which a funnel was attached was lubricated and introduced into a nostril and thus into the stomach. Morrison commented, "in comparison with the ordinary methods of feeding in these cases, (using the tube) possesses the advantage of permitting a definite amount of food to be given to a child at regular intervals, thus giving the stomach its natural periods of rest. . . . If a nourishment chart is acurately kept in these cases, the small amount actually taken is often appalling, unless tube feeding is used." He also noted that while tube feeding was best carried out by a physician, it could nevertheless be taught to any intelligent nurse or parent.

DUODENAL ALIMENTATION

In 1910 Einhorn[14] introduced a major advance in enteral nutrition. He stated that up to that time when patients were unable to take food, rectal feeding had always been used when oral or gastric feeding was impossible. He also pointed out how unsatisfactory rectal feeding had proved to be, as the materials placed in the rectum were inadequately utilized and there were problems with rectal irritation. Einhorn used a tube that he had developed as a duodenal pump for sampling duodenal contents for feeding into the duodenum or proximal jejunum. The device consisted of a rubber tube with a metal weight of 10 to 12 gm attached to its distal end. The tubing was introduced into the stomach, and feeding was begun as soon as it was in the duodenum. The tubing was left in place for 8 to 12 days. It was stated 'that the thin rubber tube did not inconvenience the patient so the patient was always ready for feeding, which was done at intervals of every two hours. After feeding, water was forced through the tube, air blown through it, and a stopcock closed.

Einhorn suggested the slow introduction of from 240 to 300 ml of food. All fluids must be at body temperature. Usually the nutritive material consisted of 240 ml of milk, one raw egg, and 15 gm of milk sugar (lactose); the mixture was well beaten and injected at body temperature. In addition, two of three reported patients were given 1 qt of physiologic saline solution daily, through the rectum according to the Murphy drip method. A third patient received water directly injected into the duodenum but very slowly, drop by drop. Einhorn detailed the outcome of the three patients, all of whom did well, and concluded that "the advantages of duodenal over rectal feeding are at once apparent; for while the rectum and colon are simply organs for the expulsion of feces and for the absorption of possibly remaining liquids, we have to deal in the duodenum with an organ where the most important digestive juices are secreted."

Einhorn's tube was rapidly adopted in the United States, and modifications of the idea were also introduced. Morgan[15] and Jones[16] reported successful use of the Einhorn tube. Morgan fed patients for up to five weeks. Jones treated patients with duodenal ulcer. Jones modified the technique by feeding drop by drop through the tube. He noticed that some patients were intolerant to the addition of milk sugar to the feeding mixtures that he used. Volumes of feeding rose from 2 oz every two hours to as much as 12 oz every two hours. In addition to milk, egg white and whole egg were included. After adaptation over a period of several days, as much as 84 oz of milk and six eggs were fed in 24 hours. On this regimen, fed at 60 to 120 drops per minute using a burette, Jones stated that his patients gained up to 5 lb in body weight in two weeks.

In 1915 Gross[17] stated "the use of the duodenal tube is not occupying the position it deserves." He introduced his own tube, a rubber tube 7 mm in diameter with a 10 to 11 gm ball on the distal end. The patient with gastric or duodenal ulcer was placed in a chair and the tube introduced in a sitting position. He stated that it took 15 to 20 minutes for the tube to reach the duodenum. The formula he fed was warm milk with 15 gm of glucose per 250 ml added first, followed by egg yolk later. He stated that cream and lactose were not well tolerated.

In 1918 Andresen[18] reported immediate jejunal feeding after gastroenterostomy. He noted that patients with pyloric stenosis from duodenal ulcer were usually 30 to 50 lb underweight and represented a very high operative risk. He used the Rehfuss gastroduodenal tube, which he passed at the time of surgery well into the jejunum; after completing the gastroenterostomy he began feeding *on the operating room table*. The formula used was peptonized milk, dextrose, and alcohol. Andresen also used the Rehfuss tube for gastric feeding preoperatively if the patient was not totally obstructed. He noted that the patient could be fed by drip into the stomach, but he preferred that a definitive amount of feeding be given by a nurse at a specific time. Jejunal feedings consisted of 200 ml of milk, 15 gm of dextrose, and 8 ml of whiskey at two-hour intervals. He stated that neither rectal infusions nor hypodermoclysis was necessary to maintain fluid balance in these patients.

Isidore Ravdin, Professor of Surgery at the University of Pennsylvania School of Medicine, was a major contributor in advancing knowledge of the importance of protein and calorie nutrition in surgical patients. In 1939 Stengel and Ravdin[19] reported on maintenance of nutrition in surgical patients with a description of an orojejunal method of feeding. The device consisted of two tubes tied together and passed nasogastrically, the longer tube being passed well into the jejunum at surgery. Later a double-lumen tube was substituted for the two tubes tied together. The principle was that of gastric emptying and simultaneous jejunal feeding. Materials fed consisted of a peptone hydrolysate, glucose, water, and salt. Stengel and Ravdin strongly recommended the use of a feeding machine to control flow over a drip. The amount of material that was fed averaged about 1500 calories per day. Later Stengel and Ravdin used the Abbott tube, a double-lumen tube but without the valves originally proposed by Abbott.

In 1939 Abbott and Rawson[20] reported on their development of a double-lumen tube for postoperative care of gastroenterostomy patients. In their initial article in 1937, they described a tube with a valve system:

an inlet valve in the stomach and an outlet valve in the jejunal tube. In 1939 they reported a double-lumen tube, the larger lumen for gastric suction and the smaller lumen for jejunal feeding. The size of the tube was 15 French, and the distal tube (12 French) extended 30 cm beyond the junction of the double-lumen tube. Abbott and Rawson reported that feeding of starved patients was begun even on the day of operation and commented that this method of feeding was more physiologic than intravenous infusions.

A year later Abbott[21] reported total fluid and nutritional maintenance by use of an intestinal tube and gave credit to Ravdin's original concept of feeding into the jejunum immediately postoperatively. He presented a case in which, with a Miller-Abbott tube in the distal small bowel to treat small intestinal obstruction, the patient was fed through the stomach, and the intestinal residual was emptied proximal to the intestinal structure through the Miller-Abbott tube. A mixture of casein hydrolysate and 5 per cent dextrose was used for the feedings.

In 1942 Bisgard[22] reported jejunal intubation through a gastrostomy for the purpose of feeding. He noted that the mortality from gastric surgery in those days was 10 to 20 per cent and believed that most of it was due to malnutrition. Using Ravdin's technique of 1939, he placed two Levin tubes in the stomach. At operation one was threaded distally 10 to 12 inches into the jejunum. The patient was started immediately postoperatively with jejunal feedings of 2 to 4 oz of pepsinized milk plus 5 gm of glucose per 100 ml. Each feeding was followed by 1 to 2 oz of isotonic saline. Bisgard stated that parenteral fluid therapy was unnecessary and added that vitamins, including vitamin B complex and C, should be placed in the tube. In the same article he reported further evolution of technique using a catheter gastrostomy with the catheter tip threaded into the jejunum and the proximal end brought through and anchored to the abdominal wall. Feedings were administered through this tube drop by drop. Suction in the stomach was provided by a nasogastric Levin tube, which was withdrawn after one or two days. Feedings by mouth began on the fourth day. The jejunal catheter was used for feeding until the seventh or eighth day if no complications occurred, and longer if necessary.

The Abbott-Rawson tube was used by Co Tui and Mulholland[23] to demonstrate the effectiveness of a high amino acid and high caloric intake in producing positive nitrogen balance following subtotal gastric resection for duodenal ulcer or carcinoma of the pylorus. In a randomized series of 19 patients, eight were treated with the then standard ward regimen of peripheral infusions of glucose and saline, with oral intake of sugar in tea and pepsinized milk begun on the sixth postoperative day. Eight were fed an average of at least 50 kcal/kg body weight; 0.6 gm of dietary nitrogen per kg of body weight per day was provided by a mixture of casein hydrolysate (Amigen) and dextrimaltose fed into the jejunal limb of the Abbott-Rawson tube, *starting within a few hours of operation.* Supplemental peripheral intravenous infusions of glucose and saline were used during the first three to four days postoperatively to maintain fluid balance as the jejunal feedings were slowly increased from 50 to 150 ml per hour. Daily nitrogen balance studies were performed on most of both series of patients. Three patients had complications that prevented adequate feeding.

The results of this study were dramatic. Patients fed high caloric and high amino acid mixtures were consistently in positive nitrogen balance, gained weight, and remained in bed less than half as long as controls. Increased urinary secretion of nitrogen in the fed patients was more than compensated for by their increased intake. The stress of surgery and minor postoperative complications was not sufficient to produce a negative nitrogen balance in the adequately fed patients.

Co Tui concluded: "A hyperalimentation regimen, consisting of high caloric and high amino acid feeding postoperatively, has been worked out, found practical, and is recommended in the routine case of gastrectomy in order to circumvent nitrogen loss, shorten convalescence, and prevent postoperative asthenia."

Another method of enteral feeding at the time of operation was used by Russian surgeons during World War II. Panikov[24] described a method of feeding wounded men at the time of surgery for penetrating wounds of the abdomen. A trocar was introduced into the proximal small bowel following repair of intra-abdominal viscera, and a high calorie food mixture consisting of milk, butter, eggs, sugar, salt, and alcohol was introduced through rubber tubing attached to the trocar. When fresh milk was not available, canned milk diluted with water was substituted. About 700 to 1000 ml of feeding was used. The opening for the trocar was closed with a pursestring suture following the feeding.

In 1947 Riegel, Rhoads, and coauthors[25] reported on studies of nutritional requirements for nitrogen balance in postoperative patients. Their patients were predominantly young males who were subjected either to craniotomy or to subtotal gastric resection for duodenal ulcer. The postgastrectomy patients were fed intrajejunally either with an Abbott-Rawson tube or by Bisgard's technique of gastrostomy and jejunal intubation. The craniotomy patients were usually fed through a Levin tube placed in the stomach. Some patients in both groups were fed by mouth. A variety of diets were used, varying from casein hydrolysate (Amigen) with dextrose to food from the metabolic kitchen.

Formal nitrogen balance studies were done on all patients for a period of five days postoperatively, and total caloric intake was also recorded. Of 18 patients who were either in nitrogen equilibrium or in positive balance, 12 received 0.3 gm of nitrogen/kg (1.88 gm of protein) and 30 to 46 kcal/kg of body weight per day. Three of these patients were fed a hospital diet supplemented by Amigen; the others were all tube-fed, into either the stomach or the jejunum. No correlation was found between nitrogen balance and age or sex, and no significant correlation existed between plasma protein concentration and either nitrogen balance or food intake. The importance of providing both a high caloric intake and a high nitrogen intake in postoperative patients to maintain nitrogen balance was stressed by the authors. The fact that this was accomplished by nasogastric, nasogastric-jejunal, and gastrojejunal tube feedings 35 years ago is pertinent to this review.

In 1952 Boles and Zollinger[26] evaluated 103 patients who had had a feeding jejunostomy placed at the time of surgery. The Stamm technique of inverting pursestring sutures was used around a 16 French catheter placed in the proximal jejunum, and the bowel was then sutured to the parietal peritoneum. Feeding was begun 8 to 12 hours postoperatively with 50 ml of 5 per cent dextrose in water per hour, 1000 ml on the first day and 2000 ml on the second day. Half-strength homogenized milk was begun on the third day; the feeding gradually progressed to 200 ml of warm whole milk every two hours. Fifteen of the 103 patients were poorly tolerant of the feedings, suffering from distention and cramps. The other patients apparently did well.[26]

Also in 1952 Fallis and Barron[27] reported 150 cases of gastric and jejunal alimentation using fine polyethylene tubes. Polyethylene tubes PE200 with an outside diameter of 1.9 mm were used. Six-foot lengths were used for the jejunum and 27-inch lengths for the gastrostomy. The method of introducing the tubes when placed nasogastrically was by attachment of a toy balloon that contained 2 to 5 ml of mercury. The balloon was attached to the end of the tubing with a catgut suture that would dissolve in the stomach or in the small bowel. The feeding formula consisted of 500 ml of homogenized milk, 175 gm of a liver protein hydrolysate, 300 gm of cerelose, a partially hydrolyzed cereal starch, 75 gm of powdered milk, and four eggs. They also provided water and electrolyte replacement.

Tube feedings were started at 30 ml every one or two hours and were gradually increased to as much as 200 ml per hour. Tincture of opium or Banthene was used for patients who had diarrhea. If feeding was continued over a prolonged period of time, liquefied and partially hydrolyzed whole foods were eventually used for feeding.

In 1954 Pareira and Elman[28] reported therapeutic nutrition of 240 patients solely by tube feedings.

Twenty patients were able to tube-feed themselves on an outpatient basis; the remainder were hospitalized. Only 42 patients were fed for less than a week; most were fed for 1 to 16 weeks, and twelve for periods of 3 to 9 months. An additional 76 patients drank the feeding mixture for periods of up to 4 weeks. The patients who were tube-fed had a variety of ailments: (1) primary malnutrition, usually from anorexia nervosa; (2) anorexia resulting from disease, trauma, burns, cerebrovascular accidents, cancer, or tuberculosis; (3) persistent anorexia following correction of the original cause of malnutrition; (4) mechanical impediments to eating; (5) depression or coma; (6) preoperative malnutrition; (7) postoperative malnutrition in patients in whom preoperative correction was not or could not be accomplished; and (8) terminal cancer, for palliation. It was also used to accelerate postoperative rehabilitation.

A 13 French polyvinyl tube with an external diameter of 2.5 mm was used. Feeding was either intermittent, using a 50-ml syringe, or continuous by drip, using a glass drip meter and an adjustable pinch clamp to regulate rate of flow. Feeding materials included dried whole milk, nonfat milk solids, calcium caseinate, dextrose, dextromaltose, vitamins and iron, and choline. The caloric density of the preparation mixed with water varied from about 1 cal/ml to as high as 3.5 cal/ml. Feedings were usually begun at half-ration for 48 hours; at times one third of the ration was used initially with time allowed for adaptation. All patients were permitted to drink water as desired, or additional water was given by tube. This was particularly important when protein intake was high, as it was with the formula used. Seven per cent of the patients had diarrhea, only 2 per cent severe enough to discontinue feeding. The authors noted no difference in weight gain and positive nitrogen balance between intermittent feeding and continuous feeding by drip.

Smith and Lee[29] used tube feeding successfully to treat 11 consecutive patients with lateral duodenal fistula. They used a continuous-drip, intrajejunal infusion through a plastic feeding tube introduced into the efferent limb of the gastrojejunostomy with the aid of a string and lead shot secured to the tip of the catheter with a catgut suture. They administered a solution of partially hydrolyzed lactalbumin and dextrose, with added electrolytes, trace elements, and vitamins. The formula had a caloric density of 900 kcal/L. Starting with slow infusion, it was possible to provide all water, electrolyte, protein, and caloric requirements for the patients within three to four days entirely enterally. In all eleven patients the fistulas closed spontaneously within one month.

In 1959 Barron[30] reported an extensive experience with tube feeding at the Henry Ford Hospital. Over a ten-year period, "several hundred" patients were fed using small polyethylene catheters (PE240) introduced into the stomach through a large split catheter or rectal tube. When jejunal intubation was desired, a small balloon containing mercury was attached to the tip of the feeding catheter by means of a string that passed up through the feeding catheter and was secured at the top of it. When the balloon was in the duodenum or jejunum as determined by radiography, the string was released and passed with the balloon, leaving the catheter in the jejunum as desired.

Barron recommended feeding into the stomach whenever possible. Feedings consisted of pureed baby foods, blenderized hospital diets, and foods processed by colloid mills or industrial commutating machines to make minuscule particles. Fluids aspirated from the stomach when the feeding tube was in the jejunum were filtered and injected into the jejunal tube. The rate of feeding was controlled by a pump devised by Barron. He noted that nausea, cramps, and diarrhea were caused by too rapid feeding of these mechanically prepared polymeric foods.

In 1959 Pareira published a monograph, *Therapeutic Nutrition with Tube Feeding*, in which he summarized previous work which he, Elman, and others had done in clinical evaluation of enteral nutrition.[6] He emphasized the relationship that exists between starvation and anorexia, and the importance of breaking the cycle that leads to malnutrition by therapeutic intervention by tube feeding. He stated that tube feeding guarantees certainty of intake, with respect to both calories and balance of nutrients.

Pareira's recommendations—use of a small caliber (2.5 mm or less), soft tube, initial feeding by continuous drip or pump, the use of dilute feeding formula for several days to permit adaptation, and emphasis on the importance of access to free water for drinking or provision of extra water by tube—are all principles that are completely applicable to modern enteral nutrition. His use of home enteral nutrition for some of his patients, including patients with advanced cancer, 25 years ago set a precedent that only now is beginning to be followed by major centers concerned with nutritional support for patients with severe problems involving normal feeding.

During the 1950s, studies by Greenstein and Winitz and colleagues at the National Cancer Institute in Bethesda, Maryland, showed that rats would grow and reproduce normally on diets that were "elemental" or of defined formula in the sense that they were made up of crystalline amino acids, simple sugars, essential fatty acids, minerals, and vitamins, all of known composition.[31] These diets were subsequently studied in normal volunteers by Winitz and proved to be capable of sustaining normal body composition and weight for periods of up to 19 weeks.[32, 33]

Stephens and Randall, in 1969,[34] reported use of chemically defined diets for partial or complete nutritional support of seriously ill surgical patients. Diets were fed either nasogastrically or through a gastrostomy, using either 5 French or 8 French polyethylene infant feeding tubes. Positive nitrogen balance and, in some cases, weight gain were achieved in patients with inflammatory bowel disease or pancreatitis. A child with a tracheoesophageal-pleural-cutaneous fistula, fed by gastrostomy, experienced spontaneous closure of the fistula.

Defined formula diets were subsequently demonstrated to be of particular value for providing nutritional support to patients with gastrointestinal-cutaneous fistulas, resulting in reduction of the volume of fistula loss, as well as positive nitrogen balance and weight gain. Spontaneous closure occurred in two thirds of fistulas.[35, 36]

The use of a small feeding tube, 8 French, as a jejunostomy for prolonged nutritional support of a patient with a severe head injury was reported in 1972.[37] Defined formula diet easily passed through this tube and was used to feed the patient for more than seven months. A similar tube, used as a gastrostomy, permitted the feeding of a patient with 60 cm of jejunum terminating in a jejunostomy at home for two years, until recurrent Crohn's disease necessitated the use of home total parenteral nutrition (TPN), which has continued for seven years. There was no leakage of intestinal juice around the small tubes and no significant narrowing of the jejunum.

Total parenteral nutrition, made practical by the major contributions of Dudrick, Wilmore, and Rhoads,[38] has become the current major method of nutritional support for seriously ill patients who cannot or will not eat and drink sufficient foods to meet their needs. There is no doubt that with TPN many patients survive and many more have fewer complications and a less difficult convalescence. However, mechanical, metabolic, and septic complications of the method are significant, and the cost in terms of materials, equipment, and professional supervision is very substantial.

Enteral nutrition by tube can often meet the needs of patients who will not or cannot normally ingest what they require. Modern techniques permit access to the stomach and the small intestine, and a wide spectrum of diets permits administration of foods that can be adjusted to the degree of digestive disability that exists. The effectiveness of enteral nutrition has been scientifically validated for more than 50 years.

If the gastrointestinal tract works, at least in part, it should be used.

REFERENCES

1. Bliss, D. W.: Feeding per rectum: As illustrated in the case of the late President Garfield and others. Med. Rec., 22:64–69, 1882.
2. Jones-Humphreys, Y. M.: An easy method of feeding per rectum. Lancet, 1:366–367, 1891.
3. Brown-Séquard, C. E.: Feeding per rectum in nervous affections. Lancet, 1:144, 1878.
4. Cole, W. H., and Elman, R. (eds.): Textbook of General Surgery. Edition 5. New York and London, D. Appleton-Century Company, Inc., 1948, Chapter 8.
5. His, W.: Zur Geschichte der Magenpumpe. Med. Klin., 21:391–393, 1925.
6. Pareira, M. D.: Therapeutic Nutrition with Tube Feeding. Springfield, Illinois, Charles C Thomas, 1959.
7. Alcock, T.: On the immediate treatment of persons poisoned. Lancet, 1:372–377, 1823.
7a. Hunter, J.: A case of paralysis of the muscles of deglutition cured by an artificial mode of conveying food and medicines into the stomach. Trans. Soc. Improvement Med. Chir. Know., 1:182–188, 1793.
8. Cooper, Sir Astley: Hospital reports, November 21, 1823. Lancet, 1:275–277, 1823.
9. Reeve, J. F.: An apparatus for administering nourishment to insane persons who refuse food. Lancet, 1:520–521, 1851.
10. Clouston, T. S.: Forcible Feeding. The Lancet, 2:797–798, 1872.
11. Dukes, C.: A simple mode of feeding some patients by the nose. Lancet, 2:394–395, 1876.
12. Holt, L. E.: Gavage (forced feeding) in the treatment of acute diseases of infancy and childhood. Med. Rec., 45:524–525, 1894.
13. Morrison, W. A.: The value of the stomach-tube in feeding after intubation, based upon twenty-eight cases; also its use in post-diphtheritic paralysis. Bost. Med. Surg. J., 132:127–130, 1895.
14. Einhorn, M.: Duodenal alimentation. Med. Rec., 78:92–95, 1910.
15. Morgan, W. C.: Duodenal alimentation. Am. J. Med. Sci., 148:360–369, 1914.
16. Jones, C. R.: Duodenal feeding. Surg. Gynecol. Obstet., 22:236–240, 1916.
17. Gross, M. H., and Held, I. W.: Duodenal alimentation. J.A.M.A., 65:520–523, 1915.
18. Andresen, A. F. R.: Immediate jejunal feeding after gastroenterostomy. Ann. Surg., 67:565–566, 1918.
19. Stengel, A., Jr., and Ravdin, I. S.: The maintenance of nutrition in surgical patients with a description

of the orojejunal method of feeding. Surgery, 6:511–519, 1939.

20. Abbott, W. O., and Rawson, A. J.: A tube for use in postoperative care of gastroenterostomy patients—Correction. J.A.M.A., 112:2414, 1939.

21. Abbott, W. O.: Fluid and nutritional maintenance by the use of an intestinal tube. Ann. Surg., 112:584–593, 1940.

22. Bisgard, J. D.: Gastrostomy-jejunal intubation. Surg. Gynecol. Obstet., 74:239–241, 1942.

23. Co Tui, Wright, A. M., Mulholland, J. H., Carabba, V., Barcham, I., and Vinci, V. J.: Studies on surgical convalescence. Ann. Surg., 120:99–122, 1944.

24. Panikov, P. A.: Spasokukotski's method of feeding abdominal wounds. Am. Rev. Soviet Med., 1:32–36, 1943.

25. Riegel, C., Koop, C. E., Drew, J., Stevens, L. W., and Rhoads, J. E.: The nutritional requirements for nitrogen balance in surgical patients during the early postoperative period. J. Clin. Invest., 26:18–23, 1947.

26. Boles, T., Jr., and Zollinger, R. M.: Critical evaluation of jejunostomy. Arch. Surg., 65:358–366, 1952.

27. Fallis, L. S., and Barron, J.: Gastric and jejunal alimentation with fine polyethylene tubes. A.M.A. Arch. Surg., 65:373–381, 1952.

28. Pareira, M. D., Conrad, E. J., Hicks, W., and Elman, R.: Therapeutic nutrition with tube feeding. J.A.M.A., 156:810–816, 1954.

29. Smith, D. W., and Lee, R. M.: Nutritional management in duodenal fistula. Surg. Gynecol. Obstet., 103:666–672, 1956.

30. Barron, J.: Tube feeding of postoperative patients. Surg. Clin. North Am., 39:1481–1491, 1959.

31. Greenstein, J. P., Birnbaum, S. M., Winitz, M., and Otey, M. C.: Quantitative nutritional studies with water-soluble chemically defined diets. I. Growth, reproduction and lactation in rats. Arch. Biochem. Biophys., 72:396–416, 1957.

32. Winitz, M., Graff, J., Gallagher, N., Narkin, A., and Seedman, D. A.: Evaluation of chemical diets as nutrition for man-in-space. Nature, 205:741–743, 1965.

33. Winitz, M., Seedman, D. A., and Graff, J.: Studies in metabolic nutrition employing chemically defined diets. I. Extended feeding of normal human adult males. Am. J. Clin. Nutr., 23:525–545, 1970.

34. Stephens, R. V., and Randall, H. T.: Use of a concentrated, balanced, liquid elemental diet for nutritional management of catabolic states. Ann. Surg., 170:642–667, 1969.

35. Rocchio, M. A., Cha, C-J. M., Haas, K. F., and Randall, H. T.: Use of chemically defined diets in the management of patients with high output gastrointestinal cutaneous fistulas. Am. J. Surg., 127:148–156, 1974.

36. Rocchio, M. A., Cha, C-J. M., Haas, K. F., and Randall, H. T.: Use of chemically defined diets in the management of patients with acute inflammatory bowel disease. Am. J. Surg., 127:469–475, 1974.

37. Liffmann, K. D., and Randall, H. T.: A modified technique for creating a jejunostomy. Surg. Gynecol. Obstet., 134:663–664, 1972.

38. Dudrick, S. J., Wilmore, D. W., Vars, H. M., and Rhoads, J. E.: Long-term total parenteral nutrition with growth, development, and positive nitrogen balance. Surgery, 64:134–142, 1968.

CHAPTER 1

The Physiology of Eating

With Particular Reference to the Role of Gastrointestinal Hormones in the Regulation of Digestion

BRIAN J. ROWLANDS
THOMAS A. MILLER

The major function of the gastrointestinal tract is to transform the many varied nutrients we ingest, irrespective of their physical or chemical properties, into simpler chemical molecules that may be absorbed, assimilated, and utilized for metabolic functions in the body. In addition, the gastrointestinal tract has a protective role in detoxification and elimination of many parasites, bacteria, viruses, chemical toxins, and drugs that may be harmful to health.[1] Food is usually ingested cyclically, but the homeostatic mechanisms that ensure an adequate supply of caloric substrate, fluid and electrolyte balance, acid-base balance, and protein substrate for tissue replacement and repair operate continuously and are a function of both complex controlling mechanisms and our immediate and usual dietary intake. In disease states, normal digestive functions may be disturbed by many factors, such as anorexia, inability to swallow, vomiting, malabsorption, and coma, and this leads to changes in substrate and hormone homeostasis that may further compromise the host. Intravenous, enteral, and tube feeding techniques that bypass the regulatory mechanisms of the upper gastrointestinal tract, and deliver nutrients continuously rather than intermittently may also signficantly alter the digestive process[2-4] and lead to structural and morphologic changes in the bowel.[5] Furthermore, the composition and physical properties of the nutrients will be important determinants of their absorption and assimilation.[6] It is therefore important,

prior to considering the principles and clinical practice of enteral and tube feeding, to have a thorough understanding of the normal physiology of eating and digestion. This chapter presents an overview of the function of the gastrointestinal tract and the mechanisms responsible for the regulation of gastrointestinal secretion and motility, with particular reference to the role of gastrointestinal hormones. Important factors in the maintenance of normal growth and function of the gastrointestinal mucosa are also discussed.[7] No attempt will be made to discuss the physiologic responses to specific foodstuffs or the alterations in metabolism produced by specific disease processes within the gastrointestinal tract, as these are the subjects of subsequent chapters.

OVERVIEW OF DIGESTION

The normal daily nutrient intake of a healthy person is about 300 gm of liquid and food. During the same period, the gastrointestinal tract adds about 10,000 ml of digestive juices, all of which are subsequently reabsorbed, leaving about 200 gm of solid feces for evacuation. Several factors control the processes of secretion, motility, and absorption. These include both voluntary and involuntary control by the central and autonomic nervous systems, local metabolic and electrophysiologic controls within mucosal and smooth muscle cells, the gastrointestinal circulation, and the gastrointestinal hormones.[8] A detailed description of the mechanisms that convert complex food molecules into chemically simpler ones is beyond the scope of this chapter and may be found elsewhere,[9] but it is important to realize that the highly coordinated sequence of steps may be disrupted by disease or by surgery.[10]

Energy for secretion and absorption is obtained from local oxidation of both glucose and fat within the gastrointestinal tract.[11] Many of these processes involve the transport of a variety of ions and organic materials against electrochemical gradients which, together with the high rate of cellular turnover, involves the consumption of large amounts of energy. These mechanisms not only require a favorable energy supply but also depend on an adequate blood flow to the gastrointestinal organs. Blood flow is influenced by the overall state of the circulation of the body, the autonomic nervous system, circulating neurohumoral substances, tissue metabolites, and intrinsic vascular characteristics such as autoregulation. An increase in secretory rate usually involves an increase in cellular metabolism, causing release of dilator metabolites and an increase in blood flow to the gland.

Gastrointestinal hormones are polypeptides that are produced by the gastrointestinal cells and influence other cells within the gastrointestinal tract.[12] Their release is stimulated by feeding, digestion, and absorption (Fig. 1–1). Although numerous hormones have been identified, four are recognized to be of major physiologic importance: gastrin, secretin, cholecystokinin (CCK), and gastric inhibitory peptide (GIP). Gastrin stimulates the secretion of acid by the stomach and influences the growth of the gastrointestinal mucosa. Secretin stimulates the secretion of pancreatic juice, which is rich in water and bicarbonate. Cholecystokinin stimulates the production of pancreatic secretions and causes emptying of the gallbladder. Gastric inhibitory peptide is insulinotropic and inhibits both secretion and emptying of the stomach. Vascular function, motility, and release of gastrointestinal hormones are under the influence of the neural components of the gastrointestinal system. These consist of sympathetic and parasympathetic efferent fibers, afferent fibers from the gastrointestinal organs, and plexuses of intrinsic nerves within the walls of these or-

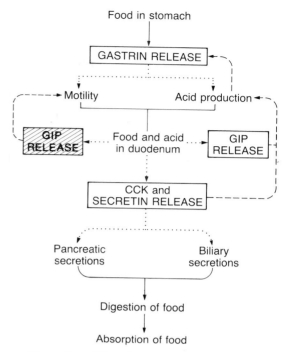

Figure 1–1. The role of four major gastrointestinal hormones in the digestion of food. *Dotted lines* represent stimulatory activity; *dashed lines* represent inhibitory activity.

gans. Afferent nerves stimulate salivary, gastric, and pancreatic secretions, the release of gastrin, and changes in the motility of smooth muscle. Factors that regulate the emptying of the stomach include the osmolality of the luminal contents, fat and protein content of the food, the level of motor activity of the stomach and duodenum, the tone of the pyloric sphincter and the extrinsic and intrinsic parasympathetic nerves, and the levels of gastrointestinal hormones such as gastrin, secretin, CCK, and GIP.[13] These hormones are also important in facilitating propulsive movement in the small bowel. Propulsive activity of the colon is less marked and is intermittent in nature.

When it is eaten, food is first mixed with saliva, which contains the enzyme amylase, which breaks down starch into smaller molecules and also helps to lubricate and macerate food during chewing. In the stomach, the oxyntic cells of the gastric mucosa actively secrete hydrochloric acid, thereby activating pepsin, an enzyme responsible for protein digestion. Subsequently, the food is mixed with biliary and pancreatic secretions in the duodenum. In their passage through the small intestine, fats, carbohydrates, and proteins are broken down into simple molecules and are absorbed through the gut wall by active transport mechanisms. Sodium is actively absorbed and is closely linked with the active transport of glucose and amino acids. Chloride and water are passively reabsorbed. This highly efficient transport system ensures that the vast majority of the daily fluid intake is reabsorbed during its passage through the bowel. Small intestinal absorption of carbohydrates depends on prior digestion of food, the integrity of the mucosa, effectiveness of the transport mechanisms for carbohydrates, intestinal transit time, and mechanical mixing by the muscular action of the intestinal wall. The average human diet contains polysaccharides and disaccharides, which are not effectively absorbed from the lumen of the gut, and which must be digested into monosaccharides by several enzymes, including salivary and pancreatic amylase and the disaccharidases, which are located in the microvilli. Eighty per cent of the carbohydrate is broken down into glucose, which is actively absorbed by a sodium-dependent transport mechanism. Protein within the lumen of the bowel is enzymatically digested into amino acids and small peptides. Tripeptides and dipeptides are actively transported by the intestinal mucosa. There are many active transport mechanisms for the individual amino acids, and these are also dependent on the presence of sodium. Fats are absorbed from the lumen of the bowel by a passive transport process. Digestion of dietary fats is mediated primarily by pancreatic lipase and related enzymes but is also dependent on emulsification of dietary lipid by bile salts. This leads to the formation of micelles, which are simple fat molecules that diffuse through the unstirred layer of chyme adjacent to the mucosa and reach the microvilli. The micelles subsequently disintegrate and their lipid components diffuse through the membrane to the inside of the mucosal cell. Some triglycerides are resynthesized from fatty acids and monoglycerides. A variety of lipid molecules are incorporated inside the cells into chylomicrons, which are soluble in the cytoplasm. Chylomicrons penetrate the basolateral membrane, enter the lymphatics, and are subsequently carried to the blood. The absorption of vitamins from the lumen of the bowel is mediated by a variety of independent mechanisms which, however, are dependent on the water- or fat-solubility of the vitamin.

PHYSIOLOGY OF DIGESTION

In this section, the fate of a single bolus of food will be reviewed, with emphasis on the role of the gastrointestinal hormones and the neuroendocrine regulation of digestion.

Mouth and Pharynx. Food is taken into the mouth, where it is chewed and mixed with salivary secretions prior to being swallowed. The amount of mastication necessary depends on the texture of the food, the dentition, and the strength of the muscles of mastication. The mouth and pharynx are lined with small salivary glands, which, together with the parotid, submandibular, and sublingual glands, produce about 1500 ml of saliva daily. The saliva is seromucoid and lubricates the food during chewing and swallowing and protects the mucosal lining of the mouth and pharynx. The serous glands, found mainly in the parotid and submandibular glands, produce amylase, which acts optimally at a pH of 6.5 to convert carbohydrate into simple disaccharides. Salivary amylase is inactivated at a pH below 4.5 so that its action ceases when the bolus of food enters the stomach. The main stimulus to the production of salivary amylase is the sight, smell, and taste of the food itself, but calcitonin, secretin, and pancreozymin can also influence the quantity and composition of saliva.[14, 15]

Esophagus. The upper and lower esophageal sphincters are normally closed but relax on swallowing to allow the bolus of food to enter the esophagus. Primary and secondary peristaltic waves then propel the bolus toward the gastroesophageal junction, just proximal to which is the lower esophageal sphincter, whose major function is to prevent reflux from the stomach. The nervous mechanisms controlling the lower esophageal sphincter are unclear, but normally a pressure of about 25 mm Hg is maintained in this area, and relaxation is initiated by passage of the bolus of food through the upper esophageal sphincter. The physiologic role of gastrointestinal hormones on the lower esophageal sphincter is also unclear, but gastrin increases pressure on the lower esophageal sphincter and secretin, cholecystokinin, glucagon, and prostaglandins all decrease pressure.[16, 17] Foodstuffs also appear to have different effects, with proteins and carbohydrates increasing sphincter tone and fats lowering it.

Stomach.[18] The stomach has four parts: the fundus, body, antrum, and pylorus. The fundus and body contain most of the cells that produce acid and pepsin, whereas the antral and pyloric cells secrete gastrin. Mucous-secreting cells are distributed throughout the stomach. The production of secretions by the gastric mucosal cells may be separated into three distinct phases: cephalic, gastric, and intestinal. In the cephalic phase, active secretion from most cells commences prior to entrance of the bolus of food into the stomach. This is the result of neurogenic stimulation, mediated through the vagus nerve and related to taste, smell, and mastication. In the gastric phase, secretion of pepsinogen begins as the bolus enters the stomach, owing mainly to vagal stimulation, but the direct action of secretin and the indirect action of gastrin also play a part. The enzyme converts large proteins into polypeptides and is maximally active at a pH of 1 to 3. Gastric juice also contains lipase, which hydrolyzes short-chain and medium-chain triglycerides found in milk, and gelatinase and urease, which partially digest gelatin and urea, respectively. The most important secretion of the stomach is hydrochloric acid, which is produced in the parietal cells. Secretion of hydrochloric acid occurs in response to eating and is mediated through the hormone gastrin. The amount of acid produced depends on the number of cells: basal secretion is 0 to 5 mEq H^+/L in health and 20 to 35 mEq H^+/L in response to histamine or pentagastrin. Gastrin produced by cells in the antrum and pylorus reaches peak elevations at 30 minutes after feeding and its rise correlates with acid production. A negative feedback mechanism inhibits the production of gastrin as the gastric acidity rises. The composition of gastric juice is dependent on the rate of secretion and on the gastric blood flow. The latter is increased by cholinergic stimulation, epinephrine, histamine, and gastrin and is reduced by vasopressin, norepinephrine, and secretin. Different foodstuffs also stimulate enzyme and acid production at different rates, but in general, maximal rates of secretion occur 45 minutes after ingestion of a bolus of food

and return to basal levels by 3 hours. Another important feature of the stomach is the gastric mucosal barrier, which prevents back-diffusion of H^+ ions into the mucosa. This barrier may be disrupted by ethanol, detergents, bile acids, lysolecithin, acetic acid, and some drugs (such as aspirin, indomethacin, and phenylbutazone), causing damage to the gastric mucosa. The intestinal phase of gastric secretion is initiated by the presence of food in the duodenum and jejunum and is mediated through the vagus nerve and gastrin.

The bolus of food, together with secretions of the stomach, form chyme, which is mixed by muscular contractions of the stomach wall, allowing initial digestion to take place. Gastric emptying of liquid food is more rapid than for solids and occurs as a result of peristalsis of the stomach wall and relaxation of the pyloric sphincter. It is under both neurogenic and hormonal control and may be influenced by the chemical nature of foodstuffs.[13] The physiologic role of gastrin, cholecystokinin, secretin, and glucagon in the regulation of gastric emptying is unclear.

Duodenum.[19] As food enters the duodenum, it meets the combined secretions of the duodenal mucosa, pancreas, liver, and gallbladder. Brunner's glands of the mucosa produce alkaline secretions with a pH of 9, which help to neutralize the acidic gastric secretions. The duodenal mucosa also produces some forms of gastrin, secretin, and CCK, which influence the secretions of organs emptying into the duodenum and inhibit gastric secretion and motility. Chyme enters the duodenum at a variable pH, but the pH and osmolality of luminal contents entering the small intestine are remarkably constant at pH 7 to 9, encouraging optimal digestion and absorption of all nutrients. Luminal acidity is the main stimulus to production of secretin whereas fat and certain amino acids (for example, tryptophan and phenylalanine) present in the duodenal chyme stimulate production of CCK.

Pancreas.[20] The pancreas produces both exocrine and endocrine secretions. The exocrine secretions are produced in the acinar cells and consist of enzyme, fluid, and electrolyte secretions. Each day when stimulated by secretin the pancreas produces about 2000 ml of secretions that are rich in bicarbonate. This alkaline secretion plays an important role in neutralizing the acid chyme delivered to the duodenum from the stomach and helps to maintain the pH of the duodenum at 7 to 9. The main enzymes produced are trypsinogen, chymotrypsinogen, amylase, and lipase. Trypsinogen and chymotrypsinogen are converted to their active forms trypsin and chymotrypsin and, along with other proteolytic enzymes, are responsible for breaking down proteins into proteoses and peptides. Amylase converts starch and glycogen into disaccharides, and lipase is essential for normal fat absorption. The production of exocrine secretions is stimulated principally by secretin and CCK, but also the vagus nerve. The endocrine secretions of the pancreas—insulin and glucagon—are important in carbohydrate homeostasis and are discussed elsewhere in this book.

Liver and Gallbladder.[21]   The liver plays a central role in substrate and hormone homeostasis, but the production of bile makes it important also in digestion and absorption. About 1000 ml of bile are produced daily in response to stimulation by gastrointestinal hormones released when food is ingested. Bile, which consists of a bile acid–independent fraction and a bile acid–dependent fraction, contains water, electrolytes, bile acids, lecithin, and cholesterol. The proportion of the constituents varies under different circumstances, but stimulation by secretin produces bile that is rich in bicarbonate ions. The enterohepatic circulation of bile acids, which ensures that the majority of bile acids are reabsorbed in the distal small bowel after they have completed their digestive function, is also an important regulator of the rate of secretion and the composition of bile. Bile is concentrated in the gallbladder, which contracts in response to hormonal stimulation, forcing bile into the duodenum through the ampulla of Vater. The main stimulus to contraction of the gallbladder is the presence of fat in the duodenum, which causes prompt release of CCK.[22] Bile functions mainly in the formation of micelles in fat digestion. Once the biliary and pancreatic secretions mix with the chyme in the duodenum, the intraluminal contents move into the small intestine, where digestion ensues rapidly.

Small Intestine.   The absorption of most protein, carbohydrates, and fats is completed within 45 minutes of the ingestion of a meal. Absorption of nutrients occurs mainly in the duodenum and proximal jejunum; little absorption, except that of fats, takes place in the distal ileum. Contractile activity of the small bowel increases after a meal in response to hormonal and vagal stimulation. In addition, intraluminal contents have a modifying effect on the production of gastric, biliary, and pancreatic secretions. Electrolyte and fluid balance are also regulated by the jejunum and ileum prior to passage of nutrients through the ileocecal valve into the colon.

Colon and Rectum.   Large quantities of fluid and electrolytes are also absorbed in the colon, which receives about 1500 ml daily from the ileum and excretes only 200 ml. Movement through the colon is slower than through the small bowel, and here the food residues are exposed to large numbers of aerobic and anaerobic bacteria, which digest some of the complex molecules of protein, fat, and carbohydrate.

GASTROINTESTINAL HORMONES

In the last decade, major advances in our understanding of the physiology of digestion have been the result of the successful isolation of the major gastrointestinal hormones, their measurement in the tissue and body fluids using radioimmunoassay, the identification of hormone-producing cells in the digestive system, and the elucidation of the mechanisms by which hormones influence gastrointestinal motility, secretion, and absorption. Twenty-eight or more peptides are known to be present in the gut and pancreas.[23–25] Four others—secretin, cholecystokinin, gastrin, and GIP—exhibit the following criteria suggested by Grossman to define them as gastrointestinal hormones:[26]

1. Stimulation of one part of the gastrointestinal tract produces a response in a distant target.
2. The effect persists after cutting all nerves connecting the site of stimulation and the target.
3. The effect is produced by an extract of the part to which the stimulus is applied.
4. The effect is produced by infusing exogenous hormone in amounts and molecular forms similar to the increase in blood concentration seen after the stimulus for endogenous release.

The gastrointestinal hormones share some common features, despite differences in chemical structure, cell of origin, and biologic activity.[23-27] They are all peptides that originate in specialized granular cells of the gastrointestinal epithelium and influence several organs in selective ways. In response to food ingestion, they are secreted in an orderly fashion in three different directions: to the blood circulation (endocrine secretion), to receptors in the neighboring cells (paracrine secretion), and to the lumen of the bowel (luminal secretion); they produce a coordinated activation and inhibition of secretion and motility in the various gastrointestinal organs. The hormones belong to two families of compounds: gastrin, including gastrin and CCK; and secretin, including secretin, GIP, vasoactive intestinal peptide (VIP), and glucagon. The hormones within these groups have similar structure and actions, but relatively small changes in their chemical composition may markedly alter their biologic activity and organ specificity. In addition, many of the hormones exist in several forms that have different potencies and are present in different amounts in the body. For example, gastrin has three major distinct forms, a 17-amino acid form called "little gastrin," a 34-amino acid form called "big gastrin," and a complex molecule called "big-big-gastrin."

A number of hormones originally isolated from the gut have subsequently been found in enteric neurons and the central nervous system, and a number of brain peptides have been found in gastrointestinal endocrine cells. It is postulated that many gastrointestinal hormones are found in both nervous and endocrine cells and are capable of functioning both as a hormone and as a neurotransmitter or modulator.[23-27] Gut endocrine cells, which contain both a peptide and an amine, belong to the amine precursor uptake and decarboxylation (APUD) system and are derived from the embryonic neural crest.[23-27] The development of our understanding of the secretion, regulation, and actions of gastrointestinal hormones has inevitably led to a reappraisal of our understanding of gastrointestinal physiology based on the classical separation of all bodily functions into those regulated by the nervous system and those by the endocrine system. Many of the digestive processes will be more readily explained by the dual role of the hormones as both hormone and neurotransmitter, and some of the more recently identified hormones will probably be shown to have major roles in the activation and inhibition of the digestive mechanisms. The important gastrointestinal hormones and their actions are summarized in Table 1–1.

Gastrin.[23-27] Gastrin is produced in the G-cells of the antral mucosa of the stomach. Three major types of gastrin have been described: "little gastrin," "big gastrin," and "big-big gastrin." The biologic activity of each is determined by the C-terminal tetrapeptide portion of the molecule. In addition, pentagastrin is a synthetic C-terminal tetrapeptide to which alanine has been added. The actions of gastrin may be regarded as physiologic or pharmacologic. The major physiologic actions are stimulation of acid secretion by the stomach and its trophic action on the mucosal lining of the stomach, small intestine, colon, and pancreas, in which gastrin can increase DNA, RNA, and protein synthesis. In addition, gastrin stimulates secretion of pepsinogen, gastric blood flow, and contraction of stomach musculature. In larger doses, its pharmacologic actions are to stimulate secretion of water, electrolyte, bicarbonate, and enzyme by the small intestine, pancreas, and liver; smooth muscle contraction of lower esophageal sphincter, gallbladder, small intestine, and colon; and the release of insulin, glucagon, and calcitonin. It also inhibits contraction of most sphincters in the gastrointestinal tract. Gastrin is produced in response to a protein-containing meal, stomach distention, and cholinergic agents. Its release is inhibited by acidification of the stomach, but vagal denervation of the stomach reduces this response. Hypergastrinemia is a characteristic of the Zollinger-Ellison syndrome, in which APUD cells in the islets of Langerhans of the pancreas produce excessive gastrin; it may also be a feature of duodenal ulceration, short bowel syndrome, hyperparathyroidism, and inadequate gastric resection with a resultant retained antrum following a Billroth II gastrectomy. In all of these conditions, duodenal ulceration is intractable and rarely responsive to medical therapy.

Cholecystokinin.[23-27] Cholecystokinin contains 33 amino acids, and its biologic activity is dependent on the C-terminal octapeptide. It is produced in the duodenum and jejunum, the major stimulus to production being the presence of fatty acids and L-isomers of amino acids in the lumen of the

Table 1–1   GASTROINTESTINAL HORMONES

HORMONE	SITE OF SECRETION	MAIN STIMULUS	MAIN ACTIONS
Gastrin	Stomach, duodenum	Proteoses and peptides	Stimulates gastric acid secretion and mucosal growth
Cholecystokinin (CCK)	Duodenum, jejunum	Fat and amino acids in duodenum	Stimulates pancreatic enzyme secretion and gallbladder contraction
Secretin	Small intestine	Duodenal acidity	Stimulates hepatic and pancreatic water and bicarbonate secretion
Gastric inhibitory peptide (GIP)	Small intestine	Carbohydrate and fat	Decreases gastric motility and stimulates insulin secretion
Vasoactive inhibitory peptide (VIP)	Small intestine, pancreas	Unknown (fat?)	Vasodilator
Glucagon	Pancreas	Plasma insulin and glucose concentrations	Stimulates hepatic glycogenolysis and inhibits motility
Enteroglucagon	Duodenum, small intestine	Carbohydrate and fat in duodenum	Inhibits motility
Pancreatic polypeptide	Pancreas	Unknown	Inhibits gallbladder contraction and pancreatic and biliary secretion
Motilin	Duodenum, small intestine	Duodenal alkalinity	Regulates motility
Somatostatin	Stomach, duodenum, small intestine, pancreas	Unknown	Regulates other hormones
Bombesin	Small intestine	Unknown	Regulates gastrin

bowel. The main physiologic action of CCK is to stimulate contraction of the gallbladder, relaxation of the ampulla of Vater, and secretion of pancreatic enzyme. It also slows gastric emptying and is trophic to the pancreas. In large doses, it is a weak stimulus to secretion of pepsinogen and acid in the stomach but will inhibit gastrin-stimulated secretion of acid. It also inhibits lower esophageal sphincter tone, stimulates colonic motility and duodenal mucosal secretions, produces satiety to food, and stimulates the release of insulin and glucagon. No diseases are known to be associated with overproduction of CCK, but a deficiency of this hormone or its release during feeding may play a role in the production of morbid obesity.[28, 29]

Secretin.[23–27]   Secretin is a polypeptide of 27 amino acids which is secreted by the S-cells of the duodenum. Its physiologic action, which is to stimulate the production of bicarbonate and water by the pancreas and liver, is dependent on the whole molecule. It is produced in response to the presence of acid in the duodenum, and as the pancreas is stimulated to produce bicarbonate, the luminal contents of the duodenum become neutralized so that production of secretin is cut off. Secretin also stimulates secretion of pepsinogen and contraction of the pyloric sphincter and inhibits gastrin-stimulated secretion of acid and contraction of the stomach. There is some synergistic action with CCK in stimulating release of pancreatic enzyme and insulin while inhibiting release of glucagon. Defective secretion of secretin may play a role in the pathogenesis of duodenal ulceration and celiac disease.

Gastric Inhibitory Peptide.[23–27, 30–32]   Gastric inhibitory peptide is produced by the K-cells of the upper small intestine and consists of 43 amino acid radicals. Its main action is to inhibit secretion of gastric acid that is stimulated by pentagastrin, gastrin, insulin, and histamine, and to inhibit secretion of pepsin. It is a potent stimulator of insulin release by the pancreas and appears to be the most important component of the entero-insular axis. Another function appears to be regulation of the delivery of the stomach contents to the small intestine so that the volume, osmolality, and pH of the luminal contents entering the jejunum do not exceed the ability of the bowel to handle them. The release of GIP appears to be biphasic and is related to its stimulation initially by glucose and subsequently by fat.

Vasoactive Intestinal Peptide.[23–27, 31–33] Vasoactive intestinal peptide contains 20 amino acids and is produced in the intestine, although the mechanism of its release is unknown. It has actions similar to those of other members of its group (secretin, glucagon). Vasoactive intestinal peptide stimulates pancreatic secretion of bicarbonate and water, release of insulin and glucagon, and production of small intestinal juice, and is capable of increasing hepatic glycogenolysis. It is also a potent vasodilator and has inotropic effects on the heart. Plasma VIP concentrations are elevated in a syndrome called pancreatic cholera, which is characterized by profuse watery diarrhea, hypokalemia, and achlorhydria.[34, 35] Excessive levels of VIP are usually associated with a VIP-producing tumor of the pancreas or sympathetic ganglia.

Glucagon and Enteroglucagon.[23–27, 31–32] Pancreatic glucagon is a single-chained polypeptide with 29 amino acids. A substance with similar physiologic and pharmacologic actions but different molecular weight, known as enteroglucagon, has been isolated from the duodenal and jejunal mucosa. Glucagon stimulates glycogenolysis and interacts with insulin to maintain carbohydrate homeostasis within the body. This aspect of the metabolic response to stress and starvation is dealt with in detail in a subsequent chapter. Glucagon and enteroglucagon have similar pharmacologic actions. They inhibit secretion of pancreatic enzyme and the motility of all parts of the bowel. They may also selectively interfere with the actions of gastrin and secretin. Enteroglucagon is stimulated by food, primarily carbohydrates and long-chained triglycerides, whereas pancreatic glucagon shows no response. Hyperglucagonemia may be related to the production of excessive quantities of the hormone by a pancreatic tumor and may give rise to weight loss, anorexia, diabetes mellitus, and skin rashes. The precise relationship between the actions of pancreatic glucagon and enteroglucagon is still not fully understood.

Other Hormones. *Pancreatic polypeptide*[23, 32] is a straight-chained polypeptide with 36 amino acids which is produced in the pancreas. Plasma concentrations rise rapidly following meals, and the most important actions are to inhibit contraction of the gallbladder and secretion of pancreatic and biliary enzymes. Its relationship to insulin and glucagon in carbohydrate metabolism is still unknown.

Motilin[23, 32] is a polypeptide with 22 amino acids which is found in the duodenum, jejunum, and upper ileum. It appears to be a regulator of gut motility and may enhance secretion of pepsin.

Somatostatin[23, 32] is a tetradecapeptide produced primarily by the hypothalamus, but it is also present in the D-cells of the antrum, upper intestine, and pancreas. It suppresses the secretion of growth hormone and thyroid-stimulating hormone and blocks the release of insulin and glucagon. It may inhibit release of gastrin and motilin, output of pancreatic enzyme and pepsin, and contraction of the gallbladder.

Bombesin[23, 32] is a peptide with 14 amino acids which is present in the gastrointestinal tract, brain, and lung. It stimulates secretion of gastric acid and release of gastrin that is independent of environmental pH and stimulates contraction of the gallbladder and secretion of pancreatic enzyme.

GASTROINTESTINAL GROWTH

Gastrointestinal hormones interact with other hormones and endocrine glands to regulate the growth of the digestive tract mucosa and the exocrine pancreas.[7] The normal development of digestive function and intestinal adaptation in response to surgery, disease, lactation, and nutrient intake involves a complex relationship between the gastrointestinal hormones and others such as growth hormones, thyroxine, and glucocorticosteroids. Normal development is also influenced by gastrointestinal secretion and the presence of specific nutrients in the lumen. The gastrointestinal mucosa has a rapid rate of turnover. Normally, proliferation and growth are balanced by exfoliation of surface cells, but disease processes may upset this balance, leading to ulceration and atrophy. Any factor influencing mucosal growth will also affect gastrointestinal function. Although nongastrointestinal hormones have been shown to alter mucosal growth, the most important influences are those factors that are stimulated by ingestion and digestion of food. Experimentally, these effects can be demonstrated by weighing the gastrointestinal organs and by measuring mucosal concentrations of DNA, RNA, and protein. Starvation decreases the total population of intestinal cells and the RNA, protein, and water concentrations of individual cells.

The effects of food in the lumen may be direct or indirect. There is a continuous process of desquamation and renewal of mucosal cells which is accelerated by the ingestion of food and its passage through the gastrointestinal tract. In addition, there is a nutritional effect of absorbed foodstuffs on the absorbing cells, prior to the passage of the absorbed nutrients into the portal and systemic circulations. The indirect effects are those produced by gastrointestinal hormones, motor and secretory activity, and neural stimulation. As has been noted previously, these effects may be interrelated and may be endocrine, paracrine, or neurotransmitter in nature. The most important trophic hormone is gastrin, and its role in mucosal development and adaptation is well established. The other hormones play lesser roles. The effects of nongastrointestinal hormones on mucosal growth may be mediated and modified by gastrin and the other gastrointestinal hormones. These complex interrelationships still have not been fully elucidated, but disease and dietary manipulation may have a profound influence on the maintenance of structure and function of the gastrointestinal tract.

OTHER FACTORS AFFECTING NORMAL DIGESTION

The preceding summary of the physiology of digestion and the description of the control mechanisms involved in gastrointestinal secretion, absorption, and motility are based on the assumption that we are dealing with a normal subject with an intact gastrointestinal tract. Food intake is normally regulated by the hypothalamus, which controls the sensations of hunger, thirst, satiety, anorexia, and appetite. Many factors may disrupt the central nervous control of food intake, and the absence of intraluminal nutrients leads not only to changes in gastrointestinal secretions and motility but also to a reduction in mucosal and pancreatic mass.[36] These changes take place despite the maintenance of energy and protein intake by parenteral nutrition and are associated with changes in the tissue stores and serum levels of many of the gastrointestinal hormones.[4, 5, 36, 37] This is an important concept to appreciate when nutritional support is used in hospitalized patients. Many of the patients requiring nutritional support already have a significant reduction in endogenous tissue mass as a result of chronic failure to satisfy requirements for energy and protein due either to hypermetabolism or to disease and surgical procedures that significantly alter the absorbent capacity of the bowel. Many intravenous regimens supply nutrients continuously over a 24-hour period, but the normal pattern of ingestion and digestion is cyclical. These factors, together with the lack of intraluminal stimulation, probably account for many of the changes in secretion of gastrointestinal hormones that are now being reported in patients receiving parenteral nutrition.[2-4, 37] These responses to total parenteral nutrition have also been compared with the metabolic and hormonal consequences of nutritional support using the enteral route and have provided evidence that the better disposal of nutrients and greater weight gain in patients receiving enteral nutrition may be attributed to hormone and substrate changes that closely approximate those seen in normal postprandial human subjects and experimental animals.[2-4, 37] The efficacy and management of this route of nutrition are the subjects of the subsequent chapters of this volume, and the physiologic changes that occur in secretion, absorption, and motility of the gastrointestinal tract will depend on the chemical constituents of the nutrients, the site of delivery (for example, gastrostomy and jejunostomy), the speed of infusion (and whether it is intermittent or continuous), and the functional absorptive surface of the bowel.[6, 38] These changes have not been extensively documented nor have their long-term effects been appraised, but as technologic advances improve the safety and efficacy of enteral feeding, the study of the effects of specific nutrients on specific digestive mechanisms should enhance our understanding of normal digestive physiology.

REFERENCES

1. Schanker, L. S.: On the mechanism of absorption of drugs from the gastrointestinal tract. J. Med. Pharm. Chem., 2:343–359, 1960.
2. Lickley, H. L. A., Track, N. S., Vranic, M., and Bury, K. D.: Metabolic responses to enteral and parenteral nutrition. Am. J. Surg., 135:172–176, 1978.
3. McArdle, A. H., Palmason, C., Morency, I., and

Brown, R. A.: A rationale for enteral feeding as the preferable route of hyperalimentation. Surgery, 90:616–623, 1981.

4. Gimmon, Z., Murphy, R. F., Chen, M.-H., Nachbauer, C. A., Fischer, J. E., and Joffe, S. N.: The effect of parenteral and enteral nutrition on portal and systemic immunoreactivities of gastrin, glucagon and vasoactive intestinal polypeptide (VIP). Ann. Surg., 196:571–575, 1982.
5. Johnson, L. R., Copeland, E. M., Dudrick, S. J., Lichtenberger, L. M., and Casto, G. A.: Structural and hormonal alterations in the gastrointestinal tract of parenterally fed rats. Gastroenterology 68:1177–1183, 1975.
6. Young, E. A., Cioletti, L. A., Traylor, J. B., and Balderas, V.: Gastrointestinal response to nutrient variation of defined formula diets. J.P.E.N. 5:478–484, 1981.
7. Johnson, L. R.: Regulation of gastrointestinal growth. In Johnson, L. R. (ed.): Physiology of the Gastrointestinal Tract. New York, Raven Press, 1981, pages 169–196.
8. Floch, M. H.: The physiology of eating. In Nutrition and Diet Therapy in Gastrointestinal Disease. New York, Plenum Press, 1981, pages 3–33.
9. Davenport, H. W.: Physiology of the Digestive Tract. Edition 5. Chicago, Year Book Medical Publishers, Inc., 1982.
10. Almy, T. P.: The gastrointestinal tract in man under stress. In Sleisenger, M. H., and Fordtran, J. S. (eds.): Gastrointestinal Disease—Pathophysiology, Diagnosis, and Management. Edition 2. Philadelphia, W. B. Saunders Co., 1978, pages 3–19.
11. Gray, G. M.: Mechanisms of digestion and absorption of food. In Sleisenger, M. H., and Fordtran, J. S. (eds.): Gastrointestinal Disease—Pathophysiology, Diagnosis, and Management. Edition 2. Philadelphia, W. B. Saunders Co., 1978, pages 241–250.
12. Bloom, S. R., and Polak, J. M.: Alimentary endocrine system. In Sircus, W., and Smith, A. M. (eds.): Scientific Foundations of Gastroenterology. Philadelphia, W. B. Saunders Co. 1980, pages 101–122.
13. Cooke, A. R.: Control of gastric emptying and motility. Gastroenterology, 68:804–816, 1975.
14. Drack, G. T., Koelz, H. R., and Blum A. L: Human calcitonin stimulates salivary amylase output in man. Gut, 17:620–623, 1976.
15. Mulcahy, A. H., Fitzgerald, H. O., and McGeeney, K. F.: Secretin and pancreozymin effect on salivary amylase concentration in man. Gut, 13:850, 1972.
16. Snape, W. F., and Cohen, S.: Hormonal control of esophageal function. Arch. Intern. Med., 136:538–542, 1976.
17. Castell, D. O.: The lower esophageal sphincter: Physiologic and clinical aspects. Ann. Intern. Med., 83:390–401, 1975.
18. Grossman, M. I.: Control of gastric secretion. In Sleisenger, M. H., and Fordtran, J. S. (eds.): Gastrointestinal Disease—Pathophysiology, Diagnosis, and Management. Edition 2. Philadelphia, W. B. Saunders Co., 1978, pages 640–659.
19. Miller, L. J., Malagelada, J. R., and Go, V. L. W.: Postprandial duodenal function in man. Gut, 19:699–706, 1978.
20. Meyer, J. H.: Pancreatic physiology. In Sleisenger,

M. H., and Fordtran, J. S. (eds.): Gastrointestinal Disease—Pathophysiology, Diagnosis, and Management. Edition 2. Philadelphia, W. B. Saunders Co., 1978, pages 1398–1408.
21. Wheeler, H. O.: Bile formation and physiology of the biliary tract. In Sleisenger, M. H., and Fordtran, J. S. (eds.): Gastrointestinal Disease—Pathophysiology, Diagnosis, and Management. Edition 2. W. B. Saunders Co., Philadelphia, 1978, pages 1279–1284.
22. Banfield, W. J.: Physiology of the gallbladder. Gastroenterology, 69:770–777, 1975.
23. Walsh, J. H.: Endocrine cells of the digestive system. In Johnson, L. R. (ed.): Physiology of the Gastrointestinal Tract. New York, Raven Press, 1981, pages 59–144.
24. Rayford, P. L., Miller, T. A., and Thompson, J. C.: Secretin, cholecystokinin and new gastrointestinal hormones. N. Engl. J. Med., 294:1093–1101, 1157–1164, 1976.
25. McGuigan, J. E.: Gastrointestinal hormones. Annu. Rev. Med., 29:307–318, 1978.
26. Grossman, M. I.: Physiological effects of gastrointestinal hormones. Fed. Proc., 36:1930–1932, 1974.
27. Walsh, J. H., and Grossman, M. I.: Gastrin. N. Engl. J. Med., 292:1324–1334, 1377–1384, 1975.
28. Straus, E., and Yalow, R. S.: Cholecystokinin in the brains of obese and nonobese mice. Science, 203:68–69, 1979.
29. Domschke, S., Domschke, W., Bloom, S. R., Mitznegg, P., Mitchell, S. J., Lux, G., and Strunz, U.: Vasoactive intestinal peptide in man: Pharmacokinetics, metabolic and circulatory effects. Gut, 19:1049–1053, 1978.
30. Brown, J. C., Dryburgh, J. R., Frost, J. L., Otte, S. C., and Pederson, R. A.: Properties and actions of GIP in gut hormones. In Bloom, S. R. (ed.): Gut Hormones. London, Churchill Livingstone, 1978, pages 277–282.
31. Grossman, M. I.: Candidate hormones. Gastroenterology, 67:730–755, 1974.
32. Chey, W. Y., and You, C. H.: Newer gut hormones and hormone candidates. In Berk, J. E. (ed.): Developments in Digestive Diseases. Volume 3. Philadelphia, Lea & Febiger, 1980, pages 179–212.
33. Said, S. I.: VIP Overview. In Bloom, S. R. (ed.): Gut Hormones. London, Churchill Livingstone, 1978, pages 465–469.
34. Bloom, S. R.: VIP and watery diarrhea—VI. In Bloom, S. R. (ed.): Gut Hormones. London, Churchill Livingstone, 1978, pages 583–588.
35. Said, S. I.: VIP and watery diarrhea—IV. In Bloom, S. R. (ed.): Gut Hormones. London, Churchill Livingstone, 1978, pages 578–580.
36. Weser, E., and Kim, Y.: Nutrition and the gastrointestinal tract. In Sleisenger, M. H., and Fordtran, J. S. (eds.): Gastrointestinal Disease—Pathophysiology, Diagnosis, and Management. Edition 2. Philadelphia, W. B. Saunders Co., 1978, pages 20–52.
37. Greenberg, G. R., Wolman, S. L., Christofides, N. D., Bloom, S. R., and Jeejeebhoy, K. N.: Effect of total parenteral nutrition on gut hormone release in humans. Gastroenterology, 80:988–993, 1981.
38. Heymsfield, S. B., Horowitz, J., and Lawson, D. H.: Enteral hyperalimentation. In Berk, J. E. (ed.): Developments in Digestive Diseases. Volume 3. Philadelphia, Lea & Febiger, 1980, pages 59–83.

CHAPTER 2

Digestion and Absorption

J. ROBERTO MORAN
HARRY L. GREENE

The gastrointestinal tract is a large epithelial interface between the external and the interior environments. Its major function is the transfer of nutrients from the bowel lumen into the body. Consequently, the gastrointestinal tract must be able to convert the varied physical and chemical forms of food that are eaten into simple molecules that can be easily transferred across cell membranes. This process requires coordinated motor activity, secretion of digestive enzymes, and the presence of substances that act upon the physical properties of complex foods. In addition, intact absorptive mechanisms are necessary to accomplish this vital function. Failure of any one of these mechanisms may result in malabsorption and eventually malnutrition.

Advances in our understanding of basic physiology and biochemistry, as well as in the field of clinical nutrition, have fostered an intense interest in the development of "ideally" digestible and utilizable diets. The purpose of these diets is to provide food in a form that will give optimal nutritional support during periods of acute and chronic illness when there is damage of one or more of the gastrointestinal functions. The review of the basic mechanisms involved in the digestion, absorption, and metabolism of nutrients necessary for the *rational* use of these diets is the topic of this chapter.

ANATOMY AND PHYSIOLOGY OF THE DIGESTIVE SYSTEM

Esophagus

The esophagus is a hollow tube of striated and smooth muscle. Its length ranges from 25 to 35 cm in the adult. An accurate appraisal of the length of the adult esophagus can be made by measuring the distance from the lower wisdom teeth to the xiphisternum, with the patient lying supine with the head fully extended.[1] It is approximately 30 mm in lateral diameter and 19 mm in anteroposterior diameter. In its resting state the esophagus is collapsed; however, it is capable of distending to accommodate fluid and solid material. Both ends of the esophagus are modified to maintain closure under resting conditions. The fibers of the cricopharyngeal muscle are traditionally considered to represent the upper esophageal sphincter. Recent work supports the presence of a specialized arrangement of semicircular muscle fibers at the lower end of the esophagus.[2] This thickening, called the *gastroesophageal ring*, may represent the sphincter. The function of the lower esophageal sphincter (LES) is to allow the passage of material coming from the mouth and the prevention of regurgitation of gastric contents back into the low pressure area of the esophagus. The LES relaxation response to swallowing seems to be mediated primarily by the vagus nerve. However, a large number of humoral substances, gastrointestinal hormones, and prostaglandins have been found to alter the LES pressure.[3, 4] Among the agents that raise LES pressure are gastrin, histamine, metoclopramide, cholinergic drugs (such as bethanecol), diazepam, and protein meal. Examples of agents that lower LES pressure are glucagon, estrogens and progesterone, isoproterenol, atropine, alcohol, and fats; smoking is also known to lower LES pressure.

The present difficulty in determining the physiologic role of humoral substances on the LES reflects a similar problem for all areas of gastrointestinal smooth muscle. The gastrointestinal smooth muscle, including the esophagus and the LES, contain receptors for virtually all humoral substances identified to date. Either the gut smooth muscle is a highly complex organ regulated by literally dozens of neurohumoral substances or the smooth muscle simply contains primitive residual receptors to many substances that have little, if any, physiologic role.

Stomach

The stomach receives and stores food for a short period, mixes it with the gastric secretions, grinds the mixture to semifluid consistency, and delivers it to the duodenum in an orderly and almost continuous fashion. The two main functions of the stomach relate to its motor activity and secretion of substances that aid in digestion.

Secretory Functions. The human stomach secretes sodium, potassium, hydrochloric acid, pepsinogen, intrinsic factor, and mucus into the gastric lumen and gastrin into the blood. These highly acidic secretions participate in some breakdown of proteins (pepsinogen is activated to the proteolytic enzyme pepsin), but most importantly they dissolve soluble foods and bring the ingested material close to the osmolality of plasma. Bactericidal action is prominent, as gastric juice has a pH of about 1.0. Intrinsic factor, which is essential for absorption of vitamin B_{12} in the ileum, is secreted in relatively large amounts by the gastric mucosa.

Acid Secretion. Acid secretion (basal or fasting) varies over time and usually represents 5 to 10 per cent of maximal rates. A circadian rhythm has been found in fasting subjects, with highest output in the early morning and the lowest output in the late evening hours. The factors responsible for basal secretion are probably connected with the spontaneous release of small amounts of gastrin and tonic vagal stimulation.

The major physiologic stimulant to acid secretion by the oxyntic, or parietal, cells is the ingestion of meals. Stimulated secretion is subdivided somewhat arbitrarily into cephalic, gastric, and intestinal phases.[5] The cephalic phase begins with the sight, smell, taste, and chewing of appetizing food; the gastric phase begins when food enters the stomach; and the intestinal phase begins when food components begin to enter the intestine. Obviously these phases overlap. The mechanisms that mediate these phases are multiple, and several mechanisms may be operating during the same period.

The cephalic phase is mediated entirely by the vagal nerves and is, therefore, abolished by proximal gastric vagotomy. Acetylcholine is the principal chemical messenger. At present, there is conflicting information on the contribution of gastrin to this phase.[6-8]

Two factors are known to be operative when food is present in the stomach: gastric distention and chemical stimulation of gastrin release. Distention of the stomach results in a small but significant stimulation of acid secretion. Presumably this is mediated by cholinergic reflexes conveyed by both intramural and long vagovagal pathways.[9] When various food components were studied for acid-stimulating activity, amino acids and partially digested protein were found to be effective while glucose and fat caused no stimulation.[10] The increase in gastrin accounted for most of the observed acid secretory response. Of the specific amino acids tested, phenylalanine and tryptophan were the most potent releasers of gastrin and stimulants of acid secretion in humans.[11] Chemical stimulation, however, is not entirely mediated by gastrin; caffeine and alcohol stimulate acid secretion without an increase in gastrin in humans.[12]

Food substances entering the intestine may cause stimulation or inhibition of gastric secretion. An as yet unidentified intestinal hormone, enterooxyntin, has been proposed as the mediator of the intestinal phase of gastric acid secretion, but it is possible that absorbed amino acids also act directly on the oxyntic cells. The evidence is that amino acids induce similar increments in acid secretion, whether given by duodenal perfusion or intravenous infusion.[13] Konturek et al. found that histidine, phenylalanine, glycine, tryptophan, and alanine were the most potent stimulants when infused into dogs.[14] The release of inhibitory peptides (that is, enteroglucagon, vasoactive intestinal peptide, and gastric inhibitory polypeptide) from the intestinal mucosa has been postulated as the mechanism by which fat in the proximal intestine inhibits gastric acid secretions.[15] This suggested mechanism has not yet been verified in humans. Another moderately potent inhibitor of acid secretion is hypertonic glucose, which has been found to be effective when given intravenously, orally, or intraduodenally.

Besides acetylcholine and gastrin, histamine is another of the best-defined chemical messengers that regulate acid secretion. It appears to act also at a separate receptor on the oxyntic cells, and potentiating interactions have been reported to occur with the other secretagogues. Factors regulating histamine release have not been defined, but studies with H_2-receptor antagonists leave little doubt that histamine has an important role in acid secretion.

Pepsin. Pepsin is secreted by gastric peptic (or chief) cells as a precursor zymogen, pepsinogen. These cells release stored pepsinogen on stimulation by the same secretagogues that stimulate acid—histamine, gastrin, and especially acetylcholine as well as secretin. Only acetylcholine and secretin stimulate peptic cells to synthesize and secrete new pepsinogen, however. The inactive pepsinogen released is activated by gastric acid and the optimal pH is 2. In addition, pepsin itself activates pepsinogen (Fig. 2–1). Although pepsinogen is released during feeding and digestion by vagal stimulation and gastrin, activation to pepsin is delayed until the simultaneously stimulated gastric acid is able to overcome food buffers, especially protein. Then pepsin is activated and begins digestion of protein. Pepsin digestion of protein is incomplete, cleaving at aromatic amino acid residues to yield various peptides. As stomach contents pass into the duodenum, pepsin is inactivated by the more alkaline pH present there (see Fig. 2–1).

Motor Functions. The stomach is required to adapt to an ingested meal in two ways: It must relax to receive a volume sometimes exceeding a liter in a matter of minutes, and it must initiate and maintain coordinated peristaltic activity to mix and slowly empty its contents into the small intestine.

Proximal gastric relaxation occurs with each swallow as well as in response to distention during filling. This response, called *receptive relaxation*, leads to an increase in volume with little rise in intragastric pressure. This response appears, at least in part, to be a centrally vagal mediated reflex, since vagotomy decreases distensibility of the proximal stomach. The lower, or distal, half of the stomach, which is considerably more motile than the proximal part, mixes and empties the meal. Smooth muscle cells of the outer longitudinal layers of the wall of the distal stomach possess a membrane that depolarizes and repolarizes rhythmically. Gastrin can increase motility by increasing the frequency of depolarization; however, activity is decreased by vagotomy, catecholamines, and secretin. Mechanical contractions of gastric smooth muscle bear a definite relation to this electrical activity. There appears to be an organized phase lag in the depolarization of various sites of the distal stomach; not all sites depolarize simultaneously. The mid-point of the greater curvature is considered to behave like the pacemaker of the stomach. The coordination of phase lag assures that the peristaltic waves will proceed smoothly from greater curvature to the pylorus.

Emptying of the Stomach. The emptying of the stomach is influenced by a complex set of hormonal[16] and neural[17] mechanisms, whose complexity makes it difficult to assess their relative importance. In practice, however, the physical and chemical properties of the ingested meal seem likely to be the dominant factors in regulating emptying.

After ingestion of a liquid meal, the normal stomach empties in an exponential pattern, as regulated by the proximal stomach. When emptying of discrete solid particles is examined, emptying patterns are approximately linear with time and are regulated by

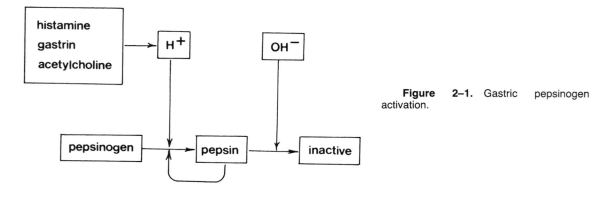

Figure 2–1. Gastric pepsinogen activation.

the antrum. Thus, with a mixed meal containing both solid and liquid components, there are two patterns of emptying, with the liquid emptying more rapidly than the solid (Fig. 2–2). The following are other factors that may also influence gastric emptying.

Osmolality. Osmoreceptors that appear to be situated in the jejunum rather than in the duodenum affect gastric emptying rate. Solutions that are either hyperosmolar or hypo-osmolar to extracellular physiologic tonicity cause slower gastric emptying than the corresponding isotonic solution.

Acid. Intraduodenal acid retards gastric emptying, the magnitude of the effect being proportional to the concentration of the acid.

Fats. Fatty acids with chain lengths of 12 and 14 carbon atoms are potent inhibitors of gastric emptying. Less slowing is brought about by fatty acids with a chain length of 16 to 18 carbon atoms. Unsaturated fats retard emptying more than do saturated fats.[18]

Amino Acids. Although recent work has suggested that tryptophan is a potent inhibitor of gastric emptying, the effect of other amino acids appears to be related more to osmotic changes than to a specific action of the amino acid.[19]

Energy Density. Hunt and Stubbs observed that the higher the energy density, the slower the emptying.[20] Whether or not this is further evidence of the existence of any form of sensory system is a matter of debate.

Temperature. The rate of emptying of solutions that are colder or warmer than body temperature is slower than that of fluids at body temperature.

Posture. Posture influences gastric emptying to some extent. Liquids are emptied more rapidly when a subject is in a sitting position or is lying on the right side. With a solid meal, emptying in normal subjects is much the same as in the erect or recumbent position.

Pathologic Conditions. Gastric stasis has been described in many pathologic situations—for example, iron-deficiency anemia, brain tumors or injury, "cast syndrome," diabetes, various fractures, gastric carcinoma, hepatic coma, hepatitis, hypocalcemia, hypokalemia, irradiation, malnutrition, pancreatitis, peritonitis, sepsis, uremia, and vagotomy. In many of these conditions, the mechanism by which gastric emptying is delayed is assumed to be a reflex inhibition of gastric peristalsis, but there is little formal proof.

Drugs. Pharmacologic modification of gastric emptying probably occurs in more clinical situations than are generally recognized, although relatively few are of practical importance.[21] Narcotic analgesics such as morphine and meperidine (Demerol) profoundly inhibit gastric emptying. Anticholinergic drugs inhibit antral peristalsis and delay emptying; however, when these are given orally in conventional therapeutic doses, this effect appears to have little clinical significance. Metoclopramide accelerates gastric emptying, possibly by facilitating release of acetylcholine by postganglionic parasympathetic neurons.[22] The action of metoclopramide is antagonized by anticholinergic drugs and narcotics. Some reports suggest that oral administration of the drug has no effect on normal gastric emptying; however, there is no doubt of its effectiveness when gastric stasis is present.

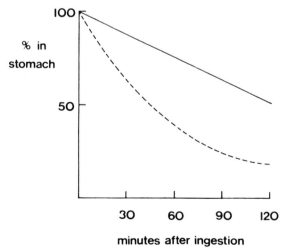

Figure 2–2. Typical gastric emptying patterns in a normal subject given a mixed meal containing both solid particles *(solid line)* and fluid *(broken line)*. (*From* Heading, R.C.: Gastric motility and emptying. *In* Sincus, W., and Smith, A. N. (eds.): The Scientific Foundations of Gastroenterology. Philadelphia, W. B. Saunders Co., 1980, p. 292, with permission.)

Small Intestine

Histology. The length of the small intestine in the newborn infant is about 200 cm. It elongates with age, so that by adulthood the length ranges from 700 to 800 cm. While the intestine grows in length, it also grows in diameter. Therefore, at birth, the calculated surface area of the intestine is about 950 sq cm and increases to about 7600 sq cm by adulthood. A normal 4-kg infant ingests about 500 calories/day. If the average adult requires 2200 cal. of intake, simple mathematics shows that an infant has only 2 sq cm of small intestine to absorb 1 cal., whereas the adult has about 3.5 sq cm. This difference accounts for what can be called the *intestinal reserve capacity* of an adult. Almost half of an adult's intestine can be removed before the efficiency of absorption approximates that of the infant's intestine. For this reason, infants do not tolerate intestinal surgery as well as adults. On the other hand, the infant, by virtue of his growth potential, has the ability to increase the length of the intestine, whereas the adult does not. The adult who has 90 per cent of his gut removed surgically may not survive, whereas the infant will increase the length of the remaining segment as he grows in height, and eventually, a relatively normal intestinal tract might develop.[23]

The luminal surface of the small intestine is so organized that the surface area available for contact with intestinal contents is greatly amplified by readily visible spiral or circular concentric folds called *plicae circulares*, most prominent in the distal duodenum and proximal jejunum. The plicae are covered by another series of infoldings called *villi* that in turn are covered by epithelial cells (Fig. 2–3). At low magnifications in the scanning electron microscope, the over-all villous pattern can be seen (Fig. 2–4). While finger villi are regarded as the norm, leaf-shaped and tongue-shaped villi are not unusual. Epithelial cells migrate from the crypts to the tip of the villi and as migration progresses, maturation and differentiation of cell functions occur (Fig. 2–5). The principal cells of the villi, generally termed *enterocytes*, have as their most distinctive feature the apical striated border composed of microvilli (Fig. 2–6). This striated border provides the vast digestive-absorptive surface area essential for nutrition. The study of these structural features is often helpful in determining the causes of inadequate absorption of nutrients (Table 2–1; Figs. 2–7 and 2–8).

The Digestive-Absorptive Sequence. After a meal, digestion and absorption of nutrients by the small intestine provide the material for normal metabolism and growth. Digestion is the process by which the large molecules in the diet are broken down into smaller ones acceptable to the enterocytes. In the case of fat it also includes coverting water-insoluble sustances into water-soluble ones. Absorption is the process by which the contents of the small bowel enter the mucosal epithelial cells and eventually the portal vein or the lymphatics. This is represented in Figure 2–9 in a way that emphasizes that digestion or reduction of molecular size does not stop at the surface of the enterocyte. It is known, for example, that hydrolysis of the polyglutamate form of dietary folate occurs at this site.

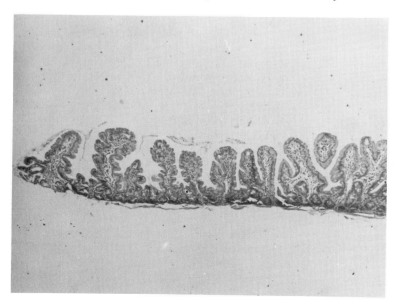

Figure 2–3. Light microscopy of normal intestinal mucosa.

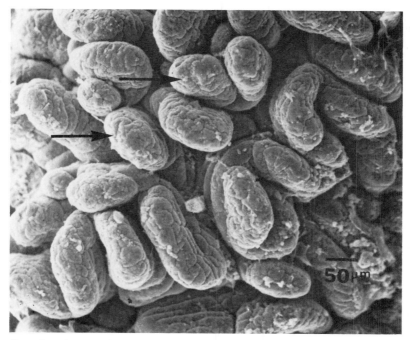

Figure 2–4. Scanning electron micrograph of normal intestinal epithelium. *Arrows* point to normal villi.

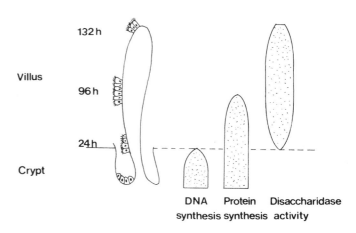

Figure 2–5. Correlation of functional activities with location of epithelial cells of the crypt-villus unit. The position of the shaded areas locates the site of the particular activity and the width denotes relative amount of each functional parameter. Note the tendency for sequential DNA synthesis, protein synthesis and appearance of disaccharide activity to occur as crypt cells migrate and mature morphologically. (*From* Gray, G. M.: Carbohydrate digestion and absorption: Role of the small intestine. N. Engl. J. Med., *292*:1225–1230, 1975, with permission.)

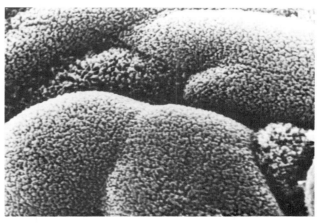

Figure 2–6. Scanning electron micrograph of microvilli of the intestinal epithelium.

Table 2–1 STRUCTURAL ABNORMALITIES OF THE SMALL BOWEL IN INADEQUATE ABSORPTION OF NUTRIENTS

USUALLY DIAGNOSTIC
Celiac disease

POSSIBLY DIAGNOSTIC
Whipple's disease
Lymphoma
Lymphangiectasia
Crohn's disease
Abetalipoproteinemia

USUALLY NONSPECIFIC
Tropical sprue
Malnutrition
Viral enteritis

Determinants of Absorption. Substances that cross the membrane of the enterocyte may do so by one of three mechanisms: simple diffusion, facilitated diffusion, or active transport (Table 2–2). The importance of these mechanisms is related to the transport kinetics—that is, an active transport mechanism is capable of saturation and sensitive to competition. Thus, if an actively absorbed substance is present in excess, the mechanism becomes overloaded and the actual absorption site then moves distally. Also, if two substances that are actively absorbed by the same mechanism are present simultaneously, competition will cause each to be absorbed less efficiently and, again, the absorption site moves distally.

Some of the other factors that determine where in the small bowel a substance is ab-

sorbed, as well as how much of it is absorbed, are as follows.

Physicochemical State. Physicochemical state is an important determinant of the site of absorption. For example, because fat and fat-soluble substances require preliminary interaction with bile to render them water-soluble, they tend to be absorbed farther down the jejunum. In contrast, water-soluble substances are already in a solubilized state and tend to be absorbed higher up (Fig. 2–10). The obvious exceptions to this are vitamin B_{12} and bile salts, both of which are actively absorbed over a relatively limited area of the terminal ileum.

Molecular Weight and Osmolarity. Molecular weight determines the rate of absorption of some substances. The more complex a molecule, and hence the greater the preliminary reduction in molecular weight that is necessary, the more distal is the absorption site. Osmolarity also has a profound effect on absorption: for example, a meal of high osmolarity is absorbed more distally than one of lower osmolarity.[24]

Of the many physiologic factors that influence the efficiency of absorption, blood supply to the intestine is one of the most important. Hormones such as cholecystokinin, pancreozymin, and secretin increase blood flow and, therefore, enhance absorption; exercise and shock impair absorption by diverting blood away from the gut. Only recently it has been found that adjacent to all biologic membranes there is a layer of relatively unstirred water, through which movement of solute molecules is determined only

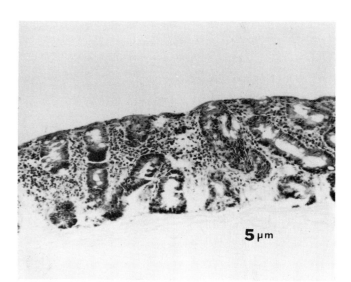

Figure 2–7. Severe villous atrophy in a patient with celiac disease.

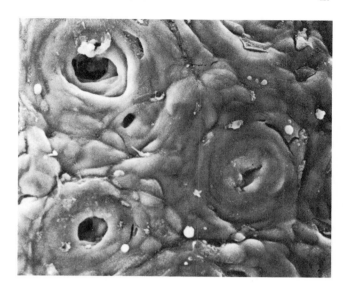

Figure 2–8. Scanning electron micrograph showing severe villous atrophy in a patient with malabsorption syndrome due to celiac disease.

Figure 2–9. The digestive absorptive process. (*From* Ward, M.: Assessment of function. *In* Sincus, W., and Smith, A. N. (eds.): The Scientific Foundations of Gastroenterology. Philadelphia, W. B. Saunders Co., 1980, p. 427, with permission.)

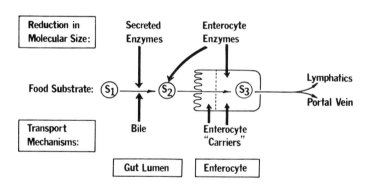

Table 2–2   CHARACTERISTICS OF TRANSPORT MECHANISMS

CHARACTERISTIC	ACTIVE TRANSPORT	PASSIVE TRANSPORT	
		Facilitated Diffusion	*Simple Diffusion*
Carrier involved	Yes	Yes	No
Competition for transport between substrates	Yes	Yes	No
Transport kinetics	Saturation	Saturation	No saturation
Energy dependent	Yes	No	No
Transport against electrochemical gradient	Yes	No	No

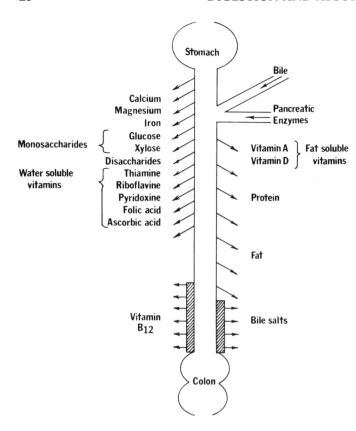

Figure 2–10. The sites of absorption. (*From* Booth, C. C.: Effect of location along the small intestine on absorption of nutrients. *In* Code, C. F., and Heidel, W. (eds.): Handbook of Physiology, Section 6, Alimentary Canal, Volume III, Intestinal Absorption. Baltimore, Williams and Wilkins, 1968, pp. 1513–1527, with permission.)

by diffusional forces. Such a layer exerts a major portion of the total resistance encountered by molecules during its passage from the intestinal lumen into the cell interior and constitutes the rate-limiting step to uptake of long-chain fatty acids and cholesterol by the enterocyte.[25]

Absorption is therefore directed toward the provision of adequate nutrition. However, the nutritional status will be controlled not only by the physicochemical limits of absorptive capacity which have been outlined, but also by daily intake, the size of body stores, the rates of metabolic utilization, and excretion by extragastrointestinal routes.

DIGESTION AND TRANSPORT OF NUTRIENTS

We will now discuss our current understanding of the mechanisms of digestion and absorption of carbohydrates, lipids, minerals, and vitamins. The digestion and transport of protein will be discussed in Chapter 3.

Lipids

Terminology

Ninety-six per cent or more of the 60 to 100 gm of fat ingested daily in the Western diet is absorbed. In the normal adult bowel, the percentage is similar even for large intakes of 300 to 500 gm. Triglycerides constitute approximately 90 per cent of the fat ingested; the remaining 10 per cent comprises cholesterol, phospholipids, and plant sterols.

The triglyceride molecule consists of glycerol and three ester-linked, usually different, fatty acids (Fig. 2–11). The majority of the triglycerides contain long-chain fatty acids (14 to 24 carbon atoms); of these, fatty acids with 16 or 18 carbon atoms predominate. A few dietary triglycerides contain fatty acids of 8 to 12 carbon atoms. These medium-chain triglycerides (MCT) derive their special effects from the fact that they are digested and metabolized differently from long-chain triglycerides (LCT).

Fatty acids may be separated into two categories according to the presence or absence of reactive (unsaturated or "double-

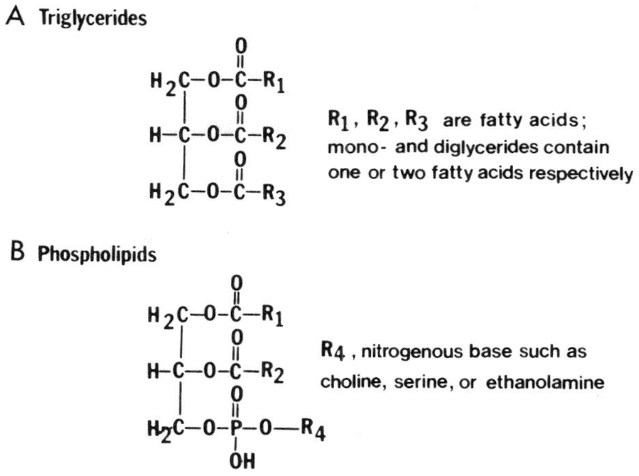

A Triglycerides

$$H_2C-O-\overset{\overset{O}{\|}}{C}-R_1$$
$$H-C-O-\overset{\overset{O}{\|}}{C}-R_2$$
$$H_2C-O-\overset{\overset{O}{\|}}{C}-R_3$$

R_1, R_2, R_3 are fatty acids; mono- and diglycerides contain one or two fatty acids respectively

Figure 2–11. Chemical structure of triglyceride and phospholipids.

B Phospholipids

$$H_2C-O-\overset{\overset{O}{\|}}{C}-R_1$$
$$H-C-O-\overset{\overset{O}{\|}}{C}-R_2$$
$$H_2C-O-\overset{\overset{O}{\|}}{P}-O-R_4$$
$$OH$$

R_4, nitrogenous base such as choline, serine, or ethanolamine

bond") linkages between the carbon atoms. Saturated fatty acids, those devoid of double bonds, are more stable chemically and account for much of the firmness of fats at room temperature. Unsaturated fatty acids contain one or more reactive ("double-bond") linkages. The carbon atoms of fatty acids are numbered either from the carboxyl group (Δ numbering system) or from the carbon atom farthest from the carboxyl group (n or ω numbering system), as seen in Figure 2–12. Both numbering systems are currently in use; however, the n or ω designation is used in describing fatty acid lengthening and desaturation reactions. For example, the monounsaturated oleic acid is abbreviated 18:1 ω 9 (or 18:1 n-9). This indicates that the acid contains 18 carbon atoms and one unsaturated double bond that is located 9 carbon atoms away from the ω-carbon atom. In this system, only the first double bond from the ω terminus is listed. Therefore, in 20:4 ω 6 (arachidonic acid), the first of the four double bonds present is 6 carbons away from the ω terminus. Of special interest are linoleic acid (18:2 ω 6) and linolenic acid (18:2 ω 3), which are considered to be essential fatty acids, as mammals cannot desaturate beyond the ω 9 position.

Phospholipids (see Fig. 2–11) are also derivatives of glycerol, differing only in that the 3-position carbon is esterified to phosphoric acid, which in turn is linked to a nitrogen-containing base such as serine, choline, or ethanolamine. These phospholipids are derived both from the diet and from the bile and are important for solubilization of the lipid products of fatty digestion.

Cholesterol is prevalent in the Western diet and is the most commonly identified sterol in the animal kingdom (Fig. 2–13). Some of the cholesterol present in the diet is esterified—that is, the OH group that projects from C_3 is attached to a fatty acid residue in ester linkage. Bile acids are the endproducts of cholesterol metabolism, formed by the reaction of the carboxyl group with sodium or the amino acids taurine and glycine. Conjugation with an amino acid makes the bile acids more soluble in the contents of the jejunal lumen.

Intraluminal Digestion

The first step in the digestion of the relatively water-insoluble fats is the formation of an emulsion. It is thought that the forceful contractions of the pyloric antrum of the

ω-Terminus	CH$_3$–	CH$_2$–	CH$_2$–	CH$_2$–	CH$_2$–	CH$_2$–	CH$_2$–	CH$_2$–	CH$_2$–	COOH	Carboxyl Terminus
Δ Numbering	10	9	8	7	6	5	4	3	2	1	
n, or ω Numbering	1	2	3	4	5	6	7	8	9	10	

Figure 2–12. Nomenclature of fatty acids.

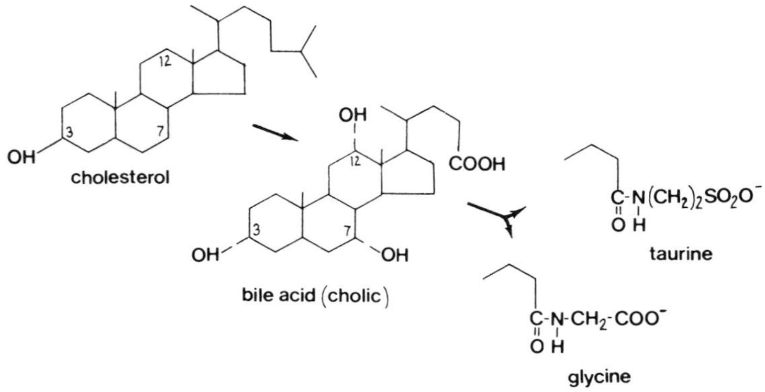

Figure 2–13. Chemical structure of cholesterol and bile acids.

stomach contribute to emulsification, which is further assisted by the addition of bile (owing to its bile acid content) in the duodenum. Before emulsification by bile salts, the fat globules have an average diameter of about 1000 Å. After bile salt emulsification, the average diameter is reduced to about 50 Å. This reduction in particle size amplifies the surface area for the enzymatic action that follows.[26]

The second step in lipid digestion is the hydrolysis of fats by lipases. Some lipolysis takes place in the stomach by the action of a lipase originated from the lingual serous glands located in the back of the tongue. This lingual lipase is more active in hydrolyzing medium-chain and short-chain triglycerides and attacks the bonds at the 3 and 1 positions; the end product of this reaction is a mixture of monoglycerides and diglycerides, glycerol, and fatty acids.[27]

The bulk of fat digestion, however, takes place in the proximal small intestine under the action of pancreatic lipase. The amount of pancreatic lipase activity in the intestinal contents of humans is very high.

It is estimated that a normal person has, in theory, the capability to digest 140 gm of fat/minute.[28] This water-soluble, negatively charged lipase does not penetrate the fat but acts upon the triglyceride at the oil-water interface. Lipase has no requirement for bile salt and functions with an optimal pH of approximately 8 to 9. However, after a meal, bile salts reach a certain concentration and spontaneously form negatively charged spherical aggregates known as micelles. At this critical micellar concentration, bile salts prevent lipase from reaching the substrate, possibly by electrostatic repulsion.[29]

The lipase activity is restored in the presence of a polypeptide cofactor, colipase (Fig. 2–14), which is secreted by the pancreas with lipase in roughly equivalent amounts. It is believed that colipase binds to triglyceride in the presence of bile salts; lipase then binds to colipase at the substrate interface and hydrolysis begins. Recent evidence indicates that colipase is secreted in a procolipase form.[30] Procolipase (102 to 107 amino acids) will not bind to phospholipid-coated triglyceride emulsions even in the

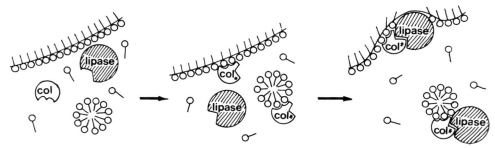

Figure 2–14. Role of colipase in the fixation of lipase to a hydrophilic interface (micelle or triglyceride interface coated with an amphipath). Col* designates the cofactor form in which a binding site for lipase has been created by previous absorption to micelle or interface. (*From* Desnuelle, P.: The lipase-colipase system. *In* Rommel, K., and Goebell, H. (eds.): Lipid Absorption: Biochemical and Clinical Aspects. Lancaster, England, MTP Press, Ltd., 1976, pp. 23–26, with permission.)

presence of bile salt micelles.[31] The inhibition of hydrolysis appears to be caused by a lack of binding of procolipase to the emulsion.[31] However, limited proteolysis of procolipase by trypsin converts it to a form (96 amino acid residues) that binds to phospholipid-covered triglyceride and makes it available for pancreatic lipase hydrolysis. This finding may have great significance to our understanding of dietary lipid digestion, as triglyceride droplets in natural foods possess a phospholipid envelope and mammalian bile is rich in phospholipid, which can bind to the surface of triglyceride droplets. After hydrolyzing triglycerides at the 1 and 3 positions, the end-products of these reactions is thus a mixture of 2-monoglycerides and free fatty acids.

Dietary phospholipids are hydrolyzed at the 2 position by pancreatic phospholipase A_2. This enzyme is secreted in pancreatic juice as an inactive proenzyme and, after removal of seven amino acid residues by trypsin, can hydrolyze lipid substrates. For the hydrolysis of the long-chain dietary phospholipids, pancreatic phospholipase A_2 has an absolute requirement for calcium and bile salts, and the products of its action are one molecule of lysophospholipid and one molecule of free fatty acid.[32]

The hydrolysis of cholesterol esters appears to be important for the absorption of cholesterol. This is carried out by pancreatic cholesterol esterase, which seems to be the same enzyme known as pancreatic nonspecific lipase. Concentrations of bile salts within the range found in intestinal lumina promote hydrolysis as well as protect the enzyme from proteolytic digestion.[33]

The products of pancreatic lipase, phospholipase, and cholesterol esterase incorporate into a shell of bile salts to form a particle called the *mixed micelle* (Fig. 2–15). For a micelle having some 33 bile salt molecules in its outer shell, some 47 fatty acid or monoglyceride molecules will be incorporated in its interior. Another five molecules of lysolecithin, two molecules of cholesterol, and perhaps a molecule of a fat-soluble vitamin will be added to the interior during digestion of phospholipid and cholesterol ester. The bile salt molecules are all oriented with their conjugated, charged ends at the micellar surface, where they interact with the polar solutes and solvents of intestinal chyme. The uncharged, hydrophobic tails of the bile salt molecules are packed in the micelle interior along with the hydrophobic tails of fatty acids, monoglycerides (mostly 2-monoglyceride), lysolecithin (mostly 2-lysolecithin), cholesterol, and the fat-soluble vitamins. The micelle is stablized by the negative charges carried mainly by conjugated bile salt molecules.

The micelle is important because it serves as an essential vehicle for diffusion of the lipid products to the site of absorption. The region through which the micelle diffuses is the unstirred water layer adjacent to the brush border. Even with the most vigorous peristalsis, this thin (about 0.25 mm) layer of fluid between the microvilli and in the glycocalyx cannot be mixed with chyme in the intestinal lumen. The micelle can diffuse through this unstirred layer because the micelle is a stable, charged particle. Although the lipid contents of the micelle have smaller molecular sizes, they are virtually insoluble and unstable in the unstirred layer (see Fig. 2–15).

The micelle itself is not absorbed. The lipid molecules it contains are just soluble

micelle

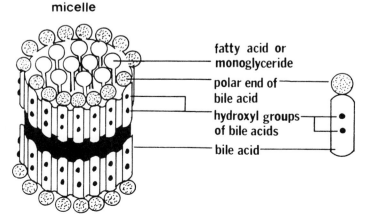

Figure 2–15. Cross section of a proposed model for the bile salt-polar lipid micelle. The center is composed of polar lipid liquid paraffin chains, and these hydrocarbon chains are chiefly responsible for the solvent capacity of the bile salt-polar lipid micelle. (*From* Brooks, F. P.: Mechanisms of digestion and absorption. *In* Sincus, W., and Smith, A. (eds.): Scientific Foundations of Gastroenterology. Philadelphia, W. B. Saunders Company, 1980, p. 395, with permission.)

fatty acid or monoglyceride

polar end of bile acid

hydroxyl groups of bile acids

bile acid

enough in the unstirred layer so that they can be released as free molecules for final absorption as they come in direct contact with the lipid components of the brush border membrane. Once that contact is established, lipids can be readily absorbed by passive transport. The release from the micelle is a passive consequence of the equilibrium that exists across the micellar surface.

The bile salts do not follow the lipid contents in absorption. When all the products of lipolysis are absorbed, the bile salt shell decomposes and the bile salts diffuse back through the unstirred layer to the lumen, where they reform new micelles with lipid constituents. Ultimately, after all the lipid has been absorbed, the conjugated bile salts themselves are actively absorbed in the ileum and into the enterohepatic circulation.

The passage through the unstirred water layer is the limiting factor in the absorption of long-chain fatty acids and monoglycerides, cholesterol, lysolecithin, and the fat-soluble vitamins. Short-chain and medium-chain fatty acids and glycerol are sufficiently soluble in the watery chyme so that they can diffuse through the unstirred layer without the assistance of the micelle. Their absorption is less limited by the unstirred layer.

Formation of Chylomicrons

After the passive absorption of the lipid constituents through the microvillous membrane, the lipids are processed within the intestinal mucosal cell. This processing consists of the resynthesis of triglyceride from absorbed fatty acids and monoglycerides and the packaging of triglycerides and other absorbed lipids into particles called *chylomicrons*. Like micelles, chylomicrons stabilize lipids in a watery medium, in this case the water within the cell. They have an outer coat of negatively charged betalipoprotein, which is analogous to the bile salts of micelles. Cellular processing and chylomicron formation maintain low cellular concentrations of the absorbed lipids. Thus their concentration gradients for passive absorption across the microvillous membrane are maintained. The nascent chylomicrons finally gain access to the lymphatics and are transported to the systemic venous system through the thoracic duct.

Mesenteric lymph chylomicrons are the major vehicles by which dietary fats are transported from the gut. However, short-chain and medium-chain triglycerides are absorbed directly into the portal blood and require neither micelles nor chylomicrons. The stages of fat digestion are summarized in Figure 2–16.

Carbohydrates

Dietary carbohydrate in the usual Western diet consists of starch (60 per cent), sucrose (30 per cent), and lactose (10 per cent). Starch comprises a mixture of amylose and amylopectin. Amylose consists of long linear chains of glucose molecules linked together through an oxygen atom between the first and the fourth carbon atoms (Fig. 2–17).

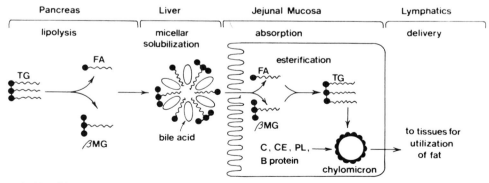

Figure 2–16. Diagrammatic representation of the major steps in the digestion and absorption of dietary fat. These include: (1) the lipolysis of dietary triglyceride *(TG)* by pancreatic enzymes; (2) micellar solubilization of the resulting long chain fatty acids *(FA)* and β-monoglycerides *(βMG)* by bile acids secreted into the intestinal lumen by the liver; (3) absorption of the fatty acids and β-monoglyceride into the mucosal cell with subsequent reesterification and formation of chylomicrons; and (4) movement of the chylomicrons from the mucosal cell into the intestinal lymphatic system. During the process of chylomicron formation small amounts of cholesterol *(C)*, cholesterol ester *(CE)*, and phospholipid *(PL)* as well as triglyceride are incorporated into this specific lipoprotein fraction. (*From* Wilson, F. A., and Dietschy, J. M.: Differential diagnostic approach to clinical problems of malabsorption. Gastroenterology, *61*:911–931, 1971, with permission.)

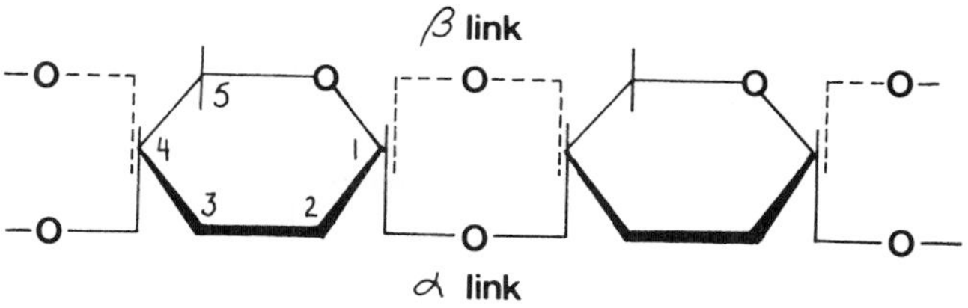

Figure 2–17. Importance of oxygen linkage for polysaccharide hydrolysis by α-amylase. Two adjacent glucose residues are shown joined by either an α- or β-link. α-Amylase can hydrolyze the α-linked polysaccharide *(solid lines)* amylose, but has no activity against the β-linked isomer *(broken line)* cellulose.

The linkage between glucose molecules is very important for specificity of the hydrolytic enzymes. Thus cellulose, a beta-linked polysaccharide isomer of amylose, cannot be hydrolyzed by intraluminal enzymes and is considered to be in the general category of dietary fiber.

The alpha-4 linkages are also present in amylopectin, but there are also branching points where the glucose molecules are linked between the first and the sixth carbon atoms (Fig. 2–18). Glycogen has a structure analogous to amylopectin and is hydrolyzed similarly.

Sucrose is a disaccharide formed by one molecule of glucose and one molecule of fructose joined by an alpha-link. Lactose, the principal carbohydrate in milk, is also a disaccharide formed by one molecule of glucose and one molecule of galactose joined by a beta-link.

Intraluminal Digestion

The digestion of starch begins in the oral cavity. Although theoretically, salivary amylase might be expected to produce some digestion of starch, only minimal starch is hydrolyzed before it reaches the duodenum.[34] There, pancreatic alpha-amylase is secreted in a fully active form and requires only a suitable pH (6 to 7) and the presence of chloride ion.

Amylase is produced in excess by the pancreas. Therefore, patients with severe pancreatic insufficiency have little evidence of impaired starch digestion even when lipid and protein digestion and absorption are grossly deficient. Alpha-amylase cleaves to the interior of the 1,4 links of starch. However, it is incapable of splitting the alpha-1,6 linkages of amylopectin and has little specificity for the alpha-1,4 links around that branching point. Thus, after complete digestion of starch in the duodenum, the final products presented to the intestinal surface are maltose, maltotriose, and alpha-limit dextrines (Fig. 2–18). Because alpha-amylase is an endoenzyme, very little free glucose is released during the intraluminal digestion of starch.

No enzymes secreted into the intestinal lumen are capable of hydrolyzing sucrose or lactose. These disaccharides along with the oligosaccharides from starch hydrolysis are cleaved by brush border enzymes.

Digestion at the Intestinal Surface

The process of surface digestion of oligosaccharides and disaccharides takes place primarily in the upper and mid jejunum. The products of starch digestion, along with the disaccharides sucrose and lactose, are hydrolyzed by constituent enzymes of the intestinal brush border whose active sites

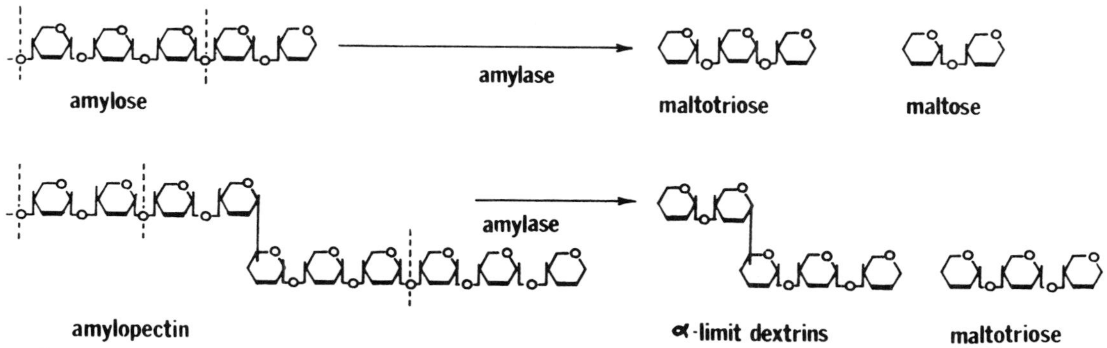

Figure 2–18. Action of pancreatic α-amylase on linear (amylose) and branched (amylopectin) forms of starch. *Horizontal links* denote -1,4 linkages and *vertical links* indicate α-1,6 linkages.

are exposed to the intestinal lumen (Fig. 2–19). It is now known that alpha-dextrins are cleaved by the complimentary action of the alpha-glucosidases, alpha-dextrinase (commonly called isomaltase), glucoamylase, and sucrase.[35] Maltose and maltotriose appear to be attacked by both glucoamylase and sucrase.

Sucrose is cleaved by sucrase, its respective alpha-glucosidase, Lactose is cleaved by lactase, the only beta-galactosidase present in the intestine.

The rate of hydrolysis by the alpha-glucosidases is highly efficient so that surface digestion is not the rate-limiting step for the overall assimilation of carbohydrate. Instead, the transport process seems to constitute the slowest step. On the other hand, lactose hydrolysis is a relatively slow process; in this instance, surface hydrolysis appears to be rate-limiting for lactose assimilation. Furthermore, in many of the world's population groups, such as African and American Black, Oriental, and Indian, lactase activity decreases substantially after 5 years of age, so that lactose cannot serve as a suitable nutrient owing to its maldigestion at the intestinal surface by some individuals.

Transport of the Final Monosaccharides

In the healthy gastrointestinal tract, carbohydrates are absorbed almost exclusively as monosaccharides. In patients with low or deficient levels of corresponding disaccharidase activity, considerable amounts of lactose or sucrose may be absorbed, but the major part of absorbed disaccharides is excreted unchanged in the urine. Moderate amounts of maltose, however, can be metabolized by the liver.[37] The monosaccharides released during digestion cannot traverse the hydrophobic brush border membrane unless they come in contact with the appropriate specific transport processes. Glucose and galactose share a common active transport mechanism that requires an expenditure of energy, is dependent on the sodium ion, and demonstrates saturation kinetics.[38] Fructose is transported largely by facilitated diffusion; it enters the mucosal cell on the basis of its concentration gradient across the cell membrane. The fructose and glucose moieties of sucrose may be absorbed more efficiently than free fructose or glucose (see Fig. 2–19).

The transport mechanisms are believed to involve the action of membrane "carriers." The nature of these carriers is not clearly elucidated, but they are characterized by their ability to move water-soluble solutes across membranes at rates higher than expected from passive diffusion. The glucose carrier has a high affinity for glucose and galactose and can transport the two sugars against steep concentration gradients.[39] The uptake of these monosaccharides is directly coupled to the absorption of sodium and will be discussed in detail under sodium absorption.

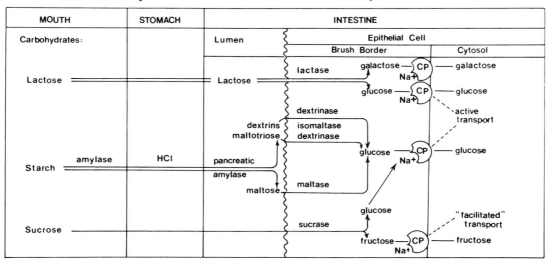

Figure 2–19. Loci of secretion of carbohydrate digesting enzymes. (*From* Greene, H. L.: Gastrointestinal development. *In* Johnson, J. R., Moore, W. M., and Jeffries, J. E. (eds.): Children Are Different: Developmental Physiology. Edition 2. Columbus, Ohio, Ross Laboratories, 1978; with permission.)

Because the assimilation of carbohydrate must occur sequentially by intraluminal digestion of starch followed by hydrolysis of oligomers at the intestinal surface and culminating in transport of specific hexoses across the intestine, a defect at any stage of assimilation can cause an osmotic diarrhea produced by the unabsorbed carbohydrates that remain in the intestinal lumen. These carbohydrate moieties attract water by osmosis to maintain an intraluminal osmolality equal to that in extracellular fluids, and the osmotic force is further increased by virtue of bacterial metabolism in the lower ileum and colon to yield fragments of 2 or 3 carbons. There is also an increased production of hydrogen and carbon dioxide gases as a result of metabolism of the undigested carbohydrate. As a consequence, patients complain of abdominal fullness and distention followed by nausea, increased flatus production, and a watery diarrhea that occurs minutes to several hours after ingestion of 10 to 50 gm of the offending carbohydrate. Children may develop more severe nausea and vomiting.

Carbohydrate intolerance is nearly always related to a defect in intestinal surface digestion of an oligosaccharide or disaccharide, but starch intolerance is rare. This is probably because the quantity of pancreatic alpha-amylase in the intestinal lumen is at least tenfold greater than that required for optimal intraluminal digestion of starch to its final oligosaccharide products.[40]

Water and Electrolytes

The total load of water and minerals in the diet and secretions that is presented to the intestines is surprisingly large; but the contribution of the diet is small when compared with that of endogenous secretions. It is estimated that for an adult, of the 8 L that reach the upper small intestine every day, only 2 L are of dietary origin. Saliva, gastric juice, bile, and pancreatic juice contribute roughly 75 per cent of the total.[41]

The small bowel absorbs about 7 L per day, leaving only about 1 to 1.5 L to enter the cecum. The colon, in turn, absorbs the vast majority of fluid that reaches it, and only 100 to 200 ml of water is passed in the stools per day (Table 2–3).

The small bowel mucosa is freely permeable to water and fairly freely permeable to electrolytes. This allows the osmotic pressure of the intestinal contents to equilibrate with that of plasma. The loss of intestinal fluids (through a fistula, for example) approximates the electrolyte content of plasma.

The colon has a remarkable capacity for conservation. Despite the relatively high concentrations of electrolytes in feces, the amounts lost each day are trivial because of the small volume of stool. These trivial losses help explain the capacity of humans to survive on an extremely low intake of salt. As one might predict, patients who have had a colectomy are less able to conserve enteric losses of electrolytes.

Average values of water and electrolyte turnover in the colon are summarized in Table 2–3. It is difficult to calculate the bicarbonate losses in the stool because a variable proportion is dissipated as carbon dioxide by organic acids generated in the colon. The mechanisms of absorption of water and minerals are discussed below.

Mechanisms of Absorption

The small bowel epithelium is categorized as "leaky" because it is characterized by low and often negligible transepithelial electrical potential differences and very high passive permeabilities to small ions and water. These properties allow this epithe-

Table 2–3 DAILY TURNOVER OF WATER AND ELECTROLYTES BY THE COLON

	ENTERING COLON		LEAVING COLON IN STOOL	
	Concentration (mEq/L)	Amount (ml or mEq)	Concentration (mEq/L)	Amount (ml or mEq)
Water	—	1500	—	100
Na	140	210	40	4
K	6	9	90	9
Cl	70	105	16	2
HCO_3	50	75	—	—

lium to absorb large quantities of salt and water in isotonic proportion.

It appears that absorption of Na and Cl by the small intestine can be accounted for by the following three processes.

1. Na absorption is directly coupled to the absorption of organic solutes such as glucose, amino acids, water-soluble vitamins, and bile salts (by the ileum only). "Carrier" molecules couple the entry of Na and the solute S into the cell (Fig. 2–20). Once inside the cell, Na is extruded against chemical and electrical potential differences existing across the basolateral membrane. Energy required to accomplish this exit is derived from ATP hydrolysis generated by the enzyme Na-K-ATPase. The flow of S from the cell across the basolateral membrane is from a region of higher concentration to one of lower concentration and thus does not require metabolic energy. Recent studies suggest that this movement of sugars across the basolateral membrane is a carrier-mediated "facilitated diffusion" process.[42]

2. The bulk of Na and Cl absorption is the result of a neutral process whose overall effect is the one-for-one transport of Na and Cl (Fig. 2–21). The downhill movement of Na facilitates the uphill movement of Cl, as in the case of nonelectrolytes. Increased intracellular levels of cAMP inhibit this process. Na is extruded from the cell by the same pump mechanism at the basolateral membrane. The exit of Cl is by means of an electrochemical potential difference. However, it appears that the permeability of the basolateral membrane to Cl is not sufficiently high to permit exit by simple electro-diffusion, and at present the precise mechanism of Cl exit is unclear.

3. Finally, there is an electrogenic mechanism that operates in the distal small intestine. The Na-K-ATPase pump maintains a low Na intracellular concentration and an electrically negative potential difference with respect to the intraluminal contents. These differences drive Na intracellularly by simple electrodiffusion.

The transfer of water across the intestinal mucosa is an entirely passive process. During the transfer of solutes by the active processes of absorption described, the luminal solution tends to become hypotonic compared with intestinal fluid and water moves along this osmotic pressure gradient following the solute. Water moves in either direction according to osmotic pressure gradients and when solute accumulates in the lumen, water enters from intestinal fluid until osmotic equilibration occurs.

The colon transforms semiliquid ileal materials to semisolid stool and in doing so creates very large ionic concentration gradients across its mucosa. Na and Cl are actively absorbed and K is secreted into the lumen by a combination of active secretion in exchange for some of the Na absorbed and secretion in mucus. Since the colonic epithelia has a much lower passive permeability to ions and water than does the small intestine, the differences in concentration created by these active transport processes are not easily dissipated by simple diffusion back across the mucosa. Thus stool concentrations of electrolytes are quite different from plasma concentrations (see Table 2–3).

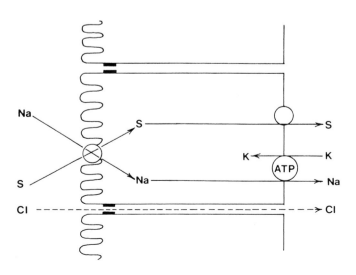

Figure 2–20. Cellular model for Na-coupled absorption of organic solutes (S) by the small intestine. S. hexoses, L-amino acids, water-soluble vitamins, bile salts (ileum). ATP required to extrude intracellular Na is generated by Na-K-ATPase.

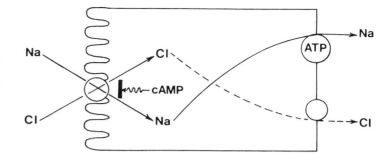

Figure 2–21. Cellular model for neutral NaCl cotransport by the small intestine. Increased intracellular levels of cAMP inhibit this process.

Absorption of Iron. Humans and other mammals maintain a relatively constant body concentration of iron throughout life. This is accomplished by remaining in positive iron balance during the growing years and establishing an equilibrium between absorption and loss during adult life. The active regulatory mechanism that keys this delicate balance is the absorptive process carried out by the small intestine, by which the mucosa remains attuned to current body requirements for iron.

While the exact mechanisms regulating iron transport across the intestinal mucosa are unknown, many factors affecting iron absorption have been studied.[43, 44] Knowledge to date indicates that the amount of iron absorbed depends on: (1) the amount of inorganic (non–heme) iron ingested, (2) the interaction of dietary components with the pool of this non–heme iron, (3) the amount of heme iron in the diet, and (4) the level of iron stores of the individual. The first three factors combine to determine the availability of dietary iron. The latter factor determines how much of that available iron will be absorbed. In food, the inorganic iron consists mainly of ferric (Fe^{+3}) complexes. Ferric iron is quite insoluble in aqueous solutions more alkaline than pH 3 unless it is chelated or reduced to the ferrous (Fe^{+2}) form. Gastric hydrochloric acid solubilizes ferric iron and makes it available for chelation with substances (such as peptides and polysaccharides) that keep iron dissolved and allow its absorption in the alkaline environment of the small intestine. Ascorbic acid and other agents reduce Fe^{+3} to Fe^{+2}.

Ferrous components are more easily absorbed because they form chelates, which are soluble in both acidic and slightly alkaline environments. Certain sugars and amino acids decrease both the precipitation and the polymerization of iron in aqueous solutions. However, other agents commonly found in the diet such as carbonates, oxalates, phosphates, phytates, tannates, and food additives such as EDTA, combine with irons to form insoluble precipitates and macromolecules that are poorly absorbed. Thus the absorption of inorganic iron from bread and vegetables is low compared with the amount absorbed from meat products, which contain an abundance of amino acids that are released by proteolytic digestion.[45, 46]

Organic iron from hemoglobin and myoglobin is absorbed from food more effectively than inorganic iron and seemingly in a different manner. The heme is taken up as such by the intestinal cells; subsequently the iron is released from the porphyrin in the intestinal mucosa and enters the circulation as iron. Unlike inorganic iron, the absorption of heme iron is independent of pH and not affected by substances that enhance or diminish the absorption of inorganic iron. The absorption of purified heme is poor, however, because iron porphyrins form polymers that have a reduced absorbability; this polymer formation does not occur in the presence of globin degradation products and certain amino acids.[47]

While anatomic and histologic alterations that decrease the effective absorption surface area of the duodenum and jejunum (for example, intestinal resections) are sometimes significant, the effectiveness of the mucosal cells in regulating iron absorption seems more important. Mucosal cells contain variable amounts of iron derived from both the diet and body stores. This deposit regulates, within limits, the quantity of available intraluminal iron that enters the cells. While it appears that the total quantity of iron in the mucosa may play a role in the absorption of iron, the amount of this iron bound to mucosal receptors that facilitate absorption probably plays a more important role. Various proteins seem to be involved in the transport of iron throughout the mucosal cells. One of them, the so-called mucosal metal-binding protein,[48] readily binds iron and lead and, to a lesser extent, calcium. This intestinal mucosal protein seems to provide an explanation for competition that exists for absorption between various divalent metals by providing a partially shared absorptive pathway.[49] Similarly, depression of iron absorption by inhibitors of protein synthesis (cycloheximide) or with protein-calorie deprivation may be due, in part, to the lack of a mucosal protein carrier.[50] This transport system and storage capacity probably regulates the absorption of small (physiologic) doses of iron. With larger (pharmacologic) doses of iron, a process suggestive of passive diffusion allows absorption of substantially larger amounts of iron.[43]

Besides tissue iron stores, the most important known stimulus to iron absorption is the rate of erythropoiesis. Accelerated production of red blood cells seems related to enhanced iron absorption, whether caused by bleeding, hemolysis, or hypoxia. Conversely, diminished erythropoiesis such as occurs with starvation or blood transfusion decreases the absorption of iron.[43] The way in which these factors inform the duodenum to transfer appropriate amounts of iron into the plasma is unknown.

Absorption of Calcium. Absorption of calcium from the intestine has been shown to comprise both passive and active processes. The passive transport predominates at concentrations about 10 mM; at lower concentrations absorption is an active process that requires the stimulus of the biologically active form of vitamin D.[51]

The secosteroid vitamin D_3 is derived from the diet and from conversion of a precursor present in the skin by the action of sunlight. After metabolic conversion of vitamin D_3 into 25-hydroxy vitamin D_3 (25 $(OH)_2$ D_3) by a liver mitochondrial enzyme, this circulating form of the secosteroid is subjected to metabolic conversion to its biologically active form, 1,25 dihydroxy vitamin D_3 (1,25 (OH_2) D_3), by mitochondrial enzymes located in the kidney cortex. The production of 1,25 $(OH)_2$ D_3 is regulated by a variety of endocrine signals, including parathyroid hormone and the "calcium needs" of the organism.

At the target intestine, 1,25 $(OH)_2$ D_3 stimulates the absorption of calcium by a mechanism analogous to that of other steroid hormones (Fig. 2–22). After formation of a complex with a highly specific cytosol receptor, 1,25 $(OH)_2$ D_3 migrates to the nucleus of the mucosal cell and stimulates messenger RNA synthesis for proteins. The most important of these proteins is the calcium-binding protein (CaBP), which directly participates in calcium intake.[52] Alkaline phosphatase and calcium-stimulated ATPase levels are also increased in the intestinal mucosa, but their role in calcium uptake has not been completely defined.

Certain dietary factors are known to affect the degree of calcium absorption from the gut. Phytates and oxalates decrease ab-

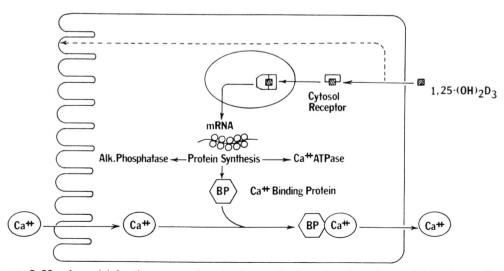

Figure 2–22. A model for the proposed molecular mechanism of action of 1-25 $(OH)_2$ vitamin D_3 on the enterocyte.

sorption by combining with calcium to form insoluble salts within the intestinal lumen. Lactose and certain amino acids enhance calcium absorption, but the mechanisms by which such enhancement occurs are unresolved.[53] The significance of these factors in influencing calcium status are believed to be minimal when a typical mixed diet is consumed. However, dietary patterns that are limited and rich in one or more of these influential components may produce a significant effect on calcium balance over time.

Bile salts increase calcium uptake presumably by forming soluble calcium complexes. On the other hand, long-chain fatty acids bind calcium as insoluble soaps, and an excess of such substances will reduce calcium absorption. Therefore, patients with steatorrhea will have impaired calcium absorption.

Absorption of Copper. Absorption of copper is regulated at the level of the intestinal mucosa, and excretion is predominantly through the intestinal tract, either through the bile or as unabsorbed copper. Urinary excretion amounts to about 1 to 2 per cent of the intake.[54]

In humans absorption occurs primarily in the stomach and duodenum. Studies in animals indicate that at least two mechanisms are concerned in copper absorption. One of these is an active process that requires energy and involves the absorption of complexes of copper and amino acids. L-amino acids facilitate copper absorption, but absorption progressively decreases with increasing molecular size of copper-amino acid complexes.[55] The other mechanism involves the binding of copper to and the successive release from macromolecular proteins. Studies in animals indicate that the protein metallothionein may not be the only protein involved in copper transfer.[56] Besides, these proteins may not be specific for copper transport, as other bivalent ions such as zinc and cadmium seem to compete for binding sites.

Besides phytates and dietary fiber, ascorbic acid is known to significantly decrease copper absorption by either interfering with the binding of copper to metallothionein or increasing the absorption and utilization of iron.

Absorption of Zinc. Zinc is well established as an essential nutrient, and signs of zinc deficiency in humans have been reported.[57] There is increasing recognition that various substances in the diet may affect the bioavailability of zinc. Of these, phytates present in whole-meal bread and soybean-based vegetable protein are the most commonly encountered.[58]

The proposed mechanism of zinc absorption include binding of zinc in the intestinal lumen to a ligand, which transports it to the mucosal surface. The zinc is then transferred to another binding site within the cell; and the protein metallothionein may be involved at this stage. Citrate,[59] prostaglandin,[60] and picolinic acid[61] have been proposed as the ligands responsible for the enhancement of zinc transport.

The site of preferential absorption in the gastrointestinal tract is still unclear, but in vitro studies have demonstrated that zinc transport is an active process that requires energy, oxygen, and sodium.[62]

Absorption of Vitamins. *B Vitamins, Vitamin C, and Folate.* Recent experimentation and reevaluation of some of the earlier work on intestinal absorption of vitamins has led to the conclusion that the small intestines of several species possess intricate transport and metabolic mechanism(s) for handling most of these nutrients. Table 2–4 summarizes some of those recent findings.[63]

Ascorbic acid, being a derivative of glucose, is transported by a sodium-dependent process resembling the mechanisms proposed for the intestinal active transport of glucose. A carrier molecule in the brush border has sites originally oriented toward the lumen which bind Na and ascorbic acid. Na is extruded by the Na-K-ATPase mechanism; after accumulating inside the cell, ascorbic acid moves by an undetermined mechanism across the basolateral cell membrane toward the blood. When high luminal concentrations of vitamin prevail (as in megavitamin therapy), the carrier mechanism becomes saturated and the additional ascorbic acid is absorbed only by simple diffusion, which proceeds at a very low rate. Thus high oral doses of ascorbic acid are likely to be incompletely absorbed by the intestine.

Thiamine transport is similar to the mechanism discussed above for ascorbic acid.[64] In addition, ethanol impairs the active, but not the passive, component of thiamine transport.[65]

Absorption of riboflavin is enhanced by the presence of bile salts in the intestinal lumen, possibly through an effect on mem-

Table 2–4   PROPERTIES OF VITAMIN TRANSPORT IN SMALL INTESTINE*

VITAMIN	SPECIES	SITE OF ABSORPTION IN INTESTINE	MECHANISM OF TRANSPORT	OTHER PROPERTIES[†]
Ascorbic acid	Human,	Ileum	Active transport	1
	guinea pig	Ileum	Active transport	1
Thiamine	Rat	Jejunum	Active transport	1,3
Riboflavin	Human	Jejunum	Facilitated diffusion	2
Niacin	Bullfrog,	Proximal	Active transport	1
	rat	Jejunum	Carrier-mediated	1,4
Vitamin B_6	Rat, hamster, human	No known preference	Simple diffusion	3,4
Folic acid (pteroylglutamic acid)				1,4
	Rat	Jejunum	Facilitated diffusion	

*Adapted from Rose, R. C.: Intestinal absorption of water-soluble vitamins. In Johnson, L. R. (ed.): Physiology of the Gastrointestinal Tract. New York, Raven Press, 1981, pages 1231–1242.

[†]Other properties: (1) Na-dependent; (2) bile salt–dependent; (3) phosphorylated; (4) metabolized other than by phosphorylation.

brane permeability or vitamin solubility in the intestinal lumen. A role of bile salts is also indicated by the impaired absorption in cases of biliary obstruction in children.[66]

Pyridoxal (PL) and pyridoxamine (PM) are the primary forms of vitamin B_6 in foods of animal origin, and pyridoxine (PN) is the major plant form. Intestinal transport is probably by simple diffusion, and the relative rates of absorption of the three forms of the vitamin appear to be PL>PN>PM.

Food folate exists as a mixture of free and conjugated forms, with the polyglutamyl conjugates predominating. There is now evidence that polyglutamyl folates undergo hydrolysis within the brush border and are split into monomers for absorption in the mucosal cell.[67] Absorption of folate takes place predominantly in the proximal jejunum. Maximal transport occurs at or near pH 6.0, whereas at pH 5.0 and 7.0 the transport decreases by half.[68] An active transport system operates at low and physiologic concentrations of substrate, whereas passive diffusion predominates at high concentrations seen with pharmacologic doses of folate.[69] Competitive inhibition of folate transport has been reported with the folate analogue methotrexate[70] and the drug sulfasalazine, an agent used for the treatment of inflammatory bowel disease.[71]

Vitamin B_{12} is mainly absorbed by active transport in the ileum. This absorption depends on several factors, the most important of which is the synthesis of gastric intrinsic factor. Gastric intrinsic factor is a glycopro-

tein that is produced by gastric oxyntic cells. It binds to vitamin B_{12} and forms a complex, which is the required substrate for ileal absorption. Besides gastric acid, pancreatic bicarbonate, trypsin, and Ca ion are required to free vitamin B_{12} from ingested proteins that block the formation of a complex with gastric intrinsic factor. Pancreatic bicarbonate and Ca ion provide the required conditions for binding of the complex to the ileal receptor. After attachment to the ileal receptor, the vitamin B_{12} is actively transported into the mucosal cell and the gastric intrinsic factor is released back into the lumen for ultimate excretion. From the mucosal cell, vitamin B_{12} is transferred to plasma proteins (transcobalamins) for delivery to peripheral tissues.

Lack of intrinsic factor as a result of pernicious anemia or total gastrectomy, the presence of bacteria in the upper small intestine that metabolize the B_{12} and render it unavailable for absorption, and ileal mucosal dysfunction due to disease, radiation, or bypass are causes of malabsorption of vitamin B_{12}.

Vitamins A, E, D, and K. In general, the fat-soluble vitamins are absorbed with fats. Vitamin A is present as retinyl ester in foods of animal origin and as beta-carotene in foods of plant origin. Retinyl ester is hydrolyzed to retinol at the brush border membrane prior to passive absorption. Inside the mucosal cell, retinol combines mainly with palmitic acid. The retinyl palmitate is incorporated into chylomicrons, which are absorbed by lymphatics. Beta-carotene is partially converted to retinol, and the remainder is incorporated directly into the chylomicrons.

Vitamin D is passively absorbed into intestinal mucosal cells, incorporated into chylomicrons, and transferred by the lymphatics to the blood.

Vitamin E is absorbed passively and relatively inefficiently in the intestine and is incorporated into chylomicrons for lymphatic transfer.

Vitamin K is unique in that it is the only vitamin that is supplied almost totally by resident bacteria in the human intestine. Like the other fat-soluble vitamins and lipids, vitamin K is passively absorbed (with carrier mediation) in the intestine, incorporated into chylomicrons, and transferred to lymph and blood.

There are many disorders that interfere with absorption of dietary fats from the lumen of the gut. Such malabsorption syndromes are also associated with loss of uptake of fat-soluble vitamins. If the disorder is prolonged, as in a chronic disease such as sprue or with long-term administration of certain drugs that interfere with absorption of fat, signs of specific vitamin deficiencies, such as decalcification of bone (avitaminosis D) or spontaneous bleeding (avitaminosis K), may occur.

REFERENCES

1. Kalloor, G. J., Deshpande, A. H., and Collis, J. L.: Observations on oesophageal length. Thorax, 31:284–288, 1976.
2. Liebermann-Meffert, D., Allgöwer, M., Schmid, P., and Blum, A. L.: Muscular equivalent of the lower esophageal sphincter. Gastroenterology, 76:31–38, 1979.
3. Cohen, S., Long, W. B., and Snape, W. J., Jr.: Gastrointestinal motility. Int. Rev. Physiol., 19:107–149, 1979.
4. Pope, C. E., II: The Esophagus. In Gitnick, G. L. (ed.): Current Gastroenterology, Vol. 1. Boston, Houghton Mifflin Medical Division, 1980, pages 1–33.
5. Soll, A. H., and Walsh, J. H.: Regulation of gastric acid secretion. Ann. Rev. Physiol., 41:35–53, 1979.
6. Moore, J. G., and Motoki, D.: Gastric secretory and humoral responses to anticipated feeding in five men. Gastroenterology, 76:71–75, 1979.
7. Feldman, M., Dickerman, R. M., McClelland, R. N., Cooper, K. A., Walsh, J. H., and Richardson, C. T.: Effect of selective proximal vagotomy on food-stimulated gastric acid secretion and gastrin release in patients with duodenal ulcer. Gastroenterology, 76:926–931, 1979.
8. Stenquist, B., Nilsson, G., Rehfeld, J. F., and Olbe, L.: Plasma gastrin concentrations following sham feeding in duodenal ulcer patients. Scand. J. Gastroenterol., 14:305–311, 1979.
9. Grötzinger, U., Bergegårdh, S., and Olbe, L.: Effect of atropine and proximal gastric vagotomy on the acid response to fundic distension in man. Gut, 18:303–310, 1977.
10. Richardson, C. T., Walsh, J. H., Hicks, M. I., and Fordtram, J. S.: Studies on the mechanism of food-stimulated gastric acid secretion in normal human subjects. J. Clin. Invest., 58:623–631, 1976.
11. Byrne, W. J., Christie, D. L., Ament, M. E., and Walsh, J. H.: Acid secretory response in man to 18 individual amino acids [Abstract]. Clin. Res., 25:108A, 1977.
12. Walsh, J. H., and Grossman, M. I.: Gastrin (Parts I and II). N. Engl. J. Med., 292:1324–1334, 1377–1384, 1975.
13. Mariano, E. C., Beloni, A., and Landor, J. H.: Some properties shared by amino acids and entero-oxyntin. Ann. Surg., 188:181–185, 1978.
14. Konturek, S. J., Tasler, J., Cieszkowski, M., and Jaworek, J.: Comparison of intravenous amino acids in the stimulation of gastric acid secretion. Gastroenterology, 75:817–824, 1978.
15. Christiansen, J., Beck, A., Fahrenkrug, J. J., Holst, J. J., Lauritsen, K., Moody, A. J., and de Muckadell, O. S.: Fat-induced jejunal inhibition of gastric acid secretion and release of pancreatic glucagon, enteroglucagon, gastric inhibitory polypeptide, and vasoactive intestinal polypeptide in man. Scand. J. Gastroenterol., 14:161–166, 1979.
16. Wingate, D.: The eupeptide system: A general theory of gastrointestinal hormones. Lancet, 1:529–532, 1976.
17. Mroz, C. T., and Kelly, K. A.: The role of the extrinsic antral nerves in the regulation of gastric emptying. Surg. Gynecol. Obstet., 145:369–377, 1977.
18. Hunt, J. N., and Knox, M. T.: A relation between the chain length of fatty acids and the slowing of gastric emptying. J. Physiol. (Lond.), 194:327–336, 1968.
19. Cooke, A. R.: Localization of receptors inhibiting gastric emptying in the gut. Gastroenterology, 72:875–880, 1977.
20. Hunt, J. N., and Stubbs, D. F.: The volume and energy content of meals as determinants of gastric emptying. J. Physiol. (Lond.), 245:209–225, 1974.
21. Nimmo, W. S.: Drugs, diseases and altered gastric emptying. Clin. Pharmacokinet., 1:189–203, 1976.
22. Schulze-Delrieu, K.: Metoclopramide. N. Engl. J. Med., 305:28–33, 1981.
23. Klish, W. J., and Putnam, T. C.: The short gut. Am. J. Dis. Child., 135:1056–1061, 1981.
24. Fordtran, J. S., and Locklear, T. W.: Ionic constituents and osmolality of gastric and smail-intestinal fluids after eating. Am. J. Dig. Dis., 11:503–521, 1966.
25. Dietschy, J. M.: General principles governing movement of lipids across biological membranes. In Dietschy, J. M., Gotto, A. M., and Ontko, J. A. (eds.): Disturbances in Lipid and Lipoprotein Metabolism. Bethesda, American Physiological Society, 1977, pages 1–28.
26. Sernka, T., and Jacobson, E.: Lipid absorption. In Sernka, T., and Jacobson E. (eds.): Gastrointestinal Physiology: The Essentials. Baltimore, Williams and Wilkins, 1979, page 139.
27. Hamosh, M.: The role of lingual lipase in neonatal fat digestion. Ciba Found. Symp., 70:69–98, 1979.

28. Patton, J. S.: Gastrointestinal lipid digestion. *In* Johnson, L. R. (ed.): Physiology of the Gastrointestinal Tract. New York, Raven Press, 1981, pages 1123–1146.

29. Borgström, B., and Erlanson, C.: Pancreatic lipase and co-lipase: Interactions and effects of bile salts and other detergents. Eur. J. Biochem., *37*:60–68, 1973.

30. Borgström, B., Wieloch, T., and Erlanson-Albertsson, C.: Evidence for a pancreatic pro-colipase and its activation by trypsin. FEBS Lett., *108*:407–410, 1979.

31. Patton, J. S., and Carey, M. C.: Inhibition of human pancreatic lipase-colipase activity by mixed bile salt-phospholipid micelles. Am. J. Physiol., *241*: G328–336, 1981.

32. deHaas, G. H., Slotboom, A. J., and Verheij, H. M.: Regulation of phospholipase A_2 activity by different lipid-water interfaces. *In* Polonovski, J. (ed.): Cholesterol Metabolism and Lipolytic Enzymes. New York, Masson Publishing, 1977, pages 191–211.

33. Kelly, L., and Newman, H. A. I.: Pancreatic sterol ester hydrolase reversal of the reaction by bile salt. Biochim. Biophys. Acta, *231*:558–560, 1971.

34. Roberts, P. J. P., and Whelan, W. J.: The mechanism of carbohydrase action: Action of human salivary α-amylase on amylopectin and glycogen. Biochem. J., *76*:246–253, 1960.

35. Gray, G. M., Lally, B. C., and Conklin, K. A.: Action of intestinal sucrase-isomaltase and its free monomers on an α-limit dextrin. J. Biol. Chem., *254*:6038–6043, 1979.

36. Greene, H. L.: Gastrointestinal development. *In* Johnson, J. R., Moore, W. M., and Jeffries, J. E. (eds.): Children are Different: Developmental Physiology. Edition 2. Columbus, Ohio, Ross Laboratories, 1978, page 151.

37. Young, J. M., and Weser, E.: The metabolism of circulating maltose in man. J. Clin. Invest., *50*:986–991, 1971.

38. Csáky, T. Z.: A possible link between active transport of electrolytes and nonelectrolytes. Fed. Proc., *22*:3–7, 1963.

39. Crane, R. K.: Na^+-dependent transport in the intestine and other animal tissues. Fed. Proc., *24*:1000–1006, 1965.

40. Fogel, M. R., and Gray, G. M.: Starch hydrolysis in man: An intraluminal process not requiring membrane digestion. J. Appl. Physiol., *35*:263–267, 1973.

41. Phillips, S. F., and Wingate, D. L.: Fluid and electrolyte fluxes in the gut. Adv. Intern. Med., *24*:429–453, 1979.

42. Kinne, R., and Kinne-Safran, E. Differentiation of cell faces in epithelia. *In* Solomon, A. K., and Karnovsky, M. (eds.): Molecular Specialization and Symmetry in Membrane Function. (Harvard Books in Biophysics, No. 2.) Cambridge, Harvard University Press, 1978, pages 272–293.

43. Conrad, M. E., and Barton, J. C.: Factors affecting iron balance. Am. J. Hematol., *10*:199–225, 1981.

44. Marx, J. J.: Iron absorption and its regulation: A review. Haematologia (Pavia), *64*:479–493, 1979.

45. Spiro, T. G., and Saltman, P.: Inorganic chemistry. *In* Jacobs, A., and Wormwood, M. (eds.): Iron in Biochemistry and Medicine. London, Academic Press, 1974, pages 1–28.

46. Van Campen, D.: Enhancement of iron absorption from ligated segments of rat intestine by histidine, cysteine, and lysine: Effects of removing ionizing groups and of stereoisomerism. J. Nutr., *103*:139–142, 1973.

47. Conrad, M. E., Weintraub, L. R., Sears, D. A., and Crosby, W. H.: Absorption of hemoglobin iron. Am. J. Physiol., *211*:1123–1127, 1966.

48. Barton, J. C., Conrad, M. E., Nuby, S., and Harrison, L.: Effects of iron on the absorption and retention of lead. J. Lab. Clin. Med., *92*:536–547, 1978.

49. Becker, G., Huebers, H., and Rummel, W.: Intestinal absorption of cobalt and iron: Mode of interaction and subcellular distribution, Blut, *38*:397–406, 1979.

50. Enwonwu, C. O., Monsen, E. R., and Jacobson, K.: Absorption of iron in protein-calorie deficient rats and immediate effects of re-feeding an adequate protein diet. Am. J. Digest. Dis., *17*:959–964, 1972.

51. Norman, A. W.: Vitamin D metabolism and calcium absorption. Am. J. Med., *67*:989–998, 1979.

52. Wasserman, R. H., Taylor, A. N., and Fullmer, C. S.: Vitamin D-induced calcium binding protein and the intestinal absorption of calcium. *In* Fraser, D. (ed.): Metabolism and Function of Vitamin D. Biochemical Society Special Publication *3*:55–74, 1974.

53. Ghishan, F. K., Stroop, S., and Meenely, R.: The effect of sugars on calcium and zinic transport in the rat during maturation. Pediatr. Res., *16*:566–568, 1982.

54. Mason, K. E.: A conspectus of research on copper metabolism and requirements of man. J. Nutr., *109*:1979–2066, 1979.

55. Kirchgessner, M., and Grassman, E.: The dynamics of copper absorption. *In* Mills, C. F. (ed.): Trace Element Metabolism in Animals. Volume I. Livingstone, Edinburgh, University Park Press, 1970, pages 277–287.

56. Mills, C. F.: Trace element interactions: Effects of dietary composition on the development of imbalance and toxicity. *In* Holkstra, W. G., Suttie, J. W., Ganther, H. E., and Mertz, W. (eds.): Trace Element Metabolism in Animals. Volume II. Baltimore, University Park Press, 1974, pages 79–90.

57. Prasad, A. S.: Deficiency of zinc in man and its toxicity. *In* Prasad, A. S., and Oberleas, D. (eds.): Trace Elements in Human Health and Disease. New York, Academic Press, 1976, page 1.

58. Oberleas, D., and Harland, B. F.: Nutritional agents which affect metabolic zinc status. *In* Brewer, G. J., and Prasad, A. S. (eds.): Zinc Metabolism: Current Aspects in Health and Disease. Progress in Clinical and Biological Research, Volume 14. New York, Alan R. Liss, 1977, pages 11–27.

59. Hurley, L. S., Lonnerdal, B., and Stanislowski, A. G.: Zinc citrate, human milk, and acrodermatitis enteropathica. Lancet, *1*:677–678, 1979.

60. Song, M. K., and Adham, N. F.: Evidence for an important role of prostaglandins E_2 and F_2 in the regulation of zinc transport in the rat. J. Nutr., *109*:2152–2159, 1979.

61. Evans, G., and Johnson, E. C.: Zinc absorption in rats fed a low-protein diet and a low-protein diet supplemented with tryptophan or picolinic acid. J. Nutr., *110*:1076–1080, 1980.

62. Kowarski, S., Blair-Stanek, C. S., and Schachter, D.: Active transport of zinc and identification of zinc-

binding protein in rat jejunal mucosa. Am. J. Physiol., 226:401–407, 1974.

63. Rose, R. C.: Intestinal absorption of water-soluble vitamins. *In* Johnson, L. R. (ed.): Physiology of the Gastrointestinal Tract. New York, Raven Press, 1981, pages 1231–1242.

64. Hoyumpa, A. M., Jr., Middleton, H. M., III, Wilson, F. A., and Schenker, S.: Thiamine transport across the rat intestine: I. Normal characteristics. Gastroenterology, 68:1218–1227, 1975.

65. Hoyumpa, A. M., Jr., Breen, K. J., Schenker, S., and Wilson, F. A.: Thiamine transport across the rat intestine: II. Effect of ethanol. J. Lab. Clin. Med., 86:803–813, 1975.

66. Jusko, W. J., Levy, G., Yaffe, S. J., and Allen, J. E.: Riboflavin absorption in children with biliary obstruction. Am. J. Dis. Child., 121:48–52, 1971.

67. Rosenberg, I. H.: Folate absorption and malabsorption. N. Engl. J. Med., 293:1303–1308, 1975.

68. Elsborg, L.: Folic acid: A new approach to the mechanism of its intestinal absorption. Dan. Med. Bull., 21:1–11, 1974.

69. Dhar, G. J., Selhub, J., Gay, C., and Rosenburg, I. H.: Characterization of the individual components of intestine folate transport [Abstract]. Gastroenterology, 72:1049, 1977.

70. Selhub, J., and Rosenberg, I. H.: Folate transport in isolated brush border membrane vesicles from rat intestine [Abstract 2066]. Fed. Proc., 39:656, 1980.

71. Dhar, G. J., Selhub, J., and Rosenburg, I. H.: Azulfidine inhibition of folic acid absorption: Confirmation of a specific saturable transport mechanism [Abstract]. Gastroenterology, 70:878, 1976.

CHAPTER 3

Peptides and Free Amino Acids

P. P. KEOHANE
D. B. A. SILK

Enteral nutrition has now become an acceptable and effective means of providing nutritional support to malnourished patients. There are now a wide variety of commercial enteric diets available, and most of these, containing whole protein as the nitrogen source, are suitable for patients with normal gastrointestinal function. In patients with severe impairment of intraluminal or mucosal absorptive capacity who may not be able to assimilate undigested nutrients, there are grounds for thinking that nutrients should be administered in the "predigested" form. Moreover, to ensure maximal absorption, the predigested nutrients should be presented to the gut mucosa in the form that allows maximal absorption. When the first chemically defined "elemental" diets were formulated, it was believed that dietary protein required complete hydrolysis to free amino acids for absorption, and thus there was little reason to believe that the free amino acid nitrogen sources contained in the diets represented anything other than the ideal nitrogen source. Recent work has shown, however, that the luminal products of protein digestion are also absorbed in the form of small peptides. Thus controversy has arisen as to whether free amino acids or oligopeptides represent the ideal nitrogen source for patients with severe impairment of absorptive capacity. It is the aim of this chapter to review our current knowledge of the processes involved in the absorption of dietary protein and to critically relate new information in this field on the formulation of the nitrogen source of chemically defined "elemental" diets.

SOURCES OF PROTEIN

Exogenous Protein. Dietary protein is derived from animal and vegetable sources and makes up 11 to 14 per cent of the average intake. In Western diets this amounts to about 70 to 100 gm of protein per day.

Endogenous Protein. Significant amounts of protein derived from endogenous sources such as gastric, biliary, pancreatic, and intestinal secretions also require assimilation by the human gastrointestinal tract. Although the initial animal studies of Nasset and coworkers suggested that the endogenous pool was considerably larger than the exogenous pool,[1, 2] more recent studies performed in humans indicate that the endogenous pool is approximately one third the size of the exogenous protein pool.[3–5]

SITE OF PROTEIN ASSIMILATION

The bulk of ingested protein appears to be absorbed in the proximal jejunum.[3–7] Small amounts reach the ileum and are absorbed at this site[7–9] and, as judged by the protein content of ileostomy effluent, absorption of protein is not completed in the small intestine.[10] The site of endogenous protein assimilation in humans has not been characterized, but recent animal studies implicate the colon as the major site.[11]

LUMINAL DIGESTION OF PROTEIN

The initial step in protein digestion is its denaturation at acid pH in the stomach by the action of several pepsins with varying substrate specificities.[12–14] Negligible amounts of free amino acids are released, and large polypeptides enter the duodenum to be further hydrolyzed by pancreatic proteolytic enzymes.

The intraluminal digestion of proteins by pancreatic proteolytic enzymes has been reviewed in some detail by Gray and Cooper[15] and the zymogen (pro-enzyme) exopeptidases, by Keller.[16] Each of the proteolytic pancreatic enzymes is secreted as an inactive precursor. Trypsinogen is then activated by contact with enterokinase, an enzyme that has been isolated in a highly purified form from the brush border membrane fraction of human intestinal mucosa.[17–19] Trypsin then hydrolyzes bonds in the other zymogens to form the active enzymes.

In addition to pancreatic proteolytic enzymes, solubilized intestinal brush border and cytoplasmic intestinal mucosal amino-oligopeptidases have been found to be present in intestinal contents.[20, 21] In the jejunum these enzymes are unlikely to have a functionally significant role in the terminal stages of protein digestion. In the ileum the activity of luminal peptidases is higher, so that significant quantities of luminal peptides may be hydrolyzed in the gut lumen rather than at the surface of ileal mucosal cells.

The products of luminal proteolysis are free amino acids and small peptides with a chain length of two to six amino acid residues.[3, 4, 8, 22] Analysis of postprandial intestinal contents aspirated from human jejunum reveals that approximately only one third of the total amino acid content exists in the free form.[8] The nature of the oligopeptides in terms of distribution of chain length frequency and amino acid composition has not yet been characterized.

TRANSPORT OF FREE AMINO ACIDS

As with glucose transport, in vitro experiments have shown that active amino acid transport is dependent on a gradient of sodium ions across the brush border membrane of intestinal epithelial cells.[23] The absorptive patterns of free amino acids in humans have been studied in some detail using various in vivo steady-state perfusion techniques. In these experiments, saturation of transport was reached with increasing solute concentration compatible with the existence in humans of carrier-mediated mechanisms for amino acid transport.[24–28] Also, different affinities of different free amino acids for these mechanisms were indicated by variations in the absorption rate of individual free amino acids when perfusion studies were performed with the use of equimolar mixtures of different acids.[24–26] To date, the absolute sodium dependency of free amino acid transport has not been demonstrated in vivo in humans.[29]

The results of competition studies in animals have indicated the likely existence of three major group-specific active transport systems:[30] (1) monoamino monocarboxylic (neutral amino acids), (2) dibasic amino acids and cystine, and (3) dicarboxylic (acidic) amino acids. This is complicated by species differences and by the fact that certain amino acids (for example, glycine, proline, and hydroxyproline) may be transported by more than one mechanism. The in vitro studies of amino acid transport in patients with Hartnup disease and cystinuria have firmly established the existence of the first two mechanisms.[29, 31, 32]

INTESTINAL HANDLING OF PEPTIDES: HISTORICAL ASPECTS

Nineteenth-century physiologists believed that dietary protein was absorbed in the form of polypeptides, a view that seemed to be confirmed when Nolf[33] and Messerli[34] showed that "peptones" produced by tryptic hydrolysis of protein disappeared from the lumen of the small intestine more rapidly than did equivalent amounts of free amino acids. When Cohnheim[35] demonstrated that intestinal juice was capable of hydrolyzing peptones to amino acids, some early workers suggested that protein must be hydrolyzed to amino acids before being absorbed. This hypothesis gained popularity when all known free amino acids were detected in intestinal contents during protein absorption in vivo[36–38] and when studies in vivo showed that complete hydrolysates of protein (consisting of free amino acids) disappeared rapidly from the lumen of the small intestine.[39, 40] When it was found that only amino acids could be isolated from the portal circulation during protein absorption,[41] the idea that protein was completely hydrolyzed to amino acids within the intestinal lumen became the classic view of protein absorption.[42] This view was held despite later observations that intraluminal peptidase activity was insufficient to account for the absorption of peptone in the form of free amino acids.[43] The final vindication of the classic view of protein absorption appeared to be provided by the demonstration, with the use of ion exchange chromatography, that only free amino acids appeared in peripheral plasma after protein was administered to human subjects.[44]

Fisher[45] strongly criticized the classic view of protein absorption. He pointed out that it had previously been shown that more than 200 hours were required for the liberation of 90 per cent of the amino acids from different proteins subjected to successive action of pepsin, trypsin, and erepsin and made the following statement: " . . . even on the most generous assumption the time course of liberation of amino nitrogen is too slow to fit with the view that protein must be digested to amino acids before they are absorbed." He suggested that the idea of absorption of protein in the form of peptides deserved serious consideration.

MUCOSAL TRANSPORT OF PEPTIDES

Initial experiments in vitro with dipeptides showed that small quantities of intact glycylglycine and glycyl-L-leucine crossed the intestinal wall.[37] Similar observations were made when glycylglycine was studied in vitro.[47] Newey and Smyth[48-50] demonstrated that dipeptides could be taken up intact by intestinal mucosa and concluded that the products of protein digestion could be transported into the mucosal cell in the form of oligopeptides as well as amino acids. The concept of intact peptide uptake as a second mode of protein absorption, although not disputed, was not thought to be quantitatively significant, as it seemed much more likely that absorption of peptides, analogous to disaccharides, would involve brush border hydrolysis with subsequent absorption of the released amino acids by amino acid transport systems.

The modern era of our knowledge of peptide absorption stems from the results of oral load experiments in humans carried out by Matthews and his colleagues.[51] They found that a given quantity of glycine was absorbed faster when administered orally as the dipeptide or tripeptide than it was in the free form. It was concluded that the glycine peptides were transported unhydrolyzed into the mucosal cell because if hydrolysis had preceded uptake, then at best the net rates of glycine transport from the free and peptide forms would have been the same. In light of more recent data on perfusion showing more rapid transport of glucose from maltose in vivo,[52-55] their data were perhaps somewhat overinterpreted. Nonetheless, their conclusions provided a powerful stimulus for further research in this area, which has subsequently provided unequivocal evidence for the existence in humans of peptide transport systems that are distinct from those used by free amino acids.

EVIDENCE FOR INTESTINAL TRANSPORT OF UNHYDROLYZED PEPTIDES

Of all the experimental data available in favor of dipeptide transport in human intestine, the most persuasive are still derived from experiments performed in patients with Hartnup disease and cystinuria. The intestinal transport defect for neutral amino acids in Hartnup disease and dibasic amino acids in cystinuria has been reviewed in detail.[29, 56] Despite these transport defects, the affected amino acids were shown to be absorbed normally or near normally if presented to the mucosa in the form of homologous or mixed dipeptides.[57-61]

If any of the dipeptides administered to these patients had been hydrolyzed to a substantial degree in the bulk phase of the gut lumen, or by brush border peptidases before transport of released amino acid by specific active transport processes, then absorption of the affected amino acids would not have occurred. This was clearly not the case in these experiments.

Additional evidence supporting the existence of intact dipeptide transport in human small intestine has included the following facts. First, the known competition between free amino acids for mucosal uptake is absent or greatly reduced when solutions of dipeptides instead of corresponding free amino acid mixtures are presented to the mucosa for absorption.[31, 32] Second, in most studies of peptide transport, faster rates of uptake of at least one of the constituent residues have been observed from dipeptides than from corresponding free amino acid solutions.[31, 32, 62, 63] Although this line of evidence is open to some criticism because the same phenomenon has been observed with disaccharides,[52–55] which are hydrolyzed at the brush border and not transported intact, the kinetic advantage conferred by dipeptides on amino acid transport has been a consistent finding and of much greater magnitude and has been observed during perfusion of dipeptide substrates known to have a low affinity for human brush border peptidase.[64, 65] Third, acidic pH abolishes the hydrolysis of dipeptides by brush border peptidases[66] but reduces only by 40 per cent the uptake of two glycine-containing dipeptides.[67] The last study cited is open to some criticism because of uncertainty of the effect that acidification of the bulk luminal phase has on unstirred layer pH.

APPEARANCE OF FREE AMINO ACIDS DURING ASSIMILATION OF DIPEPTIDE

A consistent finding during uptake experiments with dipeptides in vivo and in vitro has been the detection of free amino acids in media bathing the mucosal preparations.[24, 33, 62, 63] The rate of appearance of free amino acids during assimilation of different dipeptides varies,[65, 68] and substantially faster rates of appearance have been observed during ileal than jejunal experiments.[68, 69]

Peptidase activity in the mucosal media has been shown to be insufficient to account for the appearance of more than a small proportion of the released products of hydrolysis,[68–71] which implies that analogous to disaccharide transport, a close relationship exists between the mucosal hydrolysis and transport of dipeptides.

Numerous animal studies show that there are two distinct groups of mucosal peptidases, one located within the cytoplasmic compartment and another at the brush border of the cell.[72–80] Results of human studies indicate a similar subcellular distribution.[64, 81–83] It follows, therefore, that the appearance of free amino acids during dipeptide perfusion is likely to result from either (1) hydrolysis of proportions of dipeptides by brush border enzymes before transport has occurred or (2) hydrolysis of dipeptides by cytoplasmic peptidases after absorption, a process that would need to be followed by efflux of released free amino acids back out of the cell, across the unstirred water layer into the bulk phase of the gut lumen. For the following two reasons, the first explanation seems more probable.

First, the differential rate of appearance of free amino acids during assimilation of different dipeptides correlates well with the specific activity of brush border, and not cytoplasmic, peptidases.[84] Second, the appearance rates of hydrolytic products are greater during tripeptide than dipeptide assimilation,[70, 71] and mucosal brush border peptidases have a higher specific activity against tripeptides than dipeptides. To date, there is no available experimental evidence to favor the second explanation.

POSTULATED RELATIONSHIPS BETWEEN MUCOSAL HYDROLYSIS AND TRANSPORT OF DIPEPTIDES

One scheme proposes that all dipeptide presented to the mucosa for absorption is hydrolyzed by brush border peptidases, followed by absorption of the liberated amino acids by group-specific free amino acid transport mechanisms. Although it adequately explains the appearance of free amino acids during dipeptide assimilation, this scheme is not in keeping with the observations of normal uptake of dipeptides in patients with cystinuria and Hartnup disease, who have complete intestinal transport defects for free amino acids, nor could it explain the avoidance of competition for mucosal uptake between dipeptide-bound amino acids.

The second scheme proposes that all dipeptide presented to the mucosa for absorption is transported intact and hydrolyzed by cytoplasmic peptidases. Such a scheme would be in keeping with the evidence supporting transport of unhydrolyzed dipeptides in cystinuria and Hartnup disease but would not explain the back diffusion of free amino acids, which as discussed above are most likely to be released after the hydrolysis of dipeptides by brush border peptidases.

Considering all the available experimental data as a whole, certain features would be compatible with either of the schemes. It seems most likely, therefore, that a dual hypothesis is applicable.[31, 32, 62] Thus, those dipeptides with a high affinity for brush border peptidases would be predominantly handled according to the first scheme (brush border hydrolysis followed by uptake of liberated amino acids), whereas greater proportions of those with a low affinity for brush border peptidases would be handled according to the second scheme (transport of unhydrolyzed peptide).

Although there is as yet little experimental evidence to support it, another model, one that proposes that brush border membrane hydrolysis of a dipeptide is followed by uptake of amino acids by carrier mechanisms available only to amino acids liberated by the action of these enzymes, requires consideration. It is essentially analogous to the concept of hydrolase-related transport proposed by Crane and colleagues for sugar transport.[85–87] Its application to dipeptide transport has one theoretical drawback, however, because in contrast to disaccharides, hydrolysis of at least some dipeptides by brush border peptidase is likely to be a rate-limiting step in absorption.

ASSIMILATION OF TRIPEPTIDE

All evidence points to the fact that tripeptides are assimilated by mammalian small intestine in a fashion similar to the assimilation of dipeptides. Like dipeptides, most tripeptides have been shown to confer a kinetic advantage on amino acid uptake.[70, 71] Evidence for uptake of unhydrolyzed tripeptide is obtained from the isolation of Gly-Sar-Sar from the intracellular compartment during uptake studies with hamster jejunum in vitro.[88] When model tripeptides with a low affinity for brush border peptidases were studied, low concentrations of hydrolysis products were detected in media bathing the mucosa.[71, 88] In contrast, higher concentrations were generated during intestinal assimilation of tripeptides with high affinities for these enzymes.[70, 71] As with dipeptides, therefore, a dual mechanism for the intestinal handling of tripeptides may be proposed, and again the quantitative importance of the brush border hydrolysis versus intact transport mechanisms is likely to be dictated by the affinity of the tripeptide substrate for the brush border peptidases.

CHARACTERISTICS OF DIPEPTIDE AND TRIPEPTIDE TRANSPORT

It now appears certain that the transport system or systems utilized for absorption of unhydrolyzed peptides are distinct from those used for absorption of free amino acids. This conclusion is based first on the results of investigations in patients with inherited disorders of amino acid transport, in which normal or near normal uptake of dipeptides was demonstrated despite the transport defects for the affected free amino acids. In addition, there is now a good deal of evidence showing that the addition of high concentrations of free amino acids to peptide solutions does not significantly inhibit the intestinal uptake of dipeptides or tripeptides. Peptides studied in this way include Gly-Pro,[89] Gly-Gly,[90] carnosine,[91] Gly-Sar,[92] Gly-Sar-Sar,[93] Leu-Gly, and Leu-Gly-Gly.[94] In a number of experiments some inhibition of uptake of amino acid residues from peptides by free amino acids has been observed.[68, 68a] These effects most likely arose either because of the effect of the inhibitory amino acid on uptake of free amino acids liberated after peptide hydrolysis by brush border peptidases or as a result of a direct inhibitory effect of free amino acids on the activity of brush border peptidases.[95]

The kinetics of transport of several dipeptides and tripeptides has now been studied in some detail. Addison et al.[92] initially showed that Gly-Sar was transported into everted rings of hamster jejunum against both a chemical and electrochemical gradient by an energy-dependent and sodium-dependent process. Subsequent work in vitro with this dipeptide[96] as well as with carnosine[91] and the tripeptide Gly-Sar-Sar[88] showed that influx was a saturable process. Uptake of beta-Ala-Gly-Gly was not found to be saturable, although uptake appeared to be an energy- and sodium-dependent process.[88]

The kinetics of peptide transport has not been extensively investigated in humans, mainly because of the expense of purchasing sufficient amounts of model peptides and because there are no complete data available on the uptake of tripeptides over a wide range of substrate concentrations. Saturation has been reached, however, during intestinal perfusion in vivo of increasing substrate concentrations of the three dipeptides so far studied.[68, 90, 97]

When uptake of Gly-Sar, Glu-Glu,[98] and Lys-Lys[99] was studied in vitro under conditions designed to minimize brush border hydrolysis and over a wider range of concentrations, influx was not found to conform to simple Michaelis-Menten kinetics, suggesting that two distinct components were involved in transport. Working on the premise that a substrate whose transport is mediated and therefore saturable may be treated as a competitive inhibitor of its own transport[100, 101] and that any component of transport remaining at infinitely high concentrations of inhibitor must be nonmediated, Matthews and coworkers have identified a significant nonmediated or simple diffusional system of peptide transport, which at 10 mmol/L accounted for up to 46 per cent of total transport.[97, 98]

The conclusions that significant components of dipeptide may be transported by simple diffusion, especially at high luminal concentrations, is reminiscent of the comparable claims of Levin and coworkers for glucose transport. These workers described a method for distinguishing between electrogenic (active carrier–mediated) and nonelectrogenic (presumed to represent the simple diffusional component of transport) components of glucose transport[102–105] and claimed that up to 50 per cent of glucose could be absorbed during normal digestion by passive diffusion. Despite those claims that significant proportions of glucose are transported by passive diffusion, Batt and Peters[106] achieved 95 per cent inhibition of galactose uptake with phlorhizin during galactose perfusion studies in rat jejunum in vivo, findings which in fact suggest that there is not significant passive transfer component of galactose uptake.

An alternative means of verifying the existence of a passive diffusional component of transport would be to study intestinal absorption in conditions in which there is a genetic deletion of the carrier-mediated component. At first sight there does seem to be some verification of the concept, for it has proved difficult to identify convincingly the transport defect for lysine in homozygous cystinuria after oral administration of large lysine loads.[31, 107] A number of other studies, however, argue convincingly against any physiologically significant simple diffusional component of either hexose or amino acid transport. Thus, in two patients with congenital glucose-galactose malabsorption, lit-

tle or no glucose was absorbed during intestinal perfusion of high concentrations of glucose, maltose, or sucrose,[108, 109] and little or no amino acid was absorbed during intestinal perfusion of lysine and arginine in cystinuria.[59, 61]

One possibility not yet considered is that the experimental technique used by Matthews et al.[98] to characterize the simple diffusional component of peptide transport exaggerates its true physiologic significance. Thus all computations of the component were derived from uptake experiments performed at acid pH in vitro, and it should be appreciated that the permeability of the cell membranes of intestinal mucosal preparations markedly increases as soon as the tissue is removed from the animal.[110] It seems, therefore, that this phenomenon could substantially increase simple diffusion of any water-soluble solute during uptake experiments in vitro. The identification of the simple diffusional component of transport during uptake of peptides in vitro has, however, proved to be an essential prerequisite of the experiments performed to elucidate the number of operative carrier-mediated peptide transport systems.

Some caution is required before finally accepting the Na dependency of peptide transport, for although there seems little doubt of its importance during uptake of peptides in vitro in hamster and rat intestine,[29] Rubino et al.[89] showed appreciable influx of Gly-Pro into rabbit ileal mucosa in vitro after Na replacement. Cheeseman and Parsons[111] reported that transport of Gly-Leu by the small intestine of *Rana pipiens* in vivo was unaffected by replacement of intraluminal Na by K. Thus it is clear that there are species differences in respect of the Na dependency of peptide uptake. The Na dependency of peptide transport in humans has not yet been fully investigated.

SINGLE OR MULTIPLE PEPTIDE TRANSPORT SYSTEMS?

One question that has not yet been finally settled is whether all 400 possible dipeptides are transported by a common peptide transport system, or whether the 8000 tripeptides are also absorbed by this or an alternative system.

Initial competition experiments in vitro with carnosine as a model peptide suggested the existence of multiple peptide transport systems because uptake was inhibited by dipeptides containing neutral amino acid residues but not by those containing either dibasic or acidic amino acid residues.[112] The existence of more than one peptide transport system was also suggested by Lane, Silk, and Clark,[113] who failed to demonstrate inhibition of Gly-Pro uptake by Pro-Gly, and by Fairclough, Silk, Clark, Matthews, Marrs, Burston and Clegg,[114] who showed that Gly-Gly inhibited human jejunal uptake of only two (ser and Glu) of 15 peptide-bound residues of a partial enzymic hydrolysate of casein.

Different results, interpreted as being indicative of a single broad-specificity peptide transport system in monkey intestine, were reported by Das and Radhakrishnan.[115] Uptake of Gly-Leu by monkey intestine was inhibited by a comprehensive range of dipeptides containing N-terminal and COOH-terminal neutral, dibasic, and acidic amino acid residues. It was of interest though that Gly-Gly and the acidic dipeptides were relatively poor inhibitors. In preliminary studies with human intestinal tissue, Glu-Glu, Gly-Pro, and Pro-Gly were also found to be poor inhibitors of Gly-Leu uptake. Since there appears to be agreement that at least some dipeptides, namely Gly-Gly and Glu-Glu, are relatively poor inhibitors of uptake of model dipeptides containing neutral amino acid residues, the existence of more than one peptide transport system still appears to be a possibility.

In a number of respects, interpretation of the experimental data derived from the above experiments is quite difficult. Thus, with the exception of the experiments with carnosine, most experiments were carried out under conditions in which brush border peptide hydrolysis was operative, so that inhibition of uptake of both free and peptide-bound residues was being investigated. A number of experiments are of limited value, for they were performed with a single concentration of inhibitor.[113, 114] Finally, problems arise when interpreting the early competition experiments in vitro, in view of the findings of Matthews et al.[98] showing that peptide uptake in vitro occurs via carrier-mediated and simple diffusional processes.

In their most recently published studies, Matthews and coworkers appear to have overcome all these problems and, contrary to the tentative conclusions drawn from earlier work, their evidence indicates that carrier-mediated uptake of a neutral dipeptide (Gly-Sar) is inhibited by both an acidic (Glu-Glu)[98] and a dibasic (Lys-Lys) peptide.[99] Further work is needed to substantiate the view that a single carrier-mediated transport system is involved in translocating all unhydrolyzed dipeptides across the microvillous membrane of the mammalian enterocyte.

The question of whether unhydrolyzed dipeptides and tripeptides are transported by a single carrier-mediated transport process has not been studied in much detail. In the only experiments designed to answer this question, Gly-Sar and Gly-Sar-Sar were used as model peptides and the experimental data were in keeping with the fact that the dipeptide and tripeptide utilized a single carrier during uptake into rings of everted hamster jejunum in vitro.[96]

TETRAPEPTIDE TRANSPORT

Intestinal uptake of few tetrapeptides has been studied. Uptake of Gly-Sar-Sar-Sar by hamster jejunum in vitro was very poor, with no evidence of significant hydrolysis or carrier-mediated transport.[88] Rapid assimilation of the tetrapeptide Gly-Leu-Gly-Gly was noted by Smithson and Gray,[116] who showed that brush border hydrolysis to Leu-Gly-Gly was a prerequisite to intestinal uptake. Similar findings were noted by Adibi and Morse[117] for the assimilation in vivo of tetraglycine by the human jejunum, and by Burston et al.[118] for Ala-Gly-Gly-Gly assimilation by hamster rings in vitro. In light of these findings, it seemed that the brush border amino-oligopeptidases, known to have a high affinity for tetrapeptides,[64, 77, 119–121] play a pivotal role in the intestinal assimilation of tetrapeptides. Moreover, the absence of demonstrable uptake of unhydrolyzed tetrapeptide by a carrier-mediated tetrapeptide system would be in keeping with subfractionation studies showing the absence of significant cytoplasmic tetrapeptidase activity.[64, 77, 79]

The results and conclusions of the most recently reported study of tetrapeptide assimilation are, however, at variance with the above conclusions.[94] Significant cytoplasmic peptidase activity against Leu-Gly-Gly-Gly was shown, and uptake of the tetrapeptide in vivo was significantly inhibited by Gly-Pro, a model dipeptide[89, 113] known to be transported predominantly intact. Furthermore, Leu-Gly-Gly-Gly was found to confer a kinetic advantage on uptake of the leucine residue. It seems, therefore, that the intact peptide transport apparatus is capable of handling Leu-Gly-Gly-Gly and that the brush-border amino-oligopeptidase plays a complementary rather than an obligatory role in overall assimilation. Further work is needed to elucidate whether it is molecular structure of peptides (length of molecule, or width of side chains, or both) or the presence of cytoplasmic peptidase activity that dictates whether the intact peptide transport apparatus is utilized during the assimilation of tetra-, and higher, peptides.

FREE AMINO ACIDS OR PEPTIDES IN PORTAL BLOOD

The cytoplasmic peptidases of the intestinal mucosa have a high specific activity, and it has been generally assumed that the unhydrolyzed dipeptides and tripeptides that are transported into the mucosal cell are rapidly hydrolyzed to their constituent amino acids before entering the portal circulation. In keeping with this assumption is the difficulty most investigators have had in isolating unhydrolyzed peptides from their intestinal preparations during absorption experiments. (Exceptions to this have been sarcosine-containing peptides and carnosine, all of which have particularly low affinities for the cytoplasmic peptidases.)

Unhydrolyzed Gly-Gly, carnosine, anserine, and detectable amounts of hydroxyproline peptides have, however, been found in the peripheral circulation during absorption experiments.[68, 71, 122–126] These findings may well be of little overall physiologic significance because, in the case of Gly-Gly and Gly-Gly-Gly, high concentrations were instilled into the gut during intestinal perfusion in vivo[68, 71] and the others have an unusually low affinity for the cytoplasmic peptidases.

Using an isolated preparation of perfused rat intestine, Gardner[127, 128] has shown that unhydrolyzed peptides crossed the mucosa on to the serosal surface during absorption of some (soya bean and casein) but not other (lactalbumin) hydrolysates. At present these are the only data suggesting movement of unhydrolyzed and absorbed peptides on a wide scale into the portal circulation. These findings, therefore, require verification with technique in vivo. Unfortunately, in the only study designed to specifically investigate portal blood amino acid profiles during peptide absorption, protein-free samples of portal venous blood were not subjected to complete acid hydrolysis before analysis, so no account could be made of its peptide-bound amino acid content.[129]

If unhydrolyzed peptides do enter the portal circulation during assimilation of dietary protein, it seems likely that they will be efficiently utilized. Thus liver, muscle, and kidney contain substantial peptidase activities[130] and intravenously administered dipeptides are rapidly cleared from plasma.[131–133] It is also well known that peptides in parenteral nutrition fluids are efficiently assimilated in humans.[134]

NUTRITIONAL IMPORTANCE OF PEPTIDE TRANSPORT

The studies carried out in Hartnup disease and cystinuria have emphasized the nutritional importance of oligopeptide transport in these two conditions. The recently described kinetic advantage conferred by individual dipeptides, tripeptides, and tetra-peptides[94] on the intestinal assimilation of amino acid residues has been a consistent finding in most experiments and has suggested the possibility that there could be nutritional implications of peptide transport in normal human subjects. In addition, the kinetic advantage conferred by two dipeptides on intestinal assimilation of their amino acid residues has been shown in patients with untreated celiac disease who have subtotal villous atrophy of the small intestinal mucosa,[135, 136] suggesting nutritional implications in patients with impaired gastrointestinal absorptive function. As there are 400 possible dipeptides and 8000 possible tripeptides, it clearly has been impossible to assess the overall nutritional importance of peptide transport by studying the absorption characteristics of each in turn. As an alternative means of investigating the problem, native proteins have been hydrolyzed by enzymic methods under controlled in vitro conditions to yield final mixtures consisting predominantly of oligopeptides, with smaller quantities of free amino acids. Equivalent free amino acid mixtures whose composition and molar pattern simulated those of the partial enzymic hydrolysates of protein have also been prepared. Comparisons were made in humans of the extent of absorption of amino acid residues from the partial enzymic hydrolysates of whole protein and their respective equivalent free amino acid mixtures using a steady state in vivo perfusion technique.

Initial experiments were performed using two hydrolysates of casein[8, 137] and partial enzymic hydrolysates of fish protein and lactalbumin.[138, 139] Results showed that greater proportions of the infused alpha-amino acid nitrogen were absorbed from the two casein[8, 137] hydrolysates and the lactalbumin hydrolysate[138, 139] than from equivalent free amino acid mixtures. Moreover, the data highlighted the extreme variability in the extent of absorption of amino acid residues from the free amino acid mixtures.

As shown in Figure 3–1, this variability in amino acid uptake is not nearly so marked during perfusion of the protein hydrolysates, as those amino acids poorly assimilated from free amino acid solutions were absorbed to a greater extent from the protein hydrolysate solution.[137–139]

Two important points emerge from these experiments in perfusion. The first concerns the finding of a "more even" absorption of amino acid residues during perfusion of the protein hydrolysates. It has been suggested that more efficient protein synthesis is induced when amino acids are presented to the tissues at even, rather than different, rates.[140] If this is indeed the case, then there could be added advantages in administering peptides rather than amino acid mixtures, since in the case of amino acid mixtures

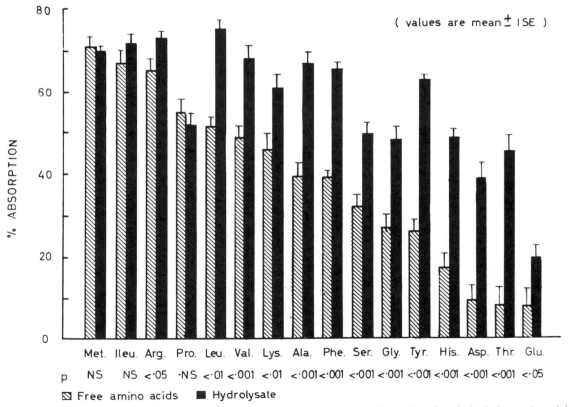

Figure 3–1. Percentage absorption of individual amino acids from casein-soy-lactalbumin hydrolysate (papain) and equivalent free amino acid mixture.

there was such a marked variation in extent of absorption of the individual amino acids.

The second point relates to the fact that in the studies with the casein and lactalbumin hydrolysates, greater proportions of infused alpha-amino nitrogen were absorbed during perfusion of the hydrolysate preparations than during perfusion of the respective free amino acid mixtures. If maximally effective absorption is required in the clinical situation, such as in patients with exocrine pancreatic insufficiency or loss of absorptive surface area due to celiac disease or intestinal resection, there would appear to be a significant advantage in administering protein hydrolysates containing oligopeptides as well as free amino acids rather than free amino acid mixtures.

RELEVANCE OF INTESTINAL PERFUSION DATA TO THE FORMULATION OF ENTERAL DIETS

The in vivo intestinal perfusion method represents an ideal experimental technique for elucidating mechanisms involved in the physiology of nutrient absorption, and indeed many of our present concepts of protein absorption in humans have come about by using this method. The technique suffers from one major disadvantage, however, in that steady states of absorption have to be reached before intestinal contents can be sampled, and practice has shown that the solute under study has to be infused at a flow rate of 15 to 20 ml/minute for a period of approximately 30 minutes before acceptable steady states of absorption are achieved. Consequently, in the perfusion experiments with the partial enzymic hydrolysates of whole protein, osmotic loads of up to 1400 μmols/minute^{-1} amino acid residue were infused. Loads such as this are in excess of those presented during constant continuous 24-hour enteral feeding (400 μmol amino acid residue/minute^{-1}),[140a] and it is not possible, therefore, to conclude that the technique of intestinal perfusion simulates normal physiologic conditions.

It may therefore be invalid to extrapolate conclusions drawn from the intestinal perfusion experiments with the protein hydrolysates and apply them to the clinical setting. This is further borne out by a recent perfusion study of the kinetics of amino acid residue absorption from a partial enzymic hydrolysate of protein in which it was shown that during infusion of low concentrations of lactalbumin hydrolysate and its equivalent free amino acid mixture (at osmotic loads much more equatable to those observed during enteral feeding), most amino acid residues were absorbed at similar rates from the two test solutions.[141] It thus seems possible that the kinetic advantage afforded by partial enzymic hydrolysates of protein on uptake of its amino acid residue is a concentration-dependent phenomenon, and one that may become apparent only during intestinal perfusion studies and not during oral or nasogastric administration. Such an explanation would certainly explain why so few differences in intestinal handling have been observed when partial enzymic hydrolysates of whole protein and their equivalent free amino acid mixtures have been administered orally in liquid test meals to normal human subjects[8, 142] and why no differences in nitrogen balance data were seen when enteral diets containing nitrogen sources based on a partial enzymic hydrolysate of lactalbumin and its equivalent free amino acid mixture were fed for a prolonged period to normal human subjects.[141]

It follows from this discussion that no firm claims can be made at present on nutritional grounds for concluding that chemically defined "elemental" diets should contain a peptide-based rather than a free amino acid–based nitrogen source. In our judgment, it will be necessary to perform careful studies on nitrogen balance and protein turnover in patients with severely impaired gastrointestinal function before any firm conclusions about the nutritional advantages of either type of predigested nitrogen source can be made.

In other important respects, though, peptide-based nitrogen sources would still appear to offer advantages over the free amino acid–based nitrogen source of the chemically defined "elemental diets." First, the cost of producing a diet containing a mixture of synthetic L-amino acids as the nitrogen source is considerably greater than that of producing a nitrogen source based on a partial enzymic of whole protein.[144] Second, the taste properties of enzymic hydrolysates of whole protein are superior to those of free amino acid mixtures.[144] The last potential advantage of peptide-based nitrogen sources relates to the reduction in diet osmolality that can be achieved by replacing a free amino acid nitrogen source with an equivalent mixture of oligopeptides. Gastrointestinal side effects, such as bloating, nausea, cramps, and diarrhea, occur in up to 30 per cent of patients receiving enteral nutrition.[144–147] Although the pathogenesis of these side effects has not been fully elucidated, evidence points to the fact that they may be due in part to the inability of the upper small intestine to handle the high osmotic load presented, particularly at the start of enteral feeding.[143]

Clinical experience has suggested that these side effects may be greatly diminished by the use of "starter" and constant infusion regimens.[148] A typical starter regimen will use "half strength" or similar concentration diet diluted with sterile water for the first two to four days, thus ensuring that reduced osmotic loads are presented to the gut during this period. Moreover, abandoning the time-honored bolus syringe feeding with its attendant side effects, including regurgitation and aspiration, for the modern constant gravity- or pump-assisted infusion through a fine bore tube would also appear to have reduced incidence of side effects.[149] In light of this experience, we believe that the incidence of gastrointestinal side effects could be reduced further still by the use of less hypertonic diets such as might be produced by replacing the free amino acid nitrogen source with an oligopeptide source.

FUTURE RESEARCH

If future clinical experience substantiates the potential advantages of an oligopeptide-based nitrogen source for chemically defined "elemental" diets, attention will need to be directed toward defining the optimal formulation. The available absorption studies of partial enzymic protein hydrolysates highlight the variability of the human small intestine in handling the different hydrolysates. We have recently shown that the absorption characteristics of hydrolysates are influenced by both starter protein composition and hydrolysis method used, although four amino acid residues (Thr, Glu, Phe, His), comprising 30 per cent of total residues, are unaffected by both factors[150] (Fig. 3–2). Peptide chain length of the hydrolysate mixtures may influence absorption. While dipeptides and tripeptides are absorbed intact, evidence has suggested that human brush border peptide hydrolysates play a pivotal and rate-limiting role in assimilation of higher peptides.[29, 63] However, since a protein hydrolysate composed of a large proportion of high molecular weight peptides will exert a lesser osmotic effect, our recent work showing that such a high molecular weight protein hydrolysate still exerted a kinetic advantage over uptake of a number of its amino acid residues is of considerable interest.[150]

Thus further research is indicated to define optimum peptide chain length and composition for maximal nitrogen absorption in

CASEIN/SOY/ LACTALBUMIN (Papain)	LACTALBUMIN II (Pancreatic)	MEAT/SOY/ LACTALBUMIN (Pancreatic)	LACTALBUMIN I (Papain)	EGG ALBUMIN (Papain)
VAL		VAL		
LYS				
GLY			GLY	
ALA			ALA	
SER	SER			
ARG	ARG			
LEU	LEU			
TYR	TYR	TYR		
ASP	ASP	ASP	ASP	
THR	THR	THR	THR	THR
GLU	GLU	GLU	GLU	GLU
PHE	PHE	PHE	PHE	PHE
HIS	HIS	HIS	HIS	HIS

Figure 3–2. Amino acid residues absorbed significantly faster ($p < 0.05$ or less) from partial protein hydrolysate compared with equivalent free AA mixtures.

patients with impaired gastrointestinal absorptive capacity.

REFERENCES

1. Nasset, E. S., Schwartz, P., and Weiss, H. V.: The digestion of proteins in vivo. J. Nutr., 56:83–94, 1955.
2. Nasset, E. S., and Ju, J. S.: Mixture of endogenous and exogenous protein in the alimentary tract. J. Nutr., 74:461–465, 1961.
3. Nixon, S. E., and Mawer, G. E.: The digestion and absorption of proteins in man. 1. The site of absorption. Br. J. Nutr., 24:227–240, 1970.
4. Nixon, S. E., and Mawer, G. E.: The digestion and absorption of proteins in man. 2. The form in which digested protein is absorbed. Br. J. Nutr., 24:241–258, 1970.
5. Johannson, C.: Studies of gastrointestinal interactions: VII. Characteristics of the absorption pattern of sugar, fat and protein from composite meals in man: A quantitative study. Scand. J. Gastroenterol., 10:33–42, 1975.
6. Borgström, B., Dahlqvist, A., Lundh, G., and Sjövall, J.: Studies of intestinal digestion and absorption in the human. J. Clin. Invest., 36:1521–1536, 1957.
7. Silk, D. B. A., Chung, Y. C., Berger, K. L., Conley, K., Beigler, M., Sleisenger, M. H., Spiller, G. A., and Kim, Y. S.: Comparison of oral feeding of peptide and amino acid meals to normal human subjects. Gut, 20:291–299, 1979.
8. Adibi, S. A., and Mercer, D. W.: Protein digestion in human intestine as reflected in luminal, mucosal and plasma amino acid concentrations after meals. J. Clin. Invest., 52:1586–1594, 1973.
9. Chung, Y. C., Kim, Y. S., Shadchehr, A., Garrido, A., MacGregor, I. L., and Sleisenger, M. H.: Protein digestion and absorption in human small intestine. Gastroenterology, 76:1415–1421, 1979.
10. Gibson, J. A., Sladen, G. E., Dawson, A. M.: Protein absorption and ammonia production: The effects of dietary protein and removal of the colon. Br. J. Nutr., 35:61–65, 1976.
11. Curtis, K. J., Kim, Y. S., Perdomo, J. M., Silk, D. B. A., and Whitehead, J. S.: Protein digestion and absorption in the rat. J. Physiol., 274:409–419, 1978.
12. Taylor, W. H.: Biochemistry of pepsins. In Handbook of Physiology, Section 6 (Volume V: Bile, Digestion, Ruminal Physiology). Washington, D.C., American Physiological Society, 1968, pages 2567–2587.
13. Turner, M. D.: Pepsinogens and pepsins. Gut, 9:134–138, 1968.
14. Whitecross, D. P., Armstrong, C., Clark, A. D., and Piper, D. W.: The pepsinogens of human gastric mucosa. Gut, 14:850–855, 1973.
15. Gray, G. M., and Cooper, H. L.: Protein digestion and absorption. Gastroenterology, 61:535–544, 1971.
16. Keller, P. J.: Pancreatic proteolytic enzymes. In Handbook of Physiology, Section 6 (Volume V: Bile, Digestion, Ruminal Physiology). Washington, D.C., American Physiological Society, 1968, pages 2605–2628.
17. Lobley, R. W., Moss, S., and Holmes, R.: Brush border localization of human enterokinase [Abstract]. Gut, 14:817, 1973.
18. Schmitz, J., Preiser, H., Maestracci, D., Ghosh, B. K., Cerda, J. J., and Crane, R. K.: Purification of the human intestinal brush border membrane. Biochim. Biophys. Acta, 323:98–112, 1973.
19. Hermon-Taylor, J., Perrin, J., Grant, D. A. W., Appleyard, A., Bubel, M., and Magee, A. I.: Immunofluorescent localisation of enterokinase in human small intestine. Gut, 18:259–265, 1977.
20. Josefsson, L., and Lindberg, T.: Intestinal dipeptidases. IX. Studies on dipeptidases of human intestinal mucosa. Acta Chem. Scand., 21:1965–1966, 1967.
21. Silk, D. B. A., Nicholson, J. A., and Kim, Y. S.: Hydrolysis of peptides within lumen of small intestine. Am. J. Physiol., 231:1323–1329, 1976.
22. Chen, M. L., Rogers, Q. R., and Harper, A. G.: Observations on protein digestion in vivo. IV. Further observations on the gastrointestinal contents of rats fed different dietary proteins. J. Nutr., 76:235–241, 1962.
23. Schultz, S. G., and Curran, P. F.: Coupled transport of sodium and organic solutes. Physiol. Rev., 50:637–718, 1970.
24. Adibi, S. A., and Gray, S. J.: Intestinal absorption of essential amino acids in man. Gastroenterology, 52:837–845, 1967.
25. Adibi, S. A., Gray, S. J., and Menden, E.: The kinetics of amino acid absorption and alteration of plasma composition of free amino acids after intestinal perfusion of amino acid mixtures. Am. J. Clin. Nutr., 20:24–33, 1967.
26. Adibi, S. A.: The influence of molecular structure of neutral amino acids on their absorption kinetics in the jejunum and ileum of human intestine in vivo. Gastroenterology, 56:903–913, 1969.
27. Adibi, S. A.: Leucine absorption rate and net movements of sodium and water in human jejunum. J. Appl. Physiol., 28:753–757, 1970.
28. Hellier, M. D., Holdsworth, C. D., and Perrett, D.: Dibasic amino acid absorption in man. Gastroenterology, 65:613–618, 1973.
29. Silk, D. B. A., and Dawson, A. M.: Intestinal absorption of carbohydrate and protein in man. In Crane, R. K. (ed.): International Review of Physiology, Volume 19, Gastrointestinal Physiology III. Baltimore, University Park Press, 1979, pages 151–204.
30. Matthews, D. M.: Proteins: Protein absorption. J. Clin. Pathol., 24[Suppl 5]:29–40, 1971.
31. Matthews, D. M.: Intestinal absorption of peptides. Physiol. Rev., 55:537–608, 1975.
32. Matthews, D. M., and Adibi, S. A.: Peptide absorption. Gastroenterology, 71:151–161, 1976.
33. Nolf, P.: Les albumoses et peptones sont-elles absorbees par l'epithelium intestinal? J. Physiol. Pathol. Generale, 9:925–938, 1907.
34. Messerli, H.: Über die Resorptionsgeschwindigkeit der Eiweisse und ihrer Abbauprodukteim Dunndarm. Biochem. Z., 54:446–473, 1913.
35. Cohnheim, O.: Die Umwandlung des Eiweiss durch die Darmwand. Hoppe Seylers Z. Physiol. Chem., 33:451–465, 1901.
36. Abderhalden, E., and Lampé, A. E.: Weiterer Beitrag zur Kenntnis des Schicksals von in den Magendarmkanal eingeführten einzelnen Amino-

säuren, Aminosäuregemischen, Peptonen und Proteinen. Hoppe Seylers Z. Physiol. Chem., 81:473–507, 1912.

37. Cohnheim, O.: Zur Frage der Eiweissresorption. III. Mitteilung. Hoppe Seylers Z. Physiol. Chem., 76:293–297, 1912.

38. Cohnheim, O.: Die Wirkung vollstandig abgebauter Nahrung auf den Verdauungskanal. Hoppe Seylers Z. Physiol. Chem., 84:419–424, 1913.

39. Cathcart, E. P., and Leathes, J. B.: On the absorption of proteids from the intestine. J. Physiol., 33:462–475, 1905.

40. Abderhalden, E., and London, E. S.: Weiterer Beitrag zur Frage nach dem Ab- und Aufbau der Proteine im tierischen Organismus. Hoppe Seylers Z. Physiol. Chem., 65:251–255, 1910.

41. Abel, J. J., Rowntree, L. G., and Turner, B. B.: On the removal of diffusable substances from the circulating blood of living animals by dialysis. II. Some constituents of the blood. J. Pharmacol. Exp. Ther., 5:611–623, 1913.

42. Verzár, F., and McDougall, E. J.: Absorption from the Intestine. London, Longmans, 1936.

43. Cajori, F. A.: The enzyme activity of dogs' intestinal juice and its relation to intestinal digestion. Am. J. Physiol., 104:659–668, 1933.

44. Stein, W. H., and Moore, S.: The free amino acids of human blood plasma. J. Biol. Chem., 211:915–926, 1954.

45. Fisher, R. B.: Protein Metabolism. London, Methuen, 1954.

46. Agar, W. T., Hird, F. J. R., and Sidhu, G. S.: The uptake of amino acids by the intestine. Biochim. Biophys. Acta, 14:80–84, 1954.

47. Wiggans, D. S., and Johnston, J. M.: The absorption of peptides. Biochim. Biophys. Acta, 32:69–73, 1959.

48. Newey, H., and Smyth, D. H.: The intestinal absorption of some dipeptides. J. Physiol. (Lond.), 145:48–56, 1959.

49. Newey, H., and Smyth, D. H.: Intracellular hydrolysis of dipeptides during intestinal absorption. J. Physiol. (Lond.), 152:367–380, 1960.

50. Newey, H., and Smyth, D. H.: Cellular mechanisms in intestinal transfer of amino acids. J. Physiol. (Lond.), 164:527–551, 1962.

51. Craft, I. L., Geddes, D., Hyde, C. W., Wise, I. J., and Matthews, D. M.: Absorption and malabsorption of glycine and glycine peptides in man. Gut, 9:425–437, 1968.

52. Cook, G. C.: Comparison of absorption rates of glucose and maltose in man in vivo. Clin. Sci., 44:425–428, 1973.

53. Fairclough, P. D., Silk, D. B. A., Webb, J. P. W., Clark, M. L., and Dawson, A. M.: A reappraisal of "osmotic" evidence for intact peptide absorbtion. Clin. Sci. Mol. Med., 53:241–248, 1977.

54. Sandle, G. I., Lobley, R. W., and Holmes, R.: Effect of maltose on the absorption of glucose in the jejunum in man [Abstract]. Gut, 18:A944–A945, 1977.

55. Jones, B. J. M., Beavis, A. K., Edgerton, D., and Silk, D. B. A.: Intestinal absorption of glucose polymers in man [Abstract]. Gut, 21:A450, 1980.

56. Milne, M. D.: Disorders of intestinal amino-acid transport. J. Clin. Pathol., 24[Suppl. 5]:41–44, 1971.

57. Asatoor, A. M., Cheng, B., Edwards, K. D. G., Lant, A. F., Matthews, D. M., Milne, M. D., Navab, F., and Richards, A. J.: Intestinal absorption of two dipeptides in Hartnup disease. Gut, 11:380–387, 1970.

58. Asatoor, A. M., Harrison, B. D. W., Milne, M. D., and Prosser, D. I.: Intestinal absorption of an arginine-containing peptide in cystinuria. Gut, 13:95–98, 1972.

59. Hellier, M. D., Holdsworth, C. D., Perett, D., and Thirumalai, C.: Intestinal dipeptide transport in normal and cystinuric subjects. Clin. Sci., 43:659–668, 1972.

60. Navab, F., and Asatoor, A. M.: Studies on intestinal absorption of amino acids and a dipeptide in a case of Hartnup disease. Gut, 11:373–379, 1970.

61. Silk, D. B. A., Perrett, D., and Clark, M. L.: Jejunal and ileal absorption of dibasic amino acids and an arginine-containing dipeptide in cystinuria. Gastroenterology, 68:1426–1432, 1975.

62. Silk, D. B. A.: Progress report: Peptide absorption in man. Gut, 15:494–501, 1974.

63. Adibi, S. A.: Intestinal phase of protein assimilation in man. Am. J. Clin. Nutr., 29(Part 1):205–215, 1976.

64. Kim, Y. S., Kim, Y. W., Sleisenger, M. H.: Studies on the properties of peptide hydrolases in the brush-border and soluble fractions of small intestinal mucosa of rat and man. Biochim. Biophys. Acta, 370:283–296, 1974.

65. Silk, D. B. A., Perrett, D., and Clark, M. L.: Intestinal transport of two dipeptides containing the same two neutral amino acids in man. Clin. Sci. Mol. Med., 45:291–299, 1973.

66. Kim, Y. S., and Brophy, E. J.: Rat intestinal brush border membrane peptidases. 1. Solubilization, purification and physicochemical properties of two different forms of the enzyme. J. Biol. Chem., 251:3199–3205, 1976.

67. Fogel, M. R., and Adibi, S. A.: Assessment of the role of brush-border peptide hydrolases in luminal disappearance of dipeptides in man. J. Lab. Clin. Med., 84:327–333, 1974.

68. Adibi, S. A.: Intestinal transport of dipeptides in man: Relative importance of hydrolysis and intact absorption. J. Clin. Invest., 50:2266–2275, 1971.

68a. Fairclough, P. D., Silk, D. B. A., Clark, M. L., Matthews, D. M., Marrs, T. C., Burston, D., and Clegg, K. M.: Unpublished data, 1982.

69. Silk, D. B. A., Webb, J. P. W., Lane, A. E., Clark, M. L., and Dawson, A. M.: Functional differentiation of human jejunum and ileum: A comparison of the handling of glucose, peptides and amino acids. Gut, 15:444–449, 1974.

70. Silk, D. B. A., Perrett, D., Webb, J. P. W., and Clark, M. L.: Absorption of two tripeptides by the human small intestine: A study using a perfusion technique. Clin. Sci. Mol. Med., 46:393–402, 1974.

71. Adibi, S. A., Morse, E. L., Masilamani, S. S., and Amin, P. M.: Evidence for two different modes of tripeptide disappearance in human intestine: Uptake by peptide carrier systems and hydrolysis by peptide hydrolases. J. Clin. Invest., 56:1355–1363, 1975.

72. Peters, T. J.: The subcellular localization of di- and tri-peptide hydrolase activity in guinea-pig small intestine. Biochem. J., 120:195–203, 1970.

73. Donlon, J., and Fottrell, P. F.: Studies on substrate

specificites and subcellular location of multiple forms of peptide hydrolases in guinea pig intestinal mucosa. Comp. Biochem. Physiol., 41(Part B):181–193, 1972.

74. Fujita, M., Parsons, D. S., and Wojnarowska, F.: Oligopeptidases of brush border membranes of rat small intestinal mucosal cells. J. Physiol. (Lond.), 227:377–394, 1972.

75. Heizer, W. D., Kerley, R. L., and Isselbacher, K. J.: Intestinal peptide hydrolases: Differences between brush border and cytoplasmic enzymes. Biochim. Biophys. Acta, 264:450–461, 1972.

76. Wojnarowska, F., and Gray, G. M.: Intestinal surface peptide hydrolases: Identification and characterization of three enzymes from rat brush border. Biochim. Biophys. Acta, 403:147–160, 1975.

77. Kim, Y. S., Brophy, E. J., and Nicholson, J. A.: Rat intestinal brush border membrane peptidases. 2. Enzymic properties, immunochemistry and interactions with lectins of two different forms of the enzyme. J. Biol. Chem., 251:3206–3212, 1976.

78. Josefsson L., Sjöström, H., and Norén, O.: Intracellular hydrolysis of peptides. In Peptide Transport and Hydrolysis. Ciba Foundation Symposium 50 (New Series): 199–207, 1977.

79. Kim, Y. S.: Intestinal mucosal hydrolysis of proteins and peptides. In Peptide Transport and Hydrolysis. Ciba Foundation Symposium 50 (New Series): 151–171, 1977.

80. Norén, O., Sjöström, H., Svensson, B., Jeppesen, L., Staun, M., and Josefsson, L.: Intestinal brush border peptidases. In Peptide Transport and Hydrolysis. Ciba Foundation Symposium 50 (New Series): 177–191, 1977.

81. Kim, Y. S., Birtwhistle, W., and Kim, Y. W.: Peptide hydrolases in the brush border and soluble fractions of small intestinal mucosa of rat and man. J. Clin. Invest., 51:1419–1430, 1972.

82. Nicholson, J. A., and Peters, T. J.: Subcellular distribution of hydrolase activities for glycine and leucine homopeptides in human jejunum. Clin. Sci. Mol. Med., 54:205–207, 1978.

83. Nicholson, J. A., and Peters, T. J.: Subcellular localization of peptidase activity in the human jejunum. Eur. J. Clin. Invest., 9:349–354, 1979.

84. Silk, D. B. A., Nicholson, J. A., and Kim, Y. S.: Relationships between mucosal hydrolysis and transport of two phenylalanine dipeptides. Gut, 17:870–876, 1976.

85. Malathi, P., Ramaswamy, K., Caspary, W. F., and Crane, R. K.: Studies on transport of glucose from disaccharides by hamster small intestine in vitro. 1. Evidence for a disaccharidase-related transport system. Biochim. Biophys. Acta, 307:613–626, 1973.

86. Ramaswamy, K., Malathi, P., Caspary, W. F., and Crane, R. K.: Studies on the transport of glucose from disaccharides by hamster small intestine in vitro. II. Characteristics of the disaccharidase-related transport system. Biochim. Biophys. Acta, 345:39–48, 1974.

87. Ramaswamy, K., Malathi, P., and Crane, R. K.: Demonstration of hydrolase-related glucose transport in brush border membrane vesicles prepared from guinea pig small intestine. Biochem. Biophys. Res. Comm., 68:162–168, 1976.

88. Addison, J. M.: Burston, D., Payne, J. W., Wilkinson, S., Matthews, D. M.: Evidence for active transport of tripeptides by hamster jejunum in vitro. Clin. Sci. Mol. Med., 49:305–312, 1975.

89. Rubino, A., Field, M., and Shwachman, H.: Intestinal transport of amino acid residues of dipeptides. 1. Influx of the glycine residue of glycyl-L-proline across mucosal border. J. Biol. Chem., 246:3542–3548, 1971.

90. Adibi, S. A., and Soleimanpour, M. R.: Functional characterization of dipeptide transport system in human jejunum. J. Clin. Invest., 53:1368–1374, 1974.

91. Matthews, D. M., Addison, J. M., and Burston, D.: Evidence for active transport of the dipeptide carnosine (B-alanyl-L-histidine) by hamster jejunum in vitro. Clin. Sci. Mol. Med., 46:693–705, 1974.

92. Addison, J. M., Burston, D., and Matthews, D. M.: Evidence for active transport of the dipeptide glycylsarcosine by hamster jejunum in vitro. Clin. Sci., 43:907–911, 1972.

93. Addison, J. M., Burston, D., Dalrymple, J. A., Matthews, D. M., Payne, J. W., Sleisenger, M. H., Wilkinson, S.: A common mechanism for transport of di- and tripeptides by hamster jejunum in vitro. Clin. Sci. Mol. Med., 49:313–322, 1975.

94. Chung, Y. C., Silk, D. B. A., and Kim, Y. S.: Intestinal transport of a tetrapeptide, L-leucylglycylglycine, in rat small intestine in vivo. Clin. Sci., 57:1–11, 1979.

95. Kim, Y. S., and Brophy, E. J.: Effect of amino acids on purified rat intestinal brush-border membrane aminooligopeptidase. Gastroenterology, 76:82–87, 1979.

96. Sleisenger, M. H., Burston, D., Dalrymple, J. A., Wilkinson, S., and Matthews, D. M.: Evidence for a single common carrier for uptake of a dipeptide and a tripeptide by hamster jejunum in vitro. Gastroenterology, 71:76–81, 1976.

97. Silk, D. B. A.: Amino acid and peptide absorption in man. In Peptide Transport and Hydrolysis. Ciba Foundation Symposium 50 (New Series):15–29, 1977.

98. Matthews, D. M., Gandy, R. H., Taylor, E., and Burston, D.: Influx of two dipeptides glycylsarcosine and L-glutamyl-L-glutamic acid into hamster jejunum in vitro. Clin. Sci., 56:15–23, 1979.

99. Taylor, E., Burston, D., and Matthews, D. M.: Influx of glycylsarcosine and L-lysyl-L-lysine into hamster jejunum in vitro. Clin. Sci., 58:221–225, 1980.

100. Neame, K. D., and Richards, T. G.: In Elementary Kinetics of Membrane Carrier Transport. Oxford, Blackwell Scientific Publications, 1972, page 53.

101. Christensen, H. N.: Biological Transport. Edition 2. Reading, Massachusetts, Benjamin, 1975, pages 112 and 136.

102. Read, N. W., Holdsworth, C. D., and Levin, R. J.: Electrical measurement of intestinal absorption of glucose in man. Lancet, 2:624–627, 1974.

103. Debnam, E. S., and Levin, R. J.: An experimental method of identifying and quantifying the active transfer electrogenic component from the diffusive component during sugar absorption measured in vivo. J. Physiol. (Lond.), 246:181–196, 1975.

104. Read, N. W., Levin, R. J., and Holdsworth, C. D.: Electrogenic glucose absorption in untreated and treated coeliac disease. Gut, 17:444–449, 1976.

105. Read, N. W., Barber, D. C., Levin, R. J., and Holdsworth, C. D.: Unstirred layer and kinetics of electrogenic glucose absorption in the human jejunum in situ. Gut, 18:865–876, 1977.

106. Batt, R. M., Peters, T. J.: Absorption of galactose by the rat small intestine in vivo: Proximal-distal kinetic gradients and a new method to express absorption per enterocyte. Clin. Sci. Mol. Med., 50:499–509, 1976.

107. Asatoor, A. M., Crouchman, M. R., Harrison, A. R., Light, F. W., Loughridge, L. W., Milne, M. D., and Richards, A. J.: Intestinal absorption of oligopeptides in cystinuria. Clin. Sci., 41:23–33, 1971.

108. Hughes, W. S., and Senior, J. R.: The glucose-galactose malabsorption syndrome in a 23-year-old woman. Gastroenterology, 68:142–145, 1975.

109. Fairclough, P. D., Clark, M. L., Dawson, A. M., Silk, D. B. A., Milla, P. J., and Harries, J. T.: Absorption of glucose and maltose in congenital glucose-galactose malabsorption. Pediatr. Res., 12:1112–1114, 1978.

110. Silk, D. B. A., and Kim, Y. S.: Release of peptide hydrolases during incubation of intact intestinal segments in vitro. J. Physiol. (Lond.), 258:489–497, 1976.

111. Cheeseman, C. I., and Parsons, D. S.: Intestinal absorption of peptides: Peptide uptake by small intestine of Rana pipiens. Biochim. Biphys. Acta, 373:523–526, 1974.

112. Addison, J. M., Matthews, D. M., and Burston, D.: Competition between carnosine and other peptides for transport by hamster jejunum in vitro. Clin. Sci. Mol. Med., 46:707–714, 1974.

113. Lane, A. E., Silk, D. B. A., and Clark, M. L.: Absorption of two proline-containing peptides by rat small intestine in vivo. J. Physiol. (Lond.), 248:143–149, 1975.

114. Fairclough, P. D., Silk, D. B. A., Clark, M. L., Matthews, D. M., Marrs, T. C., Burston, D., and Clegg, K. M.: Effect of glycylglycine on absorption from human jejunum of an amino acid mixture simulating casein and a partial enzymic hydrolysate of casein containing small peptides. Clin. Sci. Mol. Med., 53:27–33, 1977.

115. Das, M., and Radhakrishnan, A. N.: Studies on a wide-spectrum intestinal dipeptide uptake system in the monkey and in the human. Biochem. J., 146:133–139, 1975.

116. Smithson, K. W., and Gray, G. M.: Intestinal assimilation of a tetrapeptide in the rat: Obligate function of brush border membrane aminopeptidase. J. Clin. Invest., 60:665–674, 1977.

117. Adibi, S. A., and Morse, E. L.: The number of glycine residues which limits intact absorption of glycine oligopeptides in human jejunum. J. Clin. Invest., 60:1008–1016, 1977.

118. Burston, D., Taylor, E., and Matthews, D. M.: Intestinal handling of two tetrapeptides by rodent small intestine in vitro. Biochim. Biophys. Acta, 553:175–178, 1979.

119. Peters, T. J.: The hydrolysis of glycine oligopeptides by guinea-pig intestinal mucosa and by isolated brush borders. Clin. Sci. Mol. Med., 45:803–816, 1973.

120. Gray, G. M., and Santiago, N. A.: Intestinal surface amino-oligo-peptidases. 1. Isolation of two weight isomers and their subunits from rat brush border. J. Biol. Chem., 252:4922–4928, 1977.

121. Kania, R. K., Santiago, N. A., and Gray, G. M.: Intestinal surface amino-oligopeptidases. II. Substrate kinetics and topography of the active site. J. Biol. Chem., 252:4929–4934, 1977.

122. Prockop, D. J., and Sjoerdsma, A.: Significance of urinary hydroxyproline in man. J. Clin. Invest., 40:843–849, 1961.

123. Prockop, D. J., Keiser, H. R., and Sjoerdsma, A.: Gastrointestinal absorption and renal excretion of hydroxyproline peptides. Lancet, 2:527–528, 1962.

124. Perry, T. L., Hansen, S., Tischler, B., Bunting, R., and Berry, K.: Carnosinemia: A new metabolic disorder associated with neurologic disease and mental defect. N. Engl. J. Med., 277:1219–1227, 1967.

125. Hueckel, H. J., and Rogers, Q. R.: Urinary excretion of hydroxyproline-containing peptides in man, rat, hamster, dog and monkey after feeding gelatin. Comp. Biochem. Physiol., 32:7–16, 1970.

126. Peters, T. J., and MacMahon, M. T.: The absorption of glycine and glycine oligopeptides by the rat. Clin. Sci., 39:811–821, 1970.

127. Gardner, M. L. G.: Absorption of amino acids and peptides from a complex mixture in the isolated small intestine of the rat. J. Physiol. (Lond.), 253:233–256, 1975.

128. Gardner, M. L. G.: Amino acid and peptide absorption from partial digests of protein in isolated rat small intestine. J. Physiol. (Lond.), 284:83–104, 1978.

129. Sleisenger, M. H., Pelling, D., Burston, D., and Matthews, D. M.: Amino acid concentrations in portal venous plasma during absorption from the small intestine of the guinea pig of an amino acid mixture simulating casein and a partial enzymic hydrolysate of casein. Clin. Sci. Mol. Med., 52:259–267, 1977.

130. Krzysik, B. A., Peterson, J., and Adibi, S. A.: The potential of blood, liver, muscle and kidney for dipeptide hydrolysis [Abstract]. Fed. Proc., 34:466, 1975.

131. Adibi, S. A.: Clearance of dipeptides from plasma: Role of kidney and intestine. In Peptide Transport and Hydrolysis. Ciba Foundation Symposium 50 (New Series):265–280, 1977.

132. Adibi, S. A., and Krzysik, B. A.: Effect of nephrectomy and enterectomy on plasma clearance of intravenously administered dipeptides in rats. Clin. Sci. Mol. Med., 52:205–213, 1977.

133. Adibi, S. A., Krzysik, B. A., and Drash, A. I.: Metabolism of intravenously administered dipeptides in rats: Effects of amino acid pools, glucose concentration and insulin and glucagon secretion. Clin. Sci. Mol. Med., 52:193–204, 1977.

134. Lidström, F., and Wretlind, K. A. J.: Effect of dialyzed casein hydrolysate; effect of intravenous administration of a dialyzed enzymatic casein hydrolysate (Aminosol) on serum concentration and on urinary excretion of amino acids, peptides, and nitrogen. Scand. J. Clin. Lab. Invest., 4:167–178, 1952.

135. Adibi, S. A., Fogel, M. R., and Agrawal, R. M.: Comparison of free amino acid and dipeptide absorption in the jejunum of sprue patients. Gastroenterology, 67:586–591, 1974.

136. Silk, D. B. A., Kumar, P. J., Perrett, D., Clark, M. L., and Dawson, A. M.: Amino acid absorption in patients with coeliac disease and dermatitis herpetiformis. Gut, 15:1–8, 1974.

137. Silk, D. B. A., Clark, M. L., Marrs, T. C., Addison, J. M., Burston, D., Matthews, D. M., and Clegg, K. M.: Jejunal absorption of an amino acid mixture simulating casein and an enzymic hydrolysate of casein prepared for oral administration to normal adults. Br. J. Nutr., 33:95–100, 1975.

138. Fairclough, P. D.: Jejunal absorption of water and electrolytes in man: The effect of amino acids, peptides and saccharides. M.D. Thesis, University of London, 1978.

139. Silk, D. B. A., Fairclough, P. D., Clark, M. L., Hegarty, J. E., Marrs, T. C., Addison, J. M., Burston, D., Clegg, K. M., Matthews, D. M.: Uses of a peptide rather than free amino acid nitrogen source in chemically defined "elemental" diets. J. Parent. Ent. Nutr., 4:6:548–553, 1980.

140. Gitler, C.: Protein digestion and absorption in nonruminants. In Munro, H. N., Allison, J. B. (eds.): Mammalian Protein Metabolism. Volume I. New York, Academic Press, 1964, pages 35–69.

140a. Keohane, P., and Silk, D. B. A.: Unpublished observations, 1982.

141. Moriarty, K. J., Hegarty, J. E., Fairclough, P. D., et al.: Dietary nitrogen formulation: Does it really matter? [Abstract.] Gut, 22:A430, 1981.

142. Hegarty, J. E.: Amino acid and peptide absorption in man. M.D. Thesis, University of London, 1981.

143. McMichael, H. B.: Physiology of carbohydrate, electrolyte and water absorption. Res. Clin. For., 1:25, 1979.

144. Silk, D. B. A., Keohane, P. P.: Formulation of enteral diets. In Wesdorp, R., and Soeters, P. (eds.): Clinical Nutrition '81. London, Churchill Livingstone, 1982.

145. Cobb, M. L., Cartmill, A. M., and Gilsdorf, R. B.: Early post operative nutritional support using the serosal tunnel jejunostomy. J. Parent. Ent. Nutr., 5:5:397–401, 1981.

146. Powell-Tuck, J., and Goode, A. W.: Principles of enteral and parenteral nutrition. Br. J. Anaesth., 53:169–181, 1981.

147. Broom, J., and Jones, K.: Causes and prevention of diarrhoea in patients receiving enteral nutritional support. J. Hum. Nutr., 35:123–127, 1981.

148. Silk, D. B. A.: Enteral nutrition. Hosp. Update, 6:761, 1980.

149. Jones, B. J. M., Payne, S., and Silk, D. B. A.: Indications for pump-assisted enteral feeding. Lancet, 1:1057–1058, 1980.

150. Keohane, P., Brown, B., Grimble, G., and Silk, D. B. A.: The peptide nitrogen source of elemental diets: Comparisons of absorptive properties of five partial enzymic hydrolysates of whole protein. J. Parent. Ent. Nutr., 5:568, 1981.

CHAPTER 4

Hormone-Substrate Interactions

PRESTON R. BLACK
DOUGLAS W. WILMORE

Total body metabolic regulation has evolved as a result of a carefully determined set of priorities. The foremost priority is to provide an adequate quantity of glucose, which serves as an essential fuel for vital tissues such as the brain, peripheral nervous tissue, erythrocytes, and the renal medulla. To maintain normal cerebral function the brain requires 5 to 6 gm of glucose each hour, and this amount cannot be provided if arterial glucose concentration falls below a critical level. A second priority is to incorporate amino acids into the body's structural and functional proteins, which are also essential to the workings of this complex biologic unit. Net protein synthesis does not occur if glucose is deficient; amino acids will be diverted into glucose synthetic pathways to subserve this priority function. Finally, excess energy is stored as body fat when energy is plentiful. However, when requirements exceed energy intake, fat is rapidly mobilized to be utilized as a primary energy source.

This system of regulation is performed on-line, minute by minute, by interacting levels of metabolic control. On the cellular level, compartmentalization, substrate availability, and enzyme regulation are primary regulators. The mass action of substrate, frequently exerted by changes in concentration in blood and intracellular fluid, is an important regulator during the the fed state. Moreover, the presence of a substrate (such as ketone bodies during starvation) can also exert inhibitory influences on biochemical reactions. None of the events occurs, however, in an isolated setting, for substrates stimulate hormones, which then facilitate other regulatory mechanisms to aid storage or mobilization of fuel.

The word "hormone" is derived from the Greek root meaning to excite, arouse, or set into motion. It was proposed by Starling as the name for a group of chemicals that are synthesized in one cell group, travel through the bloodstream, and ultimately have an effect on another cell group. Huxley placed less emphasis on the mode of travel of these compounds and proposed that the most important function of hormones was to convey information between cell populations and thereby elicit responses beneficial to the organisms as a whole. Hence, hormones are the body's messengers. They inform the organism of alterations in the internal milieu and initiate responses necessary for preserving homeostasis. The body's rapid response to hormones makes them ideal as modulators of those systems that demand fine, but prompt changes. Insulin and glucagon, the primary regulators of energy homeostasis within the body, maintain blood glucose within narrowly defined limits. Although these hormones affect most tissues in the body, the liver, skeletal muscle, and adipose tissue are their primary target cells. Carbohydrates, lipids, protein, and their components are their major substrates.

In this chapter we will examine the hormone-target cell-substrate interactions that are central to metabolic homeostasis. A discussion of normal physiologic biochemistry will provide insight into the workings of the system during the fed and fasted states. This will be followed by a discussion of the alterations in the system caused by two perturbations frequently associated with critical illness—prolonged starvation and the stress of sepsis or injury.

THE NORMAL FEEDING-FASTING CYCLE

Since normal individuals generally eat in an episodic manner, the feeding cycle may be divided into a phase of high nutrient intake followed by a phase of fasting. For convenience, these phases are referred to as the absorptive and postabsorptive periods, respectively. Each of these periods has characteristic hormonal responses that are designed to maximize the utilization or storage of nutrients.

The Absorptive Period. During the absorptive period, food is ingested, digested, and absorbed. Usually the energy available from the consumed meal far exceeds the metabolic demands of the body. Therefore, metabolic efficiency dictates that all excess fuels be stored by the body and become available for utilization during periods of fasting.

Insulin—the "banker's hormone"—is the predominant metabolic signal during the absorptive period. After a usual meal the level of blood glucose increases. Insulin is the primary hormone elaborated to facilitate disposal of glucose into cells and to decrease plasma glucose concentration. Insulin, produced in the beta cell of the pancreas, is initially synthesized as the single-chain precursor proinsulin. Proinsulin contains a connecting peptide segment (c-peptide) that renders this molecule essentially inactive metabolically. Proteolytic cleavage of the c-peptide segment from the proinsulin molecule converts the latter into active insulin.

The rate of change and the absolute change in blood glucose concentration are the predominant factors controlling insulin secretion from the beta cell.[1] However, many additional factors are known to affect insulin release. Thus insulin secretion can be stimulated by carbohydrates other than glucose, and related substances include mannose, sorbitol, N-acetyglucosamine, glyceraldehyde, and inosine. In addition to carbohydrates, many substances of low molecular weight (such as certain amino acids, certain fatty acids, ketone bodies, and certain metabolites of intermediary metabolism) can also provoke the beta cell to release insulin.[1] More-over, insulin secretion can be modulated by neuronal stimuli by means of the sympathetic nervous system or circulating catecholamines. During the absorptive phase, however, the elevation of plasma glucose is the primary effector of insulin secretion.

The effects of insulin are tissue-specific. In adipose tissue, insulin has three, or possibly four, major actions: (1) It accelerates the transportation of glucose across the cell membrane; (2) it enhances the phosphorylation of glucose; and (3) it inhibits lipolysis. There is also an increase in the activity of lipoprotein lipase in the blood, which may be a direct effect of insulin. The net effect of all of these actions is the promotion of fat production and storage within the adipocyte and the reduction of lipolysis. Once in the adipocyte, glucose, facilitated by insulin, is catabolized to the two-carbon fragment, acetyl CoA, which is subsequently used for the synthesis of fatty acids. Glucose is also the source of L-glycerol-3-phosphate, which combines with fatty acids to form the triglycerides stored in fat cells. Finally, the reducing substances needed for fatty acid synthesis are derived from glucose through the pentose shunt.

Insulin also has three actions on skeletal muscle: It accelerates the carrier-mediated transport of glucose into the cell, enhances the synthesis of glycogen, and increases the synthesis of protein by muscle ribosomes. The net effect during the absorptive phase is for glucose to provide muscle with the energy it needs for contraction and for storage of excess glucose as glycogen, which can be used subsequently as fuel.

Of these two carcass tissues (that is, fat and skeletal muscle), it appears that the effects of insulin in promoting glucose transport are much greater on skeletal muscle than on adipose tissue. Recently reported insulin clamp experiments would suggest that the majority of nonoxidized glucose during euglycemic hyperinsulinemia is "stored" in skeletal muscle.[2]

The liver plays a central role in glucose homeostasis during the absorptive period, extracting a major portion (40 to 50 per cent) of the glucose load after an oral meal.[3] However, carrier-mediated uptake of glucose by the hepatocyte is not facilitated by the presence of high insulin concentrations.[4] Nonetheless, insulin is a very potent stimulus of glycogen synthesis and a powerful inhibitor of glycogenolysis and gluconeogenesis within the liver. The net effect of these actions is to produce significant glucose gradients across hepatic cell membranes, resulting in a rapid increase of glucose uptake by the liver. Furthermore, the hepatic response to hyperinsulinemia and hyperglycemia appears to be dependent upon the route of glucose administration.[5, 6] The hepatic extraction of glucose is several-fold higher when glucose is given orally when compared with an intravenously administered glucose load. This difference is noted even if the plasma levels of insulin are comparable in the two groups, suggesting that unknown factors (all related to intraluminal enteral feedings) play an important role in glucose disposal after enteral glucose administration. These factors appear not to be effective during intravenous glucose delivery, even if the solutions are given through the portal vein.[7] The importance of these gastrointestinal factors on protein and lipid metabolism has not been fully elucidated. It would appear, however, that delivery of nutrients through the gastrointestinal tract is not only safer, but also metabolically far more efficient.

Thus, during the absorptive period, the body's hormonal milieu is dominated by insulin, which directs ingested fuels toward intracellular translocation, or oxidation, or storage, or all three.

The Postabsorptive Period. The postabsorptive period is the period 8 to 16 hours postcibal. It has classically been that time following an overnight fast before breakfast and is best thought of as very early starvation. Insulin concentrations decline during this period, and glucagon is the dominant hormone. If insulin is the "banker's hormone," then glucagon is the "spender's hormone." Glucagon is produced in the pancreatic alpha cell and like insulin is initially synthesized as a larger precursor molecule that is selectively cleaved by proteolytic enzymes to produce the active hormone. The primary stimulus for release of glucagon is a lowering of the blood glucose concentration, although other factors, particularly neuronal stimuli, can influence secretion of glucagon.

Glucagon prevents hypoglycemia by stimulating hepatic production of glucose from the glycogen stored during the absorptive period.[8] Stimulated by glucagon, the concentration of cyclic AMP increases within the hepatocyte and glycogenolysis is enhanced. Because skeletal muscle cells lack glucose-6-phosphatase, the glucose derived from glycogen within the myocyte cannot be released into the circulation as new glucose. However, skeletal muscle supports hepatic production of glucose by releasing lactate and amino acids, which can be converted into glucose by the liver by means of gluconeogenesis. Glucagon facilitates these reactions.

The hyperglucagonemia of the postabsorptive period increases lipolysis and thereby increases the mobilization of stored fat.[8] Those tissues that do not preferentially utilize glucose as their energy source (for example, skeletal muscle) shift to fat oxidation to meet their energy demands. Additionally, the energy required by the liver for gluconeogenesis is obtained in part from the oxidation of free fatty acids.

In summary, during the postabsorptive period, the body, under the influence of glucagon, becomes a producer of glucose in order to provide glucose to those tissues that require it to meet their metabolic needs. Concurrently, utilization of glucose is minimal in those tissues that can utilize fat.

Insulin-Glucagon Interactions. While the absolute concentrations of circulating insulin and glucagon are important during the absorptive and postabsorptive periods, the interaction between the two hormones is thought to determine the overall metabolic effect.[9] For example, during the absorptive period secretion of glucagon is suppressed while that of insulin is stimulated. The net effect is that there are high concentrations of insulin and low concentrations of glucagon in the blood. Thus the total metabolic effects are primarily those mediated by insulin. During the postabsorptive period this relationship is reversed and the overall metabolic effects are those primarily mediated by glucagon. However, the basal concentrations of insulin during the postabsorptive period are sufficient to affect release of substrate from peripheral tissues to the liver. By reducing the availability of these substrates (that is, amino acids from skeletal muscle and free fatty acids from adipose tissue), insulin modulates glucose production in the postabsorptive period. Moreover, insulin is a direct antagonist of all of the effects of glucagon on the liver. Therefore, it is the ratio of the concentrations of these two hormones (the so-called insulin-glucagon ratio) that may determine the final effect on the body's metabolic processes.[9] For example, after a protein meal the reciprocal relationship usually seen between insulin and glucagon is abolished; the release of insulin parallels the secretion of glucagon. The overall effect is that insulin facilitates the incorporation of the amino acids into skeletal muscle while glucagon prevents the hypoglycemia that would result from hyperinsulinemia without concurrent ingestion of carbohydrate.

This system of bihormonal substrate control, anatomically situated within the pancreas, located within the confines of the splanchnic bed, and connected directly to the liver by the portal system, finely regulates and modulates metabolism during the fed and fasting states, maximizing efficiency at optimal safety (Fig. 4–1).

HORMONAL RESPONSE TO PROLONGED STARVATION

During long-term starvation it is essential for the body to adapt to protein and energy deprivation to increase the probability of survival. Bodily processes critical to survival must be preserved at all costs, yet the organism must continue to function. An adequate supply of protein must be available for enzymatic and neurohormonal activities, fuel must be mobilized to provide energy, and breakdown products of metabolism must be excreted. Glucose homeostasis must be maintained, and critical structural proteins and lipids (for example, enzymes, hormones, and nervous system proteolipids and lipoproteins) must be spared. Most of the energy requirements of the body must be provided by stored fat; the remaining new glucose precursors will arise from amino acids derived from skeletal muscle. Substrate-hormonal interactions during prolonged starvation favor adaptation of fat metabolism while conserving glucose and protein, thereby favoring the survival of the organism.

Metabolic Changes of Prolonged Starvation. During the latter part of the nineteenth and the early part of the twentieth centuries, extensive experimentation elucidated the adaptive changes made during starvation. It was not until newer techniques for studying hormonal physiology emerged that the mechanistic aspects of these changes were clarified. One of the earliest observations made by physiologists was that within the first few days of a fast, urinary excretion of nitrogen fell gradually, reached a plateau at about one to two weeks, and rose moderately again shortly before death.[10] Furthermore, it was demonstrated that proteins accounted for only 10 to 15 per cent of the calories expended while fasting (Table 4–1). It was found that 85 to 90 per cent of the calories utilized during a fast were derived from a nonprotein source, which was later proved to be fat.

Investigators also demonstrated that while glycogen played a significant role in the body's energetics in the postabsorptive period, these stores were gradually depleted, with little energy being derived from glycogen after a week or so of a fast.[4] New glucose was obtained primarily through gluconeogenesis. The major source of the three-carbon fragments needed in the gluconeogenic pathways was amino acids. Early in starvation these amino acids are derived from both visceral and muscle proteins; later in the fast they are derived almost exclusively from skeletal muscle proteins.[11] Rapid

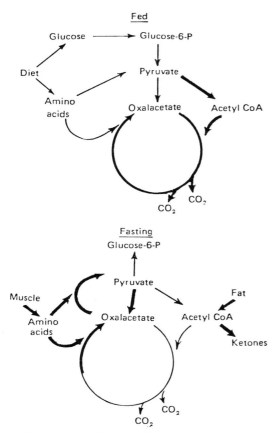

Figure 4–1. The flow of substrate during the fed and fasting states.

Table 4–1   ALTERATIONS IN SUBSTRATE UTILIZATION DURING STARVATION*

DAYS OF FAST	WEIGHT AT START OF EACH PERIOD (kg)	URINARY NITROGEN (gm/day)	CALORIC EXPENDITURE (kcal/day)	CALORIES FROM NITROGEN (%)
3 preliminary days	—	14.0	—	—
1–7	60.6	9.9	1650	15
8–14	55.1	10.3	1450	18
15–21	52.8	8.4	1290	17
22–28	50.1	7.8	1250	16
29–31	48.1	7.2	1260	15

*Adapted from Peters, J. P., and Van Slyke, D. D.: Quantitative Clinical Chemistry. Vol. I. Interpretations. Edition 2. Baltimore, Williams & Wilkins Co., 1946, page 649.

depletion of body proteins results in the rapid demise of the organism.

To conserve protein during an extended fast, most tissues in the body oxidize fat as their major energy source (Table 4–2). While the brain cannot use free fatty acids (which do not readily cross the blood-brain barrier) as an energy source, neuronal tissues adapt to use ketones, which rapidly enter the central nervous system, to provide the energy for proper function. The protein-sparing effects of ketosis are considerable. During the postabsorptive period, 2 grams of fat are used per gram of protein. Ketoadaptation results in the use of 7.5 grams of fat per gram of protein metabolized. Prior to ketoadaptation, 4.8 calories are derived from fat for every calorie derived from protein. Once the body has adapted to fat utilization, it derives 17 calories from fat for each calorie derived from protein. The overall effect is that during early starvation, about 75 gm of protein are used per day. After ketoadaptation this falls to about 20 gm per day. Therefore, ketoadaptation is essential to protein sparing during prolonged starvation.

Hormone-substrate Interaction During Prolonged Starvation. As a fast extends beyond the postabsorptive period, insulin concentrations decline below their postcibal levels; glucagon concentrations remain the same or increase slightly. The resulting lower insulin-glucagon ratio allows the effects of glucagon to become more manifest as the inhibitory effects of insulin on the glucagon-mediated responses become less pronounced. The changes in the liver, skeletal muscle, and adipose tissue evoked by these hormonal alterations are orchestrated to maximize energetic efficiency. Furthermore, as fasting continues the kidney begins to play an increasingly important role in glucose homeostasis. The hormonal influences on these tissues during a fast are such that skeletal muscle and adipose tissue supply the precursors that are subsequently used by the liver and the kidney to produce those compounds essential for energetic homeostasis. For the sake of clarity, the response of each of these tissues to hormonal stimuli will be discussed separately. However, all of these changes occur simultaneously and are integrated so that changes in one of these tissues will effect changes in the others. The changes seen as a whole will be a summation of these individual changes.

Table 4–2   BODY FUELS OXIDIZED DURING BRIEF FASTING*

DAY OF FAST	NITROGEN EXCRETION (%)	METABOLIC RATE (kcal)	FUEL METABOLIZED			PERCENTAGE OF TOTAL METABOLISM		
			Carbohydrate (gm)	Protein (gm)	Fat (gm)	Carbohydrate	Protein	Fat
1	7.1	1663	69	43	135	16.6	10.3	73.1
2	8.4	1646	42	50	142	10.2	12.2	77.6
3	11.3	1598	39	68	130	9.8	17.0	73.2
4	11.9	1524	4	71	136	1.0	18.7	80.3
5	10.4	1449	0	63	133	0	17.4	82.6
6	10.2	1441	0	61	133	0	16.9	83.1
7	9.8	1442	0	59	134	0	16.4	83.6

*Adapted from Peters, J. P., and Van Slyke, D. D.: Quantitative Clinical Chemistry. Vol. I. Interpretations. Edition 2. Baltimore, Williams & Wilkins Co., 1946, page 649.

The myocyte plays a very important role in maintaining glucose homeostasis.[11] In the presence of insulin, carrier-mediated glucose uptake by skeletal muscle is facilitated; growth hormone inhibits this process. The low serum insulin levels that accompany prolonged starvation, combined with the characteristic high levels of growth hormone during fasting, minimize glucose uptake by the myocyte. Alternatively, free fatty acid extraction by skeletal muscle is dependent primarily on concentration gradients. Consequently, the high serum levels of free fatty acids seen during fasting, combined with diminished glucose uptake, facilitates the use of fats as an energy source by the myocyte.

Skeletal muscle is also the primary source of the amino acid moieties utilized by the gluconeogenetic pathways for the production of glucose. Two important factors prevent the myocyte from directly providing glucose for utilization by the body as a whole. First, although skeletal muscle is the largest repository of glycogen in the body, the myocyte lacks the enzyme glucose-6-phosphatase. Without this enzyme, glucose-6-phosphate, which is the major product of glycogenolysis and which cannot traverse the cell membrane of the myocyte, cannot be converted to glucose. This effectively traps all of the glucose derived from glycogen inside the myocyte and forces the myocytes to use these energy stores for their own energetic needs. Additionally, skeletal muscle lacks the enzyme systems necessary for gluconeogenesis; despite the abundance of three-carbon precursors within the myocyte, they cannot be used to synthesize glucose.

Skeletal muscle plays two important roles in the body's fuel economy. Early in the fast, the hormonal milieu provides a strong stimulus for the oxidation of glucose derived from glycogen to lactate within the myocyte. The lactate is released into the circulation and subsequently is delivered to the liver, where it is converted into glucose via the Cori cycle (Fig. 4–2). The low insulin concentration, combined with falling blood amino acid levels, is a powerful stimulus for amino acid release by skeletal muscle. Following deamination in the liver, the amino acids provide the three-carbon skeletons used to produce glucose via gluconeogenesis. Finally, the utilization of ketone bodies produced by the liver facilitates conservation of skeletal muscle amino acids with more prolonged starvation. Thus, the hormone-substrate interactions in skeletal muscle during a prolonged fast encourage the myocyte to adapt to fat utilization, promote minimal usage of glucose, and enhance the release of precursors for the gluconeogenetic pathway in a carefully controlled fashion.

The primary role of adipose tissue during a fast is to provide molecules that serve as alternative fuel sources to glucose. The hormonal milieu of fasting, particularly the low insulin concentration, reverses the inhibition of lipoprotein lipase. Consequently, lipolysis is increased in the adipocyte. The free fatty acids produced by adipose tissue are then transported to the liver, skeletal muscle, and other tissues, which can use them as alternate energy sources. Importantly, the hepatocyte uses the energy resulting from the oxidation of free fatty acids to produce the energy-rich molecules essential for gluconeogenesis. Moreover, the glycerol remaining after triglyceride oxidation can be utilized by the liver as a precursor for glucose production. Additionally, the liver directs some of the free fatty acids to ketones, which provide alternate sources of energy for cerebral and other tissues that have undergone ketoadaptation. Thus, the overall effect of the hormonal milieu of fast-

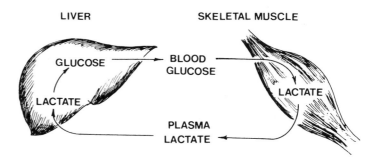

Figure 4–2. The Cori cycle. The liver utilizes lactate from skeletal muscle to produce glucose via gluconeogenesis.

LIVER SKELETAL MUSCLE

GLUCOSE → BLOOD GLUCOSE →

LACTATE

PLASMA LACTATE ←

CORI CYCLE

ing on lipid metabolism optimizes the availability of free fatty acids and other products of triglyceride oxidation to provide abundant non–glucose-derived energy for metabolic processes and thereby preserve protein stores.

The liver plays a central role as the modulator of most of the metabolic events during prolonged starvation. While skeletal muscle and adipose tissue provide the precursors for gluconeogenesis and the adipocyte provides free fatty acids as an alternate energy source, the liver coordinates the production of glucose and ketones.

The hyperglucagonemia of fasting decreases the concentration of malonyl CoA within the hepatocyte.[8] Lower levels of this substrate stimulate the oxidation of free fatty acids into acetoacetate and beta-hydroxybutyrate ("ketone bodies"). Ketones are critical to the adaptation to starvation. The reduction in glucose utilization resulting from the brain's conversion to ketones as a fuel source is highly significant and accounts for a large portion of the decrease in glucose demands during starvation. Moreover, ketones, either directly or indirectly, provide a signal to skeletal muscle to reduce amino acid release, thereby conserving protein stores.[3] Thus, the hormonal milieu responsible for the enhanced lipolysis within the adipocyte also favors the production of ketones within the liver. The result is optimal utilization of the abundant energy stores found in adipose tissue and concurrent conservation of protein mass.

The production of glucose by the hepatocyte during prolonged starvation is a finely coordinated effort between the liver and skeletal muscle involving the flux of carbon molecules for the synthesis of new glucose (Fig. 4–3). This process of gluconeogenesis within the liver is supported by energy derived from the oxidation of fat.

Although many amino acids may be used as the providers of three-carbon precursors for glucose, alanine appears to be the major gluconeogenic amino acid. Because alanine is released from skeletal muscle in quantities that exceed the amounts stored in these tissues, this amino acid is apparently produced within the myocyte. Alanine is released from the skeletal muscle and, following deamination to pyruvate within the liver, is converted to glucose. A portion of this newly produced glucose is initially oxidized to pyruvate in the myocyte. Subsequently, the pyruvate is converted to alanine by transamination, with the nitrogen moiety being provided by with the branched-chain amino acids leucine, valine, and isoleucine. Importantly, the oxidative deamination of alanine in the hepatocyte provides energy for gluconeogenesis. Thus, the alanine cycle (Fig. 4–4) is a convenient method for using muscle-derived calories from the oxidation of fat ketoacids for the resynthesis of glucose in the liver.

The Cori cycle (see Fig. 4–2) is another important pathway for producing glucose during starvation. Skeletal muscle (and other tissue such as red blood cells, the renal me-

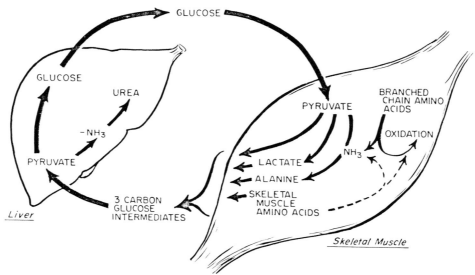

Figure 4–3. The elaboration of three-carbon precursors from skeletal muscle provides glucose precursors for hepatic gluconeogenesis during prolonged starvation.

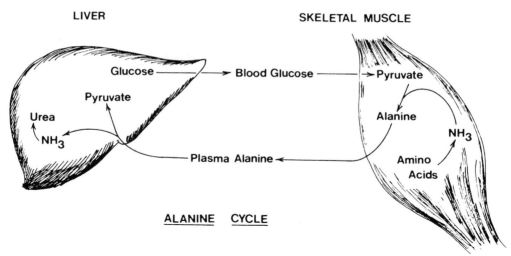

ALANINE CYCLE

Figure 4–4. The alanine cycle allows carbon chains and ammonia to be shuttled from skeletal muscle to the liver where they are used to synthesize glucose and urea, respectively.

dulla, and bone marrow) only partially oxidizes glucose to lactate and pyruvate during fasting. These intermediaries are released into the bloodstream and are subsequently reconverted into glucose in the liver. The conversion of lactate into glucose by the liver requires energy, which is derived from fat oxidation. The newly synthesized glucose is delivered to peripheral tissues, where it is used as an energy source. The net effect is that the energy derived from fat oxidation in the liver is shuttled to those tissues requiring glucose as an energy source. Thus,

the hormone-substrate interactions in the liver during fasting are such that the energy derived from fat oxidation is used to produce glucose, which can then be used by those tissues that cannot use fat as an energy source.

After 30 days of fasting, the kidney becomes an important glucose-producing organ, contributing almost one-half of the body's glucose requirements.[3] Most of the glucose synthesized by the kidney is derived from the glutamine cycle (Fig. 4–5). Glutamine, which is released by skeletal muscle,

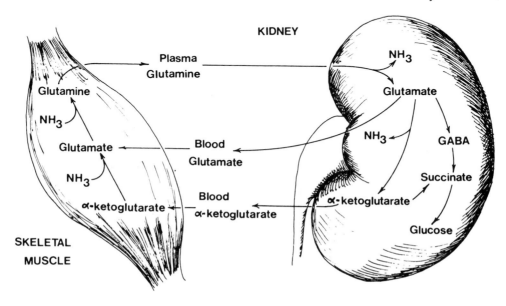

GLUTAMINE CYCLE

Figure 4–5. The glutamine cycle is a shuttle analogous to the alanine cycle which exists between skeletal muscle and the kidney. This cycle increases in importance as a fast extends beyond 30 days.

is cleaved to glutamate and ammonia within the renal parenchyma. The glutamate is deaminated to alpha-ketoglutarate, which becomes a part of the precursor pool for glucose production. Moreover, the ammonia produced in these reactions acts to neutralize the acidic by-products of metabolism by accepting hydrogen ions. This has important implications during starvation, when significant amounts of base are needed to neutralized the 10 mEq of ketoacids produced per day. Therefore, during starvation the kidney not only continues its usual role in maintaining body pH at normal levels and excreting waste products, but also becomes a major source of glucose production.

In summary, during prolonged starvation the body's hormonal milieu is characterized by high blood glucagon levels and low insulin concentrations as well as a fall in most substrate concentrations; ketones are an exception and are elevated. These alterations orchestrate changes within the liver, skeletal muscle, adipose tissue, and the kidney to maximize the probability of survival by optimizing nutrient delivery to essential organs (thus perpetuating important bodily processes) while minimizing protein losses by ketoadaptation and fat oxidation. The adaptation to fat utilization during fasting greatly reduces glucose requirements.

HORMONAL RESPONSE TO STRESS

The body's response to stress is markedly different from its response to prolonged starvation. Cuthbertson recognized two phases of the stress response: the "ebb" and "flow" phases.[12] The ebb phase is the period immediately following an injury and is characterized by cardiovascular instability, decreased peripheral perfusion, and hypometabolism. Although there is a general outpouring of hormones during this period, the ebb phase is usually accompanied by a transitory depression in the responsiveness of the target tissues to plasma hormonal concentrations. Successful resuscitation and restoration of perfusion mark the beginning of the flow phase of injury. This period is characterized by the return of tissue responsiveness to hormonal stimuli and an increase in metabolic reactions. The metabolic response to injury consists of hypermetabolism, a marked increase in glucose production, nitrogen-wasting secondary to persistent

amino acid mobilization from skeletal muscle, and a failure of ketoadaptation. These responses are mediated by complex hormonal changes elicited by the initiating stimulus (Fig. 4–6). The hormones with important metabolic implications following injury or infection include catecholamines, glucagon, insulin, glucocorticoids, and growth hormone.

Catecholamines. Catecholamines are the major mediators after significant stress. These compounds—epinephrine, which is elaborated in the adrenal medulla, and norepinephrine, found almost exclusively at sympathetic nerve endings—are synthesized from the amino acid phenylalanine and mediate a host of systemic responses following a variety of stimuli, including pain, anxiety, hypotension, hypoxia, infection, and injury. Catecholamines are essential in maintaining homeostasis following any stress. Cannon and his associates clearly demonstrated that a completely sympathectomized animal, confined to a well-controlled, warm, sheltered environment, could have a normal life span and could even reproduce.[13] However, the animal was particularly susceptible to any stressful stimulus, including hypoxia, hemorrhage, fluid restriction, and alterations in ambient temperature, and succumbed to changes that would not adversely affect an intact animal. From these experiments they concluded that catecholamine elaboration by the sympathetic nervous system following stress was essential for survival.

Early investigators also noted that although the response by any particular tissue to either epinephrine or norepinephrine was characteristic, the same tissue could react to epinephrine in a fashion that was the complete opposite of its reaction to norepinephrine. To explain these polar reactions to seemingly comparable stimuli, a dual receptor system was postulated for catecholamine responsiveness. This hypothesis was substantiated by the discovery of the epinephrine-mediated beta-adrenergic receptor and the norepinephrine-mediated alpha-adrenergic receptor. Furthermore, beta-adrenergic responses have been shown to use cyclic AMP (cAMP) as a second messenger and elicit responses by increasing intracellular concentrations of this nucleotide. However, alpha-adrenergic stimulation apparently lowers the intracellular concentration of cAMP. Thus, the divergent reactions by a single tissue to epinephrine and nor-

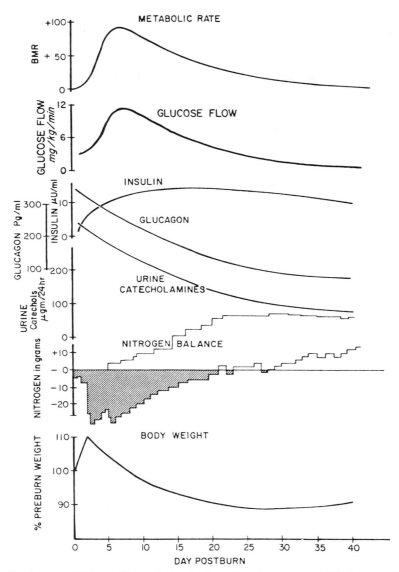

Figure 4–6. The hypermetabolism of injury during the flow phase is accompanied by increased glucose flow, negative nitrogen balance, and high levels of glucagon and catecholamines relative to insulin. The hormonal mediators return toward normal with recovery.

epinephrine could be readily explained by the difference in cellular responses to alpha-adrenergic and beta-adrenergic stimulation, although exceptions have more recently been noted to this general rule.

Catecholamines elicit numerous physiologic responses. Catecholamines maintain systemic blood pressure, control heart rate, and regulate organ perfusion. Their metabolic regulatory effects may be based in part on these activities. The adrenergic effects on metabolism are both primary and secondary. The primary effects include the direct metabolic actions of catecholamines on the liver, skeletal muscle, and adipose tissue. The secondary effects are elicited by the effects of epinephrine and norepinephrine on the pancreas, which influence the secretory activity of the alpha and beta cells, and by the effects of catecholamines on systemic perfusion.

Catecholamines stimulate gluconeogenesis and glycogenolysis within the liver, increasing the availability of glucose energy.[14] Concurrently, these hormones increase the size of the three-carbon precursor pool for glucose production by enhancing the release of lactate from skeletal muscle and by increasing free fatty acid mobilization through their actions on adipose tissue. The overall impact of the direct effects of catecholamines on these metabolically active tissues is to increase glucose production and enhance fat mobilization.

Glucagon and Insulin. The response of pancreatic beta cells to catecholamines depends on the nature of the stimulus: beta-adrenergic or alpha-adrenergic (Fig. 4–7).[15] Stimulation of the alpha-adrenergic receptors of the beta cell results in an inhibition of the release of insulin; beta-adrenergic stimulation enhances insulin secretion. This difference in response to alpha-adrenergic and beta-adrenergic stimuli is important because during the ebb phase of injury, alpha stimulation predominates and plasma insulin levels are decreased, even in the presence of hyperglycemia. During the flow phase, beta-adrenergic stimulation becomes dominant and insulin secretion normalizes or increases. Therefore, under the influence of the sympathetic discharge immediately following injury, insulin levels fall and glucose production rises, resulting in the characteristic hyperglycemia of trauma. Following resuscitation and as the patient enters the flow phase of injury, the glucose intolerance of the injured patient is not as readily explained because plasma insulin concentrations are normal or even elevated.[16] These findings suggest that there is a defect in target tissue responsiveness to insulin—that is, a peripheral tissue insensitivity to insulin. The exact nature of this defect has not been clearly elucidated but may explain the ab-

normal glucose tolerance curves noted in the injured patient during the flow phase.

The secretion of glucagon by the pancreatic alpha cell is not affected by alpha-adrenergic stimulation.[17] Beta-adrenergic stimulation, however, increases the elaboration of glucagon. Furthermore, the alpha cell production of glucagon appears to become insensitive to plasma glucose concentrations following injury. Therefore, glucagon concentrations are elevated during both phases of injury. Moreover, the abnormal elaboration of glucagon persists throughout hospitalization until recovery.

The alterations in pancreatic hormonal physiology elicited by the sympathetic nervous system have a profound effect on the insulin-glucagon ratio.[17] The increased glucagon levels and the normal or low insulin concentrations provide a lower insulin-glucagon ratio than normal. This change in the concentrations of insulin and glucagon is consistent with the increased production of glucose that follows stress. However, pancreatectomized animals appear to maintain a similar response, implying that the changes in glucagon and insulin secretion following injury occur in concert with other regulatory alterations.

Glucocorticoids. The plasma concentration of adrenocorticotropin (ACTH) is elevated following a variety of psychological and physiologic stresses.[18] This polypeptide is secreted by the hypothalamus and acts directly on the adrenal cortex to stimulate cortisol and corticosterone production and elaboration. Since the glucocorticoids have effects on metabolism, inflammation, and wound healing, the levels of ACTH play an impor-

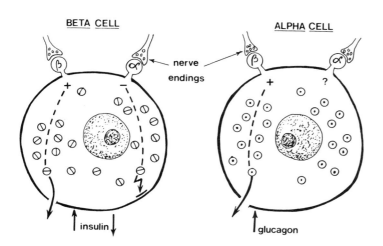

Figure 4–7. The response of pancreatic alpha and beta cells to catecholamines. Alpha-adrenergic stimulation inhibits insulin secretion while beta-adrenergic stimulation enhances insulin elaboration. Glucagon secretion is also increased by beta-adrenergic stimulation. Alpha-adrenergic stimulation apparently has no effect on alpha cell function.

tant role in the stress response. Moreover, ACTH has extra-adrenal metabolic effects including stimulating the release of free fatty acids, promoting insulin secretion, and reducing deamination of amino acids. However, the extra-adrenal effects of ACTH are overshadowed by the metabolic effects of the glucocorticoids.

The rise in ACTH, and consequently the rise in cortisol following an injury, is mediated by stimuli reaching the hypothalamus along efferent nervous tracts from impulses arising in the injured area. Hume and Egdahl demonstrated that a rise in cortisol levels was not elicited in an animal if the efferent nerves to the injured area were severed prior to the injury.[19] These studies helped to demonstrate the important role of the central nervous tissue in the acute response to trauma.

The metabolic effects of cortisol include stimulation of hepatic gluconeogenesis, mobilization of amino acids from skeletal muscle, and augmentation of alterations in fat metabolism. Cortisol stimulates hepatic gluconeogenic enzymes and thereby provides a direct signal to augment the hepatic production of glucose from three-carbon precursors. Cortisol is also essential for the mobilization of amino acids from skeletal muscle. Adrenalectomized animals, who are otherwise stable, cannot release amino acids from skeletal muscle. This defect can be corrected by the administration of cortisol. Moreover, while glucocorticoids promote amino acid release in the periphery, they enhance biosynthesis of protein by the liver. Thus, cortisol stimulates the movement of amino acids from the carcass to the viscera, where the substrate participates in the synthesis of new glucose or protein.

Growth Hormone. Human growth hormone is a major anabolic hormone. This polypeptide is elaborated by the pituitary and has its primary effect on those tissues and bodily functions that play important roles in growth. Growth hormone stimulates synthesis of collagen and bone matrix and influences the metabolism of calcium and phosphate.[20] Growth hormone also has direct effects on protein, carbohydrate, and fat metabolism. Under the influence of GH there is a generalized increase in intracellular transport of amino acids and ribosomal protein synthesis, resulting in an increase in lean body mass. Concurrently, growth hormone causes increased intracellular lipoly-

sis, stimulates a rise in plasma free fatty acids, and enhances the oxidation of fat.[20] Furthermore, growth hormone not only reduces the responsiveness of insulin to hyperglycemia, but also decreases the conversion of glucose to fat in adipose tissue. Growth hormone also inhibits the insulin-mediated facilitated uptake of glucose by skeletal muscle.

Following injury, plasma growth hormone is elevated even in the face of hyperglycemia.[18] This suggests increased stimulation of growth hormone, which overrides the glucose suppressive effects; these signals most probably arise from the hypothalamus. Exogenous growth hormone has been administered to injured patients, and many of the catabolic effects of injury could be reversed with the simultaneous administration of a high calorie–high nitrogen diet.[21]

In summary, the metabolic response to injury results in hypermetabolism, hyperglycemia, and glucose intolerance, the utilization of skeletal muscle amino acids as precursors for production of glucose and synthesis of hepatic protein, and a failure to ketoadapt. These changes explain the marked contrast between the metabolic adaptations to starvation and those following injury. What has not been clearly elucidated, however, is the afferent signal that elicits this response. Although the hormonal changes observed after an injury are well described and the nature of the alteration of target tissues to these changes is known, the precise signals that alter the hormonal and tissue responses constituting the stress response have not been determined.

REFERENCES

1. Hedeskov, C. J.: Mechanism of glucose-induced insulin secretion. Physiol. Rev., 60:442–509, 1980.
2. DeFronzo, R. A., Jacot, E., Jequier, E., Maeder, E., Wahren, J., and Felber, J. P.: The effect of insulin on the disposal of intravenous glucose: Results from indirect calorimetry and hepatic and femoral venous catheterization. Diabetes, 30:1000–1007, 1981.
3. Wilmore, D. W.: The Metabolic Management of the Critically Ill. New York Plenum Medical Book Company, 1977.
4. American College of Surgeons, Committee on Pre- and Postoperative Care. Ballinger, W. F., II, Collins, J. A., Drucker, W. R., Dudrick, S. J., and Zeppa, R. (eds.): Manual of Surgical Nutrition. Philadelphia, W. B. Saunders Company, 1975.
5. DeFronzo, R. A., Ferrannini, E., Hendler, R., Wahren, J., and Felig, P.: Influence of hyperinsuline-

mia, hyperglycemia, and the route of glucose administration on splanchnic glucose exchange. Proc. Natl. Acad. Sci., 75:5173–5177, 1978.

6. Felig, P., Wahren, J., and Hendler, R.: Influence of oral glucose ingestion on splanchnic glucose and gluconeogenic substrate metabolism in man. Diabetes, 24:468–475, 1975.

7. Lickley, H. L. A., Chisholm, D. J., Rabinovitch, A., Wexler, M., and Dupre, J.: Effects of portacaval anastomosis on glucose tolerance in the dog: Evidence of an interaction between the gut and the liver in oral glucose disposal. Metabolism, 24:1157–1168, 1975.

8. Unger, R. H., and Orci, L.: Glucagon and the A cell: Physiology and pathophysiology. N. Engl. J. Med., 304:1518–1524 and 1575–1580, 1981.

9. Unger, R. H.: Glucagon and the insulin:glucagon ratio in diabetes and other catabolic illnesses. Diabetes, 20:834, 1971.

10. Benedict, F. G.: A study of prolonged fasting. Washington, D.C., Carnegie Institute, Pub. No. 203, 1915.

11. Cahill, G. F., Jr.: Starvation in man. N. Engl. J. Med., 282:668–675, 1970.

12. Cuthbertson, D. P.: The metabolic response to injury and its nutritional implications: Retrospect and prospect. J.P.E.N., 3:108–129, 1979.

13. Cannon, W. B.: The Wisdom of the Body. New York, W. Norton, 1967.

14. Wilmore, D. W.: Carbohydrate metabolism in trauma. Clin. Endocrinol. Metab., 5:731–745, 1976.

15. Porte, D., Jr., and Robertson, R. P.: Control of insulin secretion by catecholamines, stress, and the sympathetic nervous system. Fed. Proc., 32:1792–1796, 1973.

16. Allison, S. P., Hinton, P., and Chamberlain, M. J.: Intravenous glucose tolerance, insulin, and free-fatty-acid levels in burned patients. Lancet, 2:1113–1116, 1968.

17. Iverson, J.: Adrenergic receptors and the secretion of glucagon and insulin from the isolated, perfused canine pancreas. J. Clin. Invest., 52:2102–2116, 1973.

18. Wilmore, D. W.: Hormonal responses and their effect on metabolism. Surg. Clin. North Am., 56:999–1018, 1976.

19. Hume, D. M., and Egdahl, R. H.: The importance of the brain in the endocrine response to injury. Ann. Surg., 150:697–712, 1959.

20. Daughaday, W. H., and Parker, M. L.: Human pituitary growth hormone. Ann. Rev. Med., 16:47–66, 1965.

21. Wilmore, D. W., Moylan, J. A., Jr., Briston, B. F., Mason, A. D., Jr., and Pruitt, B. A., Jr.: Anabolic effects of human growth hormone and high caloric feedings following thermal injury. Surg. Gynecol. Obstet., 138:875–884, 1974.

CHAPTER 5

Human Macronutrient Requirements

T. P. STEIN
G. M. LEVINE

Interest in human macronutrient requirements and nutrition has declined steadily since the last essential amino acid was discovered and vitamin requirements for humans were finally identified about 50 years ago. A low point was reached in about 1960. Since the qualitative human nutritional requirements were known, many believed that further investigation into the quantitative requirements would not reveal any new scientific principles. Furthermore, it appeared that the normal human diet was, in fact, rather good. The postwar economic boom and "cheap food" policies helped remove malnutrition from the view of the "man on the street" and his elected representatives.

Four events contributed to a revival of interest in human nutrition: (1) the introduction of parenteral nutrition, presenting the possibility of administering completely synthetic regimens parenterally, (2) the realization that malnutrition had not disappeared, as a sizable proportion of hospitalized patients were severely malnourished; (3) the suggestion, based on epidemiologic surveys, that certain chronic disease processes (such as atherosclerosis, cancer, and alcoholism) might have a nutritional component in their etiologies; (4) the steady accumulation of evidence that certain disease processes might have different therapeutic nutritional requirements—for example, the use of essential amino acids and ketoacids in the treatment of renal failure,[3, 4] and modified amino acid mixtures for patients in hepatic failure[5, 6]—and the suggestion that branched-chain and medium-chain triglycerides may be beneficial in sepsis.[7, 8]

Thus, human nutrition once again became an important part of the biomedical sciences. It is interesting to note that none of these advances was made by individuals whose primary training was in nutrition. Very little of the key information was actually published in the primary nutrition journals.

Our current state of knowledge allows us to recognize a good diet, but we do not know if there is such a thing as an optimal nutritional regimen, or even if this concept is valid. More and more evidence suggests that nutrition can be optimized; this may be of particular relevance to the metabolically compromised patient.

In this chapter, we shall briefly review the classic nutrition literature. To quote from another context, "Those who ignore the lessons of history are condemned to repeat it." Following this review, we shall discuss whether qualitative and quantitative macronutrient manipulation may be important in the future treatment of disease.

PROTEIN REQUIREMENTS

Human protein requirements were the subject of very intensive investigations from 1850 to about 1940. These studies were initially concerned with either documenting the quantities of food people purchased or monitoring the daily ad libitum intake records of healthy subjects. The underlying assumption was that an inner wisdom led healthy people to eat a diet matched to their

Supported by USPHS Grant No. 16658

73

requirements—that is, the body knows best. This does appear to be the case. Millions of years of evolution have led to an optimal selection and utilization of available foodstuffs.

The results of these studies tended to overestimate protein requirements, although the total energy consumption correlated well with energy demands. Presumably, the human appetite functions to limit intake when the caloric intake is excessive rather than when the protein intake is excessive—hence, the well-known feeling of satiety after a meal that is high in fats. There has been a consistent trend to reduce the human protein requirement, so that it is now about half of what was recommended in 1900.

More recently, attention has centered upon determining the lower limit for protein requirements and how these requirements relate to circumstances and the need for individual amino acids. Until very recently, the biomedical community had virtually no interest in whether these requirements differed in stress and disease states.

At present, we cannot predict individual protein needs from the wealth of in vitro biochemical knowledge available nor can we estimate amino acid needs in protein requirements from biochemical pathways. All currently available estimates of human nutritional requirements have been determined experimentally. The experimental technique typically used to determine protein requirements is the method of nitrogen balance. Although the nitrogen balance method has been much maligned, a superior method has yet to be found.

Balance studies are difficult to perform since it is necessary to monitor nitrogen intake and excretion for long periods of time. The nitrogen balance method is fraught with errors which all tend to overestimate nitrogen retention. Among these errors are the following: (1) underestimation of nitrogen excretion due to faulty or incomplete collection of all nitrogen loss from sweat, exhaled air, and so forth, and (2) incorrect measurements of intake by underestimating or overestimating the amount of food actually consumed. Furthermore, the greater the amount of nitrogen taken in, the greater the overestimate of nitrogen retention.

There is an excellent review of the early studies on human protein requirements by Irwin and Hegsted.[9] This review provides a fascinating history of how human nitrogen requirements were determined during the last century by citing over 400 references on the requirements of healthy adults, children, and lactating women, but no studies on stressed or diseased subjects.

It is highly probable that nutritional requirements of adults vary with age and state of health. In addition, biologic homogeneity cannot be assumed. Bessman has suggested that while everyone has the capacity to make the non-essential amino acids, the phenotypes and genotypes for doing so may differ among individuals.[10] Synthetic capacity may range over quite a large spectrum within a healthy population. Some individuals may barely meet their requirements for certain non-essential amino acids, while others will easily exceed them.

During stress and illness, the availability of certain non-essential amino acids may become rate-limiting for protein synthesis. This results from either increased demands or decreased amino acid synthetic capacity secondary to malnutrition. Examples of such borderline essential amino acids include histidine, which can become a true essential amino acid,[11] and arginine, as it is beneficial to add this "non-essential" amino acid to parenteral amino acid solutions.[12]

We do not know why some amino acids are essential and others are not. Neither do we know the true minimum daily requirements (MDR) of the essential amino acids. Teleologically, it can be argued that adequate amino acids were available from the diet; if mutations led to the inability to manufacture all the amino acids, it was of no consequence. Those amino acids that have important roles in intermediary metabolism, such as glutamate and aspartate, have high rates of synthesis in the body. Presumably an inadequate supply of their carbon skeletons could be lethal. In contrast, none of the carbon skeletons of the essential amino acids has quantitative (as opposed to qualitative) roles in processes other than protein synthesis.

Dietary essential amino acids replace those that are lost during metabolism. It would seem that they are lost in spite of extensive pathways for reclaiming amino acids derived from the breakdown of protein. About 80 per cent of the amino acid flux in the body is derived from protein breakdown, and the majority of these amino acids are salvaged for reincorporation into protein.[13, 14] There is a continuous demand for exogenous essential amino acids to replace those that are lost because amino acid recovery is not completely efficient. Possibly the reason for the inadvertent loss of essential amino acids is that a certain proportion of the amino acids "slips through" into the oxidative pathways instead of being salvaged for reincorporation into protein.[15] According to this argument, loss of amino acids is dependent on substrate levels and this seems to be borne out. As in starvation, protein flux is decreased and loss of nitrogen through the urine is correspondingly decreased to a minimum of 2 gm per day.[13, 16]

Thus, the MDR for an essential amino acid can be defined as the amount of that amino acid required for daily replacement of its oxidized fraction. The amount oxidized, however, depends on the protein flux, and we know only that the optimal protein flux (turnover) rate depends on nutritional status and pathophysiologic state.

A daily need for protein exists because labile or reserve proteins to fulfill the role of temporary amino acid storage depots are lacking. The body cannot store amino acids and apparently does not contain any protein whose sole function is to serve as a protein reservoir. However, under the conditions of a long-term imbalance between intake and need, proteins, such as those in muscle, are broken down to provide amino acids for proteins in tissues with higher biologic priorities. Muscle contains proteins whose function is generally not critical. Muscle is abundant in the body, and some can be spared to provide amino acids for higher priority proteins.

The two key factors in determining how protein requirements can be met are the quantity and quality of the protein source. A protein that is deficient in one or more of the essential amino acids is, by definition, of low quality. Protein synthesis requires a full complement of amino acids. If one is missing, new protein cannot be made because the metabolic pathway for protein synthesis allows no substitutions. A high-quality protein is one that has all of the amino acids in the proper proportions.

As a general rule, high-quality proteins are derived from animal sources such as albumin (egg or milk), meat, and fish. Thus, one has a choice of giving relatively small amounts of high-quality protein or large amounts of low-quality protein. In a hospitalized patient whose metabolic capacity may be compromised, the aim is to give high-quality proteins so as not to overburden the patient with metabolizing a large excess of unnecessary amino acids. Excess amino acids are toxic, and the body must maintain amino acid levels within very close limits.[17] All commercially available enteral formulations contain high-quality protein.

To the best of our knowledge, there has been no systematic attempt to establish a recommended daily allowance (RDA) for protein in hospitalized patients. Should protein RDAs be changed according to the patient's clinical status? Do certain disease states have different protein RDAs? We don't know. Currently, the general approach is to match enteral feedings to the patient's normal caloric intake and to assume that the high-quality protein it contains is sufficient. For these reasons we have appended the current RDAs for healthy Americans. What has not been shown is that the RDA for sick patients is the same as for healthy people. As previously stated, there is a suspicion that nutritional requirements may differ according to the disease state, and a start has been made in defining specific amino acid requirements in certain chronic disease states. Examples of specialized needs are discussed below.

Renal Failure. Probably the first widespread application of tailoring protein requirements to a specific disease was in patients with renal failure (creatinine clearance of less than 10 to 15 per cent of normal). Normal excretion of the end products of protein metabolism (such as urea, creatinine, and ammonia) is defective in renal failure. As a result, the consumption of protein leads to many of the symptoms and pathophysiologic changes found in uremia. However, the administration of a low-protein or no-protein diet to minimize uremia results in body-wasting.

Several therapeutic approaches have been designed to circumvent these problems. First, technology has provided us with relatively safe and efficient techniques for peritoneal and hemodialysis to remove nitrogenous wastes. Patients treated in this way are able to consume their normal dietary protein allowances. Second, several dietary regimens have been developed to specifically treat renal failure. Low-protein diets of high biologic quality have proved to be efficacious in controlling uremia and maintaining nitrogen balance.[18] These diets can delay the start of dialysis or allow less frequent dialysis in patients with renal failure.

The enteral and parenteral administration of essential amino acids has also been advocated in the treatment of acute and chronic renal failure.[19] This technique is based on the finding that uremic patients can achieve positive nitrogen balance when given essential amino acids. This allows them to use their own body nitrogen, which is contained in non-essential amino acids, for protein synthesis.[20] These essential amino acids allow for administration of a relatively low nitrogen intake and facilitate management of uremia while meeting the protein RDA. Another promising technique involves the administration of the alpha-ketoacid analogues of the essential amino acids (except for lysine and threonine, which must be administered intact).[5] Since the enzymatic machinery for transamination of the alpha-ketoacid analogues exists, patients with renal failure can transfer ammonia back into protein and thereby decrease its toxic accumulation. In most cases, dietary manipulation combined with dialysis is effective in maintaining protein synthesis.

Branched-Chain Amino Acids. During periods of inadequate caloric intake, extensive catabolism of muscle protein for gluconeogenesis occurs. This metabolic alteration is especially pronounced in patients suffering from trauma or sepsis or who are undergoing other metabolic stresses. In vitro biochemical studies by Buse,[21] Goldberg,[22] and their collaborators in the 1970s indicated that muscle was the site of oxidation for the branched-chain amino acids and that oxidation of these amino acids by muscle was a potential energy source for muscle. From these observations, others suggested that in highly stressed patients, particularly those who are septic or are victims of trauma, the oxidation of the branched-chain amino acids by muscle might be disproportionately increased with disastrous consequences to the body as the whole.[23, 24] If this disproportionate increase occurs, the body must then dispose of the other amino acids, since an incomplete mixture of amino acids is useless for protein synthesis. The residual amino acids can be disposed of only by transamination and deamination-oxidation. Their nitrogen shows up as an increased loss of nitrogen in the urine, and the carbon skeletons are either oxidized directly by entry into the Krebs cycle or are transformed to glucose by means of gluconeogenesis. The excess amino acids "push" glucose synthesis, and since gluconeogenesis is partially dependent on the level of substrate, regulation is less responsive to hormonal factors than to normal gluconeogenesis.

Thus, it has been advocated as advantageous to give supplementary branched-chain amino acids to post-trauma or septic patients to compensate for those amino acids lost by oxidation in the muscles. Supplemental branched-chain amino acids provide a full complement of amino acids for protein synthesis and permit protein synthesis to proceed at an optimal rate to respond to the stressful insult. Furthermore, correcting the imbalance would eliminate the need to dispose of the other excess amino acids.

The removal of the other excess amino acids is an important point because amino acids are toxic if allowed to accumulate. It seems that the liver's capacity to metabolize some of them, particularly the aromatic amino acids, is limited, especially in malnourished patients and in patients with hepatic insufficiency.[24, 25]

Branched-chain amino acids have been shown to have a beneficial effect on anabolism after trauma and in septic states in animals, and to improve nitrogen retention.[23, 24] Improvements are not substantial, however, and in spite of many extensive studies, there have been no claims of improved survival or shorter recovery periods as a result of supplementation with branched-chain amino acids. At present, enteral diets using branched-chain amino acids are not widely available. One of the major drawbacks is the cost of the branched-chain amino acids. However, all of this may change if current research is able to demonstrate conclusively that there is a distinct clinical, as opposed to a biochemical, benefit in giving supplemental branched-chain amino acids.

Hepatic Failure. The liver is the principal catabolic site for many amino acids and is the only organ capable of a significant degree of ureapoiesis. Several alterations in protein metabolism occur in diseases in which hepatic function is seriously impaired, such as fulminant hepatitis, cirrhosis, and portal hypertension. First, there is decreased synthesis of urea and a concomitant increase in the plasma ammonia concentration. Second, there is a change in the normal plasma amino acid profile, resulting in an increased concentration of the aromatic amino acids compared with branched-chain amino acids.[5, 6] Third, there is decreased catabolism of various amino acid degradation products, produced both endogenously and by enteric bacteria, with the accumulation of substances such as mercaptans, short-chain fatty acids, ammonia, and "false" neurotransmitters.[6]

A change also occurs in the permeability of the blood-brain barrier, which allows many of these substances to enter the nervous system, producing the characteristic changes in mentation and movement. It has been argued that these false neurotransmitters enter the nervous system and then compete with the physiologic neurotransmitters, thereby contributing to the clinical picture of hepatic encephalopathy.

For these reasons, it has been suggested that the use of a diet high in branched-chain amino acids and low in aromatic amino acids may be beneficial in the nutritional support of patients with liver disease.[6, 25] Two such enteral formulations (Hepaticaid and Travicaid) are now available in the United States. In several studies this formulation has been shown to allow positive nitrogen balance despite low overall intake of protein in patients with liver disease. However, this formulation is very expensive and whether it provides prolonged survival for patients with severe liver disease is as yet unknown.

The Elderly Patient. The elderly comprise another group of patients who may have different nutritional requirements. Nutritional studies in the elderly have not been a popular subject of investigation, although the elderly constitute a high proportion of the typical hospital population and frequently require enteral nutrition. The problem in studying ill elderly subjects is that most of them are not "normal" (or they would not be in the hospital) and suffer from a variety of other infirmities that may or may not affect nutritional requirements. If healthy elderly subjects are chosen for study, then they too may not be representative of the elderly population; they could be regarded as being physiologically younger and therefore atypical of elderly people in general. In fact, it has been suggested that one of the differences between the elderly person and the young person is the ability to

respond to stress and mobilize the enzymes necessary for a response. A recent report by Gersovitz et al.[26] suggests that the essential amino acid requirements of the elderly are higher than for young people, but their data are not conclusive. It would, however, seem quite plausible that the RDA for the healthy elderly and the hospitalized elderly may be very different from the RDA of healthy young and middle-aged adults. This subject is worthy of serious investigation particularly in view of the fact that the population of the United States is aging and the elderly comprise the bulk of the hospital population.

ENERGY SOURCES

All body processes require energy, but it is hard to give a precise definition of such a nebulous quantity as the total body energy requirement. Energy expenditure depends very much on circumstance. For example, activity or stress increases energy usage. It is difficult, therefore, to define which functions are necessary and should be included as part of the minimum daily energy requirement and which functions are unnecessary. Two extremes will illustrate this. Clearly, ion pumping for maintenance of intracellular homeostasis to prevent build-up of sodium or leakage of potassium is a critical process and there must be enough energy available to perform this in all viable cells. In contrast, if too much energy is given, then the excess energy is deposited as fat. The conversion of either glucose or fat to lipid deposits is a normal metabolic process requiring energy, but it is hard to argue that this is a critical function.

Two criteria have been accepted as defining the minimal daily energy requirement. The basal metabolic rate (BMR) is a measurement of the amount of oxygen needed and the carbon dioxide produced to provide the body with energy. The body literally obtains energy by burning glucose or other energy substrates in a sequence of chemical reactions designed to release the energy slower than simple combustion would. In the laboratory, the normal combustion of carbohydrate or fat will release energy at a rate that is uncontrolled and very fast. In the body, the process is slow and tightly controlled; the energy is released in a systematic fashion. The other method of determining the body's energy requirement is to define it as that amount of energy necessary to satisfy the body's energy needs before futile cycling. *Futile cycle* is a term that has been applied to the maintenance of metabolic pathways that break down and then resynthesize fuels to allow the body to adapt more quickly to changing metabolic requirements. The body converts food energy to work energy at an efficiency of about 60 per cent.

The unit of energy measurement is the kilocalorie (kcal) or joule (J). A kilocalorie is 1000 calories, one calorie being the amount of heat required to raise the temperature of 1 gm of water 1°C, from 14.5°C to 15.5°. Coming into use, and likely to become more popular with time, is the joule, named after one of the early pioneers of thermodynamics, J.P. Joule, who discovered the first law of thermodynamics in the 1840s. The joule is the SI (Système Internationale, or metric) unit of energy and is equivalent to 4.18 kcal.

BASAL METABOLISM

The BMR is the sum of the energy expenditure of the body at rest—that is, lying down, not doing physical work, and physiologically unstressed. Basically, it is the sum of all of the energy activities involved in the maintenance of life processes. The nervous system and brain alone account for one fifth of the basal energy expenditure, ion pumping for another 20 per cent, and other active organs, such as the liver, kidneys and heart, for much of the rest. The BMR of adults ranges from 1200 to 1800 kcal/day; values are fairly constant for any given individual. The main factors determining the BMR are body size, age, and sex. The BMR is higher in the young, but as with many other determinations of bodily functions in humans, it has not been possible to account for individual variations in the BMR, despite extensive study.

For these reasons, the RDA for energy (like that for protein) is an overestimation; they are both designed to encompass virtually the entire population and are meant to be applied in circumstances in which it is not feasible or worthwhile to determine each patient's BMR.

Even when measurement of BMR is available, it is our opinion that it is not worthwhile if the appetite mechanism is

Table 5–1 ENERGY COST OF ACTIVITIES IN RELATION TO RESTING METABOLIC RATE*

ENERGY COST ACTIVITY RATE ÷ RMR	ACTIVITY
	Resting
0.9–1.0	Sleeping, nightly average
1.0	Lying at ease, 3 to 4 hours after a meal
	Very Light Work
1.2	Sitting at ease, listening to music, reading, hand sewing, knitting
1.4	Sitting and writing, doing office desk work
1.7	Sitting, typing using electric typewriter or using desk calculator; standing and moving around an office
	Playing cards; playing woodwind instruments
1.9	Doing lower range of domestic and light industrial work
2.1	Sitting and eating; general laboratory work
	Light Work
2.3	Doing lower range of work in transportation, building trades, and mechanized agriculture; playing piano or stringed instrument; playing billiards
2.5	Doing upper range of light industrial work; horse riding at a walk
2.7	Walking 2.0 mph (3.2 km/hr) on the level
2.9	Walking 2.0 mph (3.2 km/hr) on the level, with 22 lb (10 kg) load; walking 2.5 mph (4.0 km/hr) on the level; personal care (e.g., dressing, bathing)
3.1	Playing volleyball
	Moderate Work
3.5	Walking 3.1 mph (5.0 km/hr) on the level, usual pace
3.7	Walking 3.1 mph (5.0 km/hr) on the level, with 22 lb (10 kg) load; cutting wood with power saw
4.0	Cycling at 5.5 mph (8.8 km/hr); playing with children; table tennis
4.5	Painting outside, plastering; swimming leisurely, golf, archery
5.0	Walking 2.0 mph (3.2 km/hr) up a 10% grade; dancing a waltz
6.0–6.5	Climbing stairs (70 to 80 kg person); shoveling, 18 lb (8 kg) load through 3.28 ft (1 m) ten times per minute; playing tennis; skiing downhill and using towbar uphill; cycling 10 mph (16 km/hr), usual pace
6.5–7.0	Walking 2 mph (3.2 km/hr) up a 20% grade
	Heavy Work
7.0–7.5	Digging pit in soil; weight lifting; swimming leisurely underwater wearing fins and suit

Table 5–1 *Continued*

ENERGY COST ACTIVITY RATE ÷ RMR	ACTIVITY
7.5–8.0	Doing upper range of manual work in peasant agriculture, in building, mining and steel industries; playing hockey, basketball, football
8.0–9.0	Chopping with axe, 1.25 kg head, blows/min; skiing on the level over hard snow 3.7 mph (6.0 km/hr); dancing actively, country or folk style
9.0–10.0	Cross-country running; climbing, light load and slope; swimming strenuously; boxing
10.0–15.0	Climbing, heavy load and slope; heaviest occupational work; playing football and squash
Over 15.0	Walking in loose snow with a heavy pack; skiing uphill at maximum speed; playing squash

*From Briggs, G. M., and Calloway, D. H.: Bogert's Nutrition and Physical Fitness. Edition 10. Philadelphia, W. B. Saunders Co., 1979.

functioning. The body is able to tolerate a very wide range of energy intake, manyfold in excess of the BMR without any untoward side effects, provided that energy is given enterally and not parenterally. With parenteral nutrition, the moderating effect of the gastrointestinal tract and liver is no longer present, and the effect is reduced tolerance to excessive nutritional input. Measurement of the BMR is a time-consuming, cumbersome process and is inconvenient to the patient, even if one of the newer metabolic carts is used. Furthermore, it is possible to estimate energy requirements from a patient's height, weight, and age by using an equation.

The Harris-Benedict equation and other similar equations are quite adequate for calculating clinical requirements:

$$REE \text{ for males} = 66.4230 + 13.7516W + 5.0033H - 6.7750A$$
$$REE \text{ for females} = 655.0955 + 9.6534W + 1.8496H - 4.6756A$$

where A is age in years, H is height in centimeters, W is weight in kilograms, and REE is resting energy expenditure per day.

The resting metabolism of a man of average build and weight is 1.05 kcal/kg/hour; for a typical woman it is 0.97 kcal/kg/hour. From these data, it is easy to calculate the resting energy metabolic rate. Over the last 50 or 60 years, numerous efforts have been made to determine the factors necessary to convert these basal values into values for individuals who are under stress or are active (Table 5–1).[28] In older age groups, the rate of resting metabolism has to be adjusted downward by 2 to 3 per cent per decade over age 40 (Fig. 5–1). Figures 5–2 and 5–3,

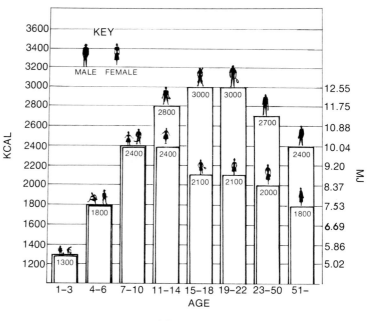

Figure 5–1. Effect of age and sex on energy needs of healthy subjects. (*From* Briggs, G. M., and Calloway, D. H.: Bogert's Nutrition and Physical Fitness. Edition 10. Philadelphia, W. B. Saunders Company, 1979, with permission.)

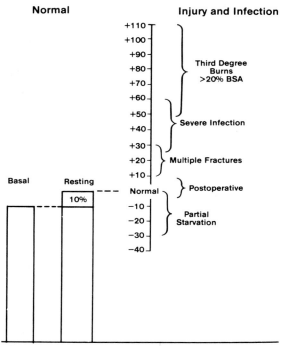

Figure 5–2. Effects of injury, sepsis, and nutritional depletion on resting energy expenditure. (*From* Kinney, J. M.: The application of indirect calorimetry to clinical studies. *In* Kinney, J. M. (ed.): Assessment of Energy Metabolism in Health and Disease. Columbus, Ohio, Ross Laboratories, 1980, with permission.)

respectively, show how the resting energy metabolic rate is increased with severity of disease for a sick or injured individual and how it changes with the clinical course. The important point about these tables and figures is that they are clinically useful. Their use provides sufficient latitude so that it is unnecessary to determine the resting energy metabolic rate of any patient receiving enteral nutrition.

Notice that the disease-related elevations are deceptively modest when compared with the activity requirements of healthy people (see Fig. 5–2 and Table 5–1). But the rate of the sick is considerable because people who engage in physical activity have frequent rest periods. In contrast, a metabolically stressed patient is continuously subjected to an increased resting energy metabolic rate. There are no rest periods from illness.

RECOMMENDED ALLOWANCES VERSUS ACTUAL NEEDS

There are many different compilations of human energy requirements. Most major countries have their own as well as that of the Food and Agriculture Organization of the World Health Organization of the United Nations. Because the United Nations is more concerned with minimal values compatible with survival in third-world countries, their estimates usually are much lower

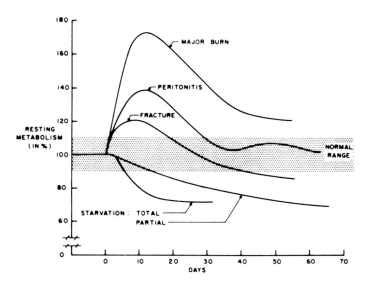

Figure 5–3. Changes in resting metabolic expenditure with time in six patient groups. (*From* Long, C. L., Schaffel, N., Geiger, J. W., et al.: Metabolic response to injury and illness: Estimation of energy and protein needs from indirect calorimetry and nitrogen balance. J.P.E.N., *3*:452–456, 1979; with permission.)

than those from developed countries. Thus the values compiled by the Food and Agriculture Organization are probably not relevant to a clinical setting.

The energy allowance set by various national and international committees are estimates intended for general use and are based on the energy needs of so-called average men and women living and working in that particular environment. For individuals who vary greatly from this norm it may be necessary to measure the BMR directly to achieve accuracy. However, the recommended allowances are above the norm, so energy is usually not a limiting factor. It is therefore not necessary to measure the energy requirements of each patient.

Even a relatively small excess of energy intake over a period of many years will lead to a steady gain in weight. This is particularly relevant in patients receiving tube feedings. Normal humans regulate their intake very precisely to maintain body weight at a constant level over a long period. These regulatory mechanisms are bypassed with tube feeding. Therefore, the possibility of overfeeding is great. If tube feeding is done for only a limited period (two to six weeks), the

net weight gain is not likely to be large and the individual will readjust to his normal weight and metabolic pattern after tube feeding. If, however, because of their other metabolic functions, particularly with regard to lipogenesis and lipid deposition in blood vessels, it may be necessary to monitor the proportion of calories derived from the three major classes of energy nutrients—that is, from carbohydrates, fats, and proteins.

Generally speaking, protein is the least desirable energy source because amino acids are needed for protein synthesis. Protein is the most expensive of the macronutrients and excess amino acids can be toxic. It is currently believed that the percentage of fat in the normal diet of Americans (40 to 45 per cent) is too high and should be reduced by 25 to 35 per cent. Therefore, it would seem that the optimal carbohydrate-to-fat ratio is probably 75 to 25.

Physicians, however, are rarely concerned with the nutritional status or nutrient requirements of normal individuals. Instead, their concern is with using normal nutritional requirements as a basis from which to predict the requirements for the sick or injured patient. With the exception of malnu-

Table 5–2   MEAN HEIGHTS, WEIGHTS, AND RECOMMENDED ENERGY INTAKES*

	AGE (yr)	WEIGHT		HEIGHT		ENERGY NEEDS		
		(kg)	(lb)	(cm)	(in)	(kcal)	(range, kcal)	(MJ)
Infants	0.0–0.5	6	13	60	24	kg × 115	(95–145)	kg × 0.48
	0.5–1.0	9	20	71	28	kg × 105	(80–135)	kg × 0.44
Children	1–3	13	29	90	35	1300	(900–1800)	5.5
	4–6	20	44	112	44	1700	(1300–2300)	7.1
	7–10	28	62	132	52	2400	(1650–3300)	10.1
Males	11–14	45	99	157	62	2700	(2000–3700)	11.3
	15–18	66	145	176	69	2800	(2100–3900)	11.8
	19–22	70	154	177	70	2900	(2500–3300)	12.2
	23–50	70	154	178	70	2700	(2300–3100)	11.3
	51–75	70	154	178	70	2400	(2000–2800)	10.1
	76+	70	154	178	70	2050	(1650–2450)	8.6
Females	11–14	46	101	157	62	2200	(1500–3000)	9.2
	15–18	55	120	163	64	2100	(1200–3000)	8.8
	19–22	55	120	163	64	2100	(1700–2500)	8.8
	23–50	55	120	163	64	2000	(1600–2400)	8.4
	51–75	55	120	163	64	1800	(1400–2200)	7.6
	76+	55	120	163	64	1600	(1200–2000)	6.7
Pregnancy						+300		
Lactation						+500		

*From Dietary Allowances Committee and Food and Nutrition Board: Recommended Dietary Allowances. Edition 9. Washington, D.C., National Academy of Sciences Press, 1980.

Table 5–3 MEAN HEIGHTS, WEIGHTS, AND RECOMMENDED INTAKE OF "HIGH-QUALITY" PROTEIN*

	AGE (yr)	WEIGHT (kg)	WEIGHT (lb)	HEIGHT (cm)	HEIGHT (in)	PROTEIN INTAKE (gm)
Infants	0.0–0.5	6	13	60	24	kg × 2.2
	0.5–1.0	9	20	71	28	kg × 2.0
Children	1–3	13	29	90	35	23
	4–6	20	44	112	44	30
	7–10	28	62	132	52	34
Males	11–14	45	99	157	62	45
	15–18	66	145	176	69	56
	19–22	70	154	177	70	56
	23–50	70	154	178	70	56
	51 +	70	154	178	70	56
Females	11–14	46	101	157	62	46
	15–18	55	120	163	64	46
	19–22	55	120	163	64	44
	23–50	55	120	163	64	44
	51 +	55	120	163	64	44
Pregnant						+30
Lactating						+20

*From Dietary Allowances Committee and Food and Nutrition Board: Recommended Dietary Allowances. Edition 9. Washington, D.C., National Academy of Sciences Press, 1980.

trition, which has been extensively studied, nutritional requirements in disease have been barely examined. An unanswered question is whether macronutrient requirements in disease and stress states are different.

CONCLUSION

One hundred years of research into the nutritional requirements of normal humans has enabled us to define the nutrient requirements of the healthy so well that totally chemically defined regimens are now commonplace. A relatively untouched area is the nutritional requirements of the ill and injured. Knowledge is still fragmentary, although there is evidence suggesting that nutritional requirements in various disease states are different. In recent years, amino acid formulations, such as those for renal failure and hepatic insufficiency, have been developed. It seems likely that the trend of tailoring specific nutrient formulations will be pursued in the future. For the present, the most recent edition of the RDA (Tables 5–2 and 5–3) and the proportionality factors for disease and stress states (Figs. 5–2 and 5–3) are the best available data.

REFERENCES

1. Dudrick, S. J., Wilmore, D. W., Vars, A. H., and Rhoads, J. E.: Long-term total parenteral nutrition with growth, development and positive nitrogen balance. Surgery, 64:134–142, 1968.
2. Bistrian, B. R., Blackburn, G. L., Vitale, J., Cochran, D., and Naylor, J.: Prevalence of malnutrition in general medical patients. J.A.M.A., 235:1567–1570, 1976.
3. Walser, M., Coulter, A. W., Dighe, S., and Crantz, F. R.: The effect of keto-analogues of essential amino acids in severe chronic uremia. J. Clin. Invest., 52:678–690, 1973.
4. Cahill, G. F., Jr.: Nitrogen versatility in bats, bears and man. N. Engl. J. Med., 290:686–687, 1974.
5. Herlong, H.F., Maddrey, W. C., and Walser, M.: The use of ornithine salts of branched-chain ketoacids in portal-systemic encephalopathy. Ann. Intern. Med., 93:545–550, 1980.
6. Fischer, J. F.: The etiology of hepatic encephalopathy—Nutritional implications. Acta Chir. Scand. [Suppl.], 507:50–68, 1981.
7. Border, J. R., Chenier, R., McMenamy, R. H., LaDuca, J., Seibel, R., Birkhahn, R., and Yu, L.: Multiple systems organ failure: Muscle fuel deficit with visceral protein malnutrition. Surg. Clin. North Am., 56:1147–1167, 1976.
8. Birkhahn, R. H., Long, C. L., and Blakemore, W. S.: New synthetic substrates for parenteral feeding. J.P.E.N., 3:346–349, 1979.
9. Irwin, M. I., and Hegsted, D. M.: A conspectus of research on protein requirements of man. J. Nutr., 101:385–429, 1971.
10. Bessman, S.: The justification theory: The essential nature of the nonessential amino acids. Nutr. Rev., 37:209–220, 1979.

11. Kopple, J. D., and Swendseid, M. E.: Evidence that histidine is an essential amino acid in normal and chronically uremic men. J. Clin. Invest., 55:881–891, 1975.
12. Seifter, E., Rettura, G., Barbul, A., and Levenson, S. M.: Arginine: An essential amino acid for injured rats. Surgery, 84:224–230, 1978.
13. Cahill, G. F., Jr.: Starvation in man. N. Engl. J. Med., 282:668–675, 1970.
14. Waterlow, J. C., and Stephen, J. M. L.: Adaptation of the rat to a low-protein diet: The effect of a reduced protein intake on the pattern of incorporation of L-^{14}C-lysine. Br. J. Nutr., 20:461–484, 1966.
15. Flatt, J. P., and Blackburn, G. L.: The metabolic fuel regulatory system: Implications for protein-sparing therapies during caloric deprivation and disease. Am. J. Clin. Nutr., 27:175–187, 1974.
16. Cahill, G. F., Jr.: Ketosis. J.P.E.N., 5:281–287, 1981.
17. Owen, O. E., Reichard, G. A., Boden, G., Patel, M. S., and Trapp, V. E.: Inter-relationships among key tissues in the utilization of metabolic substrates. In Katzen, H. M., and Mahler, R. J. (eds.): Diabetes, Obesity, and Vascular Disease: Metabolic and Molecular Interrelationships. Part 2. (Advances of Modern Nutrition Volume 2, Part 2). Washington, D.C., Hemisphere Publishing, 1978, pages 517–550.
18. Giovanetti, S., and Maggiore, O.: A low-nitrogen diet with protein of high biologic value for severe chronic uraemia. Lancet, 1:1000–1003, 1964.
19. Furst, P., Ahlberg, M., Alverstrand, A., and Bergstrom, J.: Principles of essential amino acid therapy in uremia. Am. J. Clin. Nutr., 31:1744–1755, 1978.
20. Giordano, C.: Use of exogenous and endogenous urea for protein synthesis in normal and uremic subjects. J. Lab. Clin. Med., 62:231–246, 1963.
21. Buse, M. G., and Reid, S.: Leucine: A possible regulator of protein turnover in muscle. J. Clin. Invest., 56:1250–1261, 1975.
22. Fulks, R. M., Li, J. B., and Goldberg, A. L.: Effects of insulin, glucose and amino acids on protein turnover in rat diaphragm. J. Biol. Chem., 250:290–298, 1975.
23. Blackburn, G. L., Moldawer, L. L., Usui, S., Bothe, A. Jr., O'Keefe, S. J. D., and Bistrian, B. R.: Branched chain amino acid administration and metabolism during starvation, injury and infection. Surgery, 86:307–315, 1979.
24. Freund, H., Yoshimura, N., Lunetta, L., and Fischer, J. E.: The role of the branched-chain amino acids in decreasing muscle catabolism in vivo. Surgery, 83:611–618, 1978.
25. Freund, H. R., Ryan, J. A., and Fischer, J. E.: Amino acid derrangements in patients with sepsis: Treatment with branched chain amino acid rich infusions. Ann. Surg., 188:423–430, 1978.
26. Gersovitz, M., Motil, K., Munro, H. N., Scrimshaw, N. S., and Young, V. R.: Human protein requirements: Assessment of the adequacy of the current Recommended Daily Allowance for dietary protein in elderly men and women. Am. J. Clin. Nutr., 35:6–14, 1982.
27. Briggs, G. M., and Calloway, D. H.: Bogert's Nutrition and Physical Fitness. Edition 10. Philadelphia, W. B. Saunders Company, 1979.
28. Waterlow, J. C., Garlick, P. J., and Millward, D. J.: Protein Turnover in Mammalian Tissues and the Whole Body. Amsterdam, Elsevier North Holland, 1978.

SUGGESTED READINGS

1. Dietary Allowances Committee and Food and Nutrition Board: Recommended Dietary Allowances. Edition 9. Washington, D.C., National Academy of Sciences Press, 1980.
2. Davidson, S., Passmore, R., Brock, J. E., and Truswell, A. S.: Human Nutrition and Dietetics. Edition 6. Edinburgh and New York, Churchill Livingstone, 1975.
3. Burton, B. T.: Human Nutrition. Edition 3. New York, McGraw-Hill Book Company, 1975.
4. Irwin, M. I.: Nutritional Requirements of Man: A Conspectus of Research. New York, The Nutrition Foundation, Inc., 1980.
5. Waterlow, J. C., and Stephen, J. M. L. (eds.): Nitrogen Metabolism in Man. London, Applied Science Publishers, 1981.

CHAPTER 6

Micronutrients and Enteral Nutrition

MICHAEL D. CALDWELL
CHRISTINE KENNEDY-CALDWELL

Animals fed diets containing only carbohydrate, protein, and fat cannot survive. Vitamins and certain minerals must be included to sustain life. Malnutrition has been defined as a pathologic state resulting either from a relative or an absolute deficiency or from an excess of one or more essential nutrients. This state is clinically manifested or detected by biochemical, anthropometric, topographic, or physiologic tests. Jelliffe[1] distinguishes the following four forms:

1. *Undernutrition.* The pathologic state resulting from the consumption of an inadequate quantity of food over an extended period of time. "Marasmus" and "inanition" are terms synonymous with severe undernutrition. Starvation is the long-term deprivation of food and thus the development of severe undernutrition, marasmus, or inanition.
2. *Specific Deficiency.* The pathologic state resulting from a relative or an absolute lack of an individual nutrient.
3. *Overnutrition.* The pathologic state resulting from the consumption of an excessive quantity of food and hence a caloric excess over an extended period of time.
4. *Imbalance.* The pathologic state resulting from a disproportion among essential nutrients, with or without absolute deficiency of any nutrient as determined by the requirements of a balanced diet.

The development of undernutrition requires the following sequence of events: inadequate ingestion, decreased corporeal reserves, impaired function, and anatomic lesions.

In a normal adult who maintains constant body weight, nutritional requirements are related to daily activity determined by a basal state, plus those demands created by activity, digestion, and accommodation to the nutrient environment. In the ill individual there is a reduction in physical activity, digestion, and environmental stress. However, disease, surgery, and medication frequently combine to produce inadequate ingestion, accentuate loss of corporeal reserves, and abet impaired organ function, with the resultant development of undernutrition or specific deficiency states.

NUTRIENT REQUIREMENTS

The recommended dietary allowances (RDA) are the levels of intake of essential nutrients considered, in the judgment of the Food and Nutrition Board and on the basis of available scientific knowledge, to be adequate to meet the known nutritional needs of practically all healthy persons. It is particularly important to note the following:

1. Because the human requirements for many nutrients have not been established and the essentiality of several nutrients has only recently been established, it is generally suggested that the RDA should be provided from as varied a selection of foods as practical to guarantee that possibly unrecognized nutritional needs are met.
2. The RDA are recommendations for the amounts of nutrients that should be consumed daily; they do not take into consideration losses of nutrients that occur during processing and preparation of foods.
3. The RDA should not be confused with requirements because the RDA (except for energy) are estimated to exceed the requirements of most individuals, thereby guaranteeing that the needs of nearly all individuals are met.
4. The RDA do not cover therapeutic nutritional needs, as they are intakes that meet the needs of healthy people only. As such, they may not meet requirements as affected by disease or pharmaceutical preparations.

5. The RDA are expressed by age, weight, and sex.

The problems encountered in using the RDA to determine nutrient intake include the lack of sufficient data in humans regarding nutrient requirements, the difficulty in assessing when the requirement has been met, and the difficulty in assessing absorption and processing in vivo and how these functions are affected by other nutrients. The attempted solution has been to err on the positive side to avoid even small deficits. Conditions that frequently require adjustment in dietary allowances include alterations in physiologic state; body size and sex; physical activity; climate; aging; and illness and rehabilitation.

With all of the aforementioned shortcomings duly considered, the RDA still provide the principal guidelines for nutrient intake for individuals in the continental United States using normal routes of alimentation. The advent of intravenous nutrition created a new information gap regarding the requirement of nutrients when supplied by the intravenous route. The reader should realize that much of the data concerning intravenous nutrient requirements is based on the amount of nutrients required to maintain adequate circulating concentration and that minimal investigation has been completed into the potential alteration in function or corporeal reserves by disease processes.

This chapter will examine the essential nutrients with consideration of their function. Other chapters in this text will address the potential of surgery, disease, or medication for producing nutrient dysfunction and the anatomic lesions of nutrient deficiency.

The ninth edition of the *Recommended Dietary Allowances* has abandoned the use of international units for expressing the food values for vitamins A, D, E, and K and has set forth expressions based on absolute weights. This chapter will, therefore, adhere to this standardization.

In 1967 a committee of the FAO and WHO proposed that the vitamin A value of diets be expressed as the amount of retinol plus the equivalent amount of retinol that can be obtained from the provitamins A. The total would be termed the "retinol equivalent" and would be expressed in mi-

crograms. In defining the equivalency of beta-carotene and other provitamins in terms of retinol, several assumptions were made. The efficiency of conversion of pure beta-carotene in oil when absorbed by the intestine was taken as 50 per cent. Since the provitamins are not as completely absorbed as is pure beta-carotene, a factor was chosen to account for this decreased absorption. The FAO/WHO Committee decided that 33 per cent availability from diets for beta-carotene was the best approximation that could be made for practical purposes. Thus the beta-carotene in a food would only be one-third absorbed; this in turn would be only one-half converted to retinol, giving a factor of one sixth for the overall utilization. For the other provitamins that theoretically yield only one half as much retinol as does beta-carotene, the factor is one twelfth. The total vitamin A value of a diet is calculated according to the equation shown at the bottom of the page. The resulting value of vitamin A is expressed as micrograms of retinol equivalence.

In 1970 a joint FAO/WHO report recommended expressing the intake of vitamin D as mcg of cholecalciferol rather than as international units. For conversion, the international unit is the activity of 0.025 mcg of vitamin D_3.

Only D-α-tocopherol exists naturally and is the predominant form of vitamin E in most foods. The other tocopherols and tocotrienols have no officially recognized equivalency, but a general consensus has emerged. Compared with D-α-tocopherol, the relative potencies are approximately 40 per cent for β-tocopherol, 10 per cent for γ-tocopherol, and 1 per cent for Δ-tocopherol. Only α-tocotrienol in the trienol series has significant activity, about 25 per cent that of α-tocopherol. In the 1980 edition of the *Recommended Dietary Allowances*, the designation of vitamin E activity has been changed to an expression of equivalence, with all vitamin E activity expressed relative to the naturally occurring D-α-tocopherol. The total vitamin E activity would represent the sum of the weight of D-α-tocopherol plus the weights of other tocopherols or tocotrienols after correction to their equivalency as D-α-tocopherol. In order to convert international units to α-tocopherol equivalents, the international unit value is divided by the interna-

$$\text{Vitamin A value} = \text{mcg of retinol} + \frac{\text{mcg of beta-carotene}}{6} + \frac{\text{mcg of other provitamins}}{12}$$

tional unit equivalency. The National Formulary of the American Pharmaceutical Association lists the following conversion factors: 1 mg of DL-α-tocopheryl acetate is equal to 1 IU; 1 mg of DL-α-tocopherol to 1.1 IU; 1 mg of D-α-tocopheryl acetate to 1.36 IU; and 1 mg of D-α-tocopherol to 1.49 IU. The abbreviation of "α-TE" for α-tocopherol equivalent refers only to D-α-tocopheral and not to DL-α-tocopherol.

VITAMINS

The word "vitamin" means life. Although it had been known for many years that a mere change of diet would cure certain kinds of diseases, the history of vitamins in human nutrition began in 1911 when a chemist, Casimir Funk, extracted from rice polishings a crystalline substance that was found to be capable of curing an Oriental disease called beriberi. Analysis of this crystalline substance revealed the presence of nitrogen in the form of an amine. Funk, therefore, called his extracted substance "vita-amine" or "vitamine," the root "vita" indicating that the substance was essential to life and health. In this way, the word "vitamine" was used initially with a terminal "e."[2] In his classic treatise on the etiology of deficiency diseases, Funk stated that beriberi, polyneuritis in birds, epidemic dropsy, scurvy, experimental scurvy in animals, infantile scurvy, ship beriberi, and pellagra presented with certain general characters which justified their inclusion in one group, the deficiency diseases.[3] Funk pointed out that these diseases were considered for many years either as intoxications by food or as infectious diseases, and also that two decades of experimental work were necessary to show that these diseases were caused by lack of essential substances in food and therefore that a monotonous diet should be avoided. Funk might be saddened by the findings of deficiency states in modern clinical nutrition. His summary statement in his article stated "there is no doubt that as our knowledge of the relative value of different foodstuffs increases, we will be able to prevent completely the outbreak of the latter (deficiency diseases)."[3]

The purpose of these researchers was to determine the value of different cereals as cattle feeds. Four years before Funk's discovery, a series of studies had been begun at the University of Wisconsin. McCollum participated in this early work and later transferred his studies to Johns Hopkins University. There, in collaboration with Davis,[4] he announced the discovery of a new growth factor dissolved in butter and egg yolk fat. He proved that this factor was not identical with Funk's "vitamine" by demonstrating that it did not contain nitrogen. McCollum, therefore, devised a new nomenclature and called his discovery "unidentified dietary factor, fat-soluble A." McCollum's discovery was confirmed by Osborne and Mendel,[5] who had earlier found a water-soluble growth factor in milk,[6] for which McCollum and Kennedy later suggested the name "water-soluble B."[7] As early as 1906, Hopkins had postulated the existence of growth factors effective in amounts that were far too minute to be classified as foods or nutrients. The name he suggested, "accessory factors," was unsatisfactory, as further study demonstrated that these substances were actually essential to health. Between 1911 and 1920, three of these disease-preventing and growth-promoting factors were definitely demonstrated: the anti-beriberi factor, water-soluble B; the anti-eye disease factor, fat-soluble A; and the anti-scurvy factor, water-soluble C. The terminology "unidentified dietary factors fat- or water-soluble X" was extremely cumbersome. However, Funk's "amine" suffix did not apply to compounds A or C, for neither contained nitrogen. Drummond proposed a simplification of nomenclature consisting of dropping the final "e" from Funk's "vitamine" and combining this with McCollum's alphabetical designations.[8] Therefore, unidentified dietary factors were to be called "vitamins" and distinguished by the letters "A, B, C," and so forth. By this proposal McCollum's unidentified dietary factor "fat-soluble A" was condensed to vitamin A. This suggestion was generally adopted and explains the present letter usage.

These discoveries proved that food contained substances that in very small amounts were capable of affecting growth and preventing certain types of disease. The successful isolation and synthesis of these substances showed that Funk's hypothesis—that vitamins were organic chemical compounds—was correct, even though all did not contain nitrogen. A vitamin then can be defined as an organic chemical compound whose presence in the diet is essential to the maintenance of health and growth and whose absence or inadequate supply in the diet results in the development of specific manifestations of ill health. Vitamins differ from other essential "macro" nutrients in several ways. (1) The essential amounts are far smaller than those of ordinary nutrients such as proteins, fats, carbohydrates, and minerals. (2) They are to a degree inactivated by temperature, oxidation, and other aspects of food preparation and storage. (3) They may exist in inactive forms and require special treatment to become physiologically active. Vitamins occuring in an inactive form are called provitamins. Carotene, for example, is provitamin A, and ergosterol is provitamin D_2.

For convenience, vitamins are classified according to whether they are fat-soluble or water-soluble. In addition, all of the water-soluble vitamins function as cofactors in metabolic transformations.

Fat-Soluble Vitamins

Vitamin A

Absorption and Metabolism. Although vitamin A was discovered in the early 1900s, our understanding of its metabolism and function has been greatly expanded in the last 16 years. The early work on vitamin A was reviewed by Moore in 1957.[9] Excellent reviews of the early work on the chemistry, metabolism, and dietary requirements for vitamin A are provided in the references.[10, 11]

The major sources of vitamin A for most animals are from the plant carotenoid pigments, mainly beta-carotene. Beta-carotene is converted to vitamin A primarily by the intestinal mucosa. The enzymes responsible for this conversion—beta-carotene-15,15'dioxygenase and retinaldehyde reductase—have been partially purified from intestinal mucosa.

The beta-carotene 15,15'dioxygenase is an enzyme that catalyzes the cleavage of beta-carotene at the central double bond to yield two molecules of retinaldehyde.[12] For in vitro activity, the enzyme has a nonspecific requirement for a detergent (such as bile salts) and a lipid (such as lecithin), in addition to an absolute requirement for molecular oxygen.[13] While the rat absorbs virtually no unchanged beta-carotene beyond the intestinal mucosa, several other species such as humans, cattle, and chickens absorb carotenoids intact. It is probable that these carotenoids are converted to vitamin A by a similar cleavage enzyme shown to be present in the liver.

Preformed vitamin A is obtained in the diet primarily as long-chain retinyl esters. Some of these esters are hydrolyzed while in the lumen of the intestine by the action of the pancreatic retinyl ester hydrolase.[14] Prior to absorption from the intestinal lumen, the remaining retinyl esters are hydrolyzed by brush border–bound hydrolase of the intestinal mucosa. The retinol, which is absorbed into the intestinal mucosal cell, is then rapidly reesterified. Approximately 75 per cent of the total retinyl esters are formed as esters of palmitic and stearic acids. Small amounts of retinyl oleate and linoleate are produced.[15]

Retinyl esters formed in the intestinal mucosa are transported by the lymphatic route, mainly in association with lymphatic chylomicrons. The chylomicron retinyl esters are removed from the circulation almost entirely by the liver. There is evidence to suggest that hydrolysis of retinyl esters and reesterification of retinol occur during the process of uptake and storage of vitamin A by the liver.[16]

The absorption and transport of retinoic acid are different from that of retinol or retinyl esters. While retinol and retinyl esters are transported through the lymphatic system as a component of the chylomicron, retinoic acid is transported via the portal vein. Retinoic acid is bound to serum albumin in a manner similar to other long-chain free fatty acids.[17, 18]

It has been clearly shown that the parenchymal cells contain most of the vitamin A stored in the liver under normal conditions.[19] The vitamin A is stored in the lipid droplets, primarily as a mixture of long-chain retinyl esters. Retinyl palmitate accounts for more than 50 per cent of the total, with stearyl and oleyl esters as the other main esters. The liver contains a microsomal enzyme necessary for the formation of retinyl esters.

Prior to the release of vitamin A from the liver, the retinyl esters are hydrolyzed to form retinol. A retinyl palmitate hydrolase has been characterized. The activity of this enzyme increases a hundredfold in the vitamin A–deficient rat liver, suggesting that the enzyme may play a role in the regulation of serum level of vitamin A.

Recent work in normal and vitamin

A–deficient rodents has shown that the turnover rate of labeled retinol is greater in vitamin A–sufficient rats than in vitamin A–deficient rats. The effect on turnover rate might seem to be an adaptive mechanism with the depleted animal seeking to preserve its stores of vitamin A. The fractional turnover rates (per cent of pool per hour), however, were not significantly different between vitamin A–sufficient and vitamin A–deficient animals. This finding would suggest that specific adaptive mechanisms for adjusting turnover to conserve the vitamin were not present because fraction rates remain the same in both groups.[20]

Plasma Transport and Cellular Uptake. Vitamin A is mobilized from the liver as the free alcohol retinol, which is transported bound to a specific protein, retinol-binding protein (RBP). Human retinol-binding protein contains one binding site for one molecule of retinol. The normal level of RBP in human plasma is 40 to 50 mcg per ml. Retinol-binding protein forms a highly specific protein-protein complex with plasma prealbumin. The prealbumin that binds RBP is the same protein that has been studied as a thyroxine transport protein. In the human, less than 1 per cent of the prealbumin molecules circulate with bound thyroxine; the major function of human prealbumin appears to be its role in the transport of vitamin A. The normal molar ratio of prealbumin to RBP in plasma is approximately 2.5 : 1. In addition to stabilizing the binding of retinol to RBP, the formation of the RBP-prealbumin complex decreases the glomerular filtration and renal catabolism of the small RBP molecule. This complex thereby reduces the rate of removal of vitamin A and RBP from the circulation via the kidney. The normal clearance and catabolism of RBP-bound vitamin A depends on glomerular filtration and tubular uptake of that fraction of RBP-vitamin A complex not conjugated with prealbumin.[21] Smith and Goodman calculated that the plasma clearance of RBP by the kidney in healthy subjects is approximately 8 L per day, accounting for a half-life of RBP of about 18 hours in humans. This mechanism of RBP-retinol catabolism is supported by the finding of relatively large amounts of retinol and retinoic acid in the renal tubules. In renal failure, plasma RBP and retinol increase to become equal in molarity to prealbumin. Whether this signifies

hypervitaminosis A or is merely a transport anomaly is unknown.[22, 23] It has been demonstrated that plasma levels of vitamin A take up to two years to normalize following renal transplantation.[23] This work suggests that vitamin A stores may be increased in uremia.

In vitamin A deficiency the secretion of RBP from the liver is inhibited and the apo-RBP accumulates in the liver.[24] When deficient rats are replenished with vitamin A, a rapid release of RBP into the plasma occurs.[25] In contrast to the situation in vitamin A deficiency, zinc deficiency interferes with the synthesis of RBP by the liver, rather than blocks its release.[26]

Clinical Significance of Retinol-Binding Protein in Vitamin A Transport. A variety of diseases have been shown to affect plasma levels of RBP, prealbumin, and vitamin A in humans.

In patients with hepatic disease the levels of vitamin A, RBP, and prealbumin are markedly decreased and highly correlated with each other over a wide range of concentrations. In patients with acute hepatitis, the plasma concentrations of vitamin A, RBP, and prealbumin all increase as the disease improves. The depressed level of RBP in liver disease presumably reflects decreased rates of synthesis by the diseased liver.[27]

Studies of the retinol transport system in protein calorie malnutrition demonstrated that children with kwashiorkor who were supplemented with protein and calories, but not with vitamin A, showed a marked increase in levels of RBP, prealbumin, and vitamin A. These results suggested that the low serum vitamin A levels in kwashiorkor may largely reflect a functional impairment in the hepatic release of vitamin A secondary to decreased hepatic production of vitamin A transport proteins.[28]

Clinical Studies in Vitamin A Nutrition. Two new tests for assessing vitamin A stores in cirrhotic patients have been described.[29] One method uses changes in serum retinol levels following a load of retinyl palmitate. The second involves the use of a simplified method for evaluating dark adaptation. This procedure requires less than six minutes of dark adaptation and evaluates ability to discriminate among colored standard ophthalmologic disks. This test was found to have a sensitivity of 95 per cent and specificity of 91 per cent, thus correlating well with classic dark adaptometry parameters.[30]

Depressed plasma levels of vitamin A and RBP have been reported in patients with cystic fibrosis. In these individuals, the changes in plasma vitamin A levels have been shown to correlate with zinc intake.[31, 32]

Significant vitamin A, E, or 25-hydroxy-D deficiency occurred in 76 per cent of 40 patients studied up to six years following jejunoileal bypass surgery for morbid obesity. Vitamin A levels were significantly lower in those individuals who had lost 30 per cent of their initial weight than in those who had lost less weight. Functional derangement, as measured by dark adaptometry, was found in 44 per cent of the patients studied at least 18 months after surgery.[33] These studies confirmed that the alterations in the absorbtive area or interference with bile salt metabolism produced in the gastrointestinal tract by this procedure can produce significant malabsorption of fat-soluble vitamins.

Lepromatous patients have been found to have significantly lowered vitamin A levels than did patients with tuberculoid disease. This finding seems significant since vitamin A is required for normal epithelial structure and function and can cause stimulation of the immune response.[34] It is interesting to speculate that hypovitaminosis A may play a role in the defective altered immune response and development of trophic skin ulcers in these patients, who were also noted to have low serum zinc concentration. Therefore, the metabolism of zinc must be considered before the primary role of vitamin A in this disease is defined.[34]

Vitamin A and its synthetic analogs (retinoids) have been used successfully to prevent cancer of the skin, lung, bladder, and breast in experimental animals.[35, 36] This is a pharmacologic approach to prevention of cancer by enhancement of intrinsic epithelial defense mechanisms. Synthetic retinoids appear to be superior for this purpose. Vitamin A or its derivatives appear to counteract carcinogens by inhibiting tumor promotion. A recently discovered vitamin A metabolite, 5,6-hypoxyretinoic acid, has both vitamin A and antipromotor activity.[35, 36]

Patients on oral contraceptive agents have increased plasma vitamin A concentrations.[37, 38] Estrogens increase the steady-state level of circulating RBP in the plasma, similarly to their effect on a number of other plasma proteins. The increased amount of RBP transports more vitamin A into the plasma from the liver and results in higher plasma concentrations. This phenomenon is not thought to increase the risk of vitamin A deficiency in women on oral contraceptives. Animal experiments show that the depletion rate from the liver is only slightly increased. It appears that the effect of the contraceptive is solely on the plasma level.[37, 38]

Clinical studies, animal experiments, and data from human populations suggest that hemoglobin synthesis is impaired by vitamin A deficiency.[39–41]

It has recently been demonstrated that growth hormone may have a specific effect on the storage and release of vitamin A.[42] These studies showed that vitamin A content was high in liver and low in other tissues in hypophysectomized rats. Administration of growth hormone was shown to rectify these changes. It was not determined whether growth hormone acted directly on the tissues or through somatomedin. In addition, the activities of RBP receptors and cell membranes were not studied.

High serum levels of thyroxine and triiodothyronine were observed in vitamin A–deficient rats. The levels of thyrotropin (TSH) in the pituitary and of thyrotropin-releasing hormone (TRH) in the hypothalamus were also increased, suggesting that in vitamin A deficiency the negative feedback regulation of the brain by thyroid hormone is disturbed.[43, 44]

The interrelationship of thyroid hormones with vitamin A and zinc nutritional status in patients with chronic hepatic and gastrointestinal disorders has recently been described by Morley et al., who found that serum triiodothyronine (T_3) levels and free T_3 index (FT_3I) were depressed in the patients compared with controls.[45] Retinol-binding protein and prealbumin levels correlated with both T_3 and FT_3I, whereas vitamin A levels did not. Vitamin A therapy in patients with documented vitamin A deficiency produced an increase in T_3, thyroxine (T_4), FT_3I and FT_4I, and free T_3, with a concomitant increase in RBP and no alteration in prealbumin concentrations. Zinc-deficient patients had significantly depressed T_3 and FT_3I levels and increased prolactin levels. Zinc supplementation failed to return any of these levels to normal. Vitamin A therapy in normal patients produced a transient decrease in T_3 and T_4 after one week of therapy, but after an additional two weeks, thyroid function returned to normal. These data suggested a causal relationship between the pathogenesis of deranged vitamin A and RBP metabolism and the low T_3 syndrome. Potential mechanisms include interference with T_4 entry into tissues or a direct effect on the enzymatic conversion of T_4 to T_3. Zinc is believed to be necessary for release of RBP from the liver in rats.[46] In addition, the alcohol dehydrogenase necessary for the formation of the active form of vitamin A is a zinc-dependent enzyme.

It has been proposed[47] that for vitamin A and vitamin B_{12} alone among the known micronutrients, a luxus (excessive) intake habitually exists. Evidence for this was presented by a comparison of habitual intake with recommended dietary allowance and of total body content in relation to requirements. With increasing age, both vitamins were shown to accumulate in the liver in concentrations related to dietary intake. It was shown that the loss of these vitamins from the body is exponential and related to body stores. These data were particularly challenged in relationship to the luxus state of vitamin B_{12}.[48]

Metabolic Function. Beyond its role in the visual cycle, vitamin A is known to be required for growth, reproduction, and the maintenance of life. The recent discovery of a mannosyl retinyl phosphate glycolipid suggests that vitamin A may play a primary role in the synthesis of glycoproteins.[49] This glycolipid has been shown to be a better donor of mannose to endogenous glycoproteins than GDP mannose in in vitro systems.[49a] A rat serum glycoprotein, α-1 macroglobulin, has been identified as a serum protein responding to the vitamin A status of the rat: It drops to 20 per cent of normal levels in severe vitamin A deficiency.[50] This glycoprotein is probably synthesized by the liver, contains about 2.7 per cent by weight of mannose, and may be a good candidate for mannose acceptance from mannosyl retinyl phosphate.

Specific binding proteins that bind either retinol or retinoic acid have been detected in tissues. Perinatal development of the rat is associated with tissue-specific changes in the levels of these proteins. Indirect evidence suggests that cellular-binding proteins may be involved in vitamin A action.[51] In addition to the plasma RBP and the cellular-binding proteins, Heller and associates have reported membrane proteins that specifically bind vitamin A and may have a role in the transport of retinol across the membranes.[52] It is clear that cells from two different vitamin A target tissues possess receptors for RBP on their cell surfaces. These receptors are highly specific for holo-RBP, with lower affinity for apo-RBP, thus providing a mechanism for the regulation of retinol delivery to the cells. One could readily imagine that some cells—for example, the mucus-secreting cells of the intestine—would need more; others, such as skin (a normal keratinizing tissue), would need less vitamin A. The number of receptor sites for RBP would provide such a threshold mechanism to select the right concentration of retinol accumulation within each cell type.[53, 54]

Vitamin D

In 1807 Bardsley suggested the use of cod liver oil for the treatment of demineralizing diseases of bone.[55] In 1890 Palm proposed the antirachitic properties of sunlight.

By 1919 rickets appeared in epidemic proportions in the human population of England. In this atmosphere, Sir Edward Mellanby attempted to produce rickets by nutritional means. He was successful in producing the disease in dogs maintained on a diet of oatmeal. He did not recognize the importance of the fact that the dogs were also kept in the absence of sunlight. Mellanby was inspired by McCollum's work showing that cod liver oil contained a fat-soluble substance important to the growth of rats. As a consequence, he tried this substance in his dogs and found that cod liver oil would indeed prevent and cure the disease rickets.[56] Even though Mellanby erroneously concluded that the healing of rickets was a property of the fat-soluble vitamin A, he placed the study of vitamin D deficiency in metabolic bone disease on an experimental basis. McCollum, who had discovered fat-soluble vitamin A, realized that the antirachitic activity described by Mellanby was distinct from the antixerophthalmia activity in cod liver oil. McCollum treated cod liver oil with oxygen and heat to destroy the vitamin A activity and demonstrated that the properties of cod liver oil in the prevention and cure of rickets remained. He concluded that this represented a new fat-soluble vitamin, which he called vitamin D.[57] During this era, however, Viennese and British physicians were able to cure rickets in children by simply exposing their patients to ultraviolet light from natural or artificial sources.[58] The question, therefore, was the relationship between ultraviolet light and cod liver oil in the treatment of rickets. Goldblatt and Soames[59] demonstrated that irradiation of rachitic rats with ultraviolet light produced an antirachitic substance even following hepatectomy. In the absence of irradiation, no antirachitic substance could be detected. Steenbock then suggested that ultraviolet irradiation was causing alteration of some substance in the animal and proceeded to demonstrate that ultraviolet irradiation not only of the animals but also of their food could heal or prevent rickets.[60] Subsequent work demonstrated that the activatable material was found in the nonsaponifiable fraction.[61, 62] These discoveries led to the use of ultraviolet light irradiation of such foods as milk and butter to fortify them with vitamin D and thus eliminate rickets as a major medical problem. In addition, it provided the ability to generate in the laboratory large amounts of the antirachitic substance so that it could be isolated and chemically identified. This was accomplished in 1931 by Askew,[63] who demonstrated the structure of vitamin D_2 produced by the irradiation of the plant sterol ergosterol. Although the identification of vitamin D_2 appeared to have completed the structural elucidation of the vitamin D substances, Steenbock noted that chicks did not respond as well to solutions of irradiated ergosterol as to cod liver oil.[64] Windaus and his colleagues successfully prepared an analog of ergosterol, 7-dehydrocholesterol. The irradiation of this substance produced another form of vitamin D, labeled vitamin D_3.[65] Vitamin D_3 was subsequently shown to represent the natural form of the vitamin produced in the skin upon irradiation with ultraviolet light.[66, 67] Isolation of the D vitamins in large quantities permitted their addition to food products and the production of vitamin capsules, making the D vitamins available to the clinical world for treatment of metabolic bone disease. The discovery of the vitamin D metabolites in the 1960s demonstrated the functions of vitamin D in the regulation of calcium homeostasis and phosphate metabolism.[68] A more in-depth history of the discovery of vitamin D and the actions of the vitamin D metabolites is given in a recent review by DeLuca.[69]

Physiology of Action. The function of vitamin D is to elevate plasma calcium and phosphorus to a level that will support normal bone mineralization. The maintenance of a normal plasma calcium level is also critically important in normal neuromuscular activity.

Vitamin D is required for the intestine to adjust its efficiency of calcium absorption in order to meet skeletal needs. If intestinal absorption is impaired, there is a reliance upon skeletal calcium for maintenance of normal plasma calcium concentration.[70] It is known that vitamin D stimulates the active transport of calcium and of phosphorus across the intestinal epithelium.[71-73] This stimulation involves the active form of vitamin D.[74] Parathyroid hormone indirectly stimulates the intestinal absorption of calcium by stimulating the production of 1,25-dihydroxy-vitamin D_3.[75] Talmage[76] pointed out the importance of the compartmentalization of the mineral component of bone. He emphasized the fact that the calcium of bone is separated from extracellular fluid compartment by the cellular membrane of bone. Therefore, the bone fluid compartment is dominated by the solubility of hydroxyapatite crystals found on the collagen fibrils of bone. The concentration of calcium and phosphorus in the bone fluid is below that of the extracellular fluid compartment. When calcium is needed to support serum calcium concentration, parathyroid hormone and the active form of vitamin D serve to mobilize calcium and subsequently phosphate from the bone fluid compartment into the plasma.[77, 78] This mechanism, along with the intestinal mechanism, is the principal way by which vitamin D metabolites elevate plasma calcium and plasma phosphate concentrations. Of secondary importance is the vitamin D function in the distal renal tubules to increase calcium reabsorption. Although 99 per cent of the filtered load of calcium is reabsorbed in the absence of vitamin D or parathyroid hormone, the remaining 1 per cent is under the control of these two humoral agents.[79, 80] The present known pathway for vitamin D metabolism involves an initial step in synthesis, which comes from the irradiation of 7-dehydrocholesterol in the skin to form vitamin D_3. The 7-dehydrocholesterol is abundant in the epidermis, and it has been demonstrated that ultraviolet light of an appropriate wavelength penetrates to the epidermal cells. The kinetics of the photolysis reaction suggests that no proteins or enzymes are involved in the conversion of 7-dehydrocholesterol to vitamin D_3 since the kinetics of photolysis is identical to the kinetics observed in the absence of tissue. The conversion of 7-dehydrocholesterol to vitamin D_3 involves an intermediate step involving a previtamin D form which is in equilibrium with vitamin D_3. The conversion of previtamin D to vitamin D_3 requires approximately 36 hours at body temperature to reach equilibrium.[81, 82] The input of vitamin D from the skin is a slow process that is apparently regulated only by the amount of shielding by skin pigmentation to block out ultraviolet light or by decreased exposure to ultraviolet light. The initial enzyme in the conversion pathway of vitamin D_3 to its active forms is the vitamin D_3-25-hydroxylase. This enzyme has been detected in the intestine and kidney as well as in the liver.[83] In vitro experiments, however, have demonstrated clearly that the liver carries out the major portion of the 25-hydroxylation of vitamin D.[84–86]

The final functional form of vitamin D in target tissues appears to be 1,25-dihydroxy vitamin D_3 ($1,25(OH)_2D_3$). The kidney is the sole site of production of 1,25-dihydroxy vitamin D_3.[87–89]

Other Metabolites of Vitamin D. It appears that vitamin D_2 is metabolized in an almost identical fashion to vitamin D_3.[90] However, it has been demonstrated that certain animals are able to discriminate against vitamin D_2 in terms of biologic response. Jones et al. have shown that $1,25(OH)_2$ vitamin D_2 is less effective than $1,25(OH)_2$ vitamin D_3 in stimulating intestinal calcium absorption in birds.[91] Another metabolite of vitamin D_3, 24,25-dihydroxy D_3, has been described. The enzymes that convert 25-hydroxy D_3 to 24,25-dihydroxy D_3 are located in the intestine, kidney, and cartilage. A functional role of the 25-hydroxylated metabolites of vitamin D, other than that of deactivation of vitamin D, remains in doubt.[92] There does appear to be a relationship between the serum phosphate and 24,25-dihydroxy vitamin D_3. It appears that 24,25-dihydroxy D_3 is preferentially formed when the serum phosphate is above 8 mg/dl and 1,25-dihydroxy D_3 is formed when the serum phosphate is below 8 mg/dl.[92]

Mechanism of Action of $1,25(OH)_2D$. It appears that 1,25-dihydroxy D_3 interacts with a receptorlike molecule, which may be in the cytosol or nucleus of the cell. Interaction of 1,25-dihydroxy D_3 with this receptor molecule is required for the expression of $1,25(OH)_2$ D_3 action. It is certain that $1,25(OH)_2$ D_3 must appear in the nucleus before the initiation of intestinal calcium transport. Furthermore, transcription of specific DNA is involved in the expression of $1,25(OH)_2$ D_3 action as is translation and protein synthesis. It is thought that the brush border is the site where the synthesized protein stimulates intestinal calcium transport.[93]

Vitamin D Metabolites in the Treatment of Metabolic Bone Diseases. The finding of a vitamin D endocrine system and its interrelationship with other endocrine systems has clarified several disorders of calcium and phosphorus metabolism and of metabolic bone disease. One of the diseases involving primarily a disturbance in the vitamin D system is a bone disease, renal osteodystrophy, which accompanies chronic renal failure. A major aspect of this disease appears to be the failure to produce the vitamin D hormone $1,25(OH)_2$ D_3, which is required for calcium absorption and utilization. Patients with chronic renal failure and glomerular filtration rates of less than 5 ml/min show undetectable levels of 1,25-dihydroxy D_3 in their plasma.[94, 95]

This finding probably results from a loss of renal mass and a tendency toward phosphate retention, with both factors contributing to a decreased production of $1,25(OH)_2$ D_3 during the course of development of the disease. This results in a decreased calcium absorption, and the tendency toward hypocalcemia leads to a secondary response by the parathyroid glands. The secondary hyperparathyroidism with the concomitant production of vitamin D metabolites is thought to be the mechanism for production of the diseases osteitis fibrosis cystica and osteosclerosis. In children, chronic renal failure is associated with rickets, defective bone mineralization, and poor growth.[96] Treatment with $1,25(OH)_2$ D_3 of patients with end-stage renal failure has been successful in correcting the metabolic bone disease and calcium disorders.[97, 98] The pharmacology of $1,25(OH)_2D_3$ demands that it be given in frequent small doses rather than a single large dose once daily. If small amounts are given on a more frequent basis, it is likely that these compounds will be very effective in virtually every aspect of renal osteodystrophy. Other diseases that have been well-managed with the vitamin D hormones include hypoparathyroidism and pseudohypoparathyroidism. In these diseases, either the patient has lost the ability to detect hypocalcemia (thus not increasing production of $1,25(OH)_2 D_3$) or the target organ of parathyroid hormone is resistant to the parathyroid hormone (resulting in defective synthesis of 1,25-dihydroxy D_3). These conditions are managed by the administration of $1,25(OH)_2 D_3$ and the provision of oral calcium so that plasma calcium levels can be supported from intestinal sources.[99]

Other less common diseases include the following:

1. *Vitamin D–dependent Autosomal Rickets.* This disease results from a defective 25-hydroxy D_3,1-alpha-hydroxylase and can be corrected by administering physiologic amounts of 1,25-dihydroxy D_3.[100]

2. *X-linked Hypophosphatemic Vitamin D–resistant Rickets.* This condition involves a primary defect in phosphate transport reactions and a secondary defect in the production of $1,25(OH)_2 D_3$.[101] Patients with this condition are successfully treated by the administration of oral phosphate daily plus $1,25(OH)_2 D_3$.

3. *Postmenopausal Osteoporosis.* It is known that there is a marked decrease in intestinal calcium absorption with ageing in both humans and animals.[102] This correlates with a decrease in the plasma level of $1,25(OH)_2 D_3$.[103] It has been demonstrated in postmenopausal osteoporotic women that there is an additional decrease in plasma $1,25(OH)_2 D_3$ levels, which correlates with lowered intestinal calcium absorption.[104] As a consequence, postmenopausal osteoporotic women have about 30 per cent less 1,25-dihydroxy D_3 in their plasma than do age- and sex-matched controls; in addition they have a 30 per cent decrease in their intestinal calcium absorption ability. The mechanism for the pathologic defect is thought to be a lack in sensitivity of bone to calcium mobilizing agents, giving rise to higher levels of calcium coming from bone, which in turn suppresses parathyroid secretion, thereby suppressing $1,25(OH)_2 D_3$ production and diminishing calcium absorption.[92] The administration of 1,25-dihydroxy D_3 at 0.5 μg per day to postmenopausal osteoporotic women results in increased intestinal calcium absorption.[104]

Recent investigations of the vitamin D status in patients with morbid obesity have demonstrated that the mean plasma $1,25(OH)_2 D_3$ concentrations were significantly lower in the obese individuals than in age-matched healthy controls. This study suggested that preoperative vitamin D deficiency may contribute to the postoperative development of metabolic bone disease following surgery for morbid obesity.[105]

Malabsorption of vitamin D after small bowel resection has been demonstrated to occur due to not only the interruption of the enterohepatic circulation system of bile acids but also a primary failure of the small intestine to absorb vitamin D.[106]

Vitamin D Sources and Requirements. The minimum dietary requirement for vitamin D has not been established. Since the requirement for the normal, healthy adult seems to be satisfied by nondietary sources, no dietary recommendation is generally considered necessary. A dietary intake of 400 IU for normal individuals of all ages appears to incur no risk of toxicity.[107]

Seasonal variations in vitamin D nutrition have been recently assessed by measurements of serum 25-hydroxycholecalciferol levels in outdoor workers, indoor workers, and long-term hospital inpatients. All three groups showed seasonal changes, and the outdoor workers had the highest levels at all seasons. The highest levels of 25-hydroxycholecalciferol were found in October in the indoor workers and in November in the outdoor workers; the peak in ultraviolet exposure was in July. The suggested reason for this long lag is that vitamin D continues to be formed and stored during the autumn, especially in outdoor workers.[108]

Human milk has been found to contain 40 to 50 IU/L of vitamin D activity. It has been recently shown that 75 per cent of the biologic activity of human milk is due to 25-hydroxy D_3 and that vitamin D_2, vitamin D_3, and 25-hydroxy vitamin D_3 are responsible for more than 90 per cent of the total vitamin D activity present.[109]

Vitamin E

Evans and Bishop[110] discovered that rats raised on diets lacking a fat-soluble factor did not have offspring. The females failed to carry their young to term, with death of the embryos and eventual resorption of the fetus. The female reproductive mechanisms were not damaged since adequate doses of the factor restored fertility. Male animals deprived of this factor, however, became sterile through degeneration of the germinal epithelium, and vitamin E therapy was ineffective. In 1936 Evans and the Emersons[111] gave this substance the name of alpha-tocopherol. The name is derived from "tokos" meaning "childbirth" and "pherein" meaning "to bear," the ending "ol" indicating an alcohol. In 1934 Alcott and Mattill obtained a concentrate of vitamin E from wheat germ oil which was found to have an antioxidant action as well as the effects described by Evans and Bishop.[112] The antioxidant properties of tocopherol have been amply supported.[113-117] This work has suggested to others that alpha-tocopherol may be an integral part of an enzyme system.[118-119] Vitamin E consists of two homologous series of four compounds each, the tocopherols and the tocotrienols. These compounds differ with respect to the nature of the polyisoprenoid side chain (saturated versus unsaturated) and with respect to the number and position of the methyl constituents attached to the ring system. Alpha-tocopherol is the predominant form of vitamin E in the leafy portions of plants. Seed oils, however, contain mostly non-α-tocopherols. Despite the predominance of other isomers in most humans and animal dietary ingredients, α-tocopherol is the main form found in human blood and tissues. The plasma of adult man contains primarily (90 per cent) α-tocopherol. The disparity between the proportions of dietary and tissue compounds is due to differences in turnover times and perhaps a difference in the ability of cellular components to distinguish between the compounds.

Deficiency Diseases. Vitamin E deficiency diseases in experimental animals, poultry, and livestock are now well established. Nutritional interrelationships between vitamin E, polyunsaturated fatty acids, selenium, antioxidants, sulfur amino acids, vitamin B_{12}, and prostaglandin synthesis have been noted.[120] In well-developed countries, the vitamin E intake of most populations is considered adequate for maintenance, growth, activity, and reproduction in normal individuals. Vitamin E supplementation may be required in newborn infants (particularly those who are premature or small for gestational age), in members of some low-income groups, and in individuals practicing unusual food habits that entail consumption of foods that are low in vitamin E. Several human diseases have been attributed to abnormalities in vitamin E metabolism. There are at least three special situations in which supplementary vitamin E has proved to be beneficial. One suggested usage is in the hemolytic anemia of premature infants. Owing to the poor transfer of vitamin E from the mother to a fetus across the placenta, premature and full-term newborn infants may have relatively low levels of vitamin E in both tissues and blood and develop a hemolytic anemia that responds to vitamin E supplementation.[121-125] A recent critical review by Bell and Filer and its subsequent discussion have pointed out that the usual diet of premature infants contains adequate vitamin E without supplementation.[126-128] The mechanism of action of vitamin E in the correction of the hemolytic anemia may be due either to a prevention of peroxidation of membrane lipids or to interference with the conversion of cyanocobalamin to 5'-deoxyadenosylcobalamin. The latter compound is necessary for the action of the enzyme methylmalonyl-CoA-mutase, which produces succinyl-CoA.[129] This effect would decrease the amount of succinyl-CoA available for heme synthesis. The work of Caasi et al. suggested a decrease in bone marrow of Δ-aminolevulinic acid synthetase.[130] The role of vitamin E in heme synthesis, however, remains to be elucidated.[131]

Another use for supplemental vitamin E is in the treatment of deficiencies of the vitamin caused by malabsorption of fats and oils frequently seen in postgastrectomy patients or patients with cystic fibrosis, hepatic cirrhosis, obstructive jaundice, pancreatic insufficiency, or sprue.[132, 133]

A third use for supplemental vitamin E has been suggested for patients with intermittent claudication.[134, 135] Double-blind studies have shown that this condition can be relieved by supplemental vitamin E therapy. The treatment requires 400 mg or more of vitamin E daily, and the therapy must be continued for at least three months.

Owens and Owens[136] showed a reduction in incidence of retrolental fibroplasia with vitamin E supplementation. More recently, Johnson et al.[137-139] have shown that vitamin E in pharmacologic doses not only confers partial protection of the premature infant's retina against developing retrolental fibroplasia but may also be effective in reversing established cases. These findings have been confirmed by Phelps and Rosenbaum,[140, 141] but not universally.[142, 143]

Patients with sickle cell anemia given 300 mg of vitamin E as α-tocopherol per day for 6 to 35 weeks showed a marked increase in plasma tocopherol levels from 0.7 to 2.3 mg/gm. The percentage of circulating irreversibly sickled red cells decreased from 25 per cent pretreatment to 11 per cent after administration of vitamin E. The percentage of irreversibly sickled red cells remained below pretreatment levels as long as the vitamin was administered.[144]

New Information Regarding a Metabolic Role for Vitamin E. Recent reports have linked vitamin E metabolism to that of prostaglandin metabolism. Chan and Leith reported decreased prostacyclin synthesis in aortas of vitamin E–deficient rabbits.[145] They monitored serum pyruvate kinase as evidence of vitamin E depletion-induced myopathy. In this study, the endogenous release of PGI_2 by the aorta, detected as its stable metabolite 6-keto-PGF_1, was inhibited by indomethacin and was inversely related to the size of aortic sections. Vitamin E–deficient aortas synthesized significantly less PGI_2 than did those from control animals. Repletion of deficient animals for 48 hours completely restored the prostacyclin release to a level comparable with the control values.[145] Vitamin E therapy at pharmacologic levels has been shown to decrease tissue levels of prostaglandins E_1, E_2, and F_2 in bursa and spleen of chickens.[146] Vitamin E supplementation alone, or acting synergistically with aspirin, decreases the mortality of animals injected with a lethal quantity of *Escherichia coli*. Because vitamin E has been shown to be an effective inhibitor of prostaglandin synthesis in certain tissues,[147, 148] the authors proposed that this role for vitamin E might be protective against *E. coli* infections in these animals.

Coagulopathy has been associated with vitamin E toxicity. It has been postulated that the observed coagulopathy is a result of the direct interference of vitamin E with vitamin K activity. Mellette et al. reported that the addition of large amounts of vitamin E to the diets of rats increased mortality and coagulopathy as evidenced by depressed prothrombin levels.[149] March et al.[150] reported that clotting time was lengthened in chicks fed high levels of vitamin E in the diet. In contrast, reports of large vitamin E doses in rats and humans have failed to to reveal toxic effects.[151, 152] From these and other studies it appeared clear that large doses of vitamin E did not interfere with the vitamin K–dependent coagulation factors in normal individuals. However, Corrigan and Marcus[153] observed prolonged prothrombin time and ecchymosis in a 55-year-old man taking warfarin sodium and clofibrate concomitantly with self-administration of up to 1200 IU of vitamin E per day. Discontinuation of the warfarin and vitamin E cleared the ecchymosis and reduced the prothrombin time. Subsequently the patient was again challenged with 800 IU of vitamin E for 42 days while continuing to receive 2.5 to 5 mg of warfarin sodium daily and 2 gm of clofibrate daily. A progressive increase in prothrombin time was observed. Simultaneously, levels of vitamin K–dependent coagulation factors declined, reaching a nadir by the forty-second day of vitamin E ingestion. At that point, multiple ecchymoses and hematomas appeared. Subsequently, Corrigan demonstrated that rats rendered lightly vitamin K–deficient with warfarin (0.01 mg/100 gm body weight) and given the equivalent of 1000 mg/kg of DL-α-tocopherol intramuscularly for seven days showed a marked reduction in prothrombin activity. In 12 human patients receiving warfarin, vitamin E was administered in doses of 100 or 400 mg of DL-α-tocopherol orally for four weeks. The results in these patients showed no significant change in the prothrombin time, factor 2 coagulant activity, or factor 2 antigen (by electroimmunoassay). By using a ratio of factor 2 coagulant activity to immunoreactive protein, however, significant reduction was observed when compared with pretreatment ratios. These data suggested that vitamin E acted at the step mediated by vitamin K and not in the synthesis of the factor 2 precursor.[154] Doses of vitamin E of 400 mg or less per day do not appear to induce clinical bleeding in cases of moderate vitamin K deficiency. The data suggest, however, that larger doses of vitamin E should be used with caution in such patients.

Alpha-tocopherol analogs that lack the terpenoid side chain are noncompetitive inhibitors of the beef-liver phosphodiesterases that act upon cyclic AMP and cyclic GMP. Although α-tocopherol had no effect on partially purified phosphodiesterases from beef liver, three analogs that lacked the usual polyisoprenoid chain at the 2 position were more potent noncompetitive inhibitors of the cAMP phosphodiesterase than theophylline; the analogs and theophylline were comparable but weaker inhibitors of GMP phosphodiesterase.[155] Cyclic AMP phosphodiesterase is elevated in livers from tocopherol-deficient rats, which additionally have decreased glycogen and increased serine dehydratase activity.

Chizzolini et al.[156] studied the effect of a vitamin E–deficient diet on muscular collagen in young rabbits. Intramuscular collagen content was found to increase in vitamin E–deficient rabbits both in absolute and relative values, whereas no change in urinary hydroxyproline excretion was observed. The overall solubility of intramuscular collagen was shown to be higher in the vitamin E–deficient animals and the collagen soluble in guanidine hydrochloride was richer in alpha chains. Such findings suggested that vitamin E deficiency induced the production of new intramuscular collagen.[156]

Interrelationships Between Vitamin E and Selenium. The discovery that selenium was an integral component of glutathione peroxidase illuminated some of the relationships between vitamin E and selenium in prevention of deficiency diseases of these nutrients.[157] Selenium appears to decrease vitamin E requirements in at least three ways: (1) Selenium appears to be necessary to preserve the normal integrity of the pancreas, which in turn allows normal fat digestion and thus aids vitamin E absorption. (2) Glutathione peroxidase is a selenium-dependent metalloenzyme that converts reduced glutathione to oxidized glutathione and at the same time destroys peroxides by converting them to alcohols. As a consequence, it prevents peroxidation of the polyunsaturated fatty acids of the lipid membranes of cells, thus reducing the amount of vitamin E required to maintain these membranes. (3) Selenium appears to aid in the retention of vitamin E that circulates in the blood plasma.

Vitamin E appears to decrease selenium requirements (of at least chicks) by (1) maintaining body selenium in an active form and/or preventing its loss from the body and (2) preventing the peroxidation of membrane lipids within the membrane itself, thereby decreasing the production of hydroperoxides and the need for glutathione peroxidase activity.[157]

A new method for the direct measurement of lipid peroxidation in vivo has been reported. The method relies on the quantitation of exhaled ethane and pentane, peroxidation products of linolenic and linoleic acids, respectively.[158–163] This method has been used to show that lipid peroxidation occurs in the presence of vitamin E and selenium deficiency.

Assessment of Status. Nutritional status with respect to vitamin E has traditionally been estimated from the plasma (or serum) concentration. Removal of tocopherols from the diet for two to three weeks results in a plasma vitamin E concentration of approximately one half the initial concentration. It is commonly accepted that a plasma level of total tocopherols below 0.5 mg/dl is undesirable, although this has not been shown to be associated with inadequate tissue concentrations (unless the duration of inadequate intake is one year or longer).[164] Since the bulk of plasma vitamin E is carried by lipoproteins, there is a correlation between total lipids and plasma tocopherol concentration. Therefore, conditions that alter blood lipoprotein concentrations result in abnormal plasma tocopherol concentrations. It has been suggested that a ratio of 0.8 mg of total tocopherols per gm of total plasma lipids would indicate an adequate nutritional status.[165]

Vitamin K

McFarlane and associates[166] noted that 50 per cent of chicks fed on an ether-extracted fish meal diet died from bleeding. This discovery led to the work of Dam, who noted that the subdural or muscular hemorrhages that developed in these animals could be controlled by administration of the nonsaponifiable, nonsterol fraction of hog liver fat. In these initial experiments it was shown that the addition of cholesterol, lemon juice, yeast, or cod liver oil to the diet did not decrease the incidence of hemorrhage.[167] This hemorrhagic disease was subsequently observed by others, and a period followed during which various groups attempted to identify the active component missing from the diet. Dam continued to study the distribution and lipid solubility of the active component and proposed that the antihemorrhagic vitamin of the chick was a new fat-soluble vitamin, which he called vitamin K.[167] (The letter K had not been used to describe an existing or postulated vitamin activity at the time and was also the first letter of the German word "koagulation.") In the same year that Dam reported the discovery of his new vitamin, an independent report by Almquist and Stockstead[168] stated that the hemorrhagic disease could be cured with ether extracts of alfalfa and that microbial action in fish meal and bran preparations could lead to the development of antihemorrhagic activity. In 1936 Dam demonstrated that the activity of a crude plasma prothrombin fraction was decreased when obtained from vitamin K–deficient chicks.[169] The understanding of the factors involved in the generation of thrombin from prothrombin did not develop until the mid-1950s. During the succeeding decade, factors VII, IX, and X were discovered and subsequently shown to be dependent on vitamin K for their synthesis. The elucidation of the structure of vitamin K followed rapidly. Vitamin K_1 was isolated from alfalfa and characterized as 2-methyl-3-phytyl-1,4-naphthoquinone.[170] Vitamin K_2 was shown to be very similar in structure but with the substitution of an unsaturated polyprenyl side chain. Therefore, in general, two forms of vitamin K were found in nature: K_1 in plants and K_2 secondary to bacterial synthesis. In the human, vitamin K_2 is synthesized by intestinal bacteria. Vitamin K_3 (a synthetic form of vitamin K) is used therapeutically. Although there were early suggestions that vitamin K_3 itself might be functioning as a vitamin, it is currently assumed that it is alkylated to a biologically active metabolite, either by intestinal organisms or by tissue-alkylating enzymes.

Vitamin K deficiency in the human has not been produced by administration of a vitamin K–free diet alone. It has, therefore, been assumed that the intestinal synthesis of vitamin K_2 can supply the needs of the adult human and older children under normal circumstances. Frick et al.[171] studied the vitamin K requirement of starved, debilitated, intravenously fed patients given antibiotics to decrease intestinal vitamin K synthesis. Their data indicated a requirement of approximately 1 μg of vitamin K/kg of body weight per day. These data were substantiated by the work of Doisy[172] and O'Reilly,[173] leading to the suggestion that the human requirement of vitamin K is in the range of 0.5 to 1 μg/kg/day. This amount of vitamin intake is exceeded by most diets that are in other respects nutritionally adequate, and a simple dietary deficiency appears to be of little concern.

Mechanism of Action. During the 25 years following Dam's discovery of vitamin K, knowledge regarding the biologic activity of various forms of both the vitamin and its antagonist and the significance of the vitamin in animal nutrition and human medicine has progressed to the point that it may be possible to describe the metabolic role of this vitamin at the molecular level in more detail than is possible for the other fat-soluble vitamins.

The classic defect of a vitamin K deficiency in animals is a lowered concentration of plasma prothrombin and factors VII, IX, and X. It has been shown that these proteins are synthesized in the liver in inactive precursor forms and converted to biologically active proteins by the action of vitamin K.[174, 175] It was subsequently demonstrated that these clotting factors contained residues of a previously unrecognized amino acid, γ-carboxyglutamic acid. Prothrombin contains ten residues of this amino acid.[176–178] The function of the modification of the clotting factor molecules is to allow these proteins to participate in the specific protein-calcium-phospholipid interaction essential to their biologic role. The sequence of events in vitamin K activity as far as clotting factor function is summarized in the following manner. A precursor protein for prothrombin is able to bind calcium, which in turn allows binding to a phospholipid surface for subsequent activation (cleavage) to form thrombin.

Many vitamin K–dependent proteins have been found to date.[175] The main noncollagen protein in bone (osteocalcin) has been shown to be a vitamin K–dependent γ-carboxyglutamic acid–containing protein.[179] Vitamin K–dependent proteins have now been found in kidney, placenta, lung, spleen, and associated with renal calculi and ectopic calcifications. Although it has been shown that these proteins are involved in some type of interaction with calcium or other divalent cations, unequivocal physiologic roles have not been defined for any of these non-clotting-factor, vitamin K–dependent proteins.

Theories of the mechanism of action of vitamin K are obliged to consider that the formation of the 2,3-epoxide of the vitamin is involved in the reaction.[180] Willingham and Matschiner[181] have postulated that the formation of the epoxide is an obligatory step in vitamin action with the resultant promotion of prothrombin biosynthesis. The available evidence suggests that both reactions involve some components of a microsomal redox system and that they may be somehow coupled.

Clinical Aspects. Nutritional deficiency of vitamin K has been reported in a number of studies. Kark and Lozer[182] reported four cases with generally poor nutritional state, extended prothrombin time, and a hemorrhagic syndrome, responsive to vitamin K_1 but unresponsive to vitamin C. Pineo[183] described 27 patients who developed vitamin K deficiency unexpectedly in a hospitalized environment. Of these patients 81 per cent had received antibiotics and 70 per cent were on no oral intake. All patients had marginal diets. Some had renal insufficiency and were being treated with hemodialysis. Most of these patients developed manifestations of vitamin K deficiency within seven days of admission or surgery. Ansell[184] reported 13 cases of bleeding due to vitamin K deficiency similar in background to those of Pineo et al. Ansell emphasized that postoperative patients and those with cancer or renal failure were at high risk. The triad of poor diet, injury, and antibiotic therapy—(all of which may depress or alter the protective microbiologic flora—should be considered as predisposing factors for the development of vitamin K deficiency.

Newborn infants generally require vitamin K supplementation because the placenta is a relatively poor organ for transmission of lipids and lipid-soluble nutrients, and additionally the gut is sterile during the first few days of life. In normal infants, the plasma prothrombin concentration and the concentration of other vitamin K–dependent factors may decrease to 30 per cent of normal in the second and third weeks of life. If prothrombin values fall below 10 per cent, hemorrhagic disease of the newborn appears. It has been reported that breast-fed babies are at higher risk for vitamin K deficiency than are formula-fed infants.[185] Human milk contains 1 to 2 μg/L of phylloquinone (vitamin K_1), whereas cow's milk contains 5 to 17 μg/L.[186] Because of these factors, Seeler[187] recommended that breast-fed babies receive 1 mg of phylloquinone intramuscularly at birth. Menadione (vitamin K_3) should not be given because of its propensity to bind tissue sulfhydryl groups.[188]

The bleeding tendency in uremia has been found to be associated with a decrease in the vitamin K–dependent clotting factors.[189] As noted above, Pineo found 11 to 27 cases of vitamin K deficiency associated with chronic renal disease, and Ansell noted that renal disease predisposed patients to vitamin K deficiency. It is currently unknown whether this hemorrhagic tendency represents a change in the intestinal flora or a defect in the vitamin K–dependent, peptide-bound glutamate carboxylase in liver. It is suggested that phylloquinone be given periodically to patients with chronic renal disease.

Water-Soluble Vitamins

Vitamin B_1 (Thiamine)

By the year 1878 beriberi was a devastating disease of sailors in the Japanese Navy. The average number of cases treated medically annually from 1878 to 1883 was 323.5 per 1000 men.[190] Takaki, the Director General of the Japanese Navy, was greatly impressed with the superior health of British sailors as compared with the health of the Japanese. He studied the composition of food used in the sailors' diets, replaced a part of the polished rice (which was the mainstay of the Japanese sailor) with barley, and introduced evaporated milk and wheat. These changes resulted in the eradication of beriberi from the Japanese Navy. Unfortunately, Takaki incorrectly attributed the beneficial effects of his dietary reform to the provision of a more liberal protein allowance. Around 1896 C. Eijkman, a Dutch physician attached to the military in the Dutch Indies, made a momentous (although serendipitous) discovery in the research of thiamine nutriture. While conducting investigations on fowl, he tried to economize on their diet by feeding them scraps from the wards of the military hospital to which he was attached. The scraps consisted chiefly of cooked polished rice, and the fowl developed paralysis while on this diet. When Eijkman was no longer able to feed his experimental animals on scraps, he resorted to feeding them gaba (rice still in the husk) and on this diet the animals recovered. After extensive research, Eijkman came to the conclusion that a diet of overmilled rice was the chief cause of polyneuritis in fowls and beriberi in humans. Eijkman[191] was the first to interpret correctly the connection between excessive consumption of polished rice and the cause of beriberi. He concluded that rice contained an essential nutrient found chiefly in the husk and outer layers of the grain, which were removed in polishing.

Vordermann[192] eradicated beriberi from prison populations by substituting whole rice for polished rice. Fraser and Stanton[193] confirmed the deficiency theory as the cause of beriberi in animals and humans. In 1912 Funk[194] reported the isolation of a substance from rice polishings that cured beriberi and named it "vitamine." The product Funk isolated contained little of the active principle. As a consequence, the active substance was first successfuly isolated by Jansen and Donath in 1925.[195, 196] Jansen gave the vitamin the name aneurine. This nomenclature was not accepted in the United States, and the name was eventually replaced with thiamine (thiamin). In 1934 Williams isolated enough of the vitamin to allow determination of its structure.[197]

Clinical Signs of Deficiency. Beriberi has been endemic in the Orient for over 4000 years. In general, it develops in populations whose dietary staple is polished rice. It has also been observed in individuals subsisting on unenriched white flour. The symptoms of this disease are determined by the chronicity of the deficiency and stress factors that may alter the rate of metabolism of the vitamin.[198] Individuals who subsist on a diet that offers slightly less than the thiamine requirement may become gradually deficient and a peripheral neuropathy develops. In general, the extremities of maximal use are most affected. Paresthesia, hypesthesia, anesthesia, and weakness begin in the lower extremities. The muscles are often tender and may atrophy. Subsequently foot drop may occur. If the individual's intake has been considerably less than the requirement, the deficiency will be more severe and so-called "subacute" or "wet beriberi" will develop. In these individuals cardiovascular signs and symptoms also develop. Anorexia is a common manifestation. In 1917 Eddy and Roper successfully used a solution of thiamine extracted from sheep pancreas to counteract the loss of appetite of infants suffering from malnutrition.[199] The clinical manifestations of thiamine deficiency are universally present after 30 days of decreased intake, but depletion to the point producing clinical symptoms can be produced experimentally in humans in 12 to 14 days.

The most acute type of thiamine deficiency, Wernicke's encephalopathy, occurs primarily in alcoholics and in patients with excessive vomiting. Acute administration of glucose to such severely deprived patients may precipitate the development of encephalopathy. Manifestations range from mild confusion to coma. Ophthalmoplegia, sixth nerve weakness, and lateral and/or vertical nystagmus are seen; cerebellar ataxia is often present. If the patient survives, damage to the cerebral cortex may result in a psychosis (Korsakoff's). Confabulation and impairment of retentive memory are common characteristics.[200]

In 1917 Osborne and Mendel reported that food consumption of rats was directly dependent on the amount of thiamine in the diet.[201] This led to the convention of basing the thiamine requirement on the caloric intake of mammals. A minimal requirement using this convention was demonstrated by Cowgill as follows:

Vitamin B_1 requirement (IU) = .00142 × wt (kg) × caloric intake (1 IU of thiamine = 3 μg of pure thiamine).[202] This formula gives the minimal requirement for thiamine; the optimal requirement is thought to be much greater.[203]

The early investigations into the role of thiamine in human nutrition prior to 1940 showed a link to many human ailments.[204] Thiamine was thought important not only to carbohydrate metabolism, but also as a cause of anorexia, achlorhydria, peptic ulcer disease, and constipation, in addition to the known cardiac and neurologic defects. Jolliffe detailed the signs of thiamine deficiency as related to neurologic deficits.[205]

Biologic Functions of Thiamine. The active form of thiamine in tissues is thiamine pyrophosphate. This compound functions as a coenzyme in the decarboxylation of α-keto acids and as a cofactor for the transketolase reaction in the hexose-monophosphate shunt. In thiamine deficiency, plasma levels of pyruvic and lactic acids are elevated. This fact has been explained by the role of thiamine in the decarboxylation of pyruvate to acetyl CoA (via pyruvate dehydrogenase). The decrease in energy produced from the citric acid cycle in thiamine deficiency results in stimulation of the glycolytic pathway. The greater flux through this pathway and the inhibition of pyruvate dehydrogenase activity result in increased concentrations of pyruvate and lactate in the plasma.

The transketolase reaction is important in the phosphogluconate pathway, which carries out the interconversion of 3-,4-,6-, and 7-carbon sugars. This pathway is an important source of NADPH and is a scavenger pathway for excessive ribose-5-phosphate.

Thiamine deficiency has been shown to decrease the ability of glial cells to synthesize fatty acids and cholesterol.[206] Since experimental studies in animals indicate that the site of early lesions of thiamine deficiency is in the glial cells,[207] the data provided by Volpe and Morasa suggest a biochemical basis for the changes in cellular structures seen in the neuropathy associated with thiamine deficiency.

Singh has demonstrated that thiamine deficiency induces a reduction in body weight, pancreatic protein, and digestive enzyme content in Sprague-Dawley rats while increasing protein and digestive enzyme secretion from the pancreas.[208]

Methods for Assay.   There are various methods for assay of thiamine in biologic materials, including animal and microbiologic assays. A currently accepted method evaluates erythrocyte transketolase activity following incubation of hemolyzed red cells with and without added thiamine pyrophosphate. The increase in activity with the addition of thiamine pyrophosphate is a measure of the degree to which the enzyme is unsaturated with thiamine pyrophosphate and thus an indication of the degree of thiamine deficiency.[209, 210] A recent modification, which uses leukocyte transketolase activity, seems more responsive to rapid changes in thiamine nutriture.[211]

It has been of considerable interest that chronic alcoholic patients with Wernicke-Korsakoff encephalopathy may have a reduction in plasma thiamine pyrophosphate concentrations without a change in total erythrocyte transketolase activity.[212] To explain this fact, Blass and Gibson have postulated that an abnormality in the kinetic properties in the transketolase enzyme is responsible for the relatively small population of chronic alcoholics who develop the Wernicke-Korsakoff syndrome.[213] These investigators found that although the transketolase total activity was essentially the same in fibroblasts from patients with Wernicke-Korsakoff syndrome as in those of control individuals, the Michaelis constant (K_m) for thiamine pyrophosphate for transketolase was markedly different in the two sets of fibroblasts. The patients demonstrated a K_m that was an order of magnitude greater than that in the control individuals. This phenomenon would lead to a more rapid loss of enzyme activity and subsequent thiamine depletion. This disorder also appears to be present in the transketolase from erythrocytes in patients with Wernicke-Korsakoff syndrome.[214]

Read[215] proposed that some instances of sudden infant death syndrome might result from thiamine deficiency. This hypothesis, however, has not been substantiated.[216]

Thiamine-Responsive Inborn Errors of Metabolism.   At least four diseases have been linked to thiamine-responsive inborn errors in metabolism.

1. Pyruvic acidemia, a disease characterized by elevated values of pyruvic acid in the bloodstream, can be explained by interference with pyruvate dehydrogenase activity and has been shown to be responsive to increased thiamine intake. Subacute necrotizing encephalomyelopathy (SNE) responds well to thiamine supplementation. The remissions of SNE correlate well with high thiamine levels in the cerebrospinal fluid. Several thiamine derivatives, which promote higher plasma thiamine levels, appear to be more efficacious than thiamine hydrochloride in raising the level of cerebrospinal fluid.[217]

2. Maple syrup urine disease (MSUD) has been shown to respond to pharmacologic doses of thiamine.[218, 219]

3. A thiamine-responsive megaloblastic anemia has been reported.[220, 221] The two children reported on responded to daily doses of 100 mg of thiamine hydrochloride administered parenterally. Reticulocyte count and hemoglobin markedly increased after 4 to 5 days of administration of the supplementary thiamine.

Occurrence of Thiamine Deficiency.   Thiamine deficiency detected by biochemical assay is present in 25 per cent of the alcoholics admitted to general hospitals in the United States.[222, 223] A recent review has also shown that a deficiency of thiamine and thiamine pyrophosphate is present in about 10 per cent of the elderly in the United States.[224] Alcohol intake appears to be the most important factor affecting bioavailability of thiamine at all ages. Possible interference with absorption of thiamine supplements by coffee has been reported by

Somogyi and Naegel.[225] Certain thiaminases can be reversed by supplemental thiamine.[226] It has been suggested that the deleterious effects of coffee, tea, and raw fish may be obviated by increasing thiamine supplementation in the diet.[226] This latter generality, with its obvious importance to current dietary practice, awaits elucidation.

A recent study by Wood and coworkers, using a double-blind approach to partial thiamine restriction in volunteer healthy subjects for a period of 4 to 5 weeks, demonstrated an effective method for assessing subclinical thiamine deficiency. These workers defined subclinical thiamine deficiency as a low urinary thiamine level (27 μg of thiamine per gm of creatinine) together with a thiamine pyrophosphate effect above 14.2 per cent and below 35.4 per cent.[227]

Riboflavin

On the basis of their experiments with rats on a diet of polished rice, McCollum and Davis concluded that there were only two unidentified nutrients necessary for the rat: an antineuritic substance and a pellagra-preventive factor. This theory was widely accepted for some time. The existence of still another nutrient, designated at various times as vitamin B_2, P-P, and G, was the subject of much investigation and discussion between 1919 and 1933. The term "vitamin B_2" was adopted by English investigators, while vitamin G was commonly used by American investigators. The name finally adopted was riboflavin. Although this water-soluble, yellow-green fluorescent compound had been known since the nineteenth century to be present in whey,[228] it was not isolated and shown to be a part of the vitamin B-complex until 1933.[229] In 1933 Booher[230] confirmed the fact that the growth property of whey was associated with this pigment. In 1935 the synethesis of riboflavin was accomplished by Kuhn[231] and Karrer.[232]

Other studies showed riboflavin deficiency to retard growth and cause dermatitis and cataracts in rats and to induce sudden death in dogs and rapidly acute paralysis of the main peripheral nerve trunks in chicks. Prolonged riboflavin deficiency in dogs results in neurologic abnormalities accompanied by myelin degeneration of the peripheral nerves and posterior columns of the spinal cord. In humans riboflavin deficiency results in inflammation of the lips, fissures at the mouth angles, glossitis, dermatitis, and vascularizing keratitis.[233] Kruse et al. suggested that riboflavin deficiency in humans could be diagnosed by observing corneal vascularization.[234, 235] They pointed out that the ophthalmic changes in riboflavin deficiency were those that had often been described as "toxic state," "focal infection," and "eye strain."

The first description of the clinical findings that were subsequently known as ariboflavinosis was published by Stanis in 1912.[236] An excellent comprehensive review of the medical, nutritional, physiologic, and biochemical knowledge concerning riboflavin prior to 1975 is found in a monograph by Rivlin.[237]

Hormones and drugs have been recognized as agents that regulate the absorption, utilization, metabolic transformations, binding, and excretion of riboflavin. Riboflavin must be converted into its coenzyme derivatives before it becomes fully active. Therefore, the metabolic conversion of riboflavin to its coenzymes flavin mononucleotide (FMN) and flavin adenine dinucleotide (FAD) offers an opportunity for the action of hormones and drugs to control riboflavin metabolism. In experimental animals thyroid hormone enhances the conversion of FMN and FAD.[238–240] The major site of action of thyroid hormone appears to be flavokinase, the enzyme responsible for catalyzing the formation of FMN from riboflavin. Doses of thyroxine in the physiologic range augment hepatic flavokinase in the rat.[241] Thyroid hormones also increase the activity of FAD pyrophosphorylase, which catalyzes the formation of FAD from FMN. In hypothyroidism, hepatic flavokinase activity is decreased. In addition the formation of FMN and FAD from riboflavin and the tissue concentrations of these coenzymes are reduced.[242, 243] Thyroid hormone also affects the fraction of flavins that is bound, predominantly to tissue proteins.[244] These findings indicate that thyroid hormones exert sensitive control over riboflavin metabolism. As a consequence, there may be a theoretical role for therapeutic administration of riboflavin both in hypothyroidism (due to decreased formation of the metabolically active coenzyme derivatives) and hyperthyroidism, if vitamin B_2 intake is marginal (due to the greater-than-normal conversion of riboflavin into FMN and FAD, which might decrease vitamin reserves).

Fazekas and Sandor[245] showed in experimental animals that ACTH administration greatly augments the formation of FMN and FAD from riboflavin in the adrenal cortex. Also the administration of ACTH to intact rats increased the formation of FMN from riboflavin in the kidney and liver.[246]

Tan and Trachewsky[247] demonstrated the direct effect of aldosterone in augmenting the rate of formation of the flavin coenzymes from riboflavin in the rat kidney. This effect is blocked by simultaneous treatment with the aldosterone antagonist spironolactone. These investigators were able to interfere with the sodium-conserving effect of aldosterone in the kidney by treating animals with structural analogs of riboflavin that inhibit the conversion of riboflavin to FMN. It was suggested that the role of aldosterone in increasing the tubular reabsorption in the kidney may be related to and possibly dependent upon enhancement of FMN and FAD biosynthesis.[248] The structural analogs of riboflavin that were used did not blunt the effects of aldosterone to increase potassium excretion. These findings suggested that structural analogs of riboflavin may find application in the treatment of sodium retention due to hyperaldosteronism without altering body potassium stores.

Owing to the remarkable structural similarities between riboflavin, FMN, and FAD and the phenothiazine nucleus, Pinto et al. investigated the effects of drugs of this class upon the conversion of riboflavin to FMN and FAD.[249] These studies revealed that treatment of normal rats with chlorpromazine markedly inhibited the conversion of riboflavin to FAD and antagonized thyroxine stimulation of FAD formation. Chlorpromazine appears to act as a competitive inhibitor of flavokinase.[250] Further work by these investigators demonstrated that chlorpromazine, at doses comparable to those used clinically in the treatment of psychiatric patients, alters overall riboflavin status in the rat.[251] Since preliminary evidence suggests that tricyclic antidepressants, which also have structural features in common with riboflavin, inhibit FAD formation from riboflavin in a manner similar to that of chlorpromazine, these findings suggest that treatment with psychotrophic drugs may further impair the marginal nutritional status of psychiatric patients, who in general eat poorly.

The light sensitivity of riboflavin has been known for many years. Newborn infants with hyperbilirubinemia are frequently treated with phototherapy. Many of these infants have been shown to have an elevated activity coefficient of erythrocyte glutathione reductase.[252] The longer the duration of therapy, the greater the degree of abnormality in the activity coefficient. The likelihood of decomposition of riboflavin during phototherapy suggests that administration of this vitamin may be advisable during the neonatal period. Another advantage of riboflavin supplementation may be that of stimulating photodegradation of bilirubin. Pascale et al. demonstrated, in a group of newborn infants receiving riboflavin supplementation, that the serum bilirubin decreased at a rate 50 per cent greater than in a comparable group of infants who were untreated except for the phototherapy.[253]

As with thiamine, specific binding proteins have been demonstrated for riboflavin.[254] A vital role of flavin-binding protein in the transfer of riboflavin across the placenta is suggested by the observation that passive immunization of pregnant rats (4 to 16 days) to riboflavin carrier proteins but not to ovalbumin resulted in fetal absorption.[255]

Deficiency of riboflavin has been believed by some to be associated with cataract formation.[256] This concept has been disputed in animal studies. Skalka and Prchal demonstrated no statistical evidence of increased riboflavin deficiency among idiopathic presenile patients with cataracts.[257] They concluded that riboflavin deficiency, to the extent that it occurs in racially mixed southeastern American populations composed of both rural and urban persons of generally low economic means, did not appear to be the cause of early cataract formation. They did not rule out the fact that low riboflavin intake or enzymatic abnormalities resulting in impaired riboflavin utilization could, over a period of years, lead to an increase in cataract formation, however. This conclusion is substantiated by the work of Bhat and Gopalan,[258, 259] who evaluated the possible relationship between riboflavin deficiency, galactose metabolism, and cataract formation. They concluded that riboflavin did not lead to cataract formation in rats, except those on high-galactose diets. In addition, patients with riboflavin deficiency had normal galactose metabolism. Patients with cataracts had a higher incidence of biochemical riboflavin deficiency and abnormal galactose tolerance. However, treatment with riboflavin did not improve galactose tolerance.

Recent work by Vir et al. demonstrated that riboflavin deficiency, as determined by the erythrocyte glutathione reductase activation test, was present in 26 of 60 pregnant women in their study. In comparison there was no evidence of riboflavin deficiency in 20 nonpregnant age-matched controls. The mean intake of riboflavin in the pregnant group was higher than the recommended intake and revealed a significant negative correlation with activity coefficient values during the third trimester period. There was no significant correlation of riboflavin status with outcome of pregnancy.[260] This fact is of obvious concern owing to the well-known teratogenic nature of riboflavin deficiency.[261]

Since 1943 several studies have indicated that riboflavin deficiency retards the growth of certain tumors in animals and possibly in humans,[262] limits the growth of certain types of spontaneous and transplanted cancers, and enhances azo dye carcinogenesis. Neoplasms are resistant to riboflavin depletion and maintain FAD levels. However, Morris and Robertson[263] observed that tumor growth began to decline at the same time that total riboflavin levels in tumors began to fall. In addition it has been shown that highly malignant Novikoff hepatoma grown intraperitoneally did not modify hepatic riboflavin or FMN or FAD concentrations in either normal or riboflavin-deficient rats. Lane and Smith[264] showed that riboflavin deficiency (induced by dietary means in combination with a galactoflavin) had an antitumor effect in humans, a finding that may be of value in the treatment of polycythemia vera and lymphoma. The mechanism underlining the antitumor effect of riboflavin deficiency is not totally clear.

Riboflavin has been shown to be required for the conversion of pyridoxine to pyridoxal phosphate. In riboflavin deficiency this conversion rate is low. It has been suggested that oral lesions considered characteristic of riboflavin deficiency may actually be due to cellular deficiency of pyridoxal phosphate.[265-267]

The current method of choice for estimating riboflavin nutritive is the erythrocyte glutathione measurement.[268, 269] Goodman has recently shown in experimental animal models that riboflavin deficiency is accompanied by a complex organic aciduria dominated by acidic metabolites of the substrates of FAD-dependent acyl-CoA dehydrogenases.[270] These abnormalities have not as yet been reported in riboflavin deficiency in humans.

Supplementation of riboflavin may be improved by the use of riboflavin tetrabutyrate. The half-life of this compound, which is a fat-soluble ester of riboflavin, is markedly higher than that of riboflavin in human volunteers.[271] This form of riboflavin seems to have a deposit-type action in humans and may be extremely useful clinically in situations in which daily supplementation is difficult or tissue stores are rapidly depleted. Drugs such as tetracyclines and oral contraceptives are known to have adverse effects on the riboflavin economy of the body. Therapy with riboflavin tetrabutyrate may prove useful in these situations.

Pyridoxine

The continuing search for the factors present in the vitamin B complex led to the discovery that a specific type of rat skin lesion accompanied by pink or florid dermatitis (acrodynia) resulted from lack of a factor that was first called vitamin B_6, then adermin, and subsequently pyridoxine. The presence of this vitamin was suggested by György in 1934[272] and first described as a filtrate factor I by Lepkovsky, Jukes, and Krause in 1936.[273] This factor was apparently identical to that referred to as the "Y factor" by Chick and Copping.[274] The vitamin was isolated and chemically identified in six laboratories in the same year. Lepkovsky, György, Kuhn, Ichiba, Emerson, and Keresztesy, Harris, and Folkers synthesized the vitamin in 1939.[275, 276] Several excellent reviews of vitamin B_6 metabolism are available.[277-279]

Vitamin B_6 occurs as pyridoxine, pyridoxal, pyridoxamine, and pyridoxal phosphate. Pyridoxal phosphate and, to a lesser extent, pyridoxamine are essential cofactors for many amino acid metabolizing systems including transaminases, decarboxylases, and dehydratases. Many of the neurotransmitters or inhibitors of neurotransmitters are formed by decarboxylation of amino acid derivatives. Because of its close involvement with neurotransmitters, it is not surprising to find that vitamin B_6 deficiency results in disorders of the central nervous system. In addition, pyridoxal phosphate is required in the synthesis of heme and the hemoproteins. In general, estimates of the state of pyridoxine nutriture in humans have been based on clinical signs, excretion of tryptophan metabolites, measurement of serum and erythrocyte transaminases, and the urinary excretion of pyridoxine or its metabolites.

The first evidence for the essentiality of pyridoxine for the human was reported in 1949.[280] In this report patients with poor diets were observed to have a deficiency syndrome characterized by weakness, irritability, nervousness, insomnia, and difficulty in walking. Relief was obtained within 24 hours when pyridoxine was administered. Shortly thereafter pyridoxine was reported to be effective in healing cheilosis that did not respond to riboflavin.[281] The reason for this latter effect was demonstrated 30 years later when the interrelationship between riboflavin and pyridoxine became apparent. It is now known that riboflavin is required for the conversion of pyridoxine to pyridoxal phosphate. In riboflavin deficiency, this conversion rate is low.[282]

Recent studies indicate that orolingual lesions, previously considered characteristic of riboflavin deficiency, represent cellular deficiency of pyridoxal phosphate secondary to riboflavin-controlled activation of pyridoxine and, in a significant proportion of cases, may be due to a deficiency of vitamin B_6 itself.[285, 286] Vitamin B_6 deficiency can be rapidly produced in humans within one week on a deficient diet. It can be accelerated by ingestion of various substances, such as penicillamine, desoxypyridoxine, isonicotinic hydrazide, toxopyrimidine, and cycloserine. There is a rapid reduction of blood levels of the vitamin and activity of vitamin B_6–requiring enzymes, depending on their rank order of binding capacity. Urinary excretion of B_6 vitamers is reduced as is the production of the metabolite pyridoxic acid. In addition the tryptophan loading test becomes positive with increased excretion of xanthurenic acid and 3-hydroxykynurenine. The original relationship between vitamin B_6 deficiency and xanthurenic acid excretion was determined by the findings of Lepkovsky. He observed that when slightly alkaline, the urine of pyridoxine-deficient rats was green. The urine was not green when

excreted, but became green upon contact with the iron in the metabolism cages used for these studies.[287] This precursor was later identified as xanthurenic acid, a product of tryptophan metabolism.[288] Eventually the classic test for pyridoxine nutritional status was devised. This test uses an ingested tryptophan load and collection of urine for measuring the presence of xanthurenic acid and 3-hydroxykynurenine.

Plasma levels of pyridoxal phosphate were found to be significantly lower in 22 of 31 patients with decompensated cirrhosis or subacute hepatic necrosis. Only one third of these patients responded to intravenous pyridoxal supplementation with an increase in pyridoxal phosphate. Because pyridoxic acid excretion increased after administration of both pyridoxine and pyridoxal phosphate, it was concluded that vitamin B_6 deficiency may be due to an increased rate of pyridoxal phosphate degradation.[289]

Because of the widespread distribution of vitamin B_6 among foods, major outbreaks of vitamin B_6 deficiency have not been observed throughout the world. Nevertheless, greater attention has been paid in recent years to the vitamin B_6 nutriture of humans because of the ease with which it is depleted, its participation in numerous metabolic functions, association with brain metabolism and development, apparent increased needs in pregnancy, antagonism by certain drugs and hormones, and marked losses in food processing. The bioavailability of vitamin B_6 in foods has been found to vary widely. Dietary fiber may exert a weak inhibitory effect on the utilization of the vitamin. Food processing and storage exert variable effects on the bioavailability of vitamin B_6, probably as a function of the vitamin distribution, food composition, and conditions of processing and storage.[290] A major portion of the aldehydic vitamers of vitamin B_6, mainly pyridoxal and its phosphorylated analog, react reversely with certain amino acid residues within food materials to form aldimine and aldamine compounds. A significant fraction of the aldimine (Schiff base) forms become reduced during thermal processing and thereby forms pyridoxylamino compounds, particularly with lysine, that are less biologically active.[291–293]

Rats reared on a high-protein, pyridoxine-free diet showed osteoporotic osseous changes in the tail and limb girdles with accompanying loss of O-phosphorylethanolamine (OPE) phosphorylase activity of the liver and increased urinary excretion of OPE. This finding is not surprising since OPE phosphorylase has pyridoxal phosphate as a coenzyme. The osteoporotic bone changes, however, appear to be the first report of this type of bone disease in vitamin B_6 deficiency.[294] This finding assumes clinical importance since OPE levels of urine have been shown to be high in juvenile and adult forms of the human genetic disease hypophosphatasia, which is characterized by osteoporosis and decreased serum and bone alkaline phosphatase. Osteoporotic bone changes have also been observed in cystinuria, a disease in which the defect lies in another pyridoxal phosphate enzyme, cystathionine synthetase.

Various biochemical procedures have been developed and used in the evaluation of B_6 nutritional status:[295, 296] tryptophan load test, urinary excretion of vitamin B_6, urinary excretion of 4-pyridoxic acid, blood transaminase activities, and blood vitamin B_6 concentration. Recently two new assays have been reported for measuring B_6 vitamer levels in human plasma. Guilarte and McIntyre have described a radiometric-microbiologic assay of vitamin B_6 in plasma.[297] Vanderslice et al. have recently reported methods for vitamin B_6 vitamer analysis in human plasma by using high-performance liquid chromatography.[298]

Vitamin B_{12}

In 1822 Combe reported a case of anemia which she described as due to "some disorder of the digestive and assimilative organs."[299] Because this anemia was invariably fatal it became known as "pernicious anemia." The nutritional basis of pernicious anemia was suggested by Flint in 1860.[300] It was not until 69 years later, however, that Castle demonstrated that normal human gastric secretion contained an "intrinsic factor" that combines with an "extrinsic factor" contained in animal protein to result in the absorption of the substance capable of relieving the anemia of these patients.[301] In 1948 vitamin B_{12} was isolated.[302, 303] Later that same year, Berk and associates showed that vitamin B_{12} was both the "extrinsic factor" and the "anti-pernicious anemia principle."[304]

A comprehensive review of the chemistry, causes of nutritional deficiency, nutri-

tional requirements and sources, metabolic functions, therapy, and toxicity of vitamin B_{12} is given by Herbert.[305] The work of Castle on vitamin B_{12} deficiency helped develop the concept that all vitamin deficiencies of B_{12} (or any vitamin) can be derived by one of six ways: by *inadequate* ingestion, absorption, or utilization, or by *increased* requirement, excretion, or destruction of the vitamin.[306]

Sandberg and coworkers demonstrated that although human milk from well-fed mothers contains adequate amounts of cobalamin, the vitamin may become available only if there is sufficient proteolytic enzyme to release it from binding to an R-type binder.[307] In the intestine, cobalamin is transferred from the high affinity R-protein complex to the lower affinity intrinsic factor, owing to partial degradation of an R-protein by pancreatic proteases. Intrinsic factor is not modified by these pancreatic, proteolytic enzymes. This work was stimulated by the fact that almost 50 per cent of patients suffering from exocrine pancreatic dysfunction have malabsorption of vitamin B_{12}. The defect can be partially corrected with oral administration of bicarbonate or fully corrected with pancreatic extract of trypsin or chymotrypsin given orally. It is known that these patients produce normal amounts of intrinsic factor which is physiologically active when tested in patients with pernicious anemia. It has been inferred that in the acid environment of the stomach cobalamin may preferentially bind to R-protein rather than to intrinsic factor. In the alkaline environment of the intestine, however, pancreatic proteases would partially degrade R-protein or reduce its affinity for cobalamin. This would facilitate the transfer of cobalamin from the R-protein to intrinsic factor, which would then bind it exclusively and promote absorption. In exocrine pancreatic dysfunction, R-protein would not be degraded and cobalamin would remain bound to it, resulting in malabsorption.[308, 309]

Recent developments have shown the importance of the small intestine to the vitamin B_{12} nutriture of humans. The small intestine, as well as the colon, contains microflora which synthesize significant amounts of B_{12}. Individuals subsisting on a vegetarian diet depend on this source, as well as ingested microorganisms, for their vitamin B_{12} nutriture. Since B_{12} is synthesized only by microorganisms, animals must either eat the microorganisms or absorb the vitamin synthesized by gut flora. Although human feces are a rich source of vitamin B_{12},[310] this fecal vitamin B_{12} is not available to the individual since the vitamin is absorbed in the ileum. As a consequence, animal foods are the only sources of vitamin B_{12} for man. Since vitamin B_{12} deficiency is not seen to the extent expected in vegans and vegetarians, the source of vitamin B_{12} for these individuals has presented an interesting question. It has been recently shown that the small intestine is not totally sterile,[311] that individuals subsisting on vegetarian diets have a larger growth of gastrointestinal microflora,[312] and that the microflora in the small intestine synthesize significant amounts of vitamin B_{12}.[313]

In vitamin B_{12} deficiency, megalocytic changes can be found in the small intestine epithelium in association with decreased mitoses in the crypts and shortened villi. In the vitamin B_{12} deficiency of pernicious anemia, increased intraluminal bacteria are found in the upper small intestine as a consequence of achlorhydria.[315]

Because of the complexity of the vitamin B_{12} absorption mechanism, there are many sites at which genetic defects could alter vitamin B_{12} absorption. Sophisticated diagnostic techniques have led to identification of three unique vitamin B_{12} absorptive defects, which require different methods of treatment. The areas of potential defects include synthesis and secretion of normal intrinsic factor by the gastric parietal cells, binding of dietary vitamin B_{12} to intrinsic factor, binding of the vitamin B_{12} intrinsic factor complex to ileal receptor sites, release and transfer of B_{12} across the mucosal cells, and binding of B_{12} to transcobalamin II on the serosal side. A partial differential diagnosis as to etiology of the condition may be effected by use of modifications of the Schilling test.[316] A large dose (1 mg) of nonradioactive B_{12} is injected followed by an oral dose of 2 μg of vitamin B_{12} labeled with radioactive cobalt. Urinary excretion of the radioactive vitamin B_{12} is measured over the next 24 to 48 hours. Approximately one third of the oral radioactive dose is absorbed and excreted in the urine by normal individuals. Usually less than 2 per cent of the dose is excreted in the urine of patients with pernicious anemia. A modification of the Schilling test may be carried out with radioactive vitamin B_{12} plus normal human gastric juice as source of intrinsic factor. Vitamin B_{12} mal-

absorption due to defective or insufficient production of intrinsic factor would be corrected by supplying an exogenous source of normal intrinsic factor. This procedure would not overcome vitamin B_{12} malabsorption if ileal receptor sites or mucosal mechanisms were defective. Using this method, Katz et al. have described a patient with classic symptoms of pernicious anemia due to the synthesis of an intrinsic factor that was unable to bind to ileal receptors.[317] Hakami et al. have described two infant sisters with a defect in vitamin B_{12} metabolism due to complete absence of transcobalamin II.[318] In addition, MacKenzie et al. described three brothers with symptoms of vitamin B_{12} deficiency during adolescence. These patients had a defect in B_{12} absorption which occurred *after* the intrinsic factor B_{12} complex attached to the surface of the ileal cell, and *before* the absorbed vitamin bound to transcobalamin II in portal blood. In these cases diagnosis required modification of the Schilling test and chromatographic separation of the serum vitamin B_{12} binding proteins.

A reported relationship between dietary fiber and B_{12} balance showed that inclusion of either cellulose or pectin in a fiber-free basal diet increased the rate of B_{12} excretion in feces. In addition, pectin supplement stimulated a 9- to 21-fold increase in urinary excretion of methylmalonic acid. Because the urinary excretion of methylmalonic acid is characteristic of insufficient dietary vitamin B_{12}, these experiments demonstrated that addition of either 20-50 per cent or 5-20 per cent pectin enhanced the depletion of body stores of vitamin B_{12}. Since these data were from animal studies, it would be premature to view them as clear evidence of a hazard of fiber supplementation to the general public. However, it is important to be aware of the possibility that high intake of certain fibers could aggravate a precarious B_{12} balance of individuals with a history of poor dietary intake.[319]

Other words of caution regarding common medical therapy and B_{12} metabolism have been recently reported. Carmel has recently stressed the importance of evaluating patients with mild anemia and an elevated mean red cell volume for B_{12} deficiency.[320, 321] He stressed that many physicians, house staff, and medical students may not adhere strictly to the definition of anemia (hemoglobin levels of less than 14 gm/dl in men and less than 12 gm/dl in women) and that a double-digit hemoglobin level was inappropriately comforting to these clinicians. In 11 cases described by Carmel, subnormal hemoglobin values went unattended for three months to six years before pernicious anemia was diagnosed. Three patients reported by Carmel had normal serum vitamin B_{12} levels at a point in the course of their disease, which accounted for the delay in their diagnosis. Part of the reason for this relates to artifacts in the radioimmunoassay for serum cobalamin. Since the radioimmunoassay may detect inactive analogues of cobalamin and therefore distort the assay, the microbiologic assay for B_{12} may give a more reliable result. If immunoassays are used, pure intrinsic factor should be the binder employed.[322, 323] From these studies it appeared that initially the most clinically valuable parameter was the mean corpuscular volume. Vitamin B_{12} deficiency is thought to be rare in children. In general, the megaloblastic anemia of infancy in Western countries is associated most commonly with folic acid deficiency.[324] Congenital vitamin B_{12} deficiency has been described in infants of mothers who are strict vegetarians and who fed their offspring exclusively on breast milk. The mothers in this group had mild anemia, megaloblastic bone marrow, and depressed values of vitamin B_{12} in both plasma and milk. The infants presented with the characteristic syndrome which included adequate general nutrition, skin pigmentation, apathy, retardation, involuntary movement, anemia and megaloblastosis. All of these signs were rapidly corrected by small doses of vitamin B_{12}. This syndrome was originally described in infants in Indian mothers.[325] However, the same circumstances have been described in Western countries.[326]

The anesthestic gas nitrous oxide oxidizes cobalamin and thus inactivates methionine synthetase, which requires cobalamin as a coenzyme. The effects on folates in liver, kidney, marrow, plasma, and brain in rats breathing a 1:1 nitrous oxide-to-oxygen mixture has recently been described. There is loss of folate from tissues (most marked in the liver) that affects folate polyglutamates to a greater extent than folate monoglutamate. It is suggested that these changes are due to the actions of nitrous oxide in depressing tissue uptake of folate from plasma, in promoting loss of folate in the urine, and in inhibiting synthesis of folate polyglutamate. Returning the animals to a normal atmosphere leads to restoration of most of the pre–nitrous oxide folate levels within five days. The plasma folate, which rises on exposure to nitrous oxide, falls within several hours. The restoration of tissue folates does not take place if rats are placed on a low-folate diet after withdrawal from a nitrous oxide environment. Thus, the fall in tissue folate concentration is due to a loss from the body either by excretion or increased catabolism and not to a redistribution of folate. Return of normal folate levels requires a dietary source of folate.[327] Since this anesthetic gas is commonly used, the potential of this mechanism to lead to vitamin B_{12} oxidation and subsequent depletion of human folate stores deserves careful study.[328–330]

Normal perfused rat liver or suspensions of normal rat hepatocytes metabolize histidine only to formiminoglutamate and cannot oxidize formate to carbon dioxide. The isolated organ or cells thus behave like vitamin B_{12}- or folate-deficient tissue. This has been found to be caused by lack of methionine. The deduction made from these studies is that methionine is a key factor in regulating the availability of folate. Under conditions of low levels of methionine, the folate becomes trapped as 5-methyltetrahydrofolate as in vitamin B_{12} deficiency.[331]

In a series of patients with pernicious anemia, plasma leucine levels decreased with a concomitant elevation of beta-leucine (beta-amino-isocaproic acid). It is known that cobalamin-dependent synthesis of leucine from beta-leucine occurs in rat liver and human tissues.[332] This conversion requires B_{12} for the enzyme 2,3-aminomutase. The evidence presented that the rat and man have some capacity to synthesize the essential amino acid leucine seemingly counteracts the criteria for an essential amino acid. However, Poston points out that the "concept of essentiality is one based on the maintenance of nitrogen balance; any organism which cannot supply sufficient amounts of the amino acids by means of biosynthesis may be recognized as having an essential requirement for the amino acid. The ability or lack of ability to synthesize the amino acid does not determine essentiality." The magnitude of leucine synthesis via the beta-leucine pathway in higher animals relative to the leucine requirement has not been clearly established. From the data presented the plasma level of leucine on the average dropped by one third in patients with pernicious anemia. Patients with pernicious anemia often show markedly prolonged bleeding times but only mild to moderate thrombocytopenia. Their platelets reveal functional defects. In 1943 Minot and Strauss[333] reported that thrombosis may occur after B_{12} therapy. Smith[334] observed thrombotic episodes in 2 of 9 patients who were recovering from pernicious anemia with thrombocytopenia. These reports suggested that soon after vitamin B_{12} therapy there may be an overcorrection of the clotting defect seen in pernicious anemia and greater susceptibility to thrombosis. In a retrospective study of all patients diagnosed with severe vitamin B_{12} deficiency over a 10-year period, Levine demonstrated that within two weeks after initiation of B_{12} therapy, 10 per cent (of 21 patients) had well-documented thrombotic episodes. Thus, there is considerable strong suggestive evidence that enhanced platelet responsiveness and a greater risk of thrombotic episodes may follow with vitamin B_{12} therapy for pernicious anemia. Levine felt that after vitamin B_{12} therapy a population of new platelets with greater tendency for aggregation may emerge. The platelet defect observed in pernicious anemia differs from those observed in other conditions such as uremia, myeloproliferative syndromes, or aspirin effect.

Odd-numbered fatty acids have been found in lipids of patients with deranged vitamin B_{12} utilization. Since such patients exhibit neurologic disorders, emphasis has been placed on the alterations in fatty acid content and metabolism that occur in nervous tissue during B_{12} deficiency. Propionic acid has been shown to produce odd-numbered fatty acids when nerve slices are incubated in vitro.[335, 336] These studies tend to support the possibility that accumulation of methylmalonic acid and its precursor, propionic acid, is involved in the nervous system dysfunction in vitamin B_{12} deficiency.

A search for a useful animal model for the neurologic disturbances of vitamin B_{12} deficiency has shown that the vitamin B_{12}–depleted fruit bat appears to provide a very useful model for successfully inducing neurologic changes that closely resemble the subacute combined degeneration of the spinal cord seen in pernicious anemia.[337]

Biotin

Biotin has the biologic activity previously ascribed to vitamin H (egg white injury factor). When rats consumed diets containing large amounts of uncooked egg white, they were noted to develop a syndrome known as egg white injury. This syndrome is characterized by an eczema-like dermatitis, spasticity or paralysis of the hindlimbs, and development of a "spectacle eye" lesion due to circumocular loss of hair. The lesions produced by the diet result from consumption of the protein avidin in egg white, which interacts with biotin in the food as well as biotin produced in the gut of experimental animals. Daft et al.[338] showed that therapy with crystalline biotin would prevent dermatitis, myocardial necrosis, and the other lesions in rats produced by oral sulfa-based antibiotics. These compounds have been shown to interfere with intestinal bacterial growth in the synthesis of biotin. Oppel[339] had demonstrated that biotin is synthesized by organisms in the human gastrointestinal tract. Hamm and Scott[340] demonstrated that tetracycline-based antibiotics could inhibit biotin synthesis in the intestinal tract of the rat. Boyd and Sargent[341] reported that rodents on a biotin-deficient diet were susceptible to toxic effects of large oral doses of benzyl-penicillin. Also when starch was replaced in the diet by sucrose, there was a decreased synthesis of biotin in the gastrointestinal tract. Sydenstricker[342, 343] demonstrated that feeding humans a diet rich in egg whites could produce clinical manifestations of biotin deficiency in five weeks. The human volunteers developed a fine nonpruritic dermatitis, a grayish pallor of their skin and mucosa, depression, lassitude, somnolence, muscle pains, and hyperesthesia. Later these individuals developed anorexia, nausea, dermal reticulation, anemia, hypercholesterolemia, and electrocardiographic abnormalities. All signs and symptoms disappeared within five days of parenteral biotin therapy.

The regulatory aspects of biotin coenzyme function, biotin biosynthesis, transport and metabolism, and other aspects of biotin deficiency have recently been reviewed by McCormick.[344, 345] Biotin's role in clinical medicine has been recently reviewed by Roth.[346]

Although classic biotin deficiency in the adult human has only been demonstrated by human volunteers on diets containing large amounts of egg white protein, possible biotin deficiency in adults receiving long-term total parenteral nutrition has been reported by Inis and Allardyce.[347] In this report two adult patients receiving long-term total parenteral nutrition at home presented with severe hair loss. Both patients had extensive previous gastrointestinal resections, consumed no biotin orally, and had received no biotin parenterally. Supplementation with 200 μg of biotin per day along with other B-complex vitamins resulted in gradual regrowth of healthy hair. Unfortunately, no definitive assessment of biotin status was obtained in these patients before biotin supplementation was initiated.

Prior to 1979 there had been no refined biochemical analyses of the metabolic effects of human biotin deficiency. Sweetman et al.[348] reported a case of an 11-year-old boy with hyperuricemia and mental retardation who developed alopecia totalis and a generalized erythematous scaly dermatitis. Examination of urinary organic acid excretion revealed excretion of compounds indicative of a combined deficiency of beta-methyl-crotonyl-CoA carboxylase and propionyl-CoA carboxylase. Mixed leukocyte enzyme analyses confirmed these deficiencies. Dietary assessment indicated the child had been fed raw eggs exclusively for a period of six years prior to the investigation. Treatment of this patient with 1 mg of biotin orally per day and substitution of cooked for raw eggs alleviated most of the abnormal metabolites in the urine, and resolution of the dermatitis was demonstrated within 2 days. After 6 days of treatment, the enzyme activity and the leukocyte level had returned to normal and hair growth began after two weeks. This case provided the first evidence of specific decrease in enzyme activity in a human introduced by a dietary deficiency of biotin.

There are now a number of diseases known to be attributable to deficiencies of biotin-dependent enzymes. Each of these diseases causes severe disruption in metabolism and acid-base balance.

Four potentially biotin-deficient enzyme deficiency diseases have been described in the literature: propionyl CoA carboxylase deficiency, pyruvate carboxylase deficiency, beta-methyl-crotonyl CoA carboxylase deficiency, and multiple carboxylase deficiency. Of the various biotin-dependent carboxylase deficiency diseases, only the multiple car-boxylase defects have been shown unequivocally to be biotin-responsive in vitro and in vivo.[346] Since biotin has been administered to humans in doses as high as 40 mg/day without untoward effects,[349] it is suggested that patients suspected of having any one of the four inborn errors that are potentially biotin-dependent should be treated with pharmacologic doses of biotin pending biochemical diagnosis.[346]

Biotin may be measured in biologic samples by microbiologic assays.[295] Also gas chromatographic analyses of volatile short-chain fatty acids and their derivatives in urine and plasma can be performed rapidly. This methodology can be applied to make the initial diagnosis of any of the biotin-dependent disorders.[346, 350]

Vitamin C

The earliest known account of a disease which was probably scurvy was written by the Egyptians in the Papyrus Ebers in approximately 1500 B.C.[351] The disease was described by Hippocrates in 600 B.C.[352] and by Pliny in approximately 63 A.D.[353] A chronologic view of the history of scurvy from 1541 to 1753 is given in detail in the classical reference of James Lind.[354] A review of writings on scurvy up to 1920 is given by Hess.[355]

Once it had been found that certain foods contained a factor capable of preventing or curing scurvy, extensive work was undertaken to identify the active substance. One of the major difficulties in its isolation lay in the rapid destruction of physiologic activity by oxidation.

The actual isolation of ascorbic acid was accomplished independently in 1928 by two different laboratories. Szent-Györgyi isolated "hexuronic acid" from orange juice, cabbage juice, and adrenal glands.[356] Szent-Györgyi's isolation of vitamin C was a consequence of his study of oxidation systems. In his lectures he gave the following account:

The more I learned about this new substance, the more interesting it seemed to be. Eventually, I crystallized it, that is to say, peeled it out in a pure condition which made analysis possible. It was an acid and it seemed to be related to an unknown sugar which I called 'Ignose,' the substance itself being called 'Ignosic Acid.' But the editor of the journal to whom I sent my paper did not like jokes and rejected the name. 'Godnose' being no more successful, we agreed that the child's name should be "hexuronic acid." Later, with advancing knowledge of its structure it had to be rebaptised in haste and it is now called ascorbic acid (sometimes, cevitamic acid) because it is identical with vitamin C and prevents scurvy. In this way I became a father without wishing it, the father of a vitamin. Such accidents seem to happen even in science.[357]

Chemically, L-ascorbic acid (vitamin C) is a compound with the formula $C_6H_8O_6$. Both L-ascorbic acid and dehydro-L-ascorbic acid have anti-ascorbutic activity.

Ascorbic acid is derived primarily from plant foods, especially fresh, rapidly growing fruits or vegetables. Only a few species of animals—man, monkeys, and guinea pigs—need to consume ascorbic acid in their diet. Most species are able to synthesize ascorbic acid in vivo.[358] Burns has pointed out that the basic defect in metabolism in these animals is the inability to convert L-gulonolactone to L-ascorbic acid.[359]

Despite general agreement among nutritionists that ascorbic acid prevents or cures scurvy, the actual mechanisms involved are incompletely understood. Its function in collagen formation involves growth of fibroblasts, osteoblasts, and odontoblasts as well as its role in hydroxylation of proline and lysine previously linked in a peptide bond.[360, 361] Ascorbic acid also plays a role in neurotransmitter synthesis, particularly in the formation of norepinephrine from dopamine and the conversion of tryptophan to 5-hydroxytryptophan.[362, 363] Vitamin C is a potent reducing agent and thereby enhances the absorption of iron and inhibits the absorption of copper from the digestive tract. The vitamin aids in the formation of active compounds from tetrahydrofolates.[364] Massive doses of ascorbic acid, however, may have an adverse effect on the availability of vitamin B_{12}.[365]

Clinical Aspects of Vitamin C Metabolism. A role for ascorbic acid in the regulation of lipolysis has been suggested by Tsai et al.[366] These investigators found that ascorbic acid, along with ATP and magnesium chloride ($MgCl_2$), is found to be a cofactor required for the inactivation of adipose tissue lipase. These authors also found that hydrolytic deamidization of peptides and proteins is also accelerated by ascorbic acid.

The use of massive doses of vitamin C has generated heated discussion in the scientific literature as well as in the lay press. Several reports, which were largely uncontrolled, have claimed that large daily doses of ascorbic acid can have preventative or curative benefits in a variety of clinical conditions, including upper respiratory infections. It is known that immune responses are affected by nutritional deficiency.[367] Shilotri and Bhat have examined the role of vitamin C in phagocyte function[368] and found that ascorbic acid deficiency does not alter hydrogen peroxide production or bacterial killing in leukocytes. However, massive doses of vitamin C were found to significantly impair phagocyte microbicidal activity in vitro. More recently, Kay et al.[369] have shown that in humans, ascorbic acid deficiency, even at the scorbutic level, did not alter T-cell numbers or impair in vitro T-cell function. Numerous studies have suggested that vitamin C may play an important role in determining immunologic responsiveness, however. Ascorbic acid levels in polymorphonuclear leukocytes have been shown to fall rapidly with infection, and decreased macrophage migration has been seen during vitamin C deficiency.[370] Long[371] observed a decreased humoral response to diphtheria toxoid in guinea pigs on an ascorbate-deficient diet. Anthony[372] has presented in vitro evidence that cell-mediated immunity is impaired in vitamin C deficiency. Murata[373] reported a dramatic decrease in the incidence of post-transfusion hepatitis in patients following cardiac surgery who received pre- and post-operative administration of large doses of vitamin C. A subsequent study by Knodell et al.[374] was unable to show a significant difference in the incidence of post-transfusion hepatitis or the clinical course of hepatitis following treatment with vitamin C. This latter study has recently been criticized.[375, 376]

With the claims that megadoses of vitamin C could have a positive effect on many human ailments[377–379] and the subsequent supplementation of vitamin C in megadoses, it is pertinent to study the possible side effects of large doses of vitamin C. It has been shown that megadoses of vitamin C may be detrimental to patients with a tendency to form renal stones[380–382] and to those with glucose-6-phosphate dehydrogenase deficiency,[383] gastrointestinal disturbance,[380] vitamin C-dependent syndrome,[384] inactivation of vitamin B_{12},[385] and increasing lytic sensitivity of erythrocytes to hydrogen peroxide.[386] A recent study by Chen[387] demonstrated that high supplementation of vitamin C in diets with marginally adequate vitamin E significantly increased in vitro erythrocyte hemolysis and liver lipid peroxidation, and significantly lowered erythrocyte concentration of reduced glutathione and plasma concentration of vitamin E. The effect was one of lowering the overall antioxidant potential of the animal. A small increase in vitamin E in the diet counteracted the hemolytic and peroxidative effect of the high supplements of vitamin C. A greater increase in vitamin E supplement counteracted the effect of high supplementation of vitamin C to decrease the glutathione level and plasma vitamin E concentrations. These results indicated an adverse effect of high supplementation of vitamin C on tissue antioxidant potential, an effect that may be overcome by increasing supplementation with vitamin E. The author suggested that the vitamin E requirement may be increased by increasing vitamin C supplementation.

In 1939 Sure et al.[388] demonstrated that vitamin A deficiency decreased the tissue concentration of ascorbate. Adrenal dysfunction in vitamin A–deficient rats has been reported on numerous occasions.[389] Gruber et al. have demonstrated that depletion of liver vitamin A causes a decline in hepatic synthesis of vitamin C followed by a decrease in the activity of 3-beta-hydroxysteroid dehydrogenase. The decreased activity of this enzyme diminishes steroidogenic activity, which presumably stimulates the production of ACTH, resulting in physiologic changes of hyperplasia of the glomerulosa with infiltration of the zona fasciculata and a loss of the distinct boundary between the two zones. The authors suggest that adrenal dysfunction in vitamin A deficiency can be avoided if adequate supplies of vitamin C are assured. This work casts doubts on the theory that adrenal dysfunction is a direct consequence of the reduction of dietary vitamin A in these experimental animals.

Guinea pigs with a latent, chronic ascorbic acid deficiency have been shown to accumulate serum and tissue cholesterol and have a decreased conversion of label cholesterol into bile acids. In addition, the turnover time of labeled cholesterol is decreased in these animals. These results furthered the conclusions that adequate tissue concentrations of ascorbic acid are necessary for conversion of cholesterol to bile acids.[390–393]

Milne et al. have recently examined the effects of prolonged consumption of high levels of dietary ascorbic acid on copper metabolism and cholesterol in adult monkeys fed a diet low or marginal in copper. They noted small reductions in serum copper and serum ceruloplasmin concentrations when high levels of ascorbic acid were fed. During the period of copper depletion, there was a gradual increase in serum cholesterol. When copper was added back to the diet, serum cholesterol levels stabilized or declined in the monkeys receiving the low dose of ascorbic acid. Cholesterol levels continued to increase in the group receiving the high ascorbic acid supplement (25 mg/kg body weight/day). These data suggested that high levels of ascorbic acid supplementation may make dietary copper relatively unavailable for regulating cholesterol metabolism.[394] This ascorbate-copper interaction has been suggested to involve stereo-specific postabsorption roles for L-ascorbate and the metabolism of copper.[395]

Dietary and urinary ascorbic acid studies[396, 397] have suggested that ascorbic acid deficiency occurs in alcoholics. It has been shown that the clearance of ethanol from the blood is proportional to the leukocyte ascorbic acid concentration.[398] Fazio et al.[399] have recently evaluated the acute effects of ethanol on plasma ascorbic acid in healthy subjects. When 35 gm of ethanol was ingested with ascorbic acid and breakfast, plasma ascorbic acid concentrations were significantly lower for at least 24 hours. These findings indicated that ethanol may reduce the availability of ascorbic acid from food and predispose to ascorbic acid deficiency.

Prolonged warming of meals has been shown to have deleterious effects on ascorbic acid content and iron absorption.[400] Hallberg et al. showed that meals kept warm at 75°C for four hours had a markedly reduced content of ascorbic acid. Most of this reduction occurred during the first hour. The content of ascorbate was closely correlated with non-heme iron absorption, and thus the prolonged warming of meals significantly depressed non-heme iron bioavailability. Iron bioavailability was completely restored when the ascorbate content of the meal was restored.

Oral administration of 200 mg of ascorbic acid daily for two months has been shown to restore normal chemotaxis, degranulation, and bactericidal activity to leukocytes taken from patients with Chédiak-Higashi syndrome. Improved function was accompanied by a return of the greatly elevated levels of cyclic AMP to near normal values.[401]

Altered vitamin C levels are common in both the plasma and blood white cells of institutionalized elderly people.[402] Schorah et al. have recently shown in a double-blind placebo trial of 94 elderly "long-term" inpatients known to have initially low levels of plasma and leukocyte vitamin C that at the end of two months' treatment, plasma and leukocyte vitamin C had increased considerably in those patients receiving vitamin C supplements. In this group of patients, there were slight but significant increases in the mean value for body weight, plasma albumin, and prealbumin compared with those receiving placebo therapy. There was also some clinical improvement as indicated by reduction in purpura and petechial hemorrhages in those receiving vitamin C.[403]

Measurement of Vitamin C Status. Quantitative estimation of L-ascorbic acid is generally accomplished by taking advantage of its reducing properties. A popular method is that which measures total ascorbic acid using 2,4-dinitrophenylhydrazine.[404] A summary of multiple methods for assessing vitamin C nutriture is given by Sauberlich et al.[405] A precise and specific technique employing L-ascorbic acid that has been radiolabeled for use with either ^{14}C or ^{3}H has been reported.[406]

Folic Acid

Initial reports of a disease that was probably folate deficiency were concerned with a severe form of anemia in pregnancy and the puerperium which was often fatal, especially when it resulted from several pregnancies superimposed on a bad diet.[407, 408] Evidence for the hypothesis that this anemia was different from that of B_{12} deficiency emerged from the work of Wills, who described a macrocytic anemia in Indian women, usually associated with pregnancy, that responded to therapy with a commercial preparation of autolyzed yeast.[409] Gradually, over the next few years, it became apparent that the Wills factor was actually folic acid. This conclusion was aided by the purification of pteroylglutamic acid in 1943 by Stokstad.[410] Folic acid proved to be not only the Wills' factor but also the vitamin contained in dried brewer's yeast which corrected the anemia, leukopenia, diarrhea, and gingivitis of monkeys studied by Day et al.[411] Snell and Peterson[412] showed that this compound was essential to the growth of *Lactobacillus casei* (therefore, called the "*L. casei*" factor). The term "folic acid" was given by Mitchell et al. because they found this material in a leafy vegetable (spinach).[413]

As tetrahydrofolic acid (THFA), this vitamin participates in transfers of single carbon units. Formyl, hydroxymethyl, methyl, methenyl, methylene, and formimino groups are transferred enzymatically to from THFA to other compounds. These reactions permit the degradation of histidine, the conversion of serine to glycine and of homocysteine to methionine, and the synthesis of purine and pyrimidine bases.

Folate in plasma appears to be distributed in three fractions. Free folate and that folate loosely bound to low-affinity binders are of similar magnitude; much less folate is bound to high-affinity binders. Low-affinity binding is nonspecific and is similar to nonspecific binding of bilirubin and various drugs to many different plasma proteins. The potential binding capacity is much greater than the amount of folate in serum. Current data suggest that there is only one type of high-affinity serum folate binder. These are glycoproteins with a molecular weight of 40,000. These glycoproteins are probably granulocyte-derived but modified by liver and perhaps kidney.[414] These binders carry less than 5 per cent of serum folate. The high-affinity, specific folate binder concentrations are elevated in adult females and neonates, and in pregnancy. Since the concentration of this binder is not altered in folate deficiency, it appears that these binders are induced by estrogenic hormones.[415–416] Higher levels of a folate-binding protein in human umbilical cord blood, different from that seen in maternal serum, have been observed.[417] This protein may be involved in the mechanism of increased folate uptake against a concentration gradient in the fetus. Specific folic acid–binding proteins have been detected in a variety of tissues such as serum, leukocytes, liver, kidney, intestinal epithelium, and milk. The in vitro uptake of folate by bacterial cells and rapidly dividing tumor cells has been found to be reduced when folate was bound to folic acid–binding protein from milk.[418, 419] A direct role of binders in promoting absorption of folate has been proposed but not proved.[418] In vitro uptake of folate by intestinal cells has been shown to be more efficient when folate is bound to proteins in milk. Unlike free folate, bound folate uptake is not affected by the addition of diphenylhydantoin or glucose to the medium.[420] Analysis of folic acid–binding kinetics using Scatchard and Hill plots indicates that pasteurization or subsequent processing induces alterations in binding cooperation, its pH dependence, or both. These results suggest that partial denaturation during pasteurization alters the folacin-binding characteristics and extent of molecular interaction of the folic acid–binding protein. These changes may be responsible for the reported differences between raw and pasteurized milk products and their ability to enhance folic acid absorption.[421]

Prior to the absorption of folic acid, glutamates are split off the side chain of the polyglutamate molecule by conjugases. The hydrolysis of polyglutamyl folate to simple forms has generally not been considered a rate-limiting step in the process of overall absorption of dietary folates.[422] Kesavan and Noronha have recently shown decreased hydrolysis of polyglutamyl folates in a group of aged rats.[423] These authors have suggested that dietary folates are preferentially hydrolyzed to absorbable forms by a luminal folyl conjugase of pancreatic origin. They relate that the overall enzyme levels are much lower in the pancreas of aged rats, leading to reduced availability of absorbable dietary folates and resulting in folate malabsorption in these animals. They further suggest that the intestinal mucosal conjugase does not play a significant role in the physiologic absorption of dietary folates.[423] This finding may help explain the findings by Baker et al. of an occurrence of folate deficiency in a human population over 70 years of age despite adequate dietary folate intake.[424]

Clinical Aspects of Folate Metabolism. Clinical investigation has shown that folate metabolism is affected by ethanol at the level of intestinal absorption,[425] hepatic storage,[426] and availability for hematopoiesis.[427]

Belaiche et al. have reported a folate-losing gastropathy that can produce folate deficiency in patients with giant hypertrophic gastritis (Ménétrier's disease). In these patients, the small intestine does not compensate for the gastric loss by reabsorption of that folate which has been lost from the blood into the gastric lumen.[428]

Methods of Assessing Folate Status. The dominant folate in serum and red blood cells is 5-methyltetrahydrofolate; therefore, folate assays must be capable of measuring this derivative. The only microbiologic assay that adequately measures serum and red cell folate in humans uses *L. casei*. A review of standard methods of folate assessment is given by Sauberlich et al.[429] A technique has been developed for the simultaneous radioisotope determination of serum vitamin B_{12} and folate in the same test tube.[430] A test for detection of previous deficiency in a folate-treated patient and hidden deficiency in association with iron deficiency has been described.[431, 432] This test depends on the presence of two alternative pathways for the synthesis of the nucleotide thymidylic acid which is incorporated in the DNA. Thymidylic acid can be synthesized from deoxyuridylic acid but requires sufficient folic acid in the folic acid cycle. Mammalian tissues also possess an alternative so-called salvage pathway where thymidine is incorporated into thymidylic acid directly. If adequate folic acid is present, added deoxyuridine can form thymidylic acid and thus suppress thymidine incorporation. If the thymidine is radioactively labeled, this suppression or lack thereof can be measured. This deoxyuridine suppression test does not appear to be technically complicated and is found to be very useful clinically.[433, 434]

High performance liquid chromatography has been shown to be useful in the identification of poly-gamma-glutamate chain lengths of labeled and unlabeled folates.[435]

Niacin

Pellagra was first recognized in 1735 when Casal observed the disease, which he regarded as a peculiar form of leprosy, in the town of Oviedo, Spain. The first published report was in 1755 by Thiery.[436] Thiery apparently learned about the disease from Casal. Casal's observations were not published until after his death.[437] Casal associated the disease with poverty and spoiled corn. An excellent review of the history of pellagra has been recently published.[438] The term "pellagra," or rough skin, which had been used by the peasantry in Italy to describe the symptoms, was not published until 1771 in the work of Frapolli.[439] Despite the long history of this disease, the recognition of its basis in a dietary deficiency awaited the work of Goldberger, which began in 1913.[440] In 1937 Elvehjem demonstrated that nicotinic acid could cure the manifestations of pellagra, and a direct correlation between pellagra and nicotinic acid became apparent.[441, 442] By 1946 the transformation of tryptophan to niacin was appreciated.[443]

Nicotinamide, a derivative of nicotinic acid, is a component of the coenzymes nicotinamide adenine dinucleotide (NAD) and nicotinamide adenine dinucleotide phosphate (NADP). These coenzymes (NAD and NADP) are important in oxidation-reduction reactions, particularly in the transfer of hydrogen to or from aldehydes, alcohols, and organic acids. In this capacity, NAD and NADP are necessary for oxidative catabolism of carbohydrates, proteins, and lipids. Reduced NADP (NADPH) is also necessary for the biosynthesis of fatty acids.

Estimations of niacin requirements are complicated by the conversion of tryptophan to niacin in humans, the scarcity of feeding studies with subjects on diets varied in niacin and tryptophan content, and the potential diminished availability of niacin from certain foods. In many animals the conversion of tryptophan to niacin makes a dietary supply of the vitamin unnecessary. In humans, approximately 60 mg of tryptophan ingested in the diet produces 1 mg of nicotinic acid (1 "niacin equivalent").[444]

Clinical Aspects of Niacin Nutriture. Evidence now indicates the presence in many foodstuffs of niacin-containing compounds from which niacin is not nutritionally available.[445-449] It had been demonstrated that bound niacin was ineffective in curing niacin deficiency in experimental animals. Evidence for this in humans was not as apparent, although a discrepancy had been noted between the total niacin content of the high corn diet used by Goldberger to produce experimental pellagra and the lower intake of a healthy population in North Carolina.[450] Recent investigations on the bioavailability for humans of bound niacin from wheat bran has shown bound niacin from ethanolic wheat bran extracts to be essentially unavailable for humans.[451]

An additional nutritional concept relative to niacin requirements pertains to the reported effect of a high intake of leucine in precipitating pellagra in animals. In humans, administration of leucine to normal subjects results in an increase in urinary quinolinic acid (a tryptophan metabolite) and an accompanying decrease in niacin metabolites (N-methylnicotinamide and 6-pyridone).[452] Additionally, a 10-gm daily supplement of 1-leucine decreased the ability of erythrocytes of subjects to synthesize nicotinamide nucleotides when incubated with niacin.[453] These data suggested a significant inhibitory role for leucine in niacin metabolism.

Estimation of Niacin Nutriture. Assays for niacin have employed a chemical technique in which the pyridine compound reacts with cyanogen bromide and an organic base to form a yellow color.[454, 455] Microbiologic methods that depend upon the amount of lactic acid produced by L-arabinose on a synthetic medium containing all known growth factors except niacin have been used.[456] A review of methods for assessment of niacin status is given in Sauberlich et al.[457]

Pantothenic Acid

Pantothenic acid was noted as a growth factor for yeast in 1933,[458] was isolated by Williams 6 years later,[459, 460] and was synthesized in 1940.[461]

Pantothenic acid is a part of the molecular structure of CoA and therefore is involved in the activation of a number of compounds. It participates in the formation of acyl CoA moieties. It is, therefore, involved in the formation of acetyl CoA from CoA plus acetate. This compound is important for entry of pyruvate into the tricarboxylic acid cycle and also for fatty acid synthesis and oxidation. Pantothenic acid is related to biotin through this function. It should also be noted that thiamine is involved in the formation of acetyl CoA from pyruvate. Pantothenic acid also participates in the metabolism of steroids, sterols, hormones, acetylcholine, and porphyrins.

Certain common manifestations of pantothenic acid deficiency have been described, the most common being growth failure.[462] Most animal species develop dermatitis, alterations in neuromuscular activity, and hair loss. Panthothenic acid deficiency in man is extremely rare. However, significant amounts of pantothenic acid are lost in food processing.[463] In studies designed to control dietary intake of panthothenic acid, the urinary excretion of the vitamin by man is related to dietary intake.[464-467] A review of analytical methods for assessing pantothenic acid nutriture is given by Sauberlich et al.[468] It has been shown recently that the metabolism of CoA can be affected by nutritional and hormonal changes, which have opposite effects on fatty acid synthesis and oxidation. The greater incorporation of pantothenate into liver CoA in fasted rats is the opposite of the decreased incorporation of pantothenate into 4'-phosphopantetheine in liver fatty acid synthesis.[469] These rapid shifts in the synthesis of CoA and incorporation of pantothenic acid into fatty acid synthesis appear to be among the mechanisms by which the liver can rapidly control fatty acid synthesis and oxidation. A review of the mechanisms by which co-enzyme A is synthesized from pantothenic acid in mammalian tissues is given in Abiko.[470]

REFERENCES

1. Jelliffe, D. B.: The assessment of the nutritional status of the community. World Health Organization Monograph Series, No. 53. Geneva, World Health Organization, 1966.
2. Funk, C.: On the chemical nature of the substance which cures polyneuritis in birds induced by a diet of polished rice. J. Physiol., 43:395–400, 1911.
3. Funk, C.: The etiology of deficiency disease. J. State Med., 20:341–368, 1912.
4. McCollum, E. V., and Davis, M. J.: The necessity of certain lipins in the diet during growth. J. Biol. Chem., 15:167–175, 1913.
5. Osborne, T. B., and Mendel, L. B.: Influence of butter fat on growth. J. Biol. Chem., 16:423–437, 1913.
6. Osborne, T. B., and Mendel, L. B.: Protein-free milk factor. Carnegie Yearbook, 1911.
7. McCollum, E. V., and Kennedy, C. J.: The dietary factors operating in the production of polyneuritis. J. Biol. Chem., 24:491–502, 1916.
8. Drummond, J. C.: The nomenclature of the so-called accessory food factors. Biochem. J., 14:660, 1920.
9. Moore, T.: Vitamin A. Amsterdam, Elsevier Publishing Co., 1957.
10. Olson, J. A.: The metabolism of vitamin A. Pharmacol. Rev., 19:559–596, 1967.
11. Rodriquez, M. S., and Irwin, M. I.: A conspectus of research on vitamin A requirements of man. J. Nutr., 102:909–968, 1972.
12. Goodman, D. S., and Olson, J. A.: In Clayton, R. B. (ed.): Methods in Enzymology, Steroids and Terpenoids. Volume 15. New York, Academic Press, 1969.
13. Goodman, D. S., Huang, H. S., Kanai, M., and Shiratori, T.: The enzymatic conversion of all trans-beta-carotene into retinal. J. Biol. Chem., 242:3543–3554, 1967.

14. Ganguly, J.: Absorption of vitamin Am. J. Clin. Nutr., 22:923–933, 1969.
15. Huang, H. S., and Goodman, D. S.: Vitamin A and carotenoids. I. Intestinal absorption and metabolism of vitamin A and beta-carotene in man. J. Clin. Invest., 45:1615–1623, 1966.
16. Lawrence, C. W., Crain, F. D., Lotspeich, F. J., and Krause, R. F.: Absorption, transport, and storage of retinyl-15-14C palmitate 9, 10, 3H in the rat. J. Lipid Res., 7:226–229, 1966.
17. Fidge, N. H., Shiratori, T., Ganguly, J., and Goodman, D. S.: Pathways of absorption of retinal and retinoic acid in the rat. J. Lipid Res., 9:103–109, 1968.
18. Smith, J. E., Milch, P. O., Muto, Y., and Goodman, D. S.: The plasma transport and metabolism of retinoic acid in the rat. Biochem. J., 132:821–827, 1973.
19. Hori, S. H., and Kitamura, T.: The vitamin A content and retinol esterifying activity of a Kupffer cell fraction of rat liver. J. Histochem. Cytochem., 20:811–816, 1972.
20. Lewis, K. C., Green, M. H., and Underwood, B. A.: Vitamin A turnover in rats as influenced by vitamin A status. J. Nutr., 111:1135–1144, 1981.
21. Smith, F. R., and Goodman, D. S.: The effects of diseases of the liver, thyroid and kidneys on the transport of vitamin A in human plasma. J. Clin. Invest., 50:2426–2436, 1971.
22. Ellis, S., DePalma, J., Cheng, A., Capozzalo, P., Dombeck, D., and DiScala, V. A.: Vitamin A supplements in hemodialysis patients. Nephron, 26:215–218.
23. Yatzidis, H., Digenis, P., and Koutsicos, D.: Hypervitaminosis A in chronic renal failure after transplantation. Br. Med. J., 2:1075, 1976.
24. Muto, Y., Smith, J. E., Milch, P. O., and Goodman, D. S.: Regulation of retinol binding protein metabolism by vitamin A status in the rat. J. Biol. Chem., 247:2542–2550, 1972.
25. Smith, J. E., Muto, Y., Milch, P. O., and Goodman, D. S.: The effects of chylomicron vitamin A on the metabolism of retinol-binding protein in the rat. J. Biol. Chem., 248:1544–1549, 1973.
26. Smith, J. E., Brown, E. D., and Smith, J. C., Jr.: The effect of zinc deficiency on the metabolism of retinol-binding in the rat. J. Lab. Clin. Med., 84:692–697, 1974.
27. Smith, F. R., and Goodman, D. S.: The effects of diseases of the liver, thyroid, and kidneys on the transport of vitamin A in human plasma. J. Clin. Invest., 50:2426–2436, 1971.
28. Smith, F. R., Goodman, D. S., Zaklama, M. S., Gabr, M. K., El Maraghy, S., and Patwardhan, V. N.: Serum vitamin A, retinol-binding protein, and prealbumin concentrations in protein calorie malnutrition. I. A functional defect in hepatic retinol release. Am. J. Clin. Nutr., 26:973–981, 1973.
29. Mobarhan, S., Russell, R. M., Underwood, B. A., Wallingford, J., Mathieson, R. D., and Al-Midani, H.: Evaluation of the relative dose response test for vitamin A nutriture in cirrhosis. Am. J. Clin. Nutr., 34:2264–2270, 1981.
30. Vinton, N. E., and Russell, R. M.: Evaluation of a rapid test of dark adaptation. Am. J. Clin. Nutr., 34:1961–1966, 1981.
31. Navarro, J., and Desquilbet, N.: Depressed plasma vitamin A and retinol-binding protein in cystic

fibrosis correlations with zinc deficiency. Am. J. Clin. Nutr., *34*:1439–1440, 1981.

32. Palin, D., Underwood, B. A., Denning, C. R.: The effect of oral zinc supplementation on plasma levels of vitamin A and retinol-binding in cystic fibrosis. Am. J. Clin. Nutr., *32*:1253–1259, 1979.

33. Rogers, E. L., Douglass, W., Russell, R. M., Bushman, L., Hubbard, T. B., and Iber, F. L.: Deficiency of fat-soluble vitamins after jejunoileal bypass surgery for morbid obesity. Am. J. Clin. Nutr., *33*:1208–1214, 1980.

34. Falchuk, K. R., Walker, W. A., Perrotto, J. L., and Isselbacher, K. J.: Effect of vitamin A on the systemic and local antibody responses to intragastrically administered bovine serum albumin. Infect. Immun., *17*:361–365, 1977.

35. Napoli, J. L., McCormick, A. M., Schnoes, H. K., and DeLuca, H. F.: Identification of 5,8 oxyretinoic acid isolated from small intestine of vitamin A-deficient rats dosed with retinoic acid. National Academy of Sciences USA, *75*:2603–2605, 1978.

36. Sporn, M. B., Dunlop, N. M., Newton, D. L., and Smith, J. M.: Fed. Proc., *35*:1332–1338, 1976.

37. Gal, I., Parkinson, C., and Craft, I.: Effect of oral contraceptives on human plasma vitamin A levels. Br. Med. J., *2*:436–438, 1971.

38. Supopark, W., and Olson, J. A.: Effect of Ovral, a combination type oral contraceptive agent on vitamin A metabolism in rats. Int. J. Vitam. Nutr. Res., *45*:113–123, 1975.

39. Hodges, R. E., and Canham, J. E.: *In* Hanson, R. G., and Munro, H. N. (eds.): Proceedings of a Workshop on Problems of Assessment and Alleviation of Malnutrition in the United States. Washington, D.C., U.S. Government Printing Office, 1970.

40. Sauberlich, H. E., Hodges, R. E., Wallace, D. L., Kolder, H., Canham, J. E., Hood, J., Raica, N., Jr., and Lowry, L. K.: Vitamin A metabolism and requirements in the human studied with the use of labelled retinol. Vitam. Horm., *32*:251–275, 1974.

41. Hodges, R. E., Sauberlich, H. E., Canham, J. E., Wallace, D. L., Rucker, R. B., Mejia, L. A., and Mohanram, M.: Hematopoietic studies in vitamin A deficiency. Am. J. Clin. Nutr., *31*:876–885, 1978.

42. Ahluwalia, G. S., Kaul, L., and Ahluwalia, B. S.: Evidence of facilitory effect of growth hormone on tissue vitamin A uptake in rats. J. Nutr., *110*:1185–1193, 1980.

43. Kato, J.: *In* Pasqualina, J. R. (ed.): Receptors and Mechanism of Action of Steroid Hormones. Part II. New York, Marcel Dekker, Inc., 1977.

44. Morley, J. E., Damassa, D. A., Gordon, J., Pekary, A. E., and Hershman, J. M.: Thyroid function and vitamin A deficiency. Life Sci., *22*:1901–1906, 1978.

45. Morley, J. E., Russell, R. M., Reed, A., Carney, E. A., and Hershman, J. M.: The interrelationship of thyroid hormones with vitamin A and zinc nutritional status in patients with chronic hepatitis and gastrointestinal disorders. Am. J. Clin. Nutr., *34*:1489–1495, 1981.

46. Brown, E. D., Chan, W., and Smith, J. C., Jr.: Vitamin A metabolism during the repletion of zinc deficient rats. J. Nutr., *106*:563–572, 1976.

47. McLaren, D. S.: The luxus vitamins—A and B_{12}. Am. J. Clin. Nutr., *34*:1611–1616, 1981.

48. Hall, C. A.: The luxus vitamins A and B_{12}: Reply to McLaren. Am. J. Clin. Nutr., *35*:772–774, 1982.

49. DeLuca, L., Maestri, N., Rosso, G., and Wolf, G.: Retinol glycolipids. J. Biol. Chem., *248*:641–648, 1973.

49a. Maesti, N., and DeLuca, L.: Mannose transfer from mannolipid to endogenous acceptors in hamster liver. Biochem. Biophys. Res. Commun., *53*:1344–1349, 1973.

50. Kiorpes, T. C., Molica, S. J., and Wolf, G.: A plasma glycoprotein depressed in vitamin A deficiency in the rat. Alpha 1-macroglobulin. J. Nutr., *106*:1659–1667, 1976.

51. Ong, D. E., Tsai, C-H., and Chytil, F.: Cellular retinol-binding protein and retinoic acid-binding protein in rat testes: Effect of retinol depletion. J. Nutr., *106*:204–211, 1976.

52. Heller, J.: Intracellular retinol-binding proteins from bovine pigment epithelial and photoreceptor cell fractions: Purification of high molecular weight lipoglycoproteins. J. Biol. Chem., *251*:2952–2957, 1976.

53. Rask, L., and Peterson, P. A.: In vitro uptake of vitamin A from the retinol-binding plasma protein to mucosal epithelial cells from the monkey small intestine. J. Biol. Chem., *251*:6360–6366, 1976.

54. Heller, J.: Interactions of plasma retinol-binding protein with its receptor: Specific binding of bovine and human retinol-binding protein to pigment epithelium cells from bovine eyes. J. Biol. Chem., *250*:3613–3619, 1975.

55. *In* Bennett: Treatise on the Oleum Jecoris Aselli or Cod-Liver Oil. Edinburgh, 1848.

56. Mellanby, E.: Lancet, *1*:4, 1919.

57. McCollum, E. V., Simmonds, N., Becker, J. E., and Shipley, P. G.: Studies on experimental rickets. J. Biol. Chem., *53*:293–312, 1922.

58. Huldshinsky, K.: Heilung von Rachitis durch kuenstliche Hoehensonne. Deut. Med. Wochschr., *45*:712–713, 1919.

59. Goldblatt, H., and Soames, K. M.: Studies on the fat-soluble growth-promoting factor. Biochem. J., *17*:446–453, 1923.

60. Steenbock, H., and Black, A.: Fat-soluble vitamins. J. Biol. Chem., *61*:405–422, 1924.

61. Steenbock, H., and Black, A.: Fat-soluble vitamins. J. Biol. Chem., *64*:263–298, 1925.

62. Hess, A. F., Weinstock, M., and Sherman, E.: The anti-rachitic value of irradiated cholesterol and phytosterol. J. Biol. Chem., *67*:413–423, 1926.

63. Askew, F. A., Bourdillon, R. B., Bruce, H. M., Jenkins, R. G. C., and Webster, T. A.: Distillation of vitamin D. Proc. Soc. Lond., *107*:76–90, 1931.

64. Steenbock, H., Kletzien, S. W. F., and Halpin, J. H.: The reaction of the chicken to irradiated ergosterol and irradiated yeast as contrasted with the natural vitamin D of fish liver oils. J. Biol. Chem., *97*:249–264, 1932.

65. Windaus, A., Schenck, F., and von Werder, F.: Über das antirachitisch Bestrahlungs produkt aus 7-dehydro-cholesterin. Z. Physiol. Chem., *241*:100–103, 1936.

66. Esvelt, R. P., Schnoes, H. K., and DeLuca, H. P.: Vitamin D_3 from rat skins irradiated in vitro with ultraviolet light. Arch. Biochem. Biophys., *188*:282–286, 1978.

67. Holock, M. F., Frommer, J. E., McNeill, S. C., Richtand, N. M., Henley, J. W., and Potts, J. E., Jr.: Photometabolism of 7-dehydrocholesterol to

previtamin D_3 in skin. Biochem. Biophys. Res. Commun., 76:107–114, 1977.

68. DeLuca, H. F., and Schnoes, H. K.: Metabolism and mechanism of action of vitamin D. Annu. Rev. Biochem., 45:631–666, 1976.

69. DeLuca, H. F.: The vitamin D system in the regulation of calcium and phosphorus metabolism. Nutr. Rev., 37:161–193, 1979.

70. DeLuca, H. F.: In Proceedings of the Annual Meeting of the Royal College of Physicians and Surgeons of Toronto, Canada, 1977, p. 216–225.

71. DeLuca, H. F., and Schnoes, H. K.: Metabolism and mechanism of action of vitamin D. Annu. Rev. Biochem., 45:631–666, 1976.

71a. DeLuca, H. F.: Vitamin D and calcium transport. Ann. N.Y. Acad. Sci., 307:356–376, 1978.

72. Scarpa, A., and Karafoley, E. (eds.): Ann. N.Y. Acad. Sci., 307, 1978.

73. Wasserman, R. H.: The Transfer of Calcium and Strontium Across Biological Membranes. New York, Academic Press, 1963, p. 211–228.

74. Garabedian, M., Tanaka, Y., Holock, M. F., and DeLuca, H. F.: Response of intestinal calcium mobilization to 1,25-dihydroxyvitamin D_3 in thyroparathyroidectomized rats. Endocrinology, 94:1022–1027, 1974.

75. Garabedian, M., Holick, M. F., DeLuca, H. F., and Boyle, I. T.: Control of 25-hydroxycholecalciferol metabolism by parathyroid glands. Proc. Natl. Acad. Sci. U.S.A., 69:1673–1676, 1972.

76. Talmage, R. B.: Morphological and physiological considerations in a new concept of calcium transport in bone. Am. J. Anat., 129:467–476, 1970.

77. Garabedian, M., Tanaka, Y., Holick, M. F., and DeLuca, H. F.: Response of intestinal calcium mobilization to 1,25-dihydroxyvitamin D_3 in thyroparathyroidectomized rats. Endocrinology, 94:1022–1027, 1974.

78. DeLuca, H. F., and Schnoes, H. K.: Metabolism and mechanism of action of vitamin D. Annu. Rev. Biochem., 45:631–666, 1976.

79. Sutton, R. A. L., and Dirks, J. H.: Renal handling of calcium. Fed. Proc., 37:2112–2119, 1978.

80. Steele, T. H., Engle, J. E., Tanaka, Y., Lorenc, R. S., Dudgeon, K. L., and DeLuca, H. F.: Phosphatemic action of 1,25-dihydroxyvitamin D_3. Am. J. Physiol., 229:489–495, 1975.

81. Esvelt, R. P., Schnoes, H. K., and DeLuca, H. F.: Vitamin D_3 from rat skins irradiated in vitro with ultraviolet light. Arch. Biochem. Biophys., 188:282–286, 1978.

82. Holock, M. F., Frommer, J. E., McNeill, S. C., Richtand, N. M., Henley, J. W., and Potts, J. T., Jr.: Photometabolism of 7-dehydrocholesterol to previtamin D_3 in skin. Biochem. Biophys. Res. Commun., 76:107–114, 1977.

83. Tucker, G. III, Gagnon, R. E., and Haussler, M. R.: Vitamin D_3-25-hydroxylase: Tissue occurrence and apparent lack of regulation. Arch. Biochem. Biophys., 155:47–57, 1973.

84. Ponchon, G., Kennan, A. L., and DeLuca, H. F.: Activation of vitamin D by the liver. J. Clin. Invest., 48:2032–2037, 1969.

85. Horsting, M., and DeLuca, H. F.: In vitro production of 25-hydrocholecalciferol. Biochem. Biophys. Res. Commun., 36:251–256, 1969.

86. Olson, E. B., Jr., Knutson, J. C., Bhattacharyya, M. H., and DeLuca, H. F.: The effect of hepatectomy on the synthesis of 25-hydroxyvitamin D_3.

J. Clin. Invest., 57:1213–1220, 1976.

87. Boyle, I. T., Miravet, L., Gray, R. W., Holick, M. F., and DeLuca, H. F.: The response of intestinal calcium transport to 25-hydroxy and 1,25-dihydroxy vitamin D in nephrectomized rats. Endocrinology, 90:605–608, 1972.

88. Tanaka, Y., DeLuca, H. F., Omdahl, J., and Holick, M. F.: Mechanism of action of 1,25 dihydroxycholecalciferol on intestinal calcium transport. Proc. Natl. Acad. Sci., 68:1286–1288, 1971.

89. Holick, M. F., Garabedian, M., and DeLuca, H. F.: 5,6-Trans-25-hydroxycholecalciferol: Vitamin D analog effective on intestine of anephric rats. Science, 176:1247–1248, 1972.

90. Jones, G., Schnoes, H. K., and DeLuca, H. F.: An in vitro study of vitamin D_2 hydroxylases in the chick. J. Biol. Chem., 251:24–28, 1976.

91. Jones, G., Baxter, L. A., DeLuca, H. F., and Schnoes, H. K.: Biochem. J., 15:713–716, 1976.

92. DeLuca, H. F.: The vitamin D system in the regulation of calcium and phosphorus metabolism. Nutr. Rev., 37:161–193, 1979.

93. DeLuca, H. F., Franceschi, R. T., Halloran, B. P., and Massaro, E. R.: Molecular events involved in 1,25-dihydroxyvitamin D_3 stimulation of intestinal calcium transport. Fed. Proc, 41:66–71, 1982.

94. Eisman, J. A., Hamstra, A. J., Kream, B. E., and DeLuca, H. F.: A sensitive, precise and convenient method of determination of 1,25-dihydroxyvitamin D in human plasma. Arch. Biochem. Biophys., 176:235–243, 1976.

95. Haussler, M. R., Baylink, D. J., Hughes, M. R., Brumbaugh, P. F., Wergedal, J. E., Shen, F. H., Neilsen, R. L., Counts, S. J., Bursac, K. M., and McCain, T. A.: The assay of 1-alpha,25-dihydroxyvitamin D_3: Physiologic and pathologic modulation of circulating hormone levels. Clin. Endocrinol., 5:151S–165S, 1976.

96. Chesney, R. W., Moorthy, A. V., Eisman, J. E., Jax, D. K. Mazess, R. B., and DeLuca, H. F.: Increased growth after long-term oral 1-alpha,25-vitamin D_3 in childhood renal osteodystrophy. N. Engl. J. Med., 298:238–242, 1978.

97. Brickman, A. S., Coburn, J. W., and Norman, A. W.: Action of 1,25-dihydroxycholecalciferol, a potent kidney-produced metabolite of vitamin D_3 in uremic man. N. Engl. J. Med., 287:891–895, 1972.

98. Silverberg, D. S., Bettcher, K. B., Dossetor, J. B., Overton, T. R., Holick, M. F., and DeLuca, H. F.: Effect of 1,25-dihydroxycholecalciferol in renal osteodystrophy. Can. Med. Assoc. J., 112:190–195, 1975.

99. Neer, R. M., Holick, M. F., DeLuca, H. F., and Potts, J. T., Jr.: Effects of 1-alpha-hydroxyvitamin D_3 and 1,25-dihydroxyvitamin D_3 on calcium and phosphorus metabolism in hyperparathyroidism. Metabolism, 24:1403–1413, 1975.

100. Fraser, D., Kooh, S. W., Kind, H. P., Holick, M. F., Tanaka, Y., and DeLuca, H. F.: Pathogenesis of hereditary vitamin-D-dependent rickets. An inborn error of vitamin D metabolism involving defective conversion of 25-hydroxyvitamin D to 1 alpha,25-dihydroxyvitamin D. N. Engl. J. Med., 289:817–822, 1973.

101. Scriver, C. R., Reade, T. M., DeLuca, H. F., and Hamstra, J. A. J.: Serum 1,25-dihydroxyvitamin D levels in normal subjects and in patients with hereditary rickets or bone disease. N. Engl. J. Med., 299:976–979, 1978.

102. Horst, R. L., DeLuca, H. F., and Jorgensen, N. A.: Metab. Bone Dis. Rel. Res., 1:29–33, 1978.

103. Riggs, B. L., and Gallagher, J. C.: In Norman, A. W., Schaefer, K., Coburn, J. W., DeLuca, H. F., Frazer, D., Grigoleit, H. G., and vonHerrath, D. (eds.): Vitamin D. Biochemical, Chemical and Clinical Aspects Related to Calcium Metabolism. Berlin, Walter deGruyter, Inc., 1977, p. 639–648.

104. Riggs, B. L., Gallagher, J. G., and DeLuca, H. F.: Proceedings of the Fourth International Workshop on Vitamin D. Berlin, Walter deGruyter, Inc., 1979.

105. Compston, J. E., Vedi, S., Ledger, J. E., Webb, A., Gazet, J., and Pilkington, T. R. E.: Vitamin D status and bone histomorphometry in gross obesity. Am. J. Clin. Nutr., 34:2359–2363, 1981.

106. Compston, J. E., and Creamer, B.: Plasma levels and intestinal absorption of 25-hydroxy-vitamin D in patients with small bowel resection. Gut, 18:171–175, 1977.

107. DeLuca, H. F.: Current concepts—Vitamin D. N. Engl. J. Med., 281:1103–1111, 1969.

108. Devgun, M. S., Paterson, C. R., Johnson, B. E., and Cohen, C.: Vitamin D nutrition in relation to season and occupation. Am. J. Clin. Nutr., 34:1501–1504, 1981.

109. Reeve, L. E., Chesney, R. W., and DeLuca, H. F.: Vitamin D of human milk: Identification of biologically active forms. Am. J. Clin. Nutr., 36:122–126, 1982.

110. Evans, H. M., and Bishop, K. S.: The existence of a hitherto unrecognized dietary factor essential for reproduction. Am. J. Physiol., 63:396–397, 1922.

111. Evans, H. M., Emerson, O. H., and Emerson, G. A.: The isolation from wheat germ oil of alcohol, resembling alpha tocopherol having the properties of vitamin E. J. Biol. Chem., 113:319–332, 1936.

112. Alcott, H. S., and Mattill, H. A.: Some chemical and physical properties of vitamin E. J. Biol. Chem., 104:423–435, 1934.

113. Moore, T.: The effect of vitamin E deficiency on the vitamin A reserves in the cat. Biochem. J., 34:1321–1326, 1940.

113a. Dam, H. Influence of antioxidants and redox substances on signs of vitamin E deficiency. Pharmacol. Rev., 9:1–16, 1957.

114. Hove and Harris: J. Am. Oil Chem. Soc., 28:405, 1951.

115. Tappel, A. L.: Vitamin E as the biological lipid antioxidant. Vitam. Horm., 20:493–510, 1962.

116. Whiting: Lipids, 2:109, 1967.

117. Folkers: Folkers Int. J. Vitam. Res., 39:334, 1969.

118. Boguth, W.: Aspects of the action of vitamin E. Vitam. Horm., 27:1–15, 1969.

119. Green, J., and Bunyan, J.: Vitamin E and the biological antioxidant theory. Nutr. Abstr. Rev., 39:321–345, 1969.

120. Scott, M. L.: Advances in our understanding of vitamin E. Fed. Proc., 39:2736–2739, 1980.

121. Hassan, H., Hashim, S. A., Van Itallie, T. B., and Sebrell, W. H.: Syndrome in premature infants associated with low plasma vitamin E levels and high polyunsaturated fatty acid diet. Am. J. Clin. Nutr., 19:147–157, 1966.

122. Oski, F. A., and Barness, L. A.: Vitamin E deficiency: A previously unrecognized cause of hemolytic anemia in the premature infant. J. Pediatr., 70:211–220, 1967.

123. Ritchie, J. H., Fish, M. B., McMasters, V., and Grossman, M.: Edema and hemolytic anemia in premature infants: A vitamin E deficiency syndrome. N. Engl. J. Med., 279:1185–1190, 1968.

124. Melhorn, D. K., and Gross, S.: Vitamin E dependent anemia in the premature infant. II. Relationships between gestational age and absorption of vitamin E. J. Pediatr., 79:581–588, 1971.

125. Melhorn, D. K., and Gross, S.: Vitamin E-dependent anemia in the premature infant. I. Effects of large doses of medicinal iron. J. Pediatr., 79:569–580, 1971.

126. Bell, E. F., and Filer, L. J., Jr.: The role of vitamin E in the nutrition of premature infants. Am. J. Clin. Nutr., 34:414–422, 1981.

127. Oski, F. A., and Barness, L. A.: The role of vitamin E in the nutrition of premature infants. Am. J. Clin. Nutr., 34:2599–2600, 1981.

128. Bell, E. F., and Filer, L. J., Jr.: Reply to letter by Oski & Barness. Am. J. Clin. Nutr., 34:2600–2601, 1981.

129. Pappu, A. S., Fatterpaker, P., and Sreenivasan, A: Possible interrelationship between vitamin E and B_{12} in the disturbance in methylmalonate metabolism and vitamin E deficiency. Biochem. J., 172:115–121, 1978.

130. Caasi, P. I., Hauswirth, J. W., and Nair, P. P.: Biosynthesis of heme and vitamin E deficiency. Ann. N.Y. Acad. Sci., 203:93–102, 1972.

131. Bierri, J. G.: Vitamin E in Present Knowledge in Nutrition. edition 4. New York and Washington, Nutrition Foundation, Inc., 1976, p. 98–110.

132. Binder, H. J., Herting, D. C., Hurst, V., Finch, S. C., and Spiro, H. M.: Tocopherol deficiency in man. N. Engl. J. Med., 273:1289–1297, 1965.

133. Binder, H. J., and Shapiro, H. M.: Tocopherol deficiency in man. Am. J. Clin. Nutr., 20:594–601, 1967.

134. Williams, H. T. G., Fenna, D., and Macbeth, R. A.: Alpha-tocopherol in the treatment of intermittent claudication. Surg. Gynecol. Obstet., 132:662–666, 1971.

135. Haeger, K.: Long time treatment of intermittent claudication with vitamin E. Am. J. Clin. Nutr., 27:1179–1181, 1974.

136. Owens, W. C. and Owens, E. U.: Retrolental fibroplasia in premature infants. II. Studies on the prophylaxis of the disease, the use of alpha tocopheryl acetate. Am. J. Ophthalmol., 32:1631–1637, 1949.

137. Johnson, L., Schaffer, D., and Boggs, T. R., Jr.: The premature infant, vitamin E deficiency and retrolental fibroplasia. Am. J. Clin. Nutr., 27:1158–1173, 1974.

138. Johnson, L. H., and Schaffer, D. B., Rubinstein, D., Crawford, C. S., and Boggs, T. R.: The role of vitamin E in retrolental fibroplasia. Pediatr. Res., 10:425, 1976.

139. Johnson, L., Schaffer, D., Boggs, T., Quinn, G., and Mathis, M.: Vitamin E treatment of retrolental fibroplasia grade III or worse. Pediatr. Res., 14:601, 1980.

140. Phelps, D. L., and Rosenbaum, A. L.: The role of tocopherol in oxygen-induced retinopathy: Kitten model. Pediatrics, 59:998–1005, 1977.

141. Phelps, D. L., and Rosenbaum, A. L.: Vitamin A in kitten oxygen-induced retinopathy. II. Blockage of vitreal neovascularization. Arch. Ophthal-

mol., *97*:1522–1526, 1979.

142. Curran, J. S., and Cantolino, S. J.: Vitamin E (injectable) administration in the prevention of retinopathy of prematurity: Evaluation with fluorescein angiography and fundus photography. Pediatr. Res., *12*:404, 1978.

143. McClung, H. J., Backes, C., Lavin, A., and Kerzner, B.: Prospective evaluation of vitamin E therapy in premature infants with hyaline membrane disease. Pediatr. Res., *14*:604, 1980.

144. Natta, C. L., Machlin, L. J., and Brin, M.: A decrease in irreversibly sickled erythrocytes in sickle cell anemia patients given vitamin E. Am. J. Clin. Nutr., *33*:968–970, 1980.

145. Chan, A. C., and Leith, M. K.: Decreased prostacyclin synthesis in vitamin E deficient rabbit aorta. Am. J. Clin. Nutr., *34*:2341–2347, 1981.

146. Likoff, R. O., Guptill, D. R., Lawrence, L. M., McKay, C. C., Mathias, M. M., Nockels, C. F., and Tengerdy, R. P.: Vitamin E and aspirin depress prostaglandins in protection of chickens against *Escherichia coli* infection. Am. J. Clin. Nutr., *34*:245–251, 1981.

147. Lands, W. E. M., and Rome, L. H.: Inhibition of prostaglandin biosynthesis. *In* Karen, S. M. M. (ed.): Prostaglandins: Chemical and Biochemical Aspects. Baltimore, University Park Press, 1976.

148. Machlin, J. L.: Vitamin E (Tocopherol), Oxygen and Biomembranes. New York, Elsevier, 1978, p. 179–189.

149. Mellette, S. J., and Leone, L. A.: Influence of age, sex, strain of rat and fat-soluble vitamins on hemorrhagic syndromes in rats fed irradiated beef. Fed. Proc., *19*:1045–1049, 1960.

150. March, B. E., Wong, E., Seier, L., Sim, J., and Biely, J.: Hypervitaminosis E in the chick. J. Nutr., *103*:371–377, 1973.

151. Dymsza, H. A., and Park, J.: Excess dietary vitamin E in rats. Fed. Proc., *34*:912, 1975.

152. Farell, P. M., and Willison, J. W.: Megavitamin E supplementation in man. Fed. Proc., *34*:912, 1975.

153. Corrigan, J. J., Jr., and Marcus, F. I.: Coagulopathy associated with vitamin E ingestion. J.A.M.A., *230*:1300–1301, 1974.

154. Corrigan, J. J., Jr., and Ulfers, L. L.: Effect of vitamin E on prothrombin levels and warfarin-induced vitamin K deficiency. Am. J. Clin. Nutr., *34*:1701–1705, 1981.

155. Schroder, J.: Analogs of alpha-tocopherol as inhibitors of cyclic AMP and cyclic GMP phosphodiesterases and effects of α-tocopherol deficiency on cyclic AMP controlled metabolism. Biochim. Biophys. Acta, *343*:173–181, 1974.

156. Chizzolini, R., Bracchi, P., Cabassi, E., and Maggi, E.: Effect of vitamin E deficiency on rabbit intramuscular collagen. Am. J. Clin. Nutr., *35*:1018–1022, 1982.

157. Scott, M. L.: Advances in our understanding of vitamin E. Fed. Proc., *39*:2736–2739, 1980.

158. Riley, C. A., Cohen, G., and Lieberman, M.: Ethane evolution: A new index of lipid peroxidation. Science, *183*:208–210, 1974.

159. Evans, C. D., List, D. R., Dolev, A., McConnell, D. G., and Hoffman, R. L.: Pentane from thermal decomposition of lipoxidase-derived products. Lipids, *2*:432–434, 1967.

160. Dumelin, E. E., and Tappel, A. L.: Hydrocarbon gases produced during in vitro peroxidation of polyunsaturated fatty acids and decomposition of preformed hydroperoxides. Lipids, *12*:894–900, 1977.

161. Dillard, C. J., DuMelin, E. E., and Tappel, A. L.: Effect of dietary vitamin E on expiration of pentane and ethane by the rat. Lipids, *12*:109–114, 1976.

162. Hafeman, D. G., and Hoekstra, W. G.: Protection against carbon tetrachloride–induced lipid peroxidation in the rat by dietary vitamin E, selenium, and methionine as measured by ethane evolution. J. Nutr., *107*:656–665, 1977.

163. Hafeman, D. G., and Hoekstra, W. G.: Lipid peroxidation in vivo during vitamin E and selenium deficiency in the rat as monitored by ethane evolution. J. Nutr., *107*:666–672, 1977.

164. Committee on Dietary Allowances, Committee on Interpretation of the Recommended Dietary Allowances: Recommended Dietary Allowances. Edition 8. Washington, D. C., National Academy of Sciences, 1974.

165. Horwitt, M. K., Harvey, C. C., Dahm, C. H., Jr., and Searcy, M. T.: Relationship between tocopherol and serum lipid levels for determination of nutritional adequacy. Ann. N.Y. Acad. Sci., *203*:223–236, 1972.

166. McFarlane, W. D., Graham, W. R., Jr., and Richardson, F.: The fat soluble vitamin requirements of the chick. I. The vitamin A and D content of fish meal and meat meal. Biochem. J., *25*:358–366, 1931.

167. Dam, H.: The antihaemorrhagic vitamin of the chick. Biochem. J., *21*:1273–1285, 1935.

168. Almquist, H. J., and Stockstead, E. L. R.: Dietary hemorrhagic disease in chicks. Nature (London), *136*:31, 1935.

169. Dam, H., Schonheyder, F., and Tage-Hansen, E: Studies on the mode of action of vitamin K. Biochem. J., *30*:1075–1079, 1936.

170. MacCorquodale, D. W., Cheney, L. C., Binkley, S. B., Holcomb, W. F., McKee, R. W., Thayer, S. A., and Doisy, E. A.: The constitution and synthesis of vitamin K_1. J. Biol. Chem., *131*:357–370, 1939.

171. Frick, P. G., Riedler, G., and Brogli, H.: Dose response and minimal dietary requirement for vitamin K in man. J. Appl. Physiol., *23*:387–389, 1967.

172. Doisy, E. A.: Vitamin K in human nutrition. *In* Symposium Proceedings on the Biochemistry, Assay, and Nutritional Value of Vitamin K and Related Compounds. Chicago, Association of Vitamin Chemistry, 1971, p. 79–92.

173. O'Reilly, R. A.: Vitamin K in hereditary resistance to oral anticoagulant drugs. Am. J. Physiol., *221*:1327–1330, 1971.

174. Suttie, J. W.: Vitamin K. *In* Draper, H. H. (ed.): Handbook of Lipid Research. Volume 1, New York, Plenum Press, 1978.

175. Suttie, J. W., and Jackson, C. M.: Prothrombin structure, activation and biosynthesis. Physiol. Rev., *57*:1–70, 1977.

176. Magnusson, S., Sottrup-Jensen, L., Petersen, T. E., Morris, H. R., and Dell, A.: Primary structure of the vitamin K dependent part of prothrombin. F.E.B.S. Lett., *44*:189–193, 1974.

177. Nelsestuen, G. L., Zytkovicz, T. H., and Howard, J. B.: The mode of action of vitamin K: Identification of γ-carboxyglutamic acid as a component of prothrombin. J. Biol. Chem., *249*:6347–6350, 1974.

178. Stenflo, J., Fernlund, P., Egan, W., and Roepstorff, P.: Vitamin K dependent modifications of glutamic acid residues and prothrombin. Proc. Natl. Acad. Sci. U.S.A., 71:2730–2733, 1974.

179. Hauschka, P. V., and Reid, M. L.: Vitamin K dependence of a calcium binding protein containing γ-carboxyglutamic acid in chicken bone. J. Biol. Chem., 253:9063–9068, 1978.

180. Matschiner, J. T., Bell, R. G., Amelotti, J. M., and Knauer, T. E.: Isolation and characterization of a new metabolite of phylloquinone in the rat. Biochim. Biophys. Acta, 201:309–315, 1970.

181. Willingham, A. K., and Matschiner, J. T.: Changes in phylloquinone epoxidase activity related to prothrombin synthesis and microsomal clotting activity in the rat. Biochem. J., 140:435–441, 1974.

182. Kark, R., and Lozner, E. L.: Nutritive deficiency of vitamin K in man. Lancet, 2:1162–1164, 1939.

183. Pineo, G. F., Gallus, A. S., and Hirsch, J.: Unexpected vitamin K deficiency in hospitalized patients. Can. Med. Assoc. J., 109:880–883, 1973.

184. Ansell, J. E., Kumar, R., and Deykin, D.: The spectrum of vitamin K deficiency. J.A.M.A., 238:40–42, 1977.

185. Sutherland, J. M., Glueck, H. I., and Gleser, G.: Hemorrhagic disease of the newborn. Am. J. Dis. Child., 113:524–533, 1967.

186. Shearer, M. J., Allan, V., Haroon, Y., and Barkhan, P: In Suttie, J. W. (ed.): Nutritional Aspects of Vitamin K Metabolism and Vitamin K Dependent Proteins. Baltimore, University Park Press, 1979, p. 317–327.

187. Seeler, R. A.: Vitamin K deficiency revisited. Ill. Med. J., 147:59–61, 1975.

188. Intestinal microflora, injury, and vitamin K deficiency. Nutr. Rev., 38:341–343, 1980.

189. Lewis, J. H., Zucker, M. B., and Ferguson, J. H.: Bleeding tendency in uremia. Blood, 11:1073–1076, 1956.

190. Takaki, K.: Health of the Japanese Navy. Lancet, 2:86, 1887.

191. C. Lancet, London: 218, 1097, 1930. Grijans, G.: Research on Vitamins, 1900–1911, J. Noorduyn, Gorinchem. pp. 37–38, 1935.

192. Vordermann, A. G.: Geneesk. Tjidschr. V. Ned. Ind., 1898.

193. Fraser, H., and Stanton, A. T.: Collected Papers on Beriberi. No. 17. Studies from the Institute for Medical Research in the Federation of Malay States. London, 1924.

194. Funk, C.: The etiology of the deficiency diseases. J. St. Med., 20:341–368, 1912.

195. Jansen, B.C.P., and Donath, W.E.: Mededeel. Dienst. Volksgezondbeid, Nederland Indie: I, 186, 1926.

196. Jansen, B. C. P.: Identity of vitamin B₁ and flavine and the nomenclature of vitamins. Nature, 135:267, 1935.

197. Williams, R. R., Waterman, R. E., and Keresztesy, J. C.: Larger yields of crystalline antineuritic vitamin. J. Am. Med. Soc., 56:1187, 1934.

198. Platt,: Fed. Proc., 17:8, 1958.

199. Eddy, W. H., and Roper, J. C.: The use of the pancreatic vitamin in the cases of marasmus. Am. J. Dis. Child., 14:189, 1917.

200. Victor, M., and Adams, R. D.: On the etiology of the alcoholic neurologic diseases, with special reference to the role of nutrition. Am. J. Clin. Nutr., 91:379–397, 1961.

201. Osborne, T. B., and Mendel, L. B: The role of vitamins in the diet. J. Biol. Chem., 31:149–163, 1917.

202. Cowgill, G. R.: The Human Requirement for Vitamin B₁. New Haven, Yale University Press, 1934.

203. Cowgill, G. R.: The physiology of vitamin B₁. J.A.M.A., 110:805–812, 1938.

204. Eddy, W. H.: What Are the Vitamins? New York, Reinhold Publishing Corporation, 1941.

205. Jolliffe, N., and Goodhart, R.: Beriberi in alcohol addicts. J.A.M.A., 111:380–384, 1938.

206. Volpe, J. J., and Marasa, J. C.: A role for thiamine in the regulation of fatty acid and cholesterol by a biosynthesis in cultured cells of neural origin. J. Neurochem., 30:975–981, 1978.

207. Collins, G. H.: Glial cell changes in the brain stem of thiamine deficient rats. Am. J. Pathol., 50:791–814, 1967.

208. Singh, M.: Effect of thiamin deficiency on pancreatic acinar cell function. Am. J. Clin. Nutr., 36:500–504, 1982.

209. Brin, M.: Functional evaluation of nutritional status: Thiamine in newer methods of nutritional biochemistry. In Albanese, A. A. (ed.). Volume 3. New York, Academic Press, 1967.

210. Sauberlich, H. E., Dowdy, R. P., and Skala, J. H.: Laboratory tests for the assessment of nutritional status. Florida, CRC Press Incorporated, 1979, p. 22.

211. Cheng, C. H., Koch, M., and Shank, R. E.: Leukocyte transketolase activity as an indicator of thiamin nutriture in rats. J. Nutr., 106:1678–1685, 1976.

212. McLaren, D. S., Docherty, M. A., and Boyd, D. H. A.: Plasma thiamin pyrophosphate and erythrocyte transketolase in chronic alcoholism. Am. J. Clin. Nutr., 34:1031–1033, 1981.

213. Blass, J. P., and Gibson, G. E.: Abnormality of a thiamine-requiring enzyme in patients with Wernicke-Korsakoff syndrome. N. Engl. J. Med., 297:1367–1370, 1977.

214. Blass, J. P., Gibson, G. E., and Kark, R. A: In Bubler, C. J., Fujiwara, M., and Dreyfus, N. P. M. (eds.): Pyruvate Decarboxylase Deficiency, Thiamine. New York, John Wiley & Sons, 1975, p. 321–324.

215. Read, D. J.: The aetiology of the sudden death syndrome: Current ideas on breathing and sleep and possible links to deranged thiamine neurochemistry. Aust. N. Z. J. Med., 8:322–336, 1978.

216. Peterson, D. R. Labbe, R. F., van Belle, G., and Chinn, N. M.: Erythrocyte transketolase activity and sudden infant death. Am. J. Clin. Nutr., 34:65–67, 1981.

217. Pincus, J. H., Cooper, J. R., Murphy, J. V., Rabe, E. F., Lonsdale, D., and Dunn, H. G.: Thiamine derivatives in subacute necrotizing encephalomyelopathy: A preliminary report. Pediatrics, 51:716–721, 1973.

218. Elsas, L. J., and Danner, D. J.: Effect of thiamin on normal and mutant human branch chain alpha-ketoacid dehydrogenase. In Gubler, C., Fujiwara, M., and Dreyfus, P. (eds.): Thiamine. New York, John Wiley and Sons, 1975.

219. Danner, D. J., Wheeler, F. B., Lemmon, S. K., and Elsas, L. J. II: In vivo and in vitro response of human branched chain alpha ketoacid dehydrogenase to thiamine and thiamine pyrophos-

phate. Pediatr. Res., 12:235–238, 1978.

220. Rogers, L. E., Porter, F. S., and Sidbury, J. B., Jr.: Thiamine responsive megablastic anemia. J. Pediatr., 74:495–504, 1969.

221. Viana, M. B., and Carvalho, R. I.: Thiamine responsive megablastic anemia, sensorineural deafness and diabetes mellitus, a new syndrome. J. Pediatr., 93:235–238, 1978.

222. Leevy, C. M., Baker, H., tenHove, W., Frank, O., and Cherrick, G. R.: B complex vitamins in liver disease of the alcoholic. Am. J. Clin. Nutr., 16:339–346, 1965.

223. Leevy, C. M.: Thiamine deficiency and alcoholism. Ann. N.Y. Acad. Sci., 378:316–326, 1982.

224. Iber, F. L., Blass, J. P., Brin, M., and Leevy, C. M.: Thiamin in the elderly-relation to alcoholism and to neurological degenerative disease. Am. J. Clin. Nutr., 36:1067–1082, 1982.

225. Somogyi, J. C., and Naegel, U: Antithiamine effect of coffee. Int. J. Vitam. Nutr. Res., 46:149–153, 1976.

226. Agee, C. C., and Airth, R. L.: Reversible inactivation of thiamine I of Bacillus thiaminolyticus by its primary substrate, thiamine. J. Bacteriol., 115:957, 1973.

227. Wood, B., Gijsbers, A., Good, A., Davis, S., Mulholland, J., and Breen, K.: A study of partial thiamin restriction in human volunteers. Am. J. Clin. Nutr., 33:848–861, 1980.

228. Blyth, J.: J. Chem. Soc., 35:530, 1879.

229. Kuhn, Gyorgy, and Wagner-Jauregg: Ber., 66:317, 576 and 1034, 1933.

230. Booher, L. E.: The concentration and probable chemical nature of vitamin G. J. Biol. Chem., 102:39–46, 1933.

231. Kuhn, Reinemund, Weygand, Strobell: Ber., 68: 1935.

232. Karrer, Salomon, Schoppe, and Benz: Helv. Chem. Acta, 18:1143, 1935.

233. Sebrell, W. H., and Butler, R. E.: Riboflavin deficiency in man. Publ. Health Rep., 53:2282–2284, 1938.

234. Kruse, S. E., Sydenstricker, V. P., Sebrell, W. H., and Cleckley, H. M.: Ocular manifestations of riboflavinosis. Publ. Health Rep., 55:157–169, 1940.

235. Sydenstricker, V. P., Sebrell, W. H., Cleckley, H. M., and Kruse, S. E.: J.A.M.A., 114:243, 1940.

236. Stanis: Trans. R. Soc. Trop. Med. Hyg., 5:112, 1912.

237. Rivlin, R. S. (ed.): Riboflavin. New York, Plenum Press, 1975.

238. Rivlin, R. S. (ed.): Riboflavin metabolism. N. Engl. J. Med., 283:463–472, 1970.

239. Rivlin, R. S. (ed.): Riboflavin. New York, Plenum Press, 1975, p. 393–426.

240. Fazekas, A. G. Pinto, J., Huang, Y. P., Chaudhuri, R., and Rivlin, R. S.: Age dependence of thyroxine stimulation of riboflavin incorporation into flavin coenzymes in liver and brain. Endocrinology, 102:641–648, 1978.

241. Rivlin, R. S., Fazekas, A. G., Huang, Y. P., and Chaudhuri, R. A.: In Singer, T. P. (ed.): Flavins and Flavor Proteins. Amsterdam, Elsevier, 1976, p. 747–753.

242. Domjan, G., and Kokai, K.: The flavin adenine dinucleotide (FAD) content of the rat's liver in hypothyroid state and in the liver of hypothyroid animals after in vivo thyroxine treatment.

Acta Biol. Hung., 16:237–241, 1966.

243. Rivlin, R. S.: Regulation of flavoprotein enzymes in hypothyroidism and in riboflavin deficiency. Adv. Enzyme Regul., 8:239–250, 1970.

244. Pinto, J., and Rivlin, R. S.: Regulation of formation of covalently bound flavins in liver and cerebrum by thyroid hormones. Arch. Biochem. Biophys., 194:313–320, 1979.

245. Fazekas, A. G., and Sandor, D.: In vivo effect of adrenocorticotrophin on the biosynthesis of flavin nucleotides in rat liver and kidney. Can. J. Biochem., 49:987–989, 1971.

246. Fazekas, A. G., and Sandor, D.: Studies on the biosynthesis of flavin nucleotides from 2-14-C-riboflavin by rat liver and kidney. Can. J. Biochem., 51:772–782, 1973.

247. Tan, E. L., and Trachewsky, D.: Effect of aldosterone on flavin coenzyme biosynthesis in the kidney. J. Steroid Biochem., 6:1471–1475, 1975.

248. Trachewsky, D.: Aldosterone stimulation of riboflavin incorporation into rat renal flavins coenzymes and the effect of inhibition by riboflavin analogues on sodium reabsorption. J. Clin. Invest., 62:1325–1333, 1978.

249. Pinto, J., Wolinsky, M., and Rivlin, R. S.: Chlorpromazine antagonism of thyroxine-induced flavin formation. Biochem. Pharmacol., 28:597–600, 1969.

250. Pinto, J., Wolinsky, M., and Rivlin, R. S.: Chlorpromazine antagonism of thyroxine-induced flavin formation. Biochem. Pharmacol., 28:597–600, 1979.

251. Pinto, J., Huang, Y. P., and Rivlin, R. S.: Physiological significance of inhibition of riboflavin metabolism by therapeutic doses of chlorpromazine. Clin. Res., 27:444A, 1979.

252. Gromisch, D. S., Lopez, R., Cole, H. S., and Cooperman, J. M.: Light (phototherapy)-induced riboflavin deficiency in the neonate. J. Pediatr., 90:118–122, 1977.

253. Pascale, J. A., Mins, L. C., Greenberg, M. H., Gooden, D. S., and Chronister, E.: Riboflavin and bilirubin response during phototherapy. Pediatr. Res., 10:854–856, 1976.

254. Murphy, U. S., and Idiga, P. R.: J. Biochem. Biophys., 14:118–124, 1977.

255. Adiga, P. R., and Muniyappa, K.: Estrogen induction and functional importance of carrier proteins for riboflavin and thiamine in the rat during gestation. J. Steroid Biochem., 9:829, 1978.

256. Day, P. L., Langston, W. C., and O'Brien, C. S.: Cataract and other ocular changes in vitamin G deficiency. Am. J. Ophthalmol., 14:1005–1009, 1931.

256a. Ono, S., Hira, H., Kudo, L., and Obara, K.: Some biochemical changes in lenses of riboflavin-deficient rats. J. Vitam. Nutr. Res., 14:422–426, 1976.

257. Skalka, H. W., and Prchal, J. T.: Cataracts and riboflavin deficiency. Am. J. Clin. Nutr., 34:861–863, 1981.

258. Bhat, K. S.: Riboflavin deficiency and galactose metabolism in human subjects. Nutr. Metab., 16:111–118, 1974.

259. Bhat, K. S., and Gopalan, C.: Human cataract and galactose metabolism. Nutr. Metab., 17:1–8, 1974.

260. Vir, S. C., Love, A. H. G., and Thompson, W.: Riboflavin status during pregnancy. Am. J. Clin. Nutr., 34:2699–2705, 1981.

261. Warkany, J.: In Rivlin, R. S. (ed.): Riboflavin. New York, Plenum Press, 1975, p. 279–302.

262. Rivlin, R. S.: Riboflavin and cancer: A review.

Cancer Res., 33:1977–1986, 1973.

263. Morris, H. P., and Robertson, W. V. B.: Growth rate and number of spontaneous mammary carcinomas and riboflavin concentration of liver, muscle, and tumor of C3H mice as influenced by dietary riboflavin. J. Natl. Cancer Inst., 3:479–489, 1943.

264. Lane, M., and Smith, F. E.: Induced riboflavin deficiency in treatment of patients with lymphomas and polycythemia vera. Proc. Am. Assoc. Cancer Res., 12:85, 1971.

265. Lakshmi, A. V., and Bamji, M. S.: Regulation of blood pyridoxal phosphate in riboflavin deficiency in man. Nutr. Metab., 20:228–233, 1976.

266. Iyengar, L.: Oral lesions in pregnancy. Lancet, 1:680–681, 1973.

267. Krishnaswamy, K.: Erythrocyte glutamic oxaloacetic transaminase activity in patients with oral lesions. Int. J. Vitam. Nutr. Res., 41:247–252, 1971.

268. Sauberlich, H. E., Dowdy, R. P., and Skala, J. H.: Laboratory Tests for the Assessment of Nutritional Status. Boca Raton, Florida, CRC Press Inc., 1974, p. 33.

269. Erythrocyte glutathione reductase—A measure of riboflavin nutritional status. Nutr. Rev., 30:162–164, 1972.

270. Goodman, S. I.: Organic aciduria in the riboflavin-deficient rat. Am. J. Clin. Nutr., 34:2434–2437, 1981.

271. Ramakrishanan, P., and Seth, U. K.: Serum flavin levels and urinary excretion of riboflavin and riboflavin tetrabutyrate—A comparative evaluation. Ind. J. Med. Res., 66:618–626, 1977.

272. György, P.: Vitamin B_2 and the pellagra-like dermatitis in rats. Nature, 133:498–499, 1934.

273. Liepkovsky, S., Jukes, and Krause, M. E.: J. Biol. Chem., 115:597, 1936.

274. Chick, H., and Copping, A. M.: The composite nature of the water-soluble vitamin B_1. Biochem. J., 24:1764–1779, 1930.

275. Harris, S. A., and Folkers, K.: Synthetic vitamin B. Science, 89:347, 1939.

276. Harris, S. A., and Folkers, K.: Synthesis of vitamin B_6. J. Am. Chem. Soc., 61:1245–1247, 1939.

277. International Symposium on Vitamin B_6 in honor of Professor Paul György. Vitam. Horm., 22:885, 1964.

278. Sebrell, W. H., and Harris, R. S.: The Vitamins. Volume 2. New York, Academic Press, 1968, p. 1–117.

279. Sauberlich, H. E., and Canham, J. E.: In Goodhart, S. R., and Shils, M. E. (eds.): Modern Nutrition in Health and Disease. Edition 5. Philadelphia, Lea & Febiger, 1973.

280. Spies, T. D., Bean, W. B., and Ashe, W. F.: A note on the use of vitamin B_6 in human nutrition. J.A.M.A., 112:2414, 1939.

281. Smith, S. G., and Martin, D. W.: Cheilosis successfully treated with synthetic vitamin B_6. Proc. Soc. Exp. Biol. Med., 43:660, 1940.

282. Morisue, T., Morino, Y., Sakamoto, Y., and Ichihara, K.: Enzymatic studies on pyroxidine metabolism. III. Pyroxidine phosphate oxidase. J. Biochem., 48:28–36, 1960.

283. Anderson, B. B., Saary, M., Stephens, A. D., Perry, G. M., Lersundi, I. C., and Horn, J. E.: Effect of riboflavin on red-cell metabolism of vitamin B_6. Nature, 264:574–575, 1976.

284. Lakshmi, A. B., and Bamji, M. S.: Regulation of blood pyroxidal phosphate in riboflavin deficiency in man. Nutr. Metab., 20:228–233, 1976.

285. Iyengar, L.: Oral lesions in pregnancy. Lancet, 1:680–681, 1973.

286. Krishnaswamy, K.: Erythrocyte glutamic oxaloacetic transaminase activity in patients with oral lesions. Int. J. Vitam. Nutr. Res., 41:247–252, 1971.

287. Lepkovsky, S., and Nielsen, R.: A green-pigment producing compound in urine of pyroxidine-deficient rats. J. Biol. Chem., 144:135–138, 1942.

288. Lepkovsky, S., Roboz, E., and Haagen-Smit, A. J.: Xanthenuric acid and its role in the tryptophane metabolism of pyroxidine-deficient rats. J. Biol. Chem., 149:195–201, 1943.

289. Leevy, C. M., Baker, H., tenHove, W., Frank, O., and Cherrick, G. R.: B complex vitamins in liver disease of the alcoholic. Am. J. Clin. Nutr., 16:339–346, 1965.

290. Gregory, J. F., and Kirk, J. R.: The bioavailability of vitamin B_6 in foods. Nutr. Rev., 39:1–8, 1981.

291. Gregory, J. F., and Kirk, J. R.: J. Food Sci., 42:1554–1557 and 1561, 1977.

292. Gregory, J. F., and Kirk, J. R.: J. Food Sci., 43:1585–1589, 1978.

293. Gregory, J. F., and Kirk, J. R.: Vitamin B_6 activity for rats of gamma-pyridoxyllysine bound to dietary protein. J. Nutr., 108:1192–1199, 1978.

294. Benke, P. J., Fleshood, H. L., and Pitot, H. C.: Osteoporotic bone disease in the pyroxidine-deficient rat. Biochem. Med., 6:526–535, 1972.

295. Sauberlich, H. E., Dowdy, R. P., and Skala, J. H.: Laboratory Tests for the Assessment of Nutritional Status. Boca Raton, Florida, CRC Press, 1974, p. 37–45.

296. Sauberlich, H. E., Canham, J. E., Baker, E. M., Raica, M., and Herman, Y. F.: Biochemical assessment of the nutritional status of vitamin B_6 in the human. Am. J. Clin. Nutr., 25:629–642, 1972.

297. Guilarte, T. R., and McIntyre, P. A.: Radiometric microbiologic assay of vitamin B_6: Analysis of plasma samples. J. Nutr., 111:1861–1868, 1981.

298. Vanderslice, J. T., Maire, C. E., and Beecher, G. R.: B_6 vitamer analysis in human plasma by high performance liquid chromatography: A preliminary report. Am. J. Clin. Nutr., 34:947–950, 1981.

299. Combe, J. S.: Trans. R. Med. Chir. Soc. Edinburgh, 1:194, 1822.

300. Flint: Am. Med. Times, 1:181, 1860.

301. Castle, W. B.: Observations on the etiologic relationship of achylia gastrica to pernicious anemia. Am. J. Med. Sci., 178:748–764, 1929.

302. Rickes, E. L., Brink, M. G., Koniuszy, F. R., Wood, T. R., and Folkers, K.: Crystalline vitamin B_{12}. Science, 107:396–397, 1948.

303. Smith, E. L., and Parker, L. F. J.: Purification of anti-pernicious anaemia factor. Biochem. J., 43:VIII, 1948.

304. Berk, L., Castle, W. B., Welch, A. D., Heinle, R. W., Anker, R., and Epstein, M.: Observations on the etiologic relationship of achylia gastrica to pernicious anemia. N. Engl. J. Med., 239:911–913, 1948.

305. Herbert, V.: In Goodhart, R. S., and Shills, M. E. (eds.): Modern Nutrition Health and Disease. Edition 5. Philadelphia, Lea and Febiger, 1973.

306. Herbert, V.: In Beeson, P. V. and McDermott, W. (eds.): Textbook of Medicine. Edition 14. Phila-

delphia, W. B. Saunders Co., 1975.

307. Sandberg, D. P., Bagley, J. A., and Hall, C. A.: The content, binding, and forms of vitamin B_{12} in milk. Am. J. Clin. Nutr., 34:1717–1724, 1981.

308. Allen, R. H., Seetharam, B., Podell, E., and Alpers, D. A.: Effect of proteolytic enzymes on the binding of cobalamin to R protein and intrinsic factor. J. Clin. Invest., 61:47–54, 1978.

309. Marcoullis, G., Parmentier, Y., Nicholas, J. P., Jimenez, M., and Gerard, P.: Cobalamin malabsorption due to nondegradation of R proteins in the human intestine. J. Clin. Invest., 66:430–440, 1980.

310. Girdwood, R. H.: The intestinal content in pernicious anemia of factors for the growth of Streptococcus faecalis and Lactobacillus leichmannii. Blood, 5:1009–1016, 1950.

311. Kalser, M. H., Cohen, R., Arteaga, I., Yawn, E., Mayoral, L., Hoffert, W. R., and Frazier, D.: Normal viral and bacterial flora of the human small and large intestine. N. Engl. J. Med., 274:500–505, 1966.

312. Bhat, P., Shantakumari, S., Rajan, D., Mathan, V., Kapadia, C. R., Swarnabai, C., and Baker, S. J.: Bacterial flora of the gastrointestinal tract in Southern Indian control subjects and patients with tropical sprue. Gastroenterology, 62:11–21, 1972.

313. Albert, M. J., Mathan, V. I., and Baker, S. J.: Vitamin B_{12} synthesis by human small intestinal bacteria. Nature, 283:781–782, 1980.

314. Foroozan, P., and Trier, J. S.: Mucosa of the small intestine in pernicious anemia. N. Engl. J. Med., 277:553–559, 1967.

315. Sherwood, W., Goldstein, F., Haurani, F., and Wirtz, C. W.: Studies of the small-intestinal bacterial flora and of intestinal absorption in pernicious anemia. Am. J. Digest. Dis., 9:416–425, 1964.

316. Schilling, R. F.: Intrinsic factor studies. J. Lab. Clin. Med., 42:860, 1953.

317. Katz, M., Lee, S. K., and Cooper, B. A.: Vitamin B_{12} malabsorption due to a biologically inert intrinsic factor. N. Engl. J. Med., 287:425–429, 1972.

318. Hakami, N., Nieman, P. E., Canellos, G. P., and Lazerson, J.: Neonatal megaloblastic anemia due to inherited transcobalamin II deficiency in 2 siblings. N. Engl. J. Med., 285:1163–1170, 1971.

319. Cullen, R. W., and Oace, S. M.: Methylmalonic acid and vitamin B_{12} excretion of rats consuming diets varying in cellulose and pectin. J. Nutr., 108:640–647, 1978.

320. Carmel, R.: Macrocytosis, mild anemia, and delay in the diagnosis of pernicious anemia. Arch. Intern. Med., 139:47–50, 1979.

321. Crosby, W. H.: Certain things physicians do. Arch. Intern. Med., 139:23–24, 1979.

322. Cooper, B. A., and Whitehead, V. M.: Evidence that some patients with pernicious anemia are not recognized by radiodilution assay for cobalamin in serum. N. Engl. J. Med., 299:816–818, 1978.

323. Kolhouse, J. F., Kando, H., Allen, M. C., Podell, E., and Allen, R. H.: Cobalamin analogues are present in human plasma and can mask cobalamin deficiency because current radioisotope dilution assays are not specific for true cobalamin. N. Engl. J. Med., 299:785–792, 1978.

324. Zuelzer, W. W., and Rutzky, J.: Megaloblastic anemia in infancy. Adv. Pediatr., 6:243–306, 1953.

325. Jadhav, M., Webb, J. K. G., Vaishnava, S., and Baker, S. J.: Vitamin B_{12} deficiency in Indian infants. Lancet, 2:903–907, 1962.

326. Higginbottom, M. C., Sweetman, L., and Nyhan, W. L.: A syndrome of methylmalonic aciduria, homocystinuria, megaloblastic anemia and neurologic abnormalities in a vitamin B_{12}-deficient breast-fed infant of a strict vegetarian. N. Engl. J. Med., 299:317–323, 1978.

327. Lumb, M., Perry, J., Deacon, R., and Chanarin, I.: Changes in tissue folates accompanying nitrous oxide-induced inactivation of vitamin B_{12} in the rat. Am. J. Clin. Nutr., 34:2412–2417, 1980.

327a. Lumb, M., Perry, J., Deacon, R., and Chanarin, I.: Recovery of tissue folates after inactivation of cobalamin by nitrous oxide: The significance of dietary folate. Am. J. Clin. Nutr., 34:2418–2422, 1980.

328. Chanarin, I.: Nitrous oxide and the cobalamins. Clin. Sci., 59:151–154, 1980.

329. Chanarin, I.: Cobalamins and nitrous oxide: A review. J. Clin. Pathol., 33:909–916, 1980.

330. Chanarin, I., Deacon, R., Lumb, M., and Perry, J.: Vitamin B_{12} regulates folate metabolism by the supply of formate. Lancet, 2:505–508, 1980.

331. Krebs, H., A., Hems, R., Tyler, B.: The regulation of folate and methionine metabolism. Biochem. J., 158:341–353, 1976.

332. Poston, J. M.: Cobalamin-dependent formation of leucine and beta-leucine by rat and human tissue. Chem., 255:10067–10072, 1980.

333. Minot, G. R., and Strauss, M.: In Harris, R. S., and Thimann, K. V. (eds.): Vitamins and Hormones: Advances in Research and Applications. Vol. 1. New York, Academic Press, 1943.

334. Smith, M. D., Smith, D. A., and Fletcher, M.: Haemorrhage associated with thrombocytopenia in megaloblastic anaemia. Br. Med. J., 1:982–985, 1962.

335. Frenkel, E. P.: Abnormal fatty acid metabolism in peripheral nerves of patients with pernicious anemia. J. Clin. Invest., 52:1237–1245, 1973.

336. Kishmoto, Y., Williams, M., Moser, H. W., Hignite, C., and Biemann, K.: Branched-chain and odd-numbered fatty acids and aldehydes in the nervous system of a patient with deranged vitamin B_{12} metabolism. J. Lipid Res., 14:69–77, 1973.

337. Green, R., van Tonder, S. V., Oettele, G. J., Cole, G., and Metz, J.: Neurological changes in fruit bats deficient in vitamin B_{12}. Nature, 24:148–150, 1975.

338. Daft, F. S., Ashburn, L. L., and Sebrell, W. H.: Biotin deficiency and other changes in rats given sulfanilyl-guanidine or succinyl sulfathiazole in purified diets. Science, 96:321, 1942.

339. Oppel, T. W.: Studies of biotin metabolism in man. Am. J. Med. Sci., 204:886, 1942.

340. Hamm, W. E., and Scott, K. W.: Intestinal synthesis of biotin in the rat. J. Nutr., 51:423, 1953.

341. Boyd, E. M., and Sargent, E. J.: The production of skin reactions to benzylpenicillin in animals on a biotin-deficient diet. J. New Drugs, 2:283, 1963.

342. Sydenstricker, V. P., Singal, S. A., Briggs, A. P., DeVaughn, N. M., and Isbell, H.: Preliminary observations on "egg white injury" in man and its cure with a biotin concentrate.

Science, 95:176, 1943.

343. Sydenstricker, V. P., Singal, S. A., Briggs, A. P., DeVaughn, N. M., and Isbell, H.: Observations on the "egg white injury" in man. J.A.M.A. 118:1199–1200, 1942.

344. McCormick, D. B.: Present knowledge in nutrition. Nutrition Reviews. Edition 4. New York and Washington, Nutrition Foundation, Inc., 1976.

345. McCormick, D. B.: Biotin. Nutr. Rev., 33:97–102, 1975.

346. Roth, K. S.: Biotin in clinical medicine—a review. Am. J. Clin. Nutr., 34:1967–1974, 1981.

347. Inis, S. M., and Allardyce, D. B.: Possible biotin deficiency in adults receiving long-term total parenteral nutrition. Am. J. Clin. Nutr., 37:185–187, 1983.

348. Sweetman, L., Suhr, L., and Nyhan, W. L.: Deficiencies of propionyl-CoA and 3-methylcrotonyl-CoA carboxylases in a patient with a dietary deficiency of biotin. Clin. Res., 27:118A, 1979.

349. Wolf, B., Hsai, Y. E., Boychuck, R., Sweetman, L., and Nyhan, W. L.: In vivo enzyme activation by biotin of multiple carboxylase deficiency in a neonate. Pediatr. Res., 14:529, 1980.

350. Roth, K. S., Allan, L., Yang, W., Foreman, J. W., and Dakshinamurti, K.: Serum and urinary biotin levels during treatment of holocarboxylase synthetase deficiency. Clin. Chem. Acta, 109:337–340, 1981.

351. Papyrus Ebers: Medical Writings 1550 B. C. In Chicago, Encyclopedia Britannica, 1964.

352. Hippocrates: The Genuine Works of Hippocrates. Volume I. London, Sydenham Society, 1849, pp. 196 and 267.

353. Pliny: Compages in genubers solverentur. In Major, R. H. (ed.): Classic Descriptions of Disease with Biographical Sketches of the Authors. Springfield, Illinois, Charles C Thomas, 1945.

354. Lind, J.: A Treatise on the Scurvy. London, S. Corwder, D., Wilson, G. Nicholls, T. Kidell, T. Becket, and Company, 1772.

355. Hess: Scurvy—Past and Present. Philadelphia, J. B. Lippincott, 1920.

356. Svirbely, J. L., Szent-Gyorgyi, A.: The chemical nature of vitamin C. Biochem. J., 26:865–870, 1932.

357. Szent-Gyorgyi, A.: Flexner Lectures, Series 6. Baltimore, Williams & Wilkins Company, 1939.

358. Stone, I.: On the genetic etiology of scurvy. Acta Genet. Med. Gemellol., 15:345–350, 1966.

359. Burns, J. J.: Biosynthesis of L-ascorbic acid: Basic defect in scurvy. Am. J. Med., 26:740, 1959.

360. Mussini, E., Hutton, J. J., Jr., and Udenfriend, S.: Collagen proline hydroxylase in wound healing, granuloma formation, scurvy, and growth. Science, 157:927–929, 1967.

361. On Scurvy. The Medical and Surgical History of the War of the Rebellion. Part III. Washington, D.C., U.S. Printing Office, 1888.

362. Abboud, F. M., Hood, J., Hodges, R. E., and Mayer, H. E.: Autonomic reflexes and vascular reactivity in experimental scurvy in man. J. Clin. Invest., 49:298, 1970.

363. Cooper, J. R.: The role of ascorbic acid in the oxidation of tryptophan to 5-hydroxytryptophan. Ann. N.Y. Acad. Sci., 92:208, 1961.

364. Stokes, P. L., Melikian, V., Leeming, R. L., Portman-Graham, H., Blair, J. A., and Cooke, W. T.: Folate metabolism in scurvy. Am. J. Clin. Nutr., 28:126–129, 1975.

365. Herbert V., and Jacob, E.: Destruction of vitamin B_{12} by ascorbic acid. J.A.M.A., 230:241–242, 1974.

366. Tsai, S. C., Fales, H. M., and Vaughan, M.: Inactivation of hormone-sensitive lipase from adipose tissue with adenosine triphosphate, magnesium, and ascorbic acid. J. Biol. Chem., 248:5278–5281, 1973.

367. Chandra, R. K., and Newberne, P. M.: In Nutrition, Immunity and Infection: Mechanisms of Interaction. New York, Plenum Publishing Corporation, 1977.

368. Shilotri, P. G., and Bhat, K. S.: Effect of megadoses of vitamin C on bactericidal activity of leukocytes. Am. J. Clin. Nutr., 30:1077–1081, 1977.

369. Kay, M. E., Holloway, D. E., Hutton, S. W., Bone, N. D., and Duane, W. C.: Human T-cell function in experimental ascorbic acid deficiency and spontaneous scurvy. Am. J. Clin. Nutr., 36:127–130, 1982.

370. Goetzl, E. J., Wasserman, S. I., Gigli, I., and Austin, K. F.: Enhancement of random migration and chemotactic response of human leukocytes by ascorbic acid. J. Clin. Invest., 53:813–818, 1974.

371. Long, D. A.: Ascorbic acid and the production of antibody in the guinea pig. Br. J. Exp. Pathol., 31:183–188, 1950.

372. Anthony, L. E., Kurahara, C. G., and Taylor, K. B.: Cell-mediated cytotoxicity and humoral immune response of human leukocytes by ascorbic acid. Am. J. Clin. Nutr., 32:1691–1698, 1979.

373. Murata, A., and Hasegawa, T. (ed.): Proceedings of the First Intersectional Congress of the IAMS. Volume 3. Science Council of Japan, 1975.

374. Knodell, R. G., Tate, M. A., Akl, B. F., and Wilson, J. W.: Vitamin C prophylaxis for posttransfusion hepatitis: Lack of effect in a controlled trial. Am. J. Clin. Nutr., 34:20–23, 1981.

375. Pauling, L.: Vitamin C prophylaxis for posttransfusion hepatitis. Am. J. Clin. Nutr., 34:1978–1979, 1981.

376. Sutnick, M. R.: Vitamin C prophylaxis for posttransfusion hepatitis. Am. J. Clin. Nutr., 34:1980–1981, 1981.

377. Pauling, L.: Vitamin C and the Common Cold. San Francisco, Freeman Publishers, 1970.

378. Stone, I.: In The Healing Factor—Vitamin C Against Disease. New York, Grossett and Dunlap, 1972.

379. Pauling, L.: A re-evaluation of vitamin C. In Hank, A., and Ritzel, G. (eds.): Re-Evaluation of Vitamin C. Bern, Verlag Hans Huber, 1977.

380. Barness, L. A.: In Hank, A., and Ritzel, G. (eds.): Re-Evaluation of Vitamin C. Bern, Verlag Hans Huber, 1977.

381. Stein, H. B., Hasan, A., and Fox, I. H.: Ascorbic acid-induced uricosuria: A consequence of megavitamin therapy. Ann. Intern. Med., 84:385–388, 1976.

382. Briggs, M. H., Garcia-Webb, P., and Davies, P.: Urinary oxalate and vitamin C supplements. Lancet, 2:201, 1973.

383. Campbell, G. D., Jr., Steinberg, M. N., and Bower, J. D.: Ascorbic acid-induced hemolysis in G-6-PD deficiency. Ann. Intern. Med., 82:810, 1975.

384. Cochrane, W. A.: Overnutrition in prenatal and neonatal life: A problem? Can. Med. Assoc. J., 93:893–899, 1965.

385. Herbert, B., and Jacob, E.: Destruction of vitamin B_{12} by ascorbic acid. J.A.M.A., 233:241–242, 1974.

386. Mengel C. E., and Greene, H. L., Jr.: Ascorbic acid effects on erythrocytes. Ann. Intern. Med., *84*:490, 1976.

387. Chen, L. H.: An increase in vitamin E requirement induced by high supplementation of vitamin C in rats. Am. J. Clin. Nutr., *34*:1036–1041, 1981.

388. Sure, B., Theis, R. M., and Harrelson, R. T.: Vitamin interrelationships. J. Biol. Chem., *129*:245–253, 1939.

389. Gruber, K. A., O'Brien, L. V., and Gerstner, R.: Vitamin A: Not required for adrenal steroidogenesis. Science, *191*:472–475, 1976.

394. Milne, D. B., Omaye, S. T., and Amos, W. H.: Effect of ascorbic acid on copper and cholesterol in adult cynomologus monkeys fed a diet marginal in copper. Am. J. Clin. Nutr., *34*:2389–2393, 1981.

395. DiSilvestro, R. A., and Harris, E. D.: A postabsorption effect of L-ascorbic acid on copper metabolism in chicks. J. Nutr., *11*:1964–1968, 1981.

396. Hansky, J., and Allmand, F.: Gastrointestinal bleeding: The role of vitamin C. Austral. Ann. Med., *18*:248–250, 1969.

397. Lester, D., Buccino, R., and Bizzocco, D.: The vitamin C status of alcoholics. J. Nutr., *70*:278–282, 1960.

398. Krasner, N., Dow, J., Moore, M. R., and Goldberg, A.: Ascorbic-acid saturation and ethanol metabolism. Lancet, 2:693–695, 1974.

399. Fazio, V., Flint, D. M., and Wahlqvist, M. L.: Acute effects of alcohol on plasma ascorbic acid in healthy subjects. Am. J. Clin. Nutr., *34*:2394–2396, 1981.

400. Hallberg, L., Rossander, L., Persson, H., and Svahn, E.: Deleterious effects of prolonged warming of meals on ascorbic acid content and iron absorption. Am. J. Clin. Nutr., *36*:846–850, 1982.

401. Boxer, L. A., Watanabe, A. M., Rister, M., Besch, H. R., Jr., Allen, J., and Baehner, R. L.: Correction of leukocyte function in Chediak-Higashi syndrome by ascorbate. N. Engl. J. Med., *295*:1041–1045, 1976.

402. Andrews, J., Brook, M., and Allen, M. A.: Influence of abode and season on vitamin C status of the elderly. Geront. Clin., *8*:257–266, 1966.

403. Schorah, C. J., Tormey, W. P., Brooks, G. H., Robertshaw, A. M., Young, G. A., Talukder, R., and Kelly, J. F.: The effect of vitamin C supplements on body weight, serum proteins, and general health of an elderly population. Am. J. Clin. Nutr., *34*:871–876, 1981.

404. Schaffert, R. R., and Kingsley, G. R.: A rapid simple method for the determination of reduced dehydro-, and total ascorbic acid in biological material. J. Biol. Chem., *212*:59, 1955.

405. Sauberlich, H. E., Dowdy, R. P., and Skala, J. H.: Laboratory Tests for the Assessment of Nutritional Status. Boca Raton, Florida, CRC Press, 1974.

406. Baker, E. M., Hodges, R. E., Hood, J., Sauberlich, H. E., March, S. C., and Canham, J. E.: Metabolism of 14-C and ³H-labeled L-ascorbic acid in human scurvy. Am. J. Clin. Nutr., *24*:444–454, 1971.

407. Canning: N. Engl. Q. J. Med. Surg., *1*:157, 1842.

408. Osler, W.: The severe anaemias of pregnancy and the post-mortem state. Br. Med. J., *1*:1, 1919.

409. Wills, L., Clutterbuck, P. W., and Evans, B. D. F.: A new factor in the production and cure of macrocytic anaemias and its relation to other haemopoietic principles curative in pernicious anemia. Biochem. J., *31*:2136, 1937.

410. Stokstad, E. L. R.: Some properties of a growth factor for Lactobacillus casei. J. Biol. Chem., *149*:573, 1943.

411. Day, P. L., Mims, V., Totter, J. R., Stokstad, E. L. R., Hutchings, B. L., and Sloane: The successful treatment of vitamin M deficiency in the monkey with highly purified Lactobacillus casei factor. J. Biol. Chem., *157*:423, 1945.

412. Snell, E. E., and Peterson, W. H.: Growth factors for bacteria. J. Bacteriol., *39*:273, 1940.

413. Mitchell, H. K., Snell, E. E., and Williams, R. J.: The concentration of folic acid. J. Am. Chem. Soc., *63*:2284, 1941.

414. Colman, N., and Herbert, V.: Total folate binding capacity of normal human plasma, and variations in uremia, cirrhosis, and pregnancy. Blood, *48*:911, 1976.

415. da Costa, M., and Rothenberg, S. P.: Appearance of a folate binder in leukocytes and serum of women who are pregnant or taking oral contraceptives. J. Lab. Clin. Med., *83*:207–214, 1974.

416. Fernandes-Costa, F., and Metz, J.: The specific folate-binding capacity of serum. J. Lab. Clin. Med., *98*:119–126, 1981.

417. Kamen, B. A., and Caston, J. D.: Purification of folate binding factor in normal umbilical cord serum. Proc. Natl. Acad. Sci. USA, *72*:4261–4265, 1975.

418. Ford, J. E.: Some observations on the possible nutritional significance of vitamin B_{12} and folate-binding proteins in milk. Br. J. Nutr., *31*:243–257, 1974.

419. Waxman, S., and Schriber, C.: The role of folic acid binding proteins (FABP) in the cellular uptake of folates. Proc. Soc. Exp. Biol. Med., *147*:760–764, 1974.

420. Colman, N., Hettiarachchy, N., and Herbert, V.: Detection of a milk factor that facilitates folate uptake by intestinal cells. Science, *211*:1427–1429, 1981.

421. Gregory, J. F. III: Denaturation of the folacin-binding protein in pasteurized milk products. J. Nutr., *112*:1329–1338, 1982.

422. Dahr, G. J., Selhub, J., Gay, C., and Rosenberg, I. H.: Direct in vivo demonstration of the sequence of events in intestinal polyglutamyl folate absorption. Clin. Res., *25*:309A, 1977.

423. Kesavan, V., and Noronha, J. M.: Folate malabsorption in aged rats related to low levels of pancreatic folyl conjugase. Am. J. Clin. Nutr., *37*:262–267, 1983.

424. Baker, H., Jaslow, S. P., and Frank, O.: Severe impariment of dietary folate utilization in the elderly. J. Am. Geriatr. Soc., *26*:218–221, 1978.

425. Halsted, C. H., Robles, E. A., and Mezey, E.: Decreased jejunal uptake of labeled folic acid (3H-PGA) in alcoholic patients. Role of alcohol and nutrition. N. Engl. J. Med., *285*:701–706, 1971.

426. Cherrick, G. R., Baker, H., and Frank, O.: Observations on hepatic avidity for folate in Laennec's cirrhosis. J. Lab. Clin. Med., *66*:446–451, 1965.

427. Sullivan, L. W., and Herbert, V.: Suppression of hematopoiesis by ethanol. J. Clin. Invest., *43*:2048–2062, 1964.

428. Belaiche, J., Matuchansky, C., Zittoun, J., Rambaud, J. C., Bernier, J. J., and Cattan, D.: "Folate-losing gastropathy" and intestinal folate ab-

sorption in patients with Menetrier's disease (giant hypertrophic gastritis). Am. J. Dig. Dis., 23:143–147, 1978.

429. Sauberlich, H. E., Dowdy, R. P., and Skala, J. H.: Laboratory Tests for the Assessment of Nutritional Status. Boca Raton, Florida, CRC Press, 1974.

430. Gutcho, S., and Mansback, L.: Simultaneous radioassay of serum vitamin B_{12} and folic acid. Clin. Chem., 23:1609–1614, 1977.

431. Killmann, S. A.: Effect of deoxyuridine on incorporation of tritiated thymidine: Difference between normoblasts and megaloblasts. Acta Med. Scand., 175:483–488, 1964.

432. Herbert, V., Tisman, G., Go, L. P., and Brenner, L.: The dU suppression test using ^{125}I-UdR to define biochemical megaloblastosis. Br. J. Haematol., 24:713–723, 1973.

433. Das, K. C., and Herbert, V.: The lymphocyte as a marker of past nutritional status: Persistence of abnormal lymphocyte deoxyuridine (dU) suppression test and chromosomes in patients with past deficiency of folate and vitamin B_{12}. Br. J. Haematol., 38:219–233, 1978.

434. Das, K. C., Herbert, V., Colman, N., and Longo, D. L.: Unmasking overt folate deficiency in iron-deficient subjects with neutrophil hypersegmentation: dU suppression tests on lymphocytes and bone marrow. Br. J. Haematol., 39:357–375, 1978.

435. Shane, B.: High performance liquid chromatography of folates: Identification of poly-gamma-glutamate chain lengths of labeled and unlabeled folates. Am. J. Clin. Nutr., 35:599–608, 1982.

436. Thiery, F.: DeVandermonde, 1755.

437. Casal, G.: Historia Natural y Medica de el Principado de Asturias, Madrid, 1762.

438. Sebrell, W. H., Jr.: History of pellagra. Fed. Proc., 40:1520–1522, 1981.

439. Frapolli, F.: Animadversiones in Morbum Vulgo Pelagram, Milan, 1771.

440. Goldberger, J.: The transmission of pellagra. Publ. Health Rep., 31:3159–3173, 1916.

441. Elvehjem, C. A., Madden, R. J., Strong, F. M., and Wooley, D. W.: Relation of nicotinic acid and nicotinic acid amide to canine black tongue. J. Am. Chem. Soc., 59:1767–1768, 1937.

442. Elvehjem, C. A., Madden, R. J., Strong, F. M., and Wooley, D. W.: The isolation and identification of the anti-black tongue factor. J. Biol. Chem., 123:137, 1938.

443. Krehl, W. A., Sarma, P. S., Teply, L. J., and Elvehjem, C. A.: Factors affecting the dietary niacin and tryptophane requirement of the growing rat. J. Nutr., 31:85, 1946.

444. Committee on Dietary Allowances, Committee on Interpretation of the Recommended Daily Allowances: Recommended Dietary Allowances. Edition 8. Washington, D.C., National Academy of Sciences, 1974.

445. Free and "bound" niacin for pigs. Nutr. Rev., 15:11–12, 1957.

446. Bound niacin. Nutr. Rev., 19:240–242, 1961.

447. Effect of cooking on the free niacin content of food. Nutr. Rev., 23:286–287, 1965.

448. Trigonelline as a major urinary metabolite of niacytin in the rat. Nutr. Rev., 29:260–262, 1971.

449. Forms of bound niacin in wheat. Nutr. Rev., 32:124–125, 1974.

450. Dann, W. J.: The human requirements for nicotinic acid. Fed. Proc., 3:159–161, 1944.

451. Carter, E. G. A., and Carpenter, K. J.: The bioavailability for humans of bound niacin from wheat bran. Am. J. Clin. Nutr., 36:855–861, 1982.

452. Belavady, B., Srikantia, S. G., and Gopalan, C.: The effect of the oral administration of leucine on the metabolism of tryptophan. Biochem. J., 87:652–655, 1963.

453. Raghuramulu, N., Srikantia, S. G., Narasinga Rao, B.S., and Gopalan, C.: Nicotinamide nucleotides in the erythrocytes of patients suffering from pellagra. Biochem. J., 96:837–839, 1965.

454. Swaminathan, M.: A colorimetric method for the estimation of nicotinic acid in foodstuffs. Nature, 141:830, 1938.

455. Bandier, E., and Hald, J.: A colorimetric reaction for the colorimetric estimation of nicotinic acid. Biochem. J., 33:264, 1939.

456. Snell, E. E., and Wright, L. D.: A microbiological method for the determination of nicotinic acid. J. Biol. Chem., 139:675, 1941.

457. Sauberlich, H. E., Dowdy, R. P., and Skala, J. H.: Laboratory Tests for the Assessment of Nutritional Status. Boca Raton, Florida, CRC Press, 1974.

458. Williams, R. J., Lyman, C. M., Goodyear, G. H., Truesdail, J. H., and Holliday, D.: "Pantothenic acid," a growth determinant of universal biological occurrence. J. Am. Chem. Soc., 55:2912, 1933.

459. Williams, R. J.: Pantothenic acid—a vitamin. Science, 89:486, 1939.

460. Williams, R. J., Weinstock, H. H., Jr., Rohrmann, E., Truesdail, J. H., Mitchell, H. K., and Meyer, C. E.: Pantothenic acid. II. Analysis and determination. J. Am. Chem. Soc., 61:454–457, 1939.

461. Williams, R. J., and Major, R. T.: The structure of pantothenic acid. Science, 91:246, 1940.

462. Follis: In Deficiency Disease. Springfield, Illinois, Charles C Thomas, 1958.

463. Schroeder, H. A.: Losses of vitamins and trace minerals resulting from processing and preservation of foods. Am. J. Clin. Nutr., 24:562, 1971.

464. Fox, H. M., and Linkswiler, H.: Pantothenic acid excretion on three levels of intake. J. Nutr., 74:451, 1961.

465. Pace, J. K., Stier, L. B., Taylor, D. D., and Goodman, P. S.: Metabolic patterns in preadolescent children. J. Nutr., 74:345, 1961.

466. Cohenour, S. H., and Calloway, D. H.: Blood urine, and dietary pantothenic acid levels of pregnant teenagers. Am. J. Clin. Nutr., 25:512, 1972.

467. Jellery, and Calloway: J. Nutr., 106:17, 1976.

468. Sauberlich, H. E., Dowdy, R. P., and Skala, J. H.: Laboratory Tests for the Assessment of Nutritional Status. Boca Raton, Florida, CRC Press, 1974.

469. Tweto, J., and Larrabee, A. R.: The effect of fasting on synthesis and 4'-phosphopantetheine exchange in rat liver fatty acid synthetase. J. Biol. Chem., 247:4900–4904, 1972.

470. Abiko, Y.: In Greenberg, D. M. (ed.): Metabolic Pathways. Volume 7. New York, Academic Press, 1975.

CHAPTER 7

Nutritional Assessment

GORDON P. BUZBY
JAMES L. MULLEN

Nutritional assessment is the objective evaluation of nutritional status. Until recent years it was commonly believed that nutritional deficiency states were relatively unusual in this country. When recognized, these states were primarily specific micronutrient deficiencies occurring in individuals at the lowest extreme of the socioeconomic spectrum or in individuals practicing bizarre dietary patterns. The emphasis of the American medical community on this limited view of nutritional status has been manifest in the training programs of medical professionals. Most traditional medical curricula provide for reasonable exposure to the diagnosis and treatment of rare micronutrient deficiency states, but little or no mention is made of the far more pervasive problem of diagnosing and treating protein-calorie malnutrition. Although nutritional compromise (as with anorexia and weight loss) is recognized as an accompaniment of many disorders, it has been traditionally viewed as a secondary phenomenon that will resolve spontaneously with correction of the patient's primary disorder.

In recent years several advances have provided a strong impetus to alter substantially the erroneous impression that nutrition is of limited importance in the clinical practice of medicine. First, the prevalence of nutritional deficits in hospitalized patients (particularly protein-calorie malnutrition) has been recognized to be much higher than was heretofore believed and approaches 50 per cent in most series.[1-3] Second, it is now appreciated that malnutrition, even when secondary to some other disorder, carries with it subtantial morbidity and mortality *above and beyond* that associated with the patient's primary disease.[1, 4-7] Many patients with potentially curable disorders succumb to complications of their disease or its therapy that are related directly or indirectly to

their underlying nutritional status. Finally, improved techniques for enteral and parenteral feeding have made malnutrition a uniformly treatable disorder. In most patients, improvements in nutritional status can be achieved prior to or concurrent with treatment of the patient's primary disease, if this is clinically desirable.

Recognition of the importance of nutritional status has defined the need for objective, reliable, clinically practical methods for nutritional assessment. Nutritional assessment, the first step in nutritional support, is the means by which one diagnoses, characterizes, and quantitates malnutrition and provides a mechanism to monitor the therapeutic response to nutritional support. Providing nutritional support to a patient without baseline and serial nutritional assessments is analogous to providing blood transfusions without having determined the hematocrit either before or after transfusion. Few clinicians would administer blood without objective evidence of anemia or hypovolemia. In contrast, crucial judgments regarding the need for nutritional support are frequently based on subjective impression rather than on reliable data. It is the responsibility of health care professionals in the field of clinical nutrition to establish and maintain protocols for the objective assessment of nutritional status on a hospital-wide basis.

CLINICAL APPROACH TO NUTRITIONAL ASSESSMENT

Nutritional assessment may be viewed broadly as a three-phase procedure:

Phase I   Clinical History and Physical Examination: Identification of the high-risk patient and selection of candidates for complete nutritional assessment

Phase IIa — Baseline Nutritional Assessment: Simple battery of studies to detect, characterize, and quantify suspected protein-calorie malnutrition

Phase IIb — In-depth Nutrient-specific Evaluation: Detailed biochemical evaluation of suspected specific deficiency state (usually micronutrient)

Phase III — Serial Nutritional Assessment: Monitoring therapeutic efficacy of the nutritional-support regimen

Any patient requiring hospitalization should undergo a history and physical examination that specifically seeks to uncover signs and symptoms characteristic of individuals at high risk of micronutrient or protein-calorie malnutrition. High-risk patients should be subjected to phase IIa or phase IIb testing, or both, depending on the specific risk factor(s) identified in phase I. Low-risk patients need not be subjected to more detailed baseline assessment, but the clinician is cautioned to repeat this process weekly to avoid overlooking risk factors which develop or become evident only after a period of hospitalization.

Phase I: Clinical History and Physical Examination

From a nutritional point of view, the objective of the initial history and physical examination is not to diagnose nutritional deficits but to identify patients who require more detailed assessment. In general, the clinician should sacrifice specificity for sensitivity in this initial evaluation—that is, he should have a "low threshold" for subjecting patients to more thorough assessment in order to avoid overlooking patients with subtle findings. It must be emphasized that the absence of obvious cachexia or a history of prolonged suboptimal nutrient intake does not rule out significant or even life-threatening malnutrition. Recent studies have documented the development of major metabolic and nutritional abnormalities within days of a major insult (such as trauma, onset of a major illness) in previously healthy, well-nourished individuals. It must also be emphasized that micronutrient (vitamin, mineral, trace elements) and macronutrient

Table 7–1 DISEASE STATES AND HISTORICAL FEATURES ASSOCIATED WITH MICRONUTRIENT DEFICIENCIES[24, 127–129]

DISEASE STATE OR HISTORICAL FEATURE	ASSOCIATED DEFICIENCY
Gastrointestinal Disorders	
Pancreatic insufficiency	Vitamins A, D, E, K
Gastrectomy	Vitamins A, D, E, B_{12}, folic acid, iron, calcium
Liver disease, alcoholism	Vitamins A, D, C, riboflavin, niacin, thiamine, folic acid, magnesium, zinc
Short bowel syndrome, ileal resection	Vitamins B_{12}, folic acid, calcium, magnesium
Blind loop syndrome	Vitamin B_{12}
Sprue, gluten enteropathy	Vitamin A, folic acid
Bile salt depletion, cholestyramine ingestion	Vitamins A, K
Obstructive jaundice	Vitamins A, K
Prolonged antacid therapy, peptic ulcer disease	Thiamine, vitamin C
Endocrine Disorders	
Thyrotoxicosis	Vitamins A, B_6, B_{12}, C, thiamine, folic acid
Diabetes Mellitus	Magnesium, chromium
Cardiorespiratory Disorders	
Chronic obstructive pulmonary disease	Vitamin A
Congestive heart failure	Vitamins A, C, thiamine
Cystic fibrosis	Vitamin A
Hematopoietic Disorders	
Sickle cell anemia	Folic acid
Leukemia	Folic acid
Renal Disorders	
Chronic renal failure	Magnesium, calcium, vitamin D*
Miscellaneous Disorders	
Prolonged antibiotic therapy	Vitamin K
Fever	Vitamins A, C, thiamine, riboflavin, folic acid

*Inability of renal tissue to synthesize the metabolically active form of vitamin D.

(protein-calorie) deficiencies can occur independently or simultaneously so that the clinician must specifically seek risk-factors for deficiencies of both classes of nutrients.

Micronutrient Deficiency Risk Factors. It is beyond the scope of this chapter to present a detailed description of the various micronutrient deficiency syndromes. Rather, an abbreviated screening system has been developed to use in ruling out major risk of a deficiency state or to focus attention to a specific micronutrient deficit in a given clinical setting. In Tables 7–1 and 7–2 the observed clinical finding is followed by a list of deficiency states that may be associated with it. The format of these tables reflects more closely the process of moving from a clinical observation to a biochemical diagnosis and may be more useful from a purely practical point of view.

Macronutrient Deficiency Risk Factors. In the absence of specific micronutrient deficiencies, protein-calorie malnutrition is still a common phenomenon. The prevalence of this entity in hospitalized patients dictates that clinicians be highly suspicious of its presence and do what is necessary to detect and quantitate its severity. One could argue that *all* patients sufficiently ill to require hospitalization warrant routine nutritional assessment. Although this is an extreme view, it is likely that the yield from such routine nutritional screening would be higher than the yield from many studies now performed

Table 7–2 PHYSICAL AND LABORATORY FINDINGS ASSOCIATED WITH MICRONUTRIENT DEFICIENCIES[24, 127–129]

PHYSICAL OR LABORATORY FINDING	ASSOCIATED DEFICIENCY
Mucocutaneous Organs and Hair	
Angular stomatitis, cheilosis, magenta tongue	Riboflavin
Glossitis, pellagrous dermatitis, atrophic papillae	Niacin
Xerosis, follicular hyperkeratosis	Linoleic acid
Acneiform forehead rash, nasolabial seborrhea, stomatitis	Vitamin B_6
Conjunctival and corneal xerosis, follicular hyperkeratosis, Bitot's spots, keratomalacia	Vitamin A
Petechiae, ecchymoses, swollen and hemorrhagic gums, prominent hair follicles, corkscrew hair	Vitamin C
Petechiae, ecchymoses	Vitamin K
Parakeratosis, alopecia	Zinc
Dystrophic nails (koilonychia), pale conjunctiva	Iron
Neurologic System	
Peripheral neuropathy, Wernicke's encephalopathy	Thiamine
Peripheral neuropathy, convulsive seizures, depression	Vitamin B_6
"Burning feet" syndrome	Pantothenic acid
Peripheral paresthesias, spinal cord symptoms	Vitamin B_{12}
Peripheral neuropathy, myelopathy, encephalopathy (pellagra)	Niacin
"Night blindness"	Vitamin A
Hematologic System	
Hemolytic anemia	Vitamin E
Macrocytic anemia	Vitamin B_{12}, folic acid
Microcytic and hypochromic anemia	Iron, copper
Microcytic anemia	Vitamin B_6
Coagulopathy	Vitamin K
Sideroblastic anemia, neutropenia (infants)	Copper
Thrombocytopenia	Linoleic acid
Musculoskeletal System	
Osteomalacia, tetany, rickets	Vitamin D
Tender, atrophic muscles	Thiamine
Joint pain, muscle weakness	Vitamin C
Osteopenia (infants)	Copper
Visceral Organs	
Congestive heart failure	Thiamine
Diarrhea	Folic acid, zinc, niacin
Goiter	Iodine
Hypogonadism, hepatosplenomegaly	Zinc
Other	
Anorexia, hypogeusesthesia	Zinc

routinely upon hospital admission (for example, electrocardiogram, urinalysis, serum electrolytes). Nevertheless, it is possible to establish some guidelines for selection of patients for nutritional assessment based on features of the clinical history and physical examination.

Chronic Diseases. Malignancy, kidney disease, liver disease, peptic ulcer disease, diabetes mellitus, congestive heart failure.

Digestive or Absorptive Abnormalities. Pancreatic disease, inflammatory bowel disease, short-gut syndrome (including jejuno-ileal bypass), gastrointestinal fistula, sprue, external biliary fistula, chronic diarrhea, nausea, vomiting.

Social Factors. Drug or alcohol abuse, poverty.

Dietary Factors. Fads, poor dentition.

Other Factors. Major burns, sepsis, recent surgery, pregnancy, lactation, chemotherapy, radiotherapy.

All patients with one or more of the risk factors listed above merit more detailed nutritional assessment, even if initial cursory evaluation does not point to overt protein-calorie malnutrition.

Phase II: Nutritional Assessment of the High-risk Patient

Patients identified as being at risk of nutritional deficiencies based on clinical findings should undergo more detailed nutrient-specific evaluation. For most micronutrient deficiencies, this evaluation will include some direct or indirect measure of the quantity or activity of the nutrient in some body fluid or compartment accessible to analysis (serum, urine, hair, red blood cells, and so forth). A brief summary of clinically available techniques for micronutrient analysis is provided in Table 7–3.

Patients at risk of protein-calorie malnutrition should undergo evaluation to confirm the presence of this entity, to determine its severity, and to ascertain the type of malnutrition present. There is no general agreement as to which studies most accurately characterize protein-calorie malnutrition. Most would agree, however, that these studies should include at least the following: (1) measure(s) of body weight and weight loss, (2) measure(s) of static caloric reserve (fat stores), (3) measure(s) of static protein reserve (muscle stores), (4) measure(s) of circulating protein status, and (5) measure(s) of immune status.

The particular study that best reflects the status of each of these components is open to substantial debate and may vary considerably depending upon the specific clinical situation. A variety of clinically available techniques for the measurement of each component will be discussed together with the advantages and disadvantages of each. This is followed by a summary scheme for

Table 7–3   METHODS AND STANDARDS FOR MICRONUTRIENT ANALYSIS[130, 131]

MICRONUTRIENT	SAMPLE	ASSAY	NORMAL VALUE OR RANGE
Vitamin A	Serum	Fluorometric	25–50 µgm/dl
Vitamin D (1,25(OH)$_2$D$_3$)	Serum	Radiologic after preparative chromatography	30 pg/ml ± 10 pg/ml (not affected by supplemental vitamins or exposure to sunlight)
Vitamin E	Serum	Colorimetric	0.5–1.5 mg/dl
Vitamin K		No direct method is available. For clinical purposes the one-stage test of Quick (with various modifications) for measuring plasma prothrombin time is widely used.	
Thiamine	Red cells	Enzymatic (transketolase)	Activity coefficient <1.27
Riboflavin	Red cells	Enzymatic (erythrocyte glutathione reductase)	Activity coefficient: acceptable, <1.2; deficient, >1.4
Niacin	Urine	Microbiologic	>3.0 ng/24 hr
Pantothenic acid	Urine	Microbiologic	1–15 mg/24 hr
Pyridoxine	Red cells	Enzymatic (glutamate-oxaloacetate transaminase)	EGOT index ≤1.80
Vitamin B$_{12}$	Serum	Microbiologic	200–900 pg/ml
Folic acid	Serum/red cells	Microbiologic	7–15 ng/ml; 200–900 ng/ml
Biotin	Urine	Microbiologic	6–50 µgm/24 hr
Vitamin C	Serum	Colorimetric	0.5–1.5 mg/dl
Zinc	Serum	Atomic absorption spectrophotometry	100–150 µgm/dl
Copper	Serum	Atomic absorption spectrophotometry	80–130 µgm/dl

nutritional assessment which we found useful together with a clinically applicable approach to the interpretation of a battery of nutrition studies.

Body Weight. When compared with ideal standards or usual weight, body weight may provide useful but limited information relative to overall nutritional status. Weight loss exceeding 10 per cent should alert the clinician to possible underlying nutritional compromise; weight loss exceeding 20 per cent may be a risk factor for patients undergoing major surgery.[8] Nevertheless, the use of body weight or weight loss history as an absolute screening criterion for clinically important malnutrition is frequently misleading. Significant gradual weight loss in a patient who is well adapted to inadequate caloric intake can occur through contraction of fat stores with preservation of other more crucial body compartments. That patient may tolerate a major acute insult such as surgery or sepsis remarkably well if adequate nutrition can be restored shortly after the insult. In contrast, an acutely ill patient may demonstrate marked compromise of crucial body compartments, but minimal weight change, as a result of both the acute nature of the insult and the expansion of other noncrucial compartments, especially extracellular water. It is best to consider substandard body weight (less than 80 per cent of ideal weight) and weight loss (less than 90 per cent of usual weight) as *risk factors* for malnutrition rather than *indicators* of malnu-

trition. The presence of either should induce the clinician to perform a complete nutritional assessment. However, the severity of weight loss cannot be equated with the severity of malnutrition, and the absence of *any* weight loss in no way rules out significant malnutrition. Standards for ideal body weight, established by the Metropolitan Life Insurance Company, are given in Table 7–4.

Measures of Static Caloric Reserve (Fat Stores). Fat has the greatest caloric density (calories per unit weight) of all major body tissues. Fat stores are the primary energy source during prolonged, adapted starvation. Determination of the magnitude of fat depots may permit one to estimate the duration and severity of pre-existing malnutrition and may provide an indication of a patient's caloric reserve and therefore his ability to tolerate an additional period of unstressed starvation. Reasonably accurate estimates of total body lipid content may be obtained by densitometry (usually requiring underwater weighing), isotope dilution,[9, 10] and inert gas uptake techniques.[11] Although useful in a research setting, these methods are not easily applied in a clinical setting, particularly in seriously ill patients.

Anthropometric Assessment of Body Fat. Since approximately half of total body fat is located subcutaneously in normal humans, measures of subcutaneous fat may provide a reasonable estimate of total body fat. Numerous noninvasive techniques are available for quantitative assessment of sub-

Table 7–4   IDEAL WEIGHT FOR HEIGHT*

MALES						FEMALES					
Height (cm)	Weight (kg)	Height (cm)	Weight (kg)	Height (cm)	Weight (kg)	Height (cm)	Weight (kg)	Height (cm)	Weight (kg)	Height (cm)	Weight (kg)
145	51.9	159	59.9	173	68.7	140	44.9	150	50.4	160	56.2
146	52.4	160	60.5	174	69.4	141	45.4	151	51.0	161	56.9
147	52.9	161	61.1	175	70.1	142	45.9	152	51.5	162	57.6
148	53.5	162	61.7	176	70.8	143	46.4	153	52.0	163	58.3
149	54.0	163	62.3	177	71.6	144	47.0	154	52.5	164	58.9
150	54.5	164	62.9	178	72.4	145	47.5	155	53.1	165	59.5
151	55.0	165	63.5	179	73.3	146	48.0	156	53.7	166	60.1
152	55.6	166	64.0	180	74.2	147	48.6	157	54.3	167	60.7
153	56.1	167	64.6	181	75.0	148	49.2	158	54.9	168	61.4
154	56.6	168	65.2	182	75.8	149	49.8	159	55.5	169	62.1
155	57.2	169	65.9	183	76.5						
156	57.9	170	66.6	184	77.3						
157	58.6	171	67.3	185	78.1						
158	59.3	172	68.0	186	78.9						

Modified from Jelliffe, D.: The Assessment of the Nutritional Status of the Community, with Special Reference to Field Surveys in Developing Regions of the World. Geneva, World Health Organization Monograph Series No. 53, 1966.

cutaneous fat stores. The simplest method is caliper measurement of skinfold thickness over one or more sites (for example, triceps, biceps, subscapular, abdominal, suprailiac, medial calf, anterior thigh). Subcutaneous fat as measured by skinfold thickness has been shown to correlate reasonably well with adipose content determined by densitometry, radiography, and autopsy techniques.[12, 13]

Nevertheless, estimation of subcutaneous fat and total body fat from skinfold thickness can be erroneous, with variations based on observer technique, site of measurement, position of subject (for example, erect, supine), and equipment used. Measurements made on a single subject on different days by different observers have a coefficient of variation of up to 22.6 per cent.[14] Estimation of *total body fat* from skinfolds is subject to further inaccuracies due to age, race, sex, and habitus-specific variability in topographic distribution of fat stores. Skinfold measurement at multiple sites may improve reliability,[15] and numerous formulas have been proposed to extrapolate the results of subcutaneous fat determinations to measurements of total body fat content.[16–19] These formulas attempt to relate a variety of anthropometric measurements (skinfold thicknesses, diameters, circumferences, and so forth) to actual body fat content as determined by body compositional techniques using multiple regression analysis. Several such regressions have correlation coefficients between 0.85 and 0.87, indicating that about 20 per cent of variance is not accounted for by the regression.[10]

Despite intersubject variability in topographic fat distribution, adipose tissue *losses* from subcutaneous depots during undernutrition occur proportionally.[12, 20, 21] Therefore, serial determinations of selected skinfolds can provide a good reflection of trends in the status of adipose stores in a single individual. A good correlation exists between weight change and the *sum* of triceps and subscapular skinfold thicknesses ($r = 0.75$ for males, $r = 0.74$ for females).[22, 23] These two skinfolds are relatively easy to measure, even in seriously ill patients, and are probably adequate for providing a good estimate of the qualitative status of fat depots. Percentile rankings for the sum of triceps and subscapular skinfolds are given in Table 7–5. Interpretation of the severity of fat store deficiency will vary among professionals in nutrition. In general, however, measurements below the thirty-fifth to fortieth percentile imply mild depletion, within the twenty-fifth to thirty-fifth percentile indicate moderate depletion, and below the twenty-fifth percentile denote severe depletion.[24]

Measures of Static Protein Reserve (Muscle Stores). *Anthropometric Assessment of Muscle Mass.* Approximately 60 per cent of total body protein is contained in muscle. Skeletal muscle is the major site of protein hydrolysis and is the largest donor of amino acids during undernutrition.[25] For these reasons, measures of muscle mass may provide a reasonable measure of static

Table 7–5 REFERENCE STANDARDS FOR SUM OF TRICEPS AND SUBSCAPULAR SKINFOLD*

AGE GROUP (YR)	PERCENTILE						
	5	10	25	50	75	90	95
American Men							
18–74	11.5†	13.5	19.0	26.0	34.5	44.0	51.0
18–24	10.0	12.0	15.0	21.0	30.0	41.0	51.0
25–34	11.5	13.5	19.0	26.0	35.5	45.0	54.0
35–44	12.0	15.0	21.0	28.0	36.0	44.0	48.5
45–54	13.0	15.0	21.0	28.0	37.0	46.0	53.0
55–64	12.0	14.0	20.0	26.0	34.0	44.0	48.0
65–74	11.5	14.0	19.5	26.0	34.0	42.5	49.0
American Women							
18–74	18.5	22.0	28.5	39.0	53.0	65.0	73.0
18–24	17.0	19.0	24.0	31.0	41.5	54.5	64.0
25–34	18.5	20.5	26.5	35.0	48.0	64.0	73.0
35–44	20.0	23.0	30.0	40.5	55.0	68.0	75.0
45–54	22.0	25.0	33.5	45.0	58.0	69.5	78.5
55–64	19.0	25.0	33.0	46.0	58.0	68.0	73.0
65–74	20.0	25.0	32.0	41.0	52.2	63.0	70.0

*Developed from data collected during the Health and Nutrition Examination Survey of 1971–1974.[133]
†Values are in mm.

protein reserves. Numerous biochemical and anthropometric techniques are available to estimate muscle mass. The most widely used anthropometric measure is the mid-arm muscle circumference (MAMC) and the mid-arm muscle area (MAMA). Both of these measures are derived from mid-upper arm circumference (MAC) and triceps skinfold (TSF), according to the following equations:

$$MAMC\ (cm) = MAC\ (cm) - \frac{\Pi TSF\ (mm)}{10}$$

$$MAMA\ (cm^2) = \frac{(MAMC)^2}{4\Pi}$$

Anthropometric assessment of skeletal muscle mass is subject to many errors. First, large intraobserver and interobserver errors are associated with these measurements. The combined measurement variance of skinfold thickness and arm circumference can result in up to a 33 per cent error in arm muscle area between observers and a 10 per cent error between measurements by a single observer.[24] Second, the equations presented above assume that both the arm and arm muscle compartment are circular at the point of measurement and neglect the cross-sectional area of the humerus. Heymsfield, et al. have analyzed the shape of the upper extremity by computerized axial tomography and demonstrated that the shape of the arm approximates an ellipse.[26, 27] Muscle is arranged in a clover-leaf configuration around the humerus, and subcutaneous adipose tissue is distributed asymmetrically around the arm. Third, muscle area in the upper arm may not provide an accurate indication of total body protein and correlates poorly with visceral protein levels.[28] For these reasons, anthropometric assessment can provide only a crude approximation of total body protein, although serial determinations in a single subject may be useful to follow trends in protein status. Standards for MAMC are given in Table 7–6.

Creatinine Excretion and Creatinine-Height Index. Several biochemical techniques are available for clinically assessing the adequacy of muscle protein reserves. The most widely used biochemical marker of muscle mass is the 24-hour urinary creatinine excretion. Creatinine is a product of creatine degradation. Creatine, an energy storage compound (complexed with ATP) found mainly in muscle, spontaneously dehydrates at a relatively constant rate to form creatinine. Creatinine cannot be reutilized, and its excretion in urine is proportional to muscle creatine content and therefore to total body muscle mass. A good correlation has been demonstrated between 24-hour urinary creatinine excretion and lean body mass, as measured by isotope dilution or ^{40}K total body counting.[29-31] Forbes and Bruining[32] developed the following relation between lean body mass (LBM), as measured by ^{40}K counting, and urinary creatinine excretion:

$$LBM\ (kg) = 7.38 + 0.02909\ Cr\ (mg/day) + 0.0008$$

Table 7–6 REFERENCE STANDARDS FOR MIDARM MUSCLE CIRCUMFERENCE*

AGE GROUP (YR)	PERCENTILE						
	5	10	25	50	75	90	95
	American Men						
18–74	26.4†	27.6	29.6	31.7	33.9	36.0	37.3
18–24	25.7	27.1	28.7	30.7	32.9	35.5	37.4
25–34	27.0	28.2	30.0	32.0	34.4	36.5	37.6
35–44	27.8	28.7	30.7	32.7	34.8	36.3	37.1
45–54	26.7	27.8	30.0	32.0	34.2	36.2	37.6
55–64	25.6	27.3	29.6	31.7	33.4	35.2	36.6
65–74	25.3	26.5	28.5	30.7	32.4	34.4	35.5
	American Women						
18–74	23.2	24.3	26.2	28.7	31.9	35.2	37.8
18–24	22.1	23.0	24.5	26.4	28.8	31.7	34.4
25–34	23.3	24.2	25.7	27.8	30.4	34.1	37.2
35–44	24.1	25.2	26.8	29.2	32.2	36.2	38.5
45–54	24.3	25.7	27.5	30.3	32.9	36.8	39.3
55–64	23.9	25.1	27.7	30.2	33.3	36.3	38.2
65–74	23.8	25.2	27.4	29.9	32.5	35.3	37.2

*Developed from data collected during the Health and Nutrition Examination Survey of 1971–1974.[133]
†Values are in cm.

where Cr (mg/day) is the mean 24-hour creatinine excretion on three successive days. The correlation coefficient for this regression is 0.988.

Bistrian and associates have developed a "creatinine-height index," in which the ratio between observed creatinine excretion and expected creatinine excretion for a normal adult of the same sex and height is determined.[33] Expected 24-hour creatinine excretion is calculated from the normal creatinine excretion of healthy males (23 mg/kg/day) and females (18 mg/kg/day), using the patient's ideal weight for height (from Metropolitan Life Insurance standards, assuming medium frame). It is assumed that a reduction in muscle mass produces a proportional reduction in creatinine-height index. For example, if the creatinine-height index is 50 per cent, then the patient has only 50 per cent of the normal muscle mass for a subject of this height. Creatinine-height index values between 60 per cent and 80 per cent are thought to indicate moderate depletion of muscle mass; values below 60 per cent indicate severe depletion. (Table 7–7).[34]

Several problems exist with the use of 24-hour urinary creatinine or creatinine-height index as a measure of muscle mass. Logistic difficulties in obtaining complete 24-hour urine collections may be a major problem in many clinical circumstances. Even in metabolic units, the variance in measurements of creatinine excretion may be as high as 27 per cent.[24] This may relate to the effect of dietary intake on urinary creatinine excretion. Creatinine excretion may decrease by as much as 30 per cent during consumption of creatine-free diet.[35] Further difficulties are introduced by the use of standard weight-for-height tables in predicting expected creatinine excretion. These tables do not account for variability in body habitus and normal intersubject variability in muscle mass. Age is known to be a significant factor influencing creatinine excretion. Urinary creatinine excretion decreases with increasing age,[36] so that the creatinine-height index will frequently indicate a greater degree of muscle mass depletion in the elderly than actually exists.

3-Methylhistidine Excretion. 3-Methylhistidine excretion is another biochemical means of estimating somatic protein mass. 3-Methylhistidine, an amino acid located almost exclusively in myofibrillar protein and released when this protein is degraded, cannot be recycled and is excreted in the urine.[37] The quantity of 3-methylhistidine excreted during a 24-hour period should, therefore, reflect the total amount of muscle protein that is broken down during that period of time. Several difficulties exist with this technique, however. Approximately 35 per cent of muscle protein is sarcoplasmic protein, which does not produce 3-methylhistidine when broken down. In addition, factors others than muscle mass—such as age, sex, dietary intake, and stress (trauma, infection)—have been shown to influence excretion of 3-methylhistidine. Finally, the urinary assay for 3-methylhistidine requires

Table 7–7 REFERENCE STANDARDS FOR 24-HOUR URINARY CREATININE EXCRETION[134]

MEN*		WOMEN†	
Height (cm)	Ideal Creatinine (mg)	Height (cm)	Ideal Creatinine (mg)
157.5	1288	147.3	830
160.0	1325	149.9	851
162.6	1359	152.4	875
165.1	1386	154.9	900
167.6	1426	157.5	925
170.2	1467	160.0	949
172.7	1513	162.6	977
175.3	1555	165.1	1006
177.8	1596	167.6	1044
180.3	1642	170.2	1076
182.9	1691	172.7	1109
185.4	1739	175.3	1141
188.0	1785	177.8	1174
190.5	1831	180.3	1206
193.0	1891	182.9	1240

*Creatinine coefficient = 23 mg/kg of ideal body weight.
†Creatinine coefficient = 18 mg/kg of ideal body weight.

an amino acid analyzer, which is not available in many clinical settings.

In summary, there are no methods currently available to readily assess body stores of protein in a clinical setting. The best available techniques have been described and consist of anthropometric measurements and urinary excretion of creatinine and 3-methylhistidine. Because of their limitations, these measures must be interpreted in the context of other nutritional studies. They are perhaps most useful when used in serial fashion in a single individual to indicate trends in the size of the somatic protein compartment. Several research techniques for assessment of protein reserves (for example, [40]K counting, CAT scan, and neutron activation) are currently under investigation. Some of these may prove clinically applicable and are discussed in a subsequent section of this chapter.

Measures of Circulating Protein Status (Visceral Protein). The levels of circulating serum proteins may be a useful measure of nutritional status. Although serum protein levels may or may not correlate with total body protein content, their rapid turnover and short half-life can make them sensitive indicators of acute changes in nutritional status. The level of total protein in the blood was one of the first biochemical markers recognized to be sensitive to nutritional status. Classically, the total serum protein level is reduced in kwashiorkor and remains normal in marasmus. This is not universal, however, and in some instances of advanced kwashiorkor, serum total protein may be within normal limits.[38, 39] Serum total protein reflects primarily two major components: circulating albumin and globulin. Although serum albumin levels are typically normal in marasmus and are decreased in kwashiorkor,[40] globulin levels are variable and are influenced by many factors unrelated to nutrition. Chronic infection can produce a dramatic increase in the globulin fraction (particularly immunoglobulin), which may be large enough to mask a reduction in serum albumin so that the total protein content of the serum is normal.

Serum Albumin. Albumin is a protein with a molecular weight of 65,000 and has a half-life of approximately 20 days under normal circumstances.[41] Albumin, the major protein synthesized by the liver, serves to maintain plasma oncotic pressure and functions as a carrier protein for enzymes, drugs, hormones, and trace elements.[42, 43] Chronic caloric insufficiency without marked protein insufficiency produces weight loss with maintenance of serum albumin—the classic signs of marasmus. In contrast, chronic protein deficiency (with adequate nonprotein calories) is characterized by minimal weight loss (frequently with edema) but marked hypoalbuminemia—the classic signs of kwashiorkor. This hypoalbuminemia is not a result of redistribution of albumin from the intravascular to the extravascular space. Rather, the total size of the albumin pool is decreased. Both circulating and extravascular albumin are reduced in chronic kwashiorkor to 60 per cent and 40 per cent of normal, respectively.[44] During chronic malnutrition, the rates of both synthesis and degradation of albumin appear to be decreased below normal values, but its relatively long half-life makes serum albumin a relatively poor indicator of early protein malnutrition.[45] Serum albumin concentrations greater than 3.5 gm/dl are normal, concentrations of 3.0 to 3.5 gm/dl indicate mild depletion, concentrations of 2.4 to 2.9 gm/dl moderate depletion, and concentrations of less than 2.4 gm/dl severe depletion.

Serum Transferrin. Transferrin is a glycoprotein with a molecular weight of approximately 76,000[46] and a mean serum half-life of 8.8 days.[47] It migrates electrophoretically with the beta-globulin protein fraction and is synthesized primarily in the liver. Transferrin is the carrier protein for iron in plasma. As early as 1958, a reduction in total iron-binding capacity (TIBC) was observed to accompany kwashiorkor,[48] but total iron-binding capacity is normal in the presence of marasmus.[49] With the development of radial immunodiffusion techniques in 1965,[50] the direct measurement of serum transferrin levels became possible. Prior to that time it had been assumed that the total serum iron-binding capacity was equivalent to the amount of iron required to completely saturate plasma transferrin. Although this assumption is valid in normal and iron-deficient subjects, transferrin levels measured by radial immunodiffusion are consistently lower than those calculated from iron-binding capacity in subjects with kwashiorkor, cirrhosis, and hemochromatosis.[46, 51] It has been postulated that additional iron-containing substances (such as ferritin), are present in the blood of such individuals. In 1968 Antia et al. demonstrated that serum transferrin levels were approximately one fifth of normal in Nigerian children with kwashiorkor.[52] They also demonstrated a correlation between transferrin and the severity and prognosis of the child's disease and noted improvement in transferrin levels with nutritional therapy. Studies in hospitalized patients have demonstrated a similar sensitivity of serum transferrin to nutritional status and have documented a prognostic value to this measure in these patients.[53] Because transferrin has a shorter half-life and exists in a smaller body pool than albumin, it is probably more sensitive to acute changes in the status of the visceral protein compartment.

Serum transferrin can best be measured by radial immunodiffusion, but a fairly good estimate can be obtained from total iron-binding capacity using one of several formulas. Blackburn et al.[34] have developed the following relation:

$$\text{Transferrin} = 0.8 \text{ TIBC} - 43$$

Grant et al.[24] have proposed a similar relationship:

$$\text{Transferrin} = 0.87 \text{ TIBC} + 10$$

These formulas appear most valid for nondepleted, non–iron-deficient patients and probably underestimate transferrin levels in depleted patients. The relationship between transferrin and total iron-binding capacity may vary depending upon the technique used to measure it, so each laboratory must verify the validity of such formulas in its own patient population.

The normal serum transferrin level (as measured by radial immunodiffusion) is greater than 200 mg/dl. Values between 150 and 200 mg/dl indicate mild depletion, values between 100 and 150 mg/dl moderate depletion, and values less than 100 mg/dl severe depletion.

Prealbumin and Retinol-Binding Protein. Retinol-binding protein is an alpha$_1$-globulin with a molecular weight of approximately 21,000.[54] Retinol-binding protein serves as a carrier protein for retinol in plasma and circulates in a 1-to-1 molar ratio with prealbumin.[55] It is synthesized primarily by the liver and is normally present in serum in concentrations of 40 to 50 µgm/ml.

Prealbumin, or thyroxine-binding protein, has a molecular weight of approximately 54,000. Prealbumin plays a role in the transport of thyroxine and is a carrier protein for retinol-binding protein. Prealbumin exists in plasma in concentrations of 200 to 300 µgm/ml, and the body pool of this protein is quite small.[56] The short half-lives of retinol-binding protein and prealbumin (10 hours and 24 hours, respectively) make levels of these two proteins quite sensitive to changes in protein status. Smith et al. demonstrated significant reductions in the serum concentrations of retinol-binding protein, prealbumin, and retinol in Egyptian children with kwashiorkor.[57] Repletion with a high-protein diet produced significant increases in the levels of each protein within two weeks. In a similar study, Ingenbleek[58] demonstrated a reduction in the levels of retinol-binding protein to 81 per cent of normal in 39 Senegalese children. With nutritional repletion, serum levels returned to normal within 22 days. In general, increases in retinol-binding protein and prealbumin precede corresponding changes in albumin and total protein during nutritional repletion.[59] The extreme sensitivity of both retinol-binding protein and prealbumin to any process producing a sudden demand for protein synthesis may be misleading in certain clinical situations (acute surgical stress, acute trauma). Nevertheless, it has recently been demonstrated in primates[60] that these two proteins accurately reflect the overall state of nitrogen balance during malnutrition and refeeding. This close correlation between changes in retinol-binding protein and nitrogen balance is not universal, however, and nutritional status is not the only determinant of retinol-binding protein levels in serum. For example, Venkatswamy et al.[61] have demonstrated that levels of retinol-binding protein in vitamin A-deficient Indian children do not return to normal until they have been given both vitamin A and a high protein supplement.

Measures of circulating protein status are noninvasive, simple to perform, and available in most clinical settings. The clinical relevance of these studies is discussed in a subsequent section of this chapter.

Measures of Immune Status. As early as 1944, Cannon reported an increased rate of infection in malnourished patients.[62] This relationship has been confirmed by numerous investigators[63-66] and has led to the hypothesis that malnutrition per se produces some defect in normal host defenses against infection. The complexity of the immune response and the multiple factors that can have an impact on this response make it difficult to determine the precise nature of the immune deficit in malnutrition. Immunocompetence depends upon the coordinated interaction of a complex array of cellular and humoral components, including lymphocytes, phagocytes, immunoglobulins, complement, and lymphokines. Defects in many of these components have been identified in malnourished subjects.

B-Cell–Mediated Immunity. B-lymphocytes mediate the humoral arm of the immune response. Plasma cells are derived from B-cells and synthesize the five classes of immunoglobulins: IgG, IgM, IgA, IgD, and IgE. The synthesis of immunoglobulins, however, is also dependent on other immunologic elements, and an appropriate humoral response to antigenic stimulation requires cooperation of both T-cells and accessory immune cells.[67, 68]

Determinations of serum immunoglobulin levels in malnourished subjects have produced conflicting results. Various investigators have found high, normal, or low immunoglobulin levels in both malnourished children and adults.[69–72] A major factor responsible for these disparate results may be the presence of infection in some of these subjects.[73, 74] Many of these studies were conducted in tropical or subtropical areas in which secondary infection and parasitic infestation are endemic. Cohen et al.,[75] in a study of malnourished African children, found that the immunoglobulin response to infection was of sufficient magnitude to reverse the normal serum albumin/globulin ratio and to alter total serum protein levels significantly. A second factor that may contribute to the variability of immunoglobulin levels in malnourished subjects is the rapid synthesis of immunoglobulins in response to nutritional therapy.[73] A delay in the initial assessment of immunoglobulin status until after even a brief period of nutritional support could significantly influence the "baseline" serum immunoglobulin determinations.

Despite the variability of serum immunoglobulin levels in malnutrition, several studies have revealed impaired humoral immune responsiveness in malnourished subjects. Wohl et al.[76] and Gell[77] demonstrated subnormal antibody synthesis in malnourished adults after specific antigenic challenge with typhoid antigen and tobacco mosaic virus, respectively. Hodges[78] observed decreased antibody titers to typhoid

and tetanus after dietary protein restriction in healthy human volunteers, and Law et al.[79] noted an impaired antibody response to keyhole limpet hemocyanin in malnourished patients.

Nutritional therapy has been shown to correct deficits in the humoral immune response. Reddy et al.[80] in a study of 32 Indian children with kwashiorkor, found increased antibody titers to typhoid antigen in children treated with high levels of dietary protein. Mathews et al.[81] found a similar heightened humoral response to antigenic stimulation in New Guinean children after protein supplementation, and Law et al.[79] demonstrated increases in both in vivo and in vitro tests of B-cell function in malnourished adults following nutritional repletion. From these data it appears that nutritional status and humoral immune function are related, but the precise nature of this relationship remains unclear. It has been postulated that the major changes in B-cell function seen with malnutrition may be the result of defects in T-lymphocyte function rather than of a B-cell deficit per se.[82]

T-Cell–Mediated Immunity. Thymus-derived lymphocytes (T-cells) mediate the specific cellular immune response. The thymus plays a critical role in the maturation of these cells, and the thymus gland is the most sensitive of all lymphatic tissues to malnutrition.[83] Thymic atrophy occurs in children with severe malnutrition,[84] the number of circulating T-lymphocytes is decreased in malnutrition, and the severity of this decrease parallels the degree of weight loss.[82] The number of circulating T-lymphocytes can be measured clinically by determining the number of peripheral blood lymphocytes that bear receptors for sheep red blood cells (as measured by rosette formation). In African children with protein-calorie malnutrition, Neumann et al.[85] noted more than a three-fold reduction in T-rosette formation. With 5 to 17 days of refeeding, the level of T-rosettes was restored to normal. It has been postulated that the decreased number of T-cells is probably due to either decreased maturation of precursor cells, metabolic defects limiting survival, or chromosomal defects reducing marrow production rates.[86]

Numerous functional tests are available for evaluating the status of the cell-mediated immune response. The simplest of these is the delayed cutaneous hypersensitivity reaction. This is a gross measure of the ability to respond to a challenge with one or more antigens to which the host has been previously sensitized—most commonly, tuberculin, trichophytin, mumps, and/or streptodornase. Patients with certain types of malnutrition (especially kwashiorkor) fail to respond normally to challenge with these recall antigens. Mitchell et al.[87] in 1928 demonstrated false negative reactions to tuberculin in malnourished subjects. Protein supplements (30 gm/day as skim milk) effectively restore tuberculin reactivity in malnourished children,[82] and patients with debilitating gastrointestinal disorders will demonstrate improved delayed cutaneous hypersensitivity during intravenous hyperalimentation.[79] Similarly, the anergic state associated with disseminated malignant tumors can frequently be corrected by adequate intravenous refeeding.[88]

The normal cutaneous hypersensitivity response reflects the culmination of many processes at the cellular and humoral level. The precise nature of the deficit that produces anergy in malnutrition is not known. It is likely that both the recognition arm of antigen processing and lymphoid sensitization and the response arm are impaired in the presence of malnutrition. Substantial work has been done to characterize the mechanism of anergy in malnutrition. Numerous abnormalities in T-cell function have been identified and are discussed briefly below.

The normal T-cell response to a nonspecific triggering agent (mitogen) or to a specific stimulating antigen is rapid growth and proliferation (termed *blast transformation*). In malnourished subjects, blast transformation is subnormal in response to both antigenic stimulation (mixed lymphocyte culture)[89] and nonspecific mitogen stimulation (phytohemagglutinin).[86] Likewise, the ability of T-lymphocytes to destroy target cells bearing the antigen to which the T-cell is sensitized is impaired. T-cell–mediated killing of allogeneic tumor cells by lymphocytes from malnourished mice is sensitive to deficiencies of specific nutrients. Leucine deprivation markedly impairs cytotoxicity, whereas arginine, histidine, and lysine deprivation cause only minimal impairment.[90] The relevance of these observations to anergy in malnourished humans is not known.

In addition to cytotoxic T-cells, another subpopulation of T-cells is responsible for the release of lymphokines, which elicit the response of immunologically incompetent lymphocytes, granulocytes, and monocytes. The precise role of lymphokines in producing anergy during malnutrition is not known. It has been suggested that the immunodeficiency in some agammaglobulinemic patients is due to a lymphokine defect,[82] but Meakins et al. found no such defect in traumatized and septic patients.[65]

T-cells also participate in the humoral antibody response. Antibody production by B-cells requires participation of "helper" T-cells. Kenney[91] demonstrated that protein-deficient mice show decreased antibody production to sheep erythrocytes. This defect could be corrected by transfer of T-cells but not B-cells from normal mice.[92] This implies that malnutrition may be associated with a disturbance in the ability of "helper" T-lymphocytes to provide their cooperative role in the production of an immunoglobulin by B-lymphocytes.

Thus nutritional status is an important determinant of T-lymphocyte function. A generalized depression of T-cell activity in malnourished patients results in abnormalities of both in vitro and in vivo tests. The clinical importance of these abnormalities is evidenced by the prognostic significance of cellular immunocompetence, as discussed in a subsequent section of this chapter.

Nonspecific Resistance. Numerous nonspecific immune cells participate in the response to foreign material. The functions of these cells are to process antigenic material and to modulate the activity of B- and T-lymphocytes. These cells include polymorphonuclear leukocytes, monocytes, and macrophages. Although levels of circulating neutrophils are normal in protein-calorie malnutrition, severe functional defects are common.[82] In pure malnutrition, uncomplicated by sepsis or trauma, the chemotactic response of neutrophils appears to be normal,[83] and the ability to phagocytize is unimpaired.[93] Once phagocytosis has occurred, however, the killing of *Staphylococcus* and *E. coli* by neutrophils is defective in patients with protein-calorie malnutrition.[94]

Monocytes and tissue macrophages also participate in the local inflammatory response. Edelman[95, 96] has described a delayed appearance of the macrophage/monocyte population using the Rebuck skin abrasion test, but the precise mechanism of this delayed response and its clinical importance remains to be clarified. Finally, the levels of two macrophage products, interferon and lysozyme, may be moderately decreased in nutritional deficiency.[82]

Complement. The complement system consists of a complex group of proteins. These proteins interact in sequential fashion and are an integral part of the immunologic defense system against bacterial infection. The macrophage is thought to be the major site of complement synthesis in humans.[97]

Sirisinha et al.[98] measured the serum levels of nine different complement proteins in 20 malnourished Thai children. In those with kwashiorkor, the levels of eight of nine proteins were significantly decreased when compared with levels in control subjects; only levels of C_4 remained within the normal range. In contrast, levels of only three of nine components—C_5, C_6, and C_3-proactivator—were below normal in those with marasmus. The levels of all complement proteins significantly increased with protein repletion. Similarly, Chandra[99] demonstrated decreased C_3 and serum hemolytic complement activity in 35 malnourished Indian children.

Other factors that influence serum complement levels include infection, cirrhosis, hepatitis, chronic passive hepatic congestion, schistosomiasis,[100] and perhaps cancer.[101] The multifactorial dependence of serum complement levels severely limits their value as markers of malnutrition.

Summary. From the above it is clear that malnutrition is associated with multiple defects in the immune system. The relative importance of these defects in predisposing malnourished subjects to infection is not known. Furthermore, one must also determine the importance of malnutrition per se over other concurrent conditions (such as cancer, infection, or the administration of drugs) in producing these defects. The clinical utility of selected immunologic measures as markers of malnutrition are discussed in a subsequent section.

Selection of Tests for Routine Nutritional Assessment. Given the variety of potential measures of nutritional status, the clinician must choose from these a few that are clinically applicable and suitable for incorporation into a routine nutritional assessment. The ideal test to identify protein-calorie malnutrition would have the following characteristics: (1) be consistently abnormal in patients with protein-calorie malnutrition (that is, be highly sensitive and yield few false negatives); (2) be consistently normal in patients without protein-calorie malnutrition (be highly specific and yield few false positives); (3) be unaffected by nonnutritional factors (be nutrition-specific); and (4) show normalization with adequate nutritional support (be sensitive to nutritional repletion).

No single nutritional measure consistently meets all of these criteria. In screening patients for protein-calorie malnutrition, it is necessary to use a battery of studies in order to overcome the deficiencies of any single study. To ensure its broad-based clinical applicability, the battery should be noninvasive, simple to perform, and inexpensive. Numerous schemata for nutritional assessment have been developed at various centers across the country. Clinicians at most centers have chosen to include in these schemata one or more measures from each of the five major categories previously defined: body weight, static caloric reserve, static protein reserve, circulating protein status, and immune status. The nutritional assessment battery currently used by us is provided as an example of one such approach (Table 7–8).

Table 7–8 BATTERY OF STUDIES SUITABLE FOR ROUTINE NUTRITIONAL ASSESSMENT

MEASURES OF BODY WEIGHT
  Current body weight
  Ideal body weight*
  Per cent of ideal body weight
  Usual body weight (from history)
  Per cent of usual body weight

MEASURES OF STATIC CALORIC RESERVE
  Triceps skinfold
  Subscapular skinfold
    Percentile sum of skinfolds†

MEASURES OF STATIC PROTEIN RESERVE
  Midarm muscle circumference‡
  24-Hour urinary creatinine excretion§

MEASURES OF CIRCULATING PROTEIN STATUS
  Serum albumin
  Serum transferrin

MEASURES OF IMMUNE FUNCTION
  Skin tests

*See Table 7–4
†See Table 7–5
‡See Table 7–6
§See Table 7–7; performed only in selected patients

Interpretation of Results of Nutritional Assessment. Results of nutritional assessment must be interpreted in the context of the overall clinical situation: the patient's disease, planned therapy, prognosis, current and anticipated level of nutrient intake, and so forth. For example, consider the patient with an esophageal stricture in whom nutritional assessment reveals marked depletion of static caloric and protein reserves. This patient will poorly tolerate a further period of suboptimal nutrition. If it is anticipated that an adequate intake of nutrients can be restored within a short period of time (such as by esophageal bougienage of a benign stricture), then the inadequacy of protein and calorie reserves will have little impact on the patient's clinical course and nutritional support is not indicated. In contrast, if a prolonged period of therapy is required before adequate nutrient intake is anticipated (for example, several weeks of radiotherapy to a malignant stricture), then inadequate reserves are a crucial issue and nutritional support is clearly warranted.

In recent years several investigators have attempted to determine which measures of nutritional status indicate deficits that will adversely affect a patient's clinical course. Patients in whom such deficits are identified should receive nutritional support unless adequate voluntary intake by mouth is soon anticipated. Surgery contemplated in such a patient may have to be delayed to permit preoperative nutritional support.

Prognostic Measures of Nutritional Status. Numerous nutritional measures have been shown to have prognostic significance in various clinical situations. Mullen et al.[1] examined the value of 16 nutritional and immunologic variables in predicting subsequent morbidity and mortality in surgical patients. Although only 3 per cent of patients demonstrated completely normal nutritional and immunologic profiles, only three nutritional factors examined individually were shown to correlate with outcome: serum transferrin, serum albumin, and delayed hypersensitivity reactivity. In that study, preoperative hypoalbuminemia (albumin less than 3.0 gm/dl) was associated with a 2.5-fold increase in operative complications. Similarly, serum transferrin levels of less than 220 mg/dl and skin test anergy were associated with 5-fold and 2-fold increases in morbidity, respectively. In similar studies, Kaminski[4] demonstrated a 2.5-fold increase

in mortality in patients whose serum transferrin was less than 170 mg/dl, and Seltzer[7] reported a 4-fold increase in complications and a 6-fold increase in deaths among hypoalbuminemic (less than 3.5 gm/dl) patients. When hypoalbuminemia was accompanied by lymphocytopenia (lymphocyte count less than 1500 cu mm), mortality was increased 20-fold. Harvey et al.[5] have demonstrated a correlation between mortality and serum transferrin, serum albumin, and delayed hypersensitivity reactivity. In that study, when serial skin tests remained abnormal despite adequate nutritional support, mortality was increased relative to mortality in patients who remained normal or who had improved (8 per cent versus 31 per cent). MacLean et al.[102] in 1975 reported an increased incidence of septic complications and postoperative mortality in anergic surgical patients. Meakins et al.[64] described a mortality rate of 74.4 per cent in patients who were anergic or relatively anergic and failed to improve their reactivity with appropriate therapy. This compared with a mortality rate of only 5.1 per cent in a similar group of patients who subsequently improved their cutaneous reactivity with treatment. Christou et al.[103] reported a 66 per cent septic rate and 37 per cent mortality in anergic patients whose polymorphonuclear leukocytes showed decreased chemotactic activity. No sepsis or postoperative mortality occurred in patients with normal cutaneous reactivity and with normal polymorphonuclear chemotaxis. Johnson et al.[104] demonstrated a 3-fold increase in major complications and a 9-fold increase in postoperative mortality in anergic patients as compared with relatively anergic patients and those with normal cutaneous reactivity.

Nutrition Risk Indices. Although nutritional screening techniques (skin tests, visceral proteins) accurately identify "high-risk" populations, interpretation of these studies in an individual patient can be difficult especially if one measure is abnormal while others are normal (for example, anergy in the presence of normal serum albumin and transferrin). Further, these studies do not provide a good estimate of the *magnitude* of the risk of suffering nutritionally based complications in an individual patient. Such a quantitative estimate of nutrition-related risk is especially important in surgical patients in whom it may be necessary to delay surgery to provide preoperative nutritional support. The magnitude of risk of nutritionally based operative complications must be known so that this can be weighed against the risk of delaying surgery to permit preoperative nutritional support.

In general, it is the responsibility of the surgeon to determine the risk associated with an operative delay (for example, disease progression, nosocomial infection). The Nutrition Support Team bears responsibility for quantification of nutrition-related risk. A convenient method for estimating this risk is through the use of a composite index of nutritional studies, which relates nutritional status to operative outcome. Although several such indices are available, the greatest clinical experience has probably been accumulated with the Prognostic Nutritional Index (PNI) developed at the University of Pennsylvania.[105] This index provides a quantitative estimate of the risk of operative complications for an individual patient based on his nutritional status on admission:

$$PNI\ (\%) = 158 - 16.6(ALB) - 0.78(TSF) - 0.2(TFN) - 5.8(DH)$$

where PNI is the risk of complications (%), ALB = serum albumin (gm/dl), TFN = serum transferrin (mg/dl), TSF = triceps skinfold (mm), and DH = maximal skin test reactivity to any of three recall antigens graded 0 = nonreactive, 1 = <5 mm reactivity, 2 = ≥5 mm reactivity. Calculation of the PNI in two hypothetical patients (one well-nourished, one malnourished) is shown in Figure 7–1.

The validity of the Prognostic Nutritional Index has been demonstrated in several subsequent patient populations. The initial prospective evaluation of this model was performed in 100 consecutive patients undergoing elective gastrointestinal surgery.[106] Patients were divided into low-risk (PNI<40 per cent), intermediate-risk (PNI = 40 to 49 per cent), and high-risk (PNI≥50 per cent) groups. The observed incidences of morbidity and mortality were found to increase linearly with the frequencies predicted by the PNI. In this study, 89 per cent of all complications and 93 per cent of the mortalities occurred in the 62 per cent of patients classified in the intermediate-risk and high-risk groups.

Smale et al. in 1979 found similar results in 100 patients with malignant disease prior to elective surgery.[107] To permit analysis, 46 patients were classified in the low-risk group (PNI<40 per cent) and 54 patients were placed in the high-risk group (PNI≥40 per cent). Patients in the high-risk group experienced 72 per cent of all complications and 86 per cent of the mortalities of the entire patient population.

An alternative to the PNI has been developed at the New England Deaconess Hospital.[5] Like the PNI, this index is a discriminant function relating surgical outcome to base-line nutritional status as measured by visceral protein status and immune function. This function is given by the relation:

Albumin (gm/dl) − DH − 1.7; 0 = 50% survival
DH = skin test response, graded 1 = positive, 2 = negative.

Multivariable nutritional risk indices provide a useful approach to interpretation of results of nutritional assessment studies. It is likely that additional indices will be developed relating measures of nutritional status to outcome in clinical settings other than surgery, for example, chemotherapy and renal failure.

Phase III: Serial Nutritional Assessment

A battery of studies similar to those shown in Table 7–8 are useful in defining base-line nutritional status. These studies should be repeated at one- to three-week intervals to monitor therapeutic response in patients receiving nutritional support or to assess dietary adequacy in patients not receiving nutritional support.

Patient 1: Well-Nourished

Albumin: 4.7gm/dl × 16.6	78.0
Skinfold: 14 mm × 0.78	10.9
Transferrin: 260 mg/dl × 0.20	52.0
Skin test reactive: 2 × 5.8	11.6
TOTAL	152.5

PNI = 158% − 152% = 5.5%
Predicted Risk of Complications: 5.5%

Patient 2: Malnourished

Albumin: 2.9 gm/dl × 16.6	48.1
Skinfold: 10 mm × 0.78	7.8
Transferrin: 180 mg/dl × 0.20	36.0
Skin test anergic: 0 × 5.8	0
TOTAL	91.9

PNI = 158% − 91.9 = 66.1%
Predicted Risk of Complications: 66.1%

Figure 7–1. Calculation of the prognostic nutritional index (PNI) for two hypothetical patients according to the following equation: PNI per cent = 158 − 16.6 (ALB) − 0.78 (TSF) − 0.2 (TFN) − 5.8 (DH).

Of the commonly used clinical markers of malnutrition, serum transferrin appears to be most sensitive to acute dietary manipulation. In the absence of complicating factors, nutritional support at adequate levels will produce a positive transferrin response (defined as greater than a 10 per cent increase above base line) in initially depleted patients within 4 to 10 days. In a recent study at the University of Pennsylvania,[53] patients demonstrating a positive transferrin response during a period of preoperative nutritional support showed a 5-fold reduction in operative mortality. Failure to achieve a positive transferrin response may be due to one of three causes: (1) the duration of nutritional support has been inadequate to produce repletion; (2) Calorie and/or protein provision has been inadequate to produce repletion; (3) The patient has a complicating disorder that prevents nutritional repletion.

It is recommended that serum transferrin levels be measured every seven days during nutritional support. If no transferrin response is observed with seven days of treatment, the patient is examined for complicating disorders (particularly sepsis) that may preclude nutritional repletion. In such patients, further efforts to achieve nutritional repletion will usually prove futile, and immediate measures to correct the underlying disorder (such as drainage of a septic focus) may be indicated. If no disorder preventing nutritional repletion is found, the caloric and protein requirements of the patient are reassessed and the nutritional regimen is modified to ensure its adequacy. This process is then repeated at seven-day intervals. The use of serum transferrin as a measure of short-term nutritional adequacy is supported by the recent demonstration in monkeys that serum transferrin changes during nutritional repletion correlate closely with overall nitrogen balance.[60] The additional observation that changes in serum retinol-binding protein and prealbumin correlate equally well with nitrogen balance but are more sensitive than transferrin to acute changes suggests that these markers may be superior as indicators of adequate nutritional support. The validity of these measures in a clinical setting must be documented, but this is an area of investigational promise. Other than circulating protein, measures of nutritional status commonly used in nutritional assessment change relatively slowly, even with adequate nutritional

support. It is therefore not necessary to repeat anthropometric and immunologic studies more frequently than every three weeks. The two exceptions to this are body weight, which should be determined daily to assess fluid status, and skin tests in initially anergic patients, which can be repeated at 7- to 10-day intervals until reactivity is restored.

RESEARCH TECHNIQUES IN NUTRITIONAL ASSESSMENT

Radiographic Analysis of Body Composition. As early as 1920, radiographic methods were used in the study of body composition. Garn,[108] Behnke et al.,[109] and Tanner[110] used radiographic imaging to measure fat, muscle, and bone widths in the upper and lower extremities and extrapolated these measures to estimate total body fat and lean body mass. The recent development of computerized axial tomography (CAT) has greatly increased the potential of radiographic analysis of body composition. CAT scanning may be useful in measuring the volume of adipose tissue, muscle, and viscera[26] and can provide quantitative information on the composition of these tissues.[111] This subject has recently been extensively reviewed by Heymsfield.[27] In summary, CAT scanning may be useful for the following quantifications: (1) liver triglyceride content in cases of hepatic steatosis,[112] (2) liver iron stores,[113] (3) muscle lipid content in muscular dystrophy,[114] and (4) bone density and calcium content.[115]

Radioisotopic Analysis of Body Composition. Isotope dilution techniques have long been used to assess body composition. As early as 1946, Moore and coworkers[116–118] introduced these techniques for use in determining total body content of water, sodium, and potassium. From this work came the concept of body cell mass, defined by Moore as "the oxygen-exchanging, potassium-rich, glucose-oxidizing, work-performing tissue.[118] Simplistically, the goal of nutritional support is to preserve the body cell mass. Therefore, accurate measures of body cell mass would theoretically be the ideal techniques for nutritional assessment.

There is no available method for direct measurement of the size of the body cell mass, but measurement of total body potassium provides a good approximation. Although techniques are available to determine total body potassium (^{40}K counting), measurement of exchangeable potassium is sufficiently accurate in most settings. Moore[118] has described the following relation between body cell mass (BCM) and exchangeable potassium (K_e) as measured by ^{43}K dilution:

$$BCM \text{ (gm)} = 9.14 \times K_e \text{ (mEq)}$$

Extensive work evaluating the utility of isotope dilution techniques in nutritional assessment and support has been done by Shizgal and associates.[119-121] They have developed a multiple isotope dilution technique using four isotopes (combined radiation dose, 237 millirems): ^{125}I-Albumin, ^{51}Cr-RBC's, ^{22}Na, and $^{3}H_2O$. Total exchangeable potassium is derived from exchangeable sodium (Na_e) and total body water (TBW) by the relation

$$K_e = TBW \times R - Na_e$$

where R is the ratio of sodium and potassium content divided by the water content of a whole blood sample. Shizgal has applied this method in many studies evaluating nutritional status[120] and assessing the efficacy of nutritional support.[121] In these studies, the ratio of exchangeable sodium (Na_e) to exchangeable potassium (K_e) was found to be a particularly valuable marker of malnutrition. Na_e/K_e approximates unity in well-nourished subjects (0.98 ± 0.02) and is greater than 1.22 in malnourished subjects.[122]

Isotope dilution techniques are clearly useful in a research setting. However, the radiation exposure to patient and hospital personnel may preclude widespread clinical application of these methods. Further, it has recently been shown in animal studies[123] that traditional relationships between body components (such as K:N) are not always constant but may vary in certain clinical situations including cancer and during lipid-based parenteral nutrition. In these situations, alterations in body composition markers (for example, K_e or Na_e/K_e) attributed to alterations in body cell mass may in fact represent disease-related or substrate-related effects in the presence of normal body composition.

Body Composition–Total Body Potassium (^{40}K Counting). Total body counting of potassium-40 (^{40}K) is an alternative to isotope dilution for determining total body potassium. ^{40}K is a naturally occurring radioactive isotope of potassium and accounts for 0.012 per cent of all natural potassium. Gamma emissions released by decay of ^{40}K can be detected by sensitive gamma counters,

^{40}K content of a subject can be determined, and total body potassium can be derived.

Total body potassium from total body ^{40}K counting correlates closely with exchangeable potassium, and counting error can be as low as 1.14 per cent (which in a 70-kg adult represents ± 41 mEq).[124] Since total body counting requires a specially designed, lead-enclosed counting chamber, however, its clinical utility will probably remain limited.

Neutron Activation Analysis of Body Composition. In vivo neutron activation analysis is a relatively new technique for analysis of body composition. Initally, this technique was limited to determination of total body nitrogen and potassium, but a recent description by Hill[125] expands its application to sodium, chloride, phosphorus, and calcium. In this method, the patient is radiated with high-energy neutrons (500 mrem) and then moved to a whole-body radiation counter. Over the next 30 minutes, the induced radioactivity is counted, and the complex spectrum is analyzed by a least-squares technique to give counting rates due to ^{13}N, ^{24}Na, ^{38}Cl, ^{28}Al (from phosphorus), ^{49}Ca, and ^{40}K. Total body content for each element is then calculated by use of appropriate calibration and decay factors obtained from anthropomorphic phantoms. An excellent review of this technique has recently been published by Hill.[125] Neutron activation offers an exciting opportunity to directly measure body content of many elements. Like whole body counting, however, its clinical applicability is limited by the specialized equipment required to carry out the analysis.

Biostereometrics. Biostereometrics is the spatial analysis of biologic form and may provide a method for measuring body and limb volume. In this technique, two stereo pairs of photographs of an individual are taken. Through use of a stereo plotter and computer, body volume, surface area and volumes of various segments (such as leg or arm) may be determined. This technique is sufficiently sensitive to detect the body volume increase following ingestion of 8 oz of water.[126] It may therefore be useful when used serially to detect edema and to monitor body volume changes during weight reduction, refeeding, and growth. The clinical applicability of biostereometrics has not been evaluated.

Numerous research techniques for nutritional assessment have been presented.

By no means do these represent all such techniques currently under investigation. Rather, we have chosen those techniques that we believe are most important for an understanding of current nutrition research literature and those techniques that may show clinical applicability in the future.

SUMMARY

Nutritional assessment is a science and an art that incorporates both traditional techniques and relatively new methodologies into a unified and rational approach to evaluation of nutritional status. The ultimate goal of health care professionals should be to eliminate malnutrition as a source of morbidity and mortality in their patients. The first step toward this goal is recognition of the disorder in all its forms, which is the specific and ultimate objective of nutritional assessment.

REFERENCES

1. Mullen, J. L., Gertner, M. H., Buzby, G. P., Goodhart, S. L., and Rosato, E. F.: Implications of malnutrition in surgical patient. Arch. Surg., 114:121–125, 1979.
2. Bistrian, B. R., Blackburn, G. L., Vitale, J., Cochran, D., and Naylor, J.: Prevalence of malnutrition in general medical patients. J.A.M.A., 235:1567–1570, 1976.
3. Bistrian, B. R., Blackburn, G. L., Hallowell, E., and Heddle, R.: Protein status of general surgical patients. J.A.M.A., 230:858–860, 1974.
4. Kaminski, M. V., Jr., Fitzgerald, M. J., Murphy, R. J., Pagast, P., Hoppe, M. C., Winborn, A. L., and Pluta, J.: Correlation of mortality with serum transferrin and anergy. J.P.E.N., 1(4):27A, 1977.
5. Harvey, K. B., Ruggiero, J. A., Regan, C. S., Bistrian, B. R., and Blackburn, G. L.: Hospital morbidity-mortality risk factors using nutritional assessment. Clin. Res. 26:581A, 1978.
6. Mullen, J. L., Buzby, G. P., Matthews, D. C., Smale, B. F., and Rosato, E. F.: Reduction of operative morbidity and mortality by combined preoperative and postoperative nutritional support. Ann. Surg., 192:604–613, 1980.
7. Seltzer, M. H., Bastidas, J. A., Cooper, D. M., Engler, P., Slocum, B., and Fletcher, H. S.: Instant nutritional assessment. J.P.E.N., 3:157–159, 1979.
8. Studley, H. O.: Percentage of weight loss: A basic indicator of surgical risk in patients with chronic peptic ulcer. J.A.M.A., 106:458–460, 1936.
9. Brožek, J., Grande, F., Anderson, J. T., and Keys, A.: Densitometric analysis of body composition: Revision of some quantitative assumptions. Ann. N.Y. Acad. Sci., 110:113–140, 1963.
10. Grande, F., and Keys, A.: Body weight, body composition and calorie status. In Goodhart, R. S.,

and Shils, M. E. (eds.): Modern Nutrition in Health and Disease. Edition 6. Philadelphia, Lea and Febiger, 1980, pp. 3–34.
11. Lesser, G. T., Deutsch, S., and Markofsky, J.: Use of independent measurement of body fat to evaluate overweight and underweight. Metabolism, 20:792–804, 1971.
12. Durnin, J.V.G.A., and Womersley, J.: Body fat assessed from total body density and its estimation from skinfold thickness: Measurements on 481 men and women aged from 16 to 72 years. Br. J. Nutr., 32:77–79, 1974.
13. Baker, P. T., Hunt, E. E., and Sen, T.: The growth and interrelations of skinfolds and brachial tissues in man. Am. J. Phys. Anthropol., 16:39–58, 1958.
14. Hall, J.C., O'Quigley, J., Giles, G. R., Appleton, N., and Stocks, H.: Upper limb anthropometry: The value of measurement variance studies. Am. J. Clin. Nutr., 33:1846–1851, 1980.
15. Noppa, H., Andersson, M., Bengtsson, C., Bruce, A., and Isaksson, B.: Body composition in middle-aged women with special references to the correlation between body fat mass and anthropometric data. Am. J. Clin. Nutr., 32:1388–1395, 1979.
16. Young, C. M.: Body composition and body weight: Criteria of overnutrition. Can. Med. Assoc. J., 93:900–910, 1965.
17. Jackson, A. S., and Pollock, M. L.: Generalized equations for predicting body density of men. Br. J. Nutr., 40:497–504, 1978.
18. Brožek, J.: Physique and nutritional status of adult men. Hum. Biol., 28:124–140, 1965.
19. Durnin, J. V. G. A., and Rahaman, M. M.: The assessment of the amount of fat in the human body from measurements of skinfold thickness. Br. J. Nutr., 21:681–689, 1967.
20. Allen, T. H., Peng, M. T., Chen, K. P., Huang, T. F., Chang, C., and Fang, H.S.: Prediction of total adiposity from skinfolds and the curvilinear relationship between external and internal adiposity. Metabolism, 5:346–352, 1956.
21. Edwards, D. A. W.: Differences in the distribution of subcutaneous fat with sex and maturity. Clin. Sci., 10:305–315, 1951.
22. Bray, G. A., Greenway, F. L., Molitch, M. E., Dahms, W. T., Atkinson, R. L., and Hamilton, K.: Use of anthropometric measures to assess weight loss. Am. J. Clin. Nutr., 31:769–773, 1978.
23. Bradfield, R. B., Schutz, Y., and Lechtig, A.: Skinfold changes with weight loss [Letter]. Am. J. Clin. Nutr., 32:1756, 1979.
24. Grant, J., Custer, P. B., and Thurlow, J.: Current techniques of nutritional assessment. Surg. Clin. North Am., 61:437–463, 1981.
25. Moore, F. D., and Brennan, M. F.: Surgical injury: Body composition, protein metabolism, and neuroendocrinology. In Ballinger, W. F., Collins, J. S., Drucker, W. R., Dudrick, S. J., and Zeppa, R. (eds.): Manual of Surgical Nutrition. Philadelphia, W. B. Saunders Co., 1975, pages 169–222.
26. Heymsfield, S. B., Olafson, R. P., Kutner, M. H., and Nixon, D. W.: A radiographic method of quantifying protein-calorie undernutrition. Am. J. Clin. Nutr., 32:693–702, 1979.
27. Heymsfield, S. B.: Radiographic analysis of body composition. In Levenson, S. M. (ed.): Nutritional Assessment—Present Status, Future Di-

rections, and Prospects. Columbus, Ohio, Ross Laboratories, 1981, pages 91–94.

28. Young, G. A., and Hill, G. L.: Assessment of protein-calorie malnutrition in surgical patients from plasma proteins and anthropometric measurements. Am. J. Clin. Nutr., 31:429–435, 1978.

29. Turner, W. J., and Cohn, S.: Total body potassium and 24-hour creatinine excretion in healthy males. Clin. Pharmacol. Ther., 18:405–412, 1975.

30. Muldowney, F. P., Crooks, J., and Bluhm, M. M.: The relationship of total exchangeable potassium and chloride to lean body mass, red cell mass and creatinine excretion in man. J. Clin. Invest., 36:1375–1381, 1957.

31. Boileau, R. A., Horstman, D. H., Buskirk, E. R., and Mendez, J.: The usefulness of urinary creatinine excretion in estimating body composition. Med. Sci. Sports Exerc., 4:85–90, 1972.

32. Forbes, G. B., and Bruining, G. J.: Urinary creatinine excretion and lean body mass. Am. J. Clin. Nutr., 29:1359–1366, 1976.

33. Bistrian, B. R., Blackburn, G. L., Sherman, M., and Scrimshaw, N. S.: Therapeutic index of nutritional depletion in hospitalized patients. Surg. Gynecol. Obstet., 141:512–516, 1975.

34. Blackburn, G. L., Bistrian, B. R., Maini, B. S., et al.: Nutritional and metabolic assessment of the hospitalized patient. J.P.E.N., 1:11–22, 1977.

35. Bleiler, R. E., and Schedl, H. P.: Creatinine excretion: Variability and relationships to diet and body size. J. Lab. Clin. Med., 59:945–955, 1962.

36. Rowe, J. W., Andres, R., Tobin, J. D., Norris, A. H., and Shock, N. W.: The effect of age on creatinine clearance in men: A cross-sectional and longitudinal study. J. Gerontol., 31:155–163, 1976.

37. Long, C. L., Haverberg, L. N., Young, V. R., Kinney, J. M., Munro, H. N., and Geiger, J. W.: Metabolism of 3-methylhistidine in man. Metabolism, 24:929–935, 1975.

38. Edozien, J. C.: The serum proteins in kwashiorkor. J. Pediatr., 57:594–603, 1960.

39. Butterworth, C. E., and Weinsier, R. L.: Malnutrition in hospitalized patients: Assessment and treatment. *In* Goodhart, R. S., and Shils, M. E. (eds.): Modern Nutrition in Health and Disease. Philadelphia, Lea and Febiger, 1980, pages 3–34.

40. Whitehead, R. G., Frood, J. D. L., and Poskitt, E. M. E.: Value of serum-albumin measurements in nutritional surveys: A reappraisal. Lancet, 2:287–289, 1971.

41. Rothchild, M. A., Oratz, M., and Schreiber, S. S.: Albumin synthesis. N. Engl. J. Med., 286:748–757, 1972.

42. Rothschild, M. A., Oratz, M., and Schreiber, S. S.: Serum albumin. Am. J. Dig. Dis., 14:711–744, 1969.

43. Peters, T., Jr.: Serum albumin. Adv. Clin. Chem., 13:37–111, 1970.

44. Cohen, S., and Hansen, J. D. L.: Metabolism of albumin and γ-globulin in kwashiorkor. Clin. Sci. Mol. Med., 23:351–359, 1962.

45. Picou, D., and Waterlow, J. C.: The effect of malnutrition on the metabolism of plasma albumin. Clin. Sci. Mol. Med., 22:459–468, 1962.

46. Morgan, E. H.: Transferrin and transferrin iron. *In* Jacobs, A., and Worwood, M. (eds.): Iron in Biochemistry and Medicine. London, Academic Press, 1974, pages 29–71.

47. Awai, M., and Brown, E. B.: Studies of the metab-olism of ^{131}I-labeled human transferrin. J. Lab. Clin. Med., 61:363–396, 1963.

48. Lahey, M. E., Behar, M., Viteri, F., and Scrimshaw, N. S.: Values for copper, iron, and iron-binding capacity in the serum in kwashiorkor. Pediatrics, 22:72–79, 1958.

49. El-Shobaki, F. A., El-Hawary, M. F. S., Morcos, S. R., Abdelkhalek, M. K., El-Zawahry, K., and Sakr, R.: Iron metabolism in Egyptian infants with protein-calorie deficiency. Br. J. Nutr., 28:81–89, 1972.

50. Mancini, G., Carbonara, A. O., and Heremans, J. F.: Immunochemical quantitation of antigens by single radial immunodiffusion. Immunochemistry, 2:235–254, 1965.

51. Stojceski, T. J., Malpas, J. S., and Witts, L. J.: Studies on the serum iron-binding capacity. J. Clin. Pathol., 18:446–452, 1965.

52. Antia, A. U., McFarlane, H., and Soothill, J. F.: Serum siderophilin in kwashiorkor. Arch. Dis. Child., 43:459–462, 1968.

53. Buzby, G. P., Forster, J., and Rosato, E. F.: Transferrin dynamic in total parenteral nutrition. J.P.E.N., 3:34, 1979.

54. Kanai, M., Raz, A., and Goodwin, D. S.: Retinol-binding protein: The transport protein for vitamin A in human plasma. J. Clin. Invest., 47:2025–2044, 1968.

55. Goodman, D. S.: Vitamin A transport and retinol-binding protein metabolism. Vitam. Horm., 32:167–180, 1974.

56. Oppenheimer, J. H., Surks, M. I., Bernstein, G., and Smith, J. C.: Metabolism of iodine-131-labeled thyroxine-binding prealbumin in man. Science, 149:748–751, 1965.

57. Smith, F. R., Goodman, D. S., Zaklama, M. S., Gabr, M. K., Maraghy, S. E., and Patwardham, V. N.: Serum vitamin A, retinol-binding protein, and prealbumin concentration in protein-calorie malnutrition. I. A functional defect in hepatic retinol release. Am. J. Clin. Nutr., 26:973–981, 1973.

58. Ingenbleek, Y., Van Den Schrieck, H. G., De Nayer, P., and De Visscher, M.: The role of retinol-binding protein in protein-calorie malnutrition. Metabolism, 24:633–641, 1975.

59. Smith, F. R., Goodman, D. S., Arroyave, G., and Viteri, F.: Serum vitamin A, retinol-binding protein, and prealbumin concentrations in protein-calorie malnutrition. II. Treatment including supplemental vitamin A. Am. J. Clin. Nutr., 26:982–987, 1973.

60. Smale, B. F., Hobbs, C. L., Mullen, J. L., and Rosato, E. F.: The relationship of nitrogen balance to changes in serum proteins [Abstract]. J.P.E.N., 5:558, 1981.

61. Venkataswamy, G., Glover, J., Cobby, M., and Pirie, A.: Retinol-binding protein in serum of xerophthalmic malnourished children before and after treatment at a nutrition center. Am. J. Clin. Nutr., 30:1968–1973, 1977.

62. Cannon, P. R., Wissler, R. W., Woolridge, R. L., and Benditt, E. P.: The relationship of protein deficiency to surgical infection. Ann. Surg., 120:514–525, 1944.

63. Rhoads, J. E., and Alexander, C. E.: Nutritional problems of surgical patients. Ann. N. Y. Acad. Sci., 63:268–275, 1955.

64. Meakins, J. L., Pietsch, J. B., Bubenick, O., Kelly, R., Rode, H., Gordon, J., and MacLean, L. D.:

Delayed hypersensitivity: Indicator of acquired failure of host defenses in sepsis and trauma. Ann. Surg., 186:241–250, 1977.

65. Haffejee, A. A., and Aghorn, I. B.: Nutritional status and the nonspecific cellular and humoral immune response in esophageal carcinoma. Ann. Surg., 189:475–479, 1979.

66. McFarlane, H., Reddy, S., Adcock, K. J., Adeshina, H., Cooke, A. R., and Akene, J.: Immunity, transferrin, and survival in kwashiorkor. Br. Med. J., 4:268–270, 1970.

67. Hoffman-Goetz, L., and Blackburn, G. L.: Relationship of nutrition to immunology and cancer. In Newell, G. R., and Ellison, N. M. (eds.): Nutrition and Cancer: Etiology and Treatment. (Progress in Cancer Research and Therapy, Vol. 17.)

68. Gershon, R. K.: The role of the T cell in the immune response. Adv. Exp. Med. Biol., 73(B): 3–13, 1976.

69. Aref, G. H., El-Din, M. K., Hassan, A. I., and Araby, I. I.: Immunoglobulins in kwashiorkor. J. Trop. Med. Hyg., 73:186–191, 1970.

70. Rosen, E. O., Geefhuysen, J., and Ipp, T.: Immunoglobulin levels in protein-calorie malnutrition. S. Afr. Med. J., 45:980–987, 1971.

71. Keet, M. P., and Thom, H.: Serum immunoglobulins in kwashiorkor. Arch. Dis. Child., 44:600–603, 1969.

72. El-Gholmy, A., Hashish, S., Helmy, O., Aly, R. H., and El-Gamal, Y.: A study of immunoglobulins in kwashiorkor. J. Trop. Med. Hyg., 73:192–195, 1970.

73. Faulk, W. P., Demaeyer, E. M., and Davies, A. J. S.: Some effects of malnutrition on the immune response in man. Am. J. Clin. Nutr., 27:638–646, 1974.

74. Lechtig, A., Arroyave, G., Viteri, F., and Mata, L. J.: Serum immunoglobulins in protein-calorie malnutrition in pre-school children. Arch. Latinoam. Nutr., 20:321–325, 1970.

75. Cohen, S., and Hansen, J. D. L.: Metabolism of albumin and gamma-globulin in kwashiorkor: Clin. Sci., 23:351–359, 1962.

76. Wohl, M. G., Reinhold, J. G., and Rose, S. B.: Antibody response in patients with hypoproteinemia. Arch. Intern. Med., 83:402–408, 1949.

77. Gell, P. G. H.: Serologic responses to antigenic stimuli. Medical Research Council (London) Special Report Series, 275:193–196, 1951.

78. Hodges, R. E., Bean, W. B., Ohlson, M. A., and Bleiler, R. E.: Factors affecting human antibody response. I. Effects of variations in dietary protein upon the antigenic response of men. Am. J. Clin. Nutr., 10:500–505, 1962.

79. Law, D. K., Dudrick, S. J., and Abdou, N. I.: Immunocompetence of patients with protein-calorie malnutrition: The effects of nutritional repletion. Ann. Intern. Med., 79:545–550, 1973.

80. Reddy, V., and Srikantia, S. G.: Antibody response in kwashiorkor. Indian J. Med. Res., 52:1154–1158, 1964.

81. Mathews, J. D., Whittingham, S., Mackay, I. R., and Malcolm, L. A.: Protein supplementation and enhanced antibody-producing capacity in New Guinean school children. Lancet, 2(7779):675–699, 1972.

82. Kahan, B. K.: Nutrition and host defense mechanisms. Surg. Clin. North Am., 61(3):557–570, 1981.

83. Jolly, J.: Modifications des ganglions lymphatiques à la suite de jeûne. Comp. Rend. Soc. Biol., 76:146–149, 1914.

84. Vint, F. W.: Postmortem findings in the natives of Kenya. East Afr. Med. J., 13:332–340, 1937.

85. Neumann, C. G.: Nonspecific host factors and infection in malnutrition: A review. In Suskind, R. M. (ed.): Malnutrition and the Immune Response. (Kroc Found. Series Vol. 7.) New York, Raven Press, 1977, pages 355–374.

86. Ferguson, A. C., Lawlor, G. J., Jr., Newmann, C. G., Oh, W., and Stiehm, E. R.: Decreased rosette-forming lymphocytes in malnutrition and intrauterine growth retardation. J. Pediatr., 85:717–723, 1974.

87. Mitchell, A. G., Wherry, W. B., Eddy, B., and Stevenson, F. E.: Studies in immunity. I. Nonspecific factors influencing reaction of the skin to tuberculin. Am. J. Dis. Child., 36:720–724, 1928.

88. Copeland, E. M., MacFadyen, B. V., Jr., and Dudrick, S. J.: Effect of intravenous hyperalimentation on established delayed hypersensitivity in the cancer patient. Ann. Surg., 184:60–64, 1976.

89. López, V., Davis, S. D., and Smith, N. J.: Studies in infantile marasmus. IV. Impairment of immunological responses in the marasmic pig. Pediatr. Res., 6:779–788, 1972.

90. Jose, D. G., and Good, R. A.: Quantitative effects of nutritional essential amino acid deficiency upon immune responses to tumors in mice. J. Exp. Med., 137:1–9, 1973.

91. Kenney, M. A., Roderuck, C. E., Arnrich, L., Piedad, F.: Effect of protein deficiency on the spleen and antibody formation in rats. J. Nutr., 95:173–178, 1968.

92. Mathur, M., Ramalingaswami, V., and Deo, M. G.: Influence of protein deficiency on 19S antibody-forming cells in rats and mice. J. Nutr., 102:841–846, 1972.

93. Tejada, C., Argueta, V., Sánchez, M., and Albertazzi, C.: Phagocytic and alkaline phosphatase activity of leukocytes in kwashiorkor. J. Pediatr., 64:753–761, 1964.

94. Douglas, S. D., and Schopfer, K.: The phagocyte in protein-calorie malnutrition. A review. In Suskind, R. M. (ed.): Malnutrition and the Immune Response. (Kroc Found. Series, Vol. 7.) New York, Raven Press, 1977, pages 231–243.

95. Edelman, R.: Cell-mediated immune response in protein-calorie malnutrition. A review. In Suskind, R. M. (ed.): Malnutrition and the Immune Response. (Kroc Found. Series, Vol. 7.) New York, Raven Press, 1977, pages 47–75.

96. Edelman, R., Kulapongs, P., Suskind, R. M., Olson, R. E.: Leukocyte mobilization in Thai children with kwashiorkor. In Suskind, R. M. (ed.): Malnutrition and the Immune Response. (Kroc Found. Series, Vol. 7.) New York, Raven Press, 1977, pages 265–269.

97. Stecher, V. J., and Thorbecke, G. J.: Sites of synthesis of serum proteins. I. Serum proteins produced by macrophages in vitro. J. Immunol., 99:643–652, 1967.

98. Sirisinha, S., Suskind, R., Edelman, R., Charupatana, C., and Olson, R. E.: Complement and C3-proactivator levels in children with protein-calorie malnutrition and effect of dietary treatment. Lancet, 1:1016–1020, 1973.

99. Chandra, R. K.: Serum complement and immunoconglutinin in malnutrition. Arch. Dis. Child., 50:225–229, 1975.

100. Ruddy, S., Gigli, I., and Austen, K. F.: The com-

plement system of man. N. Engl. J. Med., 287:489–495, 1972.

101. Verhaegen, H., De Cock, W., De Cree, J., and Verbruggen, F.: Increase of serum complement levels in cancer patients with progressing tumors. Cancer, 38:1608–1613, 1976.

102. MacLean, L. D., Meakins, J. L., Taguchi, M., Duigham, J. P., Dhillon, K. S., and Gordon, J.: Host resistance in sepsis and trauma. Ann. Surg., 182:207–216, 1975.

103. Christou, N. V., and Meakins, J. L.: Neutrophil function in surgical patients: Two inhibitors of granulocyte chemotaxis associated with sepsis. J. Surg. Res., 26:355–364, 1979.

104. Johnson, W. C., Ulrich, F., Meguid, M. M., Lepak, N., Bowe, P., Harris, P., Alberts, L. H., and Nabseth, D. C.: Role of delayed hypersensitivity in predicting postoperative morbidity and mortality. Am. J. Surg., 137:536–542, 1979.

105. Mullen, J. L., Buzby, G. P., Waldman, M. T., Gertner, M. H., Hobbs, C. L., and Rosato, E. F.: Prediction of operative morbidity and mortality by preoperative nutritional assessment. Surg. Forum, 30:80–82, 1979.

106. Buzby, G. P., Mullen, J. L., Matthews, D. C., Hobbs, C. L., and Rosato, E. F.: Prognostic nutritional index in gastrointestinal surgery. Am. J. Surg., 139:160–167, 1980.

107. Smale, B. F., Mullen, J. L., Buzby, G. P., and Rosato, E. F.: The efficacy of nutritional assessment and support in cancer surgery. Cancer, 47:2375–2381, 1981.

108. Garn, S. M.: Roentgenogrammetric determination of body composition. Hum. Biol., 29:337, 1957.

109. Behnke, A. R., and Siri, W. E.: The estimation of lean body weight from anthropometric and x-ray measurements. Research and Development Tech Rep USNRDL-TR-203, Biology and Medicine, 1957, pages 1–38.

110. Tanner, J. M.: The Physique of the Olympic Athlete. London, George Allen and Unwin, 1964.

111. Heymsfield, S. B., Fulenwider, T., Nordlinger, B., Barlow, R., Sones, P., and Kutner, M.: Accurate measurement of liver, kidney, and spleen volume and mass by computerized axial tomography. Ann. Intern. Med., 90:185–187, 1979.

112. Virgil, V., and Heymsfield, S.: Accurate prediction of liver fat content by computerized axial tomography (CT). Clin. Res., 27:143A, 1979.

113. Mills, S. R., Doppman, J., and Nienhuis, A. W.: Computed tomography in the diagnosis of disorders of excessive iron storage of the liver. J. Comput. Assist. Tomogr., 1:101–104, 1977.

114. Galloway, J., Heymsfield, S., and Sones, P.: Radiology. Unpublished data, 1982.

115. Ullrich, C. G., Binet, E. F., Sanecki, M. G., and Kieffer, S. A. Quantitative assessment of the lumbar spinal canal by computed tomography. Radiology, 134:137–143, 1980.

116. Moore, F. D.: Determination of total body water and solids with isotopes. Science, 104:157–160, 1946.

117. Moore, F. D.: Metabolic Care of the Surgical Patient. Philadelphia, W. B. Saunders Company, 1959.

118. Moore, F. D., Olesen, K. H., McMurray, et al.: The Body Cell Mass and Its Supporting Environ-

ment: Body Composition in Health and Disease. Philadelphia, W. B. Saunders Company, 1963.

119. Shizgal, H. M.: Body composition and nutritional support. Surg. Clin. North Am., 61:729–741, 1981.

120. Shizgal, H. M.: The effect of malnutrition on body composition. Surg. Gynecol. Obstet., 152:22–26, 1981.

121. Shizgal, H. M., and Forse, R. A.: Protein and caloric requirements with total parenteral nutrition. Ann. Surg., 192:562–569, 1980.

122. Forse, R. A., and Shizgal, H. M.: The Na_e/K_e ratio: A predictor of malnutrition. Surg. Forum, 31:89–92, 1980.

123. Buzby, G. P., Steinberg, J. J., and Giandomenico, A. R.: The effects of malnutrition, cancer, and TPN on direct and indirect measures of body composition. In press.

124. Novak, L. P.: Aging, total body potassium, fat-free mass, and cell mass in males and females between ages 18 and 85 years. J. Gerontol., 27:438–443, 1972.

125. Hill, G. L.: Use of neutron activation analysis to measure body composition in critically ill patients with nutritional and metabolic problems. In Levenson, S. M. (ed.): Nutritional Assessment—Present Status, Future Directions, and Prospects. Columbus, Ohio, Ross Laboratories, 1981.

126. Crosby, L. O.: New Horizons. Surg. Clin. North Am., 61:743–753, 1981.

127. Shils, M. E., Goodhart, R. S. (eds.): Modern Nutrition in Health and Disease. Edition 6. Philadelphia, Lea and Febiger, 1980.

128. Roe, D. A.: Drug Induced Nutritional Deficiencies. Westport Connecticut, AVI Publishing, 1976.

129. Butterworth, C. E.: Some clinical manifestations of nutritional deficiency in hospitalized patients. In Levenson, S. M. (ed.): Nutritional Assessment—Present Status, Future Directions, and Prospects. Columbus, Ohio, Ross Laboratories, 1981, pages 2–3.

130. Sauberlich, H. E., Skala, J. H., and Dowdy, R. P.: Laboratory Tests for the Assessment of Nutritional Status. Cleveland, Ohio, CRC Press, 1974.

131. Baker, H., Frank, O., and Hutner, S. H.: Vitamin analysis in medicine. In Shils, M. E., and Goodhart, R. S. (eds.): Modern Nutrition in Health and Disease. Edition 6. Philadelphia, Lea and Febiger, 1980, pages 611–640.

132. Jelliffe, D. B.: The Assessment of the Nutritional Status of the Community, with Special Reference to Field Surveys in Developing Regions of the World. Geneva, World Health Organization Monograph Series No. 53, 1966.

133. Vital and Health Statistics: Weight and Height of Adults 18–74 years of age, U.S. 1971–1974. DHEW Publication No. (PHS) 79-1659, Series 11, No. 211, Public Health Service, Washington, D.C., Government Printing Office, 1979.

134. Blackburn, G. L.: Nutritional assessment. Clinical Consultations in Nutritional Support (Chicago), 1:1–8, 1981.

135. Twomey, P., Zeigler, D., and Rombeau, J.: Utility of skin testing in nutritional assessment. A critical review. J.P.E.N., 6:50–58, 1982.

CHAPTER 8

The Use of Computers in Nutrition Support

WILLIAM P. STEFFEE

Computers have long been accepted as support devices for the delivery of health care.[1, 2] Their use in the hospital setting, whether by patient, staff, or physician, is encountered daily. Most obvious to the casual observer is the computer as an accounting device, rapidly translating services into billing statements or monitoring budgets and expenditures for segments of the medical community. One need only pause to enter a clinical laboratory to observe computers and microprocessors at work, ranging from instrument control, calculation, integration and print-out of routine laboratory studies to the more complex technologies of computerized axial tomography (CAT).

Computer-assisted medical diagnosis has been implemented to assist the practitioner in many aspects of health care.[3] Some, such as computer-assisted interpretation of electrocardiograms, have been dramatically successful. Others, particularly those related to clinical diagnosis, have been less well received, probably owing to the computer's inability to interpret or the physician's inability to accept that the computer can be programmed to understand the many nuances of medical diagnosis and therapy in the clinical setting. It is difficult indeed for a physician to accept that a "black box" can perform in that arena in which the accumulation of years of knowledge and experience finally coalesces into the science and art of medical practice.

Perhaps herein lies a unique possibility for the use of computers in nutritional support. In recent decades nutrition has been a "stepchild of the medical sciences," untaught, unappreciated, and not implemented in clinical care. The vast majority of practicing physicians must, and do, admit ignorance in matters concerning nutritional assessment and intervention. On the other hand, the near universal need for nutrition intervention in most aspects of hospital practice is rapidly becoming recognized. Initial reactions to educational efforts by pioneers in the field are eye-opening revelations to physicians when they realize that their patients are allowed to starve to death while enduring the most rigorous forms of medical therapy. These initial reactions are soon followed by demands that they be informed about when, how, and to what intensity they should intervene. Members of the medical community are suddenly faced with the realization of their inadequacies to diagnose and treat one of the most basic of medical disorders.

This dilemma, a rapidly expanding medical discipline being enforced upon an uneducated medical community, offers considerable, and heretofore unparalleled, opportunities for computer-assisted diagnosis, delivery systems, and education. The fact that the field is evolving in a truly multidisciplinary fashion with paramedical professionals expands horizons for the use of computers even more.

This chapter will provide a broad overview of potential applications of the computer. It is not meant to represent a review of the literature or to be comprehensive in scope. Many applications are currently in operation, as evidenced by ongoing efforts at several institutions. Others await refinement of techniques and development of new devices.

Five broad areas will be addressed: nutritional assessment of status and requirements, formulation of solutions, delivery of nutrients and monitoring thereof; administrative control, and education.

NUTRITIONAL ASSESSMENT

Status. Perhaps the most limiting aspect to the growth of nutrition as a credible medical entity is our near-total lack of ability to define the nutritional status of each patient with a degree of precision, sensitivity, and reproducibility to allow optimal clinical care and the conduct of prospective research. How does one put a number on cachexia? Can any combination of laboratory results be reduced into a predictive index of clinical outcome?

Current models of nutritional assessment include indices of a broad array of protein function and generally follow those suggested by Butterworth, Blackburn, and Bistrian.[4, 5] These indices have been collated by computer and the results expressed as "kwashiorkor-like" or "marasmus-like."[6] In others, such data have been statistically analyzed to generate a "prognostic index" for clinical outcome.[7] Herein lies one of the most stringent constraints of computer use. The computer-generated result is only as good as the data entered. Take, for example, changes in plasma albumin which, if low, can be indicative of protein malnutrition. In fact, it is used in all of the aforementioned assessments. Albumin concentrations alone are not reliable indicators of protein status, as many other factors influence measured levels. These factors include the patient's state of hydration; hepatic synthetic abilities other than those related to amino acid supply; abnormal losses via kidneys, gastrointestinal tract, or open wounds; albumin administration as a colloid plasma expander;

and, quite unexpectedly, quadriplegia. A computer could prompt evaluation of the patient for such conditions; should any exist, however, their contribution to the hypoalbuminemia is so ambiguous that the computer could not evaluate plasma albumin levels. The same considerations hold for loss of body weight, tests of immune function, anthropometric measurements, and others. As fast as a computer can calculate, ambiguity cannot be tolerated. Indeed, assessment of nutritional status is most difficult, and perhaps is made more unreliable if computers are used to generate numbers for statistical analysis.

Nutritional Requirements. Although computerized analysis is not precise by any standards, the computer enables us to generate estimates for total calories, protein, and fluid requirements and to revise these estimates rapidly with altered clinical status.

The formulas for calculating basal energy expenditure are reasonably well established and allow the clinician to modify nutritional prescriptions according to age, weight, height, and sex.[8] It is also accepted that the stress imposed by surgery, sepsis, or trauma induces an added fuel requirement; however, the exact magnitude of this demand is not clear. Because a computer demands clarity, an effort must be made to reduce degrees of stress to numerical values. In a recent attempt by the author,[9] degrees of stress were defined according to guidelines suggested by Kinney and associates (Fig. 8–1, Table 8–1).[10] The exact numbers are not important in this context and may, in fact, generate considerable controversy. The result, however, is the generation of guidelines for initiating therapy that have some basis in fact, rather than simply providing each patient with "3 liters per day."

Stress Code	Clinical State		
1	Basic Maintenance Without Stress		
2	Routine Surgery	Minor Sepsis	Tumor Without Therapy
3	Major Surgery	Major Sepsis	Tumor With One Surgery
4	Trauma + Surgery	Surgery + Sepsis	Tumor With Multiple Therapies
5	Trauma + Surgery + Sepsis	Third Degree Burn	Massive Tumor Load + Therapy

Figure 8–1. Relationship of stress code to clinical state.

Table 8–1 CALCULATION OF PREDICTED ENERGY REQUIREMENTS

STRESS STATUS	% INCREASE OVER BEE FOR STRESS	PREDICTED ENERGY REQUIREMENTS (% BEE)
1	10	165
2	20	180
3	30	195
4	40	210
5	50	225

BEE, basal energy expenditure

As we gain greater understanding of the specific fuel requirements for meeting the varying demands for prevention, stress, and rehabilitation, the computer can readily be utilized to adjust relative amounts of fats, carbohydrates, and synthetic fuels to meet a spectrum of requirements.

The computerized generation of protein needs is more difficult because of the additional requirements for replacement of lost protein mass and the limitations imposed by the presence of the clinical disorders of renal or hepatic dysfunction. Figure 8–2 represents an effort in this regard. Its derivation will elucidate the steps that must be taken and the difficulties that arise as assumptions are piled upon assumptions in order to reduce clinical impressions to unambiguous machine language. Estimates of adult protein requirements in health are well established[11] but are questioned as to their adequacy, even by those involved in their generation.[12] Even so, an estimate of 0.8 gm/kg ideal body weight/day would appear to be reasonable for providing for a minimally stressed adult who has no protein losses and is not in renal or hepatic failure. While not proven, it is generally accepted that stress induces enhanced protein requirements, as reflected by commercial formulations that double the "maintenance" grams nitrogen-to-calorie ratio from 1:300 to 1:150. In the context of graded stress used for the caloric prescription, we chose, quite arbitrarily, to provide graded increments according to stress up to 2.0 gm/kg.

Another commonly held assumption is that patients who are already protein-wasted require more protein for purposes of regeneration, perhaps similar to requirements during growth. In the clinical situation, we might increase protein delivery "a little" if the patient were "cachectic." Unfortunately, a computer must be informed of precisely how much to increment if body protein mass is depleted by a specific amount. Since we assume that a loss of 30 per cent of lean

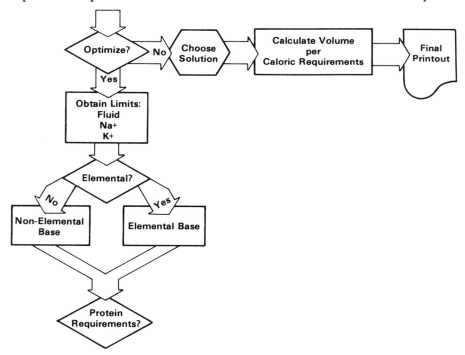

Figure 8–2. Protein requirements (gm per kg of ideal body weight) predicted by degree of stress, prior protein loss, and presence of nitrogen retention disorder.

body mass is incompatible with life, it seems reasonable to provide some margin of safety by incrementing the protein prescription after loss of only 10 per cent lean body mass. In view of the previous discussion regarding the assessment of nutritional status, how can this be accomplished?

Data have been published which indicate that the total nitrogen content of the ashed adult corpse is about 16.4 per cent of ideal body weight.[13] It is therefore necessary to define "ideal body weight." We chose to use the ideal weight for height and frame tables of the Metropolitan Life Insurance Company,[14] assuming, of course, that height measurements are obtainable and/or accurate in the clinical setting. The choice of "frame" is again quite arbitrary.

Loss of body weight cannot be simply the usual weight minus the measured weight since in many instances, particularly in patients with cancer or hypoalbuminemia, measured weight includes significant amounts of fluid or tumor mass. Estimates of this added weight must be made and subtracted from measured weight to derive a predicted "dry" weight, representing remaining body mass.

But how much of weight loss during stress is nitrogen? Whereas estimates as great as 20 per cent protein have been suggested, we chose to limit this assumption to 10 per cent of body protein. Since the average nitrogen content of protein is 16 per cent, the equation defining per cent body protein loss is as follows:

$$\text{Body Protein Loss (\%)} = \frac{\text{premorbid weight} - \text{predicted dry weight} \times 0.1 \text{ gm}}{\text{ideal body weight} \times 0.164} \times 100$$

Assuming that the number generated thus far has some validity, we can then increment the protein prescription for those who have depleted body protein, again in an arbitrary fashion.

Renal and hepatic failure have traditionally been treated with dietary protein restriction, but to what degree? To date, we have simply chosen to reduce the basal amount (stress level 1, no protein depletion) to 0.5 gm/kg body weight/day, or approximately 40 gm of protein. This assumes the protein to be of high biologic value. The prescription is incremented if enhanced stress is encountered, or if body protein depletion is present, again in arbitrary fashion.

However convenient the number generated for calorie or protein prescriptions may be, and however useful the appearance of exactness may be for convincing house staff and others to attain therapeutic goals, one must never lose sight of the assumptions that are required to allow the computer to generate estimates. Fluid and electrolyte requirements can be prescribed with more precision and will be discussed in the following segment.

FORMULATION OF SOLUTIONS

Enteral Hyperalimentation. Once "modular feeding" gains acceptance and components become available, enteral solutions can be mixed to meet the specific requirements outlined above. The computer is particularly suited to this function since its nearly unlimited memory can be utilized to generate mixes that are compatible, and at the same time meet constraints imposed to satisfy economic considerations. Until then, it can maintain a library of information relative to nutrient content of all commercially available solutions and choose the one most appropriate to meet nutrient requirements within the constraints imposed by fluid, sodium, and potassium restrictions. Figures 8–3 to 8–6 represent algorithms currently in use by our Nutrition Intervention Team. Inspection will reveal how an interactive computer system can quickly generate an optimal prescription and also print orders for safe and effective initiation of therapy. The total time required by an experienced user for generation of such orders in our system is approximately three minutes at a cost of less than one dollar.

Total Parenteral Nutrition. A currently applicable use of computers to generate orders for total parenteral nutrition (TPN) including not only calories, protein, and electrolytes, but also fluid requirements over short periods of time, meets rapidly changing metabolic demands in a safe and cost-effective manner. This assumes, of course, that adequate back-up by paramedical personnel and pharmacy is available. In most instances, solutions for TPN are prescribed using minimal variations of standard solutions to meet caloric and protein requirements. If the patient is reasonably stable, additional fluid and electrolytes need not be administered. However, in many instances, particularly when large and varying vol-

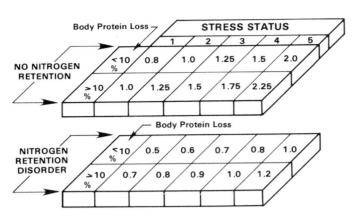

Figure 8–3. Entry into the system allows the user to choose whether the computer will seek the optimal solutions (best fit for fluid, protein, Na⁺, and K⁺ in relation to calorie need) or simply calculate volumes to meet caloric requirements for the solution of choice.

umes of fluid and electrolytes are lost by suction, fistula, or ileostomy outputs, TPN solutions are supplemented by intravenous preparations of a specially prescribed nature.

Assuming that adequate clinical data can be acquired and entered into the computer at frequent intervals, there is no reason that the computer could not generate solutions that contain appropriate amounts of glucose, fats, amino acids, and electrolytes to meet all demands, keep the clinician informed relative to trends, and offer suggestions for future formulations. A hypothetical example could be a 25-year-old male patient who has undergone extensive trauma, including multiple disruptions of bowel in-

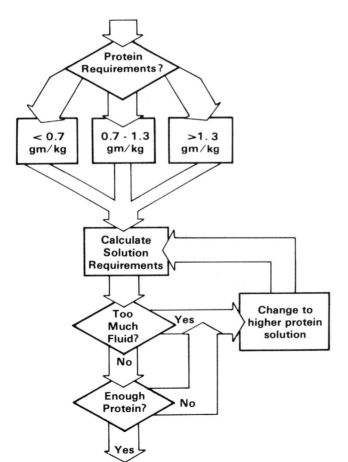

Figure 8–4. Starting with an initial solution choice based on gross protein content, the computer adjusts amounts to meet fluid constraints or moves to a solution of higher protein content.

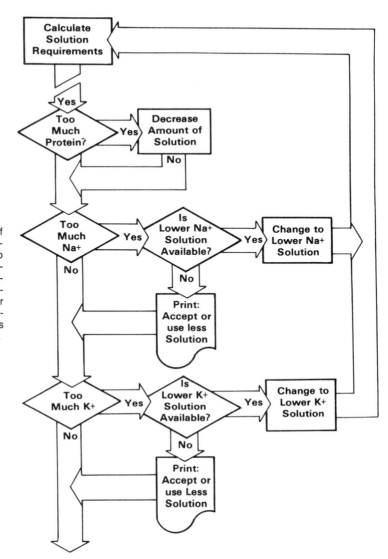

Figure 8–5. If after evaluation of all available solutions, protein still exceeds the required amount relative to fluid delivery, the total amount is decreased with the understanding that additional, concentrated, protein-free caloric source will be necessary. Similar explorations are carried out for both sodium and potassium until the best fit is identified or limitations indicated to use.

tegrity resulting in formation of a duodenal fistula, high output ileostomy, multiple long bone fractures, sepsis with fever to 105°F, and resolving obstructive nephropathy. Table 8–2 represents a computer's estimate of nutrient requirements. Outputs change rapidly (an average of 10 L daily) and include gastric suction, duodenal fistula drainage, ileostomy output, postobstructive diuresis, and insensible water losses. Initial caloric and protein requirements are estimated to be 3700 nonprotein calories and 150 gm of protein daily. To meet essential fatty acid requirements, 50 gm of intravenous fats are to be delivered daily.

Using standard TPN solutions to provide optimal delivery, 550 calories would be provided using 500 ml of 10 per cent fat emulsions. Since slightly less than the remainder would be provided by 3 L of standard 1 cal/ml TPN solutions, 4 L would be prepared and administered, or the unused balance discarded if institutional practices so dictate. Other fluids and electrolytes would be delivered using specially prepared electrolyte solutions.

In contrast, should the computer be utilized and adequate production facilities be available, 9.5 L of solution containing approximately 332 calories (95 gm of dextrose), 16 gm of amino acids per L, and replacement electrolytes could be prepared using combinations of dextrose solutions (5 to 70 per cent) and amino acid solutions (3.5 to 10

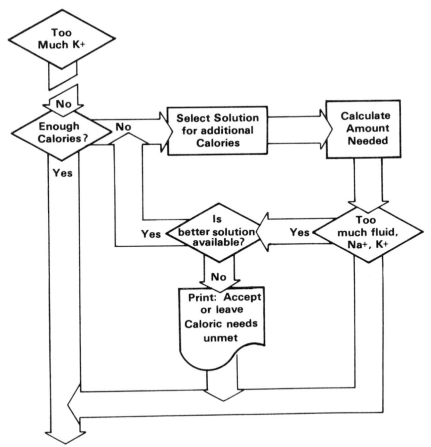

Figure 8–6. Similar searches must be conducted for caloric solutions relative to sodium and potassium content. Final output represents orders for solution delivery.

TABLE 8–2 COMPUTER ESTIMATE OF NUTRIENT REQUIREMENTS

Today's date: 17jun78
Hospital # 1234567   Room e401-1

Name Jones, John		
Age 44 years	Sex m	
Height	5 feet 4 inches	163 cm
Ideal weight	124–136 lb	56–62 kg
Premorbid weight	130 lb	59 kg
Actual weight	110 lb	50 kg
Estimated "dry" weight	108 lb	49 kg
Est. fluid/tumor load	2 lb	1 kg
Weight loss	22 lb	10 kg
Percent premorbid weight lost	16.9%	
Percent body protein lost	10.3%	
Body surface area	1.51 sq. meters	
Basal energy requirement	1396 kcal	
Ideal energy intake	2722 kcal	(46 cal/kg ideal weight)
Ideal protein intake	88.5 gm/day	(1.50 gm/kg ideal weight)
Cal/gm N ratio	192:1	

per cent) that meet constraints imposed by economic considerations.

The recent development of automated and computer-controlled admixture devices could make these formulations a reality. Use of such instrumentation will allow the formulation of complex solutions from as many as 15 base solutions within minutes, thus eliminating the need for the constant availability of highly trained pharmacists, particularly if the content of the solution is altered rapidly as a result of changing clinical responses.

Again, assuming optimal data acquisition, continuous monitoring of input and output, blood electrolyte concentrations, body weight, and body temperature, computer summaries of the impact of intervention procedures, projection of trends, and suggestions to change the solution formulation to optimize clinical outcome could be accomplished.

DELIVERY AND MONITORING

The computer is particularly applicable for controlled delivery and monitoring for effectiveness of intervention, provided that data can be acquired predictably. Results of blood tests must be entered by hand unless the hospital already has computer access to a data base generated by the clinical laboratories. If so, such data could automatically be integrated into decision-making as they enter the system, and the user could be informed of the entry of new data by notation, plots, graphs, and other indicators.

For the critically ill individual, automated bed scales are available for continuous recording of patient weight. The same is true for continuous monitoring of body temperature.

It is entirely feasible that individual pump delivery systems could be computer controlled for precise delivery of solutions. Computer access could be directly by hardware linkage to the computer, or indirectly by computer preparation of magnetic strips that could be inserted into the pump's microprocessor to generate the pump speed required for optimal delivery. Most pumps currently available have computer output connections to allow monitoring of exact amounts infused.

Whether data acquisition occurred by hand, or by direct computer linkage, computer-generated plots to define trends could be easily produced. The extensive memory capacity of the computer could be utilized advantageously, as in the following hypothetical example:

The last time this patient's weight approached this level over this time interval, serum osmolarity reached a point in 24 hours that caused concern relative to the development of a hyperosmolar syndrome. The appropriate course of action would be to increase free water delivery by making the following changes in solution composition for the next 12 hours. Do you approve?

Of no less significance would be use of the computer to monitor the effectiveness of nutritional support as patients undergo transition from one form of therapy to another. This particularly relates to the generation of daily calorie counts. The methods used can be as variable as the types of systems employed. Perhaps most applicable would be the development of menus with all items bar-coded in a manner similar to that used in supermarkets. Under each item would be printed a series of lines that would indicate to the computer the nutrient content of each item. The nurse or patient would check off the amount of each consumed, again in boxes identified by computer-readable notations. The dietitian would then need only to pass a "wand" over the menu to allow the computer to immediately document nutrient delivery, the attainment of nutrient requirements, plots of effectiveness, and suggested alternatives to boost calorie and/or protein intake, based on preferred items consumed by that particular patient in the past.

ADMINISTRATION

Many aspects relative to the administration of a nutrition support service would benefit from computerization. Most are obvious and need not be presented in detail. These would include the generation of statistics relative to the type of intervention employed, complication rates, diagnoses, cost effectiveness, and billing material. Most of these applications are merely extensions of standard hospital auditing procedures and could be applied if sufficient data are acquisitioned.

EDUCATION

A potentially exciting role for computer use in clinical nutrition relates to the recent development of two hardware devices: the microcomputer and the video disc. When combined with a television screen, the "intelligent video disc system" becomes operable.[15] Should such a system run concurrently with any of the therapeutic applications discussed above, the user could acquire near-instantaneous instruction on any point at which the user is currently operable.

Video disc technology is rapidly expanding with visual images "read" by a low-output laser beam. Under computer control, any one of 54,000 (108,000 with extended play) individual images can be found in a maximum of five seconds. That image could be viewed on the television screen as a slide, or motion could be induced by a short run as with any videotape system. The motion could proceed at normal speed, slow motion, frame by frame, or backwards, all under computer guidance. The availability of two soundtracks enables the computer to choose the educational level of audio output, depending upon the expertise of the user.

Attributes of the system include markedly expanded instructional time for users. If the disc were to be used as a "library" of slides, a total of 900 hours per disc (per side of extended play) would be available, assuming time allowance of 30 seconds per slide. In a mixed mode pattern with both slide and video, 160 hours of instructional time is a reasonable estimate.

It is proposed that an intelligent video disc system be integrated with the decision-making computer system employed in order to aid physicians and other individuals in computing status, requirements, solution formulation, delivery, monitoring, and administration. For example, let us assume that the patient described above had recovered sufficiently to allow consideration of enteral hyperalimentation and the computer suggested an elemental diet via a nasojejunal tube. At that particular point, the user could ask for instructional support. Slides listing references for use of enteral hyperalimentation in gastrointestinal fistulae could be shown with brief abstracts included. An elemental diet could be defined, the composition of commercially available solutions compared, and the rationale for computer choices given. Various types of nasojejunal tubes could be depicted, their relative merits discussed, and a brief demonstration of tube insertion shown. Depending upon the identity of the user, the soundtrack would discuss aspects of tube insertion of interest to physicians, or perhaps to nurses.

The principal advantage of this type of educational system is the instantaneous support available at the precise time of user interest. He or she would not have to perform time-consuming literature searches at the library, remember to ask a colleague, or request a filmstrip at a later date. The vast amount of storage capability could allow for an estimated 40 hours for each of four disciplines, even if information were not shared among user groups or disciplines. The potential impact of such a device on multidisciplinary education is broad indeed.

SUMMARY

For the most part, the above discussion is hypothetical at this time. However, each aspect is currently operable and could be integrated into the routine functioning of a nutrition support service. Development time is considerable. Resistance to computer use may be significant, but perhaps less so than if such systems were to be integrated into the more established medical disciplines. The disadvantages of letting the computer do the thinking and decision-making could be overcome by the advent of the intelligent video disc systems whose immediate instructional capabilities would most likely outweigh such negative effects.

REFERENCES

1. Perkins, W. J.: Biomedical Computing. Baltimore, University Park Press, 1977.
2. Proceedings of the Second Annual Symposium on Computer Application in Medical Care, November 5–9, 1978, Washington, D.C. New York, Institute of Electrical and Electronics Engineers, 1978.
3. Shortliffe, E. H.: Computer-Based Medical Consultations: MYCIN. New York, American Elsevier Publishing Company, Inc., 1976.
4. Butterworth, C. E., and Blackburn, G. L.: Hospital malnutrition. Nutr. Today, 10(2):8–18, 1975.
5. Bistrian, B. R., Blackburn, S. M., Sherman, M., and Scrimshaw, N. S.: Therapeutic index of nutritional depletion in hospitalized patients. Surg. Gynecol. Obstet., 141:512–516, 1975.
6. Blackburn, G. L., Bistrian, B. R., Maini, B. S., Schlamm, H. T., and Smith, M. F.: Nutritional

and metabolic assessment of the hospitalized patient. J.P.E.N., *1*:11–22, 1977.

7. Buzby, G. P., Mullen, J. L., Matthews, D. C., Hobbs, C. L., and Rosato, E. F.: Prognostic nutritional index in gastrointestinal surgery. Am. J. Surg., *139*:160–167, 1980.

8. Harris, J. A., and Benedict, F. G.: A Biometric Study of Basal Metabolism in Man. Washington, D.C., Carnegie Institute, 1919.

9. Geller, R. J., Blackburn, S. A., Glendon, D. H., Henneman, W. H., and Steffee, W. P.: Computer optimization of enteral hyperalimentation. J.P.E.N., *3*:79–83, 1979.

10. Kinney, J. M.: Calories, nitrogen, disease and injury relationships. *In* American Medical Association, Total Parenteral Nutrition. Acton, Massachusetts, Publishing Sciences Group, 1974, pages 81–91.

11. National Research Council, Food and Nutrition Board: Recommended Dietary Allowances. 8th revised edition. Washington, D.C., National Academy of Sciences, 1974, page 47.

12. Scrimshaw, N. S.: Through a glass darkly: Discerning the practical implications of human dietary protein-energy interrelationships. Nutr. Rev., *35*:321–337, 1977.

13. Grande, F. and Keys, A.: Body weight, body composition and calorie status. *In* Goodhart, R. S., and Shils, M. S. (eds.): Modern Nutrition in Health and Disease. Edition 5. Philadelphia, Lea & Febiger, 1973, page 9.

14. Society of Actuaries: Build and Blood Pressure Study, 1959.

15. Brown, B. R., Fowler, B., Stolurow, L. M., et al.: Instructional and Research Considerations with an Intelligent Videodisc. University of Iowa. A Presentation for the Association for Educational Data Systems. Detroit, 1979.

CHAPTER 9

The Role of the Clinical Dietitian and Modified Oral Diets

REBECCA MILLER ESVELT
SUSAN J. DEHOOG

Nutrition plays an important role in the etiology and management of many diseases that cause death and disability, including atherosclerotic vascular disease, obesity, hypertension, anemia, osteoporosis, and diabetes. Although there is a need for standardized nutritional care, it must be emphasized that each hospital has special requirements based on its particular patient population and corresponding medical and dietary staff philosophies. Thus nutritional care, just like other hospital services, has to be adapted to fit the particular characteristics of each hospital and its patients. The purpose of this chapter is to discuss the responsibilities of the clinical dietitian and the composition of special hospital diets and their indications.

THE CLINICAL DIETITIAN

The clinical dietitian is the primary practitioner of nutritional care in the hospital. Combining science and art, this professional applies nutrition and management principles in planning food intake for individuals and groups. The dietitian must consider the broader aspects of nutritional science, including the economic, social, psychologic, and physiologic relationships between humans and their food. The interaction of the clinical dietitian with the physician is based on the team concept, with the patient being the focus of the team.[1] Team members contribute a diversity of skills, knowledge, values, and attitudes to meet the patient's health care needs. The clinical dietitian's role is to evaluate the patient's nutritional status, develop and implement nutritional care plans, assess nutrient requirements, recommend nutritional prescriptions, evaluate patient tolerance of and effectiveness of nutritional care, and communicate nutritional data and information to the primary physician.[2] Clinical dietitians usually do not function as consultants in hospitals. They automatically have a responsibility to help every patient maintain and achieve optimal nutritional status. The role of the dietitian can be more precisely defined by examining how nutritional care plans are developed and implemented.

Patients at Nutritional Risk. Patient populations at risk for nutritional problems include obviously those with protein-calorie malnutrition, but also those with acute or chronic illness. In addition, certain population groups such as the obese, the cachectic, the elderly, and the adolescent with poor dietary habits are at risk.[3, 4] The nutritional screening questionnaire, shown in Figure 9–1, is useful at the time of admission to identify patients at risk who may need nutritional intervention.

The dietitian should also evaluate patients for symptoms of the following nutritional risk factors: poor appetite, anorexia nervosa, excess alcohol intake, ageusia, dysgeusia, anosmia, inadequate meals for needs, poor fitting dentures, limited or fad diets, frequent meals eaten away from home, chewing or swallowing problems, adverse food-drug interactions, and cultural or religious dietary restriction. Other risk factors include the inability to eat for more than 7 to

1. Height _____   Usual weight _____   Actual weight _____

2. Have you had a recent weight loss greater than 10 pounds within a 30 day period? Yes _____   No _____   Have you been on a weight reduction diet? Yes _____   No _____

3. Have you had surgery within the past six months? Yes _____   No _____

4. Have you had a recent illness or infection lasting 10 days or more?

   Yes _____   No _____   If yes, please specify _____.

5. Have you had a recent change in appetite? Yes _____   No _____

6. Are you on any special diet? Yes _____   No _____   If yes, what _____

   _____

7. Do you have difficulties with:

   Swallowing _____   Vomiting _____   Diarrhea _____   Chewing _____

   Nausea _____   Constipation _____   Other _____

8. Do you take any vitamin and/or mineral supplements? Yes _____   No _____

   If yes, what _____

9. Do you take any drugs/medications? Yes _____   No _____   If yes, what ____

   _____

Figure 9–1. Nutritional screening questionnaire.

10 days or maintenance on low-kilocalorie intravenous fluids for more than 10 days. These patients require prompt nutritional intervention.

Nutritional Assessment. Nutritional assessment as performed by the dietitian includes a review of dietary, social, and medical histories.[5]

Diet History. The term *diet history* refers to a review of the usual patterns of food intake and the food selection variables that dictate food intake, whereas the term *nutritional history* implies the incorporation of information from laboratory and clinical data as well as from the diet history. A diet history form providing only the most basic information is shown in Figure 9–2.

The diet history process can be conducted by collecting retrospective intake data or by summarizing current intake data.

We shall briefly review two retrospective methods and one inspective (current) approach. It should be kept in mind that whatever technique is employed, the goal is to determine the nutrient content of food intake and the appropriateness of the intake for the patient.[1]

Food Frequency Interview. The food frequency interview is a retrospective review of intake frequency of food and food supplements per day, per week, and per month. Because intake of various food items can change with the stage of an illness, food frequency forms should be completed for the period immediately prior to hospitalization (that is, during the illness) as well as for the period before the illness to arrive at an accurate dietary history. The food frequency form organizes food into groups that have nutrients in common for ease of evaluation.

Working? Yes _____ No _____ Occupation _____ Hours _____

Appetite _____ Physical Activity _____

Previous Special Diet? _____

Problems With Diet? _____

Family Members on Special Diet? _____

Cultural/Religious Practices _____

Supplements/Health Foods _____

Allergies _____

Chewing/Swallowing Problems _____

Handicaps _____

Who Shops? _____ Who Cooks? _____ For How Many? ___

Cooking Facilities _____ Refrigerator _____

Convenience Foods _____

Number of Meals Per Day _____ Number of Snacks _____

Meals Away From Home _____ Where _____

Figure 9–2. Dietary history form.

Serving size, method of cooking, and number of servings weekly are noted. Since the food frequency interview is concerned primarily with the frequency of usage of *food groups*, rather than of *specific nutrients*, it is most helpful when the focus is the diet in general rather than specific aspects of the diet.[6]

24-Hour Recall. The 24-hour recall method lists specific foods consumed in a 24-hour period. Recall data tend toward over-reporting of low intakes and under-reporting of high intakes and therefore are of limited value in evaluating an individual's true dietary intake.[7] The day chosen for recall may also be atypical; however, when both the food frequency interview and 24-hour recall are used, a more accurate estimation of the patient's dietary intake can be made.[6] This approach is termed the *cross-check*.

Diet Record. The diet record (Fig. 9–3) documents a patient's dietary intake as it occurs. Usually at least seven consecutive days are required, since one week is considered the shortest time feasible to ensure validity. The method is not suitable when symptoms or treatment of a condition affect the diet. Moreover, since the record is kept by the patient, literacy is essential.[7]

Social History. The social history evaluates the social factors that can negatively affect nutritional status. These risk factors include inadequate income, inability to buy food, living or eating alone, disabilities, old age, smoking, drug or alcohol addiction, and inadequate refrigeration or cooking facilities.

Medical History. The medical history should also be reviewed from a nutritional perspective. The dietitian should be aware of demonstrated increased metabolic states, increased nutrient losses, chronic disease, catabolic states, recent major surgery of the gastrointestinal tract, body weight 20 per cent over or under the ideal, or a recent significant weight loss or gain. General laboratory tests (such as hemoglobin and blood glucose) as well as laboratory determinations of specific nutrients (for example, iron and folic acid) should be examined, and records of body temperature, fluid intake and output, and medications are especially pertinent.[1]

INSTRUCTIONS:

Please record your intake of food and beverages for the next 7 days. Include:

1. Item consumed
2. Method of preparation
3. Amount consumed:

Liquid - cups or fluid ounces
Meat, Cheese, Fish, Poultry - in ounces, specifying if the amount given is in cooked or raw weight
Vegetables - cups or individual units (1 tomato)
Fruits - cups or individual units, including diameter of fresh fruits (apple, orange) or length (banana)
Bread - number of slices
Cereal, Pasta, Rice, Potatoes - cups
Pancakes, Waffles - number and diameter
Crackers - number
Margarine or Butter - teaspoons or pats
Dressings, Mayonnaise - teaspoons or tablespoons
Gravy - tablespoons or cups
Bacon, Sausage - number of slices or links
Jam, Jelly, Honey, Sugar, Syrup - teaspoons or tablespoons
Candy - number of bars, number and size of pieces
Jello, Pudding, Ice Cream - cups
Cookies - number
Pie, Cake - number of pieces, length and width at largest end

Record each entry as soon as possible after each meal or snack. Attempt to keep your intake as normal as possible. Do not write in last 3 columns on form.

Day # _____ *

Items Consumed	How Prepared	Amount	Protein	Fat	CHO
Breakfast _____					
Snack _____					
Lunch _____					
Snack _____					
Dinner _____					
Snack _____					

*Sample form for one day

Figure 9–3. Diet record.

Planning. Planning includes the provision of nutrient sources with food or other means. The decision made during the planning phase must be soundly based on the literature of nutritional science and medicine as well as on the patient's history. Behavioral objectives must be clearly stated to ensure success of the nutritional care plan. In some cases, the final goal of the plan is the achievement of independence in the process of food selection.

Implementation and Intervention. The process of putting the nutritional care plan into action consists of two facets: diet prescription and nutrition counseling. Diet prescription should reflect the patient's nutritional needs, be written qualitatively as well as quantitatively, and specify any current dietary deficiencies. Nutritional counseling may be described as "providing individualized professional guidance to assist a person in adjusting his daily food consumption to meet his health needs."[8] A good rapport between the dietitian and patient is essential. Once a diet is developed, the dietitian must often implement behavior modification techniques to enable the patient to comply with the nutritional program. Suggestions for procurement and preparation, as well as directions for combining or substituting nutritionally equivalent foods, must be provided. Food costs must also be considered. Finally, since any change in lifestyle, including diet, can be overwhelming to the patient and the patient's family, follow-up nutrition counseling is advised.

Reassessment. Continuous monitoring of the nutritional care plan is required to document the patient's response. Nutrient intake is evaluated through analysis of the daily calorie count. Frequent feedings or supplements should be considered if a patient is not consuming an adequate caloric intake. Serial biochemical and anthropometric assessments provide additional data to document the need for changes in the nutritional care plan. The clinical dietitian and the physician should review and interpret the data. Working together will ensure that each patient receives quality nutritional care. Nutritional care may possibly reduce the length of hospitalization and thereby reduce total health care costs.

The ultimate goal of the physician and dietitian is to maintain the patient's nutritional status after discharge. Patients may be referred to a dietitian in private practice to provide nutritional follow-up through continued teaching, assistance, and encouragement. An increasing number of communities have professionals available to provide the continuity of care required for outpatient nutritional rehabilitation.

MODIFIED HOSPITAL DIETS

Recent advances in nutrition, particularly total parenteral nutrition and tube feeding, have greatly stimulated the clinician's interest in providing optimal nutritional support for hospitalized patients. The contemporary physician must, however, be cognizant of the various oral diets as well as tube and intravenous feeding methods in order to provide optimal nutritional care.

We shall briefly review several of the most commonly used therapeutic diets. They are classified into two groups: those involving modifications in consistency and those involving modifications in nutrient intake. More detailed diet plans and rationale have been published previously[9, 10] and are available in dietetic texts. It is assumed that the clinician is familiar with the normal diet from which these special diets are derived.

Modifications in Consistency

Clear Liquid Diet. The clear liquid diet is intended to provide an oral source of fluids and small amounts of electrolytes to prevent dehydration and minimize colonic residue. It is most commonly used following certain types of surgery as an intermediate step between intravenous feedings and a full liquid or solid diet. Clear liquids may also be indicated (1) as the first step in oral feedings for fluid and electrolyte replacement in diarrheal diseases, (2) to reduce the amount of colonic residue in preparation for intestinal surgery or barium enema, or following colonic surgery, and (3) as the first step in oral alimentation in the severely debilitated patient.

The clear liquid diet includes only those foods that are liquid at room temperature, such as broth, bouillon, coffee, tea, strained fruit juices, clear or flavored gelatin, carbonated beverages, and popsicles. No milk products are included. The meal plan consists of three meals of broth, strained juice, flavored gelatin, and coffee, with juice, gelatin, or a carbonated beverage between meals and at bedtime.

This diet is highly restrictive and has little nutritive value. It is inadequate in kilocalories and all major nutrients with the possible exception of vitamin C, sodium, potassium, and water. Prolonged use of the clear liquid diet leads to weight loss, tissue wasting, and multiple nutritional deficiencies, particularly in individuals with increased caloric needs or in patients whose nutritional status is marginal. A chemically defined diet or total parenteral nutrition should be considered if clear liquids are to be maintained for longer than three days or if a patient is "at risk" nutritionally.

Full Liquid Diet. The full liquid diet is intended to provide oral nourishment to patients who are acutely ill or unable to swallow or chew solid foods. It is most commonly used in postoperative patients in the transition from clear liquids to a solid diet but is also used following surgery of the mouth, face, or neck, and in patients with mandibular fractures or esophageal strictures.

The full liquid diet includes foods that are liquid or liquefy at room temperature—for example, milk, plain frozen desserts, custards, plain puddings, fruit juices, vegetable juices, cereal gruels, broth, and eggnog made with pasteurized eggs. The meal plan consists of three meals, with gruel at breakfast and cream soups at lunch and dinner. Between-meal and bedtime snacks consisting of milkshakes, eggnog, or ice cream are also served.

The nutritional adequacy of a full liquid diet will vary with the type and quantity of food served at each institution. For example, if pureed meat soups and brewer's yeast are not included, the diet will be inadequate in folic acid, iron, and vitamin B_6.[9] Care must be taken to provide enough milk and eggs to ensure adequate protein intake. Individuals on a full liquid diet for more than three days should receive high-kilocalorie, high-protein supplements. When given a full liquid diet after surgery, some patients may be temporarily lactose-intolerant and thus suffer from nausea, vomiting, distention, or diarrhea.[11] Since the diet has a high milk content, it is rich in lactose and is therefore contraindicated in cases of lactose intolerance. The lactose content may be lowered by substituting lactose-free products.

Low-Fiber Diet. Some confusion exists as to the difference between fiber and residue. Kramer has proposed the abandonment of the term *residue* because it has two meanings: It is used to refer to fecal output as well as dietary fiber (that is, plant materials taken in through diet that are resistant to digestion).[12] As an example, prune juice yields no material residue following digestion but is still classified as a high-residue food because it contains a laxative that increases stool volume. For these reasons we refer to the "low-fiber" diet.

The purpose of the low-fiber diet is to prevent high-fiber foods from obstructing a pathologically narrow intestinal lumen.[9] Low-fiber diets decrease the weight and bulk of the stool and delay intestinal transit.[13] The diet is indicated whenever inflammatory changes have progressed to stenosis of the intestinal or esophageal lumen. Low-fiber diets are also used during the acute phases of diverticulitis, ulcerative colitis, or infectious enterocolitis. There is little evidence to support the long-term use of a low-fiber diet in the treatment of regional enteritis, ulcerative colitis, or pyloric stenosis.[9] This diet may be used as a soft diet in the transition between a completely liquid diet and a general diet in postsurgical patients.

The low-fiber diet contains a minimum of fiber and connective tissue. Because data on dietary fiber content of foods are incomplete, diets must be described in qualitative terms. Indigestible carbohydrate is reduced by using tender-cooked vegetables, ripe-canned, or well-cooked fruits and certain raw fruits and vegetables low in dietary fiber. Tender meats or meats made tender in the cooking process are used to decrease the connective tissue in the diet. There is some evidence that milk, which contains no crude fiber, may indirectly contribute to fecal residue and may, in some patients, need to be restricted to two cups per day.[9]

Since fiber-deficient diets are associated with small, infrequent stools, it has been suggested that long-term use of these diets may be associated with diverticular disease of the colon. The small compact stool causes the colon to contract more tightly, thus narrowing the lumen and increasing intraluminal pressures.[14] A low-fiber diet may also aggravate symptoms of irritable colon syndrome or diverticulitis unless the lumen of the colon is already narrowed.[14]

High-Fiber Diet. The purpose of the high-fiber diet is threefold: It increases the volume and weight of the residues that reach the distal colon, increases gastrointestinal motility, and decreases intraluminal colonic pressures. The high-fiber diet has been shown to be effective in reducing colonic pressures in diverticulosis and may maintain the size of the lumen to prevent further progression of the disease.[13] Increasing fiber intake may also benefit patients with nonobstructive constipation, irritable bowel syndrome, or any conditions that may be helped by increasing stool volume.

The diet itself contains increased amounts of cellulose, hemicellulose, lignin, and pectin to increase crude fiber to 13 or more grams per day. The general diet is modified by increasing the intake of whole grain breads and cereals, fresh fruits, and high-fiber vegetables. The caloric content of the diet is not substantially different from the general diet, since the intake of highly refined carbohydrates is reduced. Additional fluids should be encouraged.

Large amounts of dietary fiber may result in osmotic diarrhea and increased production of flatus owing to volatile fatty acids produced by intestinal bacteria. In addition, large quantities of high-fiber foods may contain insoluble phytates, which bind iron, calcium, zinc, and folate, thus preventing absorption and reducing serum levels. High-fiber diets are contraindicated in patients with stenosis of the intestinal lumen.

"Bland" Diet. The purpose of the bland diet is to relieve pain and promote healing in patients with duodenal ulcers and other gastrointestinal disorders. Historically, it has been described as a diet that is chemically and mechanically nonirritating, although there is no consensus as to which foods should be excluded. The American Dietetic Association has reviewed the available data and currently provides the following guidelines:[9]

1. The only foods shown to cause gastric irritation are black and red pepper, chili powder, caffeine, coffee, tea, decaffeinated coffee, cola beverages, cocoa, alcohol, and certain drugs. Other spices, condiments, and highly seasoned foods have not been shown to irritate the gastric mucosa, even when applied directly. Roughage or coarse foods (lettuce, nuts, fruit skins, and celery) have been excluded in some diets, but there is no evidence that these foods, when well masticated, cause any irritation to a duodenal ulcer. Milk, once thought to decrease acid secretion, may actually increase it because of its high calcium and protein content.

2. The pH of the gastric contents is increased with small-volume, frequent feedings, a regimen that offers the greatest comfort to the patient.

Based on these findings, the bland diet for patients with duodenal ulcer should exclude foods known to cause gastric irritation, be individualized to the patient's specific food intolerances and lifestyle, and utilize small volume, frequent feedings.[9]

Diet for the Dysphagic Patient. Management of the dysphagic patient requires input from the entire nutritional support team. A speech therapist or pathologist is particularly knowledgeable in dealing with dysphagia and feeding techniques. Special consideration is necessary to ensure adequate nutrition, prevent aspiration, and assist in the patient's rehabilitation. Tube feeding, although clearly indicated for some patients, does not play a role in patient rehabilitation since it cannot help patients regain the ability to swallow or feed themselves.

There are three main types of dysphagia. Mechanical dysphagia causes difficulty in moving food or liquid from the front to the back of the mouth, where it can be swallowed. Dysphagia paralytica is caused by disease or trauma to the brain stem and/or cranial nerves involved in swallowing. Pseudobulbar dysphagia is commonly brought on by stroke or damage to the upper part of the brain and cortex and often results in the inability to coordinate chewing, breathing, and swallowing.

Each type of dysphagia and each patient with dysphagia will need specialized individual care to overcome his or her difficulties. Some general guidelines for feeding these patients are presented in Figures 9–4 and 9–5. As in other diets described in this section, dietary management mainly involves modifications in consistency.

Modification of Nutrients

Kilocalorie-Restricted Diet. Kilocalorie-restricted diets are used to reduce body weight in overweight individuals. They should be part of a well-coordinated program of caloric restriction, exercise, behavior modification, and long-term guidance that will lead to new food preferences and sustained weight loss. Caloric restriction has also been shown to alleviate symptoms and

1. Proper positioning during eating is important. The patient should sit up if at all possible.

2. Special equipment, such as plate guards and built-up spoons, may need to be used. (Fig 5)

3. Sufficient time for eating must be allowed, especially in the elderly person. The patient should not be hurried while eating.

4. Small bites of food or sips of liquid should be taken, allowing sufficient time to hold food in the mouth. Food should not be washed down with liquids as the food may be aspirated.

5. When the patient is ready to swallow, he should hold his head slightly forward and hold his breath.

6. If the patient needs to be fed:

    a) Watch the thyroid cartilage (Adam's apple) to see if the patient has swallowed.

    b) Allow the patient to indicate when he is ready for the next mouthful.

    c) Converse with the patient only in regard to his condition. Communication may be distracting for patients with pseudobulbar dysphagia, but others may actually need verbal direction for eating.

Figure 9–4. Dietary guidelines for the patient with dysphagia.

7. Certain medications may affect swallowing. For example, atropine may cause the mouth to be dry, making swallowing difficult. Excessive drooling or salivation will also cause problems.

8. Some foods can be more difficult to manage than others:

    a) Milk and ice cream (i.e., uncooked milk) may produce phlegm. Cream soups and puddings are acceptable, however.

    b) Sticky foods such as mashed potatoes, fresh bread, and bananas are difficult to swallow.

    c) Dry foods (crackers) need to be moistened. Gravy can be added to potatoes and meat.

    d) Slippery foods are easier to swallow but may be difficult to control in the mouth for mastication.

    e) Pureed foods provide insufficient texture for stimulation and may be aspirated.

    f) Liquids or solid foods without flavor, or with flavors that the patient is insensitive to, will cause problems. For example, the patient may be able to drink orange juice but not water.

    g) The temperature of foods may affect the stimulation required for swallowing.

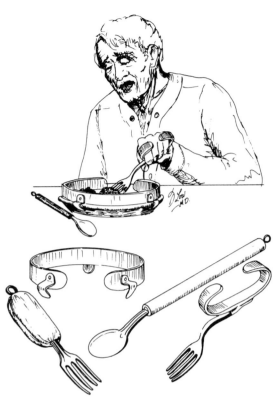

Figure 9–5. Modified feeding utensils and plate guard for dysphagic patients.

improve outcome in patients with respiratory diseases, hypertension, myocardial infarction, maturity-onset diabetes, and certain bone and joint diseases.

The diet itself should meet all other nutritional needs but is limited to a prescribed level of total kilocalories that will result in a predictable weight loss. The exchange lists, also used for diabetic diets, are used to estimate daily caloric intake. Most foods are quantity-restricted, and concentrated sources of kilocalories are eliminated. Patients should be counseled by qualified professionals who are able to tailor the diet to the individual's lifestyle, work habits, and education while satisfying nutrition requirements and providing close follow-up.

Intake of thiamine, and especially iron (which may be marginal even in a well-balanced diet), is frequently low in unbalanced fad diets. Commonly, these diets neglect major food groups and do not meet recommended dietary allowances for all nutrients. Semistarvation diets should be attempted only with close metabolic and clinical monitoring. The ketosis produced by such diets is associated with calcium depletion, dehydration, weakness, nausea, high blood uric acid levels, and kidney failure or stones in patients prone to kidney disease. Weight reduction regimens are contraindicated during pregnancy, despite the added risk of obesity.[15]

Diet for the Diabetic Patient. The most important goal of the diet for the diabetic patient is to attain and maintain ideal body weight. Individual caloric requirements depend on height, weight, age, sex, and activity level; however, important goals include meeting complete nutritional needs, maintaining normal growth and development in juveniles or in the fetus of a pregnant diabetic woman, minimizing glycosuria, and reducing elevated serum lipid levels, which are associated with the cardiovascular complications of diabetes.

Since maturity-onset diabetics are usually obese, weight reduction is of prime importance. Moreover, attaining ideal body weight alone may control mild cases. Dietary strategies for both maturity-onset and nonobese juvenile diabetics are outlined in Table 9–1.

In the diet for the diabetic patient, kilocalories, as well as protein, fat, and carbohydrate intake, are controlled. Total daily caloric intake is set at an optimal level, and the timing of meals and nutrient content should remain constant. The diet consists of a variety of foods from the normal diet which are incorporated into exchange lists. The foods within each list, in the amount given, are approximately equal in their protein, fat, and carbohydrate content. By choosing foods from these lists, a wide variety of food intake is possible.

It was once thought that the diet of an insulin-dependent diabetic should contain only moderate amounts of carbohydrates in order to control blood sugar. This resulted in a relatively high fat intake to provide caloric needs. When high fat intake was linked to cardiovascular complications, the optimal level of carbohydrate was revised upward, and current recommendations suggest carbohydrate content of 50 to 60 per cent.[9] There is actually some evidence that a higher level in patients with mild diabetes may improve glucose tolerance.[16] Concentrated sugars and sweets that are rapidly absorbed should be avoided, however, as they cause a greater and more immediate glucose response than calorically equivalent amounts of complex starches.[17]

Table 9–1   DIETARY STRATEGIES FOR THE TWO MAIN TYPES OF DIABETES

DIETARY STRATEGIES	OBESE PATIENT NOT REQUIRING INSULIN	NONOBESE PATIENT REQUIRING INSULIN
Decrease calories	Yes. Reduction of adiposity reduces hyperglycemia and reduces the insulin resistance that attends obesity.	No. Calories should not be restricted below normal levels.
Increase frequency and number of feedings	Usually no. It gives an obese patient more chances to overeat.	Yes
Meal regulation	This is not crucial if average caloric intake is reduced to provide for weight loss of 1–2 lbs/week.	Very important. Three meals with appropriate snacks are recommended.
Extra food for increased exercise	Not usually appropriate	Usually appropriate
Use of food to treat or prevent hyperglycemia	Not necessary	Important
Provide small, frequent feedings or give carbohydrate intravenously during illness	Usually not necessary because of resistance to ketosis.	Important

In planning meals for the insulin-dependent diabetic, the dietitian must also take into account the type of insulin and the amount of physical activity in order to prevent hypoglycemia. The carbohydrate intake is distributed among three meals and an evening snack consisting of protein and carbohydrate. Additional feedings may be required, depending on the peak action of the insulin.

The use of a fixed caloric intake with the food exchange system may not be appropriate for young insulin-dependent diabetics. Hypoglycemic episodes may result from variations in work, play, and exercise habits. These rigid diets also have adverse emotional and physical effects in certain patients. A more liberalized diet has been proposed which eliminates concentrated sweets and favors regularly spaced meals with snacks as needed. Exchange lists and rigid kilocalorie and carbohydrate control are deemphasized.[18] This diet should only be used once good control is established and the patient is at ideal body weight with satisfactory growth and development.

High-Kilocalorie, High-Protein Diet. The high-kilocalorie, high-protein diet has a dual purpose: It provides for nutritional rehabilitation in a malnourished patient and prevents weight loss and tissue-wasting in conditions in which calorie and protein requirements are greatly increased. In protein-calorie malnutrition, the diet should be adjusted to the needs and tolerance of the individual, with special emphasis on the kilocalorie-to-nitrogen ratio, to provide adequate calories and to ensure that protein will be used in the rebuilding of tissues rather than as an energy source. The optimal ratio is approximately 100 to 200 Kcal/gm of nitrogen in orally fed diets.

Since low serum albumin is associated with increased complications and poor outcome after surgery, this diet should also be used prior to surgery in patients with albumin levels of less than 3.5 mg/dl.[19] Additional protein and kilocalories should also be given to patients in hypermetabolic or catabolic states (for example, fever, thyrotoxicosis, and burns).

The high-protein, high-kilocalorie diet provides a level of kilocalories and protein substantially above that which is normally required. For an adult this diet may typically supply 1000 or more supplemental kilocalories and should provide a minimum of 1.5 gm protein/kg body weight.[9] Additional servings of milk, meat, and eggs are included, and high-protein, high-kilocalorie supplements are often utilized. The distribution of meals should be designed to encourage maximum food consumption by the patient. In some patients an increased number of feedings may be indicated. An extra feeding before bed, when the patient's activity level is more relaxed, is often recommended.

Possible adverse reactions to this diet include elevated lipid levels in susceptible patients, negative calcium balance, vitamin A deficiency, and hepatic coma in patients with severe hepatitis. Very high-protein diets may adversely affect calcium balance, resulting in increased urinary calcium excretion. The mechanism for this calcium loss is unknown.[20] A high-protein diet also results in a greater demand by the body for vitamin A. In patients with kwashiorkor, the liver stores of vitamin A are low, and special care should be taken to provide a sufficient intake of this vitamin.[21]

This diet is contraindicated in patients with hepatic coma, hyperammonemia, uremia, or an impaired renal glomerular filtration rate.

Sodium-Restricted Diet. The purpose of a sodium-restricted diet is to restore normal sodium balance by causing a loss of excess sodium and water from extracellular fluid compartments. Normally, sodium loads are excreted in the urine, but in certain conditions the body's homeostatic mechanisms break down, resulting in sodium and water retention.

Sodium-restricted diets are used in liver disease, hypertension, congestive heart failure, renal disease, and prolonged adrenocortical steroid therapy. The portal hypertension and hypoalbuminemia of advanced liver disease reduce plasma colloid osmotic pressure and impair the body's control of sodium and water excretion, resulting in ascites. Restriction of dietary sodium has proved to be an effective method of promoting diuresis.

In the hypertensive patient, sodium restriction acts in a manner similar to diuretic drugs, although some forms of hypertension respond to sodium restriction less favorably than others. In particular, primary aldosteronism, hypervolemic essential hypertension, and hypertension associated with chronic renal parenchymal disease benefit from negative sodium and water balance.[9]

In congestive heart failure, sodium retention and peripheral edema occur as a result of impaired cardiac output. Potent diuretics have decreased the need for severe dietary restrictions; thus a diet containing 90 mEq (2100 mg) of sodium is probably sufficiently restrictive for most patients. In patients with refractory pulmonary edema, however—particularly if potent diuretics are not used—sodium intakes of less than 22 mEq (500 mg) may be necessary.[22]

In renal disease complicated by edema or moderate hypertension (occurring most often in glomerulonephritis), sodium intake should be restricted to 40 to 90 mEq (900 to 2100 mg) daily. Sodium restriction may not be required in other forms of kidney disease. In nephrotic syndrome, sodium retention and edema may be caused by low albumin levels. Some patients may lose the capacity to excrete sodium while on a high sodium intake and lose the capacity to conserve sodium while on a low intake. Restrictions should be imposed on the basis of urinary sodium output, blood pressure, and weight changes. It may be more important to restore serum proteins through an adequate diet than to restrict sodium.[9]

Foods allowed in a sodium-restricted diet vary with the level of restriction. Foods containing large amounts of natural sodium or commercially processed foods with added sodium are either eliminated or restricted. Fruits are generally unrestricted, as they contain little sodium. Exchange lists are available from the American Heart Association to aid in planning all levels of sodium restriction. Advances in drug therapy have reduced the need for extremely low-sodium diets. When renal function is sufficient to permit a diuretic to be effective, severe sodium restriction is unnecessary. Many low-sodium diets are unpalatable, difficult to follow, and are associated with a very low rate of patient compliance. The use of mild and moderate restrictions of sodium is helpful, however, in patients receiving diuretics. Dosage can be reduced, thereby reducing diuretic-related side effects. In general, a sodium intake of 85 to 87 mEq (2000 mg) will enhance the effectiveness of diuretic agents in the treatment of some forms of hypertension.

Severe sodium restrictions should be used with caution. In some patients, an abrupt change from a normal sodium intake to a severe restriction may lead to sodium depletion, particularly in patients with chronic renal insufficiency. Age also affects renal sodium transport mechanisms, making the elderly more vulnerable to an abrupt withdrawal of sodium. Symptoms of sodium depletion include muscle cramps, convulsions, hypovolemia, hypotension, and in patients with renal disease, a deterioration of renal function.

Sodium restriction is contraindicated in uncomplicated renal disease (that is, in the absence of hypertension and edema), normal pregnancy, and myxedema, and in ileostomized patients.

Fat-Restricted Diet. Fat-restricted diets are used to treat steatorrhea in disorders causing impaired fat digestion, absorption, or transport. In chronic pancreatitis, fat restriction is used in conjunction with enzyme replacement to control steatorrhea and fat-soluble vitamin losses. To promote weight gain and maximum nutrient intake, the patient should be given the maximum amount of fat he can tolerate without increased steatorrhea or pain. Initial restriction is usually 50 gm/day or less. This is gradually increased until the limits of tolerance are reached. Medium-chain triglycerides may also be used to increase fat intake.

Fat malabsorption may also occur as a complication of cirrhosis, intestinal bypass surgery, gastrectomy, and short-gut syndrome. Fat balance studies and serum carotene levels can indicate the presence of fat malabsorption. In many of these patients fat malabsorption is only temporary.

The rationale for using low-fat diets in gallbladder disease is controversial. Although fatty acids stimulate the gallbladder to contract (by the release of cholecystokinin), so also do amino acids. It has been suggested that patients with gallbladder disease are no less tolerant of fried foods than are normals.[23] There is also little reason to restrict fat intake in cholecystectomized patients.

In the fat-restricted diet, all forms of fat are restricted and no attempt is made to differentiate among the various forms. In diets that are moderately fat-restrictive, only skim milk or buttermilk is used and whole milk cheeses are avoided. Plain breads, cereals, and vegetables are allowed, as are fruits and seasonings. Desserts are restricted to those low in fat. Lean meats, fish, and poultry are allowed in calculated amounts. Foods high in fat (for example, butter and cream) are restricted by using an exchange system to comply with the required level of restriction.

This diet should produce no adverse reactions as long as total caloric intake is adequate, and sufficient fat is included to prevent essential fatty acid deficiency.

SUMMARY

The dietitian is often the only person with formal training in nutrition in most hospitals. Among the dietitian's responsibilities are recognizing patients at nutritional risk, participating in nutritional assessment, and ensuring that the patient receives the most appropriate diet for his or her disease. Many patients require special diets at various stages of the disease process. These diets usually involve either a modification in consistency or a modification in nutrient intake.

REFERENCES

1. Mason, W., Wenberg, B. G., and Welsch, P. K.: The Dynamics of Clinical Dietetics. New York, J. Wiley and Sons, 1977.
2. Jenson, T. G., and Brooks, B. J.: Marketing strategy: A key leverage point for dietitians. J. Am. Diet. Assoc., 79:267–273, 1981.
3. Butterworth, C. E., Jr.: The skeleton in the hospital closet. Nutr. Today., 9(2):4–8, 1974.
4. Blackburn, G. L., and Bistrian, B.: Iatrogenic malnutrition II: Report from Boston. Nutr. Today, 9(3):30, 1974.
5. Grant, T. A.: Nutritional Assessment Guidelines. Edition 2. Seattle, 1979.
6. Morgan, R. W., Jain, M., Miller, A. B., Choi, N. W., Matthews, V., Munan, L., Burch, J. D., Feather, J., Howe, G. R., and Kelly, A.: A comparison of dietary methods in epidemiologic studies. Am. J. Epidemiol., 107:488–498, 1978.
7. Garsovitz, M., Madden, J. P., and Smiciklas-Wright, H.: Validity of the 24-hour dietary recall and seven-day record for group comparisons. J. Am. Diet. Assoc., 73:48–55, 1978.
8. American Dietetic Association, Diet Therapy Section Committee: Guidelines for diet counseling. J. Am. Diet. Assoc., 66:571–575, 1975.
9. American Dietetic Association: Handbook of Clinical Dietetics. New Haven, Connecticut, Yale University Press, 1981.
10. Goodhart, R. S., and Shils, M. E.: Modern Nutrition in Health and Disease. Edition 6. Philadelphia, Lea and Febiger, 1980.
11. Randall, H. T.: Enteric feeding. In American College of Surgeons, Committee on Pre- and Postoperative Care. Manual of Surgical Nutrition. Philadelphia, W. B. Saunders Company, 1975.
12. Kramer, P.: The meaning of high and low residue diets. Gastroenterology, 47:649–652, 1964.
13. Parks, T. G.: The role of dietary fibre in the prevention and treatment of diseases of the colon. Proc. R. Soc. Med. (Lond.), 66:681–683, 1973.
14. Painter, N. S., and Burkitt, D. P. Diverticular disease of the colon: A deficiency disease of Western civilization. Br. Med. J., 2:450–454, 1971.
15. National Research Council, Food and Nutrition Board, Committee on Maternal Nutrition: Maternal Nutrition and the Course of Pregnancy. Washington, D.C., National Academy of Sciences, 1970.
16. Brunzell, J. D., Lerner, R. L., Porte, D., Jr., and Bierman, E. L.: Effect of a fat free, high carbohydrate diet on diabetic subjects with fasting hyperglycemia. Diabetes, 23:128–142, 1974.
17. Crapo, P. A., Reavan, G., and Olefsky, J.: Plasma glucose and insulin responses to orally administered simple and complex carbohydrates. Diabetes, 25:741–747, 1976.
18. Schmitt, B. D.: An argument for the unmeasured diet in juvenile diabetes mellitus. Clin. Pediatr., 14:68–73, 1975.

19. Hickman, D. M., Miller, R. A., Rombeau, J. L., Twomey, P. L., and Frey, C. F.: Serum albumin and body weight as predictors of postoperative course in colorectal cancer. J.P.E.N., 4:314–316, 1980.
20. Margen, S., Chu, J. Y., Kaufman, N. A., and Calloway, D. H.: Studies in calcium metabolism. I. The calciuretic effect of dietary protein. Am. J. Clin. Nutr., 27:584–589, 1974.
21. Roels, W. A., and Lui, N. S. T.: Vitamin A and carotene. In Goodhart, R. S., and Shils, M. E. (eds.): Modern Nutrition in Health and Disease. Edition 5. Philadelphia, Lea and Febiger, 1973.
22. Kark, R. M., and Oyama, J. H.: Nutrition and cardiovascular-renal diseases. In Goodhart, R. S., and Shils, M. E. (eds.): Modern Nutrition in Health and Disease. Edition 5. Philadelphia, Lea and Febiger, 1973.
23. Price, W. H.: Gallbladder dyspepsia. Br. Med. J., 2(5350):138–141, 1963.
24. DeHoog, S. J.: Clinical Nutrition Syllabus for Physicians. Redmond, Washington, 1982.
25. U.S. Department of Health, Education and Welfare, First Health and Examination Survey: Anthropometrics and Clinical Findings. DHEW Publication Number (HSN) 72-8130, 1972.
26. Halpern, S. L. (ed.): Quick Reference to Clinical Nutrition. Philadelphia, J. B. Lippincott, 1979.
27. American Dietetic Association: Costs and Benefits of Nutritional Care, Phase I. Chicago, American Dietetic Association, 1979.

CHAPTER 10

Formulas

MAUREEN M. MACBURNEY
LORRAINE SEE YOUNG

The marked growth of commercial nutritional formulas over the past decade has stemmed from a heightened awareness of health care providers of the nutritional needs of patients and the development of smaller, safer, and more comfortable feeding tubes. Formulas have advanced significantly from the "home"-blenderized whole food diets, and they now range from blenderized diets to highly refined, "predigested" nutrients in combination or in isolated form.

Formulas may be complete diets, providing an individual's total nutrient needs solely by the administration of adequate amounts of the formula. Formulas may also be modular components, providing one or more nutrients to supplement another diet or formula, or combined together to make a modular formula (see chapter on Modular Feeding).

In all situations, however, the nutritional requirements of the patient must be kept uppermost in mind. Whether utilizing a formula as a complete diet or as a supplement, the specific requirements for water, calories, protein, electrolytes, vitamins, and minerals must first be determined. The patient's disease process may influence not only these requirements but also the ability to digest and absorb certain nutrients.

Commercial Formula versus Blenderized Food Formula. The use of non-commercial blenderized food for tube feedings has certain advantages over commercial formulas. Carbohydrate, protein, fat, and fluid may be specifically formulated, but there is less flexibility with its vitamin, mineral, and electrolyte content. In addition, blenderized food may be less costly than commercial formulas. However, there are many problems associated with its preparation and administration. Foods prepared in a blender generally yield a viscous solution that can be administered only through a large-bore feeding tube. Other problems include bacterial growth, settling out of the solid components, and potential inconsistency of nutrient composition.[1] The use of blenderized food tube feeding may be contraindicated in patients with deficits in digestion or absorption who require varying degrees of predigested nutrients. On the other hand, commercial formulas provide a sterile, homogeneous solution that is suitable for small-bore feeding tubes and insures a fixed nutrient profile in the form of intact or predigested nutrients.

The decision to use tube feedings is dependent upon a patient's ability to ingest adequate nutrients and the functional capacity of the gastrointestinal tract. The sites of tube feeding commonly used today are nasogastric, cervical esophagostomy, gastrostomy, duodenostomy, nasoduodenal, nasojejunal, and jejunostomy.[2] The final location of the tip of tubes placed through these routes is either the stomach or small bowel.

The selection and administration of a formula require a thorough knowledge of formula composition as well as normal and abnormal digestive and absorptive processes. The type and quantity of each nutritional source determine the degree of absorption and tolerance to the formula (that is, intact protein versus hydrolyzed protein), and its physical characteristics, such as osmolality. The following issues must be assessed simultaneously for appropriate formula selection. (1) What is the patient's digestive and absorptive capacity? (2) What effect will the physical characteristic of the formula selected have on gastrointestinal function?

For example, pancreatic insufficiency may dictate the need for a low-fat formula. However, the chosen formula may be hypertonic and poorly tolerated in a patient sensitive to an osmotic load. It is difficult to isolate the effects of nutrient composition and physical characteristics.

NUTRITIONAL COMPOSITION

Carbohydrate

From 45 to 50 per cent of the calories in the American diet is carbohydrate in the form of starch, sucrose, and lactose. In the normal intestine, 80 per cent of all ingested carbohydrate is hydrolyzed and absorbed as the monosaccharide glucose. Glucose is the major carbohydrate of human metabolism, and it is the only circulating carbohydrate within the body. Except for small amounts of galactose and fructose, it is the major product of carbohydrate digestion. Carbohydrates contribute 4 kcal/gm.

With the exception of lactose, carbohydrate is the most easily digested and absorbed component of most commercial formulas today. As detailed in Chapter 2, digestion and absorption of carbohydrate are mainly dependent upon the integrity of the small bowel. Among formulas, the two main differences in carbohydrate are form and concentration (Tables 10–1 and 10–2). The form, ranging from starch to simple glucose, contributes to the characteristics of osmolality, sweetness, and digestibility. Generally, the larger carbohydrate molecules exert less osmotic pressure, taste less sweet, and require more digestion than shorter ones.

Starch.   Starch is composed of glucose chains in straight (amylose) and branched (amylopectin) configurations, varying in length from 400 to many thousands of glu-

cose molecules.[3] In commercial formulas, starch is supplied from cereal solids and food starch, with some contribution from fruits and vegetables in commercial blenderized diets. (see Table 10–1). Intraluminally, starch is hydrolyzed by the pancreatic enzyme alpha-amylase to dextrin, maltose, and isomaltose. Starch intolerance is rare owing to the adequate levels of this enzyme even in severe pancreatic disease (see Chapter 2).[4-6] Because of its high molecular weight, carbohydrate in the form of starch contributes little to the osmolality of the formula. Although starch is well tolerated and easily digested by most patients, its relative insolubility makes it difficult to use in most formulas.

Polysaccharides/Oligosaccharides.   The hydrolysis of starch results in glucose polymers of intermediate chain lengths, dextrins, maltose, and, ultimately, glucose (see Table 10–2). Polysaccharides are glucose polymers greater than 10 units in length; oligosaccharides are glucose polymers from 2 to 10 units in length.[7] The hydrolysis of starch to polysaccharides and oligosaccharides increases its solubility in solution; however, the more extensively the starch is hydrolyzed toward glucose, the greater the osmolality and the sweeter the taste. One common source of carbohydrate prepared by this technique is corn syrup solid, which when hydrolyzed yields high percentages of glucose, maltose, isomaltose, and triose.

Another carbohydrate source commonly referred to as glucose polymers, maltodextrins, polysaccharides, or oligosaccharides is prepared by a more limited starch hydrolysis, which yields a higher percentage of polysaccharides and medium-length oligosaccharides. There are several advantages to

---

Table 10–1   COMMON SOURCES OF CARBOHYDRATE IN COMMERCIAL FORMULAS

STARCH (Polysaccharides)
  Hydrolyzed cereal solids
  Pureed green beans, peas, carrots
  Modified food starch
  Tapioca starch
	DISACCHARIDES
	  Sucrose
	  Lactose (nonfat and whole milk)
	  Maltose (by-product of starch and oligosaccharide
	    digestion)

GLUCOSE POLYMERS*
  Glucose oligosaccharides
  Glucose polysaccharides[†]
  Glucose polymers[†]
  Maltodextrins
  Corn syrup
  Corn syrup solids
	MONOSACCHARIDES
	  Glucose (dextrose)
	  Fructose

*Prepared by the partial hydrolysis of corn starch
[†]May contain chain lengths greater than 10 glucose units

Table 10–2 CATEGORIZATION OF CARBOHYDRATE FORMS

	NO. OF SACCHARIDE UNITS	EXAMPLE
Monosaccharide	1	Glucose (fructose-galactose)
Disaccharide	2	Sucrose (glucose-fructose)
		Lactose (glucose-galactose)
		Maltose (glucose-glucose)
Oligosaccharides	2–10	Alpha-limit dextrins
		Maltotriose
		Glucose oligosaccharides
		Maltodextrins
Polysaccharides	10	
Homosaccharides (one type of monosaccharide unit)		Starch
		Glycogen

using glucose polymers in formula. First, their molecular weight is approximately 1000, making them more soluble in solution than starch, but contributing five times less than pure glucose (molecular weight, 180) to the osmotic load of a formula. Second, glucose polymers are rapidly hydrolyzed in the intestine by the same pancreatic enzymes that hydrolyze starch molecules. It has been demonstrated in rats that these polymers are absorbed as rapidly as glucose but result in lower luminal osmolality than glucose solutions of the same weight. Thus higher concentrations of calories in the form of glucose polymers may be administered with fewer of the side effects attributed to hypertonic glucose.[8, 9] Like starch, intolerance to glucose polymers is rare; however, the final hydrolysis of starch or glucose polymers to glucose from maltose and isomaltose is dependent upon the enzyme activity of the brush border and small bowel function. As detailed in Chapter 2, carbohydrate intolerance is almost "always related to a defect in the intestinal surface digestion of oligosaccharides or disaccharides."[4, 5]

Disaccharides. The disaccharides found in normal diets and formulas are lactose, sucrose, and the by-product of partial starch digestion, dextrins, and maltose. These disaccharides require the action of specific disaccharidases (Fig. 2–19) in the brush border of the small bowel mucosa for hydrolysis to their monosaccharide components—glucose, galactose, and fructose—before being absorbed (see Table 10–2).[4, 5] In healthy tissue maltose and sucrose are hydrolyzed rapidly; lactose is hydrolyzed slowly, at approximately 50 per cent the rate of maltose and sucrose. Primary disaccharidase deficiencies are rare. However, secondary deficiencies with associated carbohydrate malabsorption

will occur in conditions in which there is disruption of the small bowel mucosa and/or a decrease in enzyme concentration. Secondary disaccharidase deficiencies have been observed in tropical sprue, celiac sprue, enteric infections, nonspecific enteritis, acute viral hepatitis, cholera, ulcerative colitis, malnutrition, and fasting.[10–15] The degree to which these conditions impair enzyme concentration and, therefore, hydrolytic activity is outlined in Table 10–3.

The presence or addition of disaccharides to formula will increase the osmotic concentration, as they are much smaller molecules than the glucose polymers.

Lactose. Lactase deficiency is the most prevalent of the disaccharidase deficiencies and has been categorized into primary, secondary, and relative deficiencies (Table 10–4).[16]

Primary lactase deficiency is common in certain racial and ethnic groups, particularly blacks, Orientals, Indians, and Jews (see Table 10–4). The degree of lactose intolerance is variable. Occasionally patients who are able to tolerate small amounts of lactose in their normal diet may become markedly symptomatic when large amounts are administered. For example, milk-based formulas provide 80 to 210 gm of lactose per 24 hours compared with normal lactose intakes of 12 gm per 24 hours.[17]

Secondary lactase deficiency, like all disaccharidase deficiencies, occurs in diseases that affect small bowel integrity or enzyme concentration (see Table 10–4). Lactase deficiency, however, is the most prevalent in this category. Recovery may require weeks to months and may last indefinitely.[10, 12, 14, 18]

Relative lactase deficiency describes a deficiency due to decreased absorptive surface and/or increased transit time. In this

Table 10–3   INCIDENCE OF DISACCHARIDASE DEFICIENCY IN VARIOUS DISEASES*

CONDITION	PATIENTS BELOW NORMAL (%)		
	Lactase	*Sucrase*	*Maltase*
Celiac sprue			
Mild	25	0	0
Moderate	100	80	20
Severe	100	100	75
Celiac sprue, treated			
Excellent response	29	0	0
Good response	100	100	43
Fair response	100	86	43
Kwashiorkor			
Acute	80	50	30
Past history of	—	—	—
Tropical sprue	100	65	68
Cholera			
Acute	86	57	20
Convalescent	86	0	0
Gastroenteritis			
Acute	100	43	57
Convalescent	100	0	0
Infant diarrhea, acute	45	27	18

Adapted from Gray, G. M.: Disaccharidases of the small intestine in selected diseases. *In* Altman, P. L., and Katz, D. D. (eds.): Human Health and Disease (Biological Handbooks, II). Bethesda, Federation of American Societies for Experimental Biology, 1977, pages 124–125.

setting, lactose concentration in tissues may be normal, but total surface area decreases, as in short bowel syndrome, or the length of time of exposure to enzymatic action is decreased, as with rapid gastric emptying.[16, 18]

Glucose. Formulas that contain pure glucose as their sole source of carbohydrate will be very sweet and hypertonic. Digestive

Table 10–4   LACTASE DEFICIENCY*

PRIMARY
  Congenital
  Racial-ethnic

SECONDARY: MUCOSAL DAMAGE;
ENZYME DEFICIENCY
  Protein-calorie malnutrition
  Infections (acute gastroenteritis, cholera, giardiasis)
  Drugs (neomycin, colchicine)
  Radiation enteritis
  Ulcerative colitis
  Fasting
  Tropical sprue
  Celiac sprue

RELATIVE DEFICIENCY
  Short bowel
  Gastric surgery

Adapted from Disaccharidase deficiencies. Mayo Clin. Proc., 48:648–652, 1973.

capacity does not impair glucose utilization since it does not require hydrolysis; however, tolerance to glucose loads may be limited by the absorptive capacity of the small bowel. Impaired glucose absorption has also been observed in children with protein-calorie malnutrition.[13]

Carbohydrate Malabsorption. The symptoms of carbohydrate malabsorption—watery diarrhea, abdominal cramps, flatulence, fullness, nausea, stool with a pH of less than 6[19] and a positive Clinitest on stool—are caused by fermentation of the unabsorbed saccharides by intestinal bacteria and subsequent increased osmotic load within the intestinal lumen. The excess carbon dioxide, hydrogen, and fatty acids produced lead to flatulence, cramping, and diarrhea.[19]

Protein

The protein content is the most critical component of enteral formulas, as protein is required for the maintenance of the body cell mass and is necessary for virtually all major bodily functions. Nearly one half of the dry weight of a typical animal cell is protein. Structural components of the cell, antibodies, and many of the hormones are proteins. As much as 90 per cent of cellular proteins are enzymes upon which fundamental cellular function depends.[20]

The protein molecule is a polymer of amino acids joined in peptide linkages. Peptide structures of less than 100 amino acids in length are sometimes classified as polypeptides rather than proteins. Twenty different amino acids occur in various spatial configurations and are fundamental units of protein structure.[20] The crucial component of protein is nitrogen, which comprises approximately 16 per cent of the protein (1 gm of nitrogen equals 6.25 gm of protein). Most naturally occurring amino acids are of the L-configuration, although D-amino acids may play a role (as yet undefined) in mammalian metabolism.

Protein in enteral formulas may be in the form of intact protein, protein partially hydrolyzed into smaller polypeptide fragments (oligopeptides, dipeptides, and tripeptides) or crystalline L-amino acids. Intact protein and hydrolysates require further digestion in the small intestine to peptides (specifically dipeptides and tripeptides) and free amino acids. Protein digestion begins in the stomach with the action of pepsins and continues in the proximal small intestine by the specific action of the pancreatic enzymes trypsin, chymotrypsin, aminopeptidases, and carboxypeptidases. Absorption of peptides and amino acids occurs primarily in the upper small intestine by active transport. Amino acid absorption requires the presence of the sodium ion; dipeptides, tripeptides, and oligopeptides have specific carrier systems that do not require sodium (Fig. 10–1).[21] In the

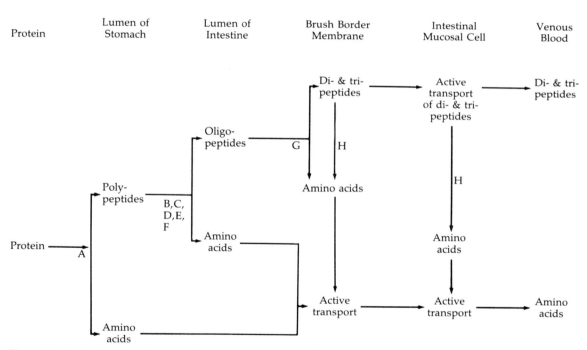

Figure 10–1. Protein digestion and absorption. Enzyme Key:
A = pepsin A (hydrolyzes peptide bonds in which an aromatic acid is present).
B = trypsin (hydrolyzes peptide bonds to which L-arginine or L-lysine contributes the carbonyl group).
C = chymotrypsin (hydrolyzes peptide bonds in which an aromatic amino acid contributes the carbonyl group).
D = elastase (hydrolyzes peptide bonds in which an aliphatic amino acid contributes the carbonyl group).
E = carboxypeptidase A (acts on those linkages in which a non-basic amino acid, particularly a neutral aromatic amino acid, is C-terminal and has a free carboxyl group).
F = carboxypeptidase B (acts on those linkages in which a basic amino acid is C-terminal and has a free carboxyl group).
G = oligopeptidases (aminopeptidases) of brush border, most active against peptides containing bulky aliphatic or aromatic amino acids.
H = di- and tri-peptidases; 15% in brush border, 85% in cytosol.
(*Adapted from* Matthews, D. M.: Intestinal absorption of peptides. Physiol. Rev., 55(4):537–608, 1975.)

normal small intestine, amino acids, dipeptides, and tripeptides are absorbed rapidly. Protein digestion and absorption are discussed in detail in another chapter.

A knowledge of the source (for example, casein, lactalbumin, egg white) and form (intact protein, hydrolyzed protein, or amino acids) of the protein in various formulas is essential when prescribing diets for individuals with defects in either protein digestion (that is, pancreatic insufficiency) or absorption (mucosal damage or short bowel syndrome).

Importance of the Quality of Protein. With the many protein sources utilized in formulas, it is necessary to be familiar with the quality of the protein, especially when feeding infants and children. Protein quality depends upon its amino acid profile, and the quality of the protein source will affect overall protein requirements.

The utilization of dietary protein is partly determined by the concentrations and relative proportions of the essential amino acids. The optimal proportions of these essential amino acids have been estimated in the FAO/WHO Report, and from this an ideal protein for nutritional purposes has been defined (Table 10–5).[22] In order to promote tissue restitution in traumatized, catabolic, or seriously undernourished patients, the essential amino acid intake must be at least 40 per cent of the total amino acid intake.[23]

The most frequently used method for evaluating the quality of a specific protein is determination of its biologic value (BV). This is a measure of the nitrogen (N) retained for growth or maintenance and is expressed as nitrogen retained divided by nitrogen absorbed.[24]

$$BV = \frac{\text{dietary N} - (\text{urinary N} + \text{fecal N})}{\text{dietary N} - \text{fecal N}} \times 100$$

Thus, measuring BV involves measuring the intake of N from protein and the output of N in the feces and the urine. In general, the lower the biologic value, the greater the amount of protein required to achieve nitrogen equilibrium (Table 10–6).[25] The nonessential amino acid content is higher in proteins with a low biologic value. Table 10–7 lists the BVs of the proteins commonly found in formulas.[26]

Another common and simple measurement used to evaluate protein quality is the amino acid profile or chemical score. This method compares the amino acid composition of a food with that of a high-quality protein, such as egg, or to a specified amino acid reference protein (FAO/WHO).[22] It is calculated by using the following equation:

$$\text{Chemical score} = \frac{\text{essential/total essential amino acids (product)}}{\text{essential/total essential amino acids (egg)}} \times 100$$

Table 10–5 ESSENTIAL AMINO ACIDS AND PROTEIN REQUIREMENTS FOR HUMANS OF VARIOUS AGES

REQUIREMENT (MG/KG BODY WEIGHT)	INFANTS	CHILDREN (10–12 YEARS)	ADULTS
Histidine	28	0	0
Isoleucine	70	30	10
Leucine	161	45	14
Lysine	103	60	12
Methionine and Cystine	58	27	13
Phenylalanine and Tyrosine	125	27	14
Threonine	87	35	7
Tryptophan	17	4	3.5
Valine	93	33	10
Total Essential Amino Acids	742	261	83.5
Total Protein Requirements	1700	700	570
Essential Amino Acids as Per Cent of Total	43%	36%	15%

*Adapted from Joint FAO/WHO Expert Committee Report: Energy and Protein Requirements. WHO Technical Report Series, No. 522. Geneva, WHO, 1973.

Table 10–6   EFFECT OF PROTEIN QUALITY
ON PROTEIN REQUIREMENTS*

SOURCE OF PROTEIN	BIOLOGIC VALUE	RELATIVE PROTEIN REQUIRED FOR EQUILIBRIUM (gm protein/day)
Milk (casein)	74	22.4
Soy flour	65	23.4
Soy-white flour	55	27.4
White flour	41	38.7

*Adapted from Bricker, M., Mitchell, H. H., and Kinsman, G. M.: The protein requirements of adult human subjects in terms of the protein contained in individual food and food combinations. J. Nutr., 30:269–283, 1945.

The protein quality of any formula must be critically analyzed before being prescribed in hospitalized patients. This is highlighted in a recent study by Marable et al., in which the chemical score was used to assess protein adequacy. A number of supplements and meal replacements were analyzed and grouped into predigested protein products and non-predigested protein products. The non-predigested products provided an amino acid distribution similar to that of egg and to the suggested patterns of amino acids for adults. The predigested protein products, however, had an unbalanced amino acid distribution with a high concentration of proline, hydroxyproline, and glycine, and lower levels of essential amino acids. Predigested protein products consequently had a low chemical score. When consumed at a level to provide the adult allowance for protein, these products failed to meet the suggested requirements for some essential amino acids.[27]

Table 10–7   BIOLOGIC VALUE OF PROTEINS FOUND IN COMMERCIAL FORMULAS*

PROTEIN SOURCE	BIOLOGIC VALUE
Lactalbumin with methionine	130
Egg, whole	100
Milk, cow	90
Fish	85
Lactalbumin	84
Beef	76
Soybeans	75
Casein	72

*Adapted from Oser, B. L.: Method for integrating essential amino acid content in the nutritional evaluation of protein. J. Am. Diet. Assoc., 27:396–402, 1951.

Most methods for evaluation of protein quality are based on the amount of nitrogen retained in the body or the essential amino acid profile. In addition to BV and chemical score, other methods for measuring and assessing the quality of a protein include the protein efficiency ratio (PER), net protein utilization (NPU), and the slope ratio assay.[28–30]

Amino acid imbalances, antagonisms, and toxicities are also major concerns. The lack of one essential amino acid will result in an imbalance that can result in growth failure. Amino acid antagonisms can occur among amino acids that are structurally related—that is, excess amounts of one of the branched-chain amino acids can depress the utilization of the other two.[31] Toxicity can also occur when disproportionate amounts of amino acids are administered.[32]

Most of the formulas on the market contain proteins of high quality, so this issue should not be a major concern.

Protein quality is only of clinical significance in adults with a limited protein intake. Proteins of high biologic value would be most beneficial in promoting nitrogen equilibrium in these patients. Dietitians can easily calculate the percentage of essential to nonessential amino acids in a certain formula after obtaining the amino acid profiles from the respective companies.

In disease states, such as hepatic or renal failure, specialized amino acid patterns have been designed to enhance protein utilization and minimize toxicities from excess protein intake. For example, for the patient with renal disease, formulas consisting of high percentages of essential amino acids are available; in the patient with hepatic failure, formulas with high levels of branched-chain to aromatic amino acids are available (see Table 10–11).

Physical Characteristics of Protein. The proteins available in nutritional formulas can be divided into three major categories depending on the degree of digestion required: (1) intact proteins; (2) hydrolyzed protein or partially digested protein (containing various percentages of dipeptides, tripeptides, oligopeptides, and crystalline amino acids); and (3) those formulas containing pure crystalline amino acids. Table 10–8 lists the forms of protein that are found in current formulas on the market.

Intact proteins are proteins in their complete and original forms as found in whole

Table 10–8 COMMON SOURCES OF PROTEIN IN COMMERCIAL FORMULAS

INTACT PROTEIN	HYDROLYZED PROTEIN	CRYSTALLINE AMINO ACIDS
Pureed beef	Casein	L-amino acids
Egg white solids	Whey, soy or meat protein	
Soy protein isolates	Lactalbumin	
Casein isolates	Collagen	
Lactalbumin		
Whey		
Nonfat and whole dry milk		
Na^+ and Ca^{++} caseinates		

foods. They will require complete digestion to smaller peptides and free amino acids before they are absorbed from the gastrointestinal tract. Protein isolates such as lactalbumin and caseinate salts are intact proteins that have been separated from their original source. For example, lactalbumin is a protein derived from whey. Intact proteins do not add appreciably to the osmolality of the formula but do require normal levels of pancreatic enzymes for complete digestion.

Hydrolyzed proteins are protein sources that have been enzymatically hydrolyzed to smaller peptide fragments and to free amino acids. Dipeptides, tripeptides, and free amino acids are absorbed directly into the bloodstream; however, larger peptides must undergo further hydrolysis before absorption can occur. As the protein molecules become smaller, they contribute more to the osmotic load. Protein hydrolysates often require the addition of free amino acids to enhance protein quality. The three most commonly added are methionine, tyrosine, and tryptophan. Protein hydrolysates are useful in situations in which there is reduced absorptive surface area, as in celiac sprue or short bowel syndrome. They are also useful in selective disorders of amino acid transport, as in Hartnup disease, cystinuria, and exocrine pancreatic insufficiency (Table 10–9).[33]

The third source of protein in formulas is pure *crystalline amino acids*. They require no further digestion in the gastrointestinal tract and are absorbed via active transport mechanisms. Owing to their small size, these particles contribute significantly to the osmolality of the formula and may adversely affect the taste. Crystalline amino acids are best utilized in designing formulas for patients with hepatic or renal failure.

Fat

Fat comprises 40 to 45 per cent of calories in the normal American diet, mainly in the form of long-chain triglycerides (LCT). The major sources of fat in standard formulas are butterfat from milk in lactose-based formula), corn, soy, safflower or sunflower oils, the medium-chain triglycerides (MCT), lecithin, and monoglycerides and diglycerides. The major role of fat in a formula is in providing a concentrated energy source (9 kcal/gm).

Because fat is insoluble in water, its digestion and absorption are complex processes. Before absorption can occur, fat must be emulsified and hydrolyzed to free fatty acids and 2-monoglycerides with the subsequent formation of micelles. These processes require the action of both bile acids and pancreatic enzymes. Once absorbed into the intestinal cell, the free fatty acids and monoglycerides are then reesterified into

Table 10–9 INDICATIONS FOR THE USE OF ENTERAL PROTEIN SOURCES

INTACT PROTEIN
Normal pancreatic enzyme levels
Normal small bowel absorptive capacity

PROTEIN HYDROLYSATES
Reduced absorptive surface
   Celiac sprue
   Short bowel syndrome
   Malnutrition
Selective disorders of amino acid transport
   Cystinuria
   Hartnup disease
Exocrine pancreatic insufficiency
   Chronic pancreatitis
   Pancreatectomy

CRYSTALLINE AMINO ACIDS
Hepatic failure
Renal failure

triglycerides and phospholipids, formed into chylomicrons, and transported to the bloodstream via the lymphatic circulation. Fat digestion and absorption are described in detail in Chapter 2. Disruption at any point of this process—due to inadequate absorptive surface area, bile acid or pancreatic insufficiency, inflammatory bowel disease, enteritis, or bacterial overgrowth—can result in the maldigestion or malabsorption of fat.[4] Adequate fat intake is important, however, because in addition to providing energy, fat also provides essential fatty acids and serves as a carrier for the fat-soluble vitamins. Fat also enhances the flavor and palatability of a formula, yet it does not increase the formula's osmolality.

Essential Fatty Acids. Because vegetable oils are a rich source of essential fatty acids[34] (Table 10–10), deficiency is unlikely in most patients receiving enteral formula.[34] However, essential fatty acid deficiency has been documented in conjunction with parenteral nutrition, long-term low-fat or fat-free elemental diets, and in diets containing only medium-chain triglycerides as the fat source.[35–37] The estimated requirement for essential fatty acids, specifically linoleic acid, is approximately 3 to 4 per cent of the total calories.[38–40]

Medium-Chain Triglycerides. An alternative to long-chain triglycerides in formulas is medium-chain triglycerides (MCT). Medium-chain triglycerides are prepared by the fractionation of coconut oil and are composed of triglycerides of 6 to 12 carbons, predominately C8 (octanoic) and C10 (decanoic). They do not contain the essential fatty acid, linoleic acid. Medium-chain triglycerides provide 8.2 to 8.4 kcal/gm. Their use in formulas is advantageous for several reasons. First, MCT are more water-soluble than long-chain triglycerides (LCT). Second, intraluminal hydrolysis of MCT occurs more rapidly and more completely than the hydrolysis of long-chain triglycerides. Third, MCT require little or no pancreatic lipase activity or bile salts for substantial absorption to occur. In fact, some MCT hydrolysis occurs within the intestinal mucosa itself. Fourth, MCT are transported directly into the blood via the portal system, thus eliminating the complex digestive and absorptive process required by LCT. The use of MCT is specifically indicated in the following disorders of fat absorption and lymphatic drainage from the intestine: malabsorption (tropical and non-tropical sprue, celiac disease, postgastrectomy, small bowel resection, blind loop syndrome, diabetic steatorrhea, chronic liver disease), pancreatic insufficiency, biliary atresia, chyluria, chylous fistulas, protein-losing enteropathy, and fat-induced hyperlipidemia.[41, 42]

Medium-chain triglycerides are rapidly hydrolyzed intraluminally, causing an increase in the osmotic concentration. When adding MCT oil to a diet, it should be introduced gradually to avoid the side effects of nausea, vomiting, abdominal distention, or diarrhea, which are occasionally observed with its administration.[42]

The metabolic side effects observed with the use of MCT oil are related to its extensive oxidation within the liver. The fatty acids from MCT are oxidized to energy, CO_2, and ketone bodies; this may induce ketogenesis in normals.[41, 42] In cirrhotic patients or in patients with portacaval shunts, the liver's diminished capacity to oxidize fatty acids from MCT results in elevated serum levels of octanoate, which may lead to increased mental impairment.[41]

Medium-chain triglycerides are most often used in combination with LCT in formulas today. This combination provides essential fatty acids via the LCT yet retains the advantages of the easy digestibility and absorption of the MCT.

Although MCT and LCT will compete for absorption, the administration of MCT in conjunction with LCT actually increases the total intestinal absorption of both over that obtained when one or the other is administered alone. As the percentage of MCT in relation to LCT is increased, a larger portion of the fat absorption as MCT will occur.[43, 44]

Table 10–10 LINOLEIC ACID CONTENT IN COMMONLY USED VEGETABLE OILS*

	LINOLEIC ACID (gm/100 gm)
Corn oil	58
Sesame oil	74.1
Partially hydrogenated soybean oil	39.4 (51, not hydrogenated)
Sunflower oil	65.7
Safflower oil	74.1

*Adapted from Composition of Foods, Fats, and Oils. Agriculture Handbook No. 8-4. United States Department of Agriculture, 1979.

Vitamins and Minerals

Commercial formulas that are nutritionally complete are designed to provide adequate vitamins and minerals when caloric requirements are met. Low caloric intakes or diluted formulas should be assessed for vitamin and mineral adequacy. Deficient formulas may be supplemented easily with addition of liquid vitamin and mineral preparations.

Some otherwise complete formulas do not contain vitamin K. Deficiency of this vitamin is rare in patients receiving enteral nutrition because it is synthesized by the gut flora; however, a weekly supplementation has been recommended.[45] Vitamin K supplementation may also be required in diseases associated with fat malabsorption (for example, biliary obstruction and short bowel syndrome). Alternatively, vitamin K may interfere with the activity of the oral anticoagulant warfarin; patients receiving warfarin should be assessed for total vitamin K intake.[46]

PHYSICAL CHARACTERISTICS

Once a formula has been selected for patient use based upon nutritional requirements and gastrointestinal function, there are certain physical characteristics of formulas that may affect tolerance. The major symptoms of tube feeding intolerance are gastric retention and diarrhea or constipation. These symptoms are often unrelated to the formula itself and may be the result of inappropriate administration techniques or drug interactions. They may also be due to an intolerance to some characteristic of the formula such as osmolality, nutrient density, caloric density, pH, or residue content.

Osmolality. One of the most important physical characteristics of a formula is its osmolality. Osmolality is a function of the number and size of molecular and ionic particles present in a given volume. These particles include electrolytes, minerals, carbohydrates, and proteins or amino acids. *Osmolality* is measured by determining the degree of depression of the freezing point by a solute per kilogram of water. *Osmolarity*, in contrast, refers to the degree of depression produced by the solute per liter of solution. For dilute solutions there is little difference between osmolality and osmolarity, but for concentrated solutions, osmolarity may be only 80 per cent of the osmolality. Osmolality is the generally preferred term.[47]

Within a solution, electrolytes exert a relatively major effect on osmolality owing to their small size and property of dissociation (that is, NaCl yields Na^+ and Cl^-) in solution. Large molecular weight carbohydrates such as starch and glucose polymers exert less osmotic pressure in a solution than sucrose or glucose. Proteins are very large molecules that exert little or no effect in solution until they are hydrolyzed, as in formulas containing partially hydrolyzed proteins. Because of their relatively small size, amino acids will contribute significantly to osmotic pressure. The more predigested the components of the formula are, the higher the osmolality of that formula.

How does osmolality influence formula feeding tolerance? First, gastric emptying is slowed by solutions with osmotic pressures higher or lower than 200 mOsm;[4] the higher the osmolality, the greater the inhibitory effect. Thus hypertonic formulas fed into the stomach, especially by bolus, may cause gastric retention, nausea, and vomiting. This effect is believed to be regulated by osmoreceptors in the duodenum.

In addition to delayed gastric emptying, hypertonic solutions may cause severe diarrhea, electrolyte depletion, and dehydration. Within the duodenum, solutions are adjusted to isotonic levels by increasing or decreasing their water content. Hypertonic solutions may cause large fluid shifts into the small bowel. Even the osmolality of an isotonic formula may rapidly increase as the intestinal enzymes hydrolyze its components into smaller molecules.[48] In the poorly functioning gut or with rapid administration of a hypertonic formula, such an osmotic load may not be tolerated.

Osmolality may affect the solute load and water requirements within the body as well. The major constituent of a formula that will contribute to the solute load within the body is protein as its breakdown product urea; the electrolytes sodium, potassium, and chloride, however, will also add to the total solute load that must be excreted by the kidneys. Thus collectively they make up the "renal solute load." Formulas that produce a large renal solute load may lead to clinical dehydration, as assessed by serum and urine concentrations of electrolytes, blood urea nitrogen (BUN), and serum and urine osmolality. Hyperosmolality exists in the extracellular fluid when the concentrations of solutes are increased above the normal range (280 to 320 mOsm). In contrast, hypo-osmolality occurs when there is too much water per solute in extracellular fluid.

Schoolman divides the syndrome of hyperosmolarity (this term is used when discussing the effect of osmolality on body functioning) into three etiologic categories: primary dehydration, central nervous system disorder (that is, a hypothalamic lesion), and the recovery phase of diabetic acidosis.[49] Primary dehydration is the category relevant to the use of formula feeding. Dehydration occurs because the kidneys are only able to concentrate urine to a certain degree (about 1300 mOsm/kg of urine in normal, healthy adults). Thus there is an obligatory loss of water with each unit of solute.[50] As a formula becomes more concentrated (increased protein, electrolytes), the patient requires more water.

It is estimated that 40 to 60 ml is the minimal amount of water necessary to excrete 1 gm of nitrogen.[51] The major (80 per cent) nitrogenous end product is urea; every gram of dietary nitrogen leads to the formation of about 2 gm of urea. If the patient eats 100 gm of protein per day, there will be 30 gm of urea generated to excrete; this is equivalent to about 500 mOsm.[52] Under normal circumstances, the body will respond to a restriction of fluid, in light of a high protein intake, by excreting a urine as concentrated as possible. The urinary excretion of sodium and chloride is also decreased. This is caused by a decreased extracellular fluid volume and will exacerbate the hyperosmolar state.[53] Figure 10–2 outlines the course of events leading to the hyperosmolar syndrome and the methods of treatment.

Case examples of dehydration and hyperosmolarity associated with high-protein tube feedings have been reported by Engel and Jaeger,[54] Wilson and Meinert,[50] Cramer et al.,[55] Gault et al.,[56] and more recently by Taitz and Byers.[57] In most of these cases the dehydration or negative water balance was due to the increased renal solute load secondary to a protein intake of 150 to 200 gm/day in 2000 to 3000 ml of fluid. The solute load delivered to these patients was increased further owing to liberal amounts of sodium and potassium in the formula.

The renal solute load from a high-protein tube feeding may be further increased

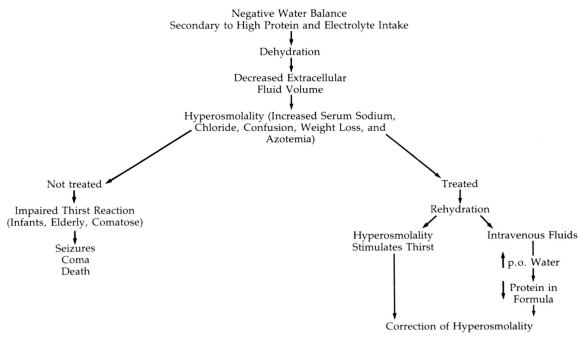

Figure 10–2. Genesis and treatment of hyperosmolality. (*Adapted from* Wilson, W. S., and Meinert, J. K.: Extracellular hyperosmolarity secondary to high protein nasogastric tube feeding. Ann. Intern. Med., *47*:585, 590, 1957.)

Table 10–11 NUTRITIONAL VALUES OF COMMERCIAL FORMULAS (PER 1000 ML)

	Vit A (IU)	Vit D (IU)	Vit E (IU)	Vit K (mcg)	Vit C (mg)	Folic Acid (mg)	Thiamine (mg)	Riboflavin (mg)	B6 (mg)	B12 (mcg)	Niacin (mg)	Choline (mg)	Biotin (mg)	Pantothenic Acid (mg)	Sodium (mEq)	Potassium (mEq)	Chloride (mEq)	Calcium (gm)	Phosphorus (gm)	Magnesium (mg)	Iodine (mcg)	Manganese (mg)	Copper (mg)	Zinc (mg)	Iron (mg)
Complete B	3332	268	20	N/A	60	.27	1.5	1.7	2.0	4.0	13.3	200	.2	6.7	55.2	35.6	24.8	.68	1.32	268	100	2.7	1.3	10	12
Formula 2	2500	240	21	N/A	39	.2	.8	.9	1.4	3.0	10	N/A	N/A	4.8	26.1	45	53.6	.72	.56	100	75	.2	1.0	7.5	12.6
Complete B Modified	3332	268	20	68	60	.3	1.5	1.7	2.0	4.0	13.3	200	.2	6.7	29.6	36	13.6	.68	.9	268	100	2.7	1.3	10	12
Vitaneed	2500	200	30	150	150	.2	1.5	1.7	2.0	6.0	20	150	.15	5	21.7	32	23.9	.5	.5	200	75	2.5	1.0	15	9
Meritene Powder	4813	385	29	77	58	.4	1.5	2.6	1.9	6.9	19.2	212	.29	9.6	46.9	71.9	61.9	2.2	1.9	385	145	3.9	1.9	14.4	17.3
Meritene Liquid	4000	320	24	N/A	72	.3	1.8	2.1	2.5	5.0	16	80	.24	8.0	38.4	40.8	45	1.2	1.2	320	120	3.2	1.6	12	14.4
Sustacal Powder	4706	375	28	N/A	56	.4	1.4	1.7	2.0	5.6	19.7	N/A	.28	9.9	40.5	65.6	38.2	1.6	1.3	380	141	2.7	2.0	14	17
Sustagen Powder	5202	417	47	260	300	.4	4.0	4.5	5.2	15.8	52	521	.3	26	54.3	85.4	79.2	3.3	2.5	417	156	5.2	2.1	20	19
Sustacal Pudding	3128	250	19	N/A	38	.3	1.0	1.1	1.0	4.0	13.0	N/A	.2	6.0	18.3	36.4	24.8	.9	.9	250	94	2.8	1.0	9.0	11.3
Forta Pudding	3332	268	20	N/A	60	.3	1.0	1.1	1.3	4.0	13.2	100	.2	6.6	38.2	30.8	23.7	.8	.8	268	240	2.6	1.3	12	12
Precision Isotonic	3199	257	19	67	60	.3	1.4	1.7	1.9	3.8	12.7	64	.2	6.5	33.4	24.6	28.9	.7	.7	257	100	2.6	1.3	9.6	11.5
Precision LR Diet	2916	235	18	59	53	.3	1.3	1.5	1.8	3.5	11.7	59	.2	5.8	30.5	22.4	31.5	.6	.6	234	88	2.3	1.2	8.8	10.5
Precision HN Diet	1750	140	11	35	32	.1	.8	.9	1.1	2.1	7.2	31	.1	3.5	42.7	23.1	33.6	.4	.4	140	53	1.4	.7	5.3	6.3
Citrotein	5208	417	31	N/A	234	.8	3.1	3.5	4.2	12.5	41.7	35	.6	21	29.7	17.2	26.6	1.0	1.0	416	156	5.2	2.1	15.6	37.5
Sustacal Liquid	4640	370	28	24	56	.4	1.4	1.7	1.9	6.0	19.0	235	.3	9.7	40	53	44	1.0	.9	380	140	3.0	1.9	14.0	17.0
Sustacal HC	4224	338	25	211	76	.5	1.9	2.2	2.5	7.6	25.0	211	.4	13	36.7	38	36	8.5	8.5	333	127	2.5	1.7	12.5	15
Isocal	2640	210	40	132	160	.2	2.1	2.0	3.0	8.0	26	264	.2	13	23.1	33.8	29.6	.6	.5	210	80	3.0	1.0	10	10
Isocal HCN	3330	267	50	167	200	.27	2.5	2.9	3.3	10	33.3	333	.2	16.7	35	36	34	.67	.67	267	100	3.3	2.0	20	12
Portagen	7813	781	31	156	81	.16	1.56	1.9	2.1	6.25	21	130	.08	10.4	20.4	32.1	24.2	.94	.70	208	73	3.1	1.6	9.4	18.8

Table 10-11 *(Continued)* NUTRITIONAL VALUES OF COMMERCIAL FORMULAS (PER 1000 ML)

	Vit A (IU)	Vit D (IU)	Vit E (IU)	Vit K (mcg)	Vit C (mg)	Folic Acid (mg)	Thiamine (mg)	Riboflavin (mg)	B6 (mg)	B12 (mcg)	Niacin (mg)	Choline (mg)	Biotin (mg)	Pantothenic Acid (mg)	Sodium (mEq)	Potassium (mEq)	Chloride (mEq)	Calcium (gm)	Phosphorus (gm)	Magnesium (mg)	Iodine (mcg)	Manganese (mg)	Copper (mg)	Zinc (mg)	Iron (mg)
Renu	2500	200	30	150	150	.2	1.5	1.7	2.0	6.0	20	250	.15	5.0	21.7	32	24	.5	.5	200	75	2.5	1.0	15	9
Magnacal	5000	400	60	30	300	.4	3.0	3.4	4.0	12	40	500	.3	10	43.5	32	26.8	1.0	1.0	400	150	5.0	2.0	30	18
Ensure	2642	211	32	148	158	.211	1.6	1.8	2.1	6.3	21	528	.16	5.3	32.2	32.5	29.9	.53	.53	210	79.2	2.1	1.1	15.8	9.5
Ensure Plus	2642	211	48	210	159	.211	2.6	2.8	3.2	9.5	31.7	528	.32	8.6	46.1	48.6	44.8	.63	.63	317	106	2.1	1.6	23.4	14.3
Osmolite	2642	211	32	148	158	.211	1.6	1.8	2.1	6.3	21.1	528	.16	5.3	23.4	27.1	22.6	.53	.53	210	79.2	2.1	1.1	15.8	9.5
Travasorb Ready to Use	2638	211	32	1013	160	.21	1.6	1.8	2.1	6.3	21.1	527	.15	5.3	32.3	32.5	29.9	.528	.528	211	80	2.1	1.1	15.9	9.5
Travasorb MCT 1 Kcal/Ml	2500	200	30	950	150	.2	1.5	1.7	2.0	6.0	20	225	.15	5.0	15.2	44.6	34.4	.5	.5	200	75	2.0	1.0	15	9
Vipep	2500	200	15	75	45	.2	.75	.85	1.0	3.0	10	142.5	.15	5.0	32.6	21.8	48	.6	.5	200	75	1.25	1.0	7.5	9
Criticare HN	2640	211	40	132	159	.21	2.0	2.3	2.6	7.9	26.4	264	.16	13.2	27.6	34	30	.528	.528	210	79	2.6	1.1	10.5	9.5
Vital HN	3333	264	40	185	60	.27	1.0	1.1	1.45	3.9	13.2	132	.2	6.6	16.7	29.8	18.8	.66	.66	264	99	2.47	1.32	9.9	11.8
Travasorb Std	2500	200	15	75	45	.2	.75	.85	1.0	3.0	10.0	144	.15	5.0	40	29.9	42.3	.5	.5	200	75	1.3	1.0	7.5	9.0
Travasorb HN	2500	200	15	75	45	.2	.75	.85	1.0	3.0	10.0	144	.15	5.0	15.2	44.5	34.3	.5	.5	200	75	1.3	1.0	7.5	9.0
Vivonex	2778	222	16.7	37	33	.22	.83	.94	1.1	3.3	11.1	41	.17	5.6	20.4	30	20.4	.56	.56	222	83	1.6	1.1	8.3	10
Vivonex HN	1666	133	10	22.3	20	.133	.5	.56	.666	2.0	6.66	74	.10	3.3	23	30	23.1	.33	.33	133	50	.94	.67	5.0	6.0
Travasorb Renal	---	---	---	---	43.2	.05	.72	.82	4.9	---	9.6	193	.144	2.7	---	---	---	---	---	---	---	---	---	---	---
Amin Aid	---	---	---	---	---	---	---	---	---	---	---	---	---	---	< 20	< 8	---	---	---	---	---	---	---	---	---
Amin Aid Pudding 5oz.	---	---	---	---	---	---	---	---	---	---	---	---	---	---	< 11	< 2	---	---	---	---	---	---	---	---	---
Travasorb Hepatus	486RE	195	4.95TE	51	44	.195	.68	.78	1.07	1.43	8.7	195	.073	2.6	19.4	29.3	19.4	.39	.48	189	73	1.2	.97	7.3	8.7
Hepatic Aid	---	---	---	---	---	---	---	---	---	---	---	---	---	---	14.2	---	---	---	---	---	---	---	---	---	---
Hepatic Aid Pudding	---	---	---	---	---	---	---	---	---	---	---	---	---	---	< 11	< 2	---	---	---	---	---	---	---	---	---

Table 10–12 NUTRITIONAL VALUES OF COMMERCIAL FORMULAS (PER 1000 ML)

I. Complete Diets - Intact Nutrients

A. Blenderized Diets - Indications: normal GI tract, tube feeding only, high residue.

Manufacturer	Product	Carbohydrate Sources	Protein Sources	Fat Sources	Kcal/Ml	mOsm/L	CHO GMS	PRO GMS	Fat GMS	Comments
1. Doyle	Complete B	cereal maltodextrin fruit and vegetable puree	beef, non-fat dry milk	corn oil	1.07	405	128	43	43	Contains lactase
2. Cutter	Formula-2	sucrose fruit and vegetable puree cereal, wheat flour	beef, eggs, milk	corn oil	1.0	435	123	38	40	Contains lactase
3. Doyle	Complete-B Modified	hydrolyzed cereal solids vegetable puree	beef, calcium caseinate	corn oil	1.07	300	140	43	37	
4. Organon	Vitaneed	maltodextrin vegetable puree	beef, sodium and calcium caseinate	soy oil	1.0	375	125	35	40	

B. Milk Based Diets - Contain lactose, high residue. Indications: lactose tolerant, normal GI tract, oral or tube feeding.

Manufacturer	Product	Carbohydrate Sources	Protein Sources	Fat Sources	Kcal/Ml	mOsm/L	CHO GMS	PRO GMS	Fat GMS	Comments
5. Doyle	Meritene Powder	corn syrup solids lactose	non-fat dry milk calcium caseinate	butterfat	1.06	690	119	69	35	Prepared with whole milk
6. Doyle	Meritene Liquid	sucrose, corn syrup solids	skim milk sodium caseinate	corn oil	0.96	505	115	58	32	
7. Mead Johnson	Sustacal Powder	sucrose corn syrup solids	non-fat dry milk	butterfat	1.01	625	136	61	25	Prepared with whole milk
8. Mead Johnson	Sustagen Powder	corn syrup solids dextrose	non-fat milk whole milk calcium caseinate	butterfat	1.82		314	111	16	Osmolality depends upon concentration.
9. Mead Johnson	Sustacal Pudding	sucrose modified food starch lactose	non-fat dry milk	soy oil	1.60	N/A	133	28	39	Values per 1000 Kcal
10. Ross	Forta Pudding	sucrose modified food starch lactose	non-fat dry milk	soy oil	1.70	N/A	136	27	39	Values per 1000 Kcal.

Table 10–12 *(Continued)* NUTRITIONAL VALUES OF COMMERCIAL FORMULAS (PER 1000 ML)

I. Complete Diets – Intact Nutrients

C. Lactose Free – Low residue. Indications: lactose intolerant (primary, secondary, relative), osmotic sensitivity, low-residue.

Manufacturer	Product	Carbohydrate Sources	Protein Sources	Fat Sources	Kcal/Ml	mOsm/L	CHO GMS	PRO GMS	Fat GMS	Comments
11. Doyle	Precision Isotonic	glucose oligo-saccharides, sucrose	egg white solids	soy oil	0.96	300	144	29	30	
12. Doyle	Precision LR Diet	maltodextrins sucrose	egg white solids	MCT oil soy oil	1.1	510	249	26	1.6	Low fat
13. Doyle	Precision HN Diet	maltodextrins sucrose	egg white solids	MCT oil soy oil	1.05	525	217	44	1.3	Low fat
14. Doyle	Citrotein	sucrose maltodextrins	egg white solids	soy oil	0.66	495	121	40	1.7	Low fat
15. Mead Johnson	Sustacal	sucrose corn syrup	calcium and sodium caseinate soy protein isolate	soy oil	1.0	625	138	60	23	High protein Flavored
16. Mead Johnson	Sustacal HC	corn syrup solids sucrose	calcium and sodium caseinate	soy oil	1.5	650	190	61	57	High protein
17. Mead Johnson	Isocal	maltodextrins	calcium and sodium caseinate soy protein isolate	soy oil MCT oil	1.06	300	132	34	44	
18. Mead Johnson	Isocal HCN	corn syrup	calcium and sodium caseinate soy protein isolate	MCT oil soy oil	2	740	225	75	91	High CHO High PRO
19. Mead Johnson	Portagen	corn syrup solids	sodium caseinate	MCT oil corn oil	1.0	158	115	35	48	MCT oil diet.
20. Organon	Renu	maltodextrins sucrose	sodium and calcium caseinate	soy oil	1.0	300	125	35	40	
21. Organon	Magnacal	maltodextrins	sodium and calcium caseinate	soy oil	2.0	590	250	70	80	High CHO High PRO
22. Ross	Ensure	corn syrup solids sucrose	sodium and calcium caseinate	corn oil	1.06	450	145	37	37	
23. Ross	Ensure Plus	corn syrup solids sucrose	sodium and calcium caseinate soy protein isolate	corn oil	1.5	600	200	55	53	
24. Ross	Osmolite	corn syrup solids	sodium and calcium caseinate soy protein isolate	corn oil MCT oil soy oil	1.06	300	145	37	38	
25. Travenol	Travasorb Liquid	sucrose corn syrup solids	soy protein isolate	soy oil	1.06	450	144	37	37	
26. Travenol	Travasorb MCT (Powder)	corn syrup solids	lactalbumin	MCT oil sunflower oil	1.0	250	123	49	33	MCT oil diet

Table 10-12 NUTRITIONAL VALUES OF COMMERCIAL FORMULAS (PER 1000 ML)

Manufacturer	Product	Carbohydrate Sources	Protein Sources	Fat Sources	Kcal/Ml	mOsm/L	CHO GMS	PRO GMS	Fat GMS	Comments
II. Complete Diets – Hydrolyzed Protein										
Indications: low residue, malabsorption, maldigestion.										
27. Cutter	Vipep	corn syrup solids sucrose corn starch tapioca flour	fish protein	MCT oil corn oil	1.0	520	176	25	25	
28. Mead Johnson	Criticare HN	maltodextrin	casein	safflower oil	1.06	650	222	38	3.2	Low fat.
29. Ross	Vital HN	glucose oligosaccharides	soy, whey, meat	safflower oil MCT oil	1.0	460	187	41	11	
30. Travenol	Travasorb STD Powder	glucose oligosaccharides	lactalbumin	MCT oil sunflower oil	1.0	450	190	30	14	
31. Travenol	Travasorb HN Powder	glucose oligosaccharides	lactalbumin	MCT oil sunflower oil	1.0	450	175	45	14	
III. Complete Diets – Crystalline Amino Acids										
32. Eaton	Vivonex	glucose glucose oligosaccharides	crystalline amino acids	safflower oil	1.0	550	230	21	1.5	Unflavored
33. Eaton	Vivonex HN	glucose glucose oligosaccharides	crystalline amino acids	safflower oil	1.0	810	207	46	1.0	Unflavored
IV. Incomplete Diets – Crystalline Amino Acids										
Indications – specialized amino acid patterns for specific disease states.										
34. Travanol	Travasorb Renal	glucose oligosaccharides	crystalline amino acids	MCT oil sunflower oil	1.35	590	274	23.1	17.9	High essential amino acids
35. McGaw	Amin-Aid Liquid	maltodextrins sucrose	crystalline amino acids	soy oil	1.95	850	366	19	46	All essential amino acids
36. McGaw	Amin-Aid Pudding	maltodextrins sucrose	crystalline amino acids	soy oil	1.74	N/A	189	9.5	23	Per 1000 Kcal.
37. Travanol	Travasorb-Hepatic	glucose oligosaccharides sucrose	crystalline amino acids	MCT oil sunflower oil	1.1	690	213	29	15	High branched chain A.A.
38. McGaw	Hepatic-Aid Liquid	maltodextrins sucrose	crystalline amino acids	soy oil	1.7	900	289	43	36	High branched chain A.A.
39. McGaw	Hepatic-Aid Pudding	maltodextrins sucrose	crystalline amino acids	soy oil	1.7	N/A	179	25	21	Per 1000 Kcal. High branched chain A.A.

by urea generated during negative nitrogen balance seen in many acutely or chronically ill patients. In addition to increasing the renal solute load, the specific dynamic action of a high-protein intake may contribute to hyperosmolarity by causing fever and hyperventilation, thus increasing insensible water loss. The high protein intake can increase energy expenditure by as much as 30 per cent.[53, 55, 58]

It is essential to rule out other sources of water loss before incriminating tube feedings. Some clinical situations in which water loss is common include the following: surgical patients who have multiple drains contributing to losses; diarrhea; infection with fevers, particularly pneumonitis or bronchitis with tachypnea; and patients with a tracheostomy without the use of humidification. Respiratory insensible losses may be increased in the latter two instances.

Treatment and Recommendations. The treatment of hyperosmolarity is the safe and gradual restoration of the physiologic balance of serum electrolytes and water. If one proceeds too rapidly, symptoms of water intoxication, including convulsions from brain edema, may develop and are well documented in infants.[59] Therefore, rehydration should occur over a period of a few days.

The thirst reaction is important in detecting hyperosmolarity. If it is impaired, as it is in comatose patients, infants, and the elderly, persistent and progressive dehydration may develop. Hyperosmolarity and, to a lesser extent, decreased extracellular volume serve as stimuli for thirst. There is an increased output of antidiuretic hormone from the posterior pituitary in response to the hyperosmolarity. This hormone enhances conservation of water in the distal tubules of the kidney. Once maximal urine concentrating capacity is reached and further fluid conservation cannot occur, there must be an increase in fluid intake if water balance is to be restored. This can be accomplished either by intravenous administration of fluids or by the addition of extra "free water" to the tube feeding formula. Decreasing the protein load administered to the patient is also beneficial in treating hyperosmolar dehydration.

Patients requiring a high-protein intake to promote positive nitrogen balance should be supplied with adequate and sometimes large amounts of water to offset the obligatory renal water loss associated with renal nitrogen excretion. If a formula does not contain enough water, as may be the case in the formulas containing 2kcal/cc or in high-nitrogen formulas, and if a patient is unable to increase his water intake through the thirst reaction, dehydration and hyperosmolarity may develop.

Steps to prevent the hyperosmolarity associated with high-protein tube feedings include lowering the protein-to-water ratio in the formula and monitoring the patient's fluid status.[50] Fluid balance, serum electrolytes, glucose, and BUN should be monitored regularly. Monitoring of serum osmolality, urine electrolytes, urine specific gravity, urine osmolality, daily weights, daily calorie and protein intake, and the clinical status of the patient is also helpful.

Calorie-Nutrient Density. Caloric density may affect the patient's tolerance of tube feeding by its effect on gastric emptying. The greater the nutrient density (kcal/ml), the slower the emptying rate into the duodenum.[60] Nutrient density may also affect tolerance of a particular formula. First, fat is one of the most powerful inhibitors of gastric motility. High intakes of fat or rapid infusion of fat-containing formula into the duodenum can cause a significant delay in gastric emptying.[4]

Nutrient density is also a consideration when initiating enteral feedings, especially in patients whose gastrointestinal tract has not been used for an extended period or who have mucosal disease or damage. Nutrients should be introduced gradually in a diluted or low-calorie formula that does not exceed the capability of the intestinal enzymes to hydrolyze the nutrients (such as disaccharidases).[10, 12–14] This allows time for gradual restoration of enzyme concentrations and tissue growth.

pH. Solutions with a pH of less than 3.5 will reduce gastric motility.[4] This does not appear to be a major concern with most commercial formulas.

Residue. Many formulas contain little or no residue. Although this may be advantageous in the management of specific gastrointestinal disorders (for example, bowel fistula or enteritis), low-residue diets may cause constipation in some patients.

INFANT FORMULAS

During the first year of life the infant grows most rapidly. This accelerated growth rate demands a nutrient density and profile not found in adult enteral formulas. Thus, infant formulas are specially tailored to meet the unique nutritional requirements necessary to promote growth and normal development. The most ideal food item available to the infant at present continues to be human milk. It is used as a model for the formulation of most infant feedings, and it is also the standard by which all infant nutrient requirements are defined.

As defined in the Infant Formula Act of 1980, an "infant formula" is "a food which purports to be or is represented for special dietary use solely as a food for infants by reason of its simulation of human milk or its suitability as a complete or partial substitute for human milk."[61]

The American Academy of Pediatrics (AAP) Committee on Nutrition published revised standards for infant formulas in 1976.[62] Both minimum levels to prevent deficiency symptoms and maximum levels to avoid toxicity were presented. The most recent minimum and maximum nutrient requirements are listed from the Infant Formula Act of 1980 in Table 10–13. These standards apply to formulas prepared for healthy infants from birth (2.5 to 4.0 kg) to

Table 10–13　NUTRIENT LEVELS OF INFANT FORMULAS*

| | REQUIREMENTS OF THE INFANT FORMULA ACT OF 1980 | |
NUTRIENT	Minimum (per 100 kcal)	Maximum (per 100 kcal)
Protein (gm)	1.8[†]	4.5
Fat		
(gm)	3.3	6.0
(% cal)	30.0	54.0
Essential fatty acids (linoleate)		
(% cal)	2.7	
(mg)	300.0	
Vitamins		
A (IU)	250.0 (75 µg)[‡]	750.0 (225 µg)[‡]
D (IU)	40.0	100.0
K (µg)	4.0	
E (IU)	0.7 (with 0.7 IU/gm linoleic acid)	
C (ascorbic acid) (mg)	8.0	
B₁ (thiamine) (µg)	40.0	
B₂ (riboflavin) (µg)	60.0	
B₆ (pyridoxine) (µg)	35.0 (with 15 µg/gm of protein in formula)	
B₁₂ (µg)	0.15	
Niacin (µg)	250.0	
Folic acid (µg)	4.0	
Pantothenic acid (µg)	300.0	
Biotin (µg)	1.5[§]	
Choline (mg)	7.0[§]	
Inositol (mg)	4.0[§]	
Minerals		
Calcium (mg)	50.0[¶]	
Phosphorus (mg)	25.0[¶]	
Magnesium (mg)	6.0	
Iron (mg)	0.15	
Iodine (µg)	5.0	
Zinc (mg)	0.5	
Copper (µg)	60.0	
Manganese (µg)	5.0	
Sodium (mg)	20.0	60.0
Potassium (mg)	80.0	200.0
Chloride (mg)	55.0	150.0

*From Anderson, S. A., Chinn, H. I., and Fisher, K. D.: History and current status of infant formulas. Am. J. Clin. Nutr., 35:381–397, 1982; reprinted with permission.
　†The source of protein shall be at least nutritionally equivalent to casein.
　‡Retinol equivalents
　§Required to be included in this amount only in formulas that are not milk-based
　¶Calcium-to-phosphorus ratio must be no less than 1.1 or more than 2.0.

12 months of age (8 to 10 kg). A formula must contain at least the minimal amount of the specified nutrients before it can be considered an "infant formula." Fomon has recommended that all formulas, except those for specific disorders, should provide 7 to 16 per cent of calories as protein, 30 to 55 per cent as fat, and the remainder as carbohydrate.[63]

Energy Content. The caloric density of most infant formulas is 670 kcal/L (20 kcal/oz). This is consistent with the energy content of human milk. Formulas with a caloric content higher or lower than this specified level should be termed "medical formulas" and labeled accordingly. Examples of these types of formulas include a 13 kcal/oz formula, which is used as a dilute first feeding, then concentrated as tolerance dictates; or a special 24 kcal/oz formula, designed for low-birth-weight infants to meet their greater energy requirements for growth.

The two major sources of energy in formulas are carbohydrate and fat.

Carbohydrate. In human milk, lactose makes up 90 per cent of the total amount of the 6 to 7 gm of carbohydrate/100 ml, and it is the carbohydrate of choice in feeding normal full-term infants. The enzyme lactase becomes functional after the thirty-second week of gestation; its activity increases at term, especially after lactose-containing feedings are introduced.[64, 65] Preterm, low-birth-weight infants frequently exhibit difficulties digesting lactose during the first several days of life before induction of the enzyme has occurred. New formulas tailored to meet the needs of premature infants substitute up to 50 per cent of the lactose with dextrose, as glucose polymers or corn syrup solids, to prevent this lactose intolerance. Infants receiving these formulas should be monitored for symptoms of lactose intolerance such as abdominal distention, gastric aspirates, and diarrhea; stools should be tested for unabsorbed sugar with Clinitest tablets.

Some infant formulas on the market contain tapioca starch as part of their carbohydrate source. The European Society of Paediatric Gastroenterology and Nutrition (ESPGAN) recommends that the initial infant formula not contain starch because of the negligible levels and activity of amylase found both in premature and full-term infants up to one month of age.[66, 67] Some formulas (those for specific disorders, such as galactosemia) contain sucrose and/or modified food starch. Sucrose will impart a sweet taste to the formula and consequently may be associated with an increased daily consumption of formula.[68] Disaccharides and oligosaccharides are the principal carbohydrates present in all infant formulas.

Fat. The fat content in human milk varies depending on the intake of the mother and the length of lactation. The total fat content decreases over time but will increase during the day and during each feeding. On the average, however, the fat content of human milk is from 50 to 55 per cent of its calories, including 8 to 10 per cent as linoleic acid, or 2.7 to 4.5 gm of fat/100 ml. Human milk also contains cholesterol, phospholipids, and free fatty acids, including the essential fatty acids.[69] The AAP Committee on Nutrition recommends that fat provide 30 to 54 per cent of calories in commercial infant formulas. At least 2.7 per cent of the calories should be available from linoleic acid.[62]

All infants absorb fat inefficiently. The full-term infant absorbs only 90 per cent of intake, whereas the preterm infant may absorb as little as 65 to 75 per cent.[70] The fat from cow's milk is absorbed poorly. Therefore, infant formulas should contain a substantial proportion of vegetable oils (polyunsaturated fatty acids) in an effort to simulate more closely the absorptive properties of human milk. An infant formula should be designed to allow for at least 85 per cent of the ingested fat to be absorbed in a full-term infant at one year of age.[66] All infant formulas marketed in the United States contain a blend of vegetable oils as the only fat source. It is not known whether vegetable fat alone is preferable to a mixture of animal and vegetable fats as in human milk.[66]

The cholesterol content of infant formulas available in the United States is much lower than that of human milk (1 to 3 mg/100 ml as opposed to 20 to 30 mg/100 ml). The effects this may have on prevention of atherosclerotic disease have yet to be elucidated. Cholesterol is necessary for the formation of nerve tissue myelin, bile salts, and steroid hormones. Although the full-term infant can synthesize these from its own endogenous cholesterol, the preterm infant may have immature cholesterol-synthesizing systems and may be more susceptible to low intakes.[69] It may also be possible that the low or zero cholesterol intake of infants fed commercial formulas may predispose them to deficiencies in the biochemical mechanisms necessary for adequate metabolism of cholesterol later in life.

Fat malabsorption is most marked in the preterm infant. Because the total fat absorption increases as fat intake increases, high-fat formulas have been recommended for premature infants.[71] It has been observed that the addition of MCT to formulas for preterm infants enhances the absorption of total fat intake (MCT and LCT) when MCT provides 40 to 80 per cent of the total calories of fat. Fat absorption was improved to the level found in adults when 80 per cent of the fat calories was derived from MCT.[72] Along with the enhanced fat absorption using MCT, there is improved weight gain and enhanced calcium and nitrogen retention.[72, 73] Most of the formulas made specifically for feeding preterm infants contain 40 to 50 per cent of their fat calories as MCT.

Protein. The optimal protein source and concentration for growth during infancy is that which is present in human milk. The amino acid pattern of protein determines its quality. The requirements for essential amino acids are high during infancy and decrease rapidly with age. The quality of proteins is more critical in infants and small children because of the need for growth, specifically of the brain.

An amino acid pattern similar to that of human milk is optimal but difficult to attain in commercial infant formulas. Many commercial formulas are designed to mimic the amino acid profile in human milk with a whey-to-casein ratio of 60:40. Recently, however, the whey-to-casein ratio in human milk has been reassessed at 80:20.[74] The protein available in the whey fraction of cow's milk is β-lactalbumin rather than the α-lactalbumin present in human milk. Therefore, the amino acid patterns of these "humanized" formulas will never exactly match those of human milk. The true protein content of human milk is approximately 0.9 gm/100 ml at one month of lactation. Variations of this figure will occur, however, depending on the mother's dietary intake. The minimum protein requirement set by the Infant Formula Act is 1.2 gm/100 ml, and the source of protein should have a Protein Efficiency Ratio (PER) at least equal to that of casein.[61] The protein requirements of pre-

term infants are greater at 2.25 to 5 gm/kg/day. Human milk may need to be supplemented with protein, if it is to be the feeding of choice.

Soy-based formulas are used in infants who are allergic to milk proteins. They are also lactose-free and are sometimes used in feeding preterm infants who exhibit lactose intolerance. When formulas other than human milk are used, such as soy-based, a higher protein intake is necessary to meet the infant's requirements for all essential amino acids.

The limiting amino acid in soy is methionine, and it is common practice to fortify soy-based products with D,L-methionine to increase their biologic value. Graham in 1971 studied the effects on nitrogen retention of supplementing soy protein with methionine fed to infants.[75, 76] He compared his experimental soy product with and without added methionine to Prosobee, a commercial, soy-based formula enriched with methionine. In each case, methionine enhanced nitrogen retention in infants ranging in age from 6 to 23 months.

By supplementing a soybean formula with D,L-methionine, the PER could be made equivalent to that obtained with modified cow's milk as reported by Shurpalekar et al. in 1961.[77] Therefore, soy-based formulas with added D,L-methionine can meet the protein quality stipulations set in the Infant Formula Act. The effects of the long-term use of soy-based formulas on growth and development of preterm infants, however, have not been adequately studied. The soy-based products on the market contain 2.0 gm of protein/100 ml as opposed to the 1.5 to 1.7 gm/100 ml in casein- or whey-derived formulas.

Preterm infants have requirements for specific amino acids because of immaturity in enzyme systems to convert one amino acid to another. Among these amino acids are cysteine, because of a deficiency in the enzyme cystathionase necessary to convert methionine to cysteine; taurine, since taurine is synthesized from cysteine; and possibly tyrosine because of the decreased levels of phenylalanine hydroxylase. Cysteine and taurine are in higher concentrations in human milk and whey-predominant formulas. Plasma amino acid and ammonia levels are lower in infants fed these formulas instead of casein-predominant formulas, as reported by Raiha and coworkers.[78] All infants, however, grew at equal rates if they were fed 117 cal/kg/day.

There are certain metabolic disturbances that may occur secondary to the protein content of the formula. These include hyperosmolarity and prerenal azotemia due to the renal solute load of a formula. Although they are discussed in another section of this chapter, they deserve reemphasis, as infants are more sensitive to the complications of a hyperosmolar or high-protein formula than are adults.

Renal Solute Load. Infants, particularly preterm infants, have an immature renal system. This contributes, in part, to the frequent problem of hypertonic dehydration in formula-fed infants. The protein end product, urea, along with sodium, chloride, and potassium, contributes to the renal solute load of a formula. Because of the infant's inability to concentrate urine, fluid cannot be retained when an infant is subjected to one of the following: a formula with a high renal solute load, restricted water intake, diseases associated with increased extrarenal losses of water, or an environment with an excessively high temperature.[69] These factors may result in the development of hypertonic dehydration. The estimated renal solute load of human milk is 80 mOsm/L,[79] whereas most formulas contain 90 to 150 mOsm/L. Blood urea nitrogen levels in normal infants reflect the protein intake. The BUN is higher in infants fed formulas rather than human milk, owing to the higher protein content of formulas. The 24 kcal/oz formulas for preterm infants have a renal solute load of approximately 150 mOsm/L. These infants must be monitored closely for dehydration by checking daily weights, serum and urine electrolytes, serum and urine osmolality, and urine specific gravity.

In contrast to the renal solute load, a formula's osmolality will influence an infant's gastrointestinal tolerance to a formula. Formulas that contain hydrolyzed protein and/or disaccharides and monosaccharides will increase the osmolality of a formula and may cause abdominal distention, diarrhea, and vomiting. An increased incidence of necrotizing enterocolitis has been reported in low-birth-weight infants fed a formula with an osmolality of 650 mOsm/L.[80]

Vitamins and Minerals. Rather than elaborate on each vitamin and mineral in formulas, this discussion will deal with those that pose particular problems in infancy. All commercially prepared infant formulas are enriched with vitamins; however, to meet the Recommended Daily Allowance of many of them, large volumes of formula (750 ml) must be ingested, which may be difficult in small infants.

One vitamin that may need to be supplemented is vitamin D. Most commercial formulas contain 400 IU/L. Therefore, infants receiving 300 to 400 ml of formula would receive only 125 to 160 IU of vitamin D, which is much lower than the RDA of 400 IU/day. Preterm infants and infants with steatorrhea will require supplementation. The recommended intake of vitamin D for preterm infants is 600 IU/day, and no available formula meets this level at the volumes normally ingested.[81]

Another fat-soluble vitamin that may be inadequately supplemented in formulas for preterm infants is vitamin E. Full-term infants require approximately 0.3 IU of vitamin E/100 kcal and at least 0.7 IU of vitamin E/gm of linoleic acid.[62] Preterm infants, however, require at least 25 to 30 IU/day to prevent hemolytic anemia.[81–83] The reasons for the increased requirements of vitamin E in this population are threefold: (1) Absorption of vitamin E by these infants is poor because of poor fat absorption (water-soluble forms of vitamin E not yet available may improve absorption); (2) the requirement for vitamin E will increase as the level of polyunsaturated fatty acids in the diet increases; and (3) when iron levels in formulas are high (12 mg/L), the requirement for vitamin E by preterm infants increases.[84] Iron is a cofactor that catalyzes peroxidation of lipid membranes; this is most pronounced if vitamin E is not available to exert its antioxidant effect.[82] There is no formula available that contains adequate vitamin E in the volumes that preterm infants would be fed; therefore, supplementation is usually necessary.

A multivitamin supplement is required for preterm infants fed the standard 20 kcal/oz formulas. The more concentrated formulas, 24 kcal/oz, contain adequate levels of all vitamins except for vitamins D and E. Full-term infants may require a supplement of vitamin D but should receive adequate amounts of the other vitamins in the available formulas.

The mineral content of most formulas is

adequate for healthy full-term infants and will not require supplementation. There are, however, certain minerals, specifically calcium, phosphorus, iron, and zinc, which deserve special attention, particularly in preterm infants.

The calcium and phosphorus content of human milk is adequate to support body functions and to promote growth in healthy full-term infants. Formula-fed infants in the neonatal period, however, will absorb less calcium because of poor fat absorption and subsequent losses of vitamin D.[69] To compensate for this decreased absorption, the AAP has recommended that the concentration of calcium and phosphorus in formulas be increased to 1.5 times that of human milk. The calcium-to-phosphorus ratio should be no less than 1.2:1 nor greater than 2:1, the latter being the ratio in human milk.[62]

Calcium and phosphorus homeostasis is difficult to attain in preterm infants owing to their immature bone mineral stores. Two thirds of bone mineralization occurs in the third trimester of pregnancy. When this is interrupted by premature birth, it is difficult to achieve intrauterine accretion rates of these minerals with existing formulas.

Human milk contains inadequate levels of calcium and phosphorus for skeletal mineralization in preterm infants and must be supplemented if it is to be used.[85] Many of the commercial formulas available are also low in calcium and phosphorus, making rickets a common but avoidable occurrence in preterm infants. The requirements for calcium and phosphorus in this population are 210 mg/kg/day and 140 mg/kg/day, respectively, based on rates of intrauterine accretion.[81] Some of the more concentrated formulas available for preterm infants now contain these higher levels of calcium and phosphorus. To prevent precipitation of these minerals, the bottles of formula must be shaken frequently. There is also some question as to the exact amounts of minerals (specifically iron, zinc, and calcium) the infant is receiving in these concentrated premature formulas. Some proportion of each mineral adheres to the feeding apparatus prior to reaching the infant when a formula is infused continuously.[86]

Frequently, preterm infants will be fed soy-based formulas initially because they are characteristically lactose-free. These formulas, with their high levels of phytates, bind many divalent compounds, particularly phosphorus, causing decreased absorption. In a study by Shenai et al., fecal loss of phosphorus was increased in infants fed soy-based formulas.[87] Although in this study, calcium absorption was not influenced by the absence of lactose, it is known that lactose will facilitate calcium absorption.[88] Another concern with soy-based formulas is that their high protein content may increase calcium requirements since urinary calcium loss is directly proportional to protein intake.[69] With these concerns in mind, if soy-based formulas are used in preterm infants for longer than two weeks, they must be supplemented with calcium and phosphorus.

Full-term infants are born with iron stores that should last until at least four to six months of age, if the infant's mother had an adequate iron intake. Iron deficiency is uncommon in term infants fed human milk. It is more common in infants fed formulas with higher protein contents.[63] The AAP recommends that all formulas contain at least the lower level of iron found in human milk (0.15 mg/100 kcal or 1 mg/L) and that infants at risk for developing iron deficiency anemia be given an iron-supplemented formula (12 mg/L). Preterm infants, because of their minimal stores and rapid growth, should be supplemented with 1 to 2 mg/kg/day of elemental iron at or before two months of age.[84] The minimal requirement for zinc in full-term and preterm infants is approximately 0.5 mg/100 kcal (3.2 mg/L), which all currently available formulas provide. Soy-based formulas may require additional supplementation owing to the diminution of zinc absorption due to phytates.[89]

Formulas for Specific Medical Purposes

There are many infant formulas available that are designed for specific medical conditions. The most prevalent of these are inborn errors of metabolism such as maple syrup urine disease, galactosemia, phenylketonuria, and tyrosinemia. Space does not permit a discussion of each disorder. Table 10–16 lists some of the specialized formulas available to treat these rare diseases.

There are also formulas available specifically for infants with gastrointestinal dysfunction, such as malabsorption and short bowel syndrome. These formulas are similar to their counterparts for adults in that they

Table 10–14 NUTRITIONAL VALUES OF INFANT FORMULAS (PER 1000 ML)

Formula	Vit A (IU)	Vit D (IU)	Vit E (IU)	Vit K (mg)	Vit C (mg)	Folic Acid (mg)	Thiamine (mg)	Riboflavin (mg)	B6 (mg)	B12 (mcg)	Niacin (mg)	Choline (mg)	Biotin (mg)	Pantothenic Acid (mg)	Sodium (mEq)	Potassium (mEq)	Chloride (mEq)	Calcium (gm)	Phosphorus (gm)	Magnesium (mg)	Iodine (mcg)	Manganese (mg)	Copper (mg)	Zinc (mg)	Iron (mg)
Enfamil	1690	422	12.7	96	55	.1	.5	.6	.4	2.1	8.4	47.5	.016	3.17	10.1	17.3	13.3	.528	.444	47.5	69	1.0	.6	4.2	1.48
Enfamil with Iron	1690	422	12.7	96	55	.1	.5	.6	.4	2.1	8.4	47.5	.016	3.17	10.1	17.3	13.3	.528	.444	47.5	69	1.0	.6	4.2	12.7
Similac 20 Kcal/oz	2500	400	17	30	55	.1	.65	1.0	.4	1.5	7.0	102	.01	3.0	10.9	20	14.9	.51	.39	41	100	.03	.6	5.0	1.5
Similac with Iron	2500	400	17	30	55	.1	.65	1.0	.4	1.5	7.0	102	.01	3.0	10.9	20	14.9	.51	.39	41	100	.03	.6	5	12
Similac 24 LBW	3000	480	18	NA	100	.1	1.0	1.2	.5	2.0	8.4	NA	.015	3.6	16.1	30.8	24.8	.73	.56	80	120	.04	.8	8	3.0
Advance	2400	400	12	20	50	.1	.75	.9	.6	2.5	10	NA	.008	4.0	13	22	14	.51	.39	64	60	.027	.9	6.0	12
Enfamil Premature (20 cal/oz)	2080	416	13	62	56	.2	.5	.6	.4	2.0	8.3	47.5	.016	3.0	11.3	18.9	15.8	.78	.39	70	53	.17	.6	6.7	1.0
Enfamil Premature (24 cal/oz)	2496	499	16	75	68	.24	.6	.7	.5	2.5	10	57	.019	3.7	13.6	22.7	26.4	.94	.47	83	63	.2	.7	8	1.3
PM 60/40	2500	400	15	30	55	.05	.65	1.0	.3	1.5	7.3	128	.01	3.0	6.9	14.9	7.0	.4	.2	42	40	.03	.4	4.0	2.6
Special Care (20 kcal/oz)	4580	1000	25	83	250	.25	1.7	4.2	1.7	3.7	20	67	.025	12.5	12.6	21.3	15.2	1.2	.6	83	125	.17	1.7	10	2.5
Special Care (24 kcal/oz)	5500	1200	30	100	300	.3	2.0	5	2	4.5	24	80	.03	15	15.2	25.6	18.3	1.4	.72	100	150	.2	2.0	12	3
SMA	2647	423	9.5	58	58	.05	.7	1.0	.4	1.0	10.2	88	.015	2.1	6.5	14.4	10.5	.45	.33	53	69	.16	.5	3.7	13
"Preemie" SMA	3200	510	15	70	70	.1	.8	1.3	.8	2	6.3	165	.018	3.6	14	19	15	.75	.4	70	83	.2	.7	5	3
Prosobee	2112	422	10.6	106	55	.11	.53	.63	.42	2.1	8.4	52.7	.05	3.2	12.6	21	15.5	.63	.50	74	69	.2	.6	5.3	12.7
Isomil	2500	400	17	150	55	.1	.4	.6	.4	3.0	9.0	NA	.03	5.0	13	18.2	15	.7	.5	50	150	.2	.5	5.0	12
Isomil SF20	2500	400	17	150	55	.1	.4	.6	.4	3.0	9.0	NA	.03	5.0	13	18	15	.7	.5	50	150	.2	.5	5.0	12
Isomil SF Concentrate	2500	400	17	150	55	.1	.4	.6	.4	3.0	9.0	NA	.03	5.0	13	18	15	.7	.5	50	150	.2	.5	5.0	12
RCF – Module	2500	400	17	150	55	.1	.4	.6	.4	3.0	9.0	NA	.03	5.0	17	18	15	.7	.5	50	100	.2	.5	1.5	1.5
Lofenolac	1690	422	10.6	106	55	.1	.5	.6	.4	2.1	8.4	90	.05	3.17	14	18	13.3	.63	.47	74	48	1.06	.63	4.2	12.7
Nutramagin	1690	422	10.6	106	55	.1	.5	.6	.4	2.1	8.4	90	.05	3.17	14	18	13.3	.63	.47	74	48	1.06	.63	4.2	12.7
Progestimil	2090	419	15	107	54	.1	.5	.6	.4	2.0	8.4	90	.05	6.6	14	14.8	17	.60	.42	74	47	.2	.6	4.0	13
Meat Base Formula	1778	467	6	NA	60	.03	.6	1.0	.87	8.7	7.3	NA	NA	2.0	7.9	9.8	NA	1.0	.67	40	33	NA	.4	2.8	14

Table 10-15 NUTRITIONAL VALUES OF INFANT FORMULAS (PER 1000 ML)

Manufacturer	Product	Carbohydrate Sources	Protein Sources	Fat Sources	Kcal/Ml	mOsm/L	CHO GMS	PRO GMS	Fat GMS	Comments
I. Milk-Based –										
Indications: normal G.I. tract; for infants greater than 36 weeks gestation.										
1. Mead Johnson	Enfamil	lactose	nonfat milk	soy oil / coconut oil	.68	290	70	15	37	
2. Mead Johnson	Enfamil with iron	lactose	nonfat milk	soy oil / coconut oil	.68	290	70	15	37	Also available at 13 cal/oz, 24 cal/oz and 27 cal/oz dilutions.
3. Ross	Similac	lactose	nonfat milk	soy oil / coconut oil	.68	262	72.3	15.5	36.1	
4. Ross	Similac with iron	lactose	nonfat milk	soy oil / coconut oil	.68	262	72.3	15.5	36.1	
5. Ross	Similac 24 LBW	corn syrup solids / lactose	nonfat milk	soy oil / corn oil / MCT oil	.81	300	84.9	22	44.9	for feeding LBW infants (< 2500 gm)
6. Ross	Advance	corn syrup solids / lactose	nonfat milk / soy isolate	soy oil / corn oil	.54	210	55	20	27	for older infants
II. Whey Adjusted Diets –										
Indications: normal or immature G.I. tract; for infants less than 36 weeks gestation.										
7. Mead Johnson	Enfamil Premature (20 cal/oz)	corn syrup solids (60%) / lactose (40%)	whey (lactalbumin) (60%) / casein (40%)	coconut oil (20%) / corn oil (40%) / MCT oil (40%)	.68	244	74	20	34	
8. Mead Johnson	Enfamil Premature (24 cal/oz)	corn syrup solids (60%) / lactose (40%)	whey (lactalbumin) (60%) / casein (40%)	coconut oil (20%) / corn oil (40%) / MCT oil (40%)	.81	300	89	24	41	
9. Ross	PM 60/40	lactose	whey (lactalbumin) (60%) / casein (40%)	coconut oil / corn oil	.68	260	68.8	15.8	37.6	
10. Ross	Special Care (20 cal/oz)	corn syrup solids (50%) / lactose (50%)	whey lactalbumin (60%) / casein (40%)	coconut oil (20%) / corn oil (30%) / MCT oil (50%)	.68	300	71.7	18.3	36.7	
11. Ross	Special Care (24 cal/oz)	corn syrup solids (50%) / lactose (50%)	whey (lactalbumin) (60%) / casein (40%)	coconut oil (20%) / corn oil (30%) / MCT oil (50%)	.81	300	86	22	44	

Table 10-15 *(Continued)* NUTRITIONAL VALUES OF INFANT FORMULAS (PER 1000 ML)

Manufacturer	Product	Carbohydrate Sources	Protein Sources	Fat Sources	Kcal/Ml	mOsm/L	CHO GMS	PRO GMS	Fat GMS	Comments
II. Whey Adjusted Diets - Continued										
12. Wyeth	SMA	lactose	whey (lactalbumin) (60%) casein (40%)	coconut oil safflower oil soy oil	.68	296	71.8	14.9	35.9	
13. Wyeth	"Preemie" SMA	lactose (50%) dextrose polymers (50%)	whey (lactalbumin) (60%) casein (40%)	safflower oil soy oil MCT oil	.81	268	86	20	44	
III. Soy Isolate -										
Indications: cows milk intolerance; otherwise normal G.I. tract.										
14. Mead Johnson	Prosobee	corn syrup solids	soy isolate	soy oil (80%) coconut oil (20%)	.68	200	69	20	36	Lactose free
15. Ross	Isomil	corn syrup solids sucrose	soy isolate	soy oil coconut oil	.68	250	68	20	36	Lactose free
16. Ross	Isomil SF20 Ready to Feed	corn syrup solids	soy isolate	soy oil coconut oil	.68	250	68	20	36	Lactose free
17. Ross	Isomil SF Concentrated Liquid	corn syrup solids	soy isolate	soy oil coconut oil	.68	250	68	20	36	Lactose free
18. Ross	RCF	------------	soy isolate	soy oil coconut oil	.68	N/A	---	20	36	Module carbohydrate free
IV. Casein Hydrolysate -										
Indications: protein sensitivity; malabsorption; short bowel syndrome; galactosemia.										
19. Mead Johnson	Lofenolac	corn syrup solids tapioca starch	casein hydrolysate	corn oil	.68	NA	87.6	21.9	27	Lactose free, low phenylalanine for use in infants and children with PKU
20. Mead Johnson	Nutramagin	sucrose modified tapioca starch	casein hydrolysate	corn oil	.68	NA	87.6	22	26	Lactose free
21. Mead Johnson	Pregestimil	corn syrup solids (85%) modified tapioca starch (15%)	casein hydrolysate	corn oil (60%) MCT oil (40%)	.68	338	91	19	27	Lactose free
V. Meat-Based Diets -										
Indications: cows milk intolerance; galactosemia.										
22. Gerber	Meat Base Formula	cane sugar modified tapioca starch	beef hearts	sesame oil	.68	NA	63.3	28.7	33.3	Lactose free

Table 10–16   FORMULAS FOR SPECIAL MEDICAL PURPOSES*

PRODUCT	COMPANY	USE
Lofenalac	Mead Johnson	Low phenylalanine; for treatment of phenylketonuria (PKU) in infancy.
Phenylfree	Mead Johnson	Phenylalanine-free food for use in PKU; not for use in infancy.
3200-AB	Mead Johnson	Low phenylalanine, low tyrosine food powder; for treatment of tyrosinemia.
PKU Aid	Milner Scientific	Protein hydrolysate of beef serum that is phenylalanine-free; for use in treating children with PKU; little or no vitamins added.
MSUD Diet Powder	Mead Johnson	Formula powder low in branched-chain amino acids (BCAA); for maple syrup urine disease; can be used alone or as supplement to infant formula.
MSUD Aid	Milner Scientific	Mixture of crystalline L-amino acids devoid of BCAA; contains minerals and water-soluble vitamins only.
3200-K	Mead Johnson	Soy protein isolate infant formula powder without added methionine; for treatment of homocystinuria.
Low-Methionine Isomil	Ross	Soy protein isolate formula low in methionine; for use in treatment of homocystinuria.
Methionaid	Milner Scientific	Methionine-free mixture of L-amino acids, water-soluble vitamins, and minerals; for treatment of homocystinuria.
80056	Mead Johnson	Protein-free base for special diets; amino acid mixtures added to meet infants' special needs.
3232-A	Mead Johnson	Protein hydrolysate base; carbohydrate must be added.
Histinaid	Milner Scientific	L-amino acid mixture devoid of histidine and containing water-soluble vitamins and most minerals; carbohydrate, fat, and fat-soluble vitamins must be added.

Adapted from American Academy of Pediatrics, Committee on Nutrition: Special diets for infants with inborn errors of amino acid metabolism. Pediatrics, *57*:783–791, 1976.

contain predigested protein and MCT and are low in total fat content.

REFERENCES

1. Gormican, A., and Liddy, E.: Nasogastric tube feedings: Practical considerations in prescription and evaluation. Postgrad. Med., *53*(7):71–76, 1973.
2. Torosian, M. H., and Rombeau, J. L.: Feeding by tube enterostomy. Surg. Gynecol. Obstet., *150*:918–927, 1980.
3. Charley, H.: Food Science. New York, Ronald Press, 1970, pages 109–128.
4. Davenport, H. W.: Physiology of the Digestive Tract. Edition 4. Chicago, Year Book Medical Publishers, 1977.
5. Gray, G. M.: Carbohydrate digestion and absorption: Role of the small intestine. N. Engl. J. Med., *292*:1225–1230, 1975.
6. Fogel, M. R., and Gray, G. M.: Starch hydrolysis in man: An intraluminal process not requiring membrane digestion. J. Appl. Physiol., *35*:263–267, 1973.
7. Lehninger, A. L.: Sugars, storage polysaccharides, and cell walls. *In* Biochemistry: The Molecular Basis of Cell Structure and Function. Edition 2. New York, Worth Publishers, Inc. 1975, pages 249–266.
8. Polycose Monograph. Columbus, Ohio, Ross Laboratories, 1978.
9. Daum, F., Cohen, M. I., McNamara, H., Finberg, L.: Intestinal osmolality and carbohydrate absorption in rats treated with polymerized glucose. Pediatr. Res., *12*:24–26, 1978.
10. Sheehy, T. W., and Anderson, P. R.: Disaccharidase activity in normal and diseased small bowel. Lancet, *2*(7401):1–4, 1965.
11. Welsh, J. D., Zschiesche, O. M., Anderson, J., Walker, A.: Intestinal disaccharidase activity in celiac sprue (gluten-sensitive enteropathy). Arch. Intern. Med., *123*:33–38, 1969.
12. Hirschhorn, N., and Molla, A.: Reversible jejunal disaccharidase deficiency in cholera and other acute diarrheal diseases. Johns Hopkins Med. J., *125*:291–300, 1969.
13. James, W. P. T.: Intestinal absorption in protein-calorie malnutrition. Lancet, *1*(7538):333–335, 1968.
14. Knudsen, K. B., Bradley, E. M., LeCocq, F. R., Bellamy, H. M., and Welsh, J. D.: Effect of fasting and refeeding on the histology and disaccharidase activity of the human intestine. Gastroenterology, *55*:46–51, 1968.
15. Bilir, S.: Acquired disaccharide intolerance in children with malnutrition. Am. J. Clin. Nutr., *25*:664–671, 1972.
16. Newcomer, A. D.: Lactase deficiency. J. Med. Soc. N. J., *77*:127–128, 1980.
17. Walike, B. C., and Walike, J. W.: Relative lactose intolerance: A clinical study of tube-fed patients. J.A.M.A., *238*:948–951, 1977.
18. Newcomer, A. D.: Disaccharidase deficiencies. Mayo Clin. Proc., *48*:648–652, 1973.
19. Olsen, W. A.: Carbohydrate digestion and absorption. Postgrad. Med., *51*(4):149–152, 1972.
20. Pike, R. L., and Brown, M. L.: Nutrition: An Integrated Approach. Edition 2. New York, John Wiley and Sons, 1975.
21. Matthews, D. M.: Intestinal absorption of peptides. Physiol. Rev., *55*(4):537–608, 1975.
22. Joint FAO/WHO Expert Committee Report: Energy

and Protein Requirements. WHO Technical Report Series, No. 522. Geneva, WHO, 1973.

23. Steffee, C. H., Wissler, R. W., Humphrey, E. M., Benditt, E. P., Woolridge, R. W., and Cannon, P. R.: Studies in amino acid utilization. V. The determination of minimum daily essential amino acid requirements in protein-depleted adult male albino rats. J. Nutr., 40:483–497, 1950.

24. Mitchell, H. H.: A method of determining the biological value of protein. J. Biol. Chem., 58:873–903, 1924.

25. Bricker, M., Mitchell, H. H., and Kinsman, G. M.: The protein requirements of adult human subjects in terms of the protein contained in individual food and food combinations. J. Nutr., 30:269–283, 1945.

26. Oser, B. L.: Method for integrating essential amino acid content in the nutritional evaluation of protein. J. Am. Diet. Assoc., 27:396–402, 1951.

27. Marable, N. L., Hinners, M. L., Hardison, N. W., and Kehmberg, N. L.: Protein quality of supplements and meal replacements. J. Am. Diet. Assoc., 77:270–276, 1980.

28. Osborne, T. B., Mendel, L. B., and Ferry, E. L.: A method of expressing numerically the growth-promoting value of proteins. J. Biol. Chem., 37:223–229, 1919.

29. Miller, D. S., and Bender, A. E.: The determination of the net utilization of protein by a shortened method. Br. J. Nutr., 9:382–388, 1955.

30. Hegsted, D. M., and Chang, Y.: Protein utilization in growing rats at different levels of intake. J. Nutr., 87:19–25, 1965.

31. Harper, A. E., Benevenger, N. J., and Wohlhereter, R. M.: Effects of ingestion of disproportionate amounts of amino acids. Physiol. Rev., 50:428–558, 1970.

32. Crim, M. C., and Munro, H. N.: Protein and amino acid requirements and metabolism in relation to defined-formula diets. In Shils, M. E. (ed.): Defined Formula Diets for Medical Purposes. Conference on Defined Formula Diets for Medical Purposes, 1975. Chicago, American Medical Association, 1977, pages 5–14.

33. Adibi, S. A.: Intestinal transport of dipeptides in man: Relative importance of hydrolysis and intact absorption. J. Clin. Invest., 50:2266–2275, 1971.

34. Composition of Foods, Fats, and Oils. Agriculture Handbook No. 8-4. United States Department of Agriculture, 1979.

35. Dodge, J. A., and Yassa, J. G.: Essential fatty acid deficiency after prolonged treatment with elemental diet. Lancet, 2(8206):1256–1257, 1980.

36. Hirono, H., Suzuki, H., Igarashi, Y., and Konno, T.: Essential fatty acid deficiency induced by total parenteral nutrition and medium chain triglyceride feedings. Am. J. Clin. Nutr., 30(10):1670–1676, 1977.

37. Wene, J. D., Connor, W. E., DenBesten, L.: The development of essential fatty acid deficiency in healthy men fed fat-free diets intravenously and orally. J. Clin. Invest., 56:127–134, 1975.

38. Holman, R. T.: The ratio of trienoic:tetraenoic acids in tissue lipids as a measure of essential fatty acid requirement. J. Nutr., 70:405–410, 1960.

39. Adam, D. J. D., Hansen, A. E., and Wiese, H. F.: Essential fatty acids in infant nutrition. II. Effect of linoleic acid on calorie intake. J. Nutr., 66:555–564, 1958.

40. Collins, F. D., Sinclair, A. J., Royle, J. P., Coats, D. A., Maynard, A. T., and Leonard, R. F.: Plasma lipids in human linoleic acid deficiency. Nutr. Metab., 13:150–167, 1971.

41. Greenberger, N. J., Skillman, T. G.: Medium-chain triglycerides: Physiologic considerations and clinical considerations. N. Engl. J. Med., 280:1045–1058, 1969.

42. Hashim, S. A.: Medium-chain triglycerides: Clinical and metabolic aspects. J. Am. Diet. Assoc., 51:221–227, 1967.

43. Clark, S. B., and Holt, P. R.: Competition for intestinal absorption of triglycerides [Abstract]. Gastroenterology, 54:1227, 1968.

44. Sarett, H. P.: Fat absorption. In Shils, M. E. (ed.): Defined Formula Diets for Medical Purposes. Conference on Defined Formula Diets for Medical Purposes, 1975. Chicago, American Medical Association, 1977, pages 38–39.

45. Shils, M. E., et al.: Liquid formulas for oral and tube feeding. Memorial Sloan-Kettering Cancer Institute, 1979.

46. Zallman, J. A., Lee, D. P., Jeffrey, P. L.: Liquid nutrition as a cause of warfarin resistance. Am. J. Hosp. Pharm., 38:1174, 1981.

47. Anderson, S. A., Chinn, H. I., and Fisher, K. D.: History and current status of infant formulas. Am. J. Clin. Nutr., 35:381–397, 1982.

48. Cha, C. M., and Randall, H. T.: Osmolality of liquid and defined formula diets: The effects of hydrolysis by pancreatic enzymes. J.P.E.N., 5:7–10, 1981.

49. Schoolman, H., Dubin, A., and Hoffman, W.: Clinical syndromes associated with hypernatremia. Arch. Intern. Med., 95:15–23, 1955.

50. Wilson, W. S., and Meinert, J. K.: Extracellular hyperosmolarity secondary to high protein nasogastric tube feeding. Ann. Intern. Med., 47:585–590, 1957.

51. Smith, H. W.: The Kidney: Structure and Function in Health and Disease. New York, Oxford University Press, 1951, page 135.

52. Davidson, L. S. P., Passmore, R., Brock, J. F., and Truswell, A. S.: Human Nutrition and Dietetics. Edition 7. New York, Churchill Livingstone, 1979.

53. Best, C., and Taylor, N. B.: Physiological Basis of Medical Practice. Edition 5. Baltimore, Williams and Wilkins, 1950.

54. Engel, F. L., Jaeger, C.: Dehydration with hypernatremia, hyperchloremia, and azotemia complicating nasogastric tube feeding. Am. J. Med., 17:196–204, 1954.

55. Cramer, L. M., Haverback, C. Z., Smith, R. R.: Hypertonic dehydration complicating high protein nasogastric tube feeding. Med. Ann. D. C., 27:331–335, 1958.

56. Gault, M. H., Dixon, M. E., Doyle, M., and Cohen, W. M.: Hypernatremia, azotemia, and dehydration due to high-protein tube feeding. Ann. Intern. Med., 68:778–791, 1968.

57. Taitz, L. S., and Byers, H. B.: High calorie osmolar feeding and hypertonic dehydration. Arch. Dis. Child., 47:257–260, 1972.

58. Brodsky, W. A.: Problems of dehydration and starvation in postoperative care. Am. J. Surg., 90:919–923, 1955.

59. Weil, W. B., and Wallace, W. M.: Hypertonic dehydration in infancy. Pediatrics, 17:171–183, 1956.

50. Hunt, J. N., and Stubbs, D. F.: The volume and en-

ergy content of meals as determinants of gastric emptying. J. Physiol., 245:209–225, 1975.

61. United States Congress Infant Formula Act of 1980. Washington, D.C.: United States Capitol Health Documents Room. Public Law 96-359, September 26, 1980.

·62. American Academy of Pediatrics, Committee on Nutrition: Commentary on breast-feeding and infant formulas, including proposed standards for formulas. Pediatrics, 57:278–285, 1976.

63. Fomon, S. J.: Infant Nutrition. Edition 2. Philadelphia, W. B. Saunders Company, 1974.

64. Auricchio, S., Rubino, A., and Murset, G.: Intestinal glycosidase activities in the human embryo, fetus, and newborn. Pediatrics, 35:944–954, 1965.

65. Boellner, S. E., Beard, A. G., and Panos, T. C.: Impairment of intestinal hydrolysis of lactose in newborn infants. Pediatrics, 36:542–550, 1965.

66. European Society of Pediatric Gastroenterology and Nutrition, Committee on Nutrition: Guidelines on infant nutrition. I. Recommendations for the composition of an adapted formula. Acta Paediatr. Scand. [Suppl.] 262:1–20, 1977.

67. Lebenthal, E., and Lee, P. C.: Development of functional response in human exocrine pancreas. Pediatrics, 66:556–560, 1980.

68. Nisbett, R. E., and Gurwitz, S. B.: Weight, sex, and the eating behavior of human newborns. J. Comp. Physiol. Psychol., 73:245–253, 1970.

69. Brostrøm, K.: Human milk and infant formulas: Nutritional and immunological characteristics. *In* Suskind, R. M. (ed.): Textbook of Pediatric Nutrition. New York, Raven Press, 1981, pages 41–64.

70. Watkins, J. B.: Infant nutrition and the development of gastrointestinal function. *In* American Academy of Pediatrics. Committee on Nutrition: Pediatric Nutrition Handbook. Evanston, Illinois, American Academy of Pediatrics, 1979, pages 58–69.

71. Morales, S., Chung, A. W., Lewis, J. M., Massina, A., and Holt, L. E.: Absorption of fat and vitamin A in premature infants. I. Effect of different levels of fat intake on the retention of fat and vitamin A. Pediatrics, 6:86–92, 1950.

72. Tantibhedhyangkul, P., and Hashim, S. A.: Medium-chain triglyceride feeding in premature infants: Effects on fat and nitrogen absorption. Pediatrics, 55:359–370, 1975.

73. Andrews, B. F., and Lorch, V.: Improved fat and calcium absorption in low birth weight infants fed a medium-chain triglyceride containing formula [Abstract]. Pediatr. Res., 8:378, 1974.

74. Hambraeus, L., Lonnerdal, B., Forsum, E., Gebre-Medhin, M.: Nitrogen and protein components of human milk. Acta Paediatr. Scand., 67:561–565, 1978.

75. Graham, G. G.: Methionine or lysine fortification of dietary protein for infants and small children. *In* Scrimshaw, N. S., and Altschul, A. M. (eds.): Amino Acid Fortification of Protein Foods. Cambridge, MIT Press, 1971, page 222.

76. Jansen, G. R.: Amino acid fortification. *In* Bodwell,

C. E. (ed.): Evaluation of Proteins for Humans. Westport, Connecticut, AVI Publishing Company, Inc., 1977, pages 177–203.

77. Shurpalekar, S. R., Chandrasekhara, M. R., Lahery, N. L., Swaminathan, M., Indiramma, K., and Subrahmanyan, V.: Studies of milk substitutes of vegetable origin. 3. The nutritive value of spray-dried soyabean milk fortified with DL-methionine and spray-dried powder from a 2:1 blend of soyabean milk and sesame milk. Ann. Biochem. Exp. Med., 21:143–150, 1961.

78. Raiha, N. C. R., Heinonen, K., Rassin, D. K., Gaull, G. E.: Milk protein quantity and quality of low-birthweight infants. I. Metabolic responses and effects on growth. Pediatrics, 57:659–674, 1976.

79. Zeigler, E. E., and Fomon, S. J.: Fluid intake, renal solute load, and water balance in infancy. J. Pediatr., 78:561–568, 1971.

80. Book, L. S., Herbst, J. J., Atherton, S. O., Jung, A. L.: Necrotizing enterocolitis in low-birth-weight infants fed an elemental formula. J. Pediatr., 87:602–605, 1975.

81. Ziegler, E. E., Biga, R. L., and Fomon, S. J.: Nutrition requirements of the premature infant. *In* Suskind, R. M. (ed.): Textbook of Pediatric Nutrition. New York, Raven Press, 1981, pages 29–40.

82. Melhorn, D. K., Gross, S.: Vitamin E-dependent anemia in the premature infant. I. Effects of large doses of medicinal iron. J. Pediatr., 79:569–580, 1971.

83. Melhorn, D. K., Gross, S.: Vitamin E-dependent anemia in the premature infant. II. Relationships between gestational age and absorption of Vitamin E. J. Pediatr., 79:581–588, 1971.

84. American Academy of Pediatrics, Committee on Nutrition: Nutritional needs of low-birth-weight infants. Pediatrics, 60:519–530, 1977.

85. Day, G. M., Chance, G. W., Radde, I. C., Reilly, B. J., Park, E., and Sheepers, J.: Growth and mineral metabolism in very low birth weight infants. II. Effects of calcium supplementation on growth and divalent cations. Pediatr. Res., 9:568–575, 1975.

86. Antonson, D. L., Smith, J. L., Nelson, R. D., Jr., Anderson, A. K., Vanderhoof, J. A.: Vitamin and mineral content of a low-birth-weight infant formula during continuous enteral feeding [Abstract]. J.P.E.N., 5:563, 1981.

87. Shenai, J. P., Jhaveri, B. M., Reynolds, J. W., Huston, R. K., and Babson, S. G.: Nutritional balance studies in very-low-birth-weight infants: Role of soy formula. Pediatrics, 67:631–637, 1981.

88. National Diet Heart Study: Final report. Circulation, 37(Suppl. 1):1–428, 1968.

89. Prasad, A. S., and Oberleas, D.: Zinc deficiency in man. Lancet, 1(7855):463–464, 1974.

90. American Academy of Pediatrics, Committee on Nutrition: Special diets for infants with inborn errors of amino acid metabolism. Pediatrics, 57:783–791, 1976.

CHAPTER 11

Modular Feeding

MAUREEN M. MACBURNEY
DANNY O. JACOBS
KEITH N. APELGREN
GEORGE MELNIK
JOHN L. ROMBEAU

Standard nutritional formulas can successfully maintain the nutritional status of most patients. There are, however, patients for whom standard formulas may not be optimal and who might benefit from modular feedings.

A module consists of single or multiple nutrients that can be either combined to produce a nutritionally complete feeding or used individually to enhance an existing "fixed ratio" formula.[1, 2] The modular concept allows the physician to alter the ratio of a constituent nutrient without affecting other nutrients. Hence, nutritional deficits may be repleted with a module specific to the needs of individual patients.

This chapter will discuss the types of modules and the rationale and indications for their use. Further discussion will include pertinent issues in nutritional assessment, administration, and preparation. Advantages, disadvantages, complications, and patient monitoring will also be addressed.

BASIC MODULES

As a starting point, a base-line module consisting of a combination of nutrients such as fat, carbohydrate, or protein may be used. These base-line formulas are classified as modules because they are nutritionally incomplete and must be combined with other products.[3-6]

The major types of modules available for commercial use are carbohydrate, fat, and protein (Table 11–1). Vitamin, mineral, and electrolyte modules for enteral use are being developed, but they are not yet commercially available.

Some of the major carbohydrate, protein, and fat modules available for commercial use and their amino acid contents are listed in Tables 11–2 and 11–3. Vitamin, mineral, and electrolyte modules are also commercially available, although they are generally marketed as preparations for parenteral use.

Carbohydrate Modules. Carbohydrate modules differ primarily in form and concentration. The form (for example, starch or simple glucose) determines the osmolality, sweetness, and digestibility. The larger the carbohydrate molecule, the less osmotic pressure and sweetness there will be. There are four common modular sources of carbohydrate: polysaccharides and oligosaccha-

Table 11–1 CHARACTERISTICS OF SUBSTRATE MODULES

CARBOHYDRATE
Readily combines with most liquid formulas
Variable contribution to osmotic load
Variable caloric contribution
Easily digested in all forms
Low cost

FAT
May form interfaces in formula
Little contribution to osmolality
High caloric contribution
Variable digestibility
Low cost (except MCT)

PROTEIN
Insolubility of powders
Little contribution to osmolality (except crystalline amino acids)
Variable caloric contribution
Variable digestibility
High cost

Table 11–2   ENTERAL MODULES*

PRODUCT	MANUFACTURER	CHO (gm)	PRO (gm)	FAT (gm)	NA (mEq)	K (mEq)	CL (mEq)	P (mEq)	CA (mEq)	OSMOL	SOURCE
Carbohydrates											
Polycose	Ross										
Powder		250	—	—	12	neg	14	neg	neg	†	Glucose polymers
Liquid		254	—	—	13	neg	15	neg	neg	850	
Meducal	Mead Johnson										
Powder		250	—	—	6	neg	12	neg	—	†	Glucose polymers
Liquid		250	—	—	7	neg	12	neg	—	810	
SumaCal	Organon	250	—	—	14	neg	12	neg	neg	860	Glucose polymers
Hycal	Beecham-Massengill	244	—	—	3	neg	neg	2	neg		Glucose
Cal Plus	Henkel	235	—	—	12	neg				†	Glucose polymers
Sugar											
Sucrose		250	—	—	—	—	—	—	—	†	Disaccharide
Dextrose		250	—	—	—	—	—	—	—	†	Monosaccharide
Fat											
Microlipid	Organon	—	—	111	—	—	—	—	—	80	Safflower oil emulsion
Lipomul	Upjohn	—	—	111	neg	neg	neg	neg	neg		Corn oil emulsion
MCT	Mead Johnson	—	—	121	—	—	—	—	—		Fractionated coconut oil
Vegetable oil		—	—	111	—	—	—	—	—		Vegetable oil
Protein											
Casec	Mead Johnson	—	237	5	18	—	—	126	216	†	Calcium caseinate
Promix	Navaco	25	225	0	20	—	—	—	—	†	Whey
EMF	Control Drugs	42	208	0	44	4	40	9	—		Hydrolyzed collagen
Aminess Tablet	Cutter	trace	230	neg	neg	neg	neg	neg	neg	1200	Crystalline essential amino acids
Combination											
Controlyte	Doyle	143	neg	48	neg	neg		1	neg	598‡	Polysac/soybean oil
Hepatic Aid-Liquid	McGaw	175	26	22	neg	neg	neg	neg	neg	900‡	Crystalline amino acid
Travasorb (Hepatic)§	Travenol	144	28	13	18	27	18	25	18	690‡	Crystalline amino acid, glucose polymers, MCT, sunflower oil
Travasorb (Renal)	Travenol	203	17	13	neg	neg	neg	neg	neg	590‡	Crystalline amino acid, glucose polymers, sucrose, sunflower oil
Amin-Aid Liquid	McGaw	176	10	33	neg	neg	neg	neg	neg	1050‡	Crystalline amino acids, glucose polymers, soybean oil

*Per 1000 kcal
†Varies with concentration
‡At standard dilution
§Contains some vitamins

Table 11–3 AMINO ACID COMPOSITION OF ENTERAL MODULES

	AMIN-AID (per package)	HEPATIC-AID (per package)	TRAVASORB RENAL (per package)	TRAVASORB HEPATIC (per package)	AMINESS (per tablet)	CASEC (per 100 gm)	GEVERAL (per 100 gm)	PRO MIX (per 100 gm)	PROPAC (per 100 gm)
Carbohydrate (gm)	124.3	97.7	94.7	73.2	0.05	88	60.1	88	76.9
Fat (gm)	15.7	12.3	6.2	5.0	0.02	2	—	—	—
Protein	6.6	14.5	8.0	10.0	0.69	—	—	—	—
Total Nitrogen (gm)	0.8	2.23	1.26	1.55	0.088	—	—	—	—
Total Calories	665	560	467	376	3.1	—	—	—	—
Non-protein Calories	638	500	435	338	trace	—	—	—	—
Kilocalories						370	351	360	400
Amino Acids (gm)									
L-Leucine	1.1	2.008	0.74	2.0	1.1	8.80	4.97	12.8	10.6
L-Methionine	1.1	0.182	0.70	0.13	1.1	2.50	1.50	3.7	2.4
L-Phenylalanine	1.1	0.180	0.60	0.10	1.1	4.83	2.70	4.3	3.2
L-Lysine Acetate	1.1	1.575	0.78	0.21	—	7.51	4.43	10.6	8.0
L-Lysine HCl	—	—	—	1.22	—	—	—	—	—
L-Lysine (Free Base)	0.8	1.116	0.55	1.17	0.8	—	—	—	—
L-Valine	0.8	1.533	0.92	1.33	0.8	6.30	3.90	6.1	6.6
L-Isoleucine	0.7	1.643	0.62	1.67	0.7	5.01	3.30	5.8	6.2
L-Threonine	0.5	0.820	0.46	0.37	0.5	3.63	2.63	5.8	7.6
L-Tryptophan	0.25	0.120	0.20	0.10	0.25	1.12	0.63	2.5	1.9
L-Histidine	0.25	0.438	0.52	0.33	0.55	2.76	1.67	2.5	1.7
Glycine	—	1.643	0.43	0.33	—	1.73	1.67	2.3	1.9
L-Proline	—	1.460	0.46	0.73	—	10.27	7.13	6.2	6.4
L-Alanine	—	1.397	0.68	0.57	—	3.28	1.87	5.5	5.0
L-Arginine	—	1.095	0.64	1.17	—	3.54	2.20	3.5	2.8
L-Serine	—	0.912	0.43	—	—	4.40	3.97	5.1	6.1
L-Tyrosine	—	—	0.06	—	—	5.01	3.97	4.1	3.4
Cystine	—	—	—	—	—	0.26	0.20	4.1	2.3
Aspartic Acid	—	—	—	—	—	6.65	4.47	11.9	10.7
Glutamic Acid	—	—	—	—	—	21.06	14.13	18.2	17.3

rides, disaccharides, glucose polymers, and monosaccharides.

Polysaccharides have more than 10 saccharide units. Oligosaccharides are soluble polymers of glucose containing 5 or more glucose molecules. Disaccharides are composed of 2 saccharide units. Commonly used disaccharides are sucrose, lactose, and maltose. Maltose is a by-product of starch and oligosaccharide digestion. Glucose polymers are prepared by the partial hydrolysis of corn starch and include a mixture of polysaccharides, oligosaccharides, maltodextrins, corn syrup, and corn syrup solids. Glucose (dextrose) and fructose are monosaccharides commonly used in modular formulas.

Polysaccharides require pancreatic amylase to initiate digestion. Oligosaccharides are hydrolyzed by enzymes in the intestinal mucosa, and pancreatic amylase is not needed. Disaccharides require specific enzyme activity in the intestinal mucosa for hydrolysis. Monosaccharides can be absorbed directly.

In general, carbohydrates combine easily with liquid formulas and are easily digested except for starch, which is relatively insoluble. As mentioned previously, the size of the carbohydrate molecule primarily determines osmolality. Monosaccharides and disaccharides, which are relatively small molecules, significantly increase osmolality. Glucose polymers are frequently used in modular feeding because they contribute less to the osmotic load than equivalent weights of glucose or dextrose. Modules based on glucose polymers have a higher caloric density than those based on smaller carbohydrate molecules. Compared with other modules, carbohydrate modules are relatively inexpensive.

Fat Modules. Butterfat, vegetable (corn, soy, safflower, or sunflower) oils, and fat emulsions are the major sources of fat in feeding modules. These modules provide fat primarily as long-chain (more than 12 carbons) triglycerides (LCT). Another fat module is medium-chain (6 to 12 carbons) triglycerides (MCT), which are more water-soluble than LCT and are digested and absorbed more readily. The intraluminal hydrolysis of MCT is more rapid and complete than that of LCT. MCT may not require pancreatic lipase for absorption and are transported directly to the portal system. Modules based on MCT are particularly useful when there is significant fat malabsorption or maldigestion.

Fat modules that contain polyunsaturated fatty acids (for example, Microlipid or Lipomul; see Table 11–2) tend to oxidize, especially when exposed to light and warm temperatures. Antioxidants are present in the commercial formulas that contain polyunsaturated fatty acids.

Vegetable oils (LCT) are a rich source of essential fatty acids, but MCT, prepared from the fractionation of coconut oil, are not. Hence essential fatty acid deficiencies may develop when MCT are the sole source of fatty acids. Vegetable oils or MCT are the most common fat sources used in fat modules.

Fat modules are relatively insoluble; however, they contribute little to the osmolality. They may form oil-water interfaces with standard feeding formulas, but this does not impair digestion or absorption. Fat modules have high caloric densities and are concentrated energy sources. Like carbohydrate modules, fat modules are relatively inexpensive, except for those that are based on MCT.

Protein Modules. Intact protein, hydrolyzed protein, and crystalline amino acids are the three main protein sources in modular formulas. The osmolality, palatability, and nutritional value of protein modules vary with the protein source. Formulas based on intact protein are generally more palatable than those based on synthetic amino acids, which may have an unpleasant odor and taste. For this reason, synthetic amino acids are usually administered by tube.

The nutritional value of the protein source can be assessed by determining the chemical score (a comparison of the amino acid composition of the protein source with a standard amino acid pattern) and biologic value (the per cent of absorbed nitrogen retained by the body). Whereas the chemical score is a fixed number, the biologic value of a protein module may vary with the physiologic state of the patient. Modules derived from the intact proteins of casein and whey are of high biologic value. Modules based on free amino acids should have profiles modeled after these proteins.

Intact proteins such as puréed beef, egg white solids, lactalbumin, whey, and sodium and calcium caseinates require complete digestion to smaller peptides before absorption. Hydrolyzed proteins are protein sources that have been enzymatically or chemically cleaved to smaller peptides and free amino acids. Small peptides can be absorbed directly, whereas larger peptides must undergo further hydrolysis. As the protein molecules become smaller, they contribute more to the osmotic load. Common sources of hydrolyzed protein are casein, whey, soy, meat, lactalbumin, and collagen. Crystalline amino acids can be absorbed directly as they require no further digestion; however, absorption may not be as efficient as with a combination of amino acids, dipeptides and tripeptides. The small amino acid molecules significantly increase osmolality and may adversely affect taste. Protein modules are commonly based on caseinates, whey, collagen, and crystalline amino acids. Protein modules based on essential amino acids or with high ratios of branched-chain to aromatic amino acids may benefit patients with renal or hepatic insufficiency.

Protein modules are relatively insoluble, especially those produced in powder form, and are expensive as compared with fat and carbohydrate modules.

Vitamin and Mineral Modules. Vitamin and mineral modules are being developed for enteral use. In general, vitamin modules contain 100 per cent of the recommended dietary allowances (RDA) of essential vitamins for the adult population wherein they are established. Mineral modules often contain standard electrolytes such as calcium, sodium, and potassium, in addition to essential trace elements, in recommended dietary allowances.

Mineral modules that have different electrolyte contents are also being developed. For example, a sodium and potassium "restricted" module that contains 100 per cent of the RDA for trace materials could be used in patients with congestive heart failure and renal insufficiency.

RATIONALE

Modular feedings are useful in patients with highly specialized nutritional requirements or specific intolerances. Intolerance is manifested as a fixed-ratio formula incompatibility. Modular feeding with different ratios of fat to carbohydrate to protein may ameliorate or eliminate the signs and symptoms of intolerance and allow the patient to

become anabolic. One can select not only the amount of each nutrient but also the extent of nutrient predigestion—for example, whole protein versus partially hydrolyzed protein versus amino acids. Modular feeding allows great flexibility in administering the exact feeding mixture needed by a particular patient. This "prescription nutrition" has potential as a means of optimizing the patient's nutritional status within the context of specific diseases.

Modular feeding may be useful in two general situations. In institutions with small numbers of patients who require tube feeding, a wide range of fixed-ratio formulas must be purchased and stored to provide an adequate selection. Modular feeding could potentially be more cost-effective by allowing the physician to prescribe formulas that suit the patients' needs exactly from supplies in stock. The second situation for use of modular feedings is in highly specialized and homogeneous populations, such as patients with renal disease or burns. Modular feedings are theoretically ideal for these groups, as their nutritional requirements are varied.

INDICATIONS

Most patients can achieve nutritional repletion or maintenance with standard fixed-ratio formulas. Probably only a few patients who receive enteral nutrition require modular formulas.[7] In these patients, the use of a modular formula may avoid the need for parenteral nutrition. One must identify those patients who have specific metabolic or fluid imbalances that preclude the administration of standard formulas.

There are recognized subgroups of patients who may benefit from modular feedings (Table 11–4). However, this efficacy has only been investigated in nonrandomized studies.[8–10] Patients with hepatic insufficiency may require a decreased protein intake to avoid precipitating encephalopathy. Some data suggest that these patients have altered plasma aminograms with deficiencies of the branched-chain amino acids leucine, isoleucine, and valine.[11] Thus patients with liver failure, cirrhosis, and ascites may benefit from a feeding formula of high caloric density and low sodium content, enriched with branched-chain amino acids.

Smith et al. noted that formulas used to

Table 11-4   INDICATIONS AND SPECIAL REQUIREMENTS FOR MODULAR FEEDING

INDICATIONS	SPECIAL REQUIREMENTS
Hepatic failure	Protein modification (branched-chain amino acids), electrolytes, fluid
Renal failure	Protein modification (essential amino acids), renal solute load, electrolytes, fluid
Diabetes	Glucose restriction
Cardiac failure	Fluid, electrolytes
Malabsorption, short bowel syndrome	Predigested nutrients, osmotic load
Acid-base and electrolyte disorders	Electrolytes

nourish malnourished, cirrhotic, ascitic patients with protein intolerance have an excess of water, sodium, and occasionally protein.[8] Using a modular formula of high caloric density and variable sodium and protein content, they were successful in alimenting cirrhotic patients, as shown by improved serum albumin level, creatinine-height, and anthropometric measures.

Patients with acute renal insufficiency may benefit when alimented with a formula that includes essential amino acids.[6] These patients may also have specific protein, fluid, and electrolyte requirements that cannot be met with fixed-ratio formulas. As noted in the patient with hepatic disease, modular feeding will allow the enteral formulas of the patient with renal failure to be tailored to specific needs.

Other patients who might benefit from modular feedings include diabetic patients, adults and children with burns, and patients with malabsorption or short bowel syndrome.

NUTRITIONAL ASSESSMENT

Patients who receive modular formulas must undergo a thorough nutritional assessment, including serial biochemical assays and a calculation of energy expenditure. The patient must be evaluated for specific nutrient requirements. The digestive and absorptive capacity of the gastrointestinal tract must be known. Once the evaluation is completed and the route of administration chosen, a modular formula can be developed.

PREPARATION OF FEEDING MODULES

The following comments represent the experiences with modular feeding at the Philadelphia Veterans Administration Medical Center.

The pharmacist prepares the modular formula with the guidance and input of physicians, dietitians, and nurses. Care is needed to avoid critical omissions or excesses of one or more components. The key is meticulous attention to detail. Our diets are prepared by the Nutrition Support Service Pharmacist. Each formula is prepared in a color-coded container that is also used for storage. This facilitates identification of the formula by the nursing staff.

Incompatibility among formulas is perhaps best avoided by using modules marketed by the same company. This may be optimal when the patient's diet will be made from separate nutrient modules. Supplementing a fixed-ratio formula with a single nutrient module is less apt to cause incompatibilities.

Quality control may be more difficult with modular feeding than with standardized feeding because many different formulas may be in use at any one time. Quality control may mandate larger pharmaceutical staffs.

Formulas do not require sterile preparation[12, 13] but we have opted for clean handling techniques. Formulas are prepared in the pharmacy at room temperature. Our experience with modular components produced by one manufacturer indicates that mixing the protein source first ensures uniform dispersion. We use a 4-L cylindrical flask and a long pharmaceutical spatula to aid in mixing. After the protein is stirred into solution, vitamins, carbohydrates, and minerals are added; fat is the final addition. The resulting formula is placed in color-coded, sterile, plastic, 1-L bottles, which are capped and refrigerated until needed. We do not exceed a storage time of 24 hours because we believe that this decreases the likelihood of contamination and decreases oxidation in those formulas that contain polyunsaturated fatty acids. Furthermore, if the patient's requirements are changing daily, preparation of formula more than 24 hours in advance could be inappropriate and wasteful.

The stability of the final solution depends primarily on its fat content. Emulsifiers, like lecithin and carboxymethylcellulose, may be used to increase stability. Although emulsifiers are probably not needed if the fat content is no more than 30 to 40 per cent of the total energy intake, they may be necessary with higher fat contents and extended hang times. Whole or hydrolyzed proteins and complex carbohydrates will also help to stabilize the fat module.

The pH and protein source of the modular formula will influence the solubility and hence the availability of the protein components. For example, casein is best utilized at the neutral pH, whereas whey is efficiently utilized in an acid pH range. Casein-based modules are useful when high-protein feedings (more than 15 per cent of the total formula) are needed, as they tend to be less viscous than the other protein sources.

The daily diet is placed in an enteral feeding bag and administered over eight-hour intervals. We do this to maximize nursing convenience and to decrease hang times. Shortening hang times during administration may avoid rapid bacterial overgrowth.[12, 13]

COMPLICATIONS AND PREVENTION

Although the advantages of modular feeding are significant, there are potential disadvantages (Table 11–5). The intermixing of various feeding modules to produce a nutritionally complete formula requires considerable expertise in enteral feeding.[6] The

Table 11–5 MODULAR FEEDING TECHNIQUES

ADVANTAGES

Can be tailored to individual patient requirements and gastrointestinal function
May avoid parenteral nutrition in selected patients
May be cost-effective in highly selective situations

DISADVANTAGES

Requires advanced enteral expertise
Increased labor costs
Increased formula costs
Increased monitoring costs
Deficiency states if one module is disregarded
Greater potential for metabolic complications

preparation of feeding modules may be expensive, time consuming, and inconvenient. Careful technique is required to avoid deficiency states and metabolic complications.[14, 15] Each type of feeding module may be associated with particular complications (Table 11–6). Like parenteral nutrition, modular feeding is associated with complications that occur secondary to the use of isolated nutrients and to formulation errors. The safety of modular feeding is largely dependent on the expertise of the person supervising the formula.

Formulas high in carbohydrate may cause osmotic diarrhea and dehydration. In these patients, decreasing the osmolality of the feeding solution will often solve the problem. Hyperglycemia, glycosuria, and the resultant osmotic diuresis can occur secondary to excessive carbohydrate intake in patients with inadequate production of insulin. Overfeeding of carbohydrate has been associated with the development of fatty livers and an increased risk of ventilatory failure secondary to increased CO_2 production.[7] Rebound hypoglycemia may occur secondary to sudden decreases in the rate at which the formula is administered.

Fat modules that are deficient in linoleic acid (such as low-fat diets or modules in which MCT are the sole source of fat) are associated with essential fatty acid deficiencies. To prevent these deficiencies, 1 to 3 per cent of total calories should be administered as linoleic acid. Formulas that have an excess of fat can delay gastric emptying and cause diarrhea if fat is maldigested. Patients with liver insufficiency may have a decreased capacity to oxidize fatty acids from MCT.

Hyperosmolar amino acid or high-protein formulas can precipitate an osmotic diarrhea in the same manner as hyperosmolar carbohydrate formulas. Patients with inadequate fluid intakes who are given protein modules may develop prerenal azotemia.

Recently, Smith, Arteaga, and Heymsfield compared the biologic value of High Nitrogen Vivonex (Norwich—Eaton Pharmaceuticals, Norwich, New York) and solid food and predigested protein (Criticare-HN, Mead Johnson, Evansville, Indiana).[16] These diets are low in fat and contain recommended amounts of the known essential nutrients. Smith et al. were able to demonstrate poor nitrogen retention with High Nitrogen Vivonex as compared with the

Table 11–6 POTENTIAL COMPLICATIONS OF MODULAR ENTERAL NUTRITION

MODULE	POSSIBLE CAUSES	SOLUTION
Carbohydrate		
Osmotic diarrhea, dehydration	Hyperosmolar formula due to high carbohydrate level	Decrease carbohydrate intake Increase fluid intake
Hyperglycemia, glucosuria, osmotic diuresis	Excessive carbohydrate intake, inadequate insulin, underlying diabetes mellitus	Decrease carbohydrate intake Increase fat intake Administer insulin
Fatty liver	Excess carbohydrate intake or inadequate protein intake	Increase protein intake Decrease carbohydrate intake
Increased CO_2 production	Excess carbohydrate intake	Decrease carbohydrate intake Increase fat intake
Rebound hypoglycemia	Sudden changes in rate of feeding	Taper over at least 12 hours
Fat		
Essential fatty acid deficiency	Inadequate linoleic acid intake; MCT as sole source of fat	Administer 1–3% of calories as linoleic acid (LCT)
Diarrhea due to fat maldigestion	Excessive fat in formula; pancreatic or biliary insufficiency; short bowel syndrome	Decrease level of fat intake
Decreased gastric motility	Excessive per cent of calories as fat	Decrease level of fat intake
Protein		
Osmotic diarrhea	Hyperosmolar formula due to the use of amino acids	Increase fluid Decrease amino acids
Pre-renal azotemia	Excessive protein intake Inadequate non-protein calories Inadequate fluid	Decrease protein Increase non-protein calories Increase fluid
Amino acid imbalance	Inappropriate amino acid profile; altered amino acid utilization	Assure a balanced amino acid profile Utilize specialized amino acid mixtures
Vitamins		
Deficiencies	Inadequate administration in proportion to calories administered Omission in formula Increased requirements in specific disease states	Increase intake
Toxicities	Excessive administration of fat-soluble vitamins	Decrease intake
Interference with medications	Vitamin K (warfarin); folic acid (methotrexate)	Omit for selected patients

Minerals/Trace Elements		
Deficiencies	Inadequate administration (Fe, Zn, Cu, Mn, Cr, I)	Increase intake
Toxicities	Excessive administration	Decrease intake
Electrolytes		
Hypokalemia	Inadequate intake for anabolism Diuretic use Renal losses	Increase intake
Hyperkalemia	Excessive intake Renal failure	Decrease intake Monitor renal function
Hypophosphatemia	Inadequate intake for anabolism	Increase intake
Hyperphosphatemia	Excessive intake Renal failure	Decrease intake
Hypocalcemia	Inadequate intake Hypoalbuminemia Phosphorus repletion without simultaneous calcium repletion Associated hypomagnesemia	Increase intake Increase magnesium intake
Hypercalcemia	Excessive intake	Decrease intake
Hypomagnesemia	Inadequate intake for anabolism	Increase intake
Hypermagnesemia	Renal failure	Decrease intake

other diets. During the study periods, the percentage of retained nitrogen was 9 to 16 times higher with food and Criticare-HN. Furthermore, blood and urinary urea nitrogen levels were higher when the patients were given High Nitrogen Vivonex. The differences in nitrogen retention between the two synthetic amino acids were thought to be most likely secondary to their different nonessential amino acid profiles. The Criticare-HN diet had a more balanced distribution of nonessential amino acids. Thus the amino acid profile of amino acid modules should be carefully balanced to optimize nitrogen retention.

Modular feeding may cause vitamin, trace metal, and mineral deficiencies or toxicities. Intact protein modules have a significant and potentially variable mineral content, even though the protein sources are demineralized commercially. For example, modules based on casein commonly are high in calcium content. To avoid difficulties, with each adjustment in the volume, composition, and concentration of a formula, the vitamin, trace metal, and mineral content should be intermittently reassessed. Unrecognized drug-nutrient interactions can also have adverse consequences. For example, excess vitamin K in enteral feedings can interfere with the activity of coumadin.[17]

Electrolyte concentrations are the most frequently adjusted component in formulas. As is the case with parenteral nutrition, excesses and deficiencies can readily occur. Hypokalemia, hypophosphatemia, and hypomagnesemia may occur in patients who are depleted and being refed and therefore are inadequately supplemented. Patients given diuretics may also become hypokalemic. Patients with renal failure tend to develop hyperkalemia, hyperphosphatemia, and hypermagnesemia. Hypocalcemia may occur secondary to inadequate calcium intake, or to hypoalbuminemia and administration of phosphorus without concomitant repletion of calcium. These complications are less apt to occur with careful monitoring of the specific electrolyte level.

The osmolar concentration and viscosity of the final module is an important determinant of the method of delivery. Formulas of greater than 750 mOsm/L can be delivered into the stomach but may be poorly tolerated in the jejunum. The diameter of some jejunal tubes may limit the administration of modular formulas. Modules based on intact protein, for example, may be too viscous to flow easily through tubes (especially those less than 5 French) and are more likely to congeal and subsequently obstruct.

MONITORING

All patients who receive tube feedings require nutritional and metabolic monitoring. Patients who receive modular formulas, however, require more thorough monitoring, since the risks of nutrient deficiencies and imbalances, fluid and electrolyte aberrations, and formula contamination are significant. Biochemical monitoring is essential. Daily assessment of fluid and electrolyte balance, blood glucose, and blood urea nitrogen is recommended until the patient's condition stabilizes. Weekly monitoring of total protein, albumin, triglycerides, transferrin, liver function, and other indices may be necessary, depending on the patient's metabolic status. Accurate intake and output records are vital, especially when the patient is receiving a concentrated formula. Patients should be weighed daily to help monitor fluid balance. A summary of recommended tests is provided in Table 11–7. The dietitian should be responsible for reviewing formulas for nutritional adequacy. Daily calorie counts are needed to document energy and

Table 11–7   MONITORING OF THE PATIENT ON MODULAR FEEDING

*Daily**	Electrolytes
	Blood glucose
	BUN and creatinine
	Urine for sugar and acetone
	Fluid balance
	Body weight
	Calorie count
Twice Weekly	Phosphorus
	Calcium
	Magnesium
Weekly	Total protein
	Triglycerides
	Liver function tests
	Total iron-binding capacity
Monthly	Serum B_{12}, folate, zinc, iron, trace minerals, as indicated

*First week minimum

protein intake. Appropriate intakes of vitamins, minerals, and electrolytes must be ensured. During formula preparation, strict quality control must be maintained to ensure accuracy of composition. In addition, meticulous handling techniques will avoid bacterial contamination.

USE OF MODULAR FEEDINGS

Hepatic Insufficiency. Patients with hepatic failure may need protein, sodium, and fluid restrictions. Some data have suggested that these patients may benefit from parenteral formulas enriched with branched-chain amino acids.[11]

Standard feeding formulas, which generally provide large amounts of protein (approximately 35 gm/1000 kcal), may be poorly tolerated when sufficient formula is given to achieve the caloric prescription. High caloric density formulas may also have an excess of protein when these formulas provide the sole nutrient source. However, high caloric density formulas may be combined with a complex carbohydrate (such as Polycose, Ross Laboratories, Columbus, Ohio) and MCT (Mead Johnson, Evansville, Indiana) module to yield a formula that is low in protein, sodium, and free water but provides sufficient calories for protein repletion.

Renal Failure. Similarly, patients with renal failure need decreased solute loads to minimize urea formation. Urea formation may be reduced by formulas enriched in essential amino acids, which are commercially available. High caloric density formulas are also useful in these patients, who may require fluid restriction. Furthermore, these patients may benefit from formulas with increased calorie-to-nitrogen ratios and low levels of potassium. Modular formats are particularly suited to the needs of these patients. Amin-Aid (American McGaw, Irvine, California) is a high caloric density (2.0 kcal/ml), low sodium and potassium, essential amino acid base formula that can be used when temporary restriction of these nutrients is needed.[18] A low-protein formula can also be constructed using Osmolite (Ross Laboratories). Osmolite's protein source is whole casein, and 50 per cent of its fat content is LCT and 50 per cent MCT. An example of modular feeding for a patient with renal insufficiency is as follows: 960 ml of Osmolite, 310 ml of Polycose (Ross Labora-

tories), and 80 ml of Microlipid (Organon, West Orange, New Jersey).[19] This prescription provides approximately 2500 kcal and 702 mg of sodium in 1350 ml of fluid.

Cardiac Disease. Another group of patients who may benefit from modular high caloric density formulas are patients with cardiac cachexia and concomitant malabsorption. Varying the fat, carbohydrate, and protein content can have specific advantages. These patients normally need 0.6 to 1.0 gm of protein/kg body weight, approximately 0.5 ml of water/kcal administered (generally 1000 to 1500 ml), and 0.5 to 1.5 gm of sodium per day.[19] An example of a formula that meets these requirements and is appropriate for the patient who has fat and protein malabsorption in addition to congestive heart failure is as follows: 1400 ml of Vital (Ross Laboratories) and 120 ml of MCT oil. Vital is a formula that contains partially digested or hydrolyzed protein and small amounts of LCT. Thus it requires minimal digestion and provides approximately 2400 kcal, 536 mg of sodium, and 42 gm of protein in 1520 ml of fluid.

Diabetes. For diabetic patients who need concomitant fluid restriction, a different formula is needed. Providing carbohydrate in a complex form instead of as monosaccharides or disaccharides may increase glucose tolerance.[19] A typical formula is as follows: 750 ml of Polycose, 110 ml of Microlipid, and 47 gm of protein as Casec (Mead Johnson) in 200 ml of water. This formula provides 2000 nonprotein calories, 17 mEq of sodium, and 47 gm of protein in approximately 1 L of fluid. Vitamins and other minerals must be added to make this formula nutritionally complete.

These are just a few examples of the versatility of modular feedings. Formulas with many different combinations and contents can be constructed by adjusting the ratios of the various component modules.

PILOT STUDY

Recently modular feedings were used to nourish a small group of patients at the Philadelphia Veterans Administration Medical Center who were refractory to conventional fixed-formula diets. The purpose of this study was to determine the feasibility and efficacy of this method.

Five men ranging from 52 to 64 years of

age were studied in the Surgical Metabolic Unit. One had tonsillar carcinoma, two had gastric carcinoma, another was a stroke victim with an impaired gag reflex, and one had peptic ulcer disease and required surgery.

The patients were fed for 14 days with a modular diet developed by the Doyle Pharmaceutical Company (Minneapolis, Minnesota). The diet consisted of a crystalline source of amino acid, hydrolyzed egg white protein, a carbohydrate source of corn syrup solids, and a fat emulsion composed of safflower oil, MCT, and other fats. Free water and electrolytes were added to the formula to prevent imbalances. A vitamin and mineral supplement containing 100 per cent of the minimum daily adult requirements, as determined by the National Research Council, was also provided. Depending on the needs of the patient, protein comprised 8 to 15 per cent of the module, fat 38 to 43 per cent, and carbohydrate 45 to 54 per cent. The patients' daily caloric needs were determined by the Long modification of the Harris-Benedict equation.[20] Formulas were prepared daily by the nutrition support service pharmacist. Four of the five patients were fed by tube enterostomies, and one patient was fed by nasoenteric tube.

Once feedings were initiated, several nutritional indices were monitored. Body weights, nutritional intake, and fluid balance were recorded on a daily basis. Blood studies were obtained every third day. Twenty-four-hour urine collections for urea and stool nitrogen were performed on two patients. Three patients had serum transferrin determinations at the beginning and near the end of the study period.

Table 11–8 summarizes the study results. The mean caloric intake was 2448 kcal per day during the study period. Two patients lost weight and three gained weight during the study. All three patients who had serum transferrin determinations demonstrated an increased level of this protein at the end of the study. One patient with an increased serum transferrin level was in positive nitrogen balance by day 7 of the study.

Hyperkalemia developed in three patients. In two of these patients, hyperkalemia was thought to be secondary to the amount of potassium present in the protein module. In the third patient, hyperkalemia was thought to be secondary to hyporenin hypoaldosteronism. Hyperkalemia was managed by decreasing the concentration of the protein sources and modifying the vitamin and mineral modules. Two patients had diarrhea that required medication for control. No other complications were noted. It was concluded that modular feeding was a viable method of enteral alimentation.

FUTURE CONSIDERATIONS

Although modular feeding techniques have limited applications in most hospitals, some important concepts should be emphasized. First, the modulation of a fixed-ratio formula is easily achieved and may be applied in many clinical situations. Second, the concept of producing a "base-line" module is essential. Such a product would be composed of the irreducible minimum nutrients. This would eliminate much of the risk of administering inappropriate mixtures of single nutrient modules. Further modulation would be required but, in most instances, a safe starting point would be provided. Third, the principle of modular feeding is based upon the theoretical efficacy of prescription nutrition. Whether creating modular formulas from a base-line module or de novo from single nutrient modules, one is prescribing a specific product to meet the nutrient needs of a given patient.

Should feeding modules be considered nutritional formulas or pharmaceutical prep-

Table 11–8   PILOT STUDY OF MODULAR FEEDING

PATIENT	MEAN KCAL/DAY	BODY WEIGHT (KG)		SERUM TRANSFERRIN (MG/DL)		NITROGEN BALANCE (gm N/24 hr)
		Day 1	Day 14	Pre-Study	Completion of Study	
P.M.	2528	76.8	78	247	306	+2 (day 7)
G.S.	2409	54.7	54.2	—	—	—
J.H.	2505	56.8	57.3	254	303	—
T.P.	2544	79.5	77	—	—	−6.6 (day 13)
I.A.	2254	78.6	79.5	196	218 (day 10)	—

arations? The nature of the modules and the necessity of precise formulation often require that the pharmacy be involved in preparation. This is apparent when electrolytes, trace elements, specific amino acids, or pharmacologic doses of one module or another are added. The resolution of this issue is dependent upon the facilities and expertise within each institution.

As we learn more about the specific metabolic and nutrient requirements of different diseases, the advantages of prescription modular feeding may become more evident. More highly defined modules may ultimately be developed, necessitating an even greater sophistication in the understanding and use of nutrients. As modular formulas are used more frequently, protocols should be developed to ensure safety and proper monitoring techniques. These protocols could parallel those currently used for parenteral nutrition.

REFERENCES

1. Newmark, S. R., Simpson, S., Daniel, P., Sublett, D., Black, J., and Geller, R.: Nutritional support in an inpatient rehabilitation unit. Arch. Phys. Med. Rehabil., 62:634–637, 1981.
2. Griggs, B. A., Chernoff, R., Hoppe, M. C., and Wade, J.: Enteral alimentation. Presented at Third Clinical Congress of American Society for Parenteral and Enteral Nutrition, Thorofare, New Jersey, January 1979.
3. McIntire, B., and Wright, R. A.: Enteral alimentation: An update on new products. Nutr. Supp. Serv., 1(8):7, 10–12, 14, 1981.
4. Chernoff, R.: Nutritional support: formulas and delivery of enteral feeding. J. Am. Diet. Assoc., 79:426–429, 1981.
5. Matarese, L. E.: Enteral alimentation: Oral and tube feedings. Part I. Nutr. Supp. Serv., 1(8):41–42, 1981.
6. Heymsfield, S. B., Horowitz, J., and Lawson, D. H.: Enteral hyperalimentation. In Berk, J. E.

(ed.): Developments in Digestive Diseases, Volume 3. Philadelphia, Lea & Febiger, 1980, pages 59–83.
7. Freed, B. A., Hsia, B., Smith, J. P., and Kaminski, M. V.: Enteral nutrition: Frequency of formula modification. J. P. E. N., 5:40–45, 1981.
8. Smith, J., Horowitz, J., Henderson, J. M., and Heymsfield, S.: Enteral hyperalimentation in undernourished patients with cirrhosis and ascites. Am. J. Clin. Nutr., 35:56–72, 1982.
9. Coale, M. S., and Robson, J. R. K.: Dietary management of intractable diarrhea in malnourished patients. J. Am. Diet. Assoc., 76:444–450, 1980.
10. Klish, W. J., Potts, E., Ferry, G. D., and Nichols, B. L.: Modular formula: An approach to the management of infants with specific or complex food intolerances. J. Pediatr., 88:948–952, 1976.
11. Fischer, J. E., Rosen, H. M., Ebeid, A. M., James, J. H., Keane, J. M., Soeters, P. B.: The effect of normalization of plasma amino acids on hepatic encephalopathy in man. Surgery, 80:77–91, 1976.
12. Martin, D. J.: Modular tube feeding. Nutr. Supp. Serv., 1(4):40, 1981.
13. Casewell, M. W., Cooper, J. E., Webster, M.: Enteral feeds contaminated with Enterobacter cloacae as a cause of septicaemia. Br. Med. J., 282:973, 1981.
14. Vanlandingham, S., Simpson, S., Daniel, P., Newmark, S. R.: Metabolic abnormalities in patients supported with enteral tube feeding. J.P.E.N., 5:332–334, 1981.
15. Kaminski, M. V.: Enteral hyperalimentation: Prevention and treatment of complications. Nutr. Supp. Serv., 1(4):21, 1981.
16. Smith, J. E., Arteaga, C., and Heymsfield, S. B.: Increased ureagenesis and impaired nitrogen use during infusion of a synthetic amino acid formula: A controlled trial. N. Engl. J. Med., 306:1013–1018, 1982.
17. Zallman, J. A., Lee, D. P., and Jeffrey, P. L.: Liquid nutrition as a cause of warfarin resistance. Am. J. Hosp. Pharm., 38:1174, 1981.
18. Steffee, S. P.: Nutritional support in renal failure. Surg. Clin. North Am., 61:661–671, 1981.
19. Heymsfield, S. B., Smith, J., Redd, S., Whitworth, H. B., Jr.: Nutritional support in cardiac failure. Surg. Clin. North Am., 61:635–653, 1981.
20. Long, C. L., Schaffel, N., Geiger, J. W., Schiller, W. R., and Blakemore, W. S.: Metabolic response to injury and illness: Estimation of energy and protein needs from indirect calorimetry and nitrogen balance. J.P.E.N., 3:452–456, 1979.

CHAPTER 12

Defined Formula Diets: Palatability and Oral Intake

R. GREGG SETTLE

Of the three major routes available for nutritional support (oral, gastrointestinal, and intravenous), the oral route is probably the least understood and most underutilized. Nutritional support by the oral route requires that the voluntary ingestion of foodstuffs not only meet recommended dietary allowances but also correct prior deficiencies and meet the additional metabolic requirements of disease or trauma.

Palatability, the hedonic response of the individual to the flavor of the food to be ingested, is an important determinant of whether it will be consumed and in what quantity. Flavor broadly defined includes smell, taste, texture, and temperature. This chapter will briefly describe gustatory (taste) and olfactory (smell) anatomy and review studies on the palatability of defined formula diets and some factors that influence palatability and oral intake.

Olfaction. The olfactory epithelium, which contains the olfactory receptor neurons, lines the olfactory cleft: the lateral, superior, and medial walls of the uppermost passageway of the nasal cavity. Olfactory neurons are bipolar cells that serve as both the receptor organs and the primary afferent fibers. The dendritic (distal) ends give rise to cilia that project into the passageway and are bathed in mucus. The cilia are believed to contain the receptor sites that are stimulated by odorant molecules. The axons of the olfactory receptor neurons project centrally and combine into larger nerve bundles entering the cranium through a series of perforations in the bone, known as the cribriform plate. These bundles of axons form fila olfactoria, which project to the olfactory bulb, a region of complex synaptic interconnections. Most of the axons of second-order neurons in the olfactory bulb (mitral and tufted cells) project centrally as the lateral olfactory tract to various brain structures, including the anterior olfactory nucleus, olfactory tubercle, prepyriform cortex, amygdaloid complex, and transitional entorhinal cortex. Neurons in the olfactory tubercle, prepyriform cortex, and amygdaloid complex project to the hypothalamus, a region believed to be of major importance in regulating ingestive behaviors.[1] A discussion of the other central connections and centrifugal pathways to the olfactory bulb is beyond the scope of this chapter but may be found elsewhere.[2]

The olfactory system appears capable of discriminating a seemingly countless number of odors. Thus odors are generally described by the name of the object with which they are associated (for example, rose, orange, tar) rather than by a few generic names.[3]

People often refer to the entire range of flavor perceptions as "taste." However, taste usually plays a minor role in flavor perception, and much of what is considered "taste" is really olfaction. Many common foods lose their characteristic flavors when olfactory input is reduced or eliminated, as when the nostrils are held closed and inspiration is prevented, or during a cold that occludes the nasal passageway to the olfactory cleft.[4] Without smell (and without the aid of visual input), most common foods are not identifiable.[5] Without smell and vision, only texture and taste sensations are available, making it difficult to distinguish among such diverse foods as apples, potatoes, and onions.

Taste. Taste receptor cells are contained within specialized structures called taste buds. Taste buds are goblet-shaped nests of cells; the cells of the bud are arranged similarly to the segments of a grapefruit. At the apical end of the taste bud cells, microvilli project into a small opening in the epithelium at the top of the taste bud, a feature known as the "taste pore." Depending on the species and investigator, three types of taste bud cells have been described, one of which is believed to be the taste receptor cell. However, conclusions linking cell types to function are largely based on inferences from structure, and the cell types may simply represent different stages of development rather than distinct cell types.[6]

Taste buds are found on the dorsal and lateral surfaces of the tongue, the soft palate, epiglottis, pharynx, larynx, and uppermost segment of the esophagus. On the tongue, taste buds are found in three of the four morphologically distinct papillae: the *fungiform papillae,* which are shaped like button mushrooms and are found mainly on the tip and lateral edges of the dorsal surface of the tongue; the *circumvallate* (or simply *vallate*) *papillae,* which look like flat mounds surrounded by moats and are found on the posterior dorsal surface of the tongue arranged in a chevronlike row, with the more medial papillae located more posteriorly; and the *foliate papillae,* which form a set of folds on the posterior lateral surface of the tongue in some mammals but are vestigial in humans. The *filiform papillae,* which are conical and distributed over the entire dorsal surface of the tongue, contain no taste buds.

The nerve fibers that innervate the taste receptor cells form a subepithelial plexus and extend upward, winding around the taste cells and forming a synapse between the taste cells and the sensory nerve fiber. The anterior region of the tongue (the fungiform and perhaps the anterior foliate papillae) is innervated by the chorda tympani nerve, a branch of the seventh cranial (facial) nerve. Taste buds of the soft palate are innervated by the greater superficial petrosal nerve, also a branch of the seventh nerve. The posterior region of the tongue (the vallate and foliate papillae) is innervated by a lingual branch of the ninth (glossopharyn-

geal) nerve. The tenth (vagus) nerve presumably innervates the epiglottis, the entrance to the larynx, and the uppermost segment of the esophagus.[7]

Taste afferents entering via the seventh, ninth, and tenth cranial nerves terminate in the nucleus of the tractus solitarius. Secondary afferents arising from the nucleus of the tractus solitarius project to the pontine taste area located in the parabrachial nucleus of the dorsal pons. It is possible that the PTA receives primary ascending afferent fibers of the seventh, ninth, and tenth nerves as well. Afferents arising from the pontine taste area project to the thalamic taste area in the medial tip of the ventrobasal complex. Afferents arising from the pontine taste area and projecting to the thalamic taste area bifurcate and continue through the medial lemniscus to terminate in the lateral hypothalamus, the central nucleus of the amygdala, and the bed nucleus of the stria terminalis.[6] There are two thalamocortical taste nerve projection areas: TNI lies in the intraoral tactile projection area (somatosensory area I) and TNII is buried in the anterior opercular-insular cortex.[8] A discussion of other central connections and centrifugal pathways to relay nuclei is beyond the scope of this chapter but may be found elsewhere.[6]

Although the number of discriminable tastes is very large, many believe they are only combinations of four basic taste qualities (sweet, sour, salty, and bitter) or combinations of taste and odor or tactile stimulation.[9, 10]

STUDIES ON PALATABILITY

Although the literature on peroral feeding of enteral supplements makes frequent allusions to palatability as a limiting factor in their usage, relatively few palatability studies have been reported.[11–18]

Elemental Diets

Healthy Individuals. Seltzer and Quarantillo published the first study comparing the palatability of several elemental diets.[11] Sixty-four members of the Walson Army Hospital staff participated in an elemental diet "tasting" party. All diets were prepared according to the directions of the manufacturer on the afternoon before testing, stored overnight in the refrigerator, and served refrigerated. Participants were presented 10-cc samples in paper cups and were instructed to either swallow or spit out the sample and to rinse their mouths with water between samples. They rated each of the 18 diet–flavor combinations as good, fair or poor (Table 12–1).

The authors' description of "good," "fair," and "poor" is most enlightening:[11]

"Poor" usually meant that when the sample was tasted, the participant experienced a violent wave of nausea, occasionally retched, encountered tearing of the eyes, and demonstrated facial grimacing. This was a generally unpleasant experience.

"Fair" meant that the participant was able to taste or swallow the sample without most of the unpleasant reactions listed above; however, there was no real desire to consume additional quantities of the sample, as might be required to effect a therapeutic dose of calories.

"Good" was arrived at by eliminating "poor" and "fair." There were no participants who were enthusiastic about any of the samples. "Good" implied that the sample was more acceptable than the other samples, and could conceivably be ingested in sufficient quantities to supply adequate calories.

The most palatable diet (which is no longer available) managed a rating of "good" from only 28 per cent (18 of 64) of the participants while receiving a "poor" rating from

23 per cent (15 of 64). Sixty-one per cent of the 18 diet–flavor combinations each received a majority (50+ per cent) of "poor" ratings. No statistical analyses were performed, but the authors observed that in general the single fruit flavors of orange, cherry, strawberry, banana, and pineapple were accepted better than grape, tomato, and fruit combinations, and that "broths and bouillon were dismal failures."

Behl and associates undertook a large study of the ability of commercially available imitation flavors to mask the flavor or improve the acceptability of Vivonex HN.[12] The study was conducted in three phases. Various flavors and flavor combinations were compared. These studies were performed with and without the addition of Vivonex HN and with and without the addition of a sweetener (0.025 per cent sodium saccharin). Taste panels of 30 or more members of the faculty and student body of the Duquesne University School of Pharmacy participated in the various phases of the study. Subjects were given approximately 5 ml of each solution to drink through a clean straw and were asked to rate each product on a 10-point scale (10 = best, 9 = like extremely, 8 = like very much, 7 = like moderately, 6 = like slightly, 5 = neither like nor dislike, 4 = dislike slightly, 3 = dislike moderately, 2 = dislike very much, 1 = dislike extremely). Subjects were instructed to allow at least 10 minutes before tasting the next sample. Nei-

Table 12–1 PALATABILITY OF ELEMENTAL DIETS[11]

| DIET | FLAVOR | RATING (%) | | | |
		Good	Fair	Poor	% Good − % Poor
Jejunal	Orange-pineapple	28	48	23	+ 5
Vivonex HN	(with) Hawaiian Punch	20	41	39	− 19
Flexical	Banana	14	52	34	− 20
Jejunal	Cherry	14	47	39	− 25
Vivonex	Orange	9	53	38	− 29
Flexical	Orange	11	42	47	− 36
Vivonex	Strawberry	6	52	42	− 36
Flexical	Vanilla	16	30	55	− 38
WT Low Residue	Tomato	14	27	59	− 45
Vivonex	Chocolate	13	30	58	− 45
Flexical	Fruit punch	8	34	58	− 50
Jejunal	Fruit punch	3	36	61	− 58
WT Low Residue	Fruit punch	5	27	69	− 64
Vivonex	Grape	8	20	72	− 64
WT Low Residue	Chicken broth	3	19	78	− 75
Vivonex	Beef broth	0	23	88	− 88
Vivonex	Vanilla	0	8	92	− 92
WT Low Residue	Beef bouillon	0	5	95	− 95

ther the approximate temperature of the solutions nor the time period over which subjects were permitted to sample solutions was noted in the study.

After the initial screening of 16 different flavoring agents and combinations of them, the six highest-rated formulations were evaluated by a panel of 50 volunteers. The ratings of these flavors appear in Table 12–2 under the heading "Phase I." Two observations can be made: (1) Vivonex HN was unpalatable, and (2) the addition of flavoring agents significantly increased the palatability of Vivonex HN.

In Phase II of the study the effect of sweetening the solutions with saccharin was investigated for the two highest-rated single flavors and the two-flavor combination from Phase I and a three-flavor combination. The data are presented in Table 12–2 under the heading "Phase II." Again, two observations can be made: (1) Sweetening of flavor combinations containing Vivonex HN significantly increased their palatability, but the same was not true for single flavors; and (2) When mixed in water, (that is, without Vivonex HN) sweetened solutions of single flavors had higher pleasantness ratings than combination flavors. When mixed with Vivonex HN, however, the ratings for single flavors showed a sharp decline. Thus sweetened flavor combinations were more effective in masking (improving) the flavor of Vivonex HN, even though they were not inherently more palatable.

In Phase III an additional 14 flavoring agents were tested (Table 12–3). Overall, the

14 single-flavor Vivonex HN solutions were more palatable than those previously tested, and the combination-flavored Vivonex was the most palatable mixture tested during the study.

Finally, a panel evaluated the flavor of four flavor packets marketed by Eaton Laboratories for inclusion in their unflavored Vivonex HN. Data are presented in Table 12–4. The highest rating obtained for a flavor packet (4.9 ± 0.3) was lower than eight of the sweetened, flavored Vivonex HN solutions prepared by Behl and associates.[12] Also included in Table 12–4 are the rankings obtained by Seltzer and Quarantillo for flavored Vivonex Standard.[11] It is interesting that both Seltzer and Behl rank-ordered the manufacturer's flavorings similarly even though Behl used Vivonex HN and Seltzer used Vivonex Standard. They also agree that the "beef broth" flavoring was poor. However, there is one discrepancy between the studies. Seltzer and Quarantillo concluded that single-fruit flavors (such as orange, cherry, strawberry, banana, and pineapple) were more acceptable than combinations. Although this may be true for the flavorings produced by manufacturers of the diets they tested, the flavor combinations reported by Behl and colleagues received higher ratings than the single flavors.

The most recent study of the palatability of elemental diets examined form as well as flavor.[14] Two elemental diets (Flexical and Vivonex) were prepared according to package directions and combined with (a) orange Tang, (b) black cherry Jell-O, (c) grape Kool-

Table 12–2 PREFERENCE FOR FLAVORED SOLUTIONS OF VIVONEX HN TESTED IN PHASES I AND II[12]

FLAVORING AGENT(S)	PHASE I UNSWEETENED SOLUTIONS		PHASE II SWEETENED SOLUTIONS*	
	With Vivonex HN	Without Vivonex HN	With Vivonex HN	Without Vivonex HN
Orange Juice	4.34 ± 0.30[†]	5.97 ± 0.28	4.42 ± 0.31	6.94 ± 0.27
Sealva Mint #381	4.24 ± 0.29	6.66 ± 0.25	4.50 ± 0.31	8.02 ± 0.28
Cherry Mint	4.21 ± 0.29	4.90 ± 0.27	—	—
Orange Mint	4.00 ± 0.26	5.21 ± 0.29	—	—
Orange Juice and Butterscotch Maple	3.97 ± 0.26	5.41 ± 0.27	5.14 ± 0.33	5.86 ± 0.28
Butterscotch Maple	3.61 ± 0.25	5.18 ± 0.24	—	—
Orange Juice, Butterscotch Maple & Sealva Mint #381	(3.98 ± 0.54)[‡]	—	5.88 ± 0.34	6.14 ± 0.27
No flavoring	1.75 ± 0.15	—	?	—

*0.025% sodium saccharin concentration
[†]Values reported are means ± standard error of the mean.
[‡]From Phase II

Table 12–3 PREFERENCE FOR SWEETENED FLAVORED VIVONEX HN SOLUTIONS TESTED IN PHASE III[12]

FLAVORING AGENT(S)	SOLUTIONS WITH VIVONEX HN	SOLUTIONS WITHOUT VIVONEX HN
Rum	5.50 ± 0.29*	7.09 ± 0.23
Strawberry	5.47 ± 0.49	6.66 ± 0.43
Raspberry #21820 (Fritzsche)	5.44 ± 0.40	6.25 ± 0.35
Raspberry (Durkee)	5.25 ± 0.34	7.47 ± 0.26
Banana	5.09 ± 0.31	6.88 ± 0.29
Chocolate #23437	4.94 ± 0.32	—
Vanilla	4.81 ± 0.33	—
Almond Extract	4.78 ± 0.37	—
Butter	4.78 ± 0.33	—
Maple Vanilla #21712	4.78 ± 0.38	—
Coffee #22637	4.38 ± 0.46	—
Maplein Maple	4.03 ± 0.44	—
Coconut #19947	3.47 ± 0.45	—
Wine Raspberry #23295	3.41 ± 0.35	—
Rum, Strawberry and Raspberry #21820	6.34 ± 0.33	6.78 ± 0.21

*Values reported are means ± standard error of the mean.

Aid, and (d) strawberry flavor packet. The diets with Jell-O, Kool Aid, and the flavor packet were mixed, strained, refrigerated, and served at room temperature in 60-ml samples. The Tang samples were mixed, strained, divided into 30-ml aliquots, and served frozen. Seventy subjects—nutrition-related students and professionals—evaluated each sample. Water was used to rinse between samples to remove any lingering aftertaste. Participants rated samples on the basis of appearance, flavor, texture/consistency, and overall acceptability and palatability, using a 7-point scale (1 = extremely unacceptable, 2 = very unacceptable, 3 = moderately unacceptable, 4 = neither acceptable nor unacceptable, 5 = moderately acceptable, 6 = very acceptable, 7 = extremely acceptable).

Table 12–4 PREFERENCE FOR VIVONEX HN SOLUTION FLAVORED BY EATON "FLAVOR PACKETS,"[12] AND FLAVORED VIVONEX STANDARD SOLUTIONS[11]

FLAVORING	VIVONEX HN (X̄ ± SD)	VIVONEX STANDARD (RANK)
Orange	4.94 ± 0.30	1
Grape	4.69 ± 0.34	2
Vanilla	3.46 ± 0.36	4
Beef Broth	1.43 ± 0.10	3

The authors collapsed ratings into two categories—"unacceptable" (ratings of 1, 2, or 3) and "acceptable" (ratings of 5, 6, or 7). The data (Fig. 12–1) showed the following: 1) The Vivonex samples were scored significantly higher in overall acceptability and palatability than Flexical for all preparations. 2) The black cherry Jell-O form of the elemental diets was rated significantly higher in overall acceptability and palatability than the other forms. The data suggested that flavor was the most important component of overall acceptability and palatability. To determine which components (appearance, flavor, and texture/consistency) contributed to the prediction of overall acceptability, we performed a multiple regression analysis on these data.* Of these three components, only flavor acceptability contributed significantly to the prediction of overall acceptability. The earlier study of Seltzer and Quarantillo,[11] which found orange-flavored Vivonex and Flexical to be about equal in overall acceptability and vanilla-flavored Flexical more acceptable than vanilla-flavored Vivonex, is in general agreement with that of Harrah and coworkers.[14]

Cancer Patients. DeWys and Herbst examined the palatability of four orange-flavored diets—three elemental diets (Vivonex HN, Vivonex Standard, and WT Low Residue) and one intact-protein, lactose-free diet (Precision LR)—and one vanilla-flavored, milk-based diet (Meritene) using a panel of 25 metastatic cancer patients.[13] Patients were given 5-cc samples of each supplement and asked to rate the taste of the supplement on a 7-point scale (−3 = very bad taste, −2 = moderately bad taste, −1 = mildly bad taste, 0 = indifferent taste, +1 = mildly good taste, +2 = moderately good taste and +3 = very good taste). The authors did not mention the temperature of the solutions. The data (Table 12–5) showed that the supplement with intact protein was rated higher than the elemental diets. Meritene was rated sig-

*For this analysis, the dependent variable (the value we were attempting to predict) was the percentage of overall acceptability, and the independent variables (the values we used to predict this) were the percentages of acceptable appearance, flavor, and texture/consistency. The small data set (there were only eight values to be predicted, the two diets multiplied by the four forms) makes this analysis tenuous. In addition, data may not meet the underlying assumptions of linear regression analysis (for example, normality and independence).

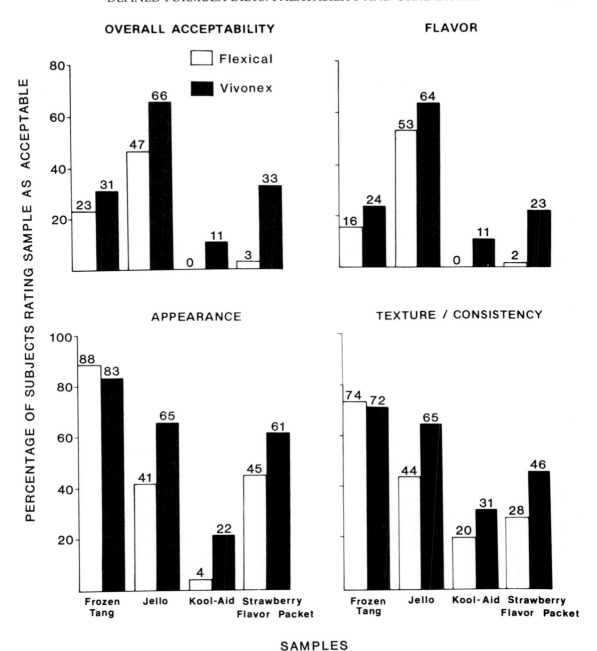

Figure 12–1. Percentage of 70 subjects rating diet samples (i.e., frozen Orange Tang, blackberry Jell-O, grape Kool-Aid, and strawberry flavor packet) as "acceptable" on the basis of overall acceptability, flavor, appearance, and texture/consistency.[14]

Table 12–5 Preference of 25 Patients with Cancer for Five Nutritional Supplements[13]

DIET	TYPE	FLAVOR	Rating* ($\bar{X} \pm SD$)
Meritene	Intact protein, milk-based	Vanilla	$+0.96 \pm 1.59$
Precision LR	Intact protein, lactose-free	Orange	-0.28 ± 1.81
Vivonex HN	Elemental	Orange	-0.32 ± 1.46
Vivonex Standard	Elemental	Orange	-1.72 ± 1.17
WT Low Residue	Elemental	Orange	-1.96 ± 1.34

*Means and standard deviations were calculated from histograms (Chart 1, DeWys and Herbst, 1977). Some of the means differ from means reported by DeWys and Herbst (1977) in their Table 1 (i.e., Meritene, $\bar{X} = +0.88$ and Vivonex HN, $\bar{X} = -0.30$).

nificantly* higher than Precision LR (and, presumably, the other supplements) and was the only diet that received a mean rating corresponding to a "good" taste. The ratings for Precision LR and Vivonex HN did not differ significantly. The ratings for Vivonex Standard and WT Low Residue were significantly lower than those for Vivonex HN and presumably for the other supplements.

The data indicate that orange-flavored supplements were not well liked and that orange-flavored Vivonex HN was superior to orange-flavored Vivonex Standard. Since Meritene was the only vanilla-flavored diet, it cannot be determined whether its higher rating was due to its milk base or to its flavoring. It is interesting that in a second panel of 25 cancer patients (Table 12–6), vanilla-flavored Meritene and vanilla-flavored Vivonex Standard did not differ significantly,[13] indicating that the flavoring, rather than the composition of the diet, was responsible for the relatively higher rating of Meritene.

Intact-Protein Supplements

Patients with Cancer. DeWys and Herbst,[13] using a second panel of 25 meta-static cancer patients and 25 "normal controls," examined five vanilla-flavored supplements, four of which were intact-protein diets and one was an "elemental" diet. The procedure was the same as that described earlier for the panel of cancer patients that rated the taste of four elemental diets and one intact-protein formula.

Data are presented in Table 12–6. These authors reported that the three most highly rated intact-protein formulas (Ensure, Nutri-1000, and Sustacal) were rated significantly higher than Meritene (intact-protein) and Vivonex Standard (elemental) by patients with cancer. Meritene and Vivonex Standard did not differ significantly from each other. They did not report any significant differences in ratings among diets by the controls, although it appears that there may be some.

DeWys and Herbst noted that the range of mean scores (Table 12–6) was narrower for patients with cancer ($+0.52$ to -1.16) than for controls ($+0.96$ to -1.88). However, their "analysis" of the data in support of this conclusion was not convincing.† In light of previous reports of "taste abnormalities" (alterations in taste thresholds) in pa-

---

*DeWys and Herbst used a Mann-Whitney U test to analyze for difference in ratings among the supplements.[13] The Mann-Whitney U test is applicable when the data (ratings) come from independent samples (different groups of subjects). Since a "panel" (a single group of subjects) rated all five supplements, the Mann-Whitney U test is inappropriate. A Friedman two-way analysis of variance would have been appropriate to determine whether the ratings for any of the supplements differed significantly from the others. A Sign test or Wilcoxon matched-pairs signed ranks test could then have been used to determine which supplements differed significantly. See Siegel (1956) for a lucid description of these and other nonparametric statistical procedures.[19]

†"Analysis of the data in [this] table (the mean ratings of cancer and control patients for the five diets) using a χ^2 test indicated a significant difference ($\chi^2 = 85.36$, 4 degrees of freedom, $p < 0.001$). Thus, the overall evaluation of nutritional supplements by patients is significantly different from the overall evaluation of some of the same supplements by a normal control population."[13]

Since there are four degrees of freedom (df = 4), and a conclusion is being drawn about a difference between patients with cancer and controls, we assume that the χ^2 is based on a 2 (cancer versus control) by 5 (diets) contingency table: df = $(2 - 1) \times (5 - 1) = 4$. Since the χ^2 test uses frequency data (the number of subjects, objects, or responses that fall into various categories), we assume that DeWys and Herbst did not actually apply the test to "the data in [the] table," which are the mean ratings of patients with cancer and controls for the five diets.[13] However, we are at a loss to determine what frequency data were used in the analysis.

Table 12–6 PREFERENCE OF 25 PATIENTS WITH CANCER AND 25 CONTROLS FOR FIVE DIETS[13]

| | | RATING | | |
| | | Patients $(\bar{X} \pm SD)$ | Controls $(\bar{X})$ | DIFFERENCE $(\bar{X}_{CA} \pm \bar{X}_{CO})$ |
DIET	FLAVOR			
Ensure	Vanilla	$+0.52 \pm 1.66$	-0.28	$+0.80$, NS
Nutri-1000	Vanilla	$+0.36 \pm 1.52$	$+0.12$	$+0.24$, NS
Sustacal	Vanilla	$+0.28 \pm 1.84$	$+0.96$	-0.68, NS
Meritene	Vanilla	-0.84 ± 1.18	-0.48	-0.36, NS
Vivonex Standard	Vanilla	-1.16 ± 1.89	-1.88	$+0.72$, $p<0.02$
GRAND MEAN		-0.17	-0.31	$+0.14$

tients with cancer and the presumed effect of these "abnormalities" on the palatability of foods and food intake.‡ It is interesting that patients with cancer were observed to give a higher rating (indicating less of an aversion) for the five diets than did the controls. Further, Vivonex Standard was the only diet for which the ratings of cancer patients and controls differed significantly, with cancer patients giving higher ratings.

One final point should not be overlooked. Vanilla-flavored Meritene was used in both panels of patients with metastatic cancer. A comparison of Tables 12–5 and 12–6 indicated a large discrepancy in the ratings of this diet between the two panels ($+0.96$ versus -0.84), which we determined was significant ($U=505.5$, $Z=3.81$, $p<.00007$). This reflects a general problem in hedonic (that is, pleasantness, degree of liking) testing. Even though the category scale (with clear verbal statements of the categories) and presumably all other procedural variables were the same, the ratings of two panels differed significantly. One possible source of this rating shift is that in the first group of diets, all of the diets were rated worse than Meritene, so Meritene "tasted good" when compared with the others. In the second group of diets, the majority of diets (three of five) "tasted" better than Meritene, so Meritene "tasted bad" when compared with the others. This is some-

times referred to as a contrast error in sensory evaluation. Practically speaking, it means that the rating may not correspond precisely to its verbal anchor.

Settle et al. recently compared pleasantness ratings for the flavor, taste, and odor of 13 intact-protein diets in 22 patients with and 38 patients without cancer. All the patients were on the Surgical Service of the Philadelphia Veterans Administration Center.[15, 16] Eight of the diets were vanilla-flavored, and five were unflavored. Pleasantness ratings of the flavor, taste, and odor were obtained using a 9-point category scale (1 = dislike extremely, 2 = dislike very much, 3 = dislike moderately, 4 = dislike slightly, 5 = neither like nor dislike, 6 = like slightly, 7 = like moderately, 8 = like very much, 9 = like extremely). The temperature of the diets was maintained at 4 to 6°C throughout testing. Each subject worked at his own pace with the majority completing the testing in about an hour. In order to assess the flavor of the diets, subjects were presented 10 cc of diet in a 1-oz plastic cup; they sampled all of it orally, expectorated the diet, and rated it. Subjects rinsed with deionized water after sampling each diet. Each diet was presented and rated twice, and the mean of these ratings was used in data analyses. The procedure for determining taste pleasantness was identical to that for flavor except that the subject wore a nose clip that occluded the nares. This reduced the contribution of olfactory stimulation from the diets. To study odor pleasantness, subjects were presented plastic cups containing 20 cc of diet. The lid of the cup was removed just before the cup was placed under the subject's nose. The subject inhaled and rated the pleasantness of the odor using the 9-point category scale. Data are presented in Figures 12–2, 12–3, and 12–4. As a group, unflavored diets were

‡As we have indicated elsewhere,[20] the miscalculation of a statistic resulted in the erroneous report of a subpopulation of cancer patients with an abnormal bitter taste threshold by DeWys and Walters (1975).[21] In addition, reports of alterations in taste thresholds in patients with cancer do not replicate each other (see Carson and Gormican, 1977;[22] DeWys and Walters, 1975;[21] Williams and Cohen, 1978).[23] Thus it has not been clearly established that patients with cancer have altered taste thresholds, much less that such alterations significantly affect the palatability of food and thus food intake.

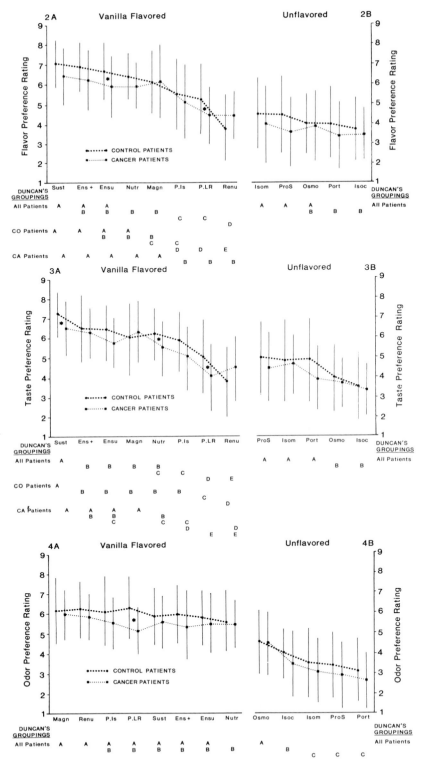

Figures 12–2, 12–3, and 12–4. Flavor (2), taste (3), and odor (4) pleasantness ratings for vanilla-flavored (A) and unflavored (B) solutions. The mean pleasantness rating (± 1 SD) is plotted for cancer (CA) and control (CO) patients for each feeding. In each figure (2A, 2B, 3A, etc.), the feedings are ordered from left to right in descending order based on the mean pleasantness rating for all 60 subjects. Asterisks (*) indicate that the mean pleasantness ratings of cancer and control patients differed significantly for that feeding. The results of Duncan's multiple range test(s) are presented below the x-axis. For a given Duncan's test (i.e., All Patients, CO or CA Patients), the mean pleasantness ratings of feedings with the same letters do not differ significantly from each other.

rated significantly lower than vanilla-flavored diets for flavor, taste, and odor. In general, patients with cancer gave lower pleasantness ratings than did patients without cancer for the flavor, taste, and odor of nearly all 13 diets. On closer examination, cancer patients gave significantly lower ratings than control patients only for the odor of vanilla-flavored diets.

For the vanilla-flavored diets, a significant correlation between the mean ratings for taste and flavor was found for both patient groups. Thus if one knew the mean taste rating of a group, one could predict the flavor rating for the group. The relationship between odor and flavor was not significant, possibly reflecting the fact that textural cues, as well as taste cues, were available during the flavor- and taste-rating tasks. Also, in odor testing, the lid was removed just as the container was being placed under the nose of the subject; thus visual cues were probably less prominent during the odor-rating task than the taste and flavor rating tasks. Therefore, taste ratings may actually reflect a complex of visual, textural, and taste stimulation (or "flavor minus odor" pleasantness*). The poor relationship between flavor and odor pleasantness ratings was surprising, since vanilla flavoring is essentially derived from its odor. During the course of testing many subjects made comments which indicated that vanilla was not the flavor they perceived; for instance, "I liked the chocolate one best," or, "The butterscotch wasn't bad." In retrospect, it would have been interesting to have asked for flavor and odor identification.

Odor pleasantness ratings were significantly correlated with flavor preference ratings for three of the unflavored diets in both patients with cancer and without cancer. This was true for only two of eight vanilla-flavored diets. Odor thus appears more important in the determination of flavor ratings of unflavored diets than of flavored diets. For the three unflavored diets, the relationship between odor and flavor ratings was stronger in cancer patients than in non-cancer patients. For patients with cancer,

odor ratings for these three diets accounted for 48 to 52 per cent of the variability in flavor ratings compared with only 21 to 30 per cent for patients without cancer.

The relationships of aging with flavor, taste, and odor pleasantness ratings were also examined in this study. Table 12–7 shows correlations of pleasantness ratings of diet with age for which both patients with and without cancer showed a correlation with p<.10. There were no diets for which taste ratings met this criteria. Only three diets (one vanilla-flavored and two unflavored) showed a significant relationship between age and flavor ratings in both groups of patients. There were four unflavored diets in which odor pleasantness ratings of both groups showed a significant relationship with age. Considering the low pleasantness ratings assigned to the odor of unflavored feedings and the published reports of reduced olfactory sensitivity with age[24, 25] (for a review, see Doty, 1979[26]), one might predict these results. That is, if older subjects were not able to smell the unpleasant odor of these diets as well as younger subjects, then their odor pleasantness ratings would be expected to be higher. It is interesting that the one unflavored feeding that did not show a relationship between odor ratings and age received the highest rating by both patient groups.

Elderly Individuals. Settle et al. compared flavor, taste, and odor pleasantness ratings in 41 elderly individuals and 43 college students.[17, 18] Procedures identical to those employed in the study of patients with cancer were used. Data are presented in Figures 12–5 to 12–7.

Elderly individuals preferred the flavor, taste, and odor of the diets significantly more than did college students. Flavor and taste pleasantness ratings paralleled each other for both elderly and young subjects; that is, the ordering of diets based on ratings were very similar for the two groups. This was not true for odor ratings. Not only did the rank ordering of vanilla-flavored diets based on odor preference ratings differ for the two groups, but the elderly group rated all diets between 5.9 and 5.3, whereas the young group gave ratings ranging from 5.7 to 4.3. Elderly individuals made fewer discriminations among vanilla-flavored diets based on odor pleasantness ratings than did young subjects.

Both elderly and young individuals

---

*Actually, we cannot rule out retronasal olfactory cues. It is possible that odors diffused from the pharynx to the nasal cavity. However, the poor correlation between taste and odor pleasantness ratings indicates that taste pleasantness ratings were probably not severely contaminated by this mechanism.

Table 12–7 CORRELATION COEFFICIENTS BETWEEN AGE AND FLAVOR AND ODOR PLEASANTNESS RATINGS OF DIETS BY PATIENTS WITH (CA) AND WITHOUT (CO) CANCER

	FLAVOR		ODOR	
	CO	CA	CO	CA
Vanilla Flavored				
Ensure	.28‡	.52†		
Unflavored				
Isocal			.54*	.57*
Isomil	.34†	.51†	.29‡	.44†
Portagen			.29‡	.52†
Prosobee	.40†	.45†	.41†	.52†

*p<.01
†p<.05
‡p<.10

showed a moderate to high correlation between flavor and taste pleasantness ratings. However, elderly individuals showed a much poorer relationship between flavor and odor ratings than did young subjects. This is consistent with the reported decline in olfactory sensitivity with age.[24-26]

In comparing the results of the two studies for taste and flavor pleasantness ratings,[16, 18] what is most striking is the similarity in the ordering of the diets of the four groups (patients with cancer, patients without cancer, elderly individuals, and college students). The largest discrepancy is in the ordering of diets based on odor ratings of vanilla-flavored diets. This is due to the narrow range of odor ratings of patients with cancer, patients without cancer, and elderly subjects compared with college students. It should be noted that the age of patients with cancer (55.0±14.3 years) and those without cancer (54.2±12.1) more closely approximates that of the elderly subjects (75.2±7.8) than that of the college students (22.8±3.2).

The effects of aging on pleasantness ratings are strikingly similar for the two studies.[16, 18] In the study of patients with cancer, Ensure was the only vanilla-flavored diet that showed a significant relationship between age and flavor ratings in both patients with and without cancer. It also showed the largest difference in flavor pleasantness ratings between elderly and young subjects. Similarly, among the unflavored diets, only Isomil and ProSobee showed a significant relationship between flavor ratings and age in both patient groups. These two diets also showed the largest differences in flavor

pleasantness ratings between elderly and young subjects. Of the unflavored feedings, only Osmolite did not show a significant relationship between odor ratings and age in both patient groups, and it showed the smallest difference between elderly and young subjects in odor pleasantness ratings.

Summary

We conclude the following from these studies: (1) The palatability of elemental diets is generally very poor. (2) Creative flavoring and/or changes in the form (for example, Jello) of elemental diets can significantly improve their palatability. (3) Unflavored intact-protein diets are generally unpalatable. (4) Vanilla-flavored, intact-protein diets are relatively palatable. (5) Elderly individuals consider intact-protein diets to be more palatable than do college-age individuals.

The work of Behl and associates[12] and Harrah and colleagues[14] clearly indicates that significant improvements can be made in palatability by modifying elemental diets. However, these modifications may significantly increase the osmolarity and alter the "elemental" quality of diets. Thus there is a need to study the physiologic consequences resulting from manipulations of form and flavor. A common scheme used for improving palatability of elemental diets without altering their "elemental" quality is serving them iced, in closed containers with straws. This effectively reduces the perceived intensity of the unpleasant odor and taste of these diets.

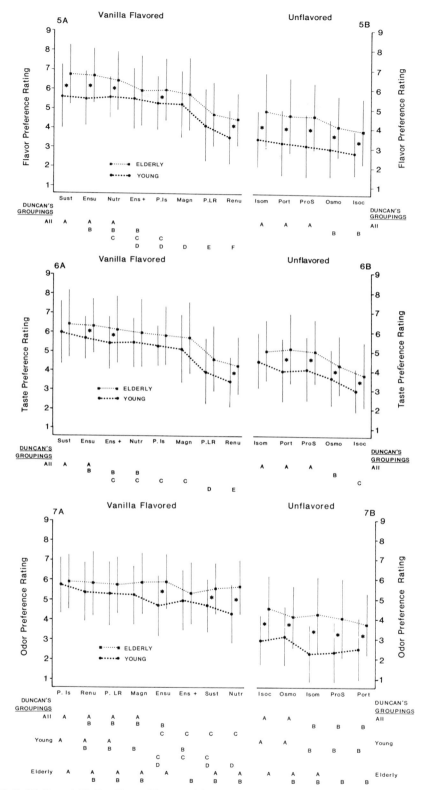

Figures 12–5, 12–6, and 12–7. Flavor (5), taste (6), and odor (7) pleasantness ratings for vanilla-flavored (A) and unflavored (B) solutions. The mean pleasantness rating (±1 SD) is plotted for elderly and young (student) subjects for each feeding. In each figure (5A, 5B, 6A, etc.), the feedings are ordered from left to right in descending order based on the mean pleasantness rating for all 84 subjects. Asterisks (*) indicate that the mean pleasantness ratings of elderly and young subjects differed significantly for that feeding. The results of Duncan's multiple range test(s) are presented below the x-axis. For a given Duncan's test (i.e., All Subjects, Young or Elderly Subjects), the mean pleasantness ratings of feedings with the same letters do not differ significantly from each other.

FACTORS INFLUENCING PALATABILITY AND ORAL INGESTION

The flavor characteristics of defined formula diets are not the sole determinant of palatability. Even the most desirable flavors are disliked by some individuals. Palatability is the individual's perception of a diet's flavor characteristics, and many factors influence an individual's perception.

Diet Repetition (Monotony). The pleasantness of a highly palatable diet can be reduced with repeated administration. Schutz and Pilgrim[27] and Siegel and Pilgrim[28] showed that monotony with food, as expressed by lowered consumption, was primarily a function of repetition. Regarding monotony and defined formula diets, two studies are of particular interest.[29, 30] Subjects were fed a defined formula diet exclusively for several weeks. Cabanac and Rabe used vanilla-flavored Renutril.[29] Intake diminished from approximately 2000 kcal to between 1000 and 1500 kcal in the first few days of the diet. The average duration of the diet was 17 days, during which there was a mean decrease in body weight of 3.13 kg.

Spiegel obtained similar results when subjects were fed ad lib with Metrecal for several weeks.[30] Although the basic Dutch chocolate flavor was alternated with strawberry, vanilla, and coffee "to relieve monotony," 9 of 12 subjects lost weight. Thus, in terms of weight loss, alternating flavors appears to be no more effective than using a single flavor. Perhaps alternating the form of the diet (for example, Jell-O, pudding, popsicle), as well as the flavor, would be more effective.

Other Factors. Monotony is only one of many factors that influence palatability and oral intake. Figure 12–8 is a schematic representation of some broadly defined influences on palatability and intake. External stimuli include the chemical constituents of a food which give rise to gustatory (taste), olfactory (smell), and trigeminal (spiciness) sensations, as well as physical properties (such as temperature, texture, visual properties). External stimuli also include other sensory stimuli in the environment (noxious odors emanating from excreta or vomitus ineffectively removed from the environment).

External stimuli interact with the organism's receptors to give rise to sensations. Thus our sensations are dependent on ac-

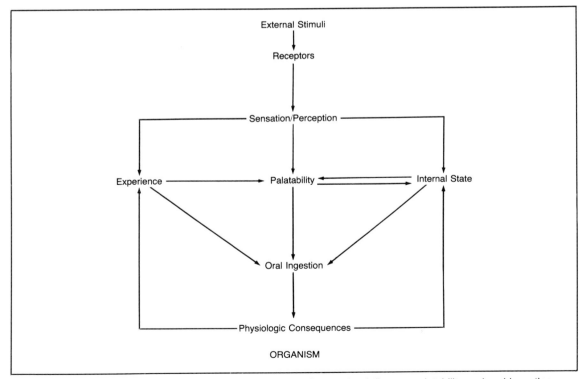

Figure 12–8. Schematic representation of some of the factors that influence palatability and oral ingestion.

cess of the stimulus to the receptors. We have all experienced the reduction in flavor of food when our nose is "stuffed-up." We cannot smell what we are eating because the stimuli cannot reach the olfactory receptors. Patients with head and neck cancer who are treated with radiation to the oropharynx complain of the blandness of food. Radiation to the oropharynx destroys taste cells, which leads to a severe reduction in taste sensitivity.[31, 32] For the interested reader, there is an impassioned description of the effect of head and neck radiation on palatability and food intake by MacCarthy and Leventhal.[33]

The sensations produced by food stimuli influence the "internal state" of the individual. The modification of the internal state of the organism with oral stimulation is referred to as "cephalic phase response." Nicolaidis[34] and Powley[35] have reviewed several preabsorptive endocrine, exocrine, and metabolic responses elicited by oral stimulation: secretion of gastric and pancreatic juices; an increase in O_2 consumption and respiratory quotient; a hyperglycemic response in fasted animals or a hypoglycemic response in fed animals; insulin release; glucagon release;[36, 37] and pancreatic polypeptide release.[38] They are thought to prepare or prime the body for transport, breakdown, and storage of incoming nutrients. Nicolaidis[39] has argued that the body's incomplete utilization of continuous intravenous infusions of a nutritionally balanced formula "is the consequence of inadequate release of insulin when sensory afferences of the orodigestive tract are eliminated." The amount of insulin released in response to a given amount of glucose varies with respect to the route of administration: oral administration results in the largest release of insulin; intragastric, the next largest; and intravenous, the smallest. This suggests that the oral route allows for the most complete utilization of a diet.

Previous experience influences the palatability and ingestion of foods. Perhaps the best established phenomenon of this type is "conditioned taste aversions," in which the ingestion of a food, if followed by nausea and other gastrointestinal symptoms within a period of several hours, results in a subsequent aversion to that food. A survey by Garb and Stunkard indicated that conditioned taste aversions are a common occurrence.[40] The phenomenon has recently been established experimentally in patients undergoing cancer chemotherapy.[41, 42] Although nausea is frequently associated with food aversions, it apparently is not a requirement.[42] Also, the avoidance of certain foods can develop as a result of discomfort unassociated with the gastrointestinal system, such avoidances occur in food allergies.[43]

On the other hand, some food preferences may result from the alleviation of a nutritional deficiency, which is a positive physiologic consequence.[44] Also, in humans, some food preferences may develop for items that are innately distasteful. For example, a shift from disliking to liking chili pepper, which is perhaps the most widely eaten spice in the world, appears to result from repeated exposure to the spice over a period of time.[45]

It is nearly self-evident that the internal state of the individual influences oral ingestion. We have all experienced loss of appetite during an illness. It has been demonstrated that insulin-induced hypoglycemia leads to gastric contractions and feelings of hunger,[46] while the injection of glucagon inhibits gastric contractions and hunger sensations.[47] Although the earlier literature stressed stimulus qualities as the major determinant of pleasantness, it has been demonstrated that the internal state of an individual modifies the perceived pleasantness of chemosensory stimuli. Olfactory and taste stimuli from foods, which are perceived as pleasant by fasting subjects, become unpleasant following the ingestion of a satiating load.[48–51]

This is not a comprehensive review of the factors that influence palatability and oral ingestion. For instance, we have not addressed the myriad of cultural, social, and environmental factors that affect food selection and intake.[9, 52] Rather, this description is intended to make the reader more aware of the complex interaction among variables that affect palatability and oral intake.

CONCLUDING REMARKS

The palatability of an oral diet involves a complex interaction among the stimulus (flavor) properties of the diet, the individual's internal state, and his previous experience. However, it is clear from the available literature that the poor flavor properties of most commercially available defined formula diets are the principal source of their poor palatability. It is unrealistic to expect patients to consume nutritionally adequate quantities of many of the defined formula diets on the market today. There is a pressing need to significantly improve the flavor characteristics, and thus palatability, of defined formula diets if they are to be effectively utilized perorally. It will also be necessary to diversify the form and flavor of diets, if peroral nutritional support is to be used for more than a brief time.

REFERENCES

1. Grossman, S. P.: Neuroanatomy of food and water intake. In Novin, D., Wyrwicka, W., and Bray, G. (eds.): Hunger: Basic Mechanisms and Clinical Implications. New York, Raven Press, 1976, pages 51–59.
2. Shepherd, G. M.: The Synaptic Organization of the Brain. New York, Oxford University Press, 1974, pages 111–144, 238–258.
3. Harper, R.: On odor classification. J. Food. Technol., 1:167, 1966.
4. Patrick, G. T.: On the confusion of tastes and odors. Psychol. Rev., 6:160, 1899.
5. Mozell, M. M., Smith, B. P., and Smith, P. E.: Nasal chemoreception in flavor identification. Arch. Otolaryngol., 90:367–373, 1969.
6. Pfaffman, C.: The vertebrate phylogeny, neural code, and integrative processes of taste. In Carterette, E. C., and Friedman, M. P.: Handbook of Perception. Volume 6. New York, Academic Press, 1978, pages 51–123.
7. Rollin, H.: Course of the peripheral gustatory nerves. Ann. Otol. Rhinol. Laryngol., 86:251–258, 1977.
8. Benjamin, R. M., and Burton, H.: Projection of taste nerve afferents to anterior opercular-insular cortex in squirrel monkey (Saimiri sciureus). Brain Res., 7:221–231, 1968.
9. Amerine, M. A., Pangborn, R. M., and Roessler, E. B.: Principles of Sensory Evaluation of Food. New York, Academic Press, 1965.
10. McBurney, D. H., and Gent, J. F.: On the nature of taste qualities. Psychol. Bull., 86:151–167, 1979.
11. Seltzer, M. H., and Quarantillo, E. P., Jr.: The taste of commercially available supplemental elemental diets. Milit. Med., 140:471–472, 1975.
12. Behl, C. R., Agarwala, B. P., Giudici, R. A., and Galinsky, A. M.: Improved taste acceptability for an oral hyperalimentation dosage form. Am. J. Hosp. Pharm., 33:1014–1017, 1976.
13. DeWys, W. D., and Herbst, S. H.: Oral feeding in the nutritional management of the cancer patient. Cancer Res., 37:2429–2431, 1977.
14. Harrah, J. D., Stephens, N. D., and Hawes, M. C.: Prospective sensory evaluation of preparatory methods of elemental diets. J.P.E.N., 4:303–306, 1980.
15. Settle, R. G., Chernoff, R., Rombeau, J. L., Hostetter, R., and Blowe, V.: Cancer patient preferences for enteral feedings [Abstract]. Am. J. Clin. Nutr., 34:648, 1981.
16. Settle, R. G., Rombeau, J. L., Blowe, V., Chernoff, R., and Meehan, K.: An evaluation of the pleas-antness of enteral feeding formulae in cancer and non-cancer patients. Unpublished data, 1982.
17. Settle, R. G., Rombeau, J. L., Chernoff, R., and Williams, G.: Pleasantness ratings of elderly individuals for enteral feedings. Am. J. Clin. Nutr., in press.
18. Settle, R. G., Williams, G., Rombeau, J. L., and Chernoff, R.: An evaluation of the pleasantness of enteral feeding formulae in elderly individuals. Unpublished data, 1982.
19. Siegel, S.: Nonparametric Statistics for the Behavioral Sciences. New York, McGraw-Hill Book Company, 1956.
20. Settle, R. G., Quinn, M. R., Brand, J. G., Kare, M. R., Mullen, J. L., and Brown, R.: Gustatory evaluation of cancer patients: Preliminary results. In van Eys, J., Nichols, B. L., Jr., and Seeling, M. S. (eds.): Nutrition and Cancer. New York, Spectrum, 1979, pages 171–185.
21. DeWys, W. D., and Walters, K.: Abnormalities of taste sensation in cancer patients. Cancer, 36:1888–1896, 1975.
22. Carson, J. A. S., and Gormican, A.: Taste acuity and food attitudes of selected patients with cancer. J. Am. Diet. Assoc., 70:361–365, 1977.
23. Williams, L. R., and Cohen, M. H.: Altered taste thresholds in lung cancer. Am. J. Clin. Nutr., 31:122–125, 1978.
24. Rovee, C. K., Cohen, R. Y., and Schlapack, W.: Life-span stability in olfactory sensitivity. Devel. Psychol., 11(3): 311–318, 1975.
25. Schiffman, S., Moss, J., Erickson, R. P.: Thresholds of food odors in the elderly. Exp. Aging Res., 2:389–398, 1976.
26. Doty, R. L.: A review of olfactory dysfunctions in man. Am. J. Otolaryngol., 1:57–79, 1979.
27. Schutz, H. G., and Pilgrim, F. J.: A field study of food monotony. Psychol. Rep., 4:559, 1958.
28. Siegel, P. S., and Pilgrim, F. J.: The effect of monotony on the acceptance of food. Am. J. Psychol., 71:756, 1958.
29. Cabanac, M., and Rabe, E. F.: Influence of a monotonous food on body weight regulation in humans. Physiol. Behav., 17(4):675–678, 1976.
30. Spiegel, T. A.: Caloric regulation of food intake in man. J. Comp. Physiol. Psychol., 84:24–37, 1973.
31. Conger, A. D.: Loss and recovery of taste acuity in patients irradiated to the oral cavity. Radiat. Res., 53:338–347, 1973.
32. Bartoshuk, L. M.: The psychophysics of taste. Am. J. Clin. Nutr., 31:1068–1077, 1978.
33. MacCarthy-Leventhal, E. M.: Post-radiation mouth blindness. Lancet, 2(7112):1138–1139, 1959.
34. Nicolaidis, S.: Early systemic responses to orogastric stimulation in the regulation of food and water balance: Functional and electrophysiological data. Ann. N.Y. Acad. Sci., 157:1176–1203, 1969.
35. Powley, T. L.: The ventromedial hypothalamic syndrome, satiety, and a cephalic phase hypothesis. Psychol. Rev., 84:89–126, 1977.
36. Nilsson, G., and Uvnäs-Wallensten, K.: Effect of teasing and sham feeding on plasma glucagon concentration in dogs. Acta Physiol. Scand., 100:298–302, 1977.
37. Steffens, A. B.: Influence of the oral cavity on insulin release in the rat. Am. J. Physiol., 230:1411–1415, 1976.
38. Taylor, I. L., Feldman, M., Richardson, C. T., and Walsh, J. H.: Gastric and cephalic stimulation of

human pancreatic polypeptide release. Gastroenterology, 75:432–437, 1978.

39. Nicolaidis, S.: Intravenous self-feeding: Long-term regulation of energy balance in rats. Science, 195:589–590, 1977.

40. Garb, J. L., and Stunkard, A. J.: Taste aversions in man. Am. J. Psychiatry., 131:1204–1207, 1974.

41. Bernstein, I. L.: Learned taste aversions in children receiving chemotherapy. Science, 200:1302–1303, 1978.

42. Bernstein, I. L., and Webster, M. M.: Learned taste aversion in humans. Physiol. Behav., 25:363–366, 1980.

43. Rozin, P.: Preference and affect in food selection. In Kroeze, J. H. (ed.): Preference Behaviour and Chemoreception: Proceedings. London, Information Retrieval, 1979.

44. Rozin, P., and Kalat, J. W.: Specific hungers and poison avoidance as adaptive specializations of learning. Psychol. Rev., 78:459–486, 1971.

45. Rozin, P., and Schiller, D.: The nature and acquisition of a preference for chili pepper by humans. Motivation and Emotion, 4:77, 1980.

46. Carlson, A. J.: The Control of Hunger in Health and Disease. Chicago, University of Chicago Press, 1916.

47. Stunkard, A. J., Van Itallie, T. B., Reis, B. B.: The mechanism of satiety: Effect of glucagon on gastric hunger contractions in man. Proc. Soc. Exp. Biol. Med., 89:258–261, 1955.

48. Declaux, R., and Cabanac, M.: Effets d'une ingestion de glucose sur la sensation et la perception d'un stimulus olfactif alimentaire. [Effect of glucose injection on the sensation and perception of an olfactory food stimulus.] C. R. Acad. Sci. [D] (Paris) 270:1006–1009, 1970.

49. Duclaux, R., Feisthauer, J., and Cabanac, M.: Effets du repas sur l'agrément d'odeurs alimentaires et nonalimentaires chez l'homme. [Effect of eating a meal on the pleasantness of food and non-food odors in man.] Physiol. Behav., 10:1029–1033, 1973.

50. Cabanac, M., Minaire, Y., and Adair, E. R.: Influence of internal factors on the pleasantness of a gustative sweet sensation. Communications in Behavioral Biology [A], 1:77–82, 1968.

51. Cabanac, M., and Duclaux, R.: Specificity of internal signals in producing satiety for taste stimuli. Nature, 227:966–967, 1970.

52. Rodin, J.: Social and immediate environmental influences on food selection. Int. J. Obes., 4:364–370, 1980.

CHAPTER 13

Enteral Delivery Systems

LORETTA FORLAW
RONNI CHERNOFF

The renaissance in clinical nutrition has heralded a renewed interest in tube feeding. In the past, enteral delivery systems have received the least attention of any aspect of tube feeding; however, new developments in materials, design, and technology have revolutionized our ability to provide this form of support. The purpose of this chapter is to discuss the background and latest developments in feeding tubes, holding devices, formula containers, and enteral pumps.

FEEDING TUBES

History. *Nasoenteric Tubes.* Devices used for artificial alimentation or forced feeding were first described in the Greco-Roman period. The "modern" experience with these devices began with Aquapendente, a monk, who used a tube made of silver for nasogastric feeding in 1617. Van HelMont produced flexible leather catheters in 1646; however, a discussion of the use of these catheters does not appear in the literature.[1, 2] The major work related to nasoenteric tube feeding in the eighteenth century was by John Hunter, who reported successful tube feeding in two patients.[3, 4] Nasogastric tubes for feeding purposes were not described in the American literature until 1879.[5] Rankin described the placement of a tube for feeding via the oral and, later, the nasal routes in an uncooperative patient in 1882.[6] The use of soft rubber tubes for gavage feeding of pediatric patients was first described in the last half of the nineteenth century.[7]

The Levin tube has been the most commonly used nasogastric tube for feeding since its introduction in 1921, and it is still an appropriate tube for gastric decompression.[8] However, a number of mechanical complications have been reported with long-term use of this tube for nasoenteric feed-

ing.[9, 10] These potential complications and the discomfort to the patient from the size and stiffness of the tube made it undesirable for feeding. In the 1950s alternatives to the Levin tube became available when polyethylene tubes were developed. Royce and Wagner advocated using polyethylene tubes for the pediatric patient.[11, 12] In 1952 Kunz suggested that polyethylene tubing could be modified with a coating of paraffin to reduce complications from the stiffness of the tube.[13] Concurrently, Fallis and Barron suggested passing polyethylene tubes into the stomach or jejunum, using a mercury-filled balloon as a weight to assist with the passage of the tube.[14] However, the mercury-filled weight was tied in place with surgical catgut, which did not remain intact in the gastrointestinal tract. A few years later, Wagner introduced a tube formed from a polyvinyl-type plastic which was more pliable than tubes of polyethylene.[15] In the late 1960s a silicone elastomer nasoenteric tube with a mercury weight was used by Keoshian.[16] Davis suggested a soft Penrose tubing to minimize the discomfort of nasal feedings.[17] The 1970s brought an influx of nasoenteric tubes made of polyurethane replacing the polyvinyl tubes. Gold beads or mercury that can be recycled may be used as weighting devices.[16, 18]

Surgically Placed Tubes. In 1918 Anderson recommended the use of the jejunostomy tube for feeding.[19] The concept of dual tubes for both decompression and feeding was described by Abbott and Rawson in 1937.[20] Feeding into the jejunum via fine polyethylene tubing inserted using a large-gauge needle was described by McDonald.[21] Delany modified this procedure in 1973, but it was Cobb who described the use of silicone, rather than polyethylene, tubing in a serosal tunnel jejunostomy.[22, 23] Moss has recently developed a dual tube for short-term use, for simultaneous feeding and decompression.[24] Recently, Rombeau has devised a silicone tube for gastrostomy decompression and jejunostomy feeding for long-term use.[25]

Present Status. *Insertion.* Methods used for the passage of nasoenteric tubes have not been widely described. Rankin reported the use of four stout men for assistance in passing the tube in an uncooperative patient.[6] Until the late 1960s, available feeding tubes were stiff enough to be passed into the cooperative patient without difficulty.

Feeding tubes made of silicone elastomer or polyurethane may require devices for stiffening them to facilitate passage. One of the older methods to aid in passage of these tubes is to wedge both a large Levin-type tube and the more flexible tube into a gelatin capsule and then allow the gelatin capsule to dissolve after the tube has passed into the gastrointestinal tract.[26] The larger tube can then be removed, leaving the smaller tube in place. Passage of the small tube inside a modified Levin tube has also been described.[27] Different types of stylets for stiffening the tubes have been used. Examples of these include gelatin-coated strings, angiographic guide wires, hydromer-coated wires, and large ribbed introducers.[28, 29]

Various weights, such as rubber finger cots filled with mercury, encapsulated mercury, gold, silicone, and tungsten, have been added to the tip of some feeding tubes to promote their passage. Tungsten weights were developed to eliminate the problems associated with the disposal of used mercury bolus tubes.[28]

Nasoenteric Tubes. *Polyurethane and Silicone Tubes.* The soft, small-bore, polyurethane or silicone elastomer nasoenteric tube, with or without a weighted bolus, is being used with increasing frequency. These tubes have several advantages over the larger-bore, stiff Levin tubes. Oropharyngeal and esophageal irritation on intubation is minimized with the silicone or polyurethane tube. The smaller, soft-bore tubes, with mercury or tungsten boluses, can be passed into the duodenum or jejunum without fluoroscopy. Use of the smaller-sized tubes may decrease the risk of aspiration because there is less compromise of the lower esophageal sphincter and thus decreased reflux of gastric contents. In addition, the patient's ability to swallow is usually not hindered by the softer tube.[28]

Polyurethane or silicone elastomer tubes come with stylets that can be inserted to stiffen the tubes and facilitate their passage. Removal of the stylet after passage of the tube is easier when the interior lumen has been lubricated.[28]

Numerous polyurethane or silicone elastomer nasoenteric tubes are now available in several sizes. Many nasoenteric tubes have entry ports that accommodate standard intravenous tubing.

Rigid Tubes or Tubes with Rigid Guides. Among the tubes currently available are those with stiff outer tubes for facilitating insertion; these are later removed, leaving an inner silicone tube in place. The Vivonex-Moss Tube is a large rigid tube that decompresses the stomach while allowing feeding through a duodenal feeding tube. The tube has three lumens, a radiographic tip, and a balloon that can be inflated and positioned at the esophagogastric junction. This tube is usually inserted at the time of surgery and removed within 48 hours. The aspiration lumen must be connected to the continuous suction to ensure appropriate decompression of the stomach.[24]

The Argyle Duo-Tube has an outer tube of polyvinylchloride for insertion and an inner tube of silicone for feeding. After insertion of the polyvinylchloride tube, the silicone catheter is expelled into the stomach by squeezing a bulb attached to the outer tube. In contrast to the Moss tube, there is no way to assure transpyloric positioning of this tube.[28]

The Cartmill tube has a spring-supported guide tube through which a radiopaque silicone tube with a lightweight bullet-shaped end is inserted. The rigid guide tube is removed once the feeding tube is advanced into the stomach. With this type of tube, a 14-gauge, 1½-inch plastic intravenous cannula is placed on the proximal end of the feeding tube to allow connection to the remainder of the enteral delivery system.[5]

The ideal nasoenteric feeding tube should be made of pliable, nonstiffening, nonleaching material. It should be the appropriate length for the feeding site, have enough strength to tolerate a pump pressure to 50 psi, and have the correct intraluminal diameter for delivery of formulas with varied viscosities; the adapter should not be compatible with intravenous tubing.

Enterostomy Tubes. Until recently the large-bore Levin tube or rubber tubing was used for feeding esophagotomies. A wide-lumen, short, silicone rubber tube designed specifically for feeding esophagotomy is now available.[30] Advantages of this tube include a flange collar for securing the tube, an attached plug for temporary closure, and a radiopaque line.

Gastrostomy tubes also made of rubber and latex are still commonly used for long-term delivery of feeding. The large-bore gastrostomy tube is more advantageous for delivery of medication and high-viscosity formulas but requires surgical placement. Foley catheters are also used with short-term Stamm gastrostomies.

In addition to the conventional jejunostomy tube of rubber or latex, two newer tubes are the K-tube and the needle catheter jejunal tube. The K-tube is a modified jejunal tube similar to the Tenckhoff or Broviac catheter but designed for jejunal feeding.[31] The needle catheter jejunostomy tube is a small polyethylene catheter introduced into the jejunum through a large bore needle or trocar. The diameters of most needle catheters do not permit the delivery of viscous formulas.[22] Polyvinyl catheters have been modified to 8-French feeding tubes that can be introduced via Jamshidi trocars and will accommodate more viscous formulas.[32]

A new variation, the Rombeau tube, is a double-lumen gastrostomy-jejunostomy tube. Made of silicone rubber, it consists of a 24-French gastric tube with a 9.6-French jejunal tube embedded within the wall of the gastric tube. The jejunal tube has a 10-gm mercury-weighted tip.[25]

HOLDING DEVICES FOR NASOENTERIC TUBES

The maintenance of nasoenteric tubes can be a major nursing problem. Skin irritation from the tape is common, and loosening of tape with accidental removal of the tube occurs frequently even in oriented, cooperative patients. Removal of the tube by confused or uncooperative patients is an even greater dilemma. Various taping methods and holding devices have been developed to address these problems. Except in diaphoretic patients, adhesive or hypoallergenic tape can be safe and effective in most patients if applied appropriately.[33]

Several devices have been designed to hold nasoenteric tubes in place in problem patients. The XOMED Naso-tube Clip is a retainer device with a self-adhesive backing. The device is taped to the forehead with the nasoenteric feeding tube placed through a slot to hold the tube firmly in place. In a study by McDonald et al., this device required changing on an average of every 12 hours and therefore was no more advantageous than adhesive or hypoallergenic tape.[34] Skin irritation from the self-adhesive backing can also be a problem.

Another type of holding device for the prevention of inadvertent removal of nasoenteric tubes is the modified nasal cannula (Fig. 13–1). A standard oxygen-nasal cannula is modified by removing the nasal tips and sleeve where the oxygen tube is attached to the cannula. An opening of the same diameter as that of the nasoenteric feeding tube made at the center of the cannula and the feeding tube is inserted, threaded through the cannula to the center opening and pulled free. The elastic strap for attachment to the cannula must be adjusted carefully to avoid skin irritation.[34] A similar device uses a rubber tourniquet approximately one inch in length and perforated at both ends. The tube is passed

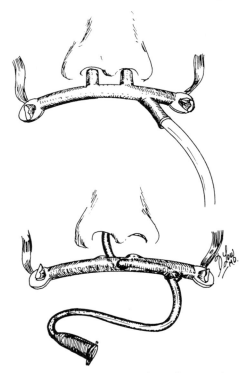

Figure 13–1. Adaptation of nasal prongs to serve as a holder for nasoenteric tubes.

through the opening in the middle, and ½-inch tape is placed at the end of the holes; the tube is then tied around the patient's head. Adhesive tape is placed near the end of the tourniquet and the end of the feeding tube is secured to the ½-inch tape.[35]

Feeding Tube Bridle. The feeding tube bridle was developed at the University of Tennessee by Dr. Wayne Luther.[36] It provides an effective method for maintaining nasoenteric tubes in patients who frequently remove them. An explanation should be given to the patient prior to placement of the bridle. It is helpful to have an assistant at the time of placement. The necessary equipment includes the primary feeding tube, two No. 5 pediatric feeding tubes (the bridle), a flashlight, tongue blade, 3–0 silk suture on a Keith needle, tincture of benzoin, ½-inch tape, and McGill forceps.

First the regular feeding tube is inserted through the most patent nostril. Proper placement of the tube in the stomach is confirmed by aspiration of the gastric contents or by obtaining an abdominal roentgenogram. The first pediatric tube is inserted into the other nostril (Fig. 13–2A) and pulled out through the mouth with the McGill forceps (Figs. 13–2,B and C). The second pediatric tube (third tube overall) is inserted into the same nostril as the regular feeding tube and pulled out through the mouth (Fig. 13–2D) as was the first pediatric tube. (Note: One pediatric tube may be used if desired; however, the adapter must be cut off.) The two ends of the pediatric tubes outside the mouth are sutured together end-on with interrupted sutures of 3–0 silk (Fig. 13–2E). One end of the pediatric tube is then pulled forward until the sutured section has been pulled completely back into the posterior pharynx and out the other nostril (Fig. 13–2,F and G). This leaves one continuous bridle. The portion of the the bridle outside the nose is then cut off to leave an approximate length of 2 inches beyond the nares. The two ends of the bridle outside the nares are then sutured together with two or three interrupted sutures (Fig. 13–2H). Tincture of benzoin is applied liberally to the bridle and the adult feeding tube. After the benzoin has dried, the three tubes are taped together with multiple strands of ½-inch tape. To prevent undue pressure on the nasal septum, the tape should not be placed too high on the bridle. Several sutures are then applied around the three tubes. The feeding tube must not be occluded with these sutures. Occasionally, these sutures and the tape may have to be reapplied.

Pediatric Devices. Two unique pediatric holding devices have been used: a modified catcher's mask for anchoring tubes[37] and an intraoral appliance for premature infants.[38] The second method utilizes a plastic mold prepared from impressions of the infant's palate. The appliance is fitted over the palate and gum and the feeding tube is manually fitted into grooves in the device. A small stainless steel tag provides an attachment loop for dental floss, which can be taped to the infant's cheek to prevent dislodgement of the tube. Both ends of the tube and the length of dental floss are taped to the infant's cheek.

FEEDING CONTAINERS

Historically, feeding containers have received little description in the literature. The pig's bladder was one of the first types of containers used for administering enteral feeding.[2] Syringelike receptacles followed, but the material from which they were made was not identified.[2] Ceramic-ware was widely used for administering feedings to infants in the late eighteenth and early nineteenth centuries;[39] however, there is no record that these devices were adapted to be used as feeding tubes. With the discovery of glass, syringelike apparatuses, including the Murphy drip bottle and Asepto syringe, were commonly used for delivery of feedings until the early 1970s. Even metal enema pails were modified for delivery of enteral formulas.

When tube feeding formulas were simply blenderized foods mixed together in the hospital kitchen, they needed to be measured by the nurses and administered by gravity boluses via syringes or funnels attached to rubber tubing. Administration of these viscous, blenderized formulas required that nurses be present throughout the feeding. With the availability of less viscous, commercially prepared feeding formulas, which could pass through intravenous tubing, the formula needed to be transferred into recycled glass bottles. During the 1960s and 1970s, bottles for administration of intravenous fluids were washed and reused for administering the tube feeding formula. When empty plastic bags de-

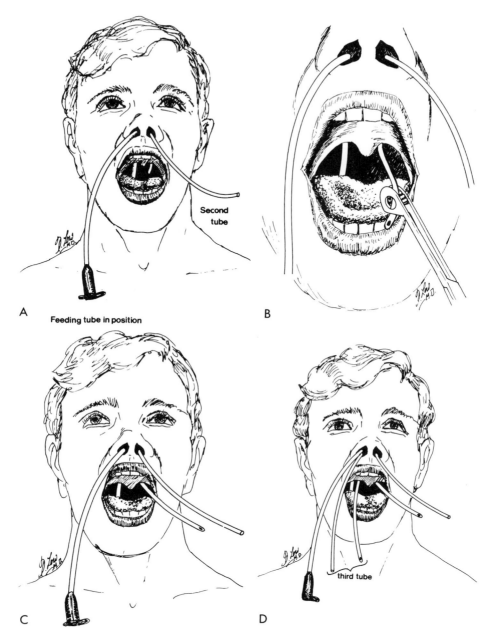

Figure 13–2. *A,* Following the insertion of the feeding tube, a No. 5 French pediatric feeding tube is inserted through the contralateral nostril into the posterior pharynx. *B,* The pediatric tube is grasped with McGill forceps and pulled out through the mouth. *C,* Exteriorization of the first pediatric tube. *D,* Insertion of another No. 5 French pediatric feeding tube (third tube) through the same nostril as the nasoenteric tube and exiting through the mouth similarly to the first pediatric tube.

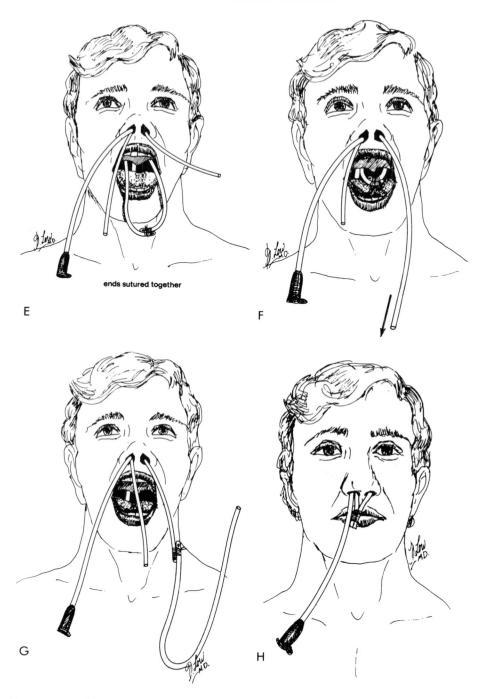

ends sutured together

E

F

G

H

Figure 13–2. *continued E,* Suturing of both ends of the pediatric tubes with 3-0 silk. *F,* Withdrawing one of the pediatric tubes back out through the nostril. *G,* Exteriorization of the sutured ends to leave one continuous pediatric tube in place for the bridle. *H,* Bridle sutured together and ready for final attachment to feeding tube.

signed for intravenous administration of fluids became available, they were also used for tube feeding.[40] Tubing used for the intravenous administration of fluids provided a screw or roller clamp for controlling the rate of flow. As a consequence, tube feedings could be administered with more control and less nursing personnel time. The intravenous tubing also had the advantage of being compatible with the pumps used for intravenous administration of fluids.

Feeding containers are currently designed with preattached tubing or can be adapted to accept standard intravenous tubing. A potential hazard associated with the use of intravenous containers and tubing is the accidental delivery of an enteral formula intravenously.[41] The introduction of opaque intravenous fat emulsions has increased the risk of this complication since the emulsions closely resemble many enteral products. Kaminski has suggested that adding food coloring to the enteral formula may decrease the risk of its being delivered intravenously.[41] Manufacturers have taken another approach, by labeling the tubing that is connected to the nasoenteric tube. Although this is helpful, at least one manufacturer labels the tube with blue lettering, which will not show up well when blue food coloring is used to color the enteral formula. Another disadvantage is that lettering on the tube is difficult to read at night with minimal light. However, the concept is appropriate and "wings" on the tubing, indicating that it is to be used for enteral feeding, may be advantageous. The optimal situation appears to be for the tubing attached to feeding bags and feeding tubes to be designed so that it will not adapt to use in intravenous systems.

Another alternative recently developed to alleviate the problem of confusion of enteral with intravenous solutions has been to package commercial tube formulas in single-serving glass bottles. These formulas are sterilely packaged with screw-off caps. In order to administer the solution to a patient, the top must be removed from the bottle and replaced with a screw-on cap with a drip chamber and attached tubing. When the cap is screwed on tightly, the bottle is inverted and the formula is ready to be fed to a patient; the tubing connectors will fit only the feeding tubes. Several types of ready-to-feed bottled formulas are prepackaged with this adaptation.[42] These bottles are available only in small volumes and are somewhat inefficient since multiple replace-

ments are required. This method of feeding is safe and acceptable for patients who are being fed intermittently; however, the continuous administration of tube feeding is becoming more popular.

Another solution to the problem of misidentification is to use containers designed specifically for enteral feedings. With the increased interest in enteral feeding in the late 1970s, manufacturers have produced feeding bags designed specifically for delivery of these formulations.

The majority of the specially designed feeding containers available today are made from medical-grade vinyl or polyvinylchloride (Table 13–1). The leaching problems associated with this material have not been investigated; however, a reduction in the delivery of specific nutrients has been reported in studies evaluating intravenous nutrition solutions.[43]

Currently, the polyvinylchloride bags, plastic irrigating containers, and semirigid containers are available in 500-, 1000-, and 1500-ml sizes. Some of these containers are made with preattached tubing and are filled from the top, whereas others are filled from the front. One of the benefits of containers designed specifically for enteral feedings is that the large filling ports allow easy transfer of solution into the containers, an advantage not available with intravenous feeding containers modified for tube feeding.

Nonrigid vinyl or vinyl-compound containers (although calibrated with measurement scales in easy-to-read marking) tend to collapse as fluid volume diminishes, thus making it difficult to estimate the volume of fluid delivered. Semirigid containers do not have this problem, but the calibration marks on these containers are difficult to read if they are not colored.

Powdered formulas that require reconstitution have to be transferred into enteral feeding containers for administration. In addition, it is often less expensive to purchase tube formulas in quart cans; therefore, formulas frequently have to be transferred into enteral feeding containers. Most formulas are sterilely packaged, and opening them for transfer increases the potential for bacterial contamination. The clinician must be aware of this as a potential problem when solutions are transferred from bulk packaging or after reconstitution or dilution into containers.[44]

An ideal enteral feeding container should be easy to fill, close, and hang. It should

Table 13–1 ENTERAL FEEDING CONTAINERS

CONTAINER/MANUFACTURER	CAPACITY	FILLING	MATERIAL	TUBING	PUMP/GRAVITY	OTHER FEATURES
Davol American Hospital Supply	1600 ml/50 ml calibrations	Top	Vinyl	48 in.	Gravity	Petcock to regulate flow
Dobhoff Enteric Feeding Bag Biosearch Medical Prods.	1000 ml/100 ml calibrations	Front		None	Both	Dual outlet ports for micro and macro administration sets; built-in sediment trap
Enteral Feeding Container Concord Laboratories	50 ml/100 ml calibrations 1000 ml/100 ml calibrations	Front	Polyvinylchloride	Optional	Gravity	Wide mouth opening with positive closure cap; tubing has drip chamber, screw clamp, male connector
Flexitainer Enteral Nutrition Container Ross Laboratories	100 ml/50 ml calibrations	Top	Polypropylene	68 in.	Both	Semi-rigid
Glass Feeding Bottle Doyle Pharmaceutical	250 ml	Prefilled	Glass	Available	Both	Compleat B
Glass Feeding Bottle Mead Johnson	8 oz	Prefilled	Glass	Available	Both	Criticare HN Isocal
Glass Feeding Bottle Ross Laboratories	8 oz	Prefilled	Glass	Available	Both	Ensure Ensure Plus Osmolite
Kangaroo Feeding Set Cheesebrough-Ponds, Inc.	1000 ml/50 ml calibrations	Top	Polyvinylchloride	Optional	Both	Wide mouth opening; tapered configuration
Keofeed Enteric Feeding Bag HEDECO Corp.	500 ml/50 ml calibrations	Top	Vinyl	Optional	Both	Tapered configuration; integral sediment trap
Keofeed Enteric Feeding Bag HEDECO Corp.	1500 ml/50 ml calibrations	Top	Vinyl	Optional	Both	Tapered configuration; integral sediment trap
Plastic Irrigating Container American McGaw	500 ml	Top	Polyolefin	Available	Both	Filled with sterile water; semi-rigid
Travenol Enteral Feeding Container Travenol Laboratories	1300 ml/50 & 100 ml calibrations	Top	Polyvinylchloride	Optional	Both	Tapered configuration
Vivonex Delivery System Norwich-Eaton	1000 ml/100 ml calibrations	Front	Polyvinylchloride	Attached	Gravity	Microdrip
Vivonex Acutrol Enteral Feeding System Norwich-Eaton	1000 ml/100 ml calibrations	Top	Polyvinylchloride	Attached	Gravity	125 ml built-in burette (25 ml calibrations)
1090 Gavage Bag Ethox Corp.	1000 ml	Front	Polyvinylchloride	Attached	Both	

also be safe, leakproof and have easy-to-read calibrations and directions for use. Finally, it should be made from a nonleaching material and should be either disposable or easy to clean.

ENTERAL FEEDING PUMPS

The use of a "stomach pump" for continuous delivery of enteral formulas was first proposed in the late nineteenth century; however, the first pump designed specifically for use with enteral tube formulas was developed by Dr. James Barron in the 1950s.[45] Tube feedings were generally fed by gravity-administered boluses, and the use of a pump for enteral feeding did not come into general usage until the early 1970s. As hyperosmolar nutrient solutions became an acceptable method for feeding patients with compromised gastrointestinal tracts, the preferred method for administration was continuous slow-drip infusion. Pumps originally designed for intravenous infusions were used because of the difficulty in controlling drip rates with screw or roller clamps on intravenous tubing.[46] Control of enteral infusions with the use of intravenous pumps has been reported frequently in the recent literature.[47–51] Continuous pump-controlled tube feedings were found to be beneficial in delivering large volumes of liquid formulas with great reliability.[52] Pumps ensure a constant rate of flow and reduce the amount of gastric pooling of solution, which are important considerations in reducing the possibility of formula aspiration.[46] With pump-controlled feeding, it has been observed that less time is required for reaching the total volume goal for most patients, with subjectively less abdominal discomfort than with bolus feeding.[50] The use of a pump for controlling enteral infusions has also reduced the incidence of osmotic diarrhea resulting from the rapid administration of hypertonic nutrient solutions.[47] This permits a more rapid advancement of enteral feeding regimens.

Intravenous pumps are a limited resource in most hospitals, and intravenous infusions retain a higher priority over pump-controlled enteral feedings because of a need for more precise regulation. The necessity of using pumps for parenteral feedings overrides the beneficial, but not the mandatory, use of pumps for controlling some methods of enteral feedings such as feeding into the jejunum. A plausible solution to the unavailability of parenteral pumps is the development of less expensive pumps for enteral feeding.

Some enteral pumps have a rotary peristaltic mechanism for delivery. The basic principle common to these pumps is a set of rollers attached to a rotating disc that alternately squeezes and releases a portion of the tubing to move fluid. Flow rate and fluid motion are determined by the speed of the rotor device and the diameter of pump chamber tubing.[53] The trend is toward manufacturing pumps that require special tubing sets for each type of enteral pump rather than pumps that accept universal tubing. This system increases cost for the consumer; however, if the extension tubing and the feeding tubes are designed differently from intravenous tubing, the possibility of accidental intravenous delivery of enteral formula will be decreased and the special sets for enteral pumps will actually be advantageous.

Another advantage of some of the enteral pumps is the alarm system. The most common systems are the empty/occlusion alarms and the low battery alarms. Enteral pumps with batteries promote mobility for patients who are ambulatory, and empty/occlusion alarms alert nurses or patients when the formula flow has stopped.

There have been only a few reports that have objectively evaluated enteral feeding pumps. In one report, enteral pumps proved efficacious for some patients who were having gastrointestinal side effects from gravity-controlled enteral feeding; such patients would have otherwise required parenteral feeding.[54] The same study found a saving of 30 minutes of nursing time per patient per day with enteral pumps. In another study, the peristaltic enteral pumps proved to be more accurate than the peristaltic infusion pumps, less accurate than the volumetric intravenous pumps, and about the same as enteral gravity drip when tested at three rates with three different types of enteral formulas.[55] The study analyzed only one of the enteral pumps, and it has been observed that other pumps are more accurate and consistent than gravity drip.

Currently available are a variety (Table 13–2) of enteral pumps that are reasonably priced and serve the needs of patients both in the hospital and at home. The ideal enteral feeding pump should be portable and inexpensive and should provide accurate delivery of formulas (Table 13–3).

Table 13–2 ENTERAL PUMPS

	FLOW RATE INCREMENTS	ACCURACY	ALARMS	POWER SOURCE	PRESSURE (psi)	HANDLE	POLE ATTACHMENT	SIZE (in.)	WEIGHT	TYPE
Biosearch Enteral Feeding Pump (Biosearch Medical Products Inc.)	20–250 ml in 10-, 25-ml increments	±10%	Empty/occlusion low battery	Electric Battery—8 hr life	6	No	Yes	3½(h) × 6(w) × 8½(d)	4½ lb	Peristaltic
Ethox/Barron Feeding Pump System (Ethox Corp.)	20–140 ml in 20-ml increments	±10%	None	Electric	28	No	No	9 × 9	6 lb	Peristaltic
Flexiflo Enteral Nutrition Pump (Ross Laboratories)	50–200 ml in 25-ml increments	±15%	None	Electric	Unknown	No	Yes	7¼(h) × 4-3/4(w) × 2½(d)	2 lb	Volumetric
Flexiflo II Enteral Nutrition Pump (Ross Laboratories)	20–250 ml*	±10%	Power on, pump on, empty/occlusion, low battery	Electric Battery—8 hour life	7.7	Shoulder strap	Yes	11(h) × 8(w) × 4½(d)	5 lb	Peristaltic
Holter Pediatric Pump 903 (Critikon)	0.33–13 ml	± 2%	None	Electric	15	Yes	Yes	2⅞(h) × 4¼(w) × 5½(d)	27 oz	Volumetric
Holter Pediatric Pump 907 (Critikon)	2.5–101 ml	± 2%	None	Electric	15	Yes	Yes	2⅞(h) × 4¼(w) × 5½(d)	27 oz	Volumetric
Kangaroo 220 Feeding Pump (Cheesebrough-Ponds Inc.)	5–295 ml in 5-ml increments	±10%	Empty/occlusion battery rate change	Electric Battery—2–3 hr life	12	Yes	Yes	6(h) × 7(w) × 5(d)	5 lb	Volumetric
Keofeed 500 Enteric Pump (HEDECO)	1–300 ml in 1-ml increments	± 5%	Empty/occlusion low battery, uncontrolled flow	Electric Battery	15	Yes	Yes	5(h) × 9(w) × 5(d)	8 lb	Volumetric
Simplicity 2100A Infusion Pump (Critikon)	1–999 ml	—	Empty/occlusion low battery	Electric Battery—4–8 hr life	19	Yes	Yes	8(h) × 7(w) × 6(d)	10 lb	Volumetric

*20–60 in 10-ml increments; 75–200 in 25-ml increments; 200–250 in 50-ml increments

Table 13–3 CHARACTERISTICS OF IDEAL ENTERAL FEEDING PUMPS

- Electrically safe
- Simple to use
- Clear instructions on pump
- Accurate to within 10% of prescribed flow rate
- Battery, minimum of 8 hours
- Alarm system
- Inexpensive
- Portable
- Quiet
- Intravenous pole attachment

SUMMARY

Equipment for the safe and effective delivery of enteral feedings is now commercially available. Tubes, holding devices, containers, and pumps are being specifically designed for enteral feeding. They have made tube feeding more comfortable and safer for the patient and more reliable and effective for the clinician. Proper selection and utilization of enteral delivery systems will greatly contribute to the overall success and accuracy of the administration of tube feeding. Interaction between nutritional support teams and industry will continue to enhance the development of high quality enteral delivery systems.

REFERENCES

1. Pareira, M. D., Conrad, E. J., Hicks, W., and Elman, R.: Therapeutic nutrition with tube feeding. J.A.M.A., 156:810–816, 1954.
2. Pareira, M. D.: Therapeutic Nutrition with Tube Feeding. Springfield, Illinois, Charles C Thomas Company, 1959.
3. Hunter, J.: Proposals for recovering persons apparently drowned. Phil. Trans. Roy. Soc. London, 66[Part 2], 1776.
4. Hunter, J.: A case of paralysis of the muscle deglutition, cured by an artificial mode of conveying food and medicines into the stomach. In The Works of John Hunter. Volume 3. London, Longman, Rees, Orme, Greene and Longman, 1837.
5. Gallagher, T. J.: On the different methods of artificial alimentation. N.Y. Med. J., 30:141–149, 1879.
6. Rankin, D. N.: Three cases of nasal alimentation. Arch. Laryngol., 3:355–358, 1882.
7. Holt, L. E.: Gavage (forced feeding) in the treatment of acute diseases of infancy and childhood. Med. Rec., 45:524–551, 1894.
8. Levin, A. L.: A new gastroduodenal catheter. J.A.M.A., 76:1007, 1921.
9. Strohl, E. L., Holinger, P. H., and Diffenbaugh, W. G.: Nasogastric intubation: Indications, complications, safeguards, and alternate procedures. Am. Surg., 24:721, 1958.
10. Hafner, C. D., Wylie, J. H., Jr., and Brush, B. E.: Complications of gastrointestinal intubation. Arch. Surg., 83:147–160, 1961.
11. Royce, S., Tepper, C., Watson, W., and Day, R.: Indwelling polyethylene nasogastric tube for feeding premature infants. Pediatrics, 8:79–81, 1951.
12. Wagner, E. A., Jones, D. V., Koch, C. A., and Smith, G. D.: Polyethylene tube feeding in premature infants. J. Pediatr., 41:79–83, 1952.
13. Kunz, H. W.: Paraffin-tipped polyethylene tubing for feeding of premature babies, infants and children. J. Pediatr., 41:84–85, 1952.
14. Fallis, L. S., and Barron, J.: Gastric and jejunal alimentation with fine polyethylene tubes. Arch. Surg., 65:373–381, 1952.
15. Wagner, E. A., Koch, C. A., and Jones, D. V.: An improved indwelling tube for feeding premature infants. J. Pediatr., 45:200–201, 1954.
16. Keoshian, L. A., and Nelsen, T. S.: A new design for a feeding tube. Plast. Reconstr. Surg., 44:508–509, 1969.
17. Davis, L. E., and Hofmann, W.: A long-term nasogastric feeding tube made from modified Penrose tubing. J.A.M.A., 209:685–686, 1969.
18. Rhea, J. W., and Kilby, J. O.: A nasojejunal tube for infant feeding. Pediatrics, 46:36–40, 1976.
19. Anderson, A. F. R.: Immediate jejunal feeding after gastro-enterostomy. Ann. Surg., 67:565–566, 1918.
20. Abbott, W. O., and Rawson, A. J.: A tube for use in the postoperative care of gastroenterostomy cases. J.A.M.A., 108:1873–1874, 1937.
21. McDonald, H. A.: Intrajejunal drip in gastric surgery. Lancet, 1:1007, 1954.
22. Delany, H. M., and Garvey, J. W.: Jejunostomy by a needle catheter technique. Surgery, 73:786–790, 1973.
23. Cobb, L. M., Cartmill, A. M., and Gilsdorf, R. B.: Early postoperative nutritional support using the serosal tunnel jejunostomy. J.P.E.N., 5(5):397–401, 1981.
24. Moss, G.: Early enteral feeding after abdominal surgery. In Dietel, M. (ed.): Nutrition in Clinical Surgery. Baltimore, Williams and Wilkins, 1980.
25. Rombeau, J. L.: Personal communication, 1981.
26. DeWys, W. D., and Kubota, T. T.: Enteral and parenteral nutrition in the care of the cancer patient. J.A.M.A., 246:1725–1727, 1981.
27. Martin, D. C.: Easy insertion of a feeding tube. Am. J. Surg., 139:728, 1980.
28. Matarese, L. E.: Enteral alimentation: Equipment—Part III. Nutr. Support Serv., 2(2):48–49, 1982.
29. Cobb, L. M., Cartmill, A. M., Barry, M., and Gilsdorf, R. B.: A tube for enteral nutrition for patients with aphagopraxia and patients with ventilator assistance. Surg. Gynecol. Obstet., 155:81–84, 1982.
30. Balkany, T. J., Jafek, B. W., and Wong, M. L.: Complications of feeding esophagotomy. Arch. Otolaryngol., 106:122–123, 1980.
31. Kaminski, M. V., and Freed, B. A.: Enteral hyperalimentation: Prevention and treatment of complications. Nutr. Support Serv. 1(4):29–35, 1981.
32. Basil, S. M.: Needle catheter jejunostomy: An approach to total enteral nutrition. Nutr. Support Serv., 1(7):31–34, 1981.
33. Cartwright, M.: Tube feeding by nasal gavage. R.N., 122(12):55–61, 1959.
34. McDonald, E., Williams, H., Daggett, M., Schut, B., Swint, E., and Buckwalter, K. C.: A comparison of four holding devices for anchoring naso-

gastric tubes. J. Neurosurg. Nurs., *14*(2):90–93, 1982.

35. Shah, N.: Method of fixing the nasogastric feeding tube. J. Laryngol. Otol., *83*:485–486, 1969.

36. Armstrong, C., Luther, W., and Sykes, T.: A technique for preventing extubation of feeding tubes. "The bridle." J.P.E.N., *4*:603, 1980.

37. Hart, J. F.: Restraining mask for children. Am. J. Nurs., *59*:1737, 1959.

38. Sullivan, P. G., and Haringman, H.: An intra-oral appliance to stabilise orogastric tube in premature infants. Lancet, *1*:416–417, 1981.

39. Morse, J. L.: Recollections and reflections on forty-five years of artificial infant feeding. J. Pediatr., *7*:303–324, 1935.

40. Page, C. P., Ryan, J. A., and Haff, R. C.: Continual catheter administration of an elemental diet. Surg. Gynecol. Obstet., *142*:184–187, 1976.

41. Kaminski, M. V.: Enteral hyperalimentation. Surg. Gynecol. Obstet., *143*:12–16, 1976.

42. Chernoff, R. (ed.): ASPEN Product Resource Manual. Edition 2. Washington, D.C., American Society of Parenteral and Enteral Nutrition, 1982.

43. Howard, L., Chu, R., Feman, S., and Wolf, B.: Vitamin A deficiency in a patient on long-term intravenous nutrition. J.P.E.N., *1*(1):10A, 1977.

44. White, W. T., III, Acuff, T. E., Jr., Sykes, T. R., and Dobbie, R. P.: Bacterial contamination of enteral nutrient solution: A preliminary report. J.P.E.N., *3*(6):459–461, 1979.

45. Champlin, L.: Enteral nutrition. Medical Products Sales *13*(2):1, 8, 28–30, 32, 35, 1982.

46. Dobbie, R. P., and Hoffmeister, J. A.: Continuous pump-tube enteric hyperalimentation. Surg. Gynecol. Obstet., *143*:273–276, 1976.

47. Freeman, J. B., and Fairfull-Smith, R. J.: Improved nitrogen equilibrium with constant infusion pumps in enteral feeding. J.P.E.N., *3*(1):27, 1979.

48. Heymsfield, S. B., Bethel, R. A., Ansley, J. D., Nixon, D. W., and Rudman, D.: Enteral hyperalimentation: An alternative to central venous hyperalimentation. Ann. Intern. Med., *90*:63–71, 1979.

49. Parker, P., Stroop, S., and Greene, H.: A controlled comparison of continuous versus intermittent feeding in the treatment of infants with intestinal disease. J. Pediatr., *99*:360–364, 1981.

50. Hiebert, J. M., Brown, A., Anderson, R. G., Halfacre, S., Rodeheaver, G. T., and Edlich, R. F.: Comparison of continuous vs. intermittent tube feeding in adult burn patients. J.P.E.N. *5*(1):73–75, 1981.

51. Kien, C. L.: Employment of a mobile infusion system for continuous ambulatory tube feeding. J.P.E.N., *5*(6):526–527, 1981.

52. Butterworth, C. E., and Weinsier, R. L.: Malnutrition in hospitalized patients: Assessment and treatment. *In* Goodhart, R. S., and Shils, M. E. (eds.): Modern Nutrition in Health and Disease. Edition 6. Philadelphia, Lea and Febiger, 1980, pages 667–684.

53. Beaumont, E.: The new IV infusion pumps. Nursing, *7*(7):31–35, 1977.

54. Jones, B. J. M., Payne, S., and Silk, D. B. A.: Indications for pump-assisted enteral feeding. Lancet, *1*:1057–1058, 1980.

55. Forlaw, L., Devlin, F. K., Rombeau, J. L., Melnik, G., and Settle, R. G.: Comparison of pumps for tube feeding [Abstract]. Am. J. Clin. Nutr., *34*:636, 1981.

CHAPTER 14

Radiologic Techniques of Gastrointestinal Intubation

GORDON K. MCLEAN

Fluoroscopically guided gastrointestinal intubation has become a routine procedure in the management of many diseases. Although usually placed for the relief of small bowel obstruction, tubes are being used increasingly for enteric alimentation as well as a variety of laboratory and radiologic tests. Traditional placement techniques have relied on both gravity and residual peristalsis to carry tubes from the stomach through the pylorus and duodenum into the small bowel. Radiologists have routinely been called on to direct small tubes by manipulating both the patient and the tube under fluoroscopy. Unfortunately, many of those patients whose need for intestinal intubation is most critical are aperistaltic, and traditional techniques of tube placement are often frustrating and unsuccessful. Since 1967, a variety of methods have been described for intubating the aperistaltic patient.[1-6] Because of the need for specialized equipment and skills, these methods did not find wide application; however, the rapid growth of interventional radiology over the past few years has changed this picture. Currently, any center with an established or developing capability in interventional radiology already has both the equipment and technical expertise needed to rapidly and safely intubate almost any portion of the bowel.

TRANSNASAL AND TRANSORAL GASTROINTESTINAL INTUBATION

Gastric Intubation

If a standard nasogastric tube is already in the stomach, it is often possible to direct a J-shaped guidewire out one of its sideholes allowing exchange for an angiographic catheter. If a nasogastric tube is not in place, a small one (such as 10 French) with an added end-hole should be passed. If the intubation is intended to be only temporary, the tube may be introduced through the mouth rather than the nose, avoiding injury to the nasopharynx. Once the tube is in the stomach, a standard angiographic guidewire is advanced through it and the tube is exchanged for either a 100-cm preformed Cobra type angiographic catheter (Cook, Bloomington, Indiana) or the MediTech steerable catheter system (MediTech, Inc., Watertown, Massachusetts).

If esophageal disease prevents free passage of the tube, the technique is modified as follows. Because esophageal intubation may be moderately painful, a mild sedative should be administered, such as diazepam, 5 mg, by slow intravenous push. The oral pharynx and proximal esophagus should also be anesthetized locally with a topical spray (for example, Cetacaine spray, Cetylite Industries, Inc., Pennsauken, New Jersey). An end-hole is cut in a nasogastric tube which is liberally coated with a water soluble lubricant, and the tube is passed through the patient's nose or mouth into the esophagus and advanced as far as possible. Once resistance is met, this tube is exchanged over a guidewire for an angiographic catheter; depending on the topography of obstruction, the catheter should be either a straight one or one with a gentle distal curve. A small amount of contrast medium is injected through the catheter to accurately outline the obstruction. If the obstruction is quite high and the risk of aspiration great, oily contrast material may be preferable; if the obstructing lesion is friable or results from recent trauma, 2 to 3 ml of water soluble contrast medium is preferable because of the risk of intravasation. Occasionally, a standard angiographic guidewire (a straight tapered wire or one with a 15-mm J curve) can be used to gently probe the obstruction and guide passage into the stomach. More often, the Lunderquist torque control guidewire should be used (Cook, Inc., Bloomington, Indiana) (Fig. 14–1). A 30- to 45-degree bend is made 1.5 cm from the wire's tip. By continuously rotating the external, coiled portion of the wire and applying only gentle forward pressure, the torque guide should rapidly find and enter the stenotic esophageal tract. The guidewire and catheter are then used in combination to cross the obstruction (Fig. 14–2). Once the catheter is beyond the obstruction, the Lunderquist torque guide is removed and a long standard guidewire is advanced well into the stomach. If it is important to demonstrate the exact limits of the obstructing lesion or define the radiographic anatomy of the esophagus distal to the obstruction, contrast material can be injected around the guidewire. To assure access through the obstructing lesion, the guidewire is left in place in the stomach and contrast material is injected through a Y adaptor or an injection hub (such as Hemostasis valve, Cordis Corporation, Miami, Florida) as the catheter is pulled up through the lesion.

Cannulating the Pylorus

In most patients, a 100-cm Cobra-type angiographic catheter can be used to cross the pylorus. The catheter is advanced along the greater curvature until its tip lies in the distal antrum and is directed up toward the pylorus. Injection of 100 to 400 cc of air through the catheter will distend the stomach, making catheter passage easier and, often, filling the duodenal bulb (Fig. 14–3). Small amounts of water soluble contrast material may also be injected intermittently to check the position of the catheter and define the topography of the gastric antrum. If a distorted gastric anatomy makes the use of an angiographic catheter awkward, the MediTech steerable catheter system may be more effective.

If the pylorus is patulous, it can be directly cannulated with standard angiographic guidewires (Fig. 14–4). Often, because of post-peptic scarring or pylorospasm, standard, flexible angiographic guidewires cannot be passed directly through the pylorus and the Lunderquist torque control guidewire should be used. A 45-degree bend is made 1.5 cm from the guide's tip and the wire is continuously rotated and advanced up to the pylorus (Fig. 14–5). Often, the catheter's position will have to be adjusted several times before the correct angle of attack is found. If the angle between the first and second portions of the duodenum is particularly acute, it may be difficult to advance the torque guide further into the duodenum. The catheter should be advanced to the tip of the torque guide and contrast material injected to confirm placement within the bulb. The torque guide should then be

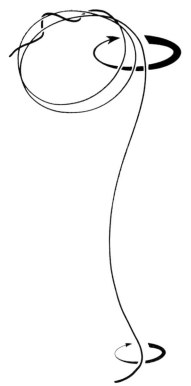

Figure 14–1. Use of the Lunderquist torque control guidewire. The Lunderquist torque control guidewire is a heavy duty, stainless steel guide with a malleable tip. The tip is shaped in accordance with the topography of the obstruction to be crossed; here, a smooth C curve has been formed. The external portion of the wire is then coiled as shown. When the external coil is rotated (*large curved arrow*) torque is transmitted to the tip, which rotates correspondingly (*small curved arrow*). A one-to-one transmission of torque is obtained no matter how many bends are made in the portion of wire between the tip and the external loop.

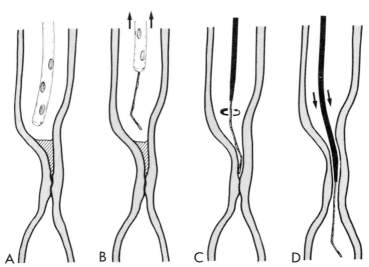

Figure 14–2. Crossing an esophageal stricture. *A*, A standard nasogastric tube with an added end-hole has been passed to the level of the obstruction. A small amount of contrast material *(hatched area)* is injected to delineate the stricture. *B*, A Lunderquist torque guide has been passed out the end-hole of the nasogastric tube; the nasogastric tube is now removed *(arrows)*. The tip of the torque control guide has been shaped in accordance with the morphology of the stricture. *C*, A standard angiographic catheter has replaced the nasogastric tube. The torque guide is being rotated continuously *(curved arrow)* while very gentle forward pressure is applied. It is the continuous rotation which allows the guidewire's tip to seek out and enter the tract through the stricture. No attempts to vigorously force the guidewire through the stricture are made, since this risks esophageal perforation. *D*, The tip of the torque guide has passed through the stricture. This is evidenced by a decrease in resistance to the passage of the guidewire as well as an obvious increase in the freedom of movement of the guide tip. The angiographic catheter can now be advanced through the lesion and into the stomach *(arrows)*.

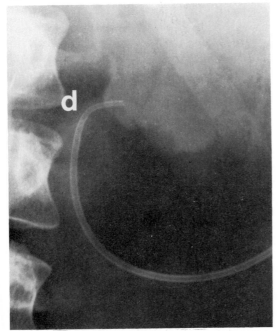

Figure 14–3. Approaching the pylorus with a Cobra catheter. A 100-cm Cobra catheter has been advanced along the greater curvature of the stomach. The preformed tip of the catheter can be seen to overlie the pylorus (note the air-filled duodenal cap (d) just beyond the tip of the catheter). If this catheter is withdrawn slightly, the tip will be directed straight up toward the pylorus.

formed into a wide C curve and reintroduced; alternatively, a 15-mm J guide may be substituted at this point.

Crossing Gastroenterostomies

Because of the more favorable angle of attack, intubation of the bowel through a gastroenterostomy usually poses fewer problems than intubation through the pylorus and duodenum. Because of the location of the anastomosis within the gastric pouch, the curve of the angiographic catheter should be less than that used to cross the pylorus. If the anastomosis is widely patent, simple torquing of the catheter and probing with a straight or J-shaped guidewire should allow rapid and selective entry into either the afferent or efferent limb of bowel (Fig. 14–6). If the anastomosis is strictured, the Lunderquist torque control guidewire should be used in the manner described previously.

Because the afferent and efferent limbs may be superimposed in the anteroposterior projection, selective intubation is usually best accomplished with the patient in a steep oblique position. A tilting fluoroscopic table is also very helpful in this setting,

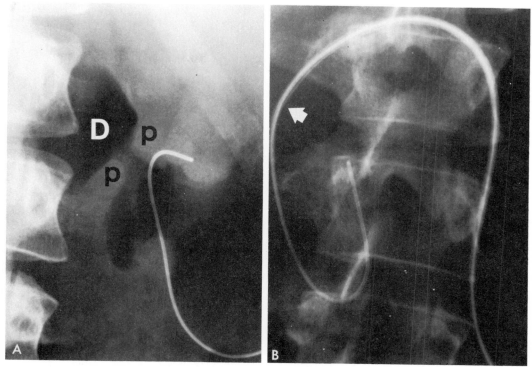

Figure 14–4.   Crossing the pylorus with a standard angiographic guidewire. *A,* The Cobra catheter has been withdrawn slightly and a standard J-curved guidewire is being advanced toward the pylorus. Here, the tip of the guide can be seen buckling through the pyloric sphincter (small p's) toward the air-filled duodenal bulb (D). *B,* The J guide has buckled completely through the pylorus and now lies in the second portion of the duodenum. Note the tip of the angiographic catheter *(arrow)* which is being advanced over the leading guidewire.

since it allows the anastomotic site to be identified with only a small volume of contrast material.

Manipulating Guidewires and Tubes Through the Bowel

The techniques described above for gaining access to the bowel are different from those employed to manipulate guidewires, catheters, and intestinal tubes through the bowel itself. Although the Lunderquist torque control guide is ideally suited to cannulating the pylorus or a stenotic anastomosis, once in the bowel its tip will repeatedly catch the valvulae conniventes, making passage difficult. The tip of the torque guide may be re-formed into a broad C curve or, preferably, a 15-mm J guide with a long tapered mandril should be substituted for the more rigid torque guide (Fig. 14–7). Similarly, preformed torque control catheters such as the Cobra catheters are not usually well suited for passage through the bowel. A long straight catheter or one with a very

gentle distal curve will pass through more easily. The distensibility of bowel coupled with its peristalsis makes passage of the catheters and guidewires through it quite different in "feel" from the passage of catheters and guidewires through the vascular tree. Often, when the catheter and guidewire are advanced externally, there is not an immediate corresponding movement of the tip. Instead, the forward pressure is gradually transmitted through the system so that the guidewire moves ahead slowly after an interval of 10 to 30 seconds.

If access to the bowel has been gained through the stomach, there is a tendency for both catheters and guidewires to coil within it. Frequent fluoroscopic checks should be made to assure that the path of the guidewire and catheter through the stomach is the straightest possible. If a large loop has formed in the stomach, pulling the guidewire and catheter back somewhat may actually help the tip to advance further in the bowel. If unusually tight bends are encountered (such as at the ligament of Treitz), reintroduction of the torque control guide-

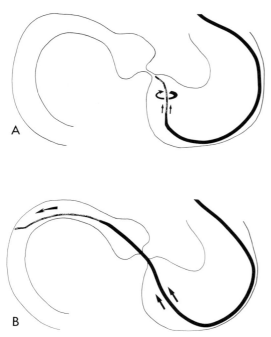

Figure 14–5. Crossing the pylorus with the Lunderquist torque guide. *A*, A 100-cm Cobra catheter lies along the greater curvature of the stomach with its tip directed toward the pylorus. A 45-degree bend has been formed 1.5 cm from the tip of a Lunderquist torque guide. The guidewire is being gently advanced out the catheter *(double arrows)* while being rotated continuously *(curved arrow)* so that its tip seeks and engages the tight pyloric canal. *B*, The torque guide has passed through the pylorus and has been advanced *(single arrow)* until its tip lodges against the duodenal wall. The guiding catheter can now be advanced over the guidewire through the pylorus *(double arrows)*.

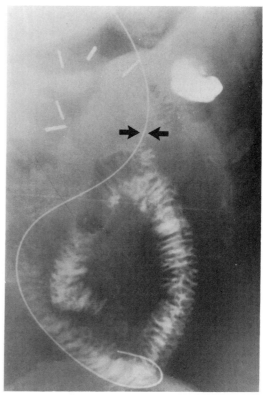

Figure 14–6. Selective intubation of an efferent loop. Placement of a jejunal feeding tube was requested for this patient because of poor gastric emptying following a subtotal gastrectomy and construction of a Billroth II anastomosis. Here, the guidewire has been placed selectively in the efferent loop. Although the site of anastomosis was too tight to prevent adequate gastric emptying *(arrows)*, it was easily crossed using standard angiographic guidewire and catheter techniques.

wire and the torqueable catheter may be necessary to negotiate difficult curves.

If a tube is being introduced for simple bowel decompression or for enteric alimentation, the tube should be advanced at least to the level of the ligament of Treitz. Preferably, the distal portion of the tube should lie beyond the ligament in the proximal jejunum. When placing the guidewire over which the final tube will be advanced, the guidewire should be placed well into the proximal jejunum. Often, tension must be applied to the guide to get a tube to advance through a tight pyloric sphincter; this tension requires pulling back some length of wire, and if the wire is not well beyond the ligament of Treitz, its stiff portion may be insufficient to carry the tube into the proximal jejunum.

TRANSSTOMAL GASTROINTESTINAL INTUBATION

Transgastrostomy Jejunal Intubation

If a feeding gastrostomy has been inserted recently, it cannot be removed and manipulations must be carried out with the tube in place. Most feeding gastrostomies are positioned so that the tip of the indwelling tube is directed up toward the gastric fundus. Although it may be possible to manipulate angiographic catheters or guidewires out an end-hole or side vent of the tube, it is usually extremely difficult to guide the catheter into the gastric antrum (Fig. 14–8A). To alter this unfavorable angle of approach to the pylorus, a guidewire is first manipulated out one of the side vents of the

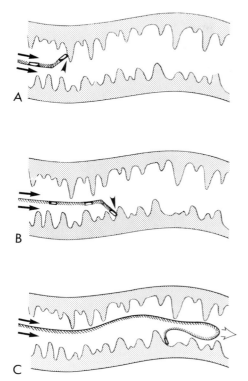

Figure 14–7. Selecting a guidewire to pass through the lumen of the bowel. *A,* The tip of a Lunderquist torque guide has been formed into a 45-degree curve. As the guidewire is advanced *(double arrows),* the rigid tip catches against one of the valvulae conniventes *(arrowhead). B,* The tip of the guide can be disengaged by simply rotating the external coiled portion of the wire. However, as the guide is advanced a short distance *(double arrows),* the tip catches again on one of the valvulae *(arrowhead).* The stiffness of this wire will cause it to catch repeatedly in the bowel, making its passage slow and difficult. *C,* Here, a 15-mm J guide is being passed through the bowel *(double arrows).* If the tip catches on one of the valvulae conniventes, the flexible portion of the mandril can buckle ahead *(open arrow),* permitting free passage through the lumen of the bowel.

gastrostomy, and 8 and 12 French Teflon biliary dilators are passed coaxially over the guide into the gastrostomy tube. While external traction is applied to the tube, the relatively rigid Teflon catheters are rotated supralaterally, changing the vector of the gastrostomy. A torque-controlled guidewire passed through the central dilator will now be directed into the gastric antrum and toward the pylorus (Fig. 14–8B). A long exchange guidewire is now placed beyond the ligament of Treitz in the usual fashion.

If the gastrostomy tube has been in place for 4 to 6 weeks, it can be removed

safely by cutting the anchoring sutures and pulling the tube directly out. Since this may be painful, mild sedation (10 mg of diazepam intramuscularly) should be used. If the gastrostomy is large (18 French or greater), torque control catheters and guidewires can be readily manipulated through it to cannulate the pylorus as described above (Fig. 14–9A). Once through the pylorus, the torque control guidewire has a tendency to catch its tip repeatedly on the valvulae conniventes, and a J guide with its long tapered inner mandril will be more effective. When the catheter has been manipulated well into the duodenum, a long, 210-cm, heavy duty exchange guidewire is placed through it into the distal duodenum or proximal jejunum. The end of the guidewire is then introduced into the jejunal catheter and brought out its hub. By applying water soluble lubricant or silicone spray to the jejunal tube, it can usually be advanced directly over the guidewire into the small bowel (Fig. 14–9B). The guidewire is then removed and the external portion of the jejunal tube is passed through a gastrostomy tube and the latter reinserted in the usual fashion. The jejunal tube should always be passed through the lumen of the gastrostomy tube, since side-by-side placement of the tube will frequently result in leakage of gastric contents (Fig. 14–9C).

In patients who have had a Billroth II anastomosis following gastric resection, the gastroenteric anastomosis usually lies directly beneath the tip of the gastrostomy tube. A preformed, head-hunter-type catheter (Simmons; SIM 2, Cook, Bloomington, Indiana) is advanced through the gastrostomy tube and re-formed in the gastric remnant. A guidewire passed through this catheter will be directed almost 180 degrees from the gastrostomy angle of entry and can be used to probe the bottom of the gastric pouch. Once the anastomosis has been traversed and the efferent loop entered, the small bowel is intubated in the usual fashion (Fig. 14–10).

Intraoperative Jejunal Intubation

The intraoperative placement of the combined gastrostomy-jejunal tube may not require fluoroscopic assistance. If general anesthesia is used and adequate access to the stomach is gained (such as construction

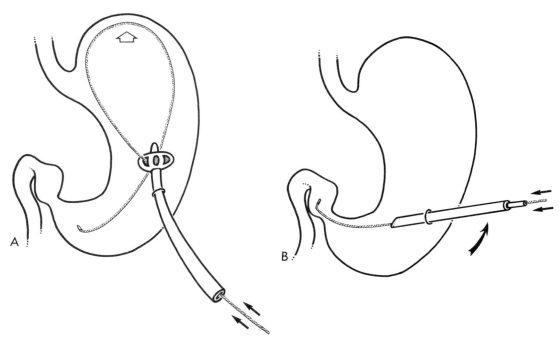

Figure 14–8. Altering an unfavorable gastrostomy angle to cannulate the pylorus. *A,* Guidewire passed through side vent of a gastrostomy tube in the usual fashion is directed toward the gastric fundus. Advancing more wire *(double arrows)* causes the guide to buckle up into the fundus *(open arrow)*. *B,* Placing rigid, coaxial Teflon dilators allows the angle of the gastrostomy to be changed. By rotating the dilators supralaterally *(curved arrow)* the guidewire may be advanced directly into the gastric antrum to the pylorus *(double arrows)*. The dilators have passed through the center of the gastrostomy tube, which is not shown in this schematic figure.

of a Janeway gastrostomy), the jejunal component of the tube may be manually passed through the pylorus and guided to the ligament of Treitz by palpation. In those patients undergoing a limited procedure under local anesthesia, C-arm fluoroscopy can be used to guide passage of the jejunal portion of the tube. Once surgical access to the stomach is gained, torque control catheters and guidewires are used as described above to cannulate the pylorus and place a long wire in the jejunum. The jejunal component of the combined tube has an end-hole passing through its mercury-weighted tip and can be passed directly over a guidewire into the jejunum. Following placement of the tip, the guidewire is removed and the remainder of the gastrostomy-jejunal tube is placed surgically in the usual fashion (Fig. 14–11).

MISCELLANEOUS ENTEROCUTANEOUS INTUBATIONS

The techniques of manipulating through the bowel are consistent no matter what the portal of entry. Successful bowel intubation can be accomplished through surgically constructed stomas or spontaneous enterocutaneous fistulas. Once access has been gained into the lumen of the bowel, floppy J-tip guides and straight catheters are used to pass through most sections of bowel, and torque control catheters and guidewires are used to negotiate unusually acute bends.

TUBE SELECTION AND PLACEMENT

Polyvinyl and polyethylene tubes are the easiest tubes to position in the bowel. Although suitable only for short-term placement, they serve a variety of therapeutic and diagnostic needs. The guidewire over which the tube will be introduced should be long enough to accommodate the entire tube externally; a 260-cm, heavy duty exchange guide is usually adequate. Using a large hole punch, an end-hole is cut in the tip of the tube. The tube is coated liberally with a water soluble lubricant and then threaded over the guidewire. Passage through the esophagus and body of the stomach is usually quite simple. If an esophageal lesion

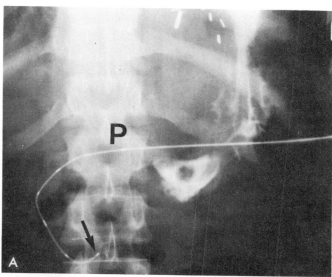

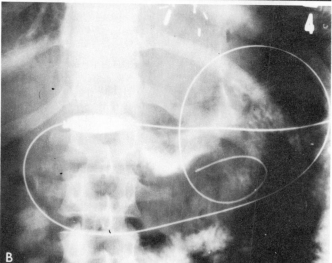

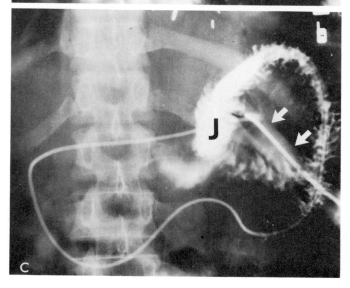

Figure 14–9. Technique of transgastrostomy jejunal intubation. *A,* Gastrostomy tube has been removed and torque-controlled guidewire has been manipulated through the pylorus (P). The guide tip *(arrow)* now lies at the junction of the second and third portion of the duodenum. *B,* Mercury-weighted tip of the jejunal catheter is advanced in over the guidewire. Here, the tip is passing through the pylorus (remainder of the tube is not radiopaque). *C,* Jejunal tube has been placed and the guidewire removed. Injection of contrast material shows infusion into the proximal jejunum (J). The gastrostomy tube *(arrows)* has been replaced.

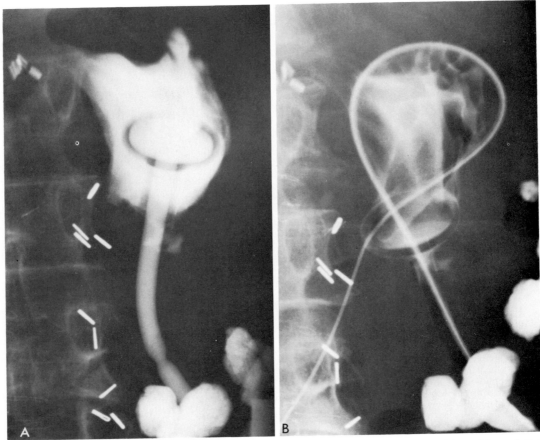

Figure 14–10. Jejunal intubation through a Billroth II anastomosis. *A*, Contrast material injected through the indwelling gastrostomy shows the area of the gastroenteric anastomosis to lie directly beneath the tip of the gastrostomy. *B*, Use of a preformed catheter has allowed the guidewire to be directed 180 degrees from its vector of entry. The guidewire has been placed in the efferent loop and will now be used to place the jejunal catheter.

prevents easy passage, the esophageal lumen can be enlarged with graded biliary dilators passed over the guidewire. If there is resistance at the pylorus, there is a tendency for both the tube and wire to buckle in the stomach; however, if sufficient length of guidewire has been advanced beyond the ligament of Treitz, there should be little difficulty in supplying sufficient tension to the wire to allow the tube to pass.

Unfortunately, the tubes that are easiest to pass into the bowel are the least well suited for long-term use. Standard polyethylene or polyvinyl nasogastric tubes, 10 to 12 French, can usually be passed with little difficulty. Standard angiographic catheters have also been used for enteric alimentation; their small size and torque control allow them to be manipulated past high grade obstructions.[7] The difficulty with all of these tubes is their lack of pliability. Over a relatively short period of time they become extremely rigid and begin to erode the bowel wall.[8, 9]

Open-ended Silastic tubes are well suited for long-term placement in the bowel. Because Silastic has a high coefficient of friction, these tubes have a tendency to bind on the guidewire and should be liberally coated with lubricant. An open-ended Silastic tube can be easily made by cutting the mercury tip from a Dobhoff catheter (Biosearch, Raritan, New Jersey).

A guidewire technique can also be used to position mercury-tipped Silastic tubes such as the Dobhoff catheter. If the patient's problem is primarily one of peristalsis and there are no tight strictures to be passed, the Dobhoff or similar catheter can often be advanced directly over a guidewire alone (Fig. 14–12). The end of the guidewire is introduced into the most distal sidehole of the catheter and brought out its hub. Water-soluble lubricant is applied liberally to the wire

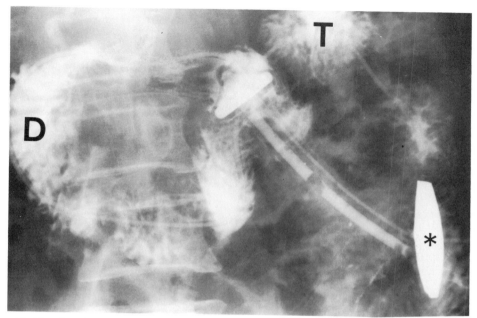

Figure 14–11. Combined gastrostomy-jejunal tube in place. The mercury-weighted tip *(asterisk)* can be seen in the first jejunal loop. The course of the jejunal catheter can be faintly seen as it passes through the duodenum (D) and beyond the ligament of Treitz (T). Contrast material also outlines the lumen of the gastrostomy component of the tube as it passes through the abdominal wall into the stomach.

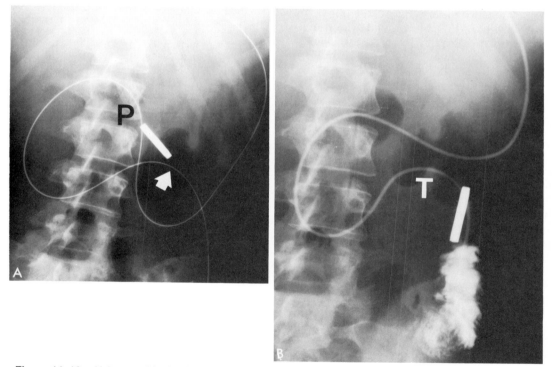

Figure 14–12. Using a guidewire for jejunal placement of Dobhoff catheter. *A,* A long (260 cm) angiographic exchange guidewire has been passed into the jejunum. Note that the wire lies well beyond the ligament of Treitz *(arrow).* The Dobhoff feeding tube is being advanced over the wire. Only the mercury-filled tip of the tube is visible radiographically; the Silastic portion of the tube is not radiopaque. Here, the mercury-filled tip is just passing through the pylorus (P). *B,* The feeding tube has been advanced beyond the ligament of Treitz (T) and the guidewire has been withdrawn. Water-soluble contrast material is injected, demonstrating the course of the Silastic tube. Note that the sideholes are infusing only into the jejunum and there is no reflux of contrast material back into the duodenum or the stomach.

and the tube is advanced over it. Generally, the best results are obtained by advancing the guidewire and catheter together as a unit and then gently pulling back on the wire. Lubricity between the guidewire and tube can be maintained if the space between the guidewire and tube is periodically injected with a silicon lubricant or "slippery water" (a mixture of one part water soluble lubricant shaken in a syringe with two parts water and rapidly injected). This injection should utilize a blunt-tipped needle to avoid injuring the fragile Silastic tube.

If there is esophageal or pyloric resistance to passage of the tube, these blunt-tipped mercury tubes can also be introduced by using an inner catheter to provide body. A polyethylene or Teflon catheter of 5 French or less is passed inside the Silastic tube and a guidewire is then passed through this inner "carrier" catheter. The tip of the carrier catheter should lie just inside the last sidehole of the mercury-tipped tube (Fig. 14–13). Removing the carrier catheter from the Silastic tube may be quite difficult because of friction between the two. The frequent injection of lubricant will allow the carrier catheter to be removed; do not remove the inner guidewire before the entire carrier catheter has been safely withdrawn.

Long tubes such as the Miller-Abbott and Cantor tubes can also be passed with guidewire techniques. Extra-long torque control guides which can be passed completely through a long tube are available (Cook, Incorporated, Bloomington, Indiana).[4] A less cumbersome technique involves passing a guidewire through a small slit cut in the side of a long tube 40 to 60 inches proximal to its tip. If the slit is cut diagonally through the tube's wall with a sharp scalpel blade, it will close following withdrawal of the guide and not leak during either suction or infusion. Specialized torque guides may be used in this fashion[1, 6] but in most cases, a standard, heavy duty, angiographic guidewire is adequate.[5]

When working through a gastrostomy tube, the size of the jejunal tube which can be placed is limited to the inner diameter of the indwelling gastrostomy. Large gastrostomy tubes will admit a standard Dobhoff catheter (8 French tubing with 18 French tip; Biosearch, Raritan, New Jersey). Smaller gastrostomies will accommodate Keofeed tubes (HEDECO, Mountainview, California) of 9.6 or 7.3 French (maximum tip diameters).

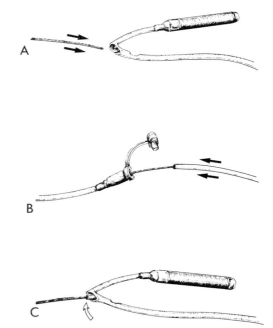

Figure 14–13. Using a "carrier" catheter to assist passage of a mercury-tipped tube. *A,* The external portion of the guidewire is introduced into the sidehole closest to the mercury-filled tip of the Silastic tube *(arrows)*. *B,* The guidewire has been passed completely through the Silastic tube, and a small catheter is advanced over the guide and into the tube *(arrows)*. Because of their low coefficient of friction, Teflon catheters make ideal "carriers"; 5 French catheters offer the advantage of accommodating heavy-duty 0.035-inch guidewires but may bind within the Silastic tube. A 4.5 French Teflon catheter passes more easily through the Silastic tubing but cannot accept a guidewire greater than 0.032 inch in diameter. *C,* The tip of the "carrier" catheter is just at the level of the last sidehole of the decompression tube *(arrow)*. With a little practice, the Silastic tube can now be advanced through tight stenoses within the lumen of the bowel. Note that if no stenosis impedes passage of the tube, the Silastic tube can usually be passed directly over the guidewire and no "carrier" catheter is necessary.

Discussion

For many years, fluoroscopy has been used to pass tubes into the duodenum and small bowel for intestinal decompression. More recently, there has been an increasing use of small bowel tubes for sampling duodenal and jejunal contents, obtaining biopsies, infusing radiopaque materials for diagnostic studies, and for enteric alimentation. Usually, specialized equipment is not needed to intubate the small bowel; in fact, the duodenum can frequently be intubated without using fluoroscopy at all.[10] When fluoroscopy and a tilting table are used, most patients can be intubated quickly and simply. However, if peristalsis is inadequate or absent, if obstructing lesions or stenoses exist within the alimentary tract, or if surgery has altered the esophageal or gastric anatomy, it may be impossible to pass a tube simply by changing the patient's position.[7, 11]

A variety of techniques for transnasal and transoral intubation of the bowel have been described previously. In 1967 Gianturco developed a guiding system which made it practical to perform hypotonic duodenography on a routine basis.[1] Since then, sets of guiding stylets and specialized guidewires have been designed to assist in the placement of small bowel tubes.[3, 4, 6] Hanafee adapted angiographic techniques to the problem of intestinal intubation by using a deflector wire system, while others have used standard angiographic guidewires to facilitate tube passage.[2, 5] The techniques described in this chapter evolved from those used routinely in the vascular, biliary, and urinary systems. With a little practice, these same maneuvers can be used to advance guidewires and tubes almost any distance into any portion of the bowel.

Enteric alimentation by transgastrostomy jejunal intubation was first described in 1942.[12] Although many of these transgastrostomy tubes will pass unaided or with the use of metaclopramide (10 mg intravenously), a substantial number will not and remain in either the stomach or the proximal duodenum (Fig. 14–14). By using the techniques described above, most simple gastrostomies can be converted to a combined jejunostomy-gastrostomy. When the need for a jejunal feeding tube is anticipated preoperatively, postoperative placement of the tube can be greatly facilitated if the surgeon places the gastrostomy so that it is directed toward the lesser curvature and antrum. The special dual lumen, Silastic gastrostomy, jejunal tube offers the most satisfactory solution to the problem, since access is gained to the stomach and the small bowel. This tube may either be placed primarily at surgery or be substituted later for a simple gastrostomy if gastric feedings prove to be ineffective and true enteric alimentation is desired.

Enthusiasm for tube placement should be tempered by the fact that iatrogenic intubation injuries are relatively common. Endoscopically, it has been found that, following gastric intubation, 60 per cent of patients sustain injury to the esophagus or hypopharynx; only 2 per cent of these intubation injuries will be clinically apparent.[9] Ulceration and mucosal bruising are commonest, but actual perforation of the hypopharynx, esophagus, or stomach may occur. The risk of intubation injury is greatest in the pediatric age group. When tubes remain in the bowel for long periods of time, their physical characteristics change. Polyvinyl and polyethylene tubes begin to discolor and

Figure 14–14. Jejunal limb of this combined gastrostomy-jejunal tube was not placed over a guide but was left in the stomach to pass spontaneously. The mercury-weighted tip has passed into the proximal jejunum, but the tube has knotted itself in the stomach *(arrow)*. Although contrast passes freely through the tube this time, the soft Silastic material is susceptible to kinking. Once the initial gastrostomy has healed, this tube will be removed and repositioned.

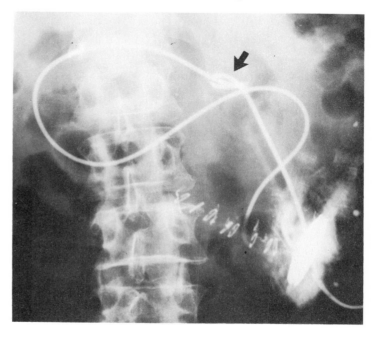

harden after as little as 6 to 12 hours in the small bowel.[8, 9] If these tubes are not changed on a regular basis, erosion and ulceration of the mucosa may eventually lead to perforation. Silastic tubes can remain safely in the bowel for long periods of time and are well tolerated by most patients. With a little practice, enough technical expertise can be gained to allow their rapid and atraumatic placement.

REFERENCES

1. Gianturco, C.: Rapid fluoroscopic duodenal intubation. Radiology, *88*:1165–1166, 1967.
2. Hanafee, W. N., and Weiner, M.: External guided passage of an intestinal intubation tube. Radiology, *89*:1100–1102, 1967.
3. Bilbao, M. K., Frische, L. H., Dotter, C. T., and Rösch, J.: Hypotonic duodenalography. Radiology, *89*:438–443, 1967.
4. Sargent, E. N., and Meyers, H. L.: Wire guide and technique for Cantor tube insertion: Rapid small bowel intubation. A.J.R., *107*:150–155, 1969.
5. Gelfand, D. W.: An easy method for passing an intestinal intubation tube under fluoroscopic guidance. Radiology, *129*:532, 1978.
6. Shipps, F. C., Sayler, C. B., Egan, J. F., Green, G. S., Weinstein, C. J., and Jones, J. M.: Fluoroscopic placement of intestinal tubes. Radiology, *132*:226–227, 1979.
7. Zornoza, J., Chuang, V. P., and Wallace, S.: Use of angiographic catheters for intestinal alimentation in patients with upper gastrointestinal obstruction. Radiology, *143*:240, 1980.
8. Siegle, R. L., Rabinowitz, J. G., and Sarasohn, C.: Intestinal perforation secondary to nasojejunal feeding tubes. AJR, *126*:1229–1232, 1976.
9. Ghahremani, G. G., Turner, M. A., and Port, R. B.: Iatrogenic intubation injuries of the upper gastrointestinal tract in adults. Gastrointest. Radiol., *5*:1–10, 1980.
10. Palmer, E. D.: Duodenal intubation. J.A.M.A., *233*:818–819, 1975.
11. Ho, C. S., Lipinski, J. K.: Selective intubation of the afferent loop. A.J.R., *130*:481–484, 1978.
12. Bisgard, J. D.: Gastrostomy-jejunal intubation. Surg. Gynecol. Obstet., *74*:239–241, 1942.
13. Hunter, T. B., Fon, G. T., and Silverstein, M. E.: Complications of intestinal tubes. Am. J. Gastroenterol., *76*:256–261, 1981.

CHAPTER 15

Feeding Methods and Gastrointestinal Function

BARBARA C. HANSEN

Centuries of trial and error have preceded the development of contemporary enteral feeding methods. As early as the twelfth century, the great Arab physician-philosopher Avenzoar of Seville reported treating palsy of the esophagus by inserting a silver or tin cannula into the patient's esophagus in order to drip liquid through it. Another report issuing from the early 1400s described the invention by Fabricius (Gerolamo Fabrizio d'Aquapendente) consisting of a silver cornucopia with its tip bent at a right angle and a silver nasal tube covered with sheep intestine for the purpose of dripping feedings through the pharynx directly into the esophagus (Fig. 15–1).

Prolonged nasogastric feeding was significantly advanced by Englishman John Hunter, who in 1790 created a tube of a fresh eel skin placed with the assistance of a flexible whalebone, thus reducing pharyngeal trauma. By 1801 a French physician, Baron D. J. Larrey, attached a funnel to a gum-elastic tube and dripped two cups of broth together with some good wine into a wounded corporal. Within 15 days both the spirits of the soldier and his strength were greatly revived. Thus, the concepts basic to the administration of enteral feedings were established. Clearly, the "gravity drip" method for the infusion of liquid diets into the esophagus or stomach has had a long history of successful use.

Tube feeding procedures continued to be refined, along with advances in the content of the liquid diet as nutritional science developed in the late 1800s and early 1900s, and as surgical efforts became increasingly aggressive. The use of nasogastric tube feeding has now been widespread for over 100 years, and this experience has led to improved nursing techniques and reduction of complications caused by improper placement, aspiration, or inappropriate nutrient composition. Nevertheless, it is only in the last 10 years that various aspects of the enteral feeding procedure have been systematically evaluated for the purpose of defining optimal methods of administration. Key aspects of the administration process, including the rate, volume, and temperature of diet infusion, have been examined for their effects on both subjective sensations and gastrointestinal function.

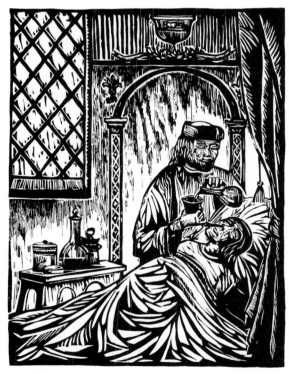

Figure 15–1. Renaissance physicians are known to have used the gravity-drip method for administering liquids to patients unable to swallow owing to paralysis, obstruction, or loss of consciousness. (*From* The Evolution of Tube Feeding. Evansville, Indiana, Mead Johnson & Company, 1964; reproduced with permission.)

TEMPERATURE OF LIQUID DIET:

Physiology and Subjective Effects

Responses of the Gastrointestinal Tract. Concern for the possible adverse effects of ingesting either very cold or very hot liquids was evidenced as early as 1884 when Jaworski described decreased tonus and peristalsis of the stomach in man following the ingestion of iced water.[1] The classic studies of gastrointestinal function by Carlson supported the finding of decreased gastric tonus and inhibition of hunger contractions following ingestion of iced water.[2] Later, using fluoroscopic methods, Todd reported that *both* hot and cold milk led to increased strength and frequency of peristalsis, with the greater and more prolonged effect induced by hot milk.[3] Both the inhibiting and the stimulatory effects were observed to be of short duration, with normal motility returning in less than 30 minutes,[3, 4] and the intragastric temperature drops produced were small.[5] Measuring the temperature of the stomach immediately before and after ingestion of an ice cold barium meal, Gershon-Cohen et al. strikingly demonstrated the capacity of the mouth, pharynx, and esophagus to rapidly heat a liquid meal.[6] As with the time course for the return of motility, temperature of the stomach returned to normal within 30 to 40 minutes. While the studies of the Gershon-Cohen group and of Carlson had suggested increased motility and emptying with cold liquids, those of Jaworski and Bisgard and Nye showed inhibition of gastric motility for 10 to 30 minutes following ingestion of cold water.[7] These discrepancies could have been due to different test liquid compositions (water, milk, barium mixture), different volumes (120 ml to unspecified amounts), and different measurement techniques (fluoroscope, intragastric balloon, aspiration of contents).

A study of the effect of the ingestion of hot and cold water on the motility of the esophagus indicates another factor which contributed in an unknown way to the results described. In this study, Winship et al. showed significant slowing and sometimes abolition of esophageal peristalsis with the oral ingestion of cold water by healthy young men.[8] Hot water, on the other hand, increased the speed of esophageal peristaltic wave propagation and reduced the duration of these rapid waves. Thus, cold water was often delayed in entering the stomach and tended to pool in the distal esophagus, whereas hot water tended to traverse the lower esophageal sphincter more rapidly than even room temperature water.

All of these studies involved the oral ingestion of liquids, thus leaving open the question of whether hot or cold fluids administered by a nasogastric tube might result in both different stimuli (colder or hotter) and different gastrointestinal responses compared with the oral route. While interest in the effects of diet temperature on gastrointestinal function has been sustained for 100 years, only in the last decade have investigators systematically examined the scientific basis for prescribing a given temperature of diet for tube feeding purposes. Many texts and hospital procedure manuals were found to make definite statements on this issue, generally (although not always) recommending that tube feeding diets be warmed to either room or body temperature,[9, 10] and sometimes stating that such fluids should *"never* be given directly from the refrigerator."[11]

Hanson had observed that nurses did not always warm the refrigerated diets prior to administration by nasogastric tube, and this led him to carry out a preliminary study in search of evidence to support or refute this practice.[12] This 1974 study used the hospital recommended procedure of gravity drip infusion of 250 to 350 ml over a period of approximately 30 minutes, and measured the temperature of the liquid diet in its reservoir, and the intragastric temperature prior to, during, and following administration of diet. His unanticipated finding was that two diets, one measured to be 5° C at initiation of administration and the other warmed to 37° C, produced almost no change in intragastric temperature. The greatest intragastric temperature drop achieved with the cold feeding was 3.7° C below baseline body temperature. The diet, warmed to body temperature prior to administration, cooled in the reservoir and tubing such that it too produced a slight drop in intragastric temperature (1.3° C below initial preinfusion level). Hanson showed that bolus tube feedings, if given over a 30 minute period, had virtually no effect on intragastric temperature, and, therefore, that neither refrigeration nor warming of a liquid diet was likely to have an important clinical effect related to temperature of administration.

In order to directly test the effects of tube feeding of various temperature diets on gastric motility, Williams and Walike chronically implanted gastric strain gauges, feeding tubes, and an intragastric thermocouple in rhesus monkeys.[13] The volume infused was approximately equivalent to a 500 ml bolus in humans, and it was administered rapidly by syringe to reproduce the maximum stimulus which could occur during the tube feeding of humans. Cold (5° to 7° C) infusions of either water or liquid diet produced contractions of slightly longer duration and resulted in a short delay in the initiation of regular digestive activity, but had no effect on the time until return of fasting-type motility after the completion of gastric emptying (Table 15–1). All observed effects were extremely small. For example, digestive-type activity was initiated within 1 minute after a warm infusion and within approximately 4 minutes after a cold infusion. Furthermore, the time to return of fasting motility, and the total gastrointestinal transit time showed no differences associated with temperature of administration. As was reported for humans by Hanson,[12] the study using rhesus monkeys showed a similar decrease in intragastric temperature even with warmed feeding, and the rapid return of intragastric temperature to normal within 15 to 20 minutes (Fig. 15–2). Thus, any clinically important effects of the temperature of an intragastric infusion are likely to be transient and probably minimal. The results of this study in an animal model were further confirmed in normal human subjects by Kagawa-Busby et al.,[14] again showing effectively no differences in patterns of gastric motility with liquid diets administered at varying temperatures, and the rapid return of intragastric temperature to normal (Fig. 15–3).

None of the above studies measured gastric emptying directly and quantitatively. Thus, it is possible that some important difference such as rapid gastric emptying during the first 5 minutes could be associated with either hot or cold feedings. The above results suggest that such future studies of emptying rate should be focused upon the first 15 minutes after infusion.

The effect of ingestion of cold (0 to 5° C), lukewarm (20 to 25° C), and hot (60 to 65° C) isotonic glycerin on splanchnic blood flow has been examined by Schofield et al.[15] No significant effects were detected for ice-cold or lukewarm infusions; however, rapid ingestion of very hot liquid produced a significant increase in splanchnic blood flow with at least a 5 minute delay in onset. The time course of this effect was not followed in detail; however, measurement at one hour showed normal blood flow.

It is well recognized that gastrointestinal function is affected by multiple stimulatory and inhibitory factors including emotional disturbances and responses to the senses of sight, taste, and smell. A few studies have looked at subjective sensations and other behavioral responses to varied diet temperatures.

Behavioral, Sensory, and Other Responses. In a study of premature infants, Holt et al. compared warmed and cold feedings (7 to 51° C) and found no significant differences in intake, weight gain, activity, vocalization, or sleep patterns, and failed to demonstrate any advantage to warming of feedings.[16] Whether there is any innate or

Table 15–1. EFFECTS OF LIQUID DIET OR WATER AT VARYING TEMPERATURES ON GASTRIC MOTILITY IN A RHESUS MONKEY

	MEAN DURATION OF CONTRACTIONS*	MEAN TIME (MIN) TO INITIATION OF DIGESTIVE MOTILITY†	MEAN TIME (MIN) TO RETURN OF FASTING MOTILITY‡
Liquid Diet Temperature			
Cold (5–7° C)	12.6	3.58	207
Room (23° C)	10.4	1.71	211
Warm (36–38° C)	9.0	0.55	171
Water Temperature			
Cold (5–7° C)	14.6	4.25	26
Room (23° C)	13.5	2.18	28
Warm (36–38° C)	10.1	0.58	29

*First 10 minutes after infusion.
†Regular three per minute contractions observed during digestion of a meal.
‡Large amplitude contractions seen only after completion of gastric emptying and return of fasting condition.

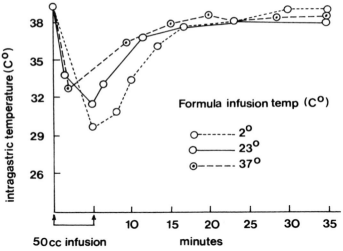

Figure 15–2. Time course for intragastric temperature change following rapid infusions of 2°, 23° and 37° C liquid diets in a rhesus monkey. (*Adapted from* Williams, K. R., and Walike, B. C.: Effect of the temperature of tube feeding on gastric motility in monkeys. Nurs. Res., *24*:4–9, 1975.)

inherent preference for cold or hot liquids was further examined in a study using rats which found temperature choice to be entirely a matter of history or conditioning.[17] Preferences were readily shifted simply by providing a different temperature liquid for a short time. Thus, there does not appear to be a psychological or sensory benefit to either warming or cooling a diet, except to the degree an association may have been developed for a particular individual. Hanson found no differences related to temperature of diet in subjective sensations such as fullness, borborygmi, cramps, or nausea in his adult human subjects.[12] The subjects of Kagawa-Busby reported only the sensation of cold in the back of the throat, associated with the cold infusions, and otherwise no differential sensations associated with temperature of diet.[14]

An interesting observation of unknown clinical importance was the finding in cats that intragastric infusion of cold water, but not of warm water, produced responses of neurons in the posterior hypothalamus.[18]

One final note relates to the possible effects on bacterial growth of warming diets to room temperature or above. To this issue should be added the potential for altering vitamin and protein when diets are overheated. While evidence is sparse, these considerations further militate against the process of warming tube feeding diets.

Thus, no evidence has yet been produced to support the desirability of warming enteral feedings prior to administration, and, furthermore, deleterious effects of administering refrigerated diets have also not been documented.

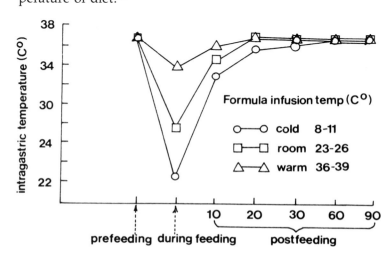

Figure 15–3. Infusion of 250 ml of liquid diet within 5 minutes at varying temperatures in six normal human volunteers. Note similarity to results in rhesus monkey shown in Figure 15–2. (*Adapted from* Kagawa-Busby, K. S., Heitkemper, M. M., Hansen, B. C., Hanson, R. L., and Vanderburg, V. V.: Effect of diet temperature on tolerance of enteral feedings. Nurs. Res., *29*:276–280, 1980.)

RATE OF ADMINISTRATION OF TUBE FEEDINGS

Intermittent or "Meal" Infusions

By far the most common method for the administration of nasogastric tube feedings has been and continues to be gravity drip delivery on an intermittent (every 3 to 6 hours) or meal-type basis. For the great majority of enterally fed patients this remains the method of choice. Indications for continuous gastric or jejunal administration are discussed in the next section.

Concern about the rate at which bolus or meal feedings should be administered has been expressed in most descriptions of tube feeding procedures.[9, 10, 11] These descriptions have primarily cautioned against too rapid a rate of infusion or infusion using the force of a syringe. Such admonitions undoubtedly arose from occasional experience in clinical situations in which a tube, not optimally placed, has induced nausea, pain, and/or vomiting caused by rapid forced distention of either the esophagus or the distal antrum or pyloric areas.

A study describing the processes and experiences of 121 patients receiving nasogastric tube feedings was carried out by a group of investigators in three states.[19] It involved a total of 1730 patient days and covered a variety of clinical settings, including private hospitals, large university medical centers, public hospitals, extended care facilities, and nursing homes, and a wide variety of patient diagnoses. Among the startling findings was the report that, with volumes per feeding approximating 300 ml, 61 per cent of all feedings were given in less than 5 minutes, and 91 per cent were administered in less than 15 minutes—this despite the usual procedural recommendation that feedings be given over no less than 30 minutes.

This report stimulated a systematic study in which rate of infusion was varied and both subjective and gastrointestinal responses monitored.[20, 21] Normal human subjects were studied using a specially constructed feeding tube which permitted precise and consistent repeated placement of a nasogastric tube, and continuous recording of gastric motility by measurement of intragastric pressure with an open-tipped cannula.[21] Rate of diet infusion of volumes ranging from 200 to 500 ml was varied from 30 to 85 ml/minute. Rate of infusion had no effect upon either the amplitude or the frequency of gastric contractions. Furthermore, there was only a small, but consistent, and therefore significant, effect of rate of administration of diet on the time lapsing after infusion prior to the return of the regular contractile activity associated with digestive motility (Fig. 15–4). Under all volumes, diets administered at rates of 60 ml/minute or less produced no untoward effects or subjective symptoms. It must be emphasized that this study carefully and consistently controlled the location of the tip of the nasogastric tube such that the tip was located 10 cm below the lower esophageal sphincter and all portals were within the body or fundus of the stomach. Rates of 85 ml/minute produced occasional adverse responses, including nausea and other subjective discomforts, although this rate had no effect for volumes of 300 ml or less.

Continuous or Pump-Controlled Infusions

Since 1976 a number of clinicians have strongly recommended the use of continuous pump-tube enteric hyperalimentation, usually into the jejunum.[22, 23] Stated advantages include use of a small-bore tube for less nasopharyngeal irritation, elimination of gastric pooling, and reduced likelihood of gastroesophageal reflux and possible aspiration. This method has been used even in patients with primary gastrointestinal disease.[24] There are undoubtedly selected clinical situations in which continuous enteral feeding is clearly advantageous. Unfortunately, to date there has been little or no research into the physiologic responses and changes induced by this procedure. A recent report has shown continuously elevated plasma insulin levels; however, effects on other gastrointestinal hormone levels have not been described.[25] Whether such sustained effects on plasma levels of hormones and substrates have any clinically important effect with long-term maintenance is not known. Deleterious effects of long-term parenteral nutrition, particularly relative to hepatic

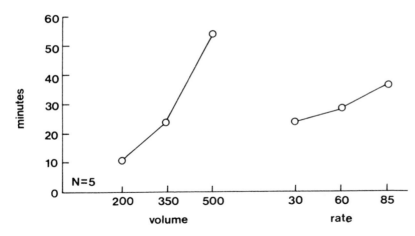

Figure 15–4. Mean time (minutes) from end of intragastric infusion of diet to beginning of regular contractile activity (digestive motility) in relation to rate and volume of infusion (N = 6 subjects). (*Adapted from* Heitkemper, M. M., Hanson, R. L., and Hansen, B. C.: Effects of rate and volume of tube feeding in normal human subjects. Commun. Nurs. Res., *10*:71–89, 1978.)

function, have been suggested; however, controlled studies comparing long-term intermittent and continuous enteral nutrition have not been reported. While short-term use is unlikely to produce untoward sequelae, the effects of continuous enteral feeding for periods of months or longer requires serious investigation.

Another study using monkeys has examined gastric motility during *combined* continuous enteral and parenteral nutrition.[26] The significant changes observed warrant further study under conditions of continuous enteral feeding to determine the nature of any sustained alterations and their possible significance.

Clinical case reports have most commonly recommended initial continuous gastric or jejunal infusion rates of 50 ml/hour, increasing each day by 25 ml/hour to a rate of 125 ml/hour or 3000 kcal/24 hours.[22, 24] Sometimes dilution to one-third or one-half is also recommended, followed by a gradual increase to full strength, 1 kcal/ml. Intragastric infusion rates have occasionally been as high as 6000 ml (or kcal) per day or 250 ml per hour. Systematic investigation of patient and diagnostic parameters associated with successful infusion rates of varying levels has not yet been carried out, and, thus, trial and error studies to find an optimal concentration and rate are considered to be necessary.[22]

VOLUME OF ENTERAL FEEDING

Perhaps the clearest finding of studies concerned with identifying the volumes of diet or total calories received by the usual

enterally fed patient is that the amount delivered has most commonly been less than that required to meet the nutritional needs of patients.[19] Furthermore, the average patient received 5 to 10 per cent less than was actually prescribed per day. Significant weight loss occurred in more than half of an unselected group of patients maintained on enteral feedings for 10 to 21 days.[19]

Intermittent or "Meal" Infusions

In a randomly selected group of patients receiving intermittent enteral feedings, frequency of feeding was directly related to total volume of diet intake over the range of two to seven feedings per day.[19] As the number of feedings was increased from seven through twelve feedings per day, the total intake per 24 hours remained approximately constant, indicating that with very frequent feedings the volume per feeding was concomitantly reduced (Table 15–2).[19] Thus, whether for clinical reasons, or because of customary practice, as the number

Table 15–2. COMPARISON BETWEEN NUMBER OF FEEDINGS PER DAY AND MEAN VOLUME OF DIET INTAKE PER 24 HOURS (N = 1394 PATIENT DAYS)

NO. OF FEEDINGS PER DAY	MEAN INTAKE PER 24 HOURS (kcal)	MEAN INTAKE PER FEEDING (kcal)
2–3	855	340
4–5	1290	285
6–7	1610	250
8–9	1615	190
10–12	1645	150

of feedings per day was increased the expected increase in the caloric load did not occur. Clearly, if optimal nutritional status is to be achieved, both volume per feeding and number of feedings per day need to be considered.

Only one study has systematically examined the effects of varying the volume of a nasogastrically administered meal on gastrointestinal function. Heitkemper et al., using normal adult volunteers, examined the effects of varying the volume of a liquid diet meal on gastric motility.[20, 21] Increasing the volume of a tube feeding from 350 to 500 ml, while controlling for rate of administration, resulted in a significant increase in the time taken for the regular digestive-type motility pattern to appear following the feedings (see Fig. 15–4). Significant differences in the frequency of gastric contractions in the immediate postinfusion period were also observed for volumes of 200, 350, and 500 ml (Fig. 15–5). This study, while clearly identifying reduced contractile activity in the early postinfusion period with increasing meal volumes, did not measure the possible resultant effects of the motility changes on gastric emptying. One must be cautious in the interpretation of these data for clinical purposes, as no deleterious effects of the 500 ml volume were observed. Thus, only further study will indicate whether infusions of volumes as large as 500 ml per meal are contraindicated. The previously mentioned study of volumes of feedings used in clinical practice suggests a need to further investigate whether practices concerning volume per meal limitations have in fact been too conservative, resulting in inadequate total caloric intakes. Alternatively, volumes exceeding 350 ml may be physiologically less well tolerated owing to possible excessive delays in gastric emptying. Where larger volumes of total intake are required, more frequent feedings while maintaining volume per feeding, or continuous infusions may be indicated.

Clinically significant gastrointestinal and metabolic problems sometimes, but not always, eliminated by modifications in the rate, concentration, and volume of the diet have included abdominal cramping, bloating, diarrhea, nausea, vomiting, fluid and electrolyte imbalances, and glucose intolerance.[27] Clearly the relatively sparse systematic investigation of the enteral feeding process has left many clinically important questions open for further study before optimal methods for the continuous or intermittent enteral infusion of nutrient loads can be defined with certainty. Until further studies are completed, the clinician might be advised to consider the following: (1) Assure that the enteral feeding prescription for each patient includes a total caloric intake adequate for the patient's needs. (2) Use volumes of 350 ml/meal infused at the rate of gravity flow and with frequency of meals adequate to meet the nutritional need. (3) Where intragastric meal feeding is not tolerated, gastric or jejunal continuous infusions are indicated, and a reasonable infusion rate may be 125 ml/hour of a 1 kcal/ml liquid diet. (4) Administer tube feedings either at room temperature or cold (refrigerated). There is no indication for warming tube feedings or for refraining from administering liquid diets straight from the refrigerator.

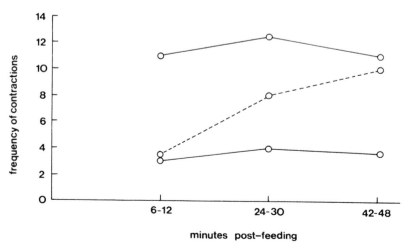

Figure 15–5. Frequency of contractions at three time periods following nasogastric liquid diet meals of varying volumes (N = 6 subjects). (*Adapted from* Heitkemper, M. M., Hanson, R. L., and Hansen, B. C.: Effects of rate and volume of tube feeding in normal human subjects. Commun. Nurs. Res., *10:*71–89, 1978.)

frequency of contractions

minutes post–feeding

REFERENCES

1. Jaworski, W.: Vergleichend experimentelle Untersuchungen ueber das Verhalten des Kissinger und Karlsbader Wassers, sowie des Karlsbader Quellsalzes im Menschlichen Magen. Deutsches Arch. f. Klin. Med., 35:38–78, 1884.
2. Carlson, A. J.: The Control of Hunger in Health and Disease. Chicago, University of Chicago Press, 1916.
3. Todd, T. W.: Behavior Patterns of the Alimentary Tract. Baltimore, Williams and Wilkins, 1930.
4. Hepburn, J. S., Eberhard, H. M., Ricketts, R., and Rieger, C. L. W.: Temperature of the gastrointestinal tract: The effect thereon of hot and cold foods and of physical therapeutic agents. Arch. Intern. Med., 52:603–615, 1933.
5. Stengel, A., and Hopkins, A. H.: A new method for determining the intragastric temperature in man, with some observations on its variations after ingestion of hot and cold liquids and during digestion. Am. J. Med. Sci., 153:101–106, 1917.
6. Gershon-Cohen, J., Shay, H., and Fels, S. S.: The relation of meal temperature to gastric motility and secretion. Am. J. Roentgenol. Radium Ther. Nucl. Med., 43:237–242, 1940.
7. Bisgard, J. D., and Nye, D.: The influence of hot and cold application upon gastric and intestinal motor activity. Surg. Gynecol. Obstet., 71:172–180, 1940.
8. Winship, D. H., Viegas de Andrade, S. R., and Zaboralske, F. F.: Influence of bolus temperature on human esophageal motor function. J. Clin. Invest., 49:243–250, 1970.
9. Brunner, L. S., and Suddarth, D. S.: Textbook of Medical-Surgical Nursing. Edition 3. Philadelphia, J. B. Lippincott Co., 1975.
10. Nursing Procedure Book of Virginia Mason Hospital. Seattle, Washington, p. 603.
11. Kintzel, K. C. (ed.): Advanced Concepts in Clinical Nursing. Philadelphia, J. B. Lippincott Co., 1971.
12. Hanson, R. L.: A study to determine the differences in effects of administering cold and warmed tube feedings. Commun. Nurs. Res., 6:136–140, 1974.
13. Williams, K. R., and Walike, B. C.: Effect of the temperature of tube feeding on gastric motility in monkeys. Nurs. Res., 24:4–9, 1975.
14. Kagawa-Busby, K. S., Heitkemper, M. M., Hansen, B. C., Hanson, R. L., and Vanderburg, V. V.: Effect of diet temperature on tolerance of enteral feedings. Nurs. Res., 29:276–280, 1980.
15. Schofield, P. F., Ingram, G., and Torrance, H. B.: The effects of the ingestion of hot and cold fluids on splanchnic blood-flow before and after gastric operations. Br. J. Surg., 53:759–760, 1966.
16. Holt, L. E. Jr., Davies, E. A., Hasselmeyer, E. G., and Adams, A. O.: A study of premature infants fed cold formulas. J. Pediatr., 61:556–561, 1962.
17. Deaux, E., and Engstrom, R.: The temperature of ingested water: Preference for cold water as an associative response. Physiol. Psychol., 1:257–260, 1973.
18. Takaori, S., Sasa, M., and Fukuda, N.: Responses of posterior hypothalamic neurons to electrical stimulation of the inferior alveolar nerve and distension of stomach with cold and warm water. Brain Res., 11:225–237, 1968.
19. Walike, B. C., Padilla, G., Bergstrom, N., Hanson, R. L., Kubo, W., Grant, M., and Wong, H. L.: Patient problems related to tube feeding. Commun. Nurs. Res., 7:89–112, 1975.
20. Heitkemper, M. M., Hansen, B. C., Hanson, R. L., and Vanderburg, V. V.: Effects of rate and volume of tube feeding on gastric motility and feeding tolerance. J.P.E.N., 1:1A, 1977.
21. Heitkemper, M. M., Hanson, R. L., and Hansen, B. C.: Effects of rate and volume of tube feeding in normal human subjects. Commun. Nurs. Res., 10:71–89, 1978.
22. Page, C. P., Ryan, J. A. Jr., and Haff, R. C.: Continual catheter administration of an elemental diet. Surg. Gynecol. Obstet., 142:184–188, 1976.
23. Dobbie, R. P., and Hoffmeister, J. A.: Continuous pump-tube enteric hyperalimentation. Surg. Gynecol. Obstet., 143:273–276, 1976.
24. Bethel, R. A., Jansen, R. D., Heymsfield, S. B., Ansley, J. D., Hersh, T., and Rudman, D.: Nasogastric hyperalimentation through a polyethylene catheter: An alternative to central venous hyperalimentation. Am. J. Clin. Nutr., 32:1112–1120, 1979.
25. Bergstrom, N., and Hansen, B. C.: Continuous and intermittent enteral feedings: Effects on 24-hour plasma glucose, insulin, glucagon and growth hormone levels. Presented at the Sixth Annual Clinical Congress of the American Society for Parenteral and Enteral Nutrition, February, 1982.
26. Hansen, B. W., DeSomery, C. H., Hagedorn, P. K., and Kalnasy, L. W.: Effects of enteral and parenteral nutrition on appetite in monkeys. J.P.E.N., 1:83–88, 1977.
27. Ryan, J. A., and McFadden, M. C.: Practical aspects of jejunal feedings. Presented at the Sixth Annual Clinical Congress of the American Society for Parenteral and Enteral Nutrition, February, 1982.

CHAPTER 16

Nasoenteric Tube Feeding

JOHN L. ROMBEAU
DANNY O. JACOBS

Nasoenteric tube feeding dates back as far as the fifteenth century. Modern usage, however, began with the efforts of Fallis and Barron (1952),[1] who developed fine polyethylene tubes for nasogastric and nasojejunal alimentation, and Pareira (1954),[2] who used nasoenteric tube feedings to nourish over 200 patients successfully. Further advances included the development of the enteral feeding pump by Barron (1959)[3] and Stephens and Randall's (1969)[4] clinical use of the elemental diet.

The current resurgence of interest in the use of nasoenteric feedings is partly due to technologic advances. Major developments have included small-bore, flexible tubes constructed of nonreactive materials (polyurethane and silicone rubber), volumetric infusion pumps, and new complete liquid diets. The new feeding tubes have obviated side effects such as rhinitis, pharyngitis, and pulmonary atelectasis associated with the previous use of larger, stiffer tubes.[5] The newer pumps allow uniform nutrient delivery and are equipped with batteries allowing the patient greater freedom of movement while being fed (see Chapter 13). The new range of liquid diets permits the individualization of feeding formulas.

This chapter discusses the rationale, assessment, indications, and methods of delivery and patient monitoring for nasoenteric tube feeding.

RATIONALE

The rationale for enteral feeding is based upon the physiologic effects of digestion and absorption, hormone-substrate interactions, safety, convenience, and economy. Since feeding into the intestine is the biologic method for alimentation, nasoenteric feeding would seem teleologically superior to alternative techniques. However, objective studies documenting this assumption are needed.

There is evidence, both theoretical and practical, suggesting that enteral feeding is superior to parenteral alimentation with regard to substrate utilization. Animal studies have shown that the intraluminal delivery of nutrients is necessary for maintaining gastrointestinal integrity.[6-8] Levine et al. reported that rats fed intravenously had lower gut weights, decreased mucosal thickness, and less mucosal protein, deoxyribonucleic acid, and disaccharidase activity than their orally fed controls. In another study, dogs that underwent jejunectomy were fed intravenously or orally. The intravenously fed dogs showed no functional adaptation of their intestine and had decreased villous height when compared with their orally fed counterparts.[7] Eastwood reported significant reductions in epithelial cell proliferation and mucosal thickness in the proximal small bowel of rabbits fed intravenously.[6]

Some studies have suggested that the morphologic changes of the intestine in response to enteral or parenteral feedings are hormonally mediated. The gut hormones cholecystokinin and gastrin have trophic effects on the gastrointestinal tract. They stimulate the following: (1) synthesis of protein, DNA, and RNA; (2) the growth of the exocrine pancreas and the mucosa of the small intestine and colon; and (3) the growth of the stomach's oxyntic glands.[9] Johnson et al. discovered that gastrin levels in parenterally fed rats were only one thirtieth of levels found in orally fed rats.[10] Others found that pentagastrin administered during parenteral feeding prevented the expected fall in small bowel weight and disaccharidase activity.[11] Johnson suggested that decreased gastrin levels were responsible for the adverse intestinal changes seen in parenterally fed animals.[10, 11] Other gut hormones such as secretin, glucagon, and cholecystokinin may also be involved.[9, 10] Based upon these studies, it seems likely that alterations in levels of gut hormones do influence gastrointestinal morphology but to our knowledge, studies in humans have yet to demonstrate abnormal levels of gastrin or other gut hormones in response to parenteral feedings.

Unlike parenteral feeding, which exposes the tissues to unmetabolized nutrients, enteral alimentation preserves the physiologic sequence of nutrient absorption, metabolism, and utilization prior to delivery to the peripheral circulation. For example, the liver and intestine are vital to fat metabolism and are the only sites of lipoprotein synthesis.[12] All water-soluble compounds absorbed by the intestine (glucose, amino acids, small peptides, and fatty acids) travel to the liver through the portal vein. Here these nutrients pass into hepatocytes and are stored, used for energy, or metabolized into other useful substances. Nutrients may be more efficiently used when the liver is the central distributing organ.[13]

The pharmacokinetics of insulin's release and substrate interactions in response to enteral or parenteral alimentation is controversial. Several authors cite a greater release of insulin in response to enteral alimentation with glucose compared with the insulin release occurring secondary to an isocaloric intravenous infusion.[13, 14] This greater insulin response following enteral feedings may result from the release of intestinal secretagogues. Higher insulin levels could lead to superior nutrient disposal in enterally fed subjects.[13, 15] This insulin response could also be harmful.[13] With continuous enteral or parenteral feeding, insulin levels could remain high and theoretically prevent the release of glycogen and fatty acids.[13, 16, 17] Excess fat and carbohydrate, stored in the liver as triglyceride and glycogen, may cause hepatomegaly, cholestasis, and impaired function as evidenced by abnormal liver function tests. Furthermore, in the presence of high insulin levels, amino acids are preferentially taken up by skeletal muscle, creating a relative substrate deficiency in the liver.[16, 17] The liver depends on the redistribution of amino acids from muscle for protein synthesis during the postabsorptive periods; the high circulating insulin levels may ultimately result in decreased levels of secretory proteins, albumin, and transferrin.

Other research has demonstrated higher insulin levels in parenterally, as compared with enterally, nourished humans. Recently, McArdle and coworkers,[18] in a prospective randomized study, compared the serum insulin levels in two groups of patients who received nearly identical feedings delivered parenterally and enterally. Significantly higher endogenous serum insulin levels were required to maintain blood glucoses within acceptable limits in the parenterally fed group than in those fed enterally. Furthermore, the insulin levels in the parenterally fed group were high enough to prevent fat mobilization and eventually decrease free fatty acid levels to zero. If circulating serum insulin levels are indeed higher in the parenterally fed patient, then this study illustrates an unfavorable physiologic consequence of parenteral feeding. Unfortunately the amount of glucose absorbed from the gastrointestinal tract was not determined. Therefore, unequal glucose loads may have accounted for the differences in serum insulin levels. Their results are in contrast to other studies that report higher insulin levels with enteral feedings.[13, 14]

To our knowledge, no study has actually demonstrated decreased metabolism of glycogen or decreased release of fatty acid in response to high circulating insulin levels. In fact, fatty acid mobilization may proceed despite high circulating insulin levels. The different insulin mechanics reported by various authors may simply be a function of the specific experimental protocols, for example, the type, rate, and total carbohydrate administered and absorbed. In summary, elevated levels of insulin in response to enteral feeding could be either beneficial if this promotes more effective nutrient disposal or harmful if fatty acid mobilization and glycogen metabolism are impaired. Adequately controlled studies with meticulous attention to glucose mechanics are needed to resolve these issues.

Safety is a major factor in support of enteral feeding. Nasoenteric alimentation avoids complications such as pneumothorax, hydrothorax, arterial puncture, catheter embolus, and sepsis that are known to be associated with central venous catheterization.[12] Thus, nasoenteric alimentation, while not without its own risks, may be safer than the parenteral technique.[12]

Finally, nasoenteric alimentation is less expensive and more convenient than total parenteral nutrition. The major difference is in the cost of the feeding solution. One liter of intravenous hyperalimentation solution at the Hospital of the University of Pennsylvania costs $90 per 1000 Kcal as compared with 90¢ for an equivalent amount of an isotonic enteral diet. Enteral nutrition does not require the extensive sterile techniques needed for parenteral feedings, and there is less need for a trained maintenance team. In addition, the minimal daily requirements of various vitamins and nutrients are established for enteral feedings, but the parenteral requirements are unknown.[14]

ASSESSMENT AND PATIENT SELECTION

Patient selection for nasoenteric feeding can be based on the algorithm in Fig. 16–1. Many apparently well-nourished individuals have adverse changes in their nutritional status after surgical stress or illness and may need nutritional support.[19] Before initiating nutritional therapy, one must first obtain

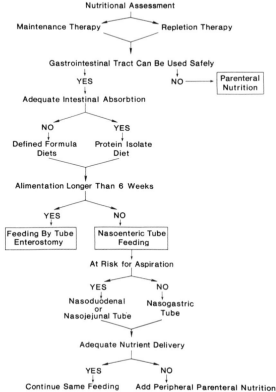

DECISION MAKING FOR NASOENTERIC FEEDING

Figure 16–1. Patient selection for nasoenteric feeding.

base-line nutritional data by taking a thorough medical history, dietary review, complete physical examination, and laboratory evaluation. To establish the need for supplementary feedings, the nutritional assessment and dietary review should demonstrate that the patient's volitional intake is insufficient for his or her caloric needs. The objectives of nutritional support must be clearly identified as to either nutritional maintenance or repletion. Although as many as 6000 Kcal per day may be administered by nasoenteric tube, the average amount delivered is 3000 Kcal per day.[20] It usually takes four to five days to reach this goal.[21, 22] Few controlled studies have evaluated the time required to reach the prescribed nutritional goal using nasoenteric feedings. A recent prospective study at the Hospital of the University of Pennsylvania and the Philadelphia Veterans Administration Medical Center reported that significantly fewer kilocalories than prescribed per day are delivered and that the actual time required to reach the caloric goal may be twice as long as commonly reported.[12] Data generated from studies by Heitkemper and associates also suggest a significant caloric deficit in most tube-fed patients.[23]

Most evidence indicates that nasoenteric feedings are generally satisfactory for maintenance nutritional therapy. However, since patients rarely tolerate more than 3000 Kcal per day nasoenterally, those patients needing repletion (more than 3000 calories per day) may need supplementary intravenous feedings to reach their nutritional goals. Peripheral intravenous alimentation is one method by which additional calories can be administered. Although the benefits of this method have not been documented with prospective randomized trials, Young and Hill have published a nonrandomized study that compared combined enteral and peripheral parenteral therapy to total parenteral nutrition.[24] Their data showed that combined therapy may be as effective as parenteral nutrition in decreasing postoperative morbidity and in achieving nitrogen and potassium balances. Central venous alimentation generally delivers a maximum of calories. This technique may be the preferred method for artificial feedings in patients who require rapid nutritional repletion.

Once volitional oral intake is shown to be inadequate, and the patient's needs are evaluated in terms of nutritional maintenance versus repletion, the route for nutrient delivery is then determined. Evaluation of the gastrointestinal tract will determine if it can be used safely. Despite the fact that the gastrointestinal tract may not be wholly "intact," a sufficient length may be available for absorption of a defined formula diet (Fig. 16–2). Winitz reported defined formula absorption with as little as 4 cm of normal small bowel between the ligament of Treitz and the ileocecal valve.[25] Freeman et al. cite the need for at least 100 cm of functioning jejunum or 150 cm of ileum, and prefer that some colon and an intact ileocecal valve be present to improve absorption.[26]

The indications for nasoenteric feedings are listed in Table 16–1. Patients with neurologic or psychological disorders preventing satisfactory oral intake and those patients with oropharyngeal or esophageal disorders who cannot eat may benefit from nasoenteric feedings. Patients with burns, certain gastrointestinal diseases, short gut, or severe malabsorption, and those undergoing chemotherapy or radiotherapy are additional candidates for this type of feeding. Nasoenteric feedings can be used in the transition from total parenteral nutrition to combined parenteral and enteral nutrition to volitional intake. This method decreases the

Table 16–1 INDICATIONS FOR NASOENTERIC TUBE FEEDING

NEUROLOGIC/PSYCHIATRIC
Cerebrovascular accidents
Neoplasms
Trauma
Inflammation
Demyelinating diseases
Severe depression
Anorexia nervosa

OROPHARYNGEAL/ESOPHAGEAL
Neoplasms
Inflammation
Trauma

GASTROINTESTINAL
Pancreatitis
Inflammatory bowel disease
Short bowel syndrome
Neonatal intestinal disease
Malabsorption
Preoperative bowel preparation
Fistulas

MISCELLANEOUS
Burn
Chemotherapy
Radiotherapy

time the patient is at risk for complications of parenteral nutrition.

Nasoenteric feedings also provide useful adjunctive therapy for patients with gastrointestinal fistulas. When high fistulas occur in the esophagus, duodenum, or proximal jejunum, tubal bypass of the fistulous tract and feeding a defined formula or other liquid diet distal to the fistula may be feasible. In the presence of a colocutaneous fistula, defined formula diets administered nasoenterally are needed. Jejunal feedings were used to treat duodenal fistula by Smith and Lee; all of their patients healed without surgery. Rocchio et al. reported that 65 per cent of 37 various gastrointestinal fistulae closed during treatment with an elemental diet.[27] Voitk et al. noted that 75 per cent of gastrointestinal fistulae closed spontaneously with tube feedings.[28]

Nasoenteric feeding is contraindicated in patients with complete gastric or intestinal obstruction. When incomplete obstruction is present, the use of nasoenteric feeding is controversial. Some authors support the use of defined formula diets in patients with incomplete obstruction of the stomach or small intestine to help decrease symptoms such as nausea, vomiting, and bloat-

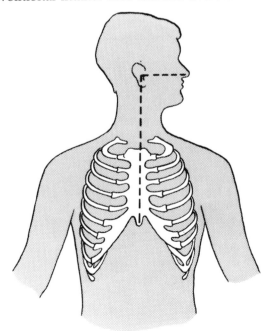

Figure 16–2. Estimating approximate length for passage of nasogastric tube. Length from tip of nose to earlobe to xiphoid process. Add an additional 50 cm.

ing.[29] Defined formula diets may possibly be used in those patients whose abdominal radiographs show no evidence of a closed loop obstruction and whose clinical condition suggests normal intestinal viability. To our knowledge, there are no controlled studies available that document the efficacy of this method. The clinician should use nasoenteric tube feeding only when the precise status of the patient's gastrointestinal tract is known. This avoids the possibility of feeding a completely obstructed patient who had been initially misdiagnosed as having a partial obstruction. Our policy has been to avoid using nasoenteric feedings in any patient with signs and symptoms of incomplete intestinal or partial gastric outlet obstruction.

Nasoenteric feeding in patients with gastroesophageal reflux and esophagitis has not, to our knowledge, been studied in a controlled fashion. This problem was seen primarily when large-bore nasogastric tubes were used. The amount of reflux, however, may not have been clinically significant.[14] The incidence of symptomatic gastroesophageal reflux in patients fed through small-bore tubes is unknown but is probably small. In those patients with severe gastroesophageal reflux, nasoenteric feedings, especially nasogastric feedings, may be contraindicated.

Nasoenteric feedings should be performed cautiously in patients with ileus. They require the clinician's careful attention because of the increased risk of complications. When the stomach fails to empty properly, as might occur postoperatively, one can avoid the risks of nausea, vomiting, or acute stomach dilatation by feeding directly into the small intestine.[13, 30] However, this may require operative or endoscopic placement of the feeding tube in the small intestine (see Chapter 17) Moss advocates the use of an esophagogastric drainage–duodenal feeding tube, which permits esophageal and gastric aspiration during duodenal feedings. Using this tube, Moss and others believe that full nutrition can be safely achieved in the immediate postoperative period.[31, 32] Studies in humans have documented the rapid achievement of positive nitrogen balance and improved wound healing when immediate postoperative feeding is done.[33] Those patients with ileus secondary to fluid and electrolyte imbalances, narcotics, infection, sepsis, or trauma are best treated by relieving the underlying condition. Nasoenteric feeding can then be started once the ileus has resolved. Patients with ileus should be monitored in an intensive care setting if nasoenteric feedings are begun. When small or large bowel ileus persists idiopathically or when the precipitating factors cannot be relieved, nasoenteric feedings should be avoided.

In certain instances the patient's primary illness may be best treated by bowel rest. For example, enteral feedings should be avoided if pancreatic or biliary stimulation is undesirable. In these patients parenteral feedings are the preferred method of therapy.

Finally, the clinician must anticipate how long the patient will require supplementary nutritional therapy. Will long-term alimentation be needed? The expected duration of treatment, as well as the patient's desires and primary disease process, will influence the type of enteral therapy chosen. Esophagostomies, gastrostomies, and jejunostomies may be performed when feasible in patients who require long-term enteral feedings (see Chapter 27). Other patients may be better served with Broviac or Hickman catheters inserted for long-term parenteral alimentation. However, it should be noted that nasoenteric tube feedings have been used for long-term alimentation in the hospital and at home with great success for periods as long as 18 months.[34–36] There is no reason why the use of nasoenteric tube feedings could not be prolonged if the patient is able to tolerate the inconvenience of the tube.

TECHNIQUES OF TUBE PLACEMENT

Until the last decade, the nasogastric tube was the mainstay of enteral feeding. Using this large-bore tube composed of rubber or plastic, however, has produced side effects of pharyngitis and otitis and may render the lower esophageal sphincter incompetent, which may increase the risk of reflux and aspiration. These problems have prompted the recent development of small-bore, flexible catheters for nasogastric and nasoduodenal use. For nasogastric feedings, several tubes are available that are nonreactive and well tolerated by the patient (see Chapter 13).

Slightly larger silicone rubber or poly-urethane tubes of approximately 105 cm in length with nonabsorbable mercury weights have been designed for passage into the duodenum. Nasoduodenal nutrient delivery may avoid some problems associated with reflux of the enteral solutions. Gustke et al. infused a nonabsorbable marker, 1 per cent polyethylene glycol, into various portions of the duodenum and proximal jejunum.[37] Si-multaneous gastric aspirations showed that the optimal tube position for minimizing re-flux through the pylorus was just distal to the ligament of Treitz (Fig. 16–3).

The supplies needed for tube insertion are as follows: feeding tube, 10- and 50-ml syringes, lubricant (water-soluble), emesis basin, stethoscope, towel or bib, tissues, al-cohol sponges, cup of water with straw, benzoin, and nonallergenic tape. The proce-dure for positioning these feeding tubes is as follows (Table 16–2): The lubricated mer-cury tip is passed through the nostril into the nasopharynx and then swallowed. In those patients who are unable to swallow, a well-lubricated arteriography guidewire (0.035 in. in diameter) can be used as an internal stylet.[38] After the tube is passed into the

Table 16–2   PROCEDURE FOR INSERTING NASOENTERIC TUBES

1. Provide privacy.
2. Explain procedure and its purpose.
3. Place patient in sitting position with neck flexed slightly and head of bed elevated to 45°.
4. Lubricate stylet and insert into feeding tube.
5. Inspect nares and determine optimal patency by having the patient breathe through one nostril while the other is occluded temporarily.
6. Estimate approximate distance for placement into the stomach by measuring the length from the tip of the nose to the earlobe and then from the earlobe to the xiphoid process. Add 50 cm to this length.
7. Lubricate the end of the tube and pass it poste-riorly. If the patient is cooperative, ask him to swal-low water to facilitate passage of the tube.
8. Once the tube is beyond the nasopharynx, allow the patient to rest.
9. Have patient flex his neck and swallow while the tube is advanced.
10. If the patient begins to cough, withdraw the tube into the nasopharynx and then reattempt passage.
11. Confirm passage in stomach by aspiration of gastric contents. If unable to aspirate gastric contents, ob-tain abdominal roentgenogram.
12. Remove stylet.
13. Secure tube to bridge of nose or upper lip with non-allergenic tape.

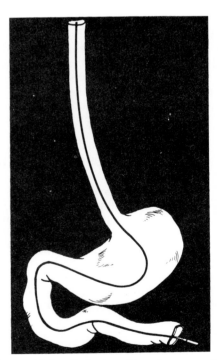

Figure 16–3. Optimal position of nasoenteric tube for patients at increased risk for aspiration.

stomach, the patient is turned on the right side so that the peristaltic motion of the stomach will propel the mercury-weighted tip through the pylorus into the duodenum. If the tube is not passed spontaneously into the duodenum after 8 to 24 hours, metoclo-pramide (10 mg every 6 hours, orally or in-travenously) may be given to stimulate gas-tric emptying. Fiberoptic endoscopy or fluoroscopic manipulation may be needed to guide the catheter through the pylorus.

When any type of nasoenteric tube is placed for enteral feeding, verification of tube location is mandatory. Simple insuffla-tion of air into the tube is not sufficient to verify the position. Auscultation over the stomach can pick up sound transmitted through a tube that has been inadvertently passed into the bronchial tree. Many of these tubes are small enough to pass through the glottis and trachea without markedly in-terfering with phonation or respiration (see Chapter 29). Enteral solutions delivered through a misplaced tube into the bronchial tree can cause severe pneumonitis and death. The simplest means of confirming proper tube placement in the gastrointestinal tract is by the aspiration of gastrointestinal contents. Because small-bore, soft tubes tend to collapse with negative pressure, a small syringe should be used. If intestinal contents cannot be aspirated through the tube, radiographic confirmation of tube location is mandatory before enteral feedings are started. Because feeding tubes are often radiopaque, a simple plain film of the abdomen may be adequate. If the exact location of the tube is still in doubt, a small amount of contrast material can be injected through the tube.

For most patients, safety demands that the patient's head be elevated at feeding time and for some period thereafter to prevent regurgitation. Nasogastric intubation, in particular, requires this, as the tube's presence through the upper and lower esophageal sphincters may render them incompetent and liable to reflux. Even the presence of a tracheostomy or endotracheal tube does not ensure against aspiration of regurgitated gastric contents into the respiratory passages. Liquid filling the pharynx will inevitably trickle past even an overinflated tube cuff and into the lung, verified by placing a bit of food coloring or methylene blue into the feeding mixture. If elevating the patient's head is not possible, an alternate site of nutrient delivery should be considered.

Difficulties of tube passage into the stomach are increased with thin, floppy tubes and in obtunded patients. Aids we have found useful include stiffeners, either inside (such as the angiography guidewire of a Keofeed stylet) or outside (Duofeed, Cartmill) the feeding tube during passage; judicious use of gravity and positioning; and designation of specially experienced and certified nursing personnel to assist in this task.

Passage of the tube through the pylorus may be needed if the patient is at increased risk for aspiration. We have found that a weighted, flexible feeding tube in the stomach (with adequate slack) passes into the duodenum within 48 hours in over 80 per cent of patients. This results from gravity alone and is enhanced by turning the patient on his right side. Of the remainder, the majority achieve passage after one or two doses of metoclopramide, 10 mg intravenously.[39] Hence our practice is to place the tube into the stomach, position the patient on his right side for several hours once or twice in the next 24 hours, then take a radi-

ograph. If the tube has not passed, metoclopramide is given while the patient is still in the Radiology department, and the film is repeated. Occasionally it is not clear from the plain film which part of the gut holds the tube (Fig. 16–4), so a small amount of contrast material can be given at that time as well (Fig. 16–5).

Comatose patients on respirators or with injuries or other problems limiting their ability to be turned to the side may achieve small bowel intubation more easily with a newly developed tube (Cartmill, Impra Inc.) which has removable rigid outer guides and an unweighted bulb tip. In one randomized trial comparing this tube with a standard weighted flexible tube (Dobhoff) in 41 patients, the stomach was more often intubated (91 per cent versus 63 per cent) and the small bowel more frequently entered (77 per cent versus 5 per cent) within 48 hours with the Cartmill tube.[40]

If the tube still has not passed through the pylorus, the aid of the fluoroscopist is enlisted. Another try at passage is made with the aid of metoclopramide and perhaps a guidewire. (The new generation of inter-

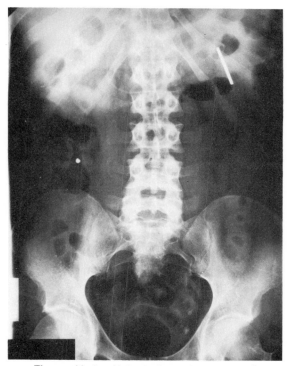

Figure 16–4. Abdominal roentgenogram demonstrates end of feeding tube within the abdomen.

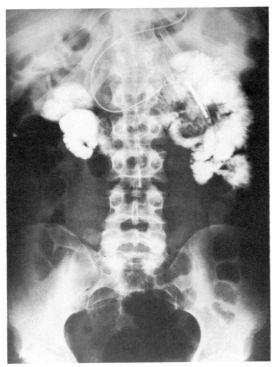

Figure 16–5. Injection of contrast material documents the position of the tube within the jejunum.

ventional radiologists take justifiable pride in their ability to cannulate almost any internal orifice.) Finally, if all else has failed and no alternative route for nutrition is appropriate, the gastrointestinal endoscopist can capture the tube tip using the biopsy forceps of the flexible endoscope (perhaps aided by a suture through the tube end) and guide the tube through the pylorus.

DELIVERY METHODS

Once the decision is made to feed a patient a specific formula using a nasoenteric tube, the clinician must decide whether to feed into the stomach or duodenum and whether to use an intermittent or continuous technique. As discussed previously, certain diseases or types of intestinal surgery may necessitate a specific feeding method and technique. For example, patients who have had a gastrectomy initially may have to be fed distal to the gastroenterostomy. Most patients, however, tolerate continuous or in-termittent feeding into the stomach or continuous feeding into the duodenum.

Intermittent Versus Continuous Feeding

The advantages of intermittent feeding are that it is convenient and inexpensive and may be more physiologic than continuous feeding. There is no need for infusion pumps or controllers and, if the nasogastric tube is of a large bore, viscous formulas or blenderized foods can flow through readily. In addition, intermittent feedings more closely simulate the normal feeding pattern and the distention caused by bolus feedings may stimulate digestion. In patients with normal gastric emptying or who are receiving home regimens, intermittent feedings may be more desirable than continuous feedings[5, 13] (see Chapter 27). Unfortunately, intermittent feedings may delay gastric emptying in the convalescent patient who has taken little food intragastrically, leading to an increased risk of aspiration.[5]

Heitkemper et al. studied the effects of rate and volume on abdominal discomfort in subjects who received intermittent nasogastric feedings.[23] Although the effects of rate and volume on gastric emptying were not studied, their report suggested that when intermittent feedings are used, formulas should not be infused at rates greater than 30 ml/min and that small volumes should be given initially.

Continuous feedings are usually necessary to deliver nutrients directly into the small intestine because it tolerates bolus feedings and sudden rate changes poorly.[5, 12, 41–43] There are several advantages to using continuous feeding, including the decreased risk of distention and aspiration.[5] Furthermore, smaller gastric residuals and improved tolerance are seen in patients who are fed continuously.[5, 44] This improved tolerance is especially important with regard to hyperosmolar formulas that may require intragastric administration by continuous infusion; they may be very poorly tolerated when delivered by an intermittent technique.

A disadvantage of continuous feedings is that the patient is "tied" to the apparatus during infusion. This can be inconvenient even if the patient is not fed continuously for 24 hours.[45] Furthermore, there is significant expense associated with the purchase of volumetric infusion pumps. This expense, however, is probably balanced by the greater security and confidence afforded by volumetric pumps.

It is not known if one technique (intermittent or continuous) is physiologically superior to the other in patients who require enteral nutritional therapy. Studies in animals have addressed this issue. Extrapolation of these data to humans, however, is difficult and perhaps physiologically and sociobiologically irrelevant for several reasons. The animal studies have concentrated on physiologic differences between those animals that were allowed to eat (or that were force-fed) a specific number of times per day (so-called meal-fed animals) and those that were allowed ad libitum access to an unlimited supply of food. Animals fed ad libitum, when left undisturbed, ate smaller amounts of food at more frequent intervals and were generally called "nibblers." Extrapolation of these animal data to humans fed three to six times daily, versus humans fed by an intermittent or continuous technique, is tenuous at best. Finally, different researchers have obtained contradictory results when studying the effects of periodic eating in the same laboratory animal.[46] Thus, there are varied opinions of the significance of the observed phenomena for the animal population itself.

Nevertheless, certain generalizations can be made. The bulk of the experimental evidence suggests that meal-fed animals seem more efficient in converting ingested foods into storage forms of energy.[47, 48] They have increased nutrient absorption, increased glucose absorption and utilization, and increased lipogenesis. The metabolic changes precipitating these phenomena primarily involve changes in carbohydrate metabolism. Studies in the rat have shown augmented activity in three basic enzyme groups: (1) those involved in the phosphorylation of glucose and its conversions to alpha-glycerophosphate and pyruvate; (2) those involved in fatty acid synthesis; and (3) those involved in the generation of NADPH for the support of fatty acid biosynthesis.[48] Although the meal composition (the fat-to-carbohydrate ratio and the type of carbohydrate administered) clearly influences these metabolic pathways, it is not the sole limiting factor. Differences in meal frequency may influence metabolic activity.[46]

Meal-fed animals may, therefore, be more efficient in converting ingested calories to stored energy in the form of body fat. Whether these differences persist in animals fed past an initial adaptation period is controversial.[46] The data, however, suggest that returning to normal or supranormal levels of caloric intake via intermittent feedings, analogous to meal feeding, may cause increased fat-to-lean body ratios.[46, 49] Furthermore, intermittent feeding may not be as efficient in repleting visceral protein stores as in patients who are fed more frequently. While intermittent "meal" feeding may be potentially harmful, it is not known if continuous feedings are necessarily superior. If smaller, more frequent meals are needed, what is the optimal number of feedings per day? Whereas the meal-fed animal may be predisposed to diabetes and have a propensity for obesity, continuously fed animals may not fare better.[46-50] Also, continuous feeding could lead to persistently elevated insulin levels and thereby decreased fat and glycogen mobilization.

Controlled prospective studies are needed to compare intermittent and continuous feeding in humans with regard to body composition, hormone-substrate interaction, and nutrient utilization. Some evidence suggests that continuous feedings are superior to intermittent feedings in terms of nutrient delivery and avoidance of gastrointestinal complications.[5, 51] Infants with various intestinal diseases had significantly greater protein synthesis and mineral absorption, associated with a greater weight gain, when fed formula intragastrically and continuously than infants fed the same formula intermittently and orally.[52] Hiebert compared continuous with intermittent tube feedings in adult burn patients.[53] Patients who received continuous feedings had significantly decreased stool frequency and required significantly less time to achieve their nutritional goals than those fed intermittently.

Data generated in a prospective study at our institution compared calorie intake with different feeding methods (Table 16–3).[54] It was found that continuous jejunal feedings were comparable to intermittent and continuous gastric feedings in terms of nutrient delivery. Intermittent jejunal feedings were inferior to other routes in a small group of patients, however, because of poor patient tolerance. Based on these findings, we use

Table 16–3   KILOCALORIES ORDERED VERSUS RECEIVED DURING DAYS 1 to 5 OF TUBE FEEDING

	GASTRIC		JEJUNAL	
	Continuous	*Intermittent*	*Continuous*	*Intermittent*
No. of Patients	17	21	11	6
Kcal Ordered*	1910 ± 208[‡§]	1388 ± 125	913 ± 196[‡]	463 ± 73
Kcal Received[†]	1515 ± 154[‡]	1161 ± 111	754 ± 136	324 ± 66
Per Cent Received or Ordered	83 ± 4.1	83 ± 3.0	87 ± 5.9	69 ± 3.6

*Kcal ordered: $F = 6.477$; d.f. = 2.44; $p < 0.005$
[†]Kcal received: $F = 5.983$; d.f. = 2.44; $p < 0.01$
[‡]$p < 0.01$
[§]$p < 0.05$

continuous delivery by pump when feeding into the jejunum and intermittent delivery for those patients who receive gastric feedings.

Stomach Versus Duodenum

The rationale for feeding into the stomach is based on several factors. First, the stomach tolerates a variety of formulas (protein isolates, crystalline amino acid, and intact protein) more readily than does the small intestine. Therefore, nasogastric feedings are versatile. Second, the stomach normally accepts high osmotic loads without cramping, distention, vomiting, diarrhea, or fluid and electrolyte shifts, all of which can occur with feedings in the small intestine. In addition, the stomach has a tremendous reservoir capacity and more readily accepts intermittent "bolus" feedings.[12] Alert patients with intact gag reflexes and no pulmonary disease generally do well with nasogastric feedings. Indeed, this route has been the traditional method for nasoenteric delivery of nutrients. Also, nasogastric tubes are more easily positioned than nasoduodenal tubes.

Nasogastric feeding, however, may increase the risk of aspiration. The actual clinical incidence of aspiration in patients who are fed nasoenterically, while probably small, is unknown. Olivares et al. reviewed 720 autopsies of neurologic patients who had been tube-fed and found a 6.5 to 12.5 per cent incidence of aspiration.[55] Their study emphasized the relationship between the use of nasogastric tube feeding and subsequent aspiration in patients with neuromotor deglutition disorders. The patients at greatest risk were those who were aged, debilitated, demented, or stuporous; had poor gag reflexes or ileus; or were immediately postoperative.

Our policy initially is to infuse intermittent feedings into the stomach at iso-osmolarity. The volume is increased over a 24- to 48-hour period until full nutrient requirements are reached. If needed, large volumes (300 to 400 ml) are delivered every three to four hours. When hyperosmolar formula is administered, the concentration is increased before the volume. If the caliber of the nasogastric tube is adequate, the prescribed volume can be delivered over 20 to 30 minutes. Diets that are too viscous to be delivered by gravity drip can be administered by volumetric infusion pump. Gastric residuals are checked before each feeding and the feeding is withheld if the residual is greater than 150 ml. Two hours later the residual is remeasured. If this residual is still greater than 150 ml, the patient may have to be evaluated for delayed gastric emptying. One should note that residuals may be difficult to check with small-bore tubes, which collapse easily with suction. Furthermore, a blenderized or viscous formula cannot be delivered through small-bore tubes. All tubes are flushed with 20 ml of water before and after each feeding.

Feeding into the duodenum or jejunum is preferred in patients with gastroparesis, delayed gastric emptying, or increased risks for aspiration, and in those who are immediately postoperative. Insertion of nasoduodenal tubes as mentioned previously may be difficult. Once the tube has reached the stomach, ideally it passes into the duodenum with peristalsis. If this does not occur, metoclopramide may be used to facilitate tube passage and promote gastric emptying.[5]

Metoclopramide, introduced in 1964 by Besancon, is a substituted benzamide with antiemetic and gastrokinetic effects.[56] The gastrokinetic effects have been described as follows: (1) an increase in resting muscle tension with increased pressure at the lower esophageal sphincter and in the gastric fundus; (2) increased peristalsis in the esophagus, antrum, and small intestine; and (3) increased coordination of mechanical activities as evidenced by relaxation of the pylorus and duodenum during contraction of the stomach.[55] The exact mechanism of metoclopramide's action is unknown. However, it contributes to accelerated esophageal clearance, increases gastric emptying of liquids and solids, and reduces the transit time in the small intestine.[57] Controlled randomized studies are needed to demonstrate the efficacy of metoclopramide as adjunctive therapy in patients with gastroparesis, ileus, and delayed gastric emptying. To date, parenteral metoclopramide has been approved only as an aid for diagnostic intubation and radiographic examination of the proximal small intestine.

A potential disadvantage of feeding into the duodenum is accidental dislodgement of the tube. Even tubes with weighted ends can reflux into the stomach with coughing or vomiting. Although the actual morbidity associated with an unknown and unsuspected change from nasoduodenal to nasogastric feeding would perhaps be minimal, there would appear to be an increased risk of aspiration. This is especially true in patients with altered gastric motility and when feedings are administered at night.[12,58]

Our policy is to start feeding into the duodenum or jejunum with a dilute formula (150 mOsm) at a rate of 50 ml/hour. In the absence of gastrointestinal side effects, or hypoalbuminemia, the rate is increased by 25 to 50 ml/hour/day until the necessary volume is reached. The osmolality is then increased until the nutrient requirements are met. Tube placement is checked and residuals measured (if possible) every four hours. Antidiarrheal agents such as paregoric-(1ml/100 ml of diet) are used if diarrhea becomes severe. Patients with refractory diarrhea or other significant gastrointestinal disturbances can often have their symptoms relieved by temporarily discontinuing the feeding. Feedings can usually be restarted in 48 hours.[12]

Monitoring

Patients who receive nasoenteric feedings require the same careful monitoring as those who receive parenteral nutrition. A protocol should be established and followed to ensure that the specified nutrtional goals are met.[12] A standard checklist is helpful in initiating and maintaining nasoenteric feeding (Fig. 16–6). This is especially relevant in institutions where individuals of varying experience are responsible for writing orders. In addition, the checklist helps to avoid the omission of important details. Careful attention to the patient's metabolic status and fluid and electrolyte balance is necessary to avoid complications. (Further discussion of the proper monitoring of patients receiving enteral feeding is included in another chapter.)

SUMMARY

There has been a renewed interest in the use of nasoenteric tube feeding due to improvements in formulas and equipment for nutrient delivery. There are specific conditions for which these feedings are preferred over other routes of nutrient administration. Enteral feedings are more physiologic, safer, as efficacious, and more cost effective than parenteral feedings.

The clinical dictum "when the gut works, and can be used safely, use it" still rings true. Many cachectic patients can be maintained or repleted with nasoenteric tube feedings. Two thirds of severely malnourished patients in the average general hospital can probably be managed with nasoenteric feeding or enteric feeding in combination with peripheral intravenous nutrition.[14] In those patients who require central venous nutrition, nasoenteric tube feedings can be used to "bridge the gap" between parenteral feeding and volitional oral intake.

Prospective, randomized, controlled studies are needed to compare the efficacy of gastric with duodenal feedings, and continuous with intermittent techniques. Intermittent feedings at rates of 30 ml/min are satisfactory for isotonic nasogastric feedings in alert, awake patients. Continuous infusion delivered with pumps are necessary when feeding directly into the small intestine.

More research is needed to determine the best preventive measures for common problems that occur with nasoenteric feedings. Metoclopramide can facilitate passage of nasoduodenal tubes through the pylorus in those patients who have delayed gastric emptying and cannot be fed into the stomach.

Feeding Tube Location: _____

Check items to be done:

_____ 1. Confirm placement of tube by aspiration of gastric contents prior to the administration of feeding. If no gastric aspirate, obtain abdominal x-ray to confirm tube location prior to administration of the feeding.

_____ 2. Elevate head of bed 45º when feeding into the stomach.

_____ 3. Name of formula _____
Volume of formula _____ ml at _____ strength to be given over _____ hours. Rate of feeding _____ ml/hour.

_____ 4. No formula to hang for more than eight (8) hours.

_____ 5. Check for residual every _____ hours for gastric feedings. Withhold feedings for _____ hours if residual is 50% greater than ordered volume. Notify physician if this occurs on two consecutive measurements of residuals.

_____ 6. Weigh patient Monday, Wednesday and Friday. Chart on graph.

_____ 7. Record intake and output daily. Chart volume of formula separately from water or other oral intake for every shift.

_____ 8. Change administration tubing and cleanse feeding bag daily.

_____ 9. Irrigate feeding tube with 20 ml of water at the completion of each intermittent feeding, when tube is disconnected, and following the delivery of crushed medications.

_____ 10. Irrigate feeding tube with 20 ml of water if feeding is stopped for any reason.

_____ 11. Calorie counts by dietitian daily for five (5) days, then once weekly.

_____ 12. Complete blood count with red cell indices, SMA-12, total iron binding capacity, serum iron, magnesium, weekly.

_____ 13. SMA-6 every Monday and Thursday.

_____ 14. 24 hour urine collection for urea to start at 8:00 AM on _____ .

_____ M.D.

Date _____

Figure 16–6. Sample orders for tube feeding.

Finally, it is necessary to establish and follow a standard protocol to ensure adequate delivery of nutrients and to achieve the specified nutritional goals safely.

REFERENCES

1. Fallis, L. S., and Barron, J.: Gastric and jejunal alimentation with fine polyethylene tubes. Arch. Surg., 65:373–381, 1952.
2. Pareira, M. D., Conrad, E. J., Hicks, W., and Elman, R.: Therapeutic nutrition with tube feeding. J.A.M.A., 156:810–816, 1954.
3. Barron, J.: Tube feeding of post-operative patients. Surg. Clin. North Am., 39:1481–1491, 1959.
4. Stephens, R. V., and Randall, H. T.: Use of a concentrated, balanced, liquid elemental diet for nutritional management of catabolic states. Ann. Surg., 170:642–667, 1969.
5. Orr, G., Wade, J., Bothe, A., and Blackburn, G. L.: Alternatives to total parenteral nutrition in the critically ill patient. Crit. Care Med., 8:29–34, 1980.
6. Eastwood, G. L.: Small bowel morphology and epithelial proliferation in intravenously alimented rabbits. Surgery, 82:613–620, 1977.
7. Feldman, E. J., Dowling, R H., McNaughton, J., and Peters, T. J.: Effects of oral versus intravenous nutrition on intestinal adaption after small bowel resection in the dog. Gastroenterology, 70:712–719, 1976.
8. Levine, G. M., Deren, J. J., Steiger, E., and Zinno,

R.: Role of oral intake in maintenance of gut mass and disaccharide activity. Gastroenterology, 67:975–982, 1974.

9. Johnson, L. R.: Gastrointestinal hormones. *In* Johnson, L. R. (ed.): Gastrointestinal Physiology. St. Louis, C. V. Mosby Company, 1977, pages 1–11.

10. Johnson, L. R., Copeland, E. M., Dudrick, S. J., Lichtenberger, L. M., and Castro, G. A.: Structural and hormonal alterations in the gastrointestinal tract of parenterally fed rats. Gastroenterology, 68:1177–1183, 1975.

11. Johnson, L. R., Lichtenberger, L. M., Copeland, E. M., Dudrick, S. J., and Castro, G. A.: Action of gastrin on gastrointestinal structure and function. Gastroenterology, 68:1184–1192, 1975.

12. Rombeau, J. L., and Barot, L. R.: Enteral nutrition therapy. Surg. Clin. North Am., 61:605–620, 1981.

13. Bothe, A., Jr., Wade, J. E., and Blackburn, G. L.: Enteral nutrition: An overview. *In* Hill, G. L. (ed.): Clinical Surgery International. Volume 2: Nutrition and the Surgical Patient. New York, Churchill Livingstone, 1981, pages 76–103.

14. Heymsfield, S. B., Bethel, R. A., Ansley, J. D., Nixon, D. W., and Rudman, D.: Enteral hyperalimentation: An alternative to central venous hyperalimentation. Ann. Intern. Med., 90:63–71, 1979.

15. Lickley, H. L. A., Track, N. S., Vranic, M., and Bury, K. D.: Metabolic responses to enteral and parenteral nutrition. Am. J. Surg., 135:172–176, 1978.

16. Blackburn, G. L., and Bistrian, B. R.: Nutritional care of the injured and/or septic patient. Surg. Clin. North Am., 56:1195–1224, 1976.

17. Flatt, J. P., and Blackburn, G. L.: The metabolic fuel regulatory system: Implications for protein-sparing therapies during caloric deprivation and disease. Am. J. Clin. Nutr., 27:175–187, 1974.

18. McArdle, A. H., Palmason, C., Morency, I., and Brown, R. A.: A rationale for enteral feeding as the preferable route for hyperalimentation. Surgery, 90:616–623, 1981.

19. Blackburn, G. L., Bistrian, B. R., Maini, B. S., Schlamm, H. T., and Smith, M. F.: Nutritional and metabolic assessment of the hospitalized patient. J.P.E.N., 1:11–22, 1977.

20. Allardyce, D. B., and Groves, A. C.: A comparison of nutritional gains resulting from intravenous and enteral feeding. Surg. Gynecol. Obstet., 139:179–184, 1974.

21. Bethel, R. A., Jansen, R. D., Heymsfield, S. B., Ansley, J. D., Hersh, T., and Rudman, D.: Nasogastric hyperalimentation through a polyethylene catheter: An alternative to central venous hyperalimentation. Am. J. Clin. Nutr., 32:1112–1120, 1979.

22. Gougeon, F. W.: Enteral hyperalimentation: A new apparatus for administration. Surgery, 79:697–701, 1976.

23. Heitkemper, M. E., Martin, D. L., Hansen, B. C., Hanson, R., and Vanderburg, V.: Rate and volume of intermittent enteral feeding. J.P.E.N., 5:125–129, 1981.

24. Young, G. A., and Hill, G. L.: A controlled study of protein-sparing after excision of the rectum. Ann. Surg., 192:183–191, 1980.

25. Winitz, M., Seedman, D. A., and Graff, J.: Studies in metabolic nutrition employing chemically defined diets. I. Extended feeding of normal human adult males. Am. J. Clin. Nutr., 23:525–545, 1970.

26. Freeman, H. J., Kim, Y. S., and Sleisenger, M. H.: Protein digestion and absorption in man: Normal mechanisms and protein-energy malnutrition. Am. J. Med., 67:1030–1036, 1979.

27. Rocchio, M. A., Chung-Ja Mo Cha, Haas, K. F., and Randall, H. T.: Use of chemically defined diets in the management of patients with acute inflammatory bowel disease. Am. J. Surg., 127:469–475, 1974.

28. Voitk, A. J., Eschave, V., Brown, R. A., McArdle, A. H., and Gurd, F. N.: Elemental diet in the treatment of fistula of the alimentary tract. Surg. Gynecol. Obstet., 137:68–72, 1973.

29. Feldtman, R. W., and Andrassy, R. J.: Meeting exception nutrition needs. 2. Elemental enteral alimentation. Postgrad. Med., 643:65–74, 1978.

30. Page, C. P., Carlton, P. K., Andrassy, R. J., Feldtman, R. W., and Shield, C. F.: Safe cost-effective postoperative nutrition: Defined formula diet via needle-catheter jejunostomy. Am. J. Surg., 138:939–945, 1979.

31. Moss, G., and Friedman, R. C.: Abdominal decompression: Increased efficiency by esophageal aspiration utilizing a new nasogastric tube. Am. J. Surg., 133:225–228, 1977.

32. Moss, G.: Postoperative decompression and feeding. Surg. Gynecol. Obstet., 122:550–554, 1977.

33. Moss, G.: Early enteral feeding after abdominal surgery. *In* Deitel, M. (ed.): Nutrition in Clinical Surgery. Baltimore, Williams & Wilkins, 1980, pages 161–170.

34. Greene, H. L., Helinek, G. L., Folk, C. C., Courtney, M., Thompson, S., MacDonell, R. C., Jr., and Lukens, J. N.: Nasogastric tube feeding at home: A method for adjunctive nutritional support of malnourished patients. Am. J. Clin. Nutr., 34:1131–1138, 1981.

35. Metz, G., Dilawari, J., and Kellock, T. D.: Simple technique for nasoenteric feeding. Lancet 2:454, 1978.

36. Newmark, S. R., Simpson, S., Beskitt, M. P., Black, J., and Sublett, D.: Home tube feeding for long-term nutritional support. J.P.E.N., 5:76–79, 1981.

37. Gustke, R. F., Varma, R. R., and Soergel, K. H.: Gastric reflux during perfusion of the small bowel. Gastroenterology, 59:890–895, 1970.

38. Bojm, M. A., and Deitel, M.: An easy method for passing fine silicone nasogastric tubes. Am. J. Surg., 143:385, 1982.

39. Christie, D. L., and Ament, M. E.: A double blind crossover study of metoclopramide versus placebo for facilitating passage of multipurpose biopsy tube. Gastroenterology, 71:726–728, 1976.

40. Cobb, L. M., Cartmill, A. M., Barry, M., and Gelsdorf, R. B.: A tube for enteral nutrition of patients with a phagopraxia and patients with ventilator assistance. Surg. Gynecol. Obstet., 155:81–84, 1982.

41. Page, C. P., Ryan, J. A., and Haff, R. C.: Continued catheter administration of an elemental diet. Surg. Gynecol. Obstet., 142:184–188, 1976.

42. Dobbie, R. P., Butterick, O. D., Jr.: Continuous pump-tube enteric hyperalimentation: Use in esophageal disease. J.P.E.N., 1:100–104, 1977.

43. Dobbie, R. P., and Hoffmeister, J. A.: Continuous pump-tube enteral hyperalimentation. Surg. Gynecol. Obstet., 143:273–276, 1976.

44. Hiebert, J. M.: Continuous nasogastric tube feeding in burn patients. Contemp. Surg., 15(3):31–41, 1979.

45. Shils, M. E.: Enteral nutrition by tube. Cancer Res., 27:2432–2439, 1977.

46. Adams, C. E., and Morgan, K. J.: Periodicity of eating: Implications for human food consumption. Nutr. Res., 1:525–550, 1981.

47. Chakrabarty, K., and Leveille, G. A.: Influence of periodicity of eating on the activity of various enzymes in the adipose tissue, liver, and muscle of the rat. J. Nutr., 96:76–82, 1968.

48. Leveille, G. A.: Adipose tissue metabolism: Influence of periodicity of eating and diet composition. Fed. Proc., 29:1294–1301, 1970.

49. Leveille, G. A., and Chakrabarty, K.: Absorption and utilizaton of glucose by meal-fed and nibbling rats. J. Nutr., 96:69–75, 1968.

50. Leveille, G. A., and Chakrabarty, K.: Diurnal variations in tissue glycogen and liver weights of meal-fed rats. J. Nutr., 93:546–554, 1967.

51. Randall, H. T.: Enteral feeding. In Ballinger, W. F. (ed.): Manual of Surgical Nutrition. Philadelphia, W. B. Saunders Company, 1975.

52. Parker, P., Stroop, S., and Green, H.: A controlled comparison of continuous versus intermittent enteral feeding in the treatment of infants with intestinal disease. J. Pediatr., 99:360–364, 1981.

53. Hiebert, J. M., Brown, A., Anderson, R. G., Halfacre, S., Rodeheaver, G. T., and Edlich, R. F.: Comparison of continuous vs intermittent tube feedings in adult burn patients. J.P.E.N., 5:73–75, 1981.

54. Evans, D., Di Sipio, M., Barot, L., and Rombeau, J.: Comparison of gastric and jejunal tube feedings. J.P.E.N., 4:79, 1980.

55. Olivares, L., Segovia, A., and Revuelta: Tube feeding and lethal aspiration in neurological patients: A review of 720 autopsy cases. Stroke, 5:654–657, 1974.

56. Schulze-Delrieu, K.: Drug therapy. Metoclopramide. N. Engl. J. Med., 305:28–33, 1981.

57. Perkel, M. S., Moore, C., Hersh, T., and Davidson, E. D.: Metoclopramide therapy in patients with delayed gastric emptying: A randomized, double-blind study. Dig. Dis. Sci., 24:662–666, 1979.

58. Rombeau, J. L., and Miller, R. A.: Nasoenteric Tube Feeding—Practical Aspects. Mountain View, California, HEDECO, 1979.

CHAPTER 17

Feeding by Tube Enterostomy

JOHN L. ROMBEAU
LENORA R. BAROT
DAVID W. LOW
PATRICK L. TWOMEY

Tube enterostomy refers to the operative placement of a tube or catheter in any segment of the gastrointestinal tract, from the pharynx to the colon. Those tubes specifically intended for delivery of nutrient preparations are generally placed in the stomach, jejunum, pharynx, or cervical esophagus (Fig. 17–1).[1] The surgical techniques employed are not new, having been pioneered in the nineteenth century and perfected in the early years of this century.[2] However, recognition of the broad spectrum of medical and surgical diseases accompanied by malnutrition and the beneficial therapeutic effects of aggressive nutritional support has been relatively recent. This has created a need for safe, reliable access to the gastrointestinal tract for enteral alimentation. Availability of effective, well-tolerated liquid formulas and improved delivery systems has also stimulated interest in using the gastrointestinal tract for nutritional support.[3] As the indications for enteral nutrition have become more clearly defined, the need for safe, long-term feeding catheter access has increased. The purpose of this chapter is to discuss the indications, surgical techniques, dietary administration, and complications of feeding by tube enterostomy.

INDICATIONS

The surgical placement of a tube or catheter into the gastrointestinal tract for nutrient delivery is indicated when the nasoenteric route is unavailable or when long-term enteral alimentation (more than four weeks) is anticipated. These tubes are placed primarily or as adjuncts to gastrointestinal surgery (Table 17–1). With certain diseases the upper gastrointestinal tract is obstructed while the small intestine and colon remain patent. This is the case with unresectable tumors of the oropharynx, esophagus, or stomach. Occasionally, benign conditions such as strictures or collagen-vascular diseases will hinder the transit of material through the esophagus. In such situations, the operative insertion of a feeding tube distal to the obstruction will allow the normal process of intestinal digestion and absorption to continue. Even if the upper gastrointestinal tract is mechanically intact, central neurologic disorders (multiple sclerosis, cerebral vascular accidents, and decreased cerebral function secondary to trauma, infection, or tumor) or primary muscular dysfunction may interfere with swallowing and reduce or prevent oral intake. For short-term enteral support in these patients, a nasoenteric tube is the preferred route (see Chapter 16). If it appears that the condition will be of a chronic nature, however, a tube enterostomy offers a more secure, manageable access site for enteral nutrition.

There are instances in which a feeding tube enterostomy is inserted as an adjunct to the primary surgery.[4] This is particularly useful when the need for nutritional support is anticipated but the oral route is unavailable, as is the case following major esophageal or gastric resections.[5] In addition, when a major segment of the small intestine is re-

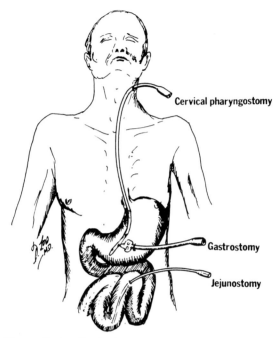

Figure 17–1. Site for feeding with tube enterostomy.

sected (because of ischemia, inflammatory bowel disease, or trauma), a tube enterostomy can be used for the infusion of defined formula diets during the period of gut adaptation. Finally, malnourished patients who are undergoing major abdominal procedures can be expected to have less than optimal oral intake for some time following surgery. If a feeding tube is placed prophylactically at

Table 17–1 INDICATIONS FOR FEEDING BY TUBE ENTEROSTOMY

Primary Tube Enterostomy
    Swallowing Dysfunction
        Central nervous system disorders
        Collagen vascular disease
        Myasthenia gravis
    Upper Gastrointestinal Obstruction
        Oropharyngeal neoplasm
        Esophageal stricture or neoplasm
        Gastric neoplasm
        Duodenal neoplasm or stricture
        Pancreatic neoplasm or stricture

Adjunctive Tube Enterostomy
    Esophagectomy
    Gastrectomy
    Pancreaticoduodenectomy
    Massive small bowel resection
    Pancreatectomy

the initial surgery, it can be used for the infusion of liquid supplements during the postoperative period and after the patient is discharged.

Gastrostomy, first performed in a human by Sedillot in 1846, is the most common method of feeding by tube enterostomy.[6] This type of tube enterostomy requires the following: (1) a stomach uninvolved by the primary disease, (2) normal gastric and duodenal emptying, (3) no significant esophageal reflux, and (4) intact gag reflexes. It is especially desirable to use the stomach because its reservoir capacity allows for intermittent bolus feeding without the need for continuous pump infusion. Aspiration pneumonia is the most serious nonsurgical complication associated with this procedure; gastrostomy is therefore contraindicated in patients at high risk for this problem.[7]

Jejunostomies were performed for feeding as early as 1885. In 1967 Rogers reintroduced the concept of jejunostomy as an adjunct to gastric surgery.[8] Jejunostomy is probably the most common tube enterostomy used for feeding in conjunction with other abdominal surgical procedures, and it is the method of choice for those patients in whom gastrostomy cannot be safely performed. Jejunostomies are preferred as adjuncts because of the ease of placement and the advantage of early feeding permitted by the rapid postoperative return of small bowel function. Fairfull-Smith and Freeman recently reported the successful initiation of feeding by jejunostomy tube in 20 patients one day following major abdominal surgery.[9] There were no complications related to the feeding tubes, and a significant improvement in nitrogen balance was observed in the enterally fed patients when compared with unfed controls.

As an adjunct to surgery for head and neck tumors or trauma to the maxillofacial region, a tube can quickly be inserted into the pharynx or cervical esophagus and passed into the stomach for feeding.[10] Royster et al. reported the use of this procedure in 52 patients undergoing maxillofacial resection. Tube feeding was initiated between the first and third postoperative days.[11] Conventional gastrostomy diets were used and there were no complications related to the feedings. Thirty patients were discharged with a tube in place for supplemental feeding at home, an additional advantage over nasogastric intubation.

SURGICAL TECHNIQUES

Gastrostomy

There are three common types of gastrostomies: Stamm, Witzel, and Janeway. In all of these procedures, an upper abdominal midline or left upper quadrant transverse incision can be used. Generally, a midline incision is preferred, as exposure is better and the exit site for the catheter can be placed laterally away from the incision. Local, regional, or general anesthesia may be used, depending upon the patient's clinical condition.

Stamm Gastrostomy. The Stamm gastrostomy is the simplest to perform. It is often used when the patient is a poor operative risk or when the need for tube feeding is only temporary. After the peritoneum is opened traction is placed on the greater omentum to bring the stomach into view. Two Babcock clamps are placed on the anterior surface of the body of the stomach and the stomach is elevated into the wound (Fig. 17–2A). A stab wound or short ½-inch incision is made between the two clamps and the gastrotomy is dilated with a Kelly clamp (Fig. 17–2B). A No. 28 Foley or mushroom catheter is inserted into the stomach and directed toward the pylorus. Several concentric pursestring sutures (2–0 chromic) are inserted at ½-inch intervals from the tube and tied down to invaginate the stomach around the tube. Once these ties are secured, the omental apron is elevated and the tube is brought through an avascular space in the omentum and exited through a stab wound in the left upper abdomen. Care must be taken to ensure that the catheter exits well away from the costal margin to avoid pain and difficulty with dressings. The tube should be placed in slight tension to bring the anterior gastric wall snugly up against the anterior parietal peritoneum. Several interrupted sutures of 2–0 silk are used to fix the stomach to the abdominal wall at the catheter exit site, and nonabsorbable suture is used to secure the catheter to the skin.

The Stamm gastrostomy is useful for continuous gastric intubation with a tube such as a mushroom, Malecot, or Foley catheter. Its advantages are simplicity of construction and ease of closure. When the need for gastrostomy has passed, removal of the tube is simple and is generally followed by prompt closure. In some situations, how-

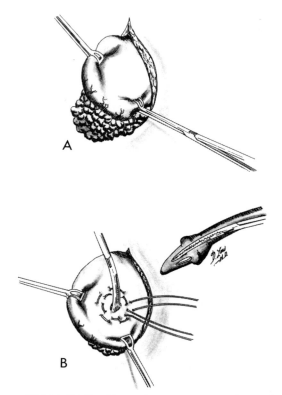

Figure 17–2. Stamm temporary gastrostomy. *A,* Fundal site for tube insertion. *B,* Tube inserted within concentric pursestring sutures. A Foley or mushroom catheter may be used.

ever, this attribute can be a disadvantage. Inadvertent removal of the tube is followed by rapid shrinkage of the cutaneous orifice in a few hours. To preserve the gastrostomy, a tube of any type must be promptly reinserted. This can be done safely with no special precautions for sterility, as long as the gastrostomy has been in place long enough to ensure fusion between the stomach and the parietal peritoneum of the abdominal wall. In patients with unimpaired healing, a period of one to two weeks is usually sufficient. The simplest method of salvaging a Stamm-type gastrostomy is reinsertion of the old tube after washing it with soap and water. Alternatively, the largest size Foley catheter that fits should be placed into the gastrostomy until a more suitable tube can be found. It is sometimes possible to dilate a contracted gastrostomy site by using progressively increasing catheter sizes or dilators of the Hegar or bougie type, augmented by a topical anesthetic if needed. It may even be possible to save a previously well-established gastrostomy that has completely healed without need for reoperation (see section on complications).

Freshly placed Stamm gastrostomies, however, require more caution in reintubation. If the surgeon has taken care to sew the stomach to the anterior abdominal wall with a ring of sutures around the gastrotomy, it may be possible to gently replace a catheter in the stomach without pushing it away from the abdominal wall. However, no feeding should be attempted until the proper intragastric location of the tube and the absence of leakage following infusion of water-soluble contrast material are confirmed radiographically. Intra-abdominal leakage of gastric contents can be lethal, especially if unrecognized in an obtunded or otherwise neurologically impaired patient. Care and conservatism are therefore in order in this situation.

Witzel Gastrostomy. A Witzel gastrostomy is similar to the Stamm gastrostomy in that a tube is inserted into the stomach in a similar fashion as described previously and secured with a pursestring suture. However, before the tube is brought through the omentum and exited from the abdomen, a seromuscular incision is made in the stomach (Fig. 17–3A) which is sewn around the tube to create a tunnel for a distance of 2 to 3 in. (Fig. 17–3B). This seromuscular tunnel, around the tube as it exits from the stomach, helps to minimize the risk of leakage when the stomach is distended or the tube is removed.

Janeway Gastrostomy. The Janeway gastrostomy is preferred when the need for permanent tube feeding is anticipated. With this type of gastrostomy, a gastric tube is created and brought through the abdominal wall to form a permanent stoma. The initial surgical approach is the same as mentioned previously, with a midline incision preferred. Once the stomach is exposed, a full-thickness rectangular flap is elevated from the anterior gastric wall with the base toward the greater curvature (Fig. 17–4A). When this is done by hand suture technique, the flap should be 5 to 6 cm wide and 12 cm long. The flap is freed by sharp dissection and bleeding is controlled with fine plain ties. The defect in the stomach is closed in two layers. The inner full-thickness layer is a simple running stitch or a Connell inverting stitch of 2–0 chromic. The seromuscular layer is closed with interrupted sutures of 2–0 silk. When the base of the flap

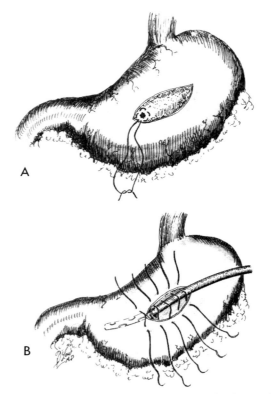

Figure 17–3. Witzel temporary gastrostomy. *A,* Three-inch tunnel created beneath serosa and muscularis. Note anchoring suture at exit site of stomach. *B,* Size 16–18 French rubber catheter with multiple openings inserted. Sutures placed for seromuscular tunnel.

is reached, a Foley catheter is inserted into the stomach (Fig. 17–4B) and the flap closed around the catheter to form a tube (Fig. 17–4C). This is a continuation of the two-layer closure of the stomach. A circumstomal incision is made in the left upper quadrant and the gastric tube is pulled through. To facilitate passage of the gastric tube through the abdominal wall, a Babcock or Allis clamp is passed through the stomal incision in a retrograde fashion to grasp the tip of the gastric tube, alone with a Kelly clamp to secure the catheter (Fig. 17–4D). When the top of the gastric tube is level with the skin the stoma is matured primarily with interrupted 3–0 chromic sutures (Fig. 17–4E). Care must be taken to ensure that there is no torsion of the tube as it passes through the abdominal wall. Tension on the tube will impair blood supply and should be avoided.

The gastric tube for the Janeway gastrostomy may also be constructed with a stapler, as described by Moss.[12] Use of the stapler considerably reduces the length of the

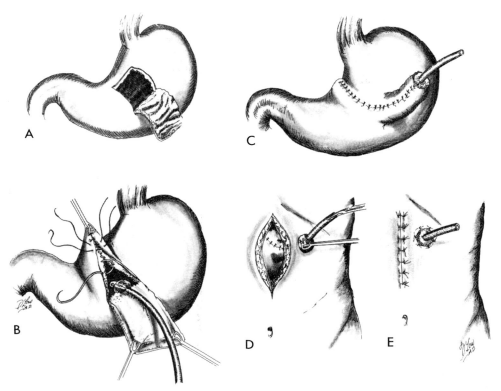

Figure 17–4. Janeway permanent gastrostomy. *A*, Rectangular flap created from anterior wall of stomach. *B*, Foley catheter inserted into gastrotomy and sutures placed to create a gastric tube. *C*, Completion of gastric tube. *D*, Gastric tube brought through abdominal wall. *E*, Creation of stoma with primary apposition with mucocutaneous sutures.

procedure. A site on the body of the stomach which affords a tube of 4 to 5 in. is chosen, and a stab wound is made through the anterior wall of the stomach several centimeters from the lesser curvature. A catheter is inserted and directed toward the greater curvature and the stomach is tented around it with Babcock clamps (Fig. 17–5*A*). A gastrointestinal stapler, which applies two double rows of staples and divides the tissue between them, is used (Fig. 17–5*B*) to separate the tube from the stomach wall (Fig. 17–5*C*). Any bleeding points along the staple line are controlled with figure-of-eight sutures of 3–0 chromic. The entire staple line is inverted with interrupted sutures of 3–0 silk (Fig. 17–5*D*). The rest of the procedure is as outlined previously. The balloon on the catheter should be inflated and the catheter attached to gravity drainage for 48 to 72 hours. If the stoma appears to be well perfused at that time, feedings can be started when the gastric drainage decreases below 300 ml/day. On the eighth to tenth postoperative day the catheter can be removed

from the gastric tube and reinserted only for nutrient infusions. Webster and Carey used a modification of this technique in 29 patients with no leaks in the suture line or peritonitis.[13] The wounds of two patients dehisced, and three patients aspirated formula. Recently we have used a special silicone rubber gastrostomy-jejunal tube in conjunction with this procedure.

A related technique, recently described by Delany and Driscoll (Fig. 17–6) employs a tube of mucosa along which passes through the abdominal wall.[14] This method has the advantage of simplicity and can even be performed under local anesthesia. Moreover, the stomach is not opened until the abdominal incision is closed, which should minimize contamination.

Complication rates as high as 10 to 35 per cent have been reported with gastrostomies.[7] This high rate is due, in part, to the poor nutritional status and multiple medical problems of these patients. Wound healing is poor, pulmonary complications are high because the patients are immobile, and in-

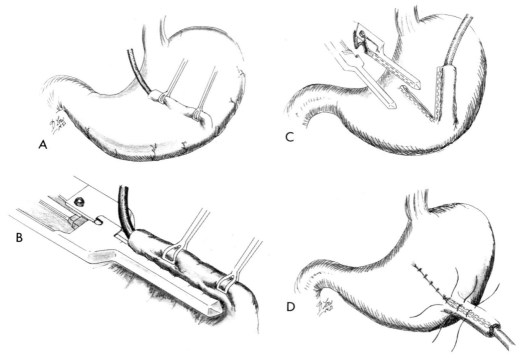

Figure 17–5. Janeway stapled permanent gastrostomy. *A*, Insertion of Foley catheter into gastrotomy and placement of Babcock clamps to create a tunnel. *B*, Placement of gastrointestinal stapler. *C*, Creation of full-thickness tunnel with stapler. *D*, Layer of interrupted seromuscular sutures covering staples.

fection is common. Technical complications are usually related to leakage around the tube, bleeding from the stomach entry site, or accidental removal of the feeding tube during the immediate postoperative period. Leakage around the tube at skin level can usually be controlled by inserting a slightly larger catheter with a balloon and taping the tube on traction.

With a Janeway gastrostomy, an inadvertently removed catheter can be gently reinserted. The most common technical problem with the Janeway gastrostomy is necrosis of the tip of the gastric tube, either from constriction at its base from the gastric closure, tension on the tube, or compression as the tube comes through the fascia. Usually only 1 cm of the distal gastric tube necroses. This is not likely to result in intraabdominal leakage, but stenosis at skin level will occur if the supporting catheter is removed. To prevent stenosis, the tube must be left in place continuously as with the Stamm and Witzel gastrostomies. In recent years the reported rate of complication associated with this technique has fallen to an acceptable level and the procedure has gained in popularity.

Although a Foley catheter can be used briefly for intragastric feeding and is available in any hospital or chronic care facility, it is not the ideal enteral feeding tube. The balloon in these catheters can be damaged by gastric secretions and its diameter can change with time as gas passes across the balloon membrane. Moreover, the balloon can act as a stimulus to gastric peristalsis. The catheter tip may be carried along to the pylorus, causing complete obstruction of the gastric outlet with occasionally serious sequelae. Preferable tubes include Malecot or mushroom catheters with perforations cut in the bulb part of the tube. Even better for intragastric feeding may be the Pezzer closed-tip catheter with extra holes cut in its bulb. The increased traction afforded by this tube will aid healing by increasing adhesion to the abdominal wall and decreasing the chance of accidental dislodgement.[15]

Jejunostomy

There are two basic types of jejunostomies used for feeding: a suberosal tunnel similar to the Witzel gastrostomy and a

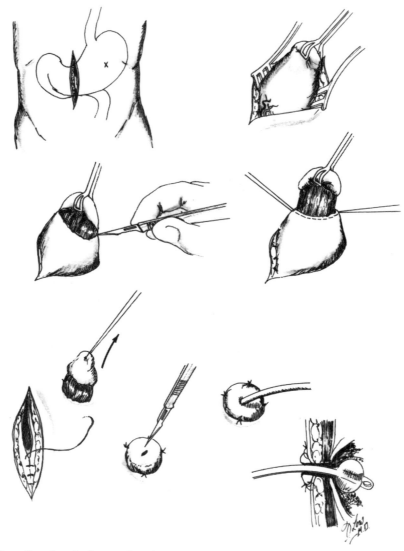

Figure 17–6. Operative steps in the creation of a mucosal gastrostomy (with permission).

needle jejunostomy that uses a catheter with a much finer gauge. The decision to use a jejunostomy rather than a gastrostomy depends on several factors: gastric function, duration of enteral support, and ambulatory status. If there is symptomatic esophagel reflux, inability to protect the airway from aspiration, ulcerative or neoplastic disease of the stomach, or impaired gastric emptying, a jejunostomy is preferable to a gastrostomy. If feedings are to be started immediately after surgery the jejunum is preferred because of its rapid return of function within 12 to 24 hours. For long-term feedings in the

ambulatory patient, a jejunostomy may be limiting because a continuous pump infusion is often required. When feeding tubes are inserted as adjuncts to major intra-abdominal operations, the jejunum is often used because of the simplicity of the procedure.

Witzel Jejunostomy. The Witzel jejunostomy is performed by first choosing a loop of jejunum 8 in. distal to the ligament of Treitz to allow easy apposition to the anterior abdominal wall (Fig. 17–7A). A small stab wound is made on the antemesenteric border, and a No. 16 catheter is introduced distally for a distance of 8 in. (Fig. 17–7B). A pursestring suture of 2–0 chromic is inserted around the tube (Fig. 17–7B) to fix it in place and the proximal 2 to 3 in. of tube are buried in a seromuscular incision as described by Marwedel (Fig. 17–7C).[16] The catheter is brought out through a stab wound in the abdominal wall and the jejunum is sutured to the anterior parietal peritoneum with several interrupted chromic sutures (Fig. 17–7D).

Needle Catheter Jejunostomy. In addition to the conventional Witzel jejunostomy, a simplified technique for needle catheter jejunostomy was described in 1973 by Delany et al.[17] A 2.75-in., 14-gauge needle of the type used for subclavian vein catheterization is inserted obliquely through the antemesenteric border of the jejunum (Fig. 17–8A) 6 in. distal to the ligament of Treitz or surgical anastomosis. A 12- to 18-in. 16-gauge polyvinyl catheter with a stylet is advanced 4 to 6 in. into the lumen (Fig. 17–8B). The needle and the stylet are withdrawn, and the catheter is secured in place with a single 4–0 silk pursestring suture (Fig. 17–8C). A separate needle is then passed into

the abdomen from the skin surface and the extraluminal portion of the catheter is passed through the needle, outside of the abdomen (Fig. 17–8D). The catheter is secured to the skin and the jejunum is tacked to the anterior parietal peritoneum of the abdominal wall at the catheter exit site (Fig. 17–8E). A defined formula diet can be infused through these catheters 24 to 48 hours after surgery if the general condition of the patient permits. It is recommended that meglumine diatriozate (Gastrografin) be injected through the catheter to verify its intraluminal position before feedings are begun. Complications associated with this technique include dislodgement of the catheter to an intraperitoneal position, early occlusion of the small-bore catheter, abdominal distention, and aspiration.[18]

Modification of the needle catheter jejunostomy was recently reported by Cobb et al. using a silicone rubber catheter (8 French) inserted through a jejunal serosal tunnel.[19] A defined formula diet was then begun in 38 patients 48 hours postoperatively with an attempt to reach full feedings by the fifth day

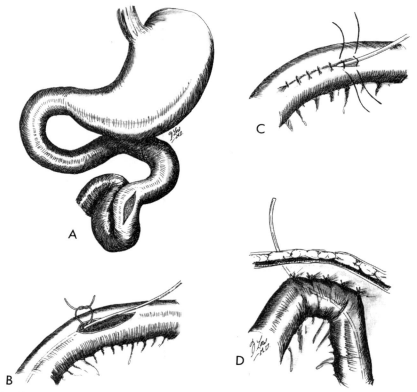

Figure 17–7. Witzel jejunostomy. *A*, Site for seromuscular tunnel approximately eight inches from the ligament of Treitz. *B*, Insertion of No. 16 French rubber catheter with anchoring suture.

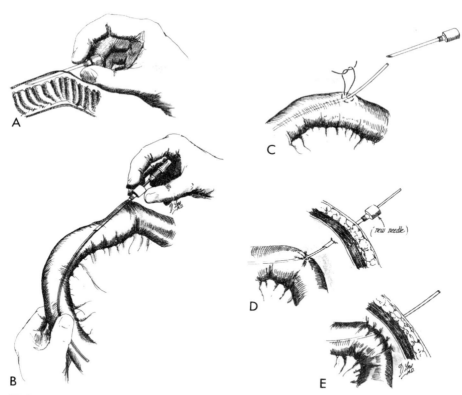

Figure 17–8. *A*, Insertion of needle within jejunal wall. *B*, Insertion of catheter with stylet through the needle into the jejunum. *C*, Removal of needle and placement of anchoring suture. *D*, Insertion of new needle through the abdominal wall for the exit of the catheter. *E*, Jejunopexy.

after surgery. There were no technical complications associated with the feeding tubes, but it was found that septic and severely malnourished patients (serum albumin <3gm/dl) tolerated early tube feeding poorly.

Roux-En-Y Jejunostomy. A permanent feeding jejunostomy can be constructed by forming a Roux-en-Y limb of proximal jejunum and bringing the free end up to skin level (Fig. 17–9). The "Y" of small bowel is needed to prevent leakage of corrosive digestive juices from the bowel lumen onto the skin. The mucosal stoma, or "bud," provides the advantage of the Janeway gastrostomy—specifically, permanence of access—even when the tube is removed for hours or days.

Gastrostomy-Jejunal Tube

For the past four years, we have been developing a new gastrostomy-jejunal feeding tube that has several advantages: It provides the option of feeding either into the stomach or jejunum; permits proximal gastric decompression to avoid the possibility of aspiration while feeding into the jejunum; allows a feeding jejunostomy to be placed under local anesthesia; provides a route to administer crushed medication; and is easily replaceable.

The double-lumen gastrostomy-jejunal tube is made of silicone rubber and consists of a 24-French gastric tube with a concentric 9.6-French jejunal tube within the wall of the gastric tube (Fig. 17–10A). The jejunal tube is 20 in. long and, regardless of the gastrotomy site, is of sufficient length to ensure positioning of the tip beyond the ligament of Treitz. A 10-g mercury weight is at the tip of the jejunal tube. The lumen through the end of the tube aids in passing the tube through the pylorus with a fluoroscopically placed guidewire if needed.

A midline or left subcostal incision may be used for tube placement. The subcostal incision must be made at least 4 cm beneath the left costal margin to ensure that the tube can exit through a separate site superior to this incision abutting against the rib margin. A standard Stamm gastrostomy is used for

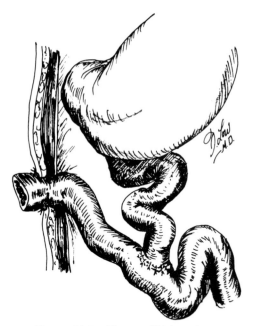

Figure 17–9. Roux-en-Y jejunostomy.

those patients who have local anesthesia. The pursestring suture is placed using 0-silk, and the mercury-weighted end of the jejunal tube is initially inserted into the stomach (Fig. 17–10B). When the jejunal tube is almost completely inserted, a closed Kelly clamp is placed through the side-hole and into the tip of the gastrostomy tube. This causes the end of the tube to elongate and facilitates insertion through the gastrotomy (Fig. 17–10C). The tube is brought out through a separate incision and the stomach is sutured to the anterior abdominal wall (Fig. 17–10D).

If local anesthesia is used, no attempt is made to guide the jejunal tube through the pylorus manually. In these patients, 10 mg of metoclopramide is slowly given intravenously to aid in the passage of the jejunal tube out of the stomach.

If general anesthesia is used, a lubricated, arteriography guidewire is placed into the jejunal tube once it has been placed into the stomach. The mercury bolus is palpated externally to the anterior wall of the prepyloric antrum, and the bolus is guided manually through the pylorus (Fig. 17–10E).

Feeding is initiated through the jejunal tube with the gastrostomy tube left to dependent drainage for at least three days.

This lessens the risk of aspiration during the immediate postoperative period and eliminates gastric distention from swallowed air. If the tube is placed as the primary operative procedure, without extensive manipulation of the small intestine, feeding may be started during the immediate postoperative period, but only through the jejunostomy tube and never through the gastrostomy tube. If the tube is placed as a procedure ancillary to a gastrectomy, esophagogastrectomy, or pancreaticoduodenectomy, for example, feeding is started when there is clinical evidence of return of peristalsis.

The diet selection and method of administration are based upon the patient's nutrient needs and absorption status as previously published.[3] The majority of our patients are fed into the jejunum with an isotonic diet, Isocal (Mead Johnson), Osmolite (Ross Laboratories), or Precision Isotonic (Doyle Pharmaceuticals) at full strength at 50 ml/hour. The diet is increased daily at a rate of 25 ml/hour. For the patient with large energy and nitrogen requirements and fluid restrictions, we have been using a new hypercaloric formula, Magnacal (Organon Pharmaceuticals) that contains 2 kcal/ml. This is started at iso-osmolar concentrations at a rate of 50 ml/hour.

The majority of our patients who receive jejunostomy feedings are fed continuously by means of a battery-driven pump. This provides temporal uniformity of administration of the formula and allows the patient mobility while being fed. Our studies on nonhuman primates have shown that continuous feeding provides a greater increase in whole-body protein synthesis than does intermittent feeding.[20] In addition, frequent gastrointestinal side effects have been noted when patients are fed into the jejunum on an intermittent schedule.[21]

Forty-five gastrostomy-jejunal tubes (HEDECO) were placed in patients at three hospitals: Philadelphia Veterans Administration Medical Center, Hospital of the University of Pennsylvania, and Martinez Veterans Administration Medical Center (Tables 17–2 and 17–3). Thirty-four of the operations were performed as a primary procedure; the tube was inserted in conjunction with an upper gastrointestinal operation in eleven patients. The most common procedure with which this tube was used was a subtotal gastrectomy and Billroth II anastomosis.

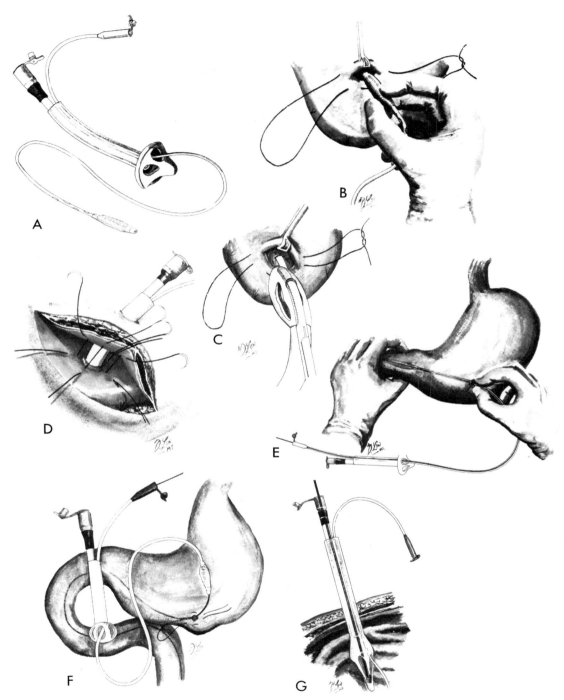

Figure 17–10. *A*, Gastrostomy-jejunal tube. *B*, Insertion of jejunal tube through the gastrotomy. *C*, Insertion of the gastrostomy tube into the stomach. A closed Kelly clamp is placed through a side hole in the tip of the tube. *D*, Exit of gastrostomy tube through separate incision and anchoring of stomach to parietal peritoneum. *E*, Manipulation of the jejunal tube through the pylorus. A lubricated guidewire is placed into the jejunal tube and the mercury bolus is palpated and guided through the pylorus. *F*, Positioning of the jejunal tube over a guidewire with the aid of intraoperative fluoroscopy. *G*, Uterine sound used as a stylet to aid in re-insertion or removal of the tube.

Of the 34 patients who had the tube inserted primarily, 17 patients had local anesthesia with or without an intercostal block, and 17 patients with general anesthesia. Of the 17 patients in whom the tube was inserted under local anesthesia, 11 had the jejunal tube guided through the pylorus intraoperatively with the aid of a fluoroscopically directed guidewire (Fig. 17–10F).[22] In the remaining six patients who had local anesthesia, the jejunal tube was initially placed into the stomach. In four of these patients the tube passed through the pylorus within 48 hours after surgery with the aid of a single dose of metoclopramide, 10 mg given intravenously. Despite proper positioning of the patient and the use of metoclopramide, the tube did not pass through the pylorus in two patients. In these patients, the jejunal tube was subsequently positioned in the jejunum in the fluoroscopy suite. All of the patients who had general anesthesia had the jejunal tube placed primarily into the jejunum as described previously.

The complications of this procedure are listed in Table 17–4. In five patients the tube was pulled out by the patient or removed inadvertently. The tube was replaced at the bedside in three of these patients with the aid of a uterine sound used for a stylet (Fig. 17–10G). One patient required reoperation. Use of the tube was discontinued in the fifth patient. Three patients had leakage of gastric contents around the tube, and one of these patients suffered a severe skin reaction. There were two instances of total obstruction of the jejunal tube. One patient had an incomplete intestinal obstruction, which was presumed to be related to the

Table 17–3 RESULTS OF GASTROSTOMY-JEJUNAL TUBE INSERTION IN 45 PATIENTS

		NO. OF PATIENTS
Primary Tube Insertion		34
Anesthesia		
Local	17	
General	17	
Adjunctive Tube Insertion		11
Type of Gastrostomy		
Stamm		36
Janeway		9

presence of the tube. One of our first patients had a wound dehiscence after the tube had been brought out through the incision. This mode of exit for the tube was then discontinued. In one patient the capsule of the mercury bolus broke while the surgeon was manually manipulating the tube through the pylorus. The mercury bolus was modified by incorporating a stronger capsule following this complication.

Two postoperative deaths occurred, both apparently unrelated to placement of the tube.

Cervical Esophagostomy and Pharyngostomy

In 1967 Graham and Royster reported a simplified technique for the insertion of a tube esophagostomy as an adjunct to head and neck surgery.[10] There were no complications in 12 patients, and the tubes were left in place for periods ranging from two

Table 17–2 DIAGNOSIS AT INSERTION OF GASTROSTOMY-JEJUNAL TUBES IN 45 PATIENTS

DIAGNOSIS	NO. OF PATIENTS
Primary Tube Insertion	
Cerebrovascular accident	25
Multiple sclerosis	3
Head injury	2
Oropharyngeal cancer	2
Esophageal cancer	2
Adjunctive Tube Insertion	
Esophageal cancer	4
Gastric cancer	4
Peptic ulcer disease	3

Table 17–4 COMPLICATIONS OF GASTROSTOMY-JEJUNAL TUBE INSERTION IN 45 PATIENTS

Major	
Incomplete obstruction of intestine	1
Wound dehiscence	1
Leakage of gastric contents with severe skin reaction	1
Minor	
Inadvertent removal of tube	5
Leakage of gastric contents without skin reaction	2
Plugging of jejunal tube	2
Breakage of mercury bolus	1

months to more than one year. A curved clamp is directed into the piriform recess through the mouth (Fig. 17–11A) on the side opposite the major surgery and pushed outward just below the cornu of the hyoid bone (Fig. 17–11B). Care must be taken in the placement of the clamp because of the anatomic proximity to the external carotid artery (Fig. 17–11C). A small skin incision is made and the underlying structures are bluntly dissected away from the tip of the clamp to avoid damage. The distal end of a nasogastric tube is pulled through the wound and passed into the stomach. The tube is then secured at the skin with a single suture (Fig. 17–11D). Laceration of the external jugular vein, local cutaneous reactions at the exit site, and temporary esophagocutaneous fistulas after tube removal have been reported.[23] The tube is easily replaced if it is removed inadvertently.

A permanent pharyngostomy can be performed as reported by Shumrick.[24] An incision is made along the anterior border of the sternocleidomastoid muscle near the superior aspect of the thyroid cartilage. The muscle and underlying carotid sheath are retracted laterally, and an incision is made in the piriform recess inferior and medial to the cornu of the hyoid bone. The mucosa is then sewn to the skin to form a permanent stoma.

A similar technique for esophageal intubation in the neck has been described by Klopp.[25] In this procedure the esophagus is approached from the left after the sternocleidomastoid muscle and underlying carotid sheath are retracted laterally. Two traction sutures are placed in the esophagus 2 to 3 cm above the clavicle, and the esophagus is opened longitudinally. To create a permanent stoma, the mucosa is sutured to the skin. As with the pharyngostomy, the tube can be simply fixed with a pursestring suture and the skin closed around it for temporary access. Complications are similar to those noted with the pharyngostomies (infection, hemorrhage, aspiration, fistula) with the additional danger of recurrent laryngeal nerve injury. This is, however, generally transient, as noted by Fitz-Hugh and Sly.[23]

Duodenostomy

The duodenum is generally not chosen as a primary site for feeding tube enterostomies because of the significant morbidity associated with leakage of bile and pancreatic juice or the establishment of a permanent duodenal fistula after tube removal. However, duodenostomy tubes are frequently placed for duodenal decompression following trauma of difficult duodenal stump closures. These tubes can be used for feeding if recovery is prolonged.[26]

DIET SELECTION AND DELIVERY TECHNIQUES

The choice of formula and delivery technique is based upon the functional status of the patient's gastrointestinal tract and the caliber and location of the tube (Fig. 17–12). Gastrostomy tubes are generally of a large enough caliber (>12 French) that the viscosity of the formula is not a problem. If the digestive and absorptive properties of the small intestine are normal, a blenderized diet or protein isolate diet can be used. Such preparations offer the advantages of decreased cost, ease of preparation, and excellent patient tolerance. If there is impairment of pancreaticobiliary function or small bowel absorption, a defined formula diet is used. In either instance, intragastric nutrient delivery offers the advantage of an intermittent bolus schedule because of the stomach's capacity as a reservoir.

Jejunostomy feeding almost always requires a continuous pump infusion because of the gastrointestinal side effects (cramping, bloating, dumping-like syndrome) that result when large volumes of hypertonic solutions are infused rapidly into the small bowel. If the tube caliber is adequate (>6 French) and intestinal function is normal, a protein isolate diet composed of intact protein, oligosaccharides, and long-chain fatty acids can be used. If the feeding catheter is small (as with the needle jejunostomy types), or if there is impairment of intestinal digestion and absorption, a defined formula diet should be used to avoid tube occlusion or nutrient malabsorption. To avoid intolerable gastrointestinal side effects, delivery schedules for jejunal feeding generally stress slow increments in volume using a dilute preparation.

COMPLICATIONS

The major complications associated with gastrostomies and jejunostomies are shown in Figures 17–13 and 17–14. Aside from the

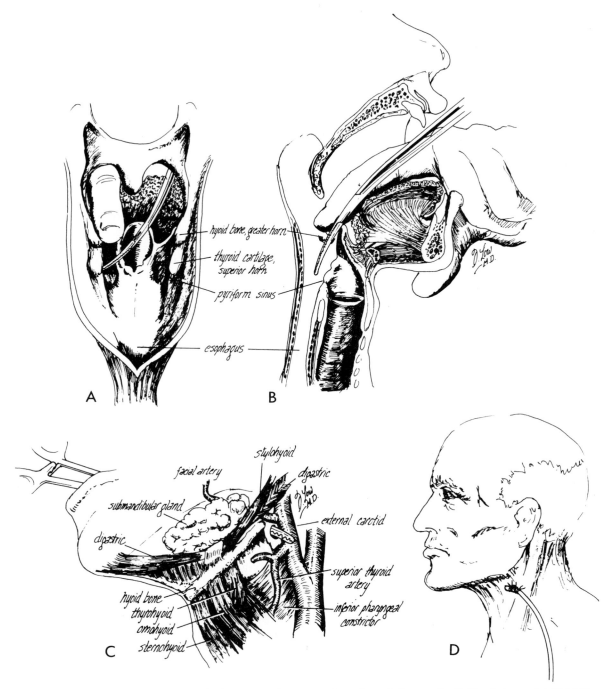

Figure 17–11.   Pharyngostomy. *A,* Placement of a curved clamp through the mouth. *B,* Tip of clamp directed just beneath the hyoid bone. *C,* Proximity of the tip of the clamp to the external carotid artery. *D,* Exit of pharyngostomy tube.

Schema for Choice of Diet and Delivery Technique

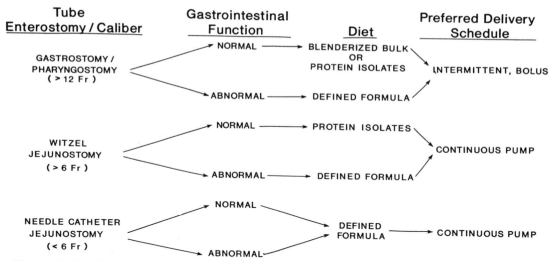

Tube Enterostomy / Caliber	Gastrointestinal Function	Diet	Preferred Delivery Schedule
GASTROSTOMY / PHARYNGOSTOMY (> 12 Fr)	NORMAL	BLENDERIZED BULK OR PROTEIN ISOLATES	INTERMITTENT, BOLUS
	ABNORMAL	DEFINED FORMULA	
WITZEL JEJUNOSTOMY (> 6 Fr)	NORMAL	PROTEIN ISOLATES	CONTINUOUS PUMP
	ABNORMAL	DEFINED FORMULA	
NEEDLE CATHETER JEJUNOSTOMY (< 6 Fr)	NORMAL	DEFINED FORMULA	CONTINUOUS PUMP
	ABNORMAL		

Figure 17–12. Choice of diet and delivery schedule based upon the caliber of the feeding tube and quality of gastrointestinal function.

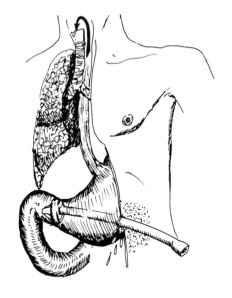

Gastrostomy Complications

Aspiration

Displacement of tube with gastric outlet obstruction

Skin excoriation

Leakage of contents intraperitoneally

Persistent fistula after tube removal

Figure 17–13. Complications associated with a feeding gastrostomy.

specific surgical complications associated with the various types of tube enterostomies described previously, the major complications are those associated with tube feeding in general (see Chapter 16), which are most commonly either gastrointestinal or metabolic. Mechanical problems associated with tube enterostomies are primarily tube obstruction, cracking, or inadvertent removal. When high viscosity feedings are used (blenderized or fiber diets), small-caliber tubes can occlude if flushing is not performed. This complication can be avoided by irrigating gastrostomy tubes with 30 ml of water after each feeding and flushing jejunostomy tubes with 15 to 20 ml of water whenever the pump infusion is stopped. When tubes have been in place for some time breakage may occur with manipulation during dressing or feeding. Gastrostomy tubes can be replaced by simply pulling out the existing catheter and inserting one of similar caliber. This should not be attempted for at least two weeks postoperatively because a firm fibrous tract and dependable adherence of the bowel to the abdominal wall may not occur for a protracted period of time in these malnourished patients. If a catheter is inadvertently removed it can usually be easily replaced within six to eight

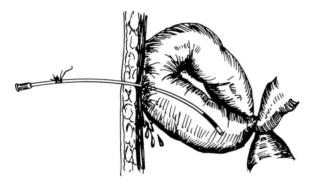

Jejunostomy Complications

Inadvertent removal or dislodgement

Leakage of contents into peritoneum

Plugging of tube

Volvulus

Diarrhea

Figure 17–14. Complications associated with a feeding jejunostomy.

hours. The tract from the stomach to the skin will close rapidly once the catheter is removed. During catheter replacement the fascial level is the point at which passage of the tube is most often inhibited. A stylet of the type used to pass urinary catheters will often add enough stiffness to the feeding tube to allow reinsertion. In patients with a Stamm gastrostomy in whom the tract has been sealed for weeks or months, a recent percutaneous technique has been described by Sacks and Glotzer for reinsertion of the gastrostomy tube.[27] The stomach is inflated with air by a nasogastric tube and a No. 18 Cournand needle inserted along the anesthetized tract into the stomach. A guidewire is introduced through the needle and successively larger dilators are threaded over the wire. The intragastric position of the dilators is verified intermittently with a 60 per cent solution of water-soluble contrast material. Finally, a 14- or 16-French Foley catheter with the tip removed is passed over the wire and into the stomach. The balloon is inflated and feedings are begun immediately.

CONCLUSIONS

Feeding by tube enterostomy is indicated in malnourished patients with functioning gastrointestinal tracts who are in need of long-term nutritional therapy. Pa-

tients with proximal obstruction of the gastrointestinal tract, thereby preventing nasoenteric intubation, or who have permanent need for enteral nutritional support are the most common candidates for primary tube enterostomies. In recent years, feeding by tube enterostomy has gained in popularity as an adjunctive procedure to gastrointestinal operations in the malnourished patient. When the procedure and choice of access site is tailored to the individual patient's needs and combined with appropriate diets and delivery schedules, the incidence of successful nutritional rehabilitation is high and the complication rate low.

REFERENCES

1. Torosian, M. H., and Rombeau, J. L.: Feeding by tube enterostomy. Surg. Gynecol. Obstet., 150:918–927, 1980.
2. Lee, R. J., and Gould, P.: Cancer of the pylorus and duodenum: Jejunostomy and death. Lancet, 2:1092, 1885.
3. Rombeau, J. L., and Barot, L. R.: Enteral nutritional therapy. Surg. Clin. North Am., 61:605–620, 1981.
4. Smith, G. K., and Farris, J. M.: Re-evaluation of temporary gastrostomy as a substitute for nasogastric suction. Am. J. Surg., 102:168–175, 1961.
5. Rogers, J. C. T.: Jejunostomy in the high risk gastrectomy patient. Surg. Gynecol. Obstet., 126:333–336, 1967.
6. Cunha, F.: Gastrostomy; Its inception and evolution. Am. J. Surg., 72:610–634, 1946.
7. Engel, S.: Gastrostomy. Surg. Clin. North Am., 49:1289–1295, 1969.
8. Sawyer, R. B.: Jejunostomy for feeding or decompression. Surg. Clin. North Am., 49:1311–1316, 1969.
9. Fairfull-Smith, R. J., and Freeman, J. B.: Immediate postoperative enteral nutrition with a nonelemental diet. J. Surg. Res., 29:236–239, 1980.
10. Graham, W. P., and Royster, H. P.: Simplified cervical esophagostomy for long-term extraoral feeding. Surg. Gynecol. Obstet., 125:127–128, 1967.
11. Royster, H. P., Noone, R. B., Graham, W. P., and Theogaraj, S. D.: Cervical pharyngostomy for feeding after maxillofacial surgery. Am. J. Surg., 116:610–614, 1968.
12. Moss, G.: A simple technique for permanent gastrostomy. Surgery, 71:369–370, 1972.
13. Webster, M. W., Carey, L. C., and Ravitch, M. M.: The permanent gastrostomy: Use of the gastrointestinal anastomotic stapler. Arch. Surg., 110:658–660, 1975.
14. Delany, H. M., and Driscoll, B.: The gastric mucosal tube: A simplified technique for permanent gastrostomy. Scientific exhibit at the American College of Surgeons Sixty-seventh Clinical Congress, San Francisco, 1981.
15. Holder, T. M., Leape, L. L., and Ashcraft, K. W.: Current concepts—Gastrostomy: Its use and dangers in pediatric patients. N. Engl. J. Med., 286:1345–47, 1972.
16. ReMine, W. H.: Carcinoma of the stomach. *In*

Maingot, R. (ed.): Abdominal Operations. New York, Appleton-Century-Crofts, 1980.

17. Delany, H. M., Carnevale, N. J., and Garvey, J. W.: Jejunostomy by a needle catheter technique. Surgery, 73:786–790, 1973.

18. Yeung, C. K., Young, G. A., Hackett, A. F., and Hill, G. L.: Fine needle catheter jejunostomy: An assessment of a new method of nutritional support after major gastrointestinal surgery. Br. J. Surg., 66:727–732, 1979.

19. Cobb, L. M., Cartmill, A. M., and Gilsdorf, R. B.: Early postoperative nutritional support using the serosal tunnel jejunostomy. J.P.E.N., 5:397–401, 1981.

20. Rombeau, J. L., Stein, T. P., and Settle, R. G.: Comparison of intermittent and continuous gastric and jejunal feeding on protein synthesis [Abstract]. Fed. Proc., 41:274, 1982.

21. Evans, D., DiSipio, M., Barot, L., Rombeau, J. L., Crosby, L. O., and Mullen, J. L.: Comparison of gastric and jejunal tube feedings [Abstract]. J.P.E.N., 4:596, 1980.

22. McLean, G. L.: Personal communication, 1983.

23. Fitz-Hugh, G. S., and Sly, D. E.: Elective cervical esophagostomy. Ann. Otol. Rhinol. Laryngol., 76:804–809, 1967.

24. Shumrick, D. A.: Pyriformsinusosotomy: A useful technique for temporary or permanent tube feeding. Arch. Surg., 94:277–279, 1967.

25. Klopp, C. T.: Cervical esophagostomy. J. Thorac. Surg., 21:490–491, 1951.

26. Oakes, D. D., and Couch, N. P.: A new use for catheter duodenostomy: Postoperative enteric alimentation. Arch. Surg., 110:845–846, 1975.

27. Sacks, B. A., and Glotzer, D. J.: Percutaneous reestablishment of feeding gastrostomies. Surgery, 85:575–576, 1979.

CHAPTER 18

The Neurologic Patient

PATRICK L. TWOMEY
JAMES N. ST. JOHN

Among the commonest indications for enteral feeding is neuromuscular disease, a broad collection of ills characterized by debility, chronicity, and the need for prolonged rehabilitation. On a typical day in our medical center, more patients receive tube feeding for neurologic indications than for any other reason. Surgical placement of long-term access to the gut for feeding is most frequently needed in neurologic patients, and the new techniques of nasoenteric feeding have been an important step forward in neurologic management. In a study of 720 patients who succumbed to neurologic diseases, over 20 per cent had required tube feeding, most of whom were patients with vascular diseases of the central nervous system.[1] In our experience the principal other categories of neurologic disease in which enteral nutritional support is needed are trauma, degenerative diseases, and neoplastic diseases.

The individual circumstances of many patients with neurologic disease can create special nutritional needs. Some patients expend vast quantities of energy through repetitive seizures, choreoathetotic movements, or decerebrate posturing. Others who are bedridden may be at particular risk for consequences of malnutrition such as pneumonia and decubitus ulcers. From the point of view of cost effectiveness, prevention of decubitus ulcers alone suffices to justify good nutritional care. Maintenance of healthy amounts of soft tissue over bony prominences not only contributes to patient comfort but also simplifies nursing management.

Even the patient's basic neurologic deficit may be influenced by his nutritional status. Often it is difficult to separate the lethargy, weakness, wasting, and apathy of devastating neurologic disease from the identical symptoms caused by starvation.

Although few scientific data on this point are available, we have been impressed that certain patients seem to brighten, take a new interest in their surroundings, and in some cases regain function with no intervention other than institution of vigorous nutritional support. The possibility that such support might be a critical therapeutic maneuver in obtunded patients was also proposed by Bryan-Brown and Savitz.[2, 3] They reported a group of patients who were comatose following craniotomy for tumor or aneurysm and in whom they diagnosed "chronic cerebral edema." All had typical findings of protein-calorie malnutrition. Four of these patients were given vigorous nutritional repletion which was followed by considerable improvement in their neurologic state. Nutritional repletion was associated with decrease in isotopic measures of the extracellular fluid, which the authors felt caused a reduction in cerebral edema.

INDICATIONS AND PREREQUISITES

Three factors enter into the decision to start enteral feeding in neurologic patients: treatable underlying disease, inability to eat, and satisfactory gut function. A fourth, the presence of recognizable malnutrition, may add to the sense of urgency for beginning support, but is not a prerequisite. Ideally, we should intervene *before* overt malnutrition occurs.

Treatable Underlying Disease. The patient with reversible or potentially reversible deficits should not be allowed to starve. Acute head injury, Guillain-Barré syndrome, and fresh stroke are examples of treatable conditions in which there is a real prospect for useful recovery, and full supportive care is indicated. Other conditions such as multiple brain metastases, diffuse hypoxic brain damage, or advanced senile dementia may not be reversible; depending on the individual circumstances, special or extraordinary measures to prolong life may not be indicated. In between is the large gray area of conditions with uncertain prognosis in patients whose prospects of benefit are unknown. In our experience, ambivalence on the part of the patient's primary decision-maker is the major cause of delay, and hence of avoidable nutritional depletion. In such situations it is helpful to recall that failure to decide is a decision in itself. We suggest that in cases of uncertainty the benefit of the doubt should be given to the patient and a trial of feeding initiated.

Inability to Eat. Poor intake results not only from depressed consciousness or difficulty in swallowing; it occurs also in alert patients who simply cannot feed themselves. Sadly, many institutions lack sufficient mealtime help to feed all patients who need assistance, even though they are alert and hungry. Other patients resist being spoon-fed, perhaps because of its profound symbolism of dependency. Tube feeding can help in all these situations. We have been pleased to observe patients whose functional status has improved during nasoenteric feeding, later feeding themselves around the tube at mealtime and finally increasing both intake and self-esteem to the point of independence. For this reason it is important to periodically retest the patient's ability to swallow and feed himself.

Satisfactory Gut Function. In contrast to other hospitalized patients at risk for serious malnutrition, the neurologic patient generally has a normal gastrointestinal tract and is an ideal candidate for enteral feeding. Some gastrointestinal problems can, however, occur. Immobility resulting from neuromuscular impairment leads to sluggish colonic function, resulting in the bane of existence of the nursing staff—fecal impaction. Ensuring adequate free water intake and encouraging movement, preferably out of bed, are the first steps in prevention. Bulk agents such as psyllium (Metamucil, Effersyllium, and others), dioctyl sodium sulfosuccinate (Colace, Senokot, and others), and high fiber foods may help but are difficult to administer by small tube because of clogging. Stimulant laxatives including milk of magnesia, cascara, phenolphthalein, magnesium citrate, and many others form the next line of defense, and can be more easily given by tube. However, stimulants engen-

der dependency, and chronic use can cause coloproctitis. Fortunately, most commercial tube feeding preparations lead to faster transit times, and even to diarrhea at the outset. The enterprising clinician can thus often "titrate" the patient to the point of proper bowel function by judicious choice of products and medications.

Special problems can occur in diseases causing impaired gut motility such as diabetes, dysautonomias, muscular dystrophies, scleroderma, and amyloidosis. In these cases, enteral feeding still may be of use, perhaps augmented with metoclopramide, bethanechol (Urecholine), or neostigmine. Usually extensive gut paralysis is a concomitant of advanced disease elsewhere, and more vigorous therapy such as total parenteral nutrition (TPN) will not be indicated. Fortunately such cases are rare.

Choice of Product. The typical neurologic patient with a normal gut has little need for "elemental diets" (Vivonex, Criticare, and others) which are of high osmolarity, low residue, and high cost.[4] In one randomized trial in patients with head injury they appeared worse, not better, than whole-protein preparations.[5] In general, adult patients with neurologic diseases do not require any special changes from the complete prepared tube feeding mixtures now available. Among the exceptions to this rule are some patients with Parkinson's disease who are receiving levodopa. Occasionally they will experience episodic loss of symptomatic control ("off-on phenomenon") which may be less severe if daily protein intake is restricted to 0.5 gm/kg/day.[6] However, increasing the medication dose or changing to a different agent should be considered in the nutritionally threatened patient before starting such a protein restriction.

Nutritional Assessment. The need for special nutritional assessment in the form of anthropometrics, specialized laboratory studies, skin testing, and the like for the average hospitalized patient is controversial.[7, 8] For neurologic patients several practical difficulties compound the problem. Even the simplest anthropometric indices such as weight or height may be difficult to determine if the patient is unable to stand, has contractures, or is comatose. Extremities affected by neuromuscular disorders undergo wasting, independent of nutritional status, making muscle circumference, skinfold thickness, and measurements of functional capacity uncertain or meaningless. The determination of "ideal body weight" for a paraplegic trauma victim or elderly hemiplegic patient suffers from lack of standards and unknown relation to outcome.

Fortunately, the decision to provide nutritional support, especially by the enteral route, can most often be made on clinical grounds alone. History, physical examination, and knowledge of the natural history of the patient's illness provide the data needed. *Changes* in weight, protein levels, or functional state, particularly in areas uninvolved with the primary neurologic disease, are useful monitors. Specifically, the finding of inability to swallow (which invariably occurs when consciousness is markedly depressed) anticipated to last more than a week or so suffices to justify tube feeding in the salvageable patient. In doubtful cases a recent history of inadequate intake provides further justification. If questions remain, we have found a simple calorie count to be the most useful special test. Depressed serum proteins (such as albumin and transferrin) are confirmatory and provide a handy index of repletion. However, shifts in water balance can confound such concentration measurements, and in any case prophylaxis is preferable to playing "nutritional catch up."

TECHNIQUES OF ENTERAL FEEDING

Two decisions must be made if the enteral route seems suitable: site of nutrient delivery and route of access. In making these decisions in neurologic patients one consideration is pivotal—the risk of aspiration.

Patients at Low Risk for Aspiration

If the patient is alert, can protect his airway, and has satisfactory pharyngeal reflexes, nutrients can be delivered directly into the stomach. This site takes advantage of the reservoir capacity of the stomach and may allow intermittent feeding by bolus to simplify nursing management. Moreover, the physiologic mixing and buffering of gastric acid by food and the metering out of gastric contents into the small bowel can minimize troublesome gastrointestinal symptoms, including distention, cramps, and diarrhea, which sometimes occur with

more distal infusion. This is a particular advantage during the start-up period.

Nasogastric Route. Selection of the route of access into the stomach depends chiefly on the expected duration of specialized feeding. For patients whose need is anticipated to last days to weeks (or in whom the duration of need for special feeding is not known), the traditional nasal route is simplest. For most patients alert enough to be fed safely by this route, a small silicone rubber catheter (number 7 to 9 French) can be passed into the stomach without special techniques. Long-term use of larger bore tubes such as a number 16 or 18 French Levin or Salem sump nasogastric tube for feeding is obsolete now that the newer soft catheters are available (see Chapter 13). An exception to this guideline might be made in patients who already have a larger tube in place to decompress the stomach in the period immediately following surgery or acute injury, and in whom this tube is to be used to check for gastrointestinal bleeding or to monitor gastric residuals during the initiation of feeding.

Gastrostomies. The most useful access route for longer term intragastric feeding (weeks to months or years) in neurologic patients is via gastrostomy. This route is generally well tolerated even by disoriented or confused patients, provides large-bore access for administration of medication, and is easily managed by semi-skilled nursing personnel in rehabilitation and extended care facilities. Indeed one of the commoner indications for construction of a gastrostomy is as an aid to institutional placement after the need for acute care hospitalization is past.

Techniques of Administration. As noted previously, intragastric feeding has the advantage of allowing bolus administration of food if the patient is not at risk for vomiting and aspiration. If the patient is able to communicate his feelings of satiety, anorexia, or gastrointestinal distress, such feeding can then be withheld or slowed. Residual gastric content should be checked before each feeding, and if more than a small amount (say 50 to 100 ml) the next feeding should be delayed. Some patients are unable to tolerate sufficient volume of feeding to meet nutritional needs with a schedule of three feedings. For them more frequent, smaller bolus feedings or continuous drip feeding is appropriate as discussed in Chapter 15.

Patients at Higher Risk of Aspiration

In the more common and more challenging situation, the neurologic patient in need of nutritional support is not able to provide adequate protection of the airway because of depressed consciousness, impaired reflexes, or weakness. The problem may be compounded by incompetence of the lower esophageal sphincter perhaps in association with hiatus hernia, by gastric atony from disease or drugs, or by gastric outlet obstruction. In the past the clinician faced the dilemma of watching malnutrition slowly progress or "taking a chance" on nasogastric feeding hoping that no regurgitation would occur.

Olivares and associates analyzed the findings of 720 autopsies of neurologic patients from two different hospitals.[1] The two institutions differed in that one used nasogastric feeding frequently (about 40 per cent) and the other, rarely (about 4 per cent). In the former institution, aspiration pneumonia was twice as common as in the latter (12 vs 6 per cent), and they concluded that this finding, a common cause of death, was clinically underdiagnosed and a serious problem in such patients.

The Three-Gate Principle. Development of techniques of small bowel feeding has changed this picture. Delivery of nutrients well downstream of the pylorus allows placement of three barriers between the food and the airway: the upper esophageal sphincter, the lower esophageal sphincter, and the pylorus (Fig. 18–1). Of course, regurgitation back into the stomach and thence into the esophagus can still occur, especially if presence of a large-bore tube renders these sphincters incompetent. Nonetheless, carefully done, small-bowel feeding greatly reduces regurgitation,[9] the greatest hazard of enteral feeding of neurologic patients.

Double Lumen Gastrostomy-Jejunal (Rombeau) Tube. For medium- to long-term access to small-bowel feeding in neurologic patients we now prefer use of the gastrostomy-jejunal tube described in Chapter 17. This tube can be placed either by temporary or permanent gastrostomy even under local anesthetic. It allows crushed medication to be placed into the stomach without fear of tube plugging, is replaceable without need for reoperation, and permits direct feeding into the small bowel. Its major

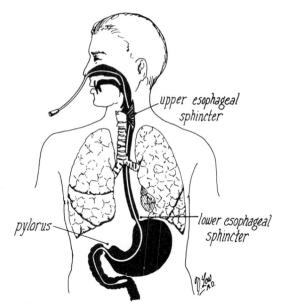

Figure 18–1. The three gates or barriers between site of nutrient delivery and the tracheobronchial tree. The more competent valves there are between the tube tip and the trachea, the safer enteral feeding will be.

advantage in the neurologic patient at risk for aspiration is the ability to use the gastric port as a vent even while feeding into the small bowel and to check occasionally for gastric residuals or tube feeding regurgitation without need to reinsert a nasogastric tube. Recent experience with this tube in 30 neurologic patients has confirmed the utility of this approach.[10]

Special Problems in Neurologic Patients

Vomiting. Since vomiting occurs in both neurologic and gastrointestinal disorders, evaluation of this symptom in enterally fed neurologic patients requires special thought. It is particularly likely to occur as a result of mass lesions of the posterior fossa which dislocate, distort, or compress the brain stem. Tumors of the cerebellum or fourth ventricle as well as mass lesions above the tentorium can cause this problem. Vomiting that occurs in the morning or without nausea is suggestive of increased intracranial pressure. This impression is confirmed by finding papilledema, cerebellar or brain stem signs, and by computed tomographic or other evidence of a mass in these areas. Therapy directed at this symptom usually consists of elimination of the offending mass lesion by surgery, radiotherapy, antibiotics, or chemotherapy. Antiemetics such as phenothiazines are also of some help.

Most of these intracranial causes of vomiting are likely to have been maximally treated prior to the initiation of enteral nutritional support. Hence, other causes need to be considered. Perhaps the commonest cause is too early or too copious feeding at a time when some degree of ileus is present (such as after trauma). Coexistent systemic or metabolic conditions such as sepsis, liver disease, or electrolyte imbalance will also occasionally prove to be at fault.

If vomiting persists without obvious cause in a bedridden patient being fed into the stomach, one should consider the possibility of an obstructive lesion at the level of the duodenum. The so-called vascular compression of the duodenum or superior mesenteric artery syndrome has been reported in patients who lie supine for long periods and lose weight, allowing the superior mesenteric vessels to obstruct the duodenum by a scissors-like compression against the aorta.[11] This syndrome has been reported following severe head injury in a patient bedridden for 16 weeks after injury and was successfully treated by nasoduodenal tube placement and nutritional repletion.[12] One of the authors (JNS) has also treated a patient with this syndrome whose symptoms developed several months following severe head injury. His protracted vomiting was initially erroneously attributed to the head injury. Simultaneous angiography and upper gastrointestinal contrast studies confirmed the diagnosis, and the symptoms resolved after several weeks of intravenous hyperalimentation. A third method of treatment, suitable in some patients, is placement in the prone position on a Stryker frame.[11] Since weight loss causing reduction of the fat about the mesenteric vessels is a common antecedent of this syndrome, it seems likely that it can be prevented in most patients by more vigorous early nutritional support.

Diarrhea. During the initiation of enteral feeding diarrhea develops in some patients, which leads the staff to curtail the feeding. This distressing development can indeed result from tube feeding, particularly if hyperosmolar (elemental or hypercaloric) products are given, or if bolus feeding in excessive amounts has been prescribed. However, diarrhea can be largely eliminated by use of isotonic, lactose-free, balanced tube feeding preparations infused continuously by pump at gradually increasing rates. Occasionally, patients may need addition of a liquid antidiarrheal such as paregoric or diphenoxylate (Lomotil). In excessive doses these agents can sometimes depress consciousness, so minimal effective doses should be used, and care should be taken not to attribute all diarrhea to tube feeding. In particular, fecal impaction must be ruled out, and more serious causes such as infection, antibiotic-induced colitis, bowel ischemia, and so on considered. With the use of techniques described in Chapter 29, we now find it rare that normal nutritional needs cannot be met by tube feeding because of diarrhea.

Regulation of Serum Osmolarity

Patients with abnormalities of the central nervous system, especially those severe enough to produce alterations in the level of consciousness, are particularly susceptible to fluid and electrolyte imbalances. Both hypertonic and hypotonic derangements of the extracellular fluid are common. Enteral feeding itself can also cause such problems, especially in patients unable to communicate their sensations of thirst or satiety. Hence the need for vigilance.

Diabetes Insipidus. Any condition that affects the neurohypophysis may produce diabetes insipidus, the state of excessive water loss via dilute urine, elevation in serum osmolarity, and deficient response of antidiuretic hormone release. Water loss in this condition may exceed 5 L/day. One third to one half of cases are primary (not associated with other abnormalities of the central nervous system); most of the remainder are due to tumors in the region of the pituitary gland or to the results of surgery for such lesions. The condition also occasionally occurs following head trauma. Most alert patients have intact thirst mechanisms and will therefore not become dehydrated. However, the comatose patient, who may also be receiving tube feedings, can become severely dehydrated in less than 12 hours. Although the large fluid losses can be replaced by means of a nasoenteric tube, if the amount exceeds 5 L/day, it is usually best to administer part of this volume intravenously. Among the effective specific treatments of diabetes insipidus are aqueous vasopressin (Pitressin) and vasopressin tannate in oil.[13]

Administration of Mannitol. In the treatment of increased intracranial pressure, the most widely used osmotic diuretic is the (nonmetabolized) sugar, mannitol. This agent predictably lowers intracranial pressure after a single dose. It may be given at the beginning of an operation or as a temporizing measure in a patient who is acutely deteriorating from an enlarging intracranial mass lesion.[14] Occasionally, repeated doses may be given over several days such as in the treatment of severely increased intracranial pressure due to head injury. Following such therapy serum osmolarity typically increases to 310 or 320 mOsm/L (normal = 280 to 305 mOsm/L). Nevertheless, within 24 to 48 hours of the last dose of mannitol, the serum osmolarity should return to normal.

Miscellaneous Causes of Hypertonicity. Hypertonic extracellular fluid develops in comatose patients for a variety of other reasons. Fluid restriction in an effort to avoid aggravation of cerebral edema commonly contributes. Hyperpyrexia and hyperpnea, frequently seen after severe head injury, also contribute to fluid losses in many cases. If unrecognized this derangement leads to further lethargy and coma, and if left untreated, renal failure, hypotension, and death can ensue.

Contribution of Enteral Feeding. Although the severity of hyperosmolar states may be aggravated by hypertonic feedings, the causes mentioned above are far more likely to be of primary importance in producing serious clinical problems. Nevertheless, use of "calorie dense" or "high nitrogen" products in this setting furthers the imbalance and demands additional free water administration. In addition, diarrhea from any cause complicates fluid and electrolyte management and confuses diagnosis. In such fluctuating metabolic states, intravenous fluid therapy will usually be required.

Hypotonic States. Hypotonicity of the extracellular fluid also frequently occurs in patients with central nervous system disease and is commonly attributed to inappropriate secretion of antidiuretic hormone or to cerebral salt wasting.[15] The administration of large quantities of electrolyte-poor solutions has also been implicated. The pathogenesis of this condition in neurologic patients remains controversial; however, when hyponatremia becomes severe, fluid intake should be limited to 500 to 1000 ml/24 hours. In this setting, the calorie dense products will help to minimize the nutritional effects of such severe restriction.

In summary, to avoid further complicating these metabolic derangements we must (1) maintain a high index of suspicion for their presence in patients with predisposing conditions, (2) monitor fluid balance with frequent specific gravity checks of urine, (3) check serum osmolarity in cases of uncertainty, and (4) tailor nutritional prescriptions in the direction of restoring homeostasis.

Stress Ulcers. As with other severe illnesses, acute neurologic disease predisposes to the development of ulcers and upper gastrointestinal hemorrhage. The data regarding the role of gastric acid output, steroid administration, and catecholamines in the development of this complication in neurologic disease are conflicting. Silen's group found that antacids were effective in reducing the incidence of gastrointestinal bleeding in critically ill patients.[16] Although this study did not include neurologic patients, similar reasoning prompts us to recommend use of antacids (such as Mylanta II, Maalox, or AlternaGEL, 30 ml every 4 hours) in acutely ill neurologic patients. Since these agents often plug smaller tubes and are of no use in the small bowel, a 14 French or larger nasogastric tube is usually needed for their administration if the patient cannot swallow. The need for antacids after the acute phase of illness is not clearly established, and in the patient who is receiving small bowel feedings, their administration is not feasible unless a second tube is inserted.

Although cimetidine (Tagamet) has proved to be effective for the treatment of gastrointestinal ulceration, its role in the *prevention* of this complication is still under investigation. Furthermore, several reports of transient metabolic encephalopathy following administration of cimetidine militate against its routine use in the patient with disease of the central nervous system,[17] particularly in states associated with an altered blood-brain barrier. Newer H_2 blockers now being developed for clinical use appear free of major side effects on the central nervous system and may be the next step in prevention of stress ulcers in neurologic patients.

SPECIFIC CLINICAL SITUATIONS

Trauma

Head Injury. A majority of patients with severe head injury require some specialized nutritional support. Standard practice has been to use nasoenteric feeding at least initially. The possible advantages of early *parenteral* nutritional support have been studied in one series of 44 patients with head injury.[18] In this prospective randomized trial, both morbidity and mortality were less in the group given TPN than in their tube-fed counterparts. This intriguing result, so far only reported in abstract form, awaits detailed reporting and confirmation by others. Pending this we feel that this use of TPN should be considered as investigational in victims of head injury with normal gastrointestinal function.

Tube insertion in the patient with a head injury may involve special hazards. Most patients with severe head injury require nasogastric or orogastric intubation on admission because of the possibility of acute gastric dilatation, vomiting, and aspiration, and for antacid administration. In patients with anterior basal skull fractures the tube may inadvertently penetrate the intracranial cavity.[19] Such penetration has been reported in at least 10 patients, and has frequently appeared to contribute to a lethal outcome (Fig. 18–2).[20] This complication is avoidable in most instances. It occurs in massive frontal trauma with epistaxis or cerebrospinal fluid rhinorrhea, and periorbital ecchymosis indicating anterior basal skull fracture. In such patients one of the following approaches should be used: oral insertion under direct vision ensuring inferior passage, or nasal insertion using a curved nasopharyngeal airway which is then removed (Fig. 18–3).[21] This latter technique is also useful in any case in which a facial injury is associated with jaw muscle rigidity, maxillary or mandibular fractures, or other conditions prohibiting the use of the oral route. The safety of both techniques is enhanced by use of a fiberoptic laryngoscope to guide tube placement and by radiographic confirmation of its location before any use of the tube.[20] Although these precautions are of primary concern to the emergency room physician, the nutrition team member who elects to change the large-bore tube for a smaller one several days later must be equally aware of this hazard.

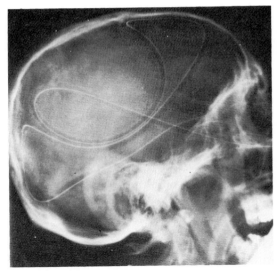

Figure 18–2. Lateral skull x-ray film following severe head injury and nasogastric tube insertion. Massive orbital hematomas and epistaxis were noted on examination. The nasogastric tube was inserted without difficulty and clear fluid returned initially after connection to suction. The drainage subsequently became bloody and the patient's responsiveness began to decrease rapidly. The tube was removed from the patient's nose (and from the intracranial cavity) about two hours after insertion; the patient expired several hours later. (*From* Fremstad, J. D., and Martin, S. H.: Lethal complication from insertion of nasogastric tube after severe basilar skull fracture. J. Trauma, *18*:820–822, 1978, with permission.)

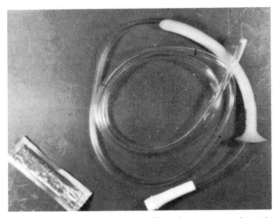

Figure 18–3. No. 18 French nasogastric tube threaded through a precurved No. 34 Davol nasopharyngeal tube. These tubes may be utilized in the "double tube" technique of nasogastric intubation. The nasopharyngeal airway (lubricated inside and out) is inserted first and then the nasogastric tube is inserted in its lumen. The former may then be removed. The preformed curve of the nasopharyngeal tube decreases the likelihood of intracranial penetration. (*From* Bouzarth, W. F., Intracranial nasogastric tube insertion. J. Trauma, *18*:818–819, 1978, with permission.)

Spinal Cord Trauma. Cord injury is occasionally an antecedent of nutritional depletion, particularly when the brain or trunk is also traumatized. In the patient with cervical spine injury, passage of nasal tubes must be done without moving the neck. In most cases the patient will be immobilized in skull tongs, halo traction, or a cervical brace, and passage of a nasal tube will not be hazardous. Rarely patients with cervical spine injuries will have an associated esophageal or hypopharyngeal injury which could be aggravated by passage of a tube through the region of injury. Clues to recognition of such an injury are development of a sticking sensation in the throat on attempts to swallow, fever, progressive cervical pain, and the finding of air in the prevertebral space on lateral cervical x-ray films.[22] Endoscopy should be considered prior to tube placement if these symptoms and findings appear.

In the period immediately after spinal cord injury, generalized ileus, often leading to acute gastric dilatation, is common. Decreased abdominal muscle tone and sphincter paralysis slow colonic transit. Tube feeding must progress slowly during this time until local gut reflexes become active. Throughout the course of upper thoracic or cervical cord injuries, vigilance must be maintained for intra-abdominal disorders such as perforated ulcer, cholecystitis, and pancreatitis, which can be particularly difficult to diagnose.[23] In the patient unable to feel abdominal pain, often the only clues will be findings such as abdominal distention, hypoactive bowel sounds, unexplained tachycardia, fever, or signs of hypovolemia. In such cases, feeding should be withheld until specific diagnostic studies have been performed.

Hydrocephalus. Impaired resorption of cerebrospinal fluid leading to hydrocephalus occurs following head injury, intracranial hemorrhage, intracranial infections, or as a result of congenital lesions. Although the process may be transient, in many cases placement of a cerebrospinal fluid (CSF) shunt is required to alleviate symptoms of headache, vomiting, and decreased mentation. In hydrocephalic patients who are obtunded or comatose, and in others with cranial nerve lesions, tube feeding is required. The majority of such patients can be managed with nasal tubes, but when surgically placed tubes are needed, special care is needed to avoid damaging or contaminating the CSF shunt. Both ventriculoatrial and ventriculoperitoneal shunt tubings (the most widely used CSF shunts) pass through the anterolateral aspect of the neck, and for this reason cervical esophagostomy or pharyngostomy should not be used, at least on the ipsilateral side. When the stomach or jejunum is used as a portal, one must ensure that the abdominal incision does not cross the path of a peritoneal catheter. Fortunately, most peritoneal catheters are introduced via a right-sided or midline incision (Fig. 18–4). This allows space for a left subcostal incision should an abdominal enterostomy be needed. Nevertheless, the peritoneal catheter may appear in the operative field, and if there is contamination of the abdominal cavity by intestinal organisms, the potential exists for ascending infection in or around the shunt tube. For this reason, the gastrostomy technique described by Delaney and Driscoll might be considered since it prevents intraoperative contamination by gastrointestinal contents (see Chapter 17).

The patient with hydrocephalus may present with vomiting as an early sign of shunt malfunction or obstruction. Usually vomiting results from impaired CSF drainage, which is manifested by neurologic deterioration, palpable malfunction of the shunt valve–reservoir device, and scan evidence of enlargement of the cerebral ventricles. Other possible intra-abdominal causes for vomiting such as volvulus and intraperitoneal pseudocysts have been reported from shunts draining into the abdomen, and should be kept in mind.[24, 25] In any case, feeding must be withheld until the cause of the vomiting is clear and the threat of aspiration removed.

Dysphagia

In most patients with neurologic disease, tube feeding is needed specifically because of inability to swallow. In head injury, stroke, motor neuron diseases, and myasthenic disorders, the impairment is usually part of a more widespread disorder. Dysphagia may, however, occur as a fairly isolated symptom.

Cranial Nerve Injuries. Following surgical transsection of the glossopharyngeal and vagus nerves, as is occasionally performed in the treatment of glossopharyngeal neuralgia, severe dysphagia commonly results.[26] Nevertheless, if the patient is carefully instructed always to direct food to the

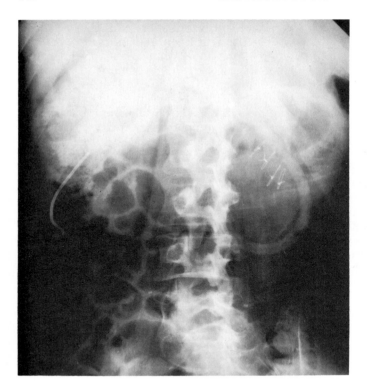

Figure 18–4. Pitfalls of gastrostomy placement in a patient with hydrocephalus. This abdominal x-ray film shows (1) a gastrostomy tube (Malecot catheter) in place on left, (2) a radiodense catheter on right (distal end of a right-sided CSF shunt), and (3) a radiodense connector in epigastric region to which a *second, radiolucent* CSF shunt catheter is connected (distal end of left-sided CSF shunt). This second shunt tubing is virtually invisible on x-ray film and could easily have been cut or contaminated during gastrostomy if special care had not been taken to avoid it.

normal side of his mouth and lean toward that side, aspiration as well as the need for enteral nutritional support should be avoidable. Patients with bilateral hypoglossal nerve injury have similar symptoms, and when this occurs, such as after bilateral carotid surgery, the patient may require endotracheal intubation to protect the airway and tube feeding for nutrition. Fortunately, this symptom almost invariably resolves within several weeks in each of these disorders.

Guillain-Barré Syndrome and Myasthenia Gravis. These illnesses may cause significant impairment of swallowing. In both diseases, it may be transient, especially when drug therapy is effective as in the case of myasthenic crises. In Guillain-Barré syndrome, dysphagia appears when the ninth and tenth cranial nerves are affected; in myasthenia the lesion is at the neuromuscular junction of the pharyngeal and laryngeal musculature. In both conditions, it is usually best to initiate nutritional support by means of a nasal tube rather than by enterostomy since the dysphagia may resolve with time.

Amyotrophic Lateral Sclerosis (Motor Neuron Disease). This disorder occasionally results in dysphagia early in the course of the illness. This may initially be managed by a diet change to semisolid foods. As the disorder progresses, some patients benefit from Teflon injection of the vocal cords or cricopharyngeal myotomy if cinefluorographic studies show trapping in the hypopharynx after swallowing.[27] In many cases, however, these measures are inadequate and either a nasal tube or enterostomy is needed.

Stroke

Isolated cranial nerve dysfunction also occurs in brain stem stroke, classically in the lateral medullary (Wallenberg) syndrome. The same advice is indicated regarding positioning and directing the food to the normal side as in peripheral nerve injury above. Bilateral lesions (usually asynchronous if survival occurs) again require tube feeding. The prognosis of patients with brain stem infarction is adversely affected by paralysis of the soft palate or disturbed sensorium, and special care in tube feeding of these patients is in order.[28]

More commonly, patients with brain infarction have cerebral hemispheric involvement. Those with dominant hemispheric stroke often suffer aphasia, obtundation, or coma in addition to hemiparesis or hemiplegia. In the patient with extensive deficits such as these, particularly in a setting of antecedent disability due to prior stroke, advanced age, or other illness, it may be prudent to observe the evolution of the present deficit before making a commitment to special nutritional support. The less severely affected can be fed by the simplest method available, using the principles described above, as soon as their general medical condition stabilizes. In most patients with recent stroke, feeding can begin at about 48 hours. In the salvageable patient without complicating conditions, delay beyond 5 days is rarely warranted.

The patient with a lesion of the nondominant hemisphere, though more likely to be alert, can have deficits of spatial orientation that make it difficult to find the food and transport it to the mouth. Often food on the left side of the tray remains untouched because the patient is unaware of its presence. Swallowing is usually unimpaired, but assistance at mealtime may be needed to prevent nutritional depletion. Failing this, tube feeding can help tide the patient over until recovery occurs.

Bilateral cerebral infarcts can produce spastic paresis of the palatal and pharyngeal muscles, part of the syndrome known as pseudobulbar palsy, with marked impairment in ability to eat. The principles of management of dysphagia noted above are also applicable here.

Dementia and Apathy. A final group of patients to be considered consists of those in whom the swallowing apparatus is intact but in whom disease, often of a degenerative nature, has eliminated the desire to eat. The decision whether to initiate tube feeding in such cases, as in any serious illness, requires consideration of numerous factors: the likelihood of recovery, the wishes of the patient if they can be learned, the wishes of the family, the availability of mealtime help to administer oral feedings, and the costs of the various options not only in money but also in morbidity. When confronted with the chronically infirm neurologic patient who has no realistic possibility of recovery, the wise clinician would do well to remember that society wants and asks him or her not only to prolong human life but also to alleviate suffering. Even if such a patient is clearly nutritionally depleted either the patient or the family may decline to accept the offer of specialized nutritional support if it means "another tube." Such withholding of possible but undesired therapy in conformity with the patient's wishes is now receiving legal and ethical support in many parts of this country. However, prudence suggests erring on the side of therapeutic optimism—in patients with possibly reversible conditions, we should consider whether malnutrition may be aggravating the disease. These are difficult questions, but the time to consider them is before complex support is begun.

CONCLUSION

We believe that neurologic patients represent the largest population of patients able to benefit from enlightened use of enteral nutritional support. Many candidates today remain untreated, in part because of lack of appreciation of the recent advances in the technology of its application. Care in selecting the patient to be treated, devising the best site and route of alimentation, choosing the nutrient source, and monitoring risks and side effects are needed here as anywhere in medicine. Such care can pay dividends in terms of improved function, more rapid healing, and the ultimate rehabilitation of many of our patients.

REFERENCES

1. Olivares, L., Segovia, A., and Revuelta, R.: Tube feeding and lethal aspiration in neurological patients: A review of 720 autopsy cases. Stroke, 5:654–657, 1974.
2. Bryan-Brown, C. W., Savitz, M. H., Elwyn, D. H., et al.: Cerebral edema unresponsive to conventional therapy in neurosurgical patients with unsuspected nutritional failure. Crit. Care Med., 1(3):125–129, 1973.
3. Savitz, M. H., Bryan-Brown, C. W., Elwyn, D. H., and Malis, L. I.: Postoperative nutritional failure and chronic cerebral edema in neurosurgical patients. Mt. Sinai J. Med., 45:394–401, 1978.
4. Koretz, R. L., and Meyer, J. H.: Elemental diets—facts and fantasies. Gastroenterology, 78:393–410, 1980.
5. Jones, D. C., Rich, A. J., Wright, P. D., and Johnston, I. D. A.: Comparison of proprietary elemental and whole-protein diets in unconscious patients with head injury. Br. Med. J., 1(6230):1493–1495, 1980.
6. Mena, I., and Cotzias, G. C.: Protein intake and treatment of Parkinson's disease with levodopa. N. Engl. J. Med., 292:181–184, 1975.

7. Twomey, P., Ziegler, D., and Rombeau, J.: Utility of skin testing in nutritional assessment: A critical review. J.P.E.N., 6:50–58, 1982.

8. Michel, L., Serrano, A., and Malt, R. A.: Nutritional support of hospitalized patients. N. Engl. J. Med., 304:1147–1152, 1981.

9. Gustke, R. F., Varma, R. R., and Soergel, K. H.: Gastric reflux during perfusion of the proximal small bowel. Gastroenterology, 59:890–895, 1970.

10. Rombeau, J. L., Twomey, P. L., McLean, G., Forlaw, L., Del Rio, D., and Caldwell, M. D.: Experience with a new gastrostomy-jejunal feeding tube. Personal communication.

11. Wayne, E., Miller, R. E., and Eiseman, B.: Duodenal obstruction by the superior mesenteric artery in bedridden combat casualties. Ann. Surg., 174:339–345, 1971.

12. Bouzarth, W. F., Crowley, J. N., and Clearfield, H. R.: Vascular compression of the duodenum following severe brain injury: Case report. J. Neurosurg., 39:405–407, 1973.

13. Randall, R. V.: Neuroendocrinology. In Youmans, J. R. (ed.): Neurological Surgery. Edition 2. Philadelphia, W. B. Saunders Co., 1982, Vol. II, pp. 931–988.

14. James, H. E., Langfitt, T. W., Kumar, V. S., and Ghostine, S. Y.: Treatment of intracranial hypertension: Analysis of 105 consecutive, continuous recordings of intracranial pressure. Acta Neurochir. (Wien), 36:189–200, 1977.

15. Nelson, P. B., Seif, S. M., Maroon, J. C., and Robinson, A. G.: Hyponatremia in intracranial disease: Perhaps not the syndrome of inappropriate secretion of antidiuretic hormone (SIADH). J. Neurosurg., 55:938–941, 1981.

16. Hastings, P. R., Skillman, J. J., Bushnell, L. S., and Silen, W.: Antacid titration in the prevention of acute gastrointestinal bleeding. N. Engl. J. Med., 298:1041–1044, 1978.

17. Schentag, J. J., Cerra, F. B., Calleri, G., DeGlopper, E., Rose, J. Q., and Bernhard, H.: Pharmacokinetic and clinical studies in patients with cimetidine-associated mental confusion. Lancet, 1(8108):177–181, 1979.

18. Twyman, D. L., Rapp, R. P., and Young, A. B.: Parenteral vs enteral feedings in severe head injury patients: A randomized study [Abstract 120]. J.P.E.N., 1981; 5:577, 1981.

19. Fremstad, J. D., and Martin, S. H.: Lethal complication from insertion of nasogastric tube after severe basilar skull fracture. J. Trauma, 18:820–822, 1978.

20. Borovich, B., Braun, J., Yosefovich, T., Guilburd, J. N., Grushkiewicz, J., and Peyser, E.: Intracranial penetration of nasogastric tube. Neurosurgery, 8:245–247, 1981.

21. Bouzarth, W. F.: Intracranial nasogastric tube insertion [Editorial]. J. Trauma, 18:818–819, 1978.

22. Pollock, R. A., Purvis, J. M., Apple, D. F., Jr., and Murray, H. H.: Esophageal and hypopharyngeal injuries in patients with cervical spine trauma. Ann. Otol. Rhinol. Laryngol., 90:323–327, 1981.

23. Carey, M. E., Nance, F. C., Kirgis, H. D., Young, H. F., Megison, L. C., Jr., and Kline, D. G.: Pancreatitis following spinal cord injury. J. Neurosurg., 47:917–922, 1977.

24. Sakoda, T. H., Maxwell, J. A., and Brackett, C. E., Jr.: Intestinal volvulus secondary to a ventriculoperitoneal shunt: Case report. J. Neurosurg., 35:95–96, 1971.

25. Latchaw, J. P., Jr., and Hahn, J. F.: Intraperitoneal pseudocyst associated with peritoneal shunt. Neurosurgery, 8:469–472, 1981.

26. St. John, J. N.: Glossopharyngeal neuralgia associated with syncope and seizures. Neurosurgery, 10:380–383, 1982.

27. McGuirt, W. F., and Blalock, D.: The otolaryngologist's role in the diagnosis and treatment of amyotrophic lateral sclerosis. Laryngoscope, 90:1496–1501, 1980.

28. Fogelholm, R., and Aho, K.: Characteristics and survival of patients with brain stem infarction. Stroke, 6:328–333, 1975.

29. Cobb, L. M., Cartmill, A. M., Barry M., and Gilsdorf, R. B.: A tube for enteral nutrition of patients with aphagopraxia and patients with ventilator assistance. Surg. Gynecol. Obstet., 155:81–84, 1982.

30. Gore, R. M., Mintzer, R. A., and Calenoff, L.: Gastrointestinal complications of spinal cord injury. Spine, 6:538–544, 1981.

CHAPTER 19

The Use of Enteral Nutrition in the Patient with Cancer

MICHAEL M. MEGUID
GREGORY E. GRAY
DANIEL DEBONIS

INDICATIONS FOR ENTERAL NUTRITION SUPPORT IN PATIENTS WITH CANCER

Protein-calorie malnutrition is a common problem among patients with cancer.[1-4] In one study of hospitalized adult cancer patients, 45 per cent had lost 10 per cent or more of their body weight, and approximately 25 per cent had lost more than 20 per cent of their body weight (Fig. 19–1).[5] Nonspecific, tumor-related starvation is the primary cause of death in many cancer patients,[6] whereas protein-calorie malnutrition is associated with a higher surgical risk.[7]

The causes of protein-calorie malnutrition in these patients are multiple; the common denominator is decreased nutrient intake. Other factors involve an altered nutrient requirement and the effects of anti-cancer therapy.[5, 8] These factors predispose the cancer patient to protein-calorie malnutrition, and indicate the need for nutritional support. Provided the gastrointestinal tract is functional, this support should be provided by the enteral route.[9, 10]

Cancer Cachexia

The marked anorexia and weight loss noted in cancer are so well recognized as to merit the term cancer cachexia (Fig. 19–2). Cancer cachexia bears no simple relationship to tumor burden, tumor cell type, or anatomic site of involvement,[11] although it is seen most commonly in patients with dis-seminated cancer or cancer of the gastrointestinal system.[12] Despite being long recognized as a common accompaniment of cancer, its etiology remains incompletely understood. Figure 19–3 shows some of the possible factors that may lead to cachexia. It is probable that cachexia results from the interaction of a number of factors, including decreased food intake secondary to anorexia, decreased digestion and absorption, and increased nutrient needs due to the autonomous tumor metabolism.

Although cachexia may be secondary to decreased intake resulting from partial or complete obstruction of the gastrointestinal tract,[12, 13] the most common causative factor is decreased nutrient intake as a result of anorexia, the cause of which currently remains unclear.[12] One possible explanation is the production by the tumor of peptides or other small molecular weight compounds which could exert their effects through the central nervous system.[14, 15] In addition, there have been reports of changes in taste perception, insulin sensitivity, as well as serum levels of lactate, fatty acids, and amino acids which may be important in regulating food intake.[16, 17] Psychological factors such as depression and fear of cancer are also important,[18] although they cannot explain the anorexia and subsequent weight loss that often appear before diagnosis.

Although most cases of cancer cachexia are associated with anorexia and decreased food intake,[12] there have been reports of weight loss in patients consuming what would appear to be adequate amounts of

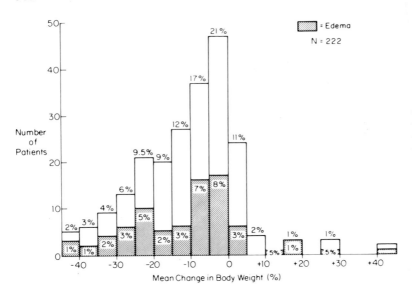

Figure 19–1. Distribution of weight change from preillness weight in hospitalized patients. Cross-hatched area in bars indicates percentage of total number of patients with some degree of edema. (*From* Shils, M. E.: Principles of nutritional therapy. Cancer, *43*:2093–2102, 1979, with permission.)

food,[19, 20] and weight loss in cancer patients has been said to be more rapid than that seen in simple starvation.[8] These observations suggest that there may be alterations in overall metabolism, but particularly that of protein and energy, contributing to the weight loss.

Changes in Energy and Nitrogen Metabolism and Their Requirements

There have been relatively few studies of energy requirements of cancer patients. Young reviewed several of these studies (Table 19–1).[20] Because of the limited information supplied in many of the papers and the numerous factors influencing the metabolic rate, he could not conclude that resting metabolism is consistently increased in cancer patients when compared with healthy controls. However, the data did suggest that resting energy metabolism is increased in many patients with Hodgkin's disease or leukemia. In addition, one study showed that increase in the resting metabolic rate paralleled exacerbation of disease and reduced food intake in some cancer patients.[21]

In comparison, studies of cancer patients who received nutritional support have noted an increased energy expenditure, probably due to the provision of nutrients stimulating basal metabolic rate.[22–25] In the absence of intense nutritional support, patients with cancer tend to be in a negative energy balance. Figure 19–4 demonstrates the markedly negative energy balance of two patients receiving relatively liberal oral energy intakes. Figure 19–5 demonstrates the high parenteral caloric intake required for a patient with a lymphoma. It has been estimated by one group of investigators that

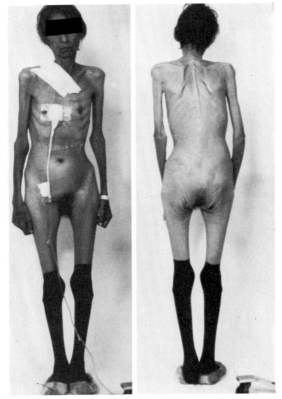

Figure 19–2. Patient with cancer cachexia.

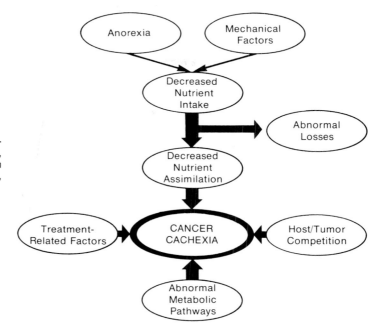

Figure 19–3. Multiple factors contributing to cancer cachexia. (*From* Buzby, G. P., and Steinberg, J. J.: Nutrition in cancer patients. Surg. Clin. North Am., *61*:691–700, 1981, with permission.)

the energy intake needed for positive nitrogen balance in the cancer patients they studied was 1.7× basal energy expenditure (BEE) if the calories were provided parenterally (without lipids) or 1.54 × BEE if provided enterally.[4]

There have been even fewer studies of protein requirements in cancer patients. Nitrogen balance studies have provided conflicting results. Nitrogen equilibrium, nitrogen loss, and nitrogen retention have all been reported, with little relationship to intake or weight changes in the patient.[4, 11] Positive nitrogen balance associated with weight loss has been attributed to retention by the tumor at the expense of the host,[4] but

more likely explanations are errors in the nitrogen balance technique[11, 26] or unmeasured loss of nitrogen.[27]

Studies of protein synthesis using isotopic techniques in muscle fibers from cancer patients demonstrate decreased synthesis and increased degradation (Fig. 19–6).[28] However, the decreased efficiency of synthesis could be overcome by increasing the amino acid supply, suggesting that higher protein intake might be advantageous in cancer patients. Similarly, the hypoalbuminemia that occurs frequently in cancer patients,[4, 25] and that is associated with decreased synthesis and increased catabolism,[11, 25] can be reversed by adequate calorie and protein intakes.[4] Hence these data suggest an increased need for protein in patients with cancer, although the exact amount and its relationship to energy needs remain to be determined. A newer metabolic approach to the study of protein metabolism uses stable isotopes and permits the assessment of changes in protein synthesis and breakdown rates of whole body proteins and amino acids.[29] The principal author is currently using this technique to further our understanding of amino acid requirements and metabolism in cancer patients.

The metabolic changes responsible for increased energy requirements are beginning to be understood. Cori cycle activity is increased in cancer patients who experience progressive weight loss,[30] but this alone does not account for sufficient energy cost to the

Table 19–1 SUMMARY OF PUBLISHED RESULTS ON THE BASAL METABOLIC RATE OF CANCER PATIENTS*

TYPE OF CANCER	BASAL METABOLIC RATE
Leukemia, 16 cases	> 20% above normal
Leukemia (myeloid and lymphocytic)	12–91% above normal
Leukemia	Increased
Chronic myelogenous leukemia	Variable
Multiple myeloma	14–60% above normal
Various cancers, 4 cases	10% above normal
Various cancers, 4 cases	0–30% above normal
Various cancers, 4 cases	Variable
Various cancers, 9 cases	Usually above normal

*Adapted from Young.[20]

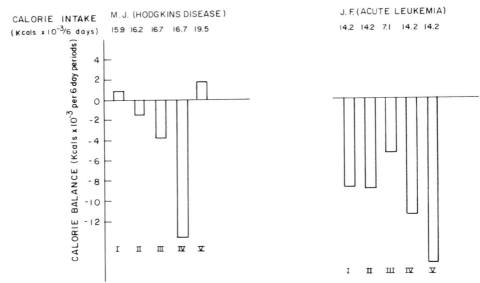

Figure 19–4.   Estimated body energy balance during cumulative six-day periods in cancer patients. (*From* Young, V. R.: Energy metabolism and requirements in the cancer patient. Cancer Res., *37*:2336–2347, 1977, with permission.)

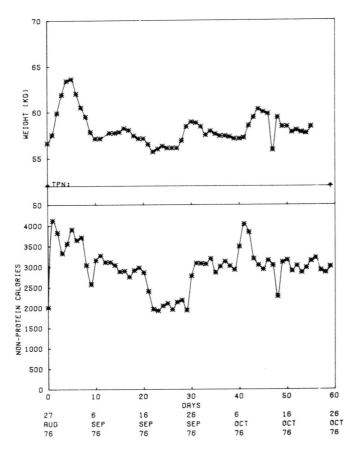

Figure 19–5. Weight changes and caloric intake of a patient with abdominal histiocytic lymphoma receiving TPN. Initial weight gain was rehydration. (*From* Brennan, M. F.: Uncomplicated starvation versus cancer cachexia. Cancer Res., *37*:2359–2365, 1977, with permission.)

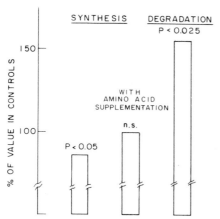

Figure 19–6. Rates of in vitro protein synthesis and degradation by muscle fibers from cancer patients, as compared with normal controls, and the effects of amino acid supplementation on synthesis. (*From* Young, V. R.: Energy metabolism and requirements in the cancer patient. Cancer Res., 37:2336–2347, 1977, with permission.)

body to cause the observed changes in energy requirements and body weight.[20]

Waterhouse and Kemperman have demonstrated that, under basal conditions, the rates of glucose and free fatty acid oxidation did not differ between patients with metastatic cancer and control subjects.[31] However, when glucose load was given, the oxidation of free fatty acids was suppressed less in the cancer patients than in healthy controls. Furthermore, there was a lower rate of glucose oxidation, while the oxidation of unlabeled gluconeogenic precursors such as alanine or acetyl-CoA was greater. If glucose is not utilized directly but is first converted to fat, this would involve a further energy cost and thus the need for a relatively high intake to meet the body's requirements.[20] However, the cost of this transformation, as with the Cori cycle, is small.[32]

The metabolic characteristics of trauma patients have been well defined,[33] and it has been found that cancer patients share some characteristics with patients subjected to trauma in that they too demonstrate increased gluconeogenesis which may not be suppressed by the provision of simple substrates.[25] As with trauma there also exists an impaired glucose tolerance caused by insulin resistance.[19, 34] Whereas the latter is thought to result from the catecholamine effects of stress in trauma patients[35] and can be reversed by beta-blockers, a similar conclusion cannot be reached in cancer patients.

Nutritional Consequence of Cancer Therapy and the Sequelae of Nutritional Support

Besides the metabolic effects of the disease itself, the cancer patient is predisposed to malnutrition as a result of therapy. Some of the more common problems and the impact of enteral nutritional support on the complications of therapy will be reviewed.

Chemotherapy. There are a number of chemotherapeutic agents in use whose effects on the alimentary tract differ (Table 19–2). Most have in common the ability to produce nausea and vomiting mediated by the chemoreceptor trigger zone in the area posterior to the fourth ventricle.[36] Nausea, vomiting, anorexia, and altered taste perception not only result in decreased oral intake, but also lead to fluid and electrolyte imbalances and weight loss. A second feature of many of these drugs is the production of mucositis and stomatitis (Fig. 19–7). The rapid turnover of cells in the gastrointestinal epithelium makes it particularly vulnerable to these agents. The resulting gastrointestinal changes lead to decreased oral intake. Decreased intestinal absorption may also occur, although this has not been systematically examined.[36] All these factors further predispose cancer patients to malnutrition.

One of the major toxic effects of chemotherapy is to the bone marrow, manifested by leukopenia, thrombocytopenia, or anemia. In severe leukopenia, infection is a serious risk and the frequency of infection has been found to be inversely proportional to the level of circulating neutrophils.[37]

Animal Studies in Nutrition and Chemotherapy. Bounous et al.[38] studied the effects of elemental diet in rats given 5-fluorouracil (5-FU), which suppresses DNA and RNA production, thereby affecting the intestinal mucosa and bone marrow. The elemental diet protected the intestinal epithelium of the rat against lesions associated with administration of 5-FU. The elemental diet was especially helpful in preventing the early drop in dipeptidase activity in the ileal mucosa induced by 5-FU.

Clinical Studies in Nutrition and Chemotherapy. In further studies by Bounous et al.,[39] an enteral diet was used in the management of the intestinal lesion produced by 5-FU in 24 patients with advanced metastatic carcinomas. The experimental group received only an enteral diet (Mead Johnson 3200 AS) for four days before and

Table 19–2 EFFECTS OF CANCER CHEMOTHERAPEUTIC AGENTS ON THE ALIMENTARY TRACT*

DRUG	NAUSEA	VOMITING	ANOREXIA	MUCOSITIS	INTESTINAL ULCERATION	ABDOMINAL PAIN	DIARRHEA	CONSTIPATION
Asparaginase	X	X	X					
BCNU	X	X	X					
Bleomycin				X				
Busulfan	X	X						
Cisplatinum	X	X	X					
Cyclophosphamide	X	X	X			X		
Cytarabine	X	X	X	X	X			
Dactinomycin	X	X	X	X		X	X	
Daunorubicin	X	X	X	X				
Doxorubicin	X	X						
Hydroxyurea	X	X		X			X	
Methotrexate	X	X	X	X	X	X		
Mithramycin	X		X				X	
Procarbazine	X	X	X		X			
Vinblastine	X	X				X		
Vincristine	X					X		X

*Adapted from Shils.[12]

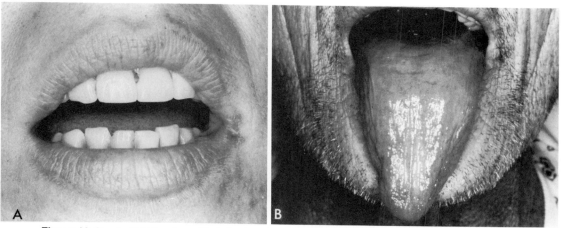

Figure 19–7. *A*, Angular stomatitis following chemotherapy. *B*, Glossitis following chemotherapy.

throughout chemotherapy. The control group was given regular hospital food ad libitum. Caloric intake was higher with the enteral diet (27.1 kcal/kg versus 20.4 kcal/kg).

Histologic abnormalities of the colonic and rectal mucosa were noted following 5-FU therapy in the control group which were not seen in similar biopsies taken from the patients on the enteral diet. These data strongly suggest that the enteral diet protected the mucosa in man, as previously shown in the rat, from the characteristic side effects of 5-FU.

Block and associates[40] reported the experience gained with the use of blenderized formula in patients with cancer cachexia suffering from a variety of disseminated, previously treated, solid tumors (seven patients) and with untreated glioblastomas (two patients). All patients suffered from anorexia. The blenderized formula (Vitaneed) was administered by continuous nasogastric infusion over a two-week period. Six of nine patients concurrently received chemotherapy.

Successful "repletion" was demonstrated in patients having a caloric input of at least 178 per cent of the BEE. This nonrandomized study suggests that an "elemental diet" is not required for repletion as is commonly believed and that a blenderized diet consisting of nutrients in a complex form was well absorbed and utilized.

Loh and colleagues[41] used Vivonex HN in seven patients with protein-calorie malnutrition and advanced carcinoma during six weeks of intensive chemotherapy (four patients also had radiotherapy). All patients had a "favorable response" to chemotherapy and appeared to tolerate therapy better,

although there were no controls for comparison. Average weight gain was 6.8 per cent. Nitrogen balance before Vivonex HN was −4.0 gm; after enteral support the mean value was +4.9 gm. Concomitantly, there were significant increases in serum albumin, blood urea nitrogen, total iron-binding capacity, and fasting blood glucose levels.

In 1977, Baker et al. reported the results of their prospective study in which patients with stages II and III breast cancer receiving adjunctive chemotherapy were given nutritional supplements.[42] The patients were generally well-nourished prior to the start of the study and were given nutritional support for three to nine months, during which time they received chemotherapy. Six patients received Isocal or Sustacal supplement, whereas six ingested only a regular diet ad libitum. The latter group was not able to meet normal protein requirements, whereas the supplement group did. There were fewer taste abnormalities in the supplement group; the control group had strong desires for cold, sweet, and protein-free drinks.

Immune competency improved in one patient in the supplement group but deteriorated in one patient in the control group. Mid-arm muscle circumference increased in three patients receiving supplement and decreased in the three control patients. The results of the study suggested that the continued deficient protein intake in the unsupplemented group over a prolonged period of time in conjunction with the postoperative chemotherapy for breast cancer eventually would lead to nutritional deterioration. To explore this hypothesis, Elkort and colleagues[43] designed a randomized prospective study to evaluate the effects of long-term (12 months) enteral nutritional support in a group of 26 ambulatory patients with stages III and IV breast cancer undergoing cytotoxic chemotherapy treatment as an adjunct to surgery.

The experimental group received 500 ml of liquid supplement on a daily basis in addition to their regular food intake. No patient required supplementation to more than 40 per cent of her caloric requirements. In comparison the control group ate ad libitum. During the chemotherapy, gastrointestinal and hematologic toxicity were comparable between the control and experimental groups.

At the end of 12 months, disease status was comparable between the two groups, and there were significant correlations between weight changes and disease status in all patients. The supplement did not influence survival: an equal number of patients in both the control and supplement groups died of disseminated cancer.

Nutritional Support During Remission Induction Therapy in Leukemia. In a retrospective study, DeVries and colleagues[45] reviewed the comparative effects of tube feeding (Nutrison RTS) versus normal hospital diet on remission induction after relapse of acute myeloid leukemia in 24 patients receiving chemotherapy. Patients were in various disease stages and nutritional status ranged from mildly depleted to normal. There were a total of 55 three-week study periods analyzed: 20 study periods in 14 patients in the tube-fed group and 35 study periods in 20 patients receiving a hospital diet. Patients with nausea or vomiting in response to chemotherapy were fed nasogastrically. No intravenous hyperalimentation was used during any study period.

The chemotherapy regimen caused bone marrow aplasia, necessitating platelet transfusions. Patients also received selective decontamination of the digestive tract to prevent infections caused by gram-negative bacteria and fungi.

During the three-week study periods, mean weight loss was 5 per cent in the hospital diet group and 1 per cent in the tube-fed group. Weight loss greater than 5 per cent of body weight was seen more frequently in the oral diet group. Malnutrition was avoided by continuous enteral feeding during these three-week periods (the amount of time required to recover from chemotherapeutic regimens).

Although nasogastric feeding is intuitively believed to be unsuited to patients with severe bone marrow depression because of the fear of hemorrhage secondary to erosion, the risk of upper digestive tract bleeding was not found to be increased with tube feeding. In both groups, the percentage of occult blood loss was high probably because of a low platelet blood count. It was not possible to assess the effects of enteral tube feeding on remission percentage because patients were in different stages of disease.

It was concluded by the authors that during a short-term catabolic state of three weeks' duration, sterile tube feeding formula by nasogastric administration can prevent severe weight loss and hypoalbuminemia in most patients. In severely granulocytopenic patients, bacteriologic control of food and the delivery system was considered mandatory.

Radiation Therapy. The effects of radiation therapy which lead to nutritional alterations are related to the region irradiated (Table 19–3). The soft tissues of the mouth and pharynx are radiosensitive. Head and neck irradiation commonly causes radiomucositis of the oropharynx leading to a decreased oral intake. Destruction of the taste buds results in abnormalities or loss of taste.[45, 46] In one study of patients receiving head and neck radiation for a six to eight week course, the average weight loss was 3.7 kg. Of these patients, 8.7 per cent lost more than 10 per cent of their body weight (Fig. 19–8).

Radiation to the thorax may cause acute dysphagia owing to inflammation of the esophageal epithelium, which typically resolves within a few weeks.[45, 46] A late effect of radiation is fibrosis and stricture formation resulting in progressive dysphagia.

The symptom complex of nausea, vomiting, and diarrhea frequently accompanies small and large bowel irradiation and may persist throughout therapy. Fat absorption is impaired, and decreased disaccharidase levels have been reported.[45] Delayed radiation-induced enteritis may follow high-dose irradiation and present with either chronic diarrhea and malabsorption or as bowel obstruction warranting further surgery (Fig. 19–9). The most commonly affected segments of the gut are the distal and terminal ileum, since these are relatively fixed and thus are exposed to higher doses of radiation. The excision of these segments of small bowel may lead to short gut syndrome,

Table 19–3   LOCALIZED EFFECTS OF RADIOTHERAPY LEADING TO
NUTRITIONAL ALTERATIONS*

REGION	ACUTE	CHRONIC
Central nervous sytem	Nausea	
Head and neck	Sore throat Dysphagia Xerostomia Mucositis Anorexia Alteration in smell Loss of taste	Ulcer Xerostomia Dental caries Osteoradionecrosis Trismus Altered taste
Thorax	Dysphagia	Fibrosis Stenosis Fistula
Abdomen-pelvis	Anorexia Nausea Vomiting Diarrhea Acute enteritis Acute colitis	Ulcer Malabsorption Diarrhea Chronic enteritis Chronic colitis

*Reproduced with permission from Donaldson and Lenon.[37]

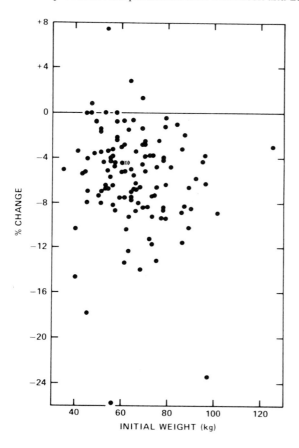

Figure 19–8. Percentage weight change in 122 adults during radiation therapy for squamous cell carcinoma of the oral cavity, oropharynx, or hypopharynx. (*From* Donaldson, S. S., and Lenon, R. A.: Alterations of nutritional status: Impact of chemotherapy and radiation therapy. Cancer, 43:2036–2052, 1979, with permission.)

which in turn has metabolic sequelae affecting the patient's nutritional status.

In one study of patients receiving a six-week course of abdominal irradiation for non-Hodgkin's lymphoma, the average weight loss was 3.4 kg, and 13 per cent lost more than 10 per cent of body weight[37, 38] (Fig. 19–10).

Nutritional Support in Animals Receiving Radiotherapy. Elson and Lamerton[47] examined the effects of low (5 per cent) and high (20 per cent) dietary protein on the response of Walker rat carcinoma-256 to whole body and local irradiation. The diets were given for seven days before the tumor was implanted.

Whole body radiation was started 24 hours later. In the first four days of treatment, the high protein group showed fast growth of tumors but thereafter they began to decrease in size. Eventually two of the tumors regressed by a shelling-out process, whereas in two other rats, tumors continued to grow rapidly and death occurred at 45 days.

In the low protein group, all but one rat showed steady tumor growth and death at 36 days. Inhibition of tumor growth was greater in the low protein group, although complete regressions did not occur. When 4000 rads of localized (not whole body) irradiation was given, complete regression occurred in 90 per cent of rats in the high protein group, and in only 15 per cent of the rats in the low protein group. The authors concluded that the low protein diet favored

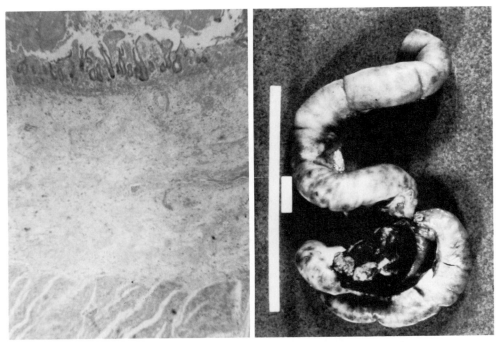

Figure 19–9. Radiation-induced enteritis. Microscopic and gross views.

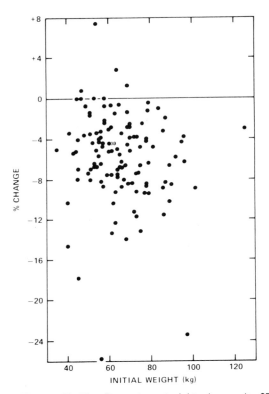

Figure 19–10. Percentage weight change in 67 adults during abdominal-pelvic radiation therapy for non-Hodgkin's lymphoma. (*From* Donaldson, S. S., and Lenon, R. A.: Alterations of nutritional status: Impact of chemotherapy and radiation therapy. Cancer, 43:2036–2052, 1979, with permission.)

initial inhibition of tumor growth, whereas cure of the animal was obtained with the high protein diet.

Hugon and Bounous[48] fed either an elemental diet (Mead Johnson 3200-AS) or a control diet (Purina Chow) or whole casein to mice given 900 rads to the abdomen. The elemental diet improved the 30-day survival rate and protected the intestinal mucosa as compared with the rats fed the control diet. Although the initial damage to the intestinal crypts from radiation was not prevented by the elemental diet, faster recovery from such lesions was observed. In the absorbing cells of the villi the initial radiation lesion was lessened by elemental diet and recovery was facilitated.

Nutritional Support in Humans Receiving Radiotherapy. In 1968 Cheraskin and associates described the effects of nutritional therapy on a study group consisting of 27 patients with squamous cell carcinomas of the cervix who received an average of 5952 rads over 37 ± 7 days.[49] The control group was 27 patients also with squamous cell carcinomas of the cervix who received no dietary counseling or nutritional supplementation. The nutritional regimens in the study were supplements of high protein, low carbohydrate, vitamins, and minerals begun one week before radiotherapy. This diet was selected because of the reduced glucose tolerance observed in patients with cervical carcinomatosis. Radiation response was judged "favorable" in only 63.3 per cent of the control group but in the majority of patients in the study group (97.5 per cent).

Bounous et al.[50] reviewed results with oral nutritional support in 18 patients receiving cobalt-60 irradiation for abdominal or pelvic malignant disease including carcinoma of the cervix (n=7), prostate (n=2), ovary (n=3), sigmoid (n=2), bladder (n=1), and pancreas (n=3). Patients assigned to the study group received an oral casein semihydrolysate containing two thirds free amino acids and one third oligopeptides (Flexical), while the control group received a normal diet.

The group receiving Flexical was given a mean dose of 4040 rads. Radiation-induced enteritis was not a problem in this group during the acute phase. Flexical also had a positive effect on body weight. Serum proteins including immunoglobulins were essentially unchanged during therapy in the study group but fell in all control patients. There was no significant difference between the two groups in peripheral blood hematocrit and red and white cell counts, while a drop in blood lymphocytes following irradiation was less in the Flexical group. Haddad et al.[59] reported in 1974 the first case of long-term (nine months) use of elemental diet in repeated subacute intestinal obstruction secondary to intensive abdominal radiation in a woman with ovarian peritoneal carcinomatosis. Recurrence occurred after hysterectomy and oophorectomy performed previously in 1967. The patient received 4100 rads to the abdominal and pelvic region, and then a central abdominal dose of 1800 rads. This irradiation caused partial obstruction of the small bowel.

A minimum residue home diet was given by nasogastric tube, and diarrhea was controlled using diphenoxylate hydrochloride. However, continued weight loss and abdominal distress resulted in the necessity for long-term use of an elemental diet. Partial obstructive symptoms recurred whenever low residue or solid foods were given. Weight gain was observed with the elemental diet.

Nealon and colleagues described a case of radiation enteritis and the use of an elemental diet in a patient with papillary adenocarcinoma of the right ovary.[52] Abdominal hysterectomy was followed by extensive radiotherapy which induced radiation enteritis in the terminal ileum. Following resec-

tion, enterocutaneous fistula and wound infection precipitated weight loss. An elemental diet (Vivonex HN, 3000 kcal/day) resulted in positive nitrogen balance and weight gain enabling fistula resection. The patient was eventually discharged and able to eat a normal diet.

In a retrospective review, Donaldson and colleagues[53] examined the management of radiation enteritis in 14 children who had received whole abdominal radiation therapy. Five of the 14 long-term survivors had developed delayed radiation injury with small bowel obstruction and severe diarrhea. Histologic appearance included severe villus blunting, lymphatic dilatation, and moderately dense inflammatory infiltrate (see Fig. 19–9). Improvement of these histologic features was noted on ingestion of a low residue, low fat diet, which was free of gluten and milk products. The mucosal pattern subsequently showed normal appearance on roentgenograms and in biopsies. No exacerbation of radiation enteritis was seen following dietary therapy.

Surgery. The patient with cancer experiences the same metabolic response to surgery as do other patients. These include increased nitrogen losses and energy requirements.[54–57] However, because cancer patients have frequently experienced significant weight loss prior to surgery, their ability to cope with these stresses is impaired.[7, 8, 47, 52]

The subsequent effects of cancer surgery on nutritional status are given in Table 19–4 and are reviewed by Shils.[12] Radical head and neck surgery, including glossectomy and mandibulectomy, often interferes with chewing and swallowing. In some cases oral feeding may be possible, whereas in other cases prolonged tube feeding may be required.

Esophagectomy may produce fat malabsorption, attributed to the accompanying bilateral vagotomy.[58] The consequences of gastrectomy are dependent on the extent of resection and include dumping syndrome, steatorrhea, and loss of intrinsic factor.[59]

The effects of intestinal resection depend on the location of the segment resected and its length.[12, 60] Although most absorption normally occurs in the proximal small bowel, the ileum adapts to absorbing these nutrients following jejunal resection.[61] However, the resection of the terminal ileum creates two particular problems. First, the ileum is the absorption site of vitamin B_{12}, and provision of intramuscular B_{12} is neces-

Table 19–4 LIST OF POTENTIAL NUTRITIONAL SEQUELAE OF SURGERY FOR CANCER CONTROL BY ANATOMIC REGION*

A. Radical resection of the oropharyngeal area
    Impaired chewing and swallowing
B. Esophagectomy and esophageal reconstruction
    Gastric stasis and hypochlorhydria secondary to
        vagotomy
    Diarrhea and steatorrhea
C. Gastrectomy
    Dumping and malabsorption
    Achlorhydria and lack of intrinsic factor
D. Intestinal resection
    Jejunum: decreased nutrient absorption
    Ileum: malabsorption of B_{12}, bile salts, and uric
        acid
    Diarrhea
    Blind loop syndrome
    Massive bowel resection—severe malabsorption
        Malnutrition
        Metabolic acidosis
    Ileostomy and colostomy
        Complications of salt and water balance
E. Pancreatectomy
    Malabsorption
    Diabetes mellitus

*Adapted from Shils.[12]

sary since body stores of B_{12} are limited. Second, the ileum is the site of bile acid resorption. The entry of bile acids into the large intestine following resection of the terminal ileum leads to diarrhea.[62] If the extent of ileal resection is less than 100 cm, the diarrhea can be controlled by cholestyramine; if it is greater than 100 cm, there is an insufficient concentration of bile salts (because of decreased enterohepatic circulation) for fat absorption, and diarrhea secondary to steatorrhea results. Massive resection of the small bowel, leaving three feet or less of small bowel, presents serious nutritional problems (Fig. 19–11).[12, 34] However, absorptive capacity generally improves with time, although fat malabsorption, and hence failure to gain weight in adults and particularly in growing children, remains a major problem.

Finally, pancreatectomy, with consequent loss of digestive enzymes, leads to malabsorption of fat and protein and consequently to a significant failure of absorption

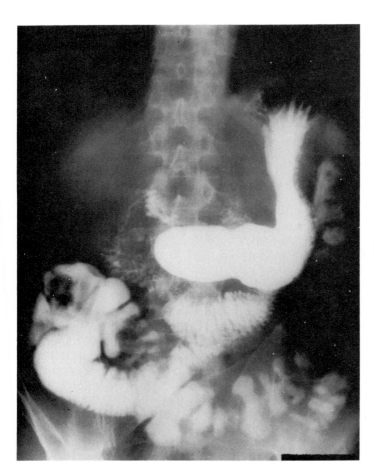

Figure 19–11. Short-gut syndrome as demonstrated by barium swallow. Transit time was 30 minutes.

of fat soluble vitamins and minerals as well. The diabetic state that may develop following pancreatectomy further complicates the nutritional management of these patients.

OBJECTIVES OF ENTERAL NUTRITION SUPPORT IN THE PATIENT WITH CANCER

The goal of enteral nutrition support is to provide sufficient calories, protein, and micronutrients by the enteral route to maintain or improve a patient's nutritional status before, during, and after therapy for cancer. There are now adequate data to show that prevention and treatment of malnutrition in cancer patients will contribute to improved outcome.[7, 63–66] Certainly, treatment of malnutrition generally results in improved physical strength,[67] functional capacity,[68] and the subjective feeling of well-being.[5] In addition, treatment can improve immune status and hypoalbuminemia,[4, 69, 70] contribute to a better surgical prognosis,[7, 8] and increase the ability of the patient to tolerate radiation and chemotherapy.[45, 46, 71–73] The complications of tube feedings are enumerated in Table 19–5.

Haffejee and Angorn[74] studied the relationship between nutritional status and the nonspecific cellular and humoral immune response in nonresectable carcinoma of the esophagus in 20 patients with protein-calorie malnutrition. Patients ate a hospital diet of 2500 kcal supplemented by Vivonex up to 3700 kcal and 20 gm of nitrogen per day delivered by nasogastric tube. The immune response was evaluated before and after nutritional support.

A reversal of negative nitrogen balance was associated with an increase in the absolute and in the T lymphocytes in particular and a significant increase in the mitogenic response to phytohemagglutinin (PHA) stimulation. The dinitrochlorobenzene (DNCB) skin test remained unreactive. Serum C_3, C_4, and C_3PA concentrations increased. Mean weight increased from 46.8 to 50.7 kg. All patients showed increased skinfold thickness and a rise in serum albumin and total iron binding capacity levels. After nutritional repletion, these patients showed the same levels of IgG and IgM but higher levels of IgA. The authors concluded that some aspects of nonspecific cellular immunity improved without therapeutic reduction in tumor load.

Rocchio et al.[75] described the use of a chemically defined diet in the management of 37 patients with high output (exceeding 200 ml/day) gastrocutaneous fistulas. In 11 patients (30 per cent) a malignant lesion was directly associated with the fistula. Sepsis was also present. Most fistulas were a result of surgery.

Elemental diet was delivered by nasogastric, gastrostomy, or jejunostomy feedings resulting in spontaneous closure in six cancer patients and enabling operative closure in one. Of the 11 cancer patients, four died.

Shils[5] has divided the objectives of nutritional support into three categories:

Supportive. To maintain good nutritional status or to rehabilitate the debilitated

Table 19–5 COMPLICATIONS OF TUBE FEEDING

TYPE OF COMPLICATION	FREQUENCY (per cent)	THERAPY
Gastrointestinal[10]		
Bloating	15	Decrease flow rate
Diarrhea and cramping	15	Decrease flow and/or concentration; consider different formula; add antidiarrheal drug
Vomiting	< 5	Decrease flow rate
Metabolic[9]		
Hyperglycemia and glucosuria	5–10	Decrease glucose concentration or administer insulin
Edema	5–10	Usually none; decrease sodium and fluid intake; use diuretics
Congestive heart failure	1–5	Decrease rate; administer diuretics and digoxin
Mechanical[64]		
Dislodged tube	45	Replace with longer caliber tube
Clogged tube lumen	< 10	Flush with water; replace tube
Pulmonary aspiration	< 10	Discontinue tube feeding
Tracheoesophageal fistula	< 1	Discontinue tube feeding and start TPN

patient while he or she awaits more definitive treatment. An example of this would be preoperative support of a malnourished patient to improve nutritional status and to lower the surgical risk.[76]

Adjunctive. Use of nutrition as part of a therapeutic program. An example would be improving the resistance to infection by improving immune status or permitting better adherence to a therapeutic regimen.[77] In a number of patients, a combination of nutritional support modalities may be used in order to achieve this goal (Fig. 19–12).

Definitive. Nutrition is the modality on which the existence of the patient depends. This can include a successfully treated patient with head and neck cancer who depends on tube feeding for nutrition, or a patient with severe enteritis who depends on an elemental diet (Fig. 19–13).

Besides the prevention and treatment of malnutrition and its sequelae in cancer patients, the use of enteral nutrition has other

specific objectives: (1) provision of amino acids to meet amino acid requirements for protein synthetic needs, (2) meeting energy requirements, (3) inducing an anabolic hormonal milieu by stimulating insulin and by inhibiting glucagon secretion, and (4) providing an adequate amount of vitamins and minerals. Specific to enteral nutrition is the maintenance of intestinal epithelium and gut organ mass (see Chapter 20). Compared with the use of total parenteral nutrition, enteral feeding is speculated to increase the mucosal weight, DNA and protein content, and enzyme activities both by direct contact and by endocrine and neurotrophic mechanisms.[78, 79]

Other objectives are prevention of radiation and chemotherapy-induced gastrointestinal toxicity. There are studies, previously mentioned, which demonstrate a beneficial effect of elemental diets in preventing radiation enteritis in patients receiving abdominal radiation and in preventing

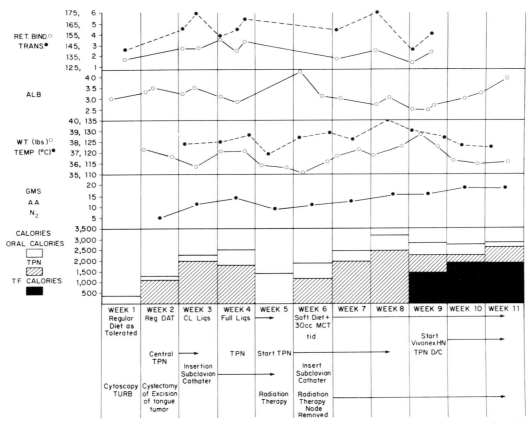

Figure 19–12. Transitional cell carcinoma of the bladder and squamous cell carcinoma of the tongue in a 64-year-old patient who received a combination of treatment methods. Nutritional status was maintained through a variety of nutritional support modalities. (Ret Bind, retinal binding protein; Trans, transferrin; Alb, albumin; TF, tube feeding; Reg, regular diet; CL, clear liquids; MCT, medium chain triglycerides.)

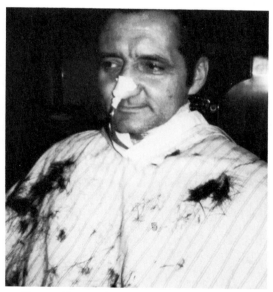

Figure 19–13. Even though nasogastric feedings were required this patient could engage in relatively normal activities such as having his hair cut.

mucosal changes induced by 5-fluorouracil, although other studies have not confirmed these findings.[45, 46, 78, 80]

An additional objective is the healing of high bowel fistulas, such as those in the esophagus, duodenum, or upper jejunum, by bypassing the fistula with a tube so that the feedings enter distally.[78]

A final objective is the treatment of malabsorption syndromes through the use of elemental diets, many of which now contain medium-chain triglycerides.

MODES OF ENTERAL SUPPORT

While the oral route is generally the route preferred by the patient, many cancer patients are unable to consume sufficient calories voluntarily either because of anorexia or because physical factors limit their ability to take foods by this route. These patients require enteral nutrition through a feeding tube. Two major techniques are used: nasoenteric tubes, which can be placed at the bedside, and ostomy tubes, which require surgical placement.

Patients with head and neck disease may demonstrate inadequate dietary intake owing to malignant disease, alcoholism, tobacco abuse, and poor oral hygiene.[81, 82] Long-term extraoral alimentation may be re-

quired following surgical procedures involving resection or during radiation therapy or chemotherapy. Radical surgical reconstruction with major regional flaps may require three to six weeks of extraoral nutritional support. Severely depleted patients may also require two to three weeks of preoperative support.

Nasogastric Tube

The feeding tube most commonly used for nasoenteric feedings is the large nasogastric tube intended and commonly used for nasogastric decompression, but commonly used instead to feed (Fig. 19–14). These hard polyvinyl tubes are generally taped to the nose, with care exercised to prevent necrosis of nasolabial cartilage (Fig. 19–15), a potentially disfiguring deformity for which the physician is medicolegally responsible. However, small caliber tubes are more comfortable, are well tolerated because of their size, and can be left in place for extended periods without the complications of the larger nasogastric tubes used in the past (Fig. 19–16).[78, 79] Difficulties with small cali-

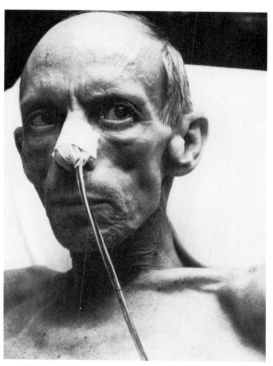

Figure 19–14. Malnourished patient being repleted with an old-fashioned large-bore feeding tube.

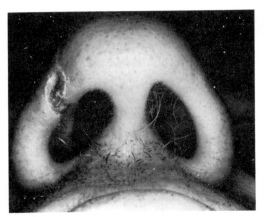

Figure 19–15. Necrosis of right nasoalar cartilage caused by pressure from a poorly taped nasogastric tube.

useful for short-term support (7 to 10 days) following surgery and is useful in uncomplicated laryngectomy with or without associated radical neck dissection.[82]

Johns,[81] in a retrospective study of 31 patients, showed that with early treatment of head and neck regions, patients are less likely to suffer nutritional depletion caused by various therapies. He recommended that nutritional support be used in palliative treatment as well as in curative therapy. Gormica and Catli[84] reported using a milk-base formula as palliative support in a 69-year-old cachectic man with extensive carcinoma of the throat. Achieving a positive nitrogen balance by the second week of nutritional support, the man was able to tolerate soft foods by mouth toward the end of his life.

Valdivieso[85] reported using a defined formula diet (Flexical) in 12 patients with head and neck cancer who failed to improve on a hospital formula of blenderized diet. The defined formula diet was well tolerated. At the end of the study seven patients had normal serum levels of protein and albumin and nine experienced weight gain. Upon discontinuation of the formula diet, all patients were restarted on hospital formula, with additional weight gain occurring in four patients and weight loss occurring in five patients.

Sobol and associates[86] described two

ber tubes include their considerable resistance to flow, necessitating either a formula of low viscosity or the use of a pump,[79] and frequent dislodgement caused by coughing.

Nasogastric feeding is the time-honored approach in these patients since the gastrointestinal tract remains intact. However, the nasogastric tube may contribute to a pooling of secretions resulting in pulmonary complications. Furthermore, presence of the nasogastric tube can be a source of direct trauma to a postoperative pharyngeal suture line.[83] In addition, the cough reflex may also be inhibited. Nasogastric feeding may be

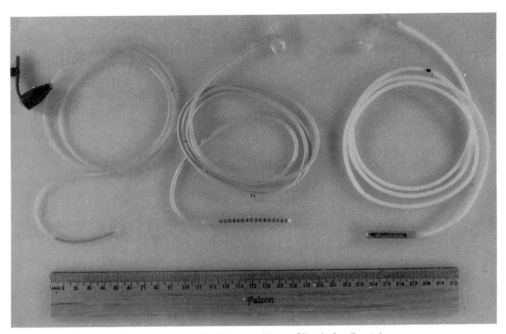

Figure 19–16. Flexible, small-bore Silastic feeding tubes.

cases of epidermoid carcinoma requiring adjunctive radiotherapy. Despite 4000 calories delivered by nasogastric feeding during radiotherapy (3000 rads), one patient continuously lost weight. In the second patient, mucositis persisted and the patient experienced discomfort from the presence of the nasogastric tube. A gastrostomy tube was placed to provide 2500 kcal/day but did not improve weight gain. Central venous hyperalimentation was started and 4000 kcal/day was given which resulted in weight gain and apparent nutritional repletion. After laryngectomy the patient was able to resume gastrostomy feeding. Thus, despite enteral feeding in the first case, there was progressive wound breakdown, flap necrosis and failure with fistulization, and malnutrition resulting in death. In the second case, nutritional salvage was achieved only with total parenteral nutrition (TPN).

Other types of upper enteric feeding routes include nasopharyngeal and esophageal, with placement of the catheter tip into the stomach, and nasogastric and nasoduodenojejunal feeding. The first three methods of feeding are the most physiologic and enable either bolus or continuous feedings to be given. The major problem associated with these techniques is aspiration, particularly in debilitated patients with depressed cough reflexes.[87, 88] To minimize the chance of aspiration, the position of the distal end of the feeding tube needs to be verified radiographically prior to feeding to ensure its placement into the stomach. It is our policy that the patient be kept in a sitting or semisitting position (30°) during and for two hours after feeding.[78, 89]

The nasogastric route is perhaps the most commonly used and may be associated with reflux when the patient returns prematurely to the supine position following feeding,[78] as the gastroesophageal sphincter is rendered incompetent by the placement of a feeding tube through it. The stomach acts as a reservoir and allows both continuous and bolus feedings. The osmolality of the solution causes relatively few problems when the feeding is infused into the stomach,[90] and this method requires somewhat less care than the use of the nasoduodenal tube.

Nasoduodenal or nasojejunal feeding in the cancer patient is associated with fewer problems from reflux,[91] although tube placement is more difficult. The solution used needs to be iso-osmolar, and must be given as a continuous infusion, since the bolus administration of hyperosmolar solution into the small intestine results in fluid and electrolyte shifts, abdominal distention, and diarrhea.[91]

In 1977 Dobbie and Butterick[92] described the use of a lactose-free formula in 14 patients with esophageal disease, most with obstruction. Ten patients had carcinoma of the esophagus; in four patients, suture line leakage and fistula formation developed postoperatively. Seven patients with nonresectable carcinoma given radiotherapy gained weight and showed improved "tolerance" to therapy. Three patients whose tumors were resected had had a significant weight loss prior to admission. Thus, operative management included transnasal passage, and manual transpyloric positioning of a small feeding tube enabled the feedings of 2400 to 3600 kcal/day, which were given as soon as normal bowel sounds were heard postoperatively. Nutritional support continued for 7 to 14 days. The patients who received nutritional support were thought to heal faster.

Four patients with postoperative fistulas of the esophagus became seriously ill and three were profoundly septic and hypoxic. All required chest tube drainage and nasogastric decompression of the stomach distal to the esophageal leakage.

The authors concluded that enteral tube feeding was a useful adjunct in the management of esophageal carcinoma in either surgical or radiation treatment. Based on the experience reported the authors claim that direct visualization of the feeding tube beyond the carcinoma at the time of initial workup had become part of their standard practice. Feeding into the proximal duodenum or jejunum was favored. An elemental diet was not essential according to the authors since the rest of the gastrointestinal tract was functional. However, the location of the feeding tube was considered to be of critical importance.

Regardless of the site of insertion of the feeding catheter, in the nutritional management of the cancer patient, it is important to confirm the location of the feeding catheter. Most of the available tubes are radiopaque, enabling rapid radiographic confirmation.[93] In the cancer patient the simple method of insufflation of air with auscultation over the epigastric region, which is so frequently used, is not sufficient to verify the tube location, as auscultation can pick up transmitted sounds from a catheter situated in the bronchial tree in a comatose patient.[91] Aspiration of stomach contents with confirmation of pH is the easiest nonradiographic method of confirming the position of the catheter. A distinct disadvantage of the nasoenteric route is that it increases upper airway resistance, thereby interfering with ventilatory exchange. This can become of consequence in a patient whose respiratory status may already be borderline. In these circumstances ostomy tubes are recommended.

Ostomy Tubes in Patients with Head and Neck Cancer

For patients who may require tube feeding for prolonged periods of time, an ostomy tube is indicated. An esophagostomy tube may be placed, under light general anesthesia, into the proximal esophagus.[94] It is a simpler procedure than a gastrostomy and can be an alternative to a jejunostomy for unobstructed patients requiring long-term tube feedings and who have had a prior subtotal gastrectomy or esophagogastrectomy.[78] It can be used with both bolus and continuous feedings and, in general, osmolality of the feeding formula is not a problem. In some instances, a permanent sinusostomy can be performed, allowing the feeding tube to be removed between meals.[93]

The anatomic position of this tube is somewhat more comfortable, although a disadvantage is that the oropharyngeal secretions are somewhat irritating to the skin. A further advantage of the use of an esophagostomy tube is that its proximity to a potentially contaminated tracheostomy site does not pose a potential source of sepsis, as might be the case with a central venous subclavian catheter. This is our standard practice in patients with head and neck cancer (Fig. 19–17).

As early as 1967 Graham and Royster[95] described the use of cervical esophagostomy for long-term feeding of 12 patients. Tube feeding of a blenderized diet was begun by the second or third postoperative day. The authors recommended the procedure after radical maxillofacial surgery and recurrent malignant growth of the oral pharyngeal area.

Aguilar et al.[96] emphasized the importance of deglutition retraining exercises, dietary modification counseling, and instructions in self-intubation in patients being rehabilitated after head and neck surgery. During a three-month program, 38 patients were counseled and trained. The authors noted that patients with combined oral-pharyngeal, pharyngeal-laryngeal, and oral-pharyngeal-laryngeal dysphagia had a poorer outcome: only four of 13 oral-pharyngeal pa-

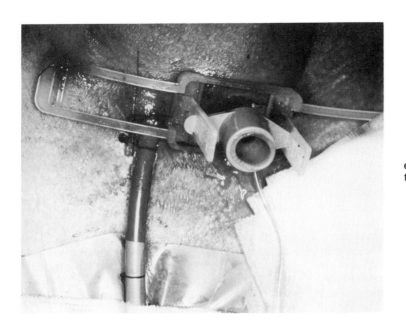

Figure 19–17. Proximity of esophagostomy feeding catheter to tracheostomy tube is shown.

tients were able to return to oral alimentation, and two patients with pharyngeal-laryngeal dysphagia required alimentation by surgical route. Of nine patients with laryngeal phase dysphagia, six resumed oral feedings. One of two patients with esophageal dysphagia secondary to stenosis, requiring repeated dilatation and eventually anastomotic revision, resumed oral feeding. The other patient had to continue nasogastric feeding.

We also find pharynogostomy tubes useful. These may be inserted quite simply under local anesthesia into the piriform sinus.[97] Nissan and colleagues[98] described piriformostomy in the treatment of malignant tumors obstructing the esophagus. In piriformostomy, indwelling nasogastric tubes are brought out through stab wounds in the piriform sinus, bypassing the nose and upper pharynx. The technique was used as early as 1958 at Barnes Hospital in St. Louis in high esophageal carcinoma.

Nissan reported his experience with the technique over a ten-year period in 13 patients with inoperable carcinoma of the esophagus or cardia, or with esophageal obstruction associated with other malignant tumors. Patients averaged 65 years of age. Some patients received radiotherapy (average dose, 2000 rads). In 7 of the 13 patients, the piriformostomy was retained until the death of the patient (mean survival, six months). In six, it was left in place until the patient could tolerate a soft or regular diet. One patient with lymphosarcoma of the esophagus was alive and free of tumor at 84 months after surgery. The method proved helpful during irradiation in the management of esophageal obstruction caused by edema. Regurgitation of saliva was avoided since a narrow passage for saliva around the tube was maintained.

Meguid and Williams[88] emphasize the practical nature of gastrostomy tube in cancer patients who are likely to require tube feedings for prolonged periods. The procedure is easily performed at the time of laparotomy. In our study of 46 tube gastrostomies, 43 were placed electively for nutritional support, using local anesthesia, by intern house staff. The method is well described and eloquently illustrated by Gross.[100] Following intestinal surgery in which a significant degree of malabsorption may arise, it is recommended that a feeding gastrostomy be included at the time of surgery.[78] Once the

wound heals, the tube can be easily replaced should the feeding tube become dislodged. One advantage of a gastrostomy tube is that it bypasses the lower esophageal sphincter, thus minimizing the risk of aspiration.[93] A further advantage is that the larger caliber tubing used allows for more viscous solutions or a blenderized diet to be used which, in general, is less expensive.[87, 100] A common mechanical problem encountered, particularly in the cancer patient requiring prolonged gastrostomy tube feeding using a Foley catheter, is deflation of the balloon with consequent dislodgement of the feeding catheter. To avert this problem, we have established the practice of suturing the tube into place (Fig. 19–18).

Gastrostomy may be particularly suited for long-term or permanent extraoral alimentation in head and neck cancer. It is a useful method of feeding in nonresectable carcinoma of the head and neck region, in

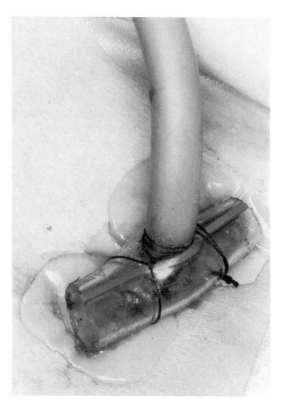

Figure 19–18. The gastrostomy tube is secured by passing the Foley catheter through the pierced segment of a large-bore catheter, which is sutured securely into place.

total obstruction to swallowing (as in carcinoma of the larynx, pharynx, thoracic, or cervical esophagus), and in the home management of pharyngocutaneous fistulas.

Widiss, Hill, and Meguid found that young patients with stable advanced cancer who have complex clinical courses frequently became hospital dependent since they require repeated, prolonged admissions for "beefing up" their nutritional state.[102]

To enable patients to be independent of hospital settings, a feeding tube gastrostomy was inserted for aggressive home total enteral feeding in 25 patients with stable advanced cancer, median age of 62 years (27 to 79 years). Gastrostomy was placed for dysphagia and inanition[92] and for salivary fistula after head and neck surgery.

During the six-month period prior to gastrostomy insertion, an average weight loss of 12.75 per cent from 134 to 117 lbs. occurred. Mean albumin and total lymphocyte count at surgery were 3.7 and 1087, respectively. Home nutritional support for a median of 94 days (18 to 1149 days) prevented further deterioration of nutritional indices and resulted in a decreased readmission rate: 20, 16, and 48 per cent were readmitted 0, 2, and 2 times, respectively, during their median survival of 176 days (33 to 1167 days).

The impact of home enteral nutritional support using gastrostomy enabled stable cancer patients to maintain their nutritional status and enjoy life independent from the hospital setting for an extended period of time.

In an additional study, Rains[103] described tube feeding at home in 10 patients aged 52 to 80 years, who were able to maintain adequate nutritional status for three to five years by gastrostomy or pharyngeal tube feeding of commercial formulas, baby food, or blenderized diets, and thus were able to live alone at home and maintain independence.

A jejunostomy tube is recommended when there is an obstruction or fistula proximally in the gastrointestinal tract. Heymsfield et al.[93] cited several advantages to this site: (1) less stomal leakage and skin erosion than with a gastrostomy; (2) less gastric and pancreatic secretion because the stomach and duodenum are bypassed; (3) less nausea, vomiting, and bloating compared with gastric or duodenal feeding; and (4) reduced risk of aspiration. In our cancer patients, we use a jejunostomy tube routinely following a Whipple procedure for cancer of the pancreas or following total gastrectomy for cancer of the stomach. As with nasoduodenal or nasojejunal feedings, a continuous infusion of isotonic formula must be used.[10, 87] One potential problem with intrajejunal feeding is the possibility that there will be inadequate mixing of the formula with bile and pancreatic enzymes, resulting in maldigestion and malabsorption.[78] This problem can be obviated by the use of an elemental diet where necessary.

The standard method of performing a jejunostomy is by the Whitzel technique, although a needle catheter jejunostomy in which a 16-gauge polyvinyl central venous catheter is passed into the jejunum through a 14-gauge needle has been recently popularized.[104] Rombeau and Barot[91] recommend that even with jejunostomy tubes, meglumin diatrizoate (Gastrografin) be injected prior to the start of feedings to ensure the intraluminal position of the catheter.

Bolus Versus Continuous Feeding in the Patient with Cancer

Among the determining factors in the choice between bolus and continuous feeding are the site of the distal end of the feeding tube, and the degree of malnutrition of the cancer patient.

Continuous feeding is required if the nutrient formula is infused distal to the duodenum. In mild to severe forms of protein-calorie malnutrition, atrophy of the gastrointestinal mucosa occurs, leading to malabsorption. In addition, with hypertonic formulas or when serious absorption problems exist, continuous feedings are preferable.[64] Other advantages of continuous feedings include the ability to administer larger daily volumes with greater facility and reliability, less chance of abdominal distention resulting in aspiration, and less chance of bacterial contamination in a closed delivery system. In contrast, the primary advantage of bolus feedings is that they allow greater patient mobility.[105] Bolus feedings are probably best reserved for gastrostomy or esophagostomy patients requiring long-term tube feedings.

In our cancer population, continuous

feeding is given either by gravity drip or with a constant infusion pump. It has been our experience that difficulties encountered with formula tolerance during continuous feedings are usually caused by uncontrolled changes in flow rate.[79]

FORMULA SELECTION AND METHODS OF FEEDING IN THE ONCOLOGIC PATIENT

In the patient with cancer, the factors that enter into the selection of an enteral nutrient product include the degree and extent of malnutrition, the energy and nitrogen requirements, and fluid tolerance. In the cancer patient, the route of feeding and site of administration may be dictated by the altered anatomy following surgery.

Johnston and associates[106] reported a randomized comparison in malnourished cancer patients of standard nutritional support versus supplemental feeding through a fine-bore nasogastric tube that was passed through an esophageal stricture secondary to squamous cell carcinoma at or below the thoracic inlet. The experimental group received 2400 ml of Isocal during radiotherapy.

Results showed a small weight gain in the experimental group while four patients in the control group lost weight. Total body potassium rose in the supplement group, but fell in controls. There was no change in triceps skinfold thickness or muscle circumference of the arms in eight patients in the supplemental group.

The efficacy of gastrostomy feeding versus total parenteral nutrition was examined by Lim and colleagues,[107] who compared the use of gastrostomy feeding versus TPN in 24 presurgical patients with esophageal carcinoma presenting with total dysphagia. These patients were randomly placed in either support group. All were dehydrated prior to the start of the study. The gastrostomy group received blenderized food, while the TPN group received a mixture of dextrose, amino acid, and fat.

The gastrostomy group had a higher nitrogen intake per kilogram of body weight and a slightly higher caloric intake. Despite this, the patients receiving TPN were in a positive nitrogen balance from the first day of nutritional support, whereas the gastrostomy fed group achieved positive nitrogen balance by the fifth day. On the sixth day, both groups had a similar nitrogen balance. Weight gain in the TPN group was gradual and by the fourth week, a gain of 6.3 per cent average was achieved. No studies of body composition were done to determine the nature of the weight gain. The gastrostomy fed group showed a decrease in weight until the thirteenth day of support, but on average gained 1 per cent of weight during the four week study period. There was no statistically significant difference in the final serum albumin level between the two groups or in operative (radical resection or palliative bypass) morbidity and mortality.

The delay in positive nitrogen balance in the gastrostomy fed group was probably caused by the need for a gradual increase in the quantity and concentration of the feedings owing to intolerance manifested secondary to atrophy of the gastrointestinal tract associated with disuse. The authors could only conclude that the use of the gastrostomy was a useful method of feeding since patients remained mobile, active, and independent, and the blenderized formula was economical relative to TPN. This study clearly underscores the physiologic limitations posed by the malnourished, atrophied gut which leads to malabsorption. This clearly dictates the choice of products.

The majority of enteral products fall into four main groups: (1) blenderized formulas; (2) milk-based formulas (including lactose-containing and lactose-free formulas); (3) elementally defined formulas; and (4) disease-related formulas. These have been discussed in detail in another section of this book. Since the patient with cancer has a high requirement for both energy and nitrogen of high biologic value, there is a trend toward the development of newer enteral products with the emphasis on the use of casein hydrolysate or whole protein as the nitrogen source instead of the use of crystalline amino acids. The rationale and the advantages of such a development are related to the higher biologic value of the nitrogen source.

It has long been clear that proteins differ in nutritional quality because of the differences in their essential amino acid content. The amount of protein needed for growth in an infant or for anabolism rises as the nutritive quality of the protein falls. Thus both the quantity and the quality of a protein are involved in determining the biologic value of proteins and their relative benefits in nitrogen accretion.[108, 109]

When we examine protein quantity, that is, protein intake and how it relates to biologic value, we find that the relationship is an inverse one.[110] When we look at the relationship between protein quality and biologic value, a curvilinear rather than linear relationship is found. As an example, the biologic value of egg protein is greater than that of wheat gluten, probably because of the different proportionality pattern of essential amino acids in these two proteins.[111, 112] Another factor that affects the biologic value of proteins is the caloric intake, because energy intake influences nitrogen metabolism. Recent studies[111] suggest that the net protein utilization (NPU) values of egg and rice protein were 44 and 33, respectively, with energy intake fixed at the maintenance level of about 35 to 40 kcal/kg. When energy intake was increased to 55 kcal/kg, the NPU values were 63 and 55 for egg and rice proteins, respectively.

Thus NPU is related to the quality of a protein, which is determined primarily by its essential amino acid composition. When single amino acids exceed certain levels in the amino acid mixture, the utilization of the dietary amino acid can be severely depressed. This phenomenon depends on various metabolic mechanisms that are classed as amino acid imbalance, amino acid antagonism, or amino acid toxicity according to the type of mechanism responsible.[113] Hence nitrogen retention is superior when whole proteins, such as cottage cheese, are given orally, than when casein hydrolysate is given intravenously, and the latter gives better nitrogen retention than intravenous crystalline amino acids.[114] The preliminary results of ongoing randomized studies at our institution in depleted cancer patients would support these observations. If our results are confirmed, it would signal a new era in the developmental field of tube feeding formulas.

Experimental Enteral Formulas to Inhibit Tumor Growth. Greenstein and coworkers[115] (cited by Lorincz, 1969) showed that by giving a synthetic diet deficient in one essential amino acid to rats, Walker carcinoma growth could be inhibited; however, most animals also suffered severe weight loss. Lorincz and colleagues used a phenylalanine-tyrosine limited diet in a series of preliminary experiments in patients with very advanced cancer and a variety of malig-

nant diseases.[115] The diet was well tolerated. In further studies a commercial preparation was used which was based on casein hydrolysates in which the phenylalanine was removed and then enriched up to 0.08 per cent. A formula that limited tyrosine as well as phenylalanine was also used. Patients were permitted supplementation with foods low in phenylalanine. The experiment was to be considered successful if growth of the tumor was retarded without lowering tumor levels of the restricted amino acid, which could cause further host catabolism. In one case history of advanced metastatic carcinoma at the terminal stage which had not responded to chemotherapy or radiotherapy, restriction of phenylalanine led to a stabilization and a subsiding of ascites and edema. With free alimentation, there was a recurrence of symptoms. In addition, two cases of mammary adenocarcinoma were presented in which moderate inhibition was achieved. Measurements of free amino acid in serum and in tumors of control and experimental groups showed that there was no change in the levels of free circulating amino acid of the tumor.

Demopoulos studied restricted intake of phenylalanine and tyrosine in five patients with pigmented malignant melanoma.[116] These tumors contain large amounts of active tyrosinase, which oxidizes tyrosine to 3,4-dihydroxyphenylalanine and which is further oxidized to DOPA quinone with oxygen coupling. Eventually DOPA quinone is further metabolized to an indole structure and polymerized into the insoluble pigment melanin. To inhibit the tyrosinase, phenylalanine and tyrosine were restricted by feeding a casein hydrolysate from which phenylalanine and tyrosine were removed. Furthermore, D-penicillamine was used to chelate copper, required by the tyrosinase. The combined minimum estimated requirements of phenylalanine and tyrosine (1000 mg) were to be supplied by fruits and vegetables.

A significant decrease in phenylalanine and tyrosine in the daily diet was accompanied by selective detrimental effects on the tumor but only when phenylalanine and tyrosine levels were decreased. In three cases abrupt cessation of tumor growth was noted, while some tumors regressed completely. One problem was that large metastases served as cryptic sources of phenylalanine and tyrosine.

Abell and coworkers[117] evaluated phenylalanine ammonia-lyase (PAL) from yeast for its chemotherapeutic potential against murine L5178 lymphoblastic leukemia maintained in specially bred mice. The enzyme was administered at concentrations of 300 units/kg. This rapidly lowered plasma phenylalanine and tyrosine and inhibited tumor growth, producing "cures" in 40 per cent of the mice. Partially purified preparations of this enzyme coupled with diets low in phenylalanine significantly increased the life span of the mice on average. The advantage to the use of PAL was that a long period of dietary restriction to reduce plasma levels was not necessary. The most outstanding results were obtained when PAL was given every eight hours for five days. However, while it maintained plasma phenylalanine at low concentration, three of seven mice died of enlarged livers; only the mouse was cured. Partially purified enzyme was less effective in retarding tumor growth than was purified enzyme.

Theuer[118] studied the effects of diets containing decreased levels of single essential amino acids on growth in normal mice and of single amino acid restriction on tumor-bearing mice and tumor growth. Restriction of tryptophan, threonine, leucine, or methionine significantly inhibited tumor growth but depressed host weight as well, whereas restriction of phenylalanine, valine, or isoleucine inhibited tumor growth but did not affect host weight. Lysine had no effect on weight gain or tumor growth.

Jose and Good[119] measured the effect of different degrees of deficiency of essential and relatively essential amino acids on specific responses to allogenic tumor cells in mice. Synthetic amino acid diets were used. Response was measured by an in vitro assay of cellular immunity. A moderate reduction of phenylalanine-tyrosine, valine, threonine, methionine-cystine, isoleucine, or tryptophan produced a profound depression of hemagglutinin and blocking of antibody responses, but cytotoxic cell-mediated immunity remained intact. Restrictions of arginine, histidine, or lysine caused only a slight depression in the immune response. Moderate leucine restriction resulted in a paradoxical depression of cytotoxic cell-mediated immunity with little effect on serum blocking activity. It was concluded that a deficiency or imbalance of essential amino acids in the diet may produce a profound depression of the immune response and apparent marked changes in immune resistance of the host to tumors. Amino acids whose restriction depressed both tumor growth and host body weight either had no demonstrable effect on immune response or depressed both cellular and humoral responses to a similar magnitude. Also, diets deficient in leucine but adequate in other amino acids may depress host immune resistance to tumors, and diets containing excess leucine may increase host resistance because of resulting isoleucine-valine deficiency.

Physiologic State of the Gastrointestinal Tract

In the presence of malabsorption resulting from surgery, radiation, or chemotherapy, an elemental diet is indicated. Medium-chain triglycerides alone (as a supplement) or as the predominant fat source in a formula are indicated in patients with fat malabsorption. In patients with lactase deficiency, either as a result of heredity or more commonly secondary to enteritis, a lactose-free formula is indicated.

Long-Term Use of Enteral Nutritional Support in Patients with Cancer

On a yearly basis, approximately 25 patients with stable advanced cancer are discharged home on enteral feeding regimens from our institution. It has been our experience that for long-term use at home, additional considerations such as convenience, availability, and cost need to be considered. Liquid, ready-to-feed products are most convenient. They can be stored at room temperature, requiring refrigeration only for the unused portion after opening.

The cost of formulas is a further consideration since third party reimbursement may not be universally applicable. In general the cost of elemental formulas is higher than that of other formulas providing comparable nutrients.

For those patients who desire to prepare their own tube feedings, several recipes are available.[120] However, a blenderized diet may be too viscous to pass readily through a small-bore feeding tube. The indication for their use is in patients with a large (18 French and upward) gastrostomy tube and an otherwise normal and well functioning gastrointestinal tract.[10]

Food Preferences and Anorexia

Anorexia and food aversions caused by taste abnormalities, nausea, generalized pain, gastritis secondary to medications, and endogenous depression are among some of the problems experienced by patients with cancer.[16-18, 121-124] Vickers et al.[88] found that many patients with cancer have a strong aversion for meats and sweet and salty foods. Unfortunately, these dietary ingredients constitute the mainstay of a regular hospital diet. Improved food acceptability was found for bitter or sour foods, fruits and vegetables, and dairy products. Taste tests have demonstrated that at least some enteral feeding formulas are acceptable to patients with cancer, although the overall taste evaluation of enteral formulas differed between cancer patients and controls.[124]

Since generalized or specific sources of pain may affect appetite, use of analgesics prior to a meal may be beneficial, and the use of antiemetics such as the phenothiazines for nausea may improve food intake.[124] Reactive depression, common in patients with cancer, may also interfere with food intake,[18] and the use of tricyclic antidepressants may be of help. Finally, there may be conditioned or social food aversions that interfere with adequate nutrient intake.

In an effort to stimulate the patient's appetite, the use of behavior modification has met with some success.[90] The patient is persuaded to participate in his own care by setting a realistic goal of nutrient intake which he must meet. Positive reinforcement is given for intakes that meet or exceed the agreed upon minimal level.

Finally, the dietitian and physician should provide the patient with guidance on the value of good nutrient intake during the treatment for cancer, information on common problems and how to manage them, and guidance on product selection. By encouraging the patient to take a more active role in his own care, and through guidance and support, the patient's appetite may improve. To reinforce these positive aspects it should be emphasized to the patient and his family that nutrition is the one area of the patient's treatment that he and his family can control.[126] To aid in this area, several helpful books have recently become available,[92-94] and a list of these publications should be made available to the patient.

Nutritional Support in Patients with Cancer—Early Studies

In the 1950s, a number of investigators reported their experience with nutritional support of the cancer patient.[130-132] Pareira and associates[130, 131] were among the early investigators to report the results of using nasogastric feeding of a milk-based formula in 240 patients, 64 of whom had cancer of the cervix, large intestine, stomach, oropharynx, tongue, pancreas, or breast. The formula consisted of powdered whole milk, calcium caseinate, dextrose, maltose, vitamins, iron, and choline, providing 3500 kcal/day and 33.6 gm of nitrogen. All patients in the larger series achieved positive nitrogen balance during the one to two weeks of nasogastric alimentation. Cancer patients who were terminally ill and who lived for more than one week after the start of tube feeding reported increased strength and weight gain. However, tube feeding did not lengthen life expectancy. The tumor seemed to grow at an equal pace with body weight gain in cases in which this could be observed.

In all cancer patients in the series, the gastrointestinal tract was intact and tolerance for the formula was as good in cancer patients as in noncancer patients. Anorexia diminished in all cancer patients except in those whose tube feeding was begun shortly before death. Appetites tended to return within one to three weeks after the start of nutritional support. Patients with noncancer cachexia showed a restoration in serum albumin concentrations, whereas 5 of 14 cancer patients in whom this was studied showed either no increase in albumin levels or a continued fall. The remaining nine cancer patients showed roughly the same gain in albumin levels as did noncancer patients. The authors concluded on the basis of the study that cancer cachexia is not due to any specific effect of cancer but to malnutrition initiated and sustained by anorexia. They proposed that hyperalimentation could break the anorexia-malnutrition cycle and induce weight gain and return of appetite, regeneration of hemoglobin and positive nitrogen balance. Only serum albumin regeneration was impaired in these patients.

Peden et al., also in the 1950s,[132] compared protein repletion in cancer and noncancer cachexia in eight patients, four of whom had various types of cancer: postradiation cervical cancer, palliative resection of carcinoma of the rectum, postoperative persistence of carcinoma of the breast, and nonresectable carcinoma of the esophagus. All four cancer patients had very advanced disease and succumbed within three days to six weeks after the study was completed. The sole food intake was a feeding mixture of known and uniform composition. In noncancer patients, nitrogen balance was always positive during the period of repletion with intake of 10 to 18 gm/day of nitrogen. Weight gain was not proportional to nitrogen intake. In cancer patients the nitrogen balance, though positive, was less in degree than in noncancer patients, possibly owing to small intakes. Weight gain was variable but less than in noncancer patients. Absolute plasma volume and total circulating plasma protein did not change appreciably in noncancer patients but significant gains in total circulating albumin were noted, largely at the expense of globulin. Cancer patients demonstrated no significant changes in red blood cell volume or total circulating hemoglobin. Only one cancer patient had a favorable albumin response. Two cancer patients had some loss of weight despite positive nitrogen balance.

Terepka et al.[133] conducted forced feeding studies in eight patients with a variety of malignant diseases: prostatic carcinoma, bladder carcinoma, sarcoma of the uterus, lymphosarcoma, monocytic leukemia, malignant melanoma, and cancer of the pancreas and bronchus. Control periods in each patient were used to establish normal eating patterns. Between control periods were periods of forced feeding in which the diet chosen by the patient was increased in nitrogen content and calories by 50 to 100 per cent. Supplementation was accomplished with concentrated oral feedings or by intubation. In general, forced feedings were not well tolerated by these patients and thus forced feeding periods were brief, varying from 8 to 12 days.

Patients generally fell into two groups in their response to tube feeding. In the first group caloric expenditure increased only slightly but calorie balances became much less negative or even slightly positive. There were no changes in basal oxygen consumption. Thus forced feeding did not significantly disturb the established host-tumor relationship in this group of patients. There was minimal clinical improvement with a return to the control state after forced feeding. In the second group, there was a marked increase in the basal metabolic rate. Caloric expenditure increased during or immediately after forced feeding, as would be expected. In this group, forced feeding disturbed the nutritional balance to the detriment of the host and the change proved to be irreversible. An acceleration of the malignant process was observed.

Balance studies demonstrated that seven of the eight patients retained more phosphorus during the forced feeding period than during the control periods. A strongly negative calcium balance was seen in four patients. More potassium was retained during forced feedings than during control periods. Intracellular fluid was accumulating during the weight gain associated with forced feeding. In three patients in whom the malignant process was accelerated during forced feeding, caloric expenditure did not return to control values after forced feeding. The nitrogen balance became more positive in forced feeding but approached equilibrium and a negative balance developed after forced feeding. Terepka concluded that sustained nitrogen repletion probably requires an attack on the tumor itself. Return to a negative nitrogen balance after forced feeding suggests that host repletion could not be sustained without concomitant anti-neoplastic therapy.

Comparative Studies of Enteral Feeding Versus TPN in Patients with Cancer

Valerio and associates[134] compared intravenous versus oral alimentation in patients receiving 4000 rads of external beam radiation to the pelvis or abdomen for adenocarcinoma or transitional cell carcinoma. Twenty patients were stratified by percentage weight loss and randomly allocated to either TPN (central catheter via subclavian puncture) or oral feeding. The TPN group received 40 to 45 kcal/kg/day over the duration of radiotherapy. The oral group (controls) received 30 to 35 kcal/kg/day with supplements when indicated. A three-day diary was used to calculate intake in the control group. The TPN group had lower serum albumin values and more patients with advanced cancer and severe weight loss. Two of these patients died during radiotherapy and three died shortly after. In the control group, three patients died after radiotherapy.

In the TPN group, despite advanced disease, a higher dose of radiotherapy was able to be given to the nine patients completing the radiotherapy; five patients had 50 per cent or more reduction in tumor bulk. In the control group, three patients had 50 per cent or more reduction. TPN patients gained an average of 2.1 kg during radiotherapy. Control patients maintained their weight. Albumin concentrations decreased slightly in both groups but there was a significant increase in transferrin levels in the TPN group only. The authors observed that patients who did not respond to nutritional support also did not respond to radiotherapy and died during treatment or succumbed rapidly after termination of intravenous hyperalimentation.

Rickard and coworkers[135] compared the effectiveness of two nutritional supplements (lactose-free Ensure Plus or lactose-containing Carnation Instant Breakfast) with TPN (FreAmine II) in nine children with Wilms' tumors who received intensive treatment including operative removal of the tumor, actinomycin D following surgery, with weekly vincristine for six weeks; doxorubicin (Adriamycin) was also used in four children, and additional radiotherapy in eight children. The sites of tumor included abdomen, liver, and lung. Although initially eight children were receiving enteral feedings, four children had to be given TPN because of a weight loss of greater than 20 per cent, weight/height ratio less than the 5th percentile, albumin less than 3.2 gm/dl, and kilocalorie intake less than 80 per cent of the RDA.

The loss of weight was 22 ± 7 (M $\pm$ SD) per cent by 26 ± 17 days from the beginning of treatment in the enteral group. All patients gained weight in the TPN group. Intake was greater in the TPN group (105 ± 9 per cent RDA versus 64 ± 27 per cent RDA). TPN restored weight for height percentile, but there was a variable effect on repletion of skinfold thickness. Patients in the TPN group who completed treatment and had no evidence of disease maintained their weight for height. The enteral group regained the lost weight by the six-month cycle of chemotherapy. TPN was recommended for children with stage IV disease, in patients with unfavorable histologic findings who received intense treatment, and in children with protein-calorie malnutrition associated with cancer cachexia. Enteral nutrition was found to be inadequate in these cases until the initial phase of treatment was completed. The authors recommended enteral or oral feeding for maintenance purposes when the patient was disease-free.

Harvey and colleagues[136] compared nutritional support using TPN (24 patients) with enteral feeding (32 patients) and combined parenteral and enteral feeding (55 patients) in cancer patients who were nutritionally assessed before receiving oncologic therapy consisting of a combination of surgery, chemotherapy, and radiotherapy. Nutritional plans were based on the extent of malnutrition, whether the gastrointestinal tract was functional, and on the patient's BEE. Enteral calories provided 150 per cent BEE and 1.2 to 1.5 gm of protein/kg/day by oral or nasogastric feedings: TPN supplied 175 per cent BEE with the same amount of protein. Patients were assessed before and after therapy to show which assessment parameters were predictive of outcome.

The results of the study show that anergy was significantly higher in patients who died. Also, serum albumin and transferrin were initially lower in these patients. Serum transferrin concentration and delayed hypersensitivity skin antigen testing were the most reliable indices of response to therapy and nutritional support. Serum albumin less than 3.0 gm/dl or total peripheral lymphocyte count of less than 900 cells/cc in the presence of enteral or parenteral support carried an unfavorable prognosis. The feeding regimen, however, did not correlate with outcome. All methods proved to be equally effective in repletion. Eighty-four per cent (27 of 32) of initially anergic patients became immunocompetent; of these, 11 per cent died. Of five remaining patients who remained anergic, mortality was 100 per cent. Thirty-nine per cent (14 of 36) of initially immune competent patients became anergic. Mortality in this group was 50 per cent. In 22 patients in whom the immune function was preserved, mortality was 14 per cent.

Lim et al.[63] provided nutritional support as either gastrostomy feedings or TPN in esophageal carcinoma. The gastrostomy group received a blenderized diet. In the TPN group, patients achieved a positive nitrogen balance from the very first day of treatment, whereas in the gastrostomy group, a positive nitrogen balance was achieved only by the fifth day. By the sixth day, both groups were in similar balance. The percentage weight gain was higher in the TPN group: a gradual increase was observed until 6.3 per cent was attained at the end of the fourth week. The gastrostomy group showed weight loss which peaked on day seven. By day 13 there was demonstrable weight gain in the group. Thus gastrostomy feeding did not produce the degree of weight gain or nitrogen balance comparable to that of TPN, but proved simpler and safer, and all patients were able to remain active and mobile. The procedure of gradually increasing formula concentration over a number of days may account for the continued weight loss in the gastrostomy group during the initial feeding period.

Skidmore and associates[137] compared intravenous and nasogastric feeding in 20 patients with head and neck cancer. In one group, beef serum protein derivative (Gastro-Caloreen) was administered nasogastrically, while in another a crystalline amino acid solution was given intravenously for one to three days before surgery. Serum urea and electrolytes were maintained in a normal range with both regimens, and all patients achieved positive nitrogen balance.

Sako and coworkers[138] reported a randomized study of 64 patients stratified by nutritional status and prognosis and randomized within each stratum to either a TPN or an enteral group. The patients had cancers of the larynx, oral cavity, oropharynx, hypopharynx, or maxillary sinus. The TPN group (30 patients) received 35 cal/kg/day in the form of 4.25 per cent crystalline amino acids and dextrose (FreAmine II) for at least 14 days postoperatively (eight received preoperative TPN also). The enteral control group (32 patients) received nasogastric feeding using liquified tube diet or ate ad libitum.

Postoperative nitrogen balance was attained in the TPN group and had a mean value of +6.65 gm. In the enteral-control group this was +3.8 gm. The changes noted in albumin, SGOT, and bilirubin were not significant between the two groups, whereas alkaline phosphatase and LDH were elevated in the TPN group only. The total red blood cell and lymphocyte counts were not significantly different between the two groups at one, two, or three weeks postoperatively.

Wound complications were not significantly different between the two groups. There was sustained difference in mean weight change in the two groups: in the TPN group 17 patients gained weight during the first week, while 11 patients lost weight. In the enteral-control group only four patients gained weight, while 26 patients lost weight. These differences were maintained even during the second and third weeks of nutritional support. Immune parameters (including recall skin antigens) were not improved in the TPN group versus the enteral-control group. There were a higher number of early deaths in the TPN group. Survival analysis showed that in the group with 0 to 6 per cent weight loss before surgery, patients receiving TPN had a lower survival curve. This was also true of the 6 to 12 per cent weight loss group and the 12 to 24 per cent weight loss group. Actual number of deaths in the TPN group exceeded the number of deaths in the enteral-control group in all three weight-loss groups, for which the authors could not offer a reason.

Ching and associates[139] reported the nutritional repletion of 45 cancer patients aged 60 to 86 years with cancer of the gastrointestinal tract (20 patients), head and neck (10 patients), lung (eight patients), breast (three patients), hematopoietic system (two patients), and metastatic melanoma (two patients). Most patients (75 per cent) had metastatic cancer and were receiving radiotherapy and/or chemotherapy as well as undergoing surgery. Nutritional support consisted of a variety of forms. Patients received either a regular hospital diet; peripheral amino acids with or without a source of nonprotein energy, Vivonex HN, or Precision HN; or a regular diet combined with either an enteral diet or TPN.

In patients undergoing surgical therapy,

serum albumin level was preserved when nutritional support was employed and Vivonex HN proved equally effective to TPN. In other therapies (radiotherapy and chemotherapy) serum albumin levels were best preserved when an adequate diet was ingested or when a regular diet was supplemented with an enteral diet. A significant decrease in serum albumin occurred during therapy in patients receiving only peripheral amino acids, TPN, or enteral diet.

Nixon and colleagues[140] performed trace element balances, and measured serum proteins, anthropometrics, and creatinine/height ratio in 15 patients with protein-calorie malnutrition of advanced cancer and in 10 undernourished controls without cancer, using TPN or enteral hyperalimentation. There were two patients with cancer of the pancreas, three with cancer of the stomach, five with cancer of the colon, three with cancer of the head and neck, and one with cancer of the lung. All had metastatic lesions to the liver, lung, or bone.

Cancer patients receiving TPN showed significantly less improvement than noncancer control patients in body weight (median increment of 5 kg versus 8.5 kg), in albumin levels (0.1 g/dl versus 0.5 g/dl), in creatinine/height ratio (4 per cent of standard versus 10 per cent of standard), and in midarm muscle area (4 per cent of standard versus 11 per cent of standard). Triceps skinfold increments were similar following therapies in the cancer and noncancer patients. Nitrogen retention was similar in the cancer and noncancer groups. The cancer patients, however, retained significantly less magnesium and phosphorus. In six cancer patients given enteral hyperalimentation, the average balance for phosphorus, potassium, sodium, chloride, and magnesium was lower compared with those obtained with TPN. In noncancer patients, enteral nutrition and TPN gave similar results both in elemental balances and in nutritional indices. In cancer subjects, there was less retention of sodium, chloride, phosphorus, potassium, and magnesium with the use of the enteral route. The retention of nitrogen, phosphorus, and calcium in abnormal ratios in cancer patients indicated that lean body mass was not being restored.

The authors suggested that the cancer cachexia was associated not only with anorexia but also with metabolic aberrations, and they concluded that their study did not support the contention that a positive nitrogen balance and weight gain in advanced cancer was representative of lean body mass.

EFFICACY OF ENTERAL FEEDING IN THE PATIENT WITH CANCER

In evaluating the efficacy of enteral nutrition in the patient with cancer, two lines of arguments need to be explored based on two conceptual assumptions.

First, if one accepts the concept that one of the "rights" of the patient with cancer is to be given a well-balanced diet appropriate to fully meet his nutrient requirements during the altered metabolic state induced by cancer and the consequences of its therapy, then much of the information discussed in the previous sections clearly supports the clinical impression. Based on data from nonrandomized studies, enteral nutrition or TPN is of benefit to the majority of patients with cancer. These data clearly show that with the provision of nutritional support, patients remain hydrated, subjectively feel better, gain weight (the quality of which is not under discussion), maintain serum albumin, can improve anergy states, and are able to complete a therapeutic modality which they otherwise would not be able to tolerate. To this end, an immense amount of energy has been spent outlining the clinical benefits of enteral nutrition for patients with cancer. Hence, enteral nutritional support is of immense, often life-saving, value to the cancer patient during the acute and stressful phase encountered during therapy.

Second, if one puts forward the concept that enteral nutritional support is a modern panacea able to cure the patient with cancer and influence survival, then one would need to review the following data of randomized prospective studies.

Elkort et al.[43] initiated a randomized prospective study designed to evaluate the effects of prolonged enteral nutritional support (12 month period) in a group of well-nourished ambulatory patients with breast cancer receiving adjunctive cytotoxic chemotherapy. The control group (23 patients) ate ad libitum, whereas the experimental group (24 patients) received free choice diet supplemented daily with 500 ml of a liquid diet

(Isocal or Sustacal) to meet their caloric requirements.

During the 12 month study period, 21 of the original 47 patients were lost from the study for a variety of reasons, leaving 14 control and 12 experimental subjects. The subjects in both groups experienced gastrointestinal toxicity to the same degree caused by chemotherapy. Hence, it was felt that improved nutritional status did not correlate with a decrease in the toxicity of chemotherapy.

The experimental group showed a significant correlation between weight change and mid-arm muscle circumference and arm circumference, indicating that the weight change represented an increase in protein when a weight gain had occurred and a loss of fat when there was a weight loss.

Nutritional support had no effect on survival since equal numbers of patients had recurrent disease or died in both groups. The authors felt that their most important observation in their study was that an increase in weight was associated with an increased risk of recurrent disease and of mortality.

Douglass et al.[141] reported the use of an elemental diet as adjuvant therapy in 30 patients with locally advanced gastrointestinal cancer with no metastases outside the radiation fields. Twenty patients had tumors of the upper abdomen: 13 had pancreatic adenocarcinomas, two had ampullary or duodenal adenocarcinoma, and five had gastric cancer. Ten patients had lower abdominal cancer and were given pelvic irradiation: five had rectosigmoidal cancer, four had rectal cancer, and one had anal cancer. Since nutritional deficits were generally greater in patients with cancer of the upper abdomen, more of these patients were included. These were all locally advanced, nonresectable or recurrent cancers. In the upper abdomen group all but one patient received adjuvant chemotherapy; in the lower abdomen group only four patients received chemotherapy.

Patients were given either a standard diet or the diet plus a daily supplement of 900 kcal in the form of Vivonex HN. Patients receiving the supplement had 50 per cent more calories per day than controls (or 37 kcal/kg/day versus 20 kcal/kg/day). The supplement group averaged 0.27 ± 0.15 gm of nitrogen; the controls averaged 0.12 ± 0.04 gm/kg/day of nitrogen. Weight loss was noted in 25 of 30 patients given abdominal radiotherapy.

There was little difference in survival between patients given a supplement and control patients. Delayed hypersensitivity skin test responses were improved in patients receiving supplementation. Delayed hypersensitivity, however, deteriorated in controls. Serum albumin levels also decreased in control patients with gastric and colonic carcinoma but were unchanged in patients in the supplement group with gastric, colorectal, and pancreatic cancer. These differences, however, were not significant.

There was no correlation between the amount of weight lost and caloric intake. Those who initially weighed greater than 90 per cent of their ideal body weight had mean survivals of eight (controls) and nine (supplement) months. Those with weight loss greater than 10 per cent below their ideal body weight showed a survival of six months (controls) and 14 months (supplement group). There were an insufficient number of patients to determine whether the difference was significant.

In a randomized study of 30 patients receiving primary radiation for epidermoid cancer of the head and neck regions, Crossland and Higgins[142] compared the benefits of a dietary supplement of 1080 kcal/day (Sustacal) with a hospital diet as tolerated. The indices followed during the six week course of radiation included weight change, dietary tolerance, serum chemistries (SMA-12), and a sense of well-being. Decreased weight loss, improved sense of well-being, maintenance of adequate serum protein levels, and satisfactory albumin levels were observed in the nutritionally supplemented group.

In another study Foster et al.[143] reviewed the effects of therapeutic irradiation with low residue diet and with a low residue diet supplemented with an elemental diet. Twelve patients received standard dietary intake in the form of reduced fiber diet and 20 patients received the low residue diet along with three packets of Vivonex HN (900 kcal). The organs affected by cancer in these patients included bladder, prostate, uterus, colon, and testis.

Significant weight loss occurred during radiotherapy in both treatment groups; the mean weight loss in controls was 1.4 kg, whereas that in the Vivonex group was 1.0 kg. Irradiation was associated with a small decrease in plasma potassium and calcium in both groups. Most patients studied were at their normal weight and were in good nutritional status before radiotherapy was started.

Brown and colleagues[144] reviewed the use of elemental diet supplementation (three packets of Vivonex HN) in 30 patients with various pelvic cancers who underwent abdominal and pelvic irradiation. The patients in this series had primarily bladder or prostatic cancer. Other patients in the series had cancer of the testis, ureter, cervix, endometrium, ovary, colon, and lymphoma.

A control group of 17 patients received a low residue diet. Twenty-one patients found Vivonex HN unacceptable because of nausea or unpalatability. In the remaining patients, an increased dietary intake did not offset the weight loss or change in stool frequency seen with abdominal radiation. The radiotherapy dose of 4000 to 6000 rads was given in a fractionated course. The complications of radiotherapy were not avoided in the group receiving elemental diet supplement.

In a similar study, Bourous et al.[40] studied the benefits of an elemental diet versus an ad libitum diet in 24 patients receiving palliative intravenous 5-fluorouracil therapy for six to nine days. The patients had advanced metastatic carcinomas. The group receiving the elemental diet experienced significantly less weight loss ($p < 0.05$) than controls and had significantly better preservation of rectal mucosa as determined by rectal biopsy than did controls.

From these and similar data, one may conclude that weight gain is almost uniformly experienced in the supplemented population. However, there are severe limitations in further interpreting these data because of the small population, the sample size, the mixed disease stages, the heterogenous diagnoses, and the use of subjects with nutritional status varying from well-fed to malnourished. The question thus asked as to whether enteral nutrition improves survival remains unanswered.

However, this may not be a pertinent question for the following reasons: one needs to view cancer as a long-term process. Thus the induction phase may be up to 25 to 30 years, the cancer in situ phase about 5 to 10 years, the invasive phase between one and five years, and the cancer dissemination phase about one to five years, depending on the tumor type. If one assumes that the average solid tumor doubling time is about 100 days, then the average tumor is diagnosed and treated between 30 and 40 doubling times (Table 19–6). Is it reasonable to expect that the provision of intense nutritional support, enterally or parenterally, for a limited time during tumor reduction therapy would influence a process initiated many years before? Current data show that survival is not affected and indeed this may well have been anticipated. A more pertinent question would be whether nutrition played a permissive or causative role during the induction phase many years before. Indeed Figure 19–19 shows the likely mechanisms by which diet influences the development of cancer.[145] However, this is not the subject we are currently addressing. The main issue is whether there is clinical benefit from enteral nutritional support to the patient with cancer during anti-cancer therapy. From the data reviewed, the overwhelming evidence would indicate the need for intense nutritional support during a time when there is a decreased voluntary nutrient intake and increased nutrient requirement secondary to the stress of the therapy, and an autonomous tumor metabolism failing to respond to starvation.

Table 19–6   NUMBER AND VOLUME OF DOUBLING TIME OF A CANCER MODEL*

No. of Doublings	0	10	20	30	40
Volume	1000 μm^3	0.001 mm^3	1 mm^3	1 cm^3	1000 cm^3
No. of Cells	1	1000	10^6	10^9	10^{12}
Diameter	10 μmm	0.124 mm	1.24 mm	1.24 cm	12.4 cm

*The assumption is made that the average solid tumor doubling time is about 100 days. Hence, the average tumor is diagnosed and treated at about 30 to 40 doubling times.

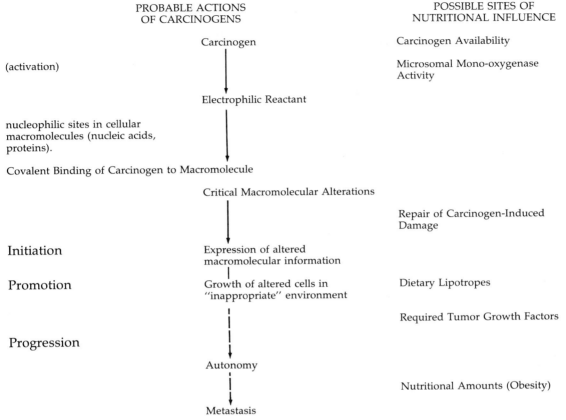

Figure 19–19. Likely mechanisms by which diet influences the development of cancer

REFERENCES

1. Van Eys, J.: Malnutrition in children with cancer: Incidence and consequences. Cancer, 43:2030–2035, 1979.
2. McLaren, D. S., Meguid, M. M.: Nutritional assessment at the crossroads. J.P.E.N., 7(4):371–379, 1983.
3. Meguid, M. M., and Howard, L. J.: The application of nutritional science to surgery. In Peters, R. M., Peacock, E. E., and Benfield, J. R. (eds.): Science Applied to Surgery. Boston, Little, Brown and Co., 1983.
4. Blackburn, G. L., Maini, B. S., Bistrian, B. R., and McDermott, W. V.: The effect of cancer on nitrogen, electrolyte, and mineral metabolism. Cancer Res., 37:2348–2353, 1977.
5. Shils, M. E.: Principles of nutritional therapy. Cancer, 43:2093–2102, 1979.
6. Warren, S.: The immediate cause of death in cancer. Am. J. Med. Sci., 184:610–615, 1932.
7. Buzby, G. P., Mullen, J. L., Matthews, D. C., et al.: Prognostic nutrition index in gastrointestinal surgery. Am. J. Surg., 139:160–167, 1979.
8. Buzby, G. P., and Steinberg, J. J.: Nutrition in cancer patients. Surg. Clin. North Am., 61:691–700, 1981.
9. Meguid, M. M.: The enteral alternative. Contemp. Surg., 13:41–52, 1978.
10. Widiss, T. L., and Meguid, M. M.: The enteral alternative: Update. Contemp. Surg., 19:75–95, 1981.
11. Costa, G.: Cachexia, the metabolic component of neoplastic diseases. Cancer Res., 37:2327–2335, 1977.
12. Shils, M. E.: Nutrition and neoplasia. In Goodhart, R. S., and Shils, M. E. (eds.): Modern Nutrition in Health and Disease, Edition 6. Philadelphia, Lea and Febiger, 1980.
13. Shils, M. E.: Nutritional problems associated with gastrointestinal and genitourinary cancer. Cancer Res., 37:2366–2372, 1977.
14. Theologides, A.: Cancer cachexia. Cancer, 43:2004–2012, 1979.
15. Theologides, A.: Anorexia-producing intermediary metabolites. Am. J. Clin. Nutr., 29:552–558, 1976.
16. DeWys, W. D.: Anorexia as a general effect of cancer. Cancer, 43:2013–2019, 1979.
17. DeWys, W. D.: Abnormalities of taste as a remote

effect of neoplasm. Ann. N.Y. Acad. Sci., *230*:427–434, 1974.

18. Schmale, A. H.: Psychological aspects of anorexia: Areas for study. Cancer, *43*:2087–2092, 1979.

19. Schein, P. S., Kisner, D., Huller, D., et al.: Cachexia of cancer: Potential role of insulin in nutritional management. Cancer, *43*:2070–2076, 1979.

20. Young, V. R.: Energy metabolism and requirements in the cancer patient. Cancer Res., *37*:2336–2347, 1977.

21. Warnold, I., Lundholm, K., and Schersten, T.: Energy balance and body composition in cancer. Cancer Res., *38*:1801–1807, 1978.

22. Watkin, D. M.: Nitrogen balance as affected by neoplastic disease and its therapy. Am. J. Clin. Nutr., *9*:446–460, 1961.

23. Waterhouse, C. L., Fenninger, L. D., and Keutman, E. H.: Nitrogen exchange and caloric expenditure in patients with malignant neoplasm. Cancer, *4*:500–514, 1951.

24. Watkin, D. M., and Steinfield, J. L.: Nutrient and energy metabolism in patients with and without cancer during hyperalimentation with fat administered intravenously. Am. J. Clin. Nutr. *16*:182–212, 1965.

25. Brennan, M. F.: Uncomplicated starvation versus cancer cachexia. Cancer Res., *37*:2359–2365, 1977.

26. Munro, H. N., and Crim, M. C.: The proteins and amino acids. *In* Goodhart, R. S., and Shils, M. E. (eds.): Modern Nutrition in Health and Disease. Edition 6. Philadelphia, Lea and Febiger, 1980.

27. Costa, G., Hooshmand, H., Martinez, A. J., et al.: Overproduction of N_2 by man: A new metabolic syndrome. Clin. Res., *22*:59a, 1974.

28. Lundholm, K., Bylund, A. C., Holm, J., and Schersten, T.: Skeletal muscle metabolism in patients with malignant tumor. Eur. J. Cancer, *12*:465–473, 1976.

29. Young, V. R., Meguid, M. M., Meredith, C., et al.: Newer knowledge of human amino acid requirements. *In* Waterlow, E. J. (ed.): Nitrogen Metabolism in Man. London, Applied Science Publisher, 1981.

30. Holroyde, C. P., Gabuzda, T. G., Putnam, R. C., et al.: Altered glucose metabolism in metastatic carcinoma. Cancer Res., *35*:3710–3714, 1975.

31. Waterhouse, C., and Kemperman, J. H.: Carbohydrate metabolism in subjects with cancer. Cancer Res., *31*:1273–1278, 1971.

32. Milligan, L. P.: Energetic efficiency and metabolic transformations. Fed. Proc., *30*:1454–1458, 1971.

33. Meguid, M. M., Brennan, M. F., Aoki, T. T., et al.: Hormone-substrate interrelationships following trauma. Arch. Surg., *109*:776–783, 1974.

34. Meguid, M. M., Aun, F., Soeldner, J. S., et al.: Insulin half-life in man after trauma. Surgery, *89*:650–653, 1981.

35. Meguid, M. M., Moore-Ede, M. C., Fitzpatrick, G., Moore, F. D.: Norepinephrine-induced insulin and substrate changes in normal man: Incomplete reversal by phenotolamine. J. Surg. Res., *18*:365–369, 1975.

36. Ohnuma, T., and Holland, J. F.: Nutritional consequences of cancer chemotherapy and immunotherapy. Cancer Res., *37*:2395–2406, 1977.

37. Carter, S. K.: Nutritional problems associated with cancer chemotherapy. *In* Newell, G. R., and Ellison, N. M. (eds.): Nutrition and Cancer: Etiology and Treatment. New York, Raven Press, 1981, pages 303–317.

38. Bounous, G., Hugon, J., and Gentile, J. M.: Elemental diet in the management of the intestinal lesion produced by 5-fluorouracil in the rat. Can. J. Surg., *14*:298–311, 1971.

39. Bounous, G., Gentile, J. M., and Hugon, J.: Elemental diet in the management of the intestinal lesion produced by 5-fluorouracil in man. Can. J. Surg., *14*:312–324, 1971.

40. Block, J. H., Chlebowski, R. T., and Herrold, J. N.: Continuous enteric alimentation with a blenderized formula in cancer cachexia. Clin. Oncol., *7*:93–98, 1981.

41. Loh, K. K., Inamasu, M. S., Melish, J., Shigemasa, S. R., Walker, J. Z., and Oishi, N.: Enteral hyperalimentation in the treatment of malnourished cancer patients [Abstract C-35]. Proc. Am. Soc. Clin. Oncol., *20*:301, 1979.

42. Baker, F., Vitale, J. J., Elkort, P., Vavrousek-Jakuba, E., and Cordano, A.: Nutritional enteral support of breast cancer patients [Abstract]. J.P.E.N., *1*:18A, 1977.

43. Elkort, R. J., Baker, F. L., Vitale, J. J., and Cordano, A.: Long-term nutritional support as an adjunct to chemotherapy for breast cancer. J.P.E.N., *5*:385–390, 1981.

44. DeVries, E. G. E., Mulder, N. H., Houwen, B., and DeVries-Hospers, H. G.: Enteral nutrition by nasogastric tube in adult patients treated with intensive chemotherapy for acute leukemia. Am. J. Clin. Nutr., *35*:1490–1496, 1982.

45. Donaldson, S. S., and Lenon, R. A.: Alterations of nutritional status: Impact of chemotherapy and radiation therapy. Cancer, *43*:2036–2052, 1979.

46. Donaldson, S. S.: Nutritional consequences of radiotherapy. Cancer Res., *37*:2407–2413, 1977.

47. Elson, L. A., and Lamerton, L. F.: The influence of the protein content of the diet on the response of Walker rat carcinoma-256 to X radiation. Br. J. Cancer, *3*:414–426, 1949.

48. Hugon, J. S., and Bounous, G.: Elemental diet in the management of the intestinal lesions produced by radiation in the mouse. Can. J. Surg., *15*:18–26, 1972.

49. Cheraskin, E., Ringsdorf, W. M., Jr., Hutchins, K., Setyaadmadja, A. T. S. H., and Wideman, G. L.: Effect of diet upon radiation response in cervical carcinoma of the uterus: A preliminary report. Acta Cytol., *12*:433–438, 1968.

50. Bounous, G., LeBel, E., Schuster, J., Gold, P., Tahan, W. T., and Bastin, E.: Dietary protection during radiation therapy. Strahlentherapie, *149*:476–483, 1975.

51. Hadda, H., Bounous, G., Tahan, W. T., Devroede, G., Beaudry, R., and Lafond, R.: Long-term nutrition with an elemental diet following intensive abdominal irradiation: Report of a case. Dis. Colon Rectum, *17*:373–376, 1974.

52. Nealon, T. F., Jr., Grossi, C. E., and Steier, M.: Use of an elemental diet to correct catabolic states prior to surgery. Ann. Surg., *180*:9–13, 1974.

53. Donaldson, S. S., Jundt, S., Ricour, C., Sarrazin, D., Lemerle, J., and Schweisguth, O.: Radiation enteritis in children. Cancer, *35*:1167–1178, 1975.

54. Brennan, M. F.: Metabolic response to surgery in the cancer patient: Consequences of aggressive

multimodality therapy. Cancer, 43:2053–2064, 1979.

55. Stein, T. P., and Buzby, G. P.: Protein metabolism in surgical patients. Surg. Clin. North Am., 61:519–527, 1981.

56. Meguid, M. M., Collier, M. D., and Howard, L. J.: Uncomplicated and stressed starvation. Surg. Clin. North Am., 62:529–543, 1981.

57. Elwyn, D. H., Kinney, J. M., and Askanazi, J.: Energy expenditure in surgical patients. Surg. Clin. North Am., 61:545–556, 1981.

58. Shils, M. D., and Gilat, T.: The effect of esophagectomy on absorption in man: Clinical and metabolic observations. Gastroenterology, 50:347–357, 1966.

59. Fein, H. D.: Nutrition in diseases of the stomach, including related areas in the esophagus and duodenum. In Goodhart, R. S., and Shils, M. E. (eds.): Modern Nutrition in Health and Disease. Edition 6. Philadelphia, Lea and Febiger, 1980.

60. Broitman, S. A., and Zamcheck, N.: Nutrition in diseases of the intestines. In Goodhart, R. S., and Shils, M. E. (eds.): Modern Nutrition in Health and Disease. Edition 6. Philadelphia, Lea and Febiger, 1980.

61. Wright, H. K., and Tilson, M. D.: Postoperative Disorders of the Gastrointestinal Tract. New York, Grune and Stratton, 1973.

62. Russell, R. I.: Clinical aspects of alterations in bile acid metabolism—the wrong bile acids in the wrong place. Scot. Med. J., 18:146–151, 1973.

63. Lim, S. T., Choa, R. G., Lam, K. K., and Ong, G. B.: Total parenteral nutrition versus gastrostomy in the preoperative preparation of patients with carcinoma of the esophagus. Br. J. Surg., 68:69–72, 1981.

64. Moghissi, K., and Tensdale, P. R.: Parenteral feeding in patients with carcinoma of the esophagus treated with surgery: Energy and nitrogen requirements. J.P.E.N., 4:371–375, 1980.

65. Meguid, M. M., and Williams, L. F.: The use of gastrostomy to correct malnutrition. Surg. Gynecol. Obstet., 149:27–32, 1979.

66. Preshaw, R. M., Attiha, R. P., and Hollingsworth, W. J.: Randomized sequential trial of parenteral nutrition in healing of colonic anastomosis in man. Can. J. Surg., 22:437–439, 1979.

67. Wood, C. D.: Postoperative exercise capacity following nutritional support with hypotonic glucose. Surg. Gynecol. Obstet., 152:39–42, 1981.

68. Klidjian, A. M., Foster, K. J., Kammerling, R. M., et al.: Relation of anthropometric and dynamometric variables to serious postoperative complications. Br. J. Med., 281:899, 1980.

69. Harvey, K. B., Bothe, A., and Blackburn, G. L.: Nutritional assessment and patient outcome during oncological therapy. Cancer, 43:2065–2069, 1979.

70. Deitel, M., Alexander, M., and Hew, L. R.: Hyperalimentation and cancer. Can. J. Surg., 23:11–14, 1980.

71. Lanzotti, V. C., Copeland, E. M., George, S. L., et al.: Cancer chemotherapeutic response and intravenous hyperalimentation. Cancer Chemother. Rep., 59:437–439, 1975.

72. Douglass, H. O., Milliron, S., Nava, H., et al.: Elemental diet as an adjuvant for patients with locally advanced gastrointestinal cancer receiving

73. Copeland, E. M., Daly, J. M., and Dudrich, S. J.: Nutrition as an adjuvant to cancer treatment in the adult. Cancer Res., 37:2451–2456, 1977.

74. Haffejee, A. A., and Angorn, I. B.: Nutritional status and the nonspecific cellular and humoral response in esophageal carcinoma. Ann. Surg., 189:475–479, 1979.

75. Rocchio, M. A., Cha, C.-J.M., Haas, K. F., and Randall, H. T.: Use of chemically defined diets in the management of patients with high output gastrocutaneous fistulas. Am. J. Surg., 127:148–156, 1974.

76. Holter, A. R., Rosen, H. M., and Fischer, J. E.: The effects of hyperalimentation on major surgery in patients with malignant disease: A prospective study. Acta Chir. Scand. [Suppl.], 466:86–87, 1976.

77. Chandra, R. K.: Immunodeficiency in undernutrition and overnutrition. Nutr. Rev., 39:225–231, 1981.

78. Shils, M. E.: Enteral nutrition by tube. Cancer Res., 37:2432–2439, 1977.

79. Heymsfield, S. B., Bethel, R. A., Ansley, J. D., et al.: Enteral hyperalimentation: An alternative to central venous hyperalimentation. Ann. Intern. Med., 90:63–71, 1979.

80. Suskind, R. M., and Gordon, D.: The use of elemental diets in the cancer patient. In Van Eys, J., Seelig, M. S., and Nichols, B. L. (eds.): Nutrition and Cancer. New York, Spectrum Publications, 1979.

81. Johns, M. E.: The nutrition problem in head and neck cancer. Otolaryngol. Head Neck Surg., 88:691–694, 1980.

82. Noone, R. B., and Graham, W. P., III: Nutritional care after head and neck surgery. Postgrad. Med., 53(7):80–86, 1973.

83. Sobol, S. M., Conoyer, J. M., Zill, R., Thawley, S. E., and Ogura, J. H.: Nutritional concepts in the management of the head and neck cancer patient. Laryngoscope, 89:962–979, 1979.

84. Gormican, A., and Catli, E.: Nutritional and clinical responses of immobilized patients to a sterile milk-base feeding. J. Chron. Dis., 25:291–303, 1972.

85. Valdivieso, M.: A defined-formula diet as exclusive source of nutrition in patients with cancer (Commentary). In Shils, M. E. (ed.): Defined Formula Diets for Medical Purposes. Chicago, American Medical Association, 1977, pages 80–85.

86. Sobol, S. M., Conoyer, J. M., and Sessions, D. G.: Enteral and parenteral nutrition in patients with head and neck cancer. Ann. Otol. Rhinol. Laryngol., 88:495–501, 1979.

87. Jeffers, S. L., Debonis, D., and Meguid, M. M.: Management of enteral feedings. Contemp. Surg., 19:19–31, 1981.

88. Olivares, L., Segovia, A., and Revueltra, R.: Tube feeding and lethal aspiration in neurological patients: A review of 720 autopsy cases. Stroke, 5:654–656, 1974.

89. Howard, L., and Meguid, M. M.: Nutritional assessment in total parenteral nutrition. Clin. Lab. Med., 1:611–630, 1981.

90. Wollard, J.: Enteral and parenteral elemental nutrition. In Wollard, J. J. (ed.): Nutritional Man-

radiation therapy: A prospectively randomized study. J.P.E.N., 2:682–686, 1978.

agement of the Cancer Patient. New York, Raven Press, 1979.

91. Rombeau, J. L., and Barot, L. R.: Enteral nutritional therapy. Surg. Clin. North Am., *61*:605–620, 1981.

92. Dobbie, R. P., and Butterick, O. D., Jr.: Continuous pump/tube enteric hyperalimentation—Use in esophageal cancer. J.P.E.N., *1*:100–104, 1977.

93. Heymsfield, S. B., Horowitz, J., and Lawson, D. H.: Enteral hyperalimentation. *In* Berk, J. E. (ed.): Developments in Digestive Diseases. Philadelphia, Lea and Febiger, 1980.

94. Bush, J.: Cervical esophagostomy to provide nutrition. Am. J. Nurs., 107–109, 1979.

95. Graham, W. P., III, and Royster, H. P.: Simplified cervical esophagostomy for long-term extraoral feeding. Surg. Gynecol. Obstet., *125*:127–128, 1967.

96. Aguilar, N. V., Olson, M. L., and Shedd, D. P.: Rehabilitation of deglutition problems in patients with head and neck cancer. Am. J. Surg., *138*:501–507, 1979.

97. Noone, R. B., and Graham, W. P.: Cervical pharyngostomy for tube feeding. J.A.M.A., *216*:334, 1971.

98. Nissan, S., Bar-Maor, J. A., and Lernau, O.: Piriformostomy in the treatment of malignant tumors obstructing the esophagus. Isr. J. Med. Sci., *16*:682–683, 1980.

99. Meguid, M. M., and Williams, L. F.: The use of gastrostomy to correct malnutrition. Surg. Gynecol. Obstet., *149*:27–32, 1979.

100. Gross, R. E.: An Atlas of Children's Surgery. Philadelphia, W. B. Saunders Co., 1970, pages 12–13.

101. Shils, M. E., Bloch, A. S., and Chernoff, R.: Liquid formulas for oral and tube feeding. Clin. Bull., *6*:151–158, 1976.

102. Widiss, T., Hill, L. R., Meguid, M. M.: Aggressive home total enteral feeding program allows independence from hospital setting in stable advanced cancer patients. J.P.E.N., *4*:596, 1980.

103. Rains, B. L.: The non-hospitalized tube-fed patient. Oncol. Nurs. Forum, *8*(2):8–13, 1981.

104. Page, C. P., Ryan, J. A., and Haff, R. L.: Enteral catheter administration of an elemental diet. Surg. Gynecol. Obstet., *142*:184–188, 1976.

105. Weinsier, R. L., and Butterworth, C. E.: Handbook of Clinical Nutrition. St. Louis, C. V. Mosby, 1981, pp. 77–79.

106. Johnston, I. D. A., Wright, P. D., Lennard, T. W. J., Calgue, M. B., Carmichael, M. J., Francis, D. M. A., and Williams, R. H. P.: Malnutrition in cancer. Clin. Oncol., *7*:83–91, 1981.

107. Lim, S. T. K., Choa, R. G., Lam, K. H., Wong, J., and Ong, G. B.: Total parenteral nutrition versus gastrostomy in the preoperative preparation of patients with carcinoma of the esophagus. Br. J. Surg., *68*:69–72, 1981.

108. Crim, M. C., and Munro, H. N. *In* Present Knowledge in Nutrition. New York, Nutrition Foundation, 1976.

109. Young, V. R., and Scrimshaw, N. S.: Nutritional evaluation of proteins and protein requirements. *In* Milner, M., Scrimshaw, N. S., and Wang, D. I. C. (eds.): Protein Resources and Technology: Status and Research Needs. Westport, Connecticut, AVI Publishing, 1978.

110. Young, V. R., and Scrimshaw, N. S.: Human proteins and amino acid metabolism and require-ments in relation to protein quality. *In* Bodwell, C. E. (ed.): Evaluation of Proteins for Humans. Westport, Connecticut, AVI Publishing, 1977.

111. Inoue, G., Fujita, Y., and Niiyama, Y.: Studies on protein requirements of young men fed egg protein and rice protein with excess and maintenance energy intake. J. Nutr., *103*:1673, 1973.

112. Young, V. R., Taylor, Y. S., Rand, W. M., and Scrimshaw, N. S.: Protein requirements of man: Efficiency of egg protein utilization at maintenance and submaintenance levels in young men. J. Nutr., *103*:1164, 1973.

113. Harper, A. E.: Amino acid requirements. *In* Munro, H. N. (ed.): Mammalian Protein Metabolism, Vol. 2. New York, Academic Press, 1964, page 87.

114. Pastel, D., Anderson, G. H., and Jeejeebhoy, K. N.: Amino acid adequacy for parenteral casein hydrolysate and oral cottage cheese in patients with gastrointestinal disease, as measured by nitrogen balance and blood aminogram. Gastroenterology, *65*:427–437, 1973.

115. Lorincz, A. B., Kutner, R. E., and Brandt, M. B.: Tumor response to phenylalanine-tyrosine-limited diets. J. Am. Diet. Assoc., *54*:198–205, 1969.

116. Demopoulos, H. B.: Effects of reducing the phenylalanine-tyrosine intake of patients with advanced malignant melanoma. Cancer, *19*:657–664, 1966.

117. Abell, C. W., Hodgins, D. S., and Stith, W. J.: An *in vivo* evaluation of the chemotherapeutic potency of phenylalanine ammonia-lyase. Cancer Res., *33*:2529–2532, 1973.

118. Theuer, R. C.: Effects of essential amino acid restriction on the growth of female C57BL mice and their implanted BW10232 adenocarcinomas. J. Nutr., *101*:223–232, 1971.

119. Jose, D. G., and Good, R. A.: Quantitative effects of nutritional essential amino acid deficiency upon immune responses to tumors in mice. J. Exp. Med., *137*:1–9, 1973.

120. Bloch, A. S., and Shils, M. E.: Appendix. *In* Goodhart, R. S., and Shils, M. E. (eds.): Modern Nutrition in Health and Disease. Edition 6. Philadelphia, Lea and Febiger, 1980.

121. Kare, M. R., and Maller, O. (eds.): The Chemical Senses and Nutrition. New York, Academic Press, 1977.

122. DeWys, W. D., and Walters, K.: Abnormalities of taste sensation in cancer patients. Cancer, *36*:1888–1896, 1975.

123. Vickers, Z. M., Nielson, S. S., and Theologides, A.: Food preferences of patients with cancer. J. Am. Diet. Assoc., *79*:443, 1981.

124. DeWys, W. D., and Herbst, S. A.: Oral feeding in the nutritional management of the cancer patient. Cancer Res., *37*:2429–2431, 1977.

125. Hoffman, P. K.: Nutritional rehabilitation: A modality of behavior modification. *In* Wollard, J. J. (ed.): Nutritional Management of the Cancer Patient, New York, Raven Press, 1979.

126. Selig, D. E.: Nutritional supplementation. *In* Wollard, J. J. (ed.): Nutritional Management of the Cancer Patient. New York, Raven Press, 1979.

127. Aker, S., and Lenssea, P.: A Guide to Good Nutrition During and After Chemotherapy and Radiation. Seattle, Washington, Fred Hutchinson Cancer Research Center, 1979.

128. Rosenbaum, E. H., Stitt, C. A., Drasin, H., and Rosenbaun, I. R.: Health Through Nutrition: A

Comprehensive Guide for the Cancer Patient. San Francisco, Alchemy Books, 1977.

129. Eating Hints: Recipes and Tips for Better Nutrition During Treatment. NIH Publication No. 80-2079. Bethesda, Maryland, National Cancer Institute, 1980.

130. Pareira, M. D., Conrad, E. J., Hicks, W., and Elman, R.: Therapeutic nutrition with tube feeding. J.A.M.A., *156*:810–816, 1954.

131. Pareira, M. D., Conrad, E. J., Hicks, W., and Elman, R.: Clinical response and changes in nitrogen balance, body weight, plasma proteins and changes in nitrogen balance, body weight, plasma proteins, and hemoglobin following tube feeding in cancer cachexia. Cancer, *8*:803–808, 1955.

132. Peden, J. C., Jr., Bond, L. F., and Maxwell, M.: Comparative protein repletion in cancer and non-cancer cachexia: With special reference to changes in blood volume and total circulating plasma protein and hemoglobin. Am. J. Clin. Nutr., *5*:305–315, 1957.

133. Terepka, A. R., and Waterhouse, C.: Metabolic observations during forced feeding of patients with cancer. Am. J. Med., *20*:225–238, 1956.

134. Valerio, D., Overett, L., Malcolm, O., and Blackburn, G. L.: Nutritional support for cancer patients receiving abdominal and pelvic radiotherapy: A randomized prospective clinical experiment of intravenous versus oral feeding. Surg. Forum, *29*:145–148, 1978.

135. Rickard, K. A., Kirksey, A., Baehner, R. L., Grosfeld, J. L., Provisor, A., Weetman, R. M., Boxer, L. A., and Ballantine, T. V. N.: Effectiveness of enteral and parenteral nutrition in the nutritional management of children with Wilms' tumor. Am. J. Clin. Nutr., *33*:2622–2629, 1980.

136. Harvey, K. B., Bothe, A., Jr., and Blackburn, G. L.: Nutritional assessment and patient outcome during oncologic therapy. Cancer, *43*:2065–2069, 1979.

137. Skidmore, F. D., Tweedle, D. E. F., Gleave, E. N., Gowland, E., and Knass, D. A.: Abnormal liver function during nutritional support in postoperative cancer patients. Ann. R. Coll. Surg. (Engl.), *61*:183–188, 1979.

138. Sako, K., Lore, J. M., Kaufman, S., Razack, M. S., Bakamjiam, V., and Reese, P.: Parenteral hyperalimentation in surgical patients with head and neck cancer: A randomized study. J. Surg. Oncol., *16*:391–402, 1981.

139. Loh, K. K., Isamasu, M. S., Melish, J., et al.: Enteral hyperalimentation in the treatment of malnourished cancer patients. Proc. Am. Soc. Clin. Oncol., *20*:301, 1979.

140. Douglass, H. O., Jr., Milliron, S., Nava, H., et al.: Randomized assessment of an elemental supplement as an adjuvant to abdominal radiotherapy in patients with gastrointestinal cancer. J.P.E.N., *1*:3A, 1977.

141. Smith, J. L., Arteaga, C., and Heymsfield, S. B.: Increased ureagenesis and impaired nitrogen use during infusion of a synthetic amino acid formula: A controlled trial. N. Engl. J. Med., *306*:1013–1018, 1982.

142. McLaren, D. S., and Meguid, M. M.: Nutritional assessment at the crossroads. J.P.E.N., *7*:575–579, 1983.

CHAPTER 20

Enteral Nutrition and Gastrointestinal Disease

JAMES BETZHOLD
LYN HOWARD

Abnormalities of nutrient absorption and assimilation are seen with many disorders of the gastrointestinal tract. It is imperative that the patient's nutritional status be maintained while treatment is under way. In some conditions enteral feeds will seem to exacerbate the underlying disease process, and a period of "bowel rest" is recommended. The use of total parenteral nutrition (TPN) has enabled physicians to better assess the benefits of bowel rest without further compromising nutritional status. The body responds differently to the delivery of nutrients by the parenteral route compared with the enteral route. Additionally, although TPN has become a relatively safe means of nutritional support, it still has a higher incidence of complications than enteral feeding, and is significantly more expensive. This chapter will attempt to assess the usefulness of enteral feedings in a wide range of gastrointestinal disorders. Three separate issues will be addressed: the role of enteral nutrition in the acceleration of healing and adaptation in the compromised gut; the evidence that modified diets may extend the benefits of enteral feeding in gastrointestinal disorders; and the data showing potential aggravation of gastrointestinal inflammation or damage by enteral feeding.

ENTERAL FEEDING AND THE ACCELERATION OF HEALING AND ADAPTATION OF THE GASTROINTESTINAL TRACT

The functional absorptive capacity of the gut depends upon the total number of villi, the number of cells per villus, and the maturational state of these epithelial cells.[1]

The number of functional epithelial cells is in turn determined by their life span and the proliferative capacity of the crypt cells. A change in any of these parameters will alter the functional capacity of the small intestine. An increase in DNA synthesis indicates an actual increase in cell number, or hyperplasia, whereas an increase in RNA synthesis relative to DNA reflects cell enlargement, or hypertrophy.

Small bowel resection in man and animals is followed by compensatory changes in the remaining gastrointestinal tract (Fig. 20–1). The changes consist of an increase in: (1) the diameter and mucosal weight of the residual bowel;[2–5] (2) the size of remaining villi,[2, 3, 5, 6] and the number of epithelial cells per villus;[3, 5, 6] (3) the size of the crypt proliferative zone and rate of migration;[3, 6] (4) the rate of epithelial cell turnover;[3] and (5) the absorptive capacity per centimeter of remaining gut for various nutrients.[7–11]

As a result of these changes the efficiency of nutrient absorption increases per centimeter of bowel length, but conversely absorption per individual mucosal cell may be less than normal, presumably because of a rapid migration of less mature cells.[5, 7, 12] DNA synthesis in crypt cells increases within a few days of bowel resection,[3, 13] suggesting that hyperplasia and other adaptive changes begin very rapidly.

Absorptive capacity for most nutrients shows a proximal-distal gradient.[5] The ileum has a greater adaptive potential, as shown by a greater increase in villus height and absorption of nutrients in residual ileum following a proximal resection, compared with the same indices in residual jejunum following a distal resection.[4, 5] In fact, compensatory bowel growth is so great that in a rat, a

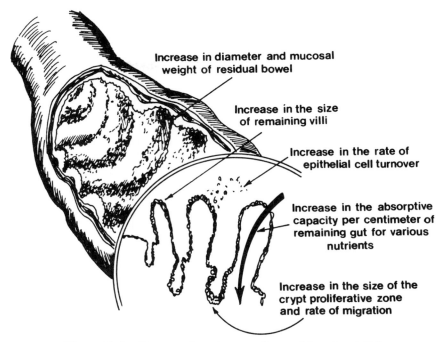

Increase in diameter and mucosal weight of residual bowel

Increase in the size of remaining villi

Increase in the rate of epithelial cell turnover

Increase in the absorptive capacity per centimeter of remaining gut for various nutrients

Increase in the size of the crypt proliferative zone and rate of migration

Figure 20–1. Compensatory changes after small bowel resection.

50 per cent proximal resection results in a total intestinal weight nine weeks later which is not significantly different from that of a sham-operated control.[4, 14] It has also been shown that residual ileal epithelial cells change their cell surface glycoprotein composition to one more characteristic of jejunal epithelial cells,[15] reflecting the fact that the adapted ileum has developed the greater absorptive capacity of the jejunum while incorporating the specialized functions of the ileum (B_{12}, bile salt absorption).

The ultimate usefulness of bowel rest as a therapeutic modality is based on the assumption that the exclusion of nutrients and secretions from the bowel is less deleterious to the underlying disease process than their continued presence. A period of bowel rest without other means of nutritional support will rapidly lead to disaccharidase deficiencies as well as diminished absorption of peptides and amino acids.[16] Similar changes may be seen in the excluded limb created by a jejunoileal bypass or Thiry-Vella fistula.[17, 18]

Levine and others have conclusively demonstrated the superiority of enteral versus parenteral feeding in the maintenance of gastrointestinal function.[19] Rats maintained on TPN for seven days show significant decreases in intestinal weight, mucosal weight,

protein and DNA content, a decrease in villus height, and a marked diminution of disaccharidase activity compared with rats fed isocaloric amounts of the same formula intragastrically. Parenterally nourished rats have fewer proliferating crypt cells than orally fed controls. They do, however, develop an increase in length of microvillus,[20] suggesting hypertrophy of existing absorptive cells.

The effect of enteral and parenteral diets on epithelial cell kinetics has not been well defined. In general, in all segments of the small intestine, enteral diets promote an acceleration in the rate of proliferation and migration of epithelial cells when compared with TPN.[21] The relationship between villus height and epithelial renewal kinetics is likewise complex. The greater villus height in parenterally fed animals may reflect the absence of mechanical abrasion by luminal contents.

The complexity of the diet has a further effect on intestinal mucosal mass. In the rat an elemental diet does not maintain body weight, mucosal weight, or DNA or protein content per segment as well as does the isocaloric quantity of rat chow;[22–24] on the other hand, the elemental diet is more effective than the same diet delivered parenterally.[22, 25, 26] In these studies the elemental diet had a lower protein content than rat chow, which may have explained some of the observed differences.

There are few data on the site of maximum protein uptake (villus or crypt cells) when the nutrient is administered by enteral versus parenteral routes. Alpers concluded that the route of administration of precursor amino acids is important in determining which portion of the villus unit takes up the label for protein synthesis.[27] L-leucine infused intravenously is incorporated into cells near the villus-crypt junction, while enteral administration is followed by heavy uptake near the villus tip. In fact intraluminal L-leucine is preferentially utilized for local protein synthesis when compared with that given intravenously.[27] This may help to explain the rapid decline in intestinal mucosal weight following several days of fasting. Sims et al. have shown that total body protein synthesis is greater when isonitrogenous isocaloric diets are given enterally rather than parenterally.[28] This probably reflects the greater stimulus to gut protein synthesis from the intraluminal route.

In 1971 Wilmore et al.[29] demonstrated a critical role for TPN during the early phases of short bowel adaptation, when oral diets induce massive diarrhea and loss of nutrients. Beagle pups with resection of 90 to 95 per cent of the small bowel had a much better chance of growth and survival if fed intravenously for a month compared with chow-fed beagle controls with resected small bowels. After one month the dogs being given TPN were successfully transferred to dog chow and at one year these dogs had intestinal weights and villus heights comparable to those of the surviving controls that were fed dog chow.

While this study and subsequent experience with patients emphasize the importance of TPN in the acute adaptive phase of short bowel management,[30–33] there are considerable data showing that enteral feeding accelerates adaptation in the resected bowel, just as it prevents the atrophy associated with bowel rest.

Levine et al.[34] demonstrated hyperplastic changes in the proximal and distal small bowel in enterally fed rats following a proximal resection, but no changes were seen in animals supported by TPN. Feldman et al.[35] corroborated these findings in dogs undergoing resection of 50 per cent of the jejunum, and noted enhanced ileal glucose absorption in enterally fed animals. In moderate jejunal resections (50 per cent),[24] macromolecular diets enhance postresectional hyperplasia to a greater extent than elemental diets. In more extreme resections (85 per cent),[36] both diets appear to be equally well absorbed. The role of early enteral nutrition following truly massive (90 to 95 per cent) small bowel resection is unclear. Studies to date demonstrating the importance of early enteral feedings have used animals undergoing lesser degrees of resection.[34, 35]

The next question is by what mechanism does enteral nutrition exert maximal bowel adaptation? Recent animal studies suggest that luminal nutrients exert this effect by one of at least three different mechanisms: tropic effects of hormones released during the digestive process, neurovascular mechanisms, and the greater dependence of gut mucosa on luminal nutrients rather than blood-borne nutrients.

Hormonal Factors

Tilson, in 1971, showed that villus hyperplasia occurred in a rat whose parabiotically joined twin was subjected to a resection of 75 per cent of the proximal small bowel.[37] Further evidence for a hormonal influence on bowel hyperplasia derives from studies using Thiry-Vella fistulas, which are isolated bowel segments with intact blood supplies. Significant bowel resection leads to villus hyperplasia in the fistula.[18, 38] Similar changes have been noted in excluded segments of bowel in animals and humans with a jejunoileal bypass.[39, 40] The literature on this point tends to suggest conflicting conclusions. Certainly there has to be a significant bowel resection to stimulate a hyperplastic response in the contiguous and bypassed segments,[18] and clearly enteral feeding is superior to parenteral feeding,[38, 40] indicating that any hormonal stimulus is best released by enteral nutrients. Studies that have shown no hyperplasia in excluded segments, or even hypoplasia, have either not involved a major resection[17, 18, 41] or have been associated with significant weight loss (patients with jejunoileal bypass) in which many components of body cell mass are depleted.[42]

It is difficult to sort out a hormonal effect from a possible tropic effect of nonhormonal enteric secretions (gastric acid, bile, pancreatic juice) or increased stimulation resulting from greater adaptive nutrient intake and hence greater nutrient availability for mucosal growth. The fact that hypertonic dextrose, which does not stimulate pancreaticobiliary secretions,[43] will induce both proximal and distal hyperplasia when infused directly into the ileum[44] strongly argues for an important hormonal influence.

A tropic influence on the bowel has been credited to many of the gut hormones. The data ascribing an influence to the different gut hormones will now be briefly reviewed.

Gastrin. Many studies point to gastrin as the major hormone that induces tropic effects in the gastrointestinal tract. Antrectomy, and hence resection of the major site of gastrin production, leads to atrophy of the oxyntic cell mucosa,[45] an effect that can be lessened by the simultaneous infusion of pentagastrin.[45] Patients with the Zollinger-Ellison syndrome, characterized by high serum levels of gastrin and increased secretion of gastric acid, may have hypertrophy of the gastric mucosa.[46]

Hypergastrinemia and increased gastric acid secretion are regularly seen following resection of the small bowel,[47–50] especially after removal of the jejunum.[47] Whether the hypergastrinemia is the result of increased production, decreased catabolism by the shortened bowel, or lack of an inhibitory substance elaborated by the small intestine remains to be established.

Exogenously administered pentagastrin will prevent the gastric and duodenal atrophy that occur in starved rats or in animals maintained on TPN.[51–53] This effect is not caused by the stimulatory effect of pentagastrin on gastric acid secretion, since histamine, which increases acid output without affecting serum gastrin levels, has no such tropic effect.[53] While gastrin appears to be important for maintenance of exocrine pancreatic function[53, 54] and gastric and duodenal mucosal mass following antral resection or starvation, its influence on small bowel hyperplasia following intestinal resection appears to be rather modest. Gastrin has some effect on duodenal hyperplasia but almost no effect on jejunal or ileal adaptation.[55, 56] In the jejunectomized rat, antrectomy does not influence ileal DNA synthesis.[57]

A number of studies have pointed to the fact that elemental diets support mucosal mass less effectively than standard diets,[21–23] and at the same time elemental diets cause a significant decrease in serum and antral gastrin levels.[58] These investigators conclude that the difference in gastrin stimulation may demonstrate the importance of this hormone for bowel adaptation. It should be recognized, however, that in these studies the diets were not isonitrogenous, and protein availability may have been the real limiting factor, restricting bowel hyperplasia.

In a series of studies of rats, Oscarson et al. altered serum gastrin levels by doing a vagotomy, vagotomy and pyloroplasty, antrectomy, or fundectomy in rats with a small bowel resection or a sham procedure.[59] There was no correlation between indices of hyperplasia and serum gastrin levels. The various gastric operations in the sham-operated animals caused profound differences in serum gastrin levels without any effect on villus height or crypt depth. Conversely, resection led to an increase in villus height and crypt death but did not correlate with serum gastrin levels. Starvation atrophy was not prevented by high levels of circulating gastrin. Tilson and colleagues have corroborated these findings in similar experiments.[60]

Johnson has proposed a role for intraluminal gastrin in enhancing mucosal growth.[61] Pharmacologic doses of gastrin infused into the rat ileum result in hyperplastic changes distally and proximal to the site of infusion. There were no changes in the duodenum, suggesting that the gastrin was not absorbed to a significant extent. Gastrin infused directly into the stomach was not followed by small bowel hyperplasia; in fact, it was rapidly destroyed. The relevance of these pharmacologic doses to physiologic bowel adaptation is not clear.

In summary, gastrin is probably an important hormone in the maintenance of gastrointestinal mucosal mass. It may have a minor role in the stomach and duodenum in promoting adaptive changes following small bowel resection, but does not appear to exert a major influence on jejunal or ileal adaptation.

Cholecystokinin. Cholecystokinin (CCK) and gastrin share common structural components. CCK is a strong stimulus to emptying of the gallbladder and a weak enhancer of gastric acid secretion, whereas gastrin exhibits the opposite effects. Johnson et al. showed that CCK exerts weak tropic influences on the stomach and duodenum.[62] CCK infused together with secretin prevented the hypoplasia and atrophy of the small bowel that occurred in parenterally alimented animals.[63, 64] Likewise, CCK stimulated absorption of galactose from the gut while TPN decreased it.[63] CCK-secretin infusions also prevent pancreatic atrophy in animals.[62]

As with gastrin, CCK may partly explain bowel hyperplasia but is not the total explanation. Weser et al. recently showed that rats with resected bowels maintained on TPN demonstrated greater hyperplasia of the small bowel when infused with octapeptide-CCK.[64] Since the hyperplastic response was even greater with intragastric feeding of rat chow,[64] CCK stimulation was not the only important difference. Hyperplasia of the small bowel promoted by CCK-secretin infusions is peculiar in that there is a partial loss of the normal proximal-distal gradient.[64] Secretin, by itself, appears to have no primary tropic effect on small bowel mucosa and may even antagonize the tropic actions of pentagastrin.[65]

Enteroglucagon. Gleeson in 1971 described a patient with a glucagon-secreting tumor.[66] Enlargement of intestinal villi developed. No studies were done to further define these changes. Serum enteroglucagon levels have recently been shown to correlate with rate of production of ileal crypt cells in a group of enterectomized rats fed by either enteral or parenteral techniques.[67] Further studies are needed to clarify a possible tropic role of enteroglucagon.

Neurovascular Influence

Vagotomy in the dog and rat leads to decreased mucosal thickness in the stomach and small bowel.[68, 69] The effect of vagotomy on food intake or volume of pancreatic secretions was not investigated. Touloukian and Spencer,[70] using the radio-rubidium distribution technique in the enterectomized rat, found increased mucosal blood flow in the ileal remnant coincident with the hyperplastic phase. These changes were not seen in the jejunal remnant, in which compensatory changes were negligible.

Luminal Influences

The proximal-distal gradient of gastrointestinal mucosal mass and enzyme activity suggest the concept of direct stimulation of

mucosal growth by luminal contents. This could reflect stimulation of pancreaticobiliary secretions or the influence of greater availability of luminal nutrients.

In 1967 Dowling and Booth reported an increase in ileal villus height and segmental glucose absorption following jejunoileal transposition,[2] but noted no histologic changes in the transplanted jejunum. Altmann and Leblond confirmed these findings in the transplanted ileum[71] but noted a decrease in the size of villi in the transplanted jejunum. Several investigators have confirmed these findings.[41, 72] Transplantation of a segment of duodenum containing the ampulla of Vater to the ileum stimulates hyperplasia of the ileal villus,[71, 73] and has also been shown to augment the distal adaptational changes seen after proximal resection.[74] When isolated pancreatic or biliary secretions are delivered through the transplanted ampulla of Vater, it is the pancreatic secretions that have a more significant effect on hyperplastic changes.[73] Interestingly, Altmann transplanted duodenum into the distal small bowel without the ampulla of Vater and showed a hyperplastic ileal response, suggesting a direct tropic influence of duodenal mucosa.[71]

Roy et al. demonstrated a decrease in proliferative pool size and rate of shedding of epithelial cells from ileal villi of rats undergoing biliary diversion, changes that were reversed by intragastric infusion of sodium taurocholate.[75] Conversely, ligation of the common bile duct will reduce but not eliminate hyperplasia following small bowel resection.[76] Thus, pancreatic and biliary secretions play a major role in the adaptational responses of the gastrointestinal tract, but other factors are also contributory. It may be the stimulation of these secretions that account for the greater adaptive response of macromolecular diets as compared with elemental diets.[22-24]

Recent animal studies suggest that luminal nutrients contribute directly to the maintenance of gastrointestinal mucosal mass. The normal proximal-distal gradient of intestinal absorptive capacity and enzyme activity may best be ascribed to the concentration of luminal nutrients presented to the bowel mucosa. Small bowel resection would expose more distally located villi to higher concentrations of nutrients with resultant hyperplasia.

It is well known that sucrase and maltase activities are profoundly influenced by the dietary content of sucrose and maltose.[77, 78] Glucose in the diet can also mildly enhance these two enzymes.[79] Lactose, on the other hand, does not appear to induce lactase in man.[77, 78] The significance of any enzyme induction in overall carbohydrate absorption is not clear, since only lactase appears to be a rate-limiting step. As mentioned earlier, bowel resection is followed by increased disaccharidase activity per unit length of gut with increased carbohydrate absorption,[2] even though there is a decreased disaccharidase-specific activity per gram of tissue,[5] reflecting immaturity of the hyperplastic villi.

Rodgers and Bochenek[80] reported an increase in the ileal activities of fatty acid CoA lipase and acyl CoA monoglyceride acyltransferase, two key enzymes in lipid re-esterification, after jejunectomy. There was an increase in enzyme activity per unit length, as well as per gram of tissue (indicating increased specific activity). Balint et al.[81] expanded on this study and showed that a diet high in fat induces more efficient absorption of triglyceride. Thus mid small bowel can show an increase in the coefficient of fat absorption from 89 per cent on ordinary rat chow (4 per cent fat by weight) to 98 per cent after four weeks on a high (45 per cent) fat diet. They noted increased dry weight of the distal jejunum and proximal ileum, but no change in DNA content, so they ascribed these changes to hypertrophy rather than to hyperplasia of the small bowel.

There is no active pathway for the de novo synthesis of purine nucleotides in the small bowel of the rat.[82] A diet containing purine will cause an increase in intestinal activity of hypoxanthine-guanine phosphoribosyl transferase, a key enzyme in the salvage pathways for purines, compared with an otherwise identical, purine-free diet. This effect was unique to the small intestine, and it was suggested that this salvage might be essential for optimal RNA synthesis and cell turnover in the bowel mucosa.

The possible importance of non-nutritive bulk was investigated by Ecknauer and colleagues in unoperated rats.[83] Rats fed chow were compared with rats receiving an elemental diet with or without added cellulose in isocaloric quantities. The chow-fed animals demonstrated greater body weights and greater villus height and crypt depth (especially proximally) than either elemental diet group. In comparing the two groups fed elemental diets there was an increase in number of mitoses per crypt in the group receiving bulk, perhaps stimulated by cell loss from mechanical trauma. Villi were shortened and broadened by the addition of bulk, but there was no change in cell number.

In animal studies, elemental diets do not support intestinal mucosal mass "as effectively" as more complex diets.[21-23] Several hypotheses have been suggested. As previously alluded to, elemental diets have a lower protein content than do standard animal diets.[23] Most investigators infuse elemental diets directly into the stomach, whereas standard diets are taken by mouth Bypassing the cephalic phase of digestion may have a deleterious effect on secretion of gastric acid,[84, 85] but this is by no means clear. Other authors have suggested that elemental diets may be absorbed over a shorter length of intestine or cause less stimulation of biliary and pancreatic secretions. These issues will be addressed later in this chapter, but briefly, there is little evidence to support either contention.

In summary, oral nutrition is essential for maintenance of normal gut mass and absorptive capacity. Although parenteral nutrition is a life-saving intervention in patients with massive resection of the small bowel and can prevent development of malnutrition, the data would suggest that constant exposure of the remaining intestine to luminal nutrients will allow maximal adaptation to take place. The relative contributions of hormonal, vascular, pancreaticobiliary, or direct nutrient mechanisms remain to be clarified. Further studies are also needed to determine what form of nutrient components are most effective.

Finally, most of the studies cited above were performed in animals. It has been suggested that human subjects are more resistant than laboratory animals to bowel atrophy occurring during TPN.[86]

CAN MODIFIED DIETS EXTEND THE BENEFITS OF ENTERAL FEEDING IN GASTROINTESTINAL DISORDERS?

Carbohydrate Modified Diets

Carbohydrate intolerance is a common occurrence during an episode of infectious gastroenteritis. Bacterial or viral invasion results in widespread epithelial cell damage, with reductions in all disaccharidases but especially lactase. Seventy-seven per cent of a large series of infants with diarrhea studied by Lifshitz and coworkers were lactose intolerant.[87] Severe intolerance was associated with prolongation of symptoms when patients were kept on a lactose-containing diet. The use of a lactose-free formula resulted in significant improvement in the diarrhea. If intolerance to other disaccharides develops,[88] substitution of a formula containing glucose or glucose polymer may be beneficial.

Fat Modified Diets

Intestinal lymphangiectasia is a protein-losing enteropathy resulting from an abnormality in lymphatic drainage. Intestinal lacteals swell and eventually rupture, with spillage of triglyceride-rich material into the intestinal lumen resulting in steatorrhea. A diet containing normal amounts of fat is soon followed by diarrhea, hypoproteinemia, and edema. A fat-free diet results in a decrease in fecal fat, increased albumin half-life, and improvement in biochemical parameters.[89, 90] Medium-chain triglycerides, which are absorbed directly into the portal system and do not utilize the lymphatic system, have also resulted in clinical remission when used as the main source of fat in the diet.[91]

Protein Modified Diets

Gluten-sensitive enteropathy is a malabsorptive disorder resulting from a toxic reaction to gliadin, a component of dietary gluten. Gluten is contained in wheat, oats, rye, and barley. Histologically in gluten-sensitive enteropathy there is patchy or diffuse mucosal damage with atrophy of villi and hypertrophy of crypts. Elimination of gluten from the diet usually leads to a sustained clinical remission. A transient intolerance to foods containing gluten occasionally occurs secondary to mucosal damage caused by cow's milk or acute gastroenteritis.[92, 93] It is not known if a gluten-free diet during acute bouts of diarrhea would prevent this condi-

tion from developing. These temporary disturbances in gluten tolerance may explain why some children with postinfectious chronic diarrhea improve on gluten-free diets but show no evidence of gliadin sensitivity when rechallenged several months later.

Adverse reactions to protein components of cow's milk occur in 0.1 to 8 per cent of all infants.[94] These reactions generally present in one of three manners: milk-induced colitis, malabsorption syndrome with chronic diarrhea and mucosal changes, and allergic gastroenteropathy. Symptoms of vomiting and diarrhea subside upon removal of the offending cow's milk antigen. The defect in the malabsorptive syndrome is probably IgG-mediated, and is generally outgrown by two to three years of age. Allergic gastroenteropathy is a lifelong IgE-mediated hypersensitivity to cow's milk protein.

Nutritional support in patients with cirrhosis of the liver is often hindered by protein intolerance and the development of hepatic encephalopathy. Traditional management includes protein restriction, although an intake of less than 40 gm/day causes negative nitrogen balance and limits any potential for hepatic healing.

Clinical severity of hepatic encephalopathy does not correlate well with plasma ammonia levels. Fischer et al. have described characteristic alterations in plasma and cerebrospinal fluid levels of certain amino acids.[95] Levels of aromatic amino acids, namely phenylalanine, tyrosine, and tryptophan, increase, whereas concentrations of the branched chain amino acids, valine, leucine, and isoleucine, fall. Levels of cerebrospinal fluid tryptophan and tyrosine can be markedly elevated even when plasma levels are normal.[96] High levels of tryptophan in the central nervous system lead to an increased production of serotonin, an inhibitory neurotransmitter. Tyrosine is a precursor for the putative adrenergic neurotransmitters, norepinephrine and dopamine. Although tyrosine is normally metabolized to catecholamines, if it accumulates in large amounts it is preferentially metabolized to octopamine, a known false neurotransmitter.[97]

The rate of transport across the blood-brain barrier of all neutral amino acids is increased in encephalopathic rats.[98] This effect may be mediated by increased plama ammonia levels, indirectly implicating the liver as an important determinant of amino acid uptake in the central nervous system.[98]

Since branched-chain amino acids and aromatic amino acids compete for the same transport system in the brain, Fischer et al. have suggested that normalization of plasma amino acid concentrations with intravenous amino acid solutions high in branched-chain amino acids and low in aromatic amino acids could normalize the encephalopathic profile and competitively inhibit brain uptake of aromatic amino acids, leading to increases in concentration of octopamine and serotonin in cerebrospinal fluid.[99] These investigators infused such a solution parenterally into a group of patients with chronic hepatic encephalopathy and improved the plasma amino acid pattern.[99] Clinical improvement was coincident with increases in plasma levels of branched-chain amino acids. Further work showed that infusions of branched-chain amino acids not only prevent the ammonia-induced uptake of aromatic amino acids in the central nervous system, but also enhance their clearance from the brain.[100] Standard amino acid solutions do not have this effect. Maddrey et al.[101] noted clinical improvement in 8 of 11 encephalopathic patients treated with oral or parenteral ketoanalogs of branched-chain amino acids plus methionine and phenylalanine; again the improvement was coincident with normalization of the plasma amino acid patterns. Freund and coworkers[102] reported a case of a 53-year-old man with chronic hepatic encephalopathy who was managed for several years with a 20-gm protein diet supplemented by a formula enriched with branched-chain amino acids; his mental status improved while on this regimen. Herlong et al.[103] in a controlled, double-blind crossover study noted clinical improvement in encephalopathic patients using ornithine salts of branched-chain amino acids, or branch-chain amino acids themselves compared with calcium salts of branched-chain amino acids or ornithine alpha-ketoglutarate. In another controlled study Michel and coworkers[104] found no benefit in using a solution rich in branched-chain amino acids compared with standard TPN solution in encephalopathic patients.

Most of the studies reporting clinical improvement used enteral formulas enriched with branched-chain amino acids, while the negative reports utilized parenteral infusions. More studies are required before these enriched formulas can be clearly recommended.

Gastrointestinal Disorders That May Benefit from Diets Modified in Several Aspects

Short Bowel Syndrome. Patients with insufficient surface area for absorption as a result of prior resections have abnormal stool losses of dietary carbohydrate, protein, and fat. Depending on the site and extent of resection, malabsorption of iron, fat-soluble vitamins (A, D, E, and K), folate, vitamin B_{12} (and other water-soluble vitamins), and bile salts may occur. A negative balance of the divalent cations calcium, magnesium, zinc, and copper may result from inadequate absorptive surface area and the formation of insoluble soaps with unabsorbed fat in the intestine.[105, 106] Unabsorbed fatty acids will induce a secretory diarrhea in the colon with loss of sodium, potassium, bicarbonate, and chloride.[107] Continued losses of nutrients leads to a compromised nutritional status with its attendant increase in morbidity.

The contribution of parenteral nutrition to the early management of short bowel syndrome and the importance of continued exposure of the gastrointestinal tract to luminal nutrients have already been discussed. Controversy still exists about the most appropriate dietary formulation to use. Ideally, a dietary preparation in a patient with short bowel syndrome should be absorbed as rapidly as possible and over a minimum of surface area. It should also provide a strong tropic stimulus to hasten adaptation. Unfortunately, no consensus has been reached as to the optimal diet.

In the normal individual, protein hydrolysis is not the rate-limiting step in its absorption. In the 1960s, investigators fed ^{15}N-labeled protein or isonitrogenous amounts of a hydrolysate of the same protein, and found appearance of the label in blood equally rapidly in both groups.[108] Other studies performed during the same period confirmed that in normal individuals absorption of protein is generally complete within the first 100 cm of jejunum, and showed that gastric emptying is the rate-limiting step.[109, 110] Adibi, in a more recent study, found whole and partially digested protein in the ileum four hours after ingestion of a meal containing bovine serum albumin.[111] No proteins or amino acids were found after a second, protein-free meal, suggesting that endogenously derived secretions were not the source of the protein found in the ileum. Chung et al.[112] using larger, more physiologic amounts of protein than earlier studies, sampled from three sites throughout the intestine. Sixty per cent of the ingested protein was absorbed before it reached the proximal jejunum, and no whole protein was seen in the distal ileum. Since some whole protein was found in the proximal ileum, it seems likely that the ileum does have a role in protein digestion and absorption. In essence, although most protein absorption occurs proximally, longer segments of bowel may be required for complete uptake.

Recent data suggest that protein absorption occurs predominantly by intact dipeptide and tripeptide absorption with subsequent intracellular hydrolysis rather than by uptake of free amino acids.[113–115] It is not known if a protein hydrolysate is absorbed over a shorter span of intestine than solid protein foods or amino acids. In dogs, solid food is not emptied from the stomach until food particles reach a size of less than 1 mm, and so normal food would probably be released and absorbed more slowly than elemental diets.[116] There are no data available comparing the length of intestine over which solid foods and elemental diets are absorbed. Experiments comparing the absorption of protein hydrolysates to isonitrogenous amino acid diets utilize techniques of intestinal perfusion that bypass the gastric phase of digestion.[117, 118] Adibi et al. have concluded that perfused amino acids are almost completely absorbed 25 cm beyond the ligament of Treitz.[117] Hecketsweiler et al. infused Vivonex or crushed food at the ligament of Treitz in human volunteers.[119] There was an increased percentage of glucose absorbed from the crushed food at 35, 70, and 105 cm distally, but no difference in the percentage of nitrogen absorbed. However, since the protein content of the crushed food was much higher than in the Vivonex, the absolute amount of nitrogen absorbed was significantly more from the crushed food. Silk and colleagues[118] perfused hydrolysates of casein and lactalbumin at the ligament of Treitz in volunteers and compared absorption of protein hydrolysate over 30 cm with that from an isonitrogenous mixture of component amino acids. His study showed greater absorption of nitrogen from the hydrolysates. Since the effects of the stomach on secretion, rate of gastric emptying, and transit time were bypassed, no firm conclusions can be reached about the relative superiority of intragastrically administered diets containing whole proteins, peptides, or amino acids in the patient with short bowel syndrome.

Ruppin et al. recently evaluated the effect of varying the carbohydrate composition of the diet on carbohydrate absorption.[120] A liquid diet was tested, using 31 per cent fat and 55 per cent carbohydrate. The carbohydrate was either all sucrose, all glucose polymer (Polycose), or equal proportions of each. Gastric emptying was most rapid with the Polycose, the least hyperosmolar solution. Although duodenal osmolarity was equivalent with all three formulations, the Polycose resulted in an increased duodenal flow rate. Sucrose was absorbed to a slightly greater extent than Polycose in the duodenum. The authors concluded that glucose polymers may be more likely to cause dumping symptoms.

Many patients with short bowel syndrome have steatorrhea from lack of absorptive surface area or decreased absorption of bile salts with subsequent inadequate luminal concentrations for micelle formation. Malabsorbed fat and deconjugated bile acids both stimulate net fluid and electrolyte secretion in the ileum and colon.[107, 121, 122] Bochenek et al. compared the use of long-chain triglycerides, micellar fat, oral bile salts, and medium-chain triglycerides in seven patients with distal small bowel resection.[123] Only the substitution of medium-chain triglyceride for long-chain triglycerides resulted in positive fluid balance and significant weight gain. Simko and colleagues[124] studied the impact of a low (64 gm/day) and high (200 gm/day) fat diet in a patient with excessive jejunostomy losses. The percentage of fat absorbed was the same in each meal, hence the absolute amount of calories absorbed increased dramatically with the high fat intake. They also noted a return to positive fluid balance and a decrease in bile acid output. Circulating levels of gastrin and glucagon were highest on the high fat intake. One point not mentioned is that the unabsorbed fatty acids will form insoluble soaps with the divalent cations, an effect that is more pronounced with increasing amounts of dietary fat.[105, 106] A more recent study by Ovesen et al. in five patients with jejunostomies and short bowel syndrome failed to substantiate any consistent beneficial effect of high fat intake (two thirds of total calories) on jejunostomy output.[125] Ostomy losses of divalent cations increased markedly with an increase in dietary fat. Ovesen also found no decrease in ostomy output with a diet high in polyunsaturated fat, even though studies have shown a more rapid absorption of unsaturated fatty acids compared with saturated fatty acids.[126]

Numerous uncontrolled reports purport to document the efficacy of elemental diets in the management of short bowel syndrome.[30-32, 36, 127-131] Simko and Lindscheer studied a number of elemental diets administered by nasogastric infusion in a patient with Crohn's disease and short bowel syndrome.[127] Positive fluid balance was achieved only with Flexical, which was also the only diet that contained significant quantities of fat. The patient had a jejunostomy and therefore the results may not be applicable to patients with an intact colon. Voitk[36] fed an elemental diet or chow to a group of rats with resection of 85 per cent of the jejunum, and noted an increased weight gain in the chow-fed animals with comparable indices of distal adaptation. Queen et al.[132] infused nonelemental or elemental formulas into a patient with short bowel syndrome and a jejunostomy. Absorption of nitrogen, calcium, and magnesium was superior with the nonelemental formulas (intact protein, complex carbohydrate, and fat). The elemental diet, which consisted of amino acids, glucose, and glucose oligosaccharides, caused net losses of calcium and magnesium. Tepas has recommended the use of a rather complicated system of feeding infants with short bowel syndrome.[31] It consists of 12 stages of graduated formula, beginning with CHO-free (soy protein isolate 3.6 per cent weight volume and soy oil 7 per cent weight/volume) and Polycose (glucose polymer) with slow increases in the amount of CHO-free and Polycose, and gradual addition of medium-chain triglyceride and sucrose. Since the dietary components are added one at a time, specific food intolerances may be rapidly recognized. This system was not compared with any simpler, easier to implement approach.

Continuous infusions of liquid diets may provoke less diarrhea than bolus infusions.[32, 33] Meals are emptied logarithmically from the stomach.[133] A continuous infusion may alter the emptying curve to one that is more linear, and thereby maintain a relatively constant rate of intestinal flow and minimize the risk of dumping symptoms.

Patients with short bowel syndrome are a heterogeneous group in which such factors as segment and length of bowel resected, presence or absence of the ileocecal valve, bacterial overgrowth, abnormal motility, and residual disease may all interact and have an influence on the pattern of malabsorption. For this reason it is difficult to make general statements about effective dietary approaches. Nonetheless several conclusions may be drawn from the available studies: (1) In the patient with a moderate amount of remaining small bowel, a standard diet will be well tolerated. (2) With severe short bowel syndrome, an initial period of TPN will maintain normal body functions and reverse any nutritional deficits. (3) Continuous infusions of liquid formulas are better tolerated than boluses. (4) Divalent cations and fat soluble vitamins must be supplemented in cases of short bowel syndrome. Parenteral injections of vitamin B_{12} are needed if the terminal ileum is resected. (5) Oral intake will accelerate the adaptation process. (6) Nonelemental diets are absorbed as well as, or better than, elemental diets. (7) Proximally absorbed water-soluble vitamins will be adequately absorbed from the diet in any patient with short bowel syndrome who can maintain his protein and energy status without parenteral support.[134]

Chemotherapy and Radiation-Induced Enteritis. Chemotherapy is commonly used in the treatment of malignant disease. Gastrointestinal side effects may limit its usefulness. Proliferating and mature enterocytes become vacuolated, flattened, and necrotic. The villi and crypts become smaller, and loss of villus architecture may occur. These changes may preclude more aggressive chemotherapeutic management, and by virtue of concomitant anorexia and malabsorption have an adverse effect on nutritional status. Elemental diets may protect against cytotoxic damage. Rats maintained on chow and given 150 mg of 5-fluorouracil (5-FU) sustained greater intestinal mucosal damage when compared with rats maintained on a protein hydrolysate formula.[135] To be effective, the elemental diet had to precede the injection of 5-FU and be continued afterward. Similar results were obtained in a human study looking at rectal mucosal abnormalities.[136] The same investigator[137] noted less decrease in total serum protein and albumin concentrations in rats given 5-FU for nine days and maintained on an elemental diet. Stanford and associates,[138] however, noted an increased incidence of diarrhea and mortality in rats given 5-FU for six days and fed a variety of elemental diets, as compared with chow-fed animals. Further studies are necessary to explain these disparate results.

Radiation injury to the small bowel frequently occurs following high doses of abdominal irradiation. Symptoms of anorexia, nausea, vomiting, and diarrhea are common. Histologic findings include severe villus blunting, lymphatic dilatation, and an inflammatory infiltrate.[139] Morgenstern and Hiatt showed in dogs with Thiry-Vella fistulas that only those segments in contact with pancreatic juice became severely damaged.[140] In studies by Hugon and Bounous, mice fed an elemental diet survived radiation better than did mice fed whole casein.[141] The mice on the elemental diet showed faster recovery of villi. Similar results were obtained by Pageau and colleagues, who also noted an increase in thymidine uptake and mitotic activity in intestinal mucosa of rats fed an elemental diet compared with those fed chow.[142] Dogs fed Vital for three days tolerated 2000 rads better than dogs fed chow, with no evidence of ileal villus damage or decreased food intake.[143] Donaldson et al. have noted clinical improvement and recovery from histologic abnormalities in children with radiation enteritis treated with a low-residue, low-fat, gluten-free, and milk-free diets.[139]

Crohn's Disease.   Twenty to thirty per cent of children with Crohn's disease have severe retardation of linear growth.[144] This may result from the high doses of steroids often necessary to control disease activity, but not uncommonly short stature is part of the initial presentation or occurs in a patient who is in clinical remission and is off steroid therapy. Kelts et al.[145] evaluated seven children with inactive Crohn's disease and growth failure and found that their caloric intake was 82 per cent of what would be expected for normal children of the same age. All endocrine studies were normal. For six to eight weeks the children received parenteral nutrition supplying 136 per cent of their "expected intake." These children all gained weight and finally showed a spurt in linear growth which continued for a while even after TPN was stopped, and the children returned to their pre-TPN low intakes. Morin et al.[146] were able to obtain similar results in four children with growth retardation and mild disease activity using a six-week course of continuous nasogastric infusion of Vivonex. Other investigators have reversed growth failure using nocturnal infusions of low-residue diets. Kirschner et al.[147] carried this idea to its logical conclusion by offering dietary counseling and liquid supplements to a group of children with Crohn's disease and growth failure. Caloric intake increased from 56 to 91 per cent of recommended for height age. None was receiving more than 10 mg of prednisone daily. Five of seven children increased their height percentile.

The available evidence would suggest that growth failure in children with Crohn's disease occurs most commonly on a nutritional basis. It has been shown in children with renal disease that a caloric intake of 67 per cent of the recommended intake results in a growth rate of 34 per cent of the expected growth rate.[148] In Crohn's disease inadequate caloric intake may result from anorexia or fear of developing abdominal pain. Energy expenditure in underweight patients with Crohn's disease is slightly increased.[149] The Boston Children's group has recently reported an increased protein turnover and high energy cost of growth in children with Crohn's disease.[150, 151]

Although release of growth hormone is normal in these children, somatomedin deficiency may be a factor in growth failure associated with Crohn's disease. Serum somatomedin levels are diminished before nutritional restitution,[152] and increase coincident with improvement in linear growth. Similar findings occur in protein-calorie malnutrition.

The use of elemental diets has also been advocated in the management of Crohn's disease with perianal involvement. Such therapy has been advocated to correct malnutrition and to present less antigen load to the colon by decreasing fecal output and fecal flora. It has been postulated that patients with Crohn's disease have a defect in clearing foreign antigens from the intestinal tract,[153] leading to inflammation and granuloma formation. Although elemental diets may diminish fecal output, it is highly questionable whether they have any effect on fecal flora.[154]

Several anecdotal reports in the literature claim a beneficial effect of an elemental diet on closure of perianal fistula or ulcer healing.[155–157] None of these studies was controlled. The major benefit of any diet may be maintenance of normal nutritional status, with reduction in fecal weight playing a secondary role. Additionally, the recent experience with the use of metronidazole in the healing of Crohn's perianal disease should relegate elemental diets to a position of secondary importance.

CAN ENTERAL FEEDINGS AGGRAVATE INFLAMMATION OF THE GASTROINTESTINAL TRACT?

The development of parenteral nutrition as a legitimate and safe means of nutritional support has enabled physicians to prescribe periods of bowel rest to minimize intraluminal secretions and nutrients. The patient's state of nutrition can be maintained or improved without the risk of nutrient-induced gastrointestinal inflammation. It is necessary to separate the impact of good nutrition from a primary role of bowel rest. In some disorders, such as necrotizing enterocolitis, bowel rest is such an established form of management that no data exist relevant to enteral feeding. In other disorders, such as pseudomembranous colitis, definitive therapy is begun soon enough to preclude a meaningful role for bowel rest. The evidence for and against bowel rest will be examined for several gastrointestinal disorders.

Disorders in Which Bowel Rest is Probably Essential

In some disorders, complete bowel rest is such an established form of therapy that studies utilizing enteral feedings are unlikely ever to be carried out. An example is necrotizing enterocolitis in infancy, a disease that almost never occurs in the absence of enteral feedings. The likelihood of bowel perforation is significant, because it precludes a trial of enteral nutrition. Toxic megacolon secondary to inflammatory bowel disease, ulcerative colitis, Crohn's disease,

and Hirschsprung's disease is another disorder in which surgical intervention often occurs, and hence bowel rest is uniformly invoked.

Disorders in Which Bowel Rest is Controversial

Acute Gastroenteritis. Cholera and several types of *Escherichia coli* produce an enterotoxin that does not cause intestinal mucosal injury but does increase local concentrations of cyclic AMP.[158] Sodium chloride absorption at the brush border is inhibited and active secretion of anions occurs from crypt cells.[158] Glucose-sodium coupled absorption remains intact allowing the patients to be rehydrated using an oral glucose-electrolyte solution.[159]

Acute gastroenteritis in this country is more likely to be caused by other bacterial or viral agents. Histologic damage to the small intestine with malabsorption of fat, disaccharides, and rarely glucose may occur.[160–162] Removal of lactose from the diet is often associated with cessation of diarrhea.[88]

What is the importance of bowel rest in acute gastroenteritis? Absorption of glucose and amino acids is reduced after several days of bowel rest even when adequate calories are supplied parenterally.[16, 163] Disaccharidase activities diminish and, furthermore, the effects of fasting and diarrhea on intestinal disaccharidase activity appear to be additive.[164] In rats, after one week of mannitol-induced diarrhea, disaccharidase levels showed an even greater dependence on substrate induction than in animals without diarrhea, an effect that was unrelated to histologic changes.[164]

Rotavirus is a very common etiologic agent in acute gastroenteritis in infancy. The mechanism of the diarrhea may be mucosal destruction followed by migration of immature enterocytes with lower disaccharidase levels and enhanced secretion of anions characteristic of crypt cells.[165, 166] In spite of the presence of these immature villus cells, these children may be successfully rehydrated with sucrose-electrolyte solutions.[167] Absorption of neutral amino acids, such as glucose, is coupled to sodium uptake, and glycine can apparently be substituted for glucose in oral rehydration solutions.[168]

In 1948, Chung reported that children with acute diarrhea fed milk and corn syrup recovered more rapidly than fasted controls, in spite of an increase in stool losses.[169] It would be interesting to compare the use of complex carbohydrates and polypeptides with traditional glucose-electrolyte solutions in the early treatment of gastroenteritis.

Exposure to cow's milk protein has caused histologic damage to the jejunum in children recovering from acute gastroenteritis.[170] Villus blunting has occurred after rechallenge with cow's milk protein as long as eight weeks after the initial episode of diarrhea, even when cow's milk had been excluded from the diet in the interim. It is suggested that cow's milk protein be excluded from the diet of all children experiencing acute gastroenteritis. The importance of acute gastroenteritis as a factor in the pathogenesis of long-term cow's milk protein intolerance remains to be investigated.

Intractable Diarrhea Syndrome. Intractable diarrhea of infancy is fortunately a rare disorder characterized by early onset, severe diarrhea of greater than three weeks' duration, and malnutrition, often partially resulting from repeated trials of bowel rest.[171] Most children will show villus atrophy with decreases in disaccharidase activity. Previously, TPN was believed to be the only appropriate form of therapy for these children.[172, 173] This was often carried out for many weeks with cautious reintroduction of formula into the diet. Hyman et al. in 1971[172] used parenteral alimentation for three weeks followed by gradual reintroduction of medium-chain triglycerides, Lactinex granules (Lactobacillus), and finally a fructose-containing formula. This approach was clinically successful; however, there were no controls to compare Hyman's formula with more standard therapy. Sherman, in 1975,[174] successfully treated 24 of 27 cases of intractable diarrhea syndrome using continuous nasogastric infusions of two thirds strength Vivonex or Vivonex HN. Greene et al.[175] compared TPN with a combination of peripheral intravenous nutrition and dilute casein hydrolysate formula given by continuous nasogastric drip. Mean duration of hospitalization was reduced in the orally fed group, but two of eight infants had to be switched to TPN after failing on oral therapy. All had severe histologic changes with decreased disaccharidase activities. The enterally fed groups showed more rapid recovery of disaccharidase levels. In a nonrandomized study, Rossi et al.[176] found that the duration of hospital stay was markedly

shortened and mucosal recovery significantly hastened in a group of infants maintained on intermittent feedings of Pregestimil compared with a regimen of TPN and continuous nasogastric Pregestimil. The TPN group, however, may have been a population with more severe malnutrition. Weight gain on Pregestimil was satisfactory at one year of age in spite of persisting mucosal abnormalities. This group of patients was somewhat atypical because of their persisting histologic damage. Thus, bowel rest has not been shown to be superior to partial enteral feeding in the intractable diarrhea syndrome. Further investigations are required to determine if more complex formulas promote more rapid healing.

Acute Episodes of Inflammatory Bowel Disease. Crohn's disease is a transmural inflammatory process that can involve any portion of the gastrointestinal tract from the mouth to the anus. It is a disease characterized by exacerbations and spontaneous improvements, making it difficult to evaluate any therapeutic regimen. Traditional management has consisted of anti-inflammatory agents, with the goal of suppressing acute inflammation. Eventually, fibrosis may occur in the chronically inflamed areas, at which point surgical resection is often necessary. Bowel rest has been recommended as a therapeutic tool because of several observations: (1) the worst symptoms develop in most patients after eating; (2) there are reports of improvement in Crohn's colitis following ileostomy,[177] and worsening after instillation of food into the isolated segment; and (3) there is a report of failure of normal neutrophil migration in Crohn's disease[153] leading to delayed removal of bacteria and ingested protein, with subsequent granuloma formation. It is believed that removal of the offending antigen may prevent further inflammation.

Several recent uncontrolled studies have examined the effect of bowel rest and TPN on the course of Crohn's disease.[178-183] Criteria for use of TPN in these series were disease unresponsive to intensive medical management. Short-term remission rates of approximately 70 per cent are described in most studies, but long-term remissions occurred in a minority of cases. Only Greenberg and colleagues[179] were able to achieve a two-year remission rate of 79 per cent for reasons that are not apparent. Surgery can be avoided in some patients, at least temporarily, and nutritional status may be improved in patients who do require surgery. Medical therapy is said to induce remissions in 70 per cent of patients with active Crohn's disease, making these uncontrolled studies difficult to interpret. Since all patients in these reports had active disease in spite of aggressive medical management, TPN and bowel rest appear to have a role in the short-term treatment of Crohn's disease, but there is probably no alteration of the long-term course of the disease.

A recent randomized, controlled study failed to demonstrate any therapeutic benefit of TPN and bowel rest in Crohn's colitis and ulcerative colitis.[184] However, preoperative nutritional repletion of malnourished patients can be accomplished.

Elemental diets have been used in an uncontrolled fashion during exacerbations of Crohn's disease as a form of physiological bowel rest. It is hypothesized that the component nutritions will be absorbed before reaching the area of inflammation and will produce minimal gastric and pancreatic secretions. But as discussed earlier, it is not known if nutrients in elemental diets are absorbed over a shorter length of bowel than in macromolecular diets, and while stool output is usually diminished, this is an inconsistent finding. Voitk and coworkers[185] used Flexical in seven patients with Crohn's disease, three of whom had short bowel syndrome after multiple resections, and four of whom had indications for surgery but were considered too cachectic to be operated upon. Nutritional status was improved in all seven subjects, but none of the patients in the unresected group escaped surgical intervention. Other studies using elemental diets have also shown nutritional improvement with inconsistent changes in disease activity.[186–189] Logan et al. showed reduced gastrointestinal protein losses in seven patients with jejunoileal Crohn's disease fed an elemental diet.[190] This may be one explanation for the observed nutritional improvement. While newly diagnosed cases have a high likelihood of achieving remission on an elemental diet as their sole therapy,[191] these patients are likely to improve on standard medical management also, which emphasizes the need for randomized clinical trials.

While elemental diets are not of proven therapeutic benefit in inflammatory bowel disease, they have also not been associated with exacerbation of symptoms. One rationale for their use, in addition to their low bulk, is that they are free of lactose. Several groups have reported a 50 per cent incidence of lactose intolerance in patients with ulcerative colitis.[192, 193] Intolerance to lactose seemed to correlate with disease activity. Lactose intolerance was less common in a Danish study which found lactose malabsorption in only 9 per cent of patients with ulcerative colitis and in 6 per cent of patients with Crohn's disease.[194] Four of seven lactose-deficient subjects experienced an improvement in their diarrhea on a lactose-free diet. However, it is worth noting that 7 of 21 lactose-tolerant patients also improved on a milk-free diet. A recent study by Kirschner[195] in children and adolescents with inflammatory bowel disease used the lactose breath hydrogen assay to document lactose malabsorption. When ethnic factors were considered, there was no higher incidence of lactose malabsorption in these patients than in a control population. Based on these reports, it would seem prudent to undertake a trial of a milk-free diet in any patient with inflammatory bowel disease whose symptoms are not totally responsive to standard therapy.

In summary, bowel rest with parenteral nutritional support appears to have no therapeutic benefit in ulcerative colitis except in patients requiring preoperative nutritional buildup. In Crohn's disease bowel rest appears to be of benefit in selected patients. Further studies are required to determine which patients are most likely to respond to this expensive means of nutritional repletion. Elemental diets are useful in some early cases of Crohn's disease, but studies are needed to compare this approach with standard low-residue diets and medical management. If beneficial, the use of elemental diets may be an intriguing means of investigating the effect of long-term partial bowel rest on the ultimate prognosis of Crohn's disease.

Pancreatitis. Bowel rest with TPN is used in patients with pancreatitis because it is assumed that the continued secretion of enzymes and fluid by an inflamed pancreas is deleterious, and that TPN does not induce pancreatic secretions. Traditional management consists of nasogastric suction to remove gastric acid as a stimulus to pancreatic secretion and pharmacologic suppression of gastric acid secretion.

Intravenously administered amino acids stimulate gastric acid secretion to a minor degree.[196] TPN has been reported to cause slight stimulation of pancreatic secretion in one study,[197] and slight inhibition in two others.[198, 199] The changes were minor in either case, and the known association of pancreatic atrophy with prolonged TPN implies that, at the least, TPN causes less pancreatic secretion than orally ingested food. The remaining question is, does continued pancreatic secretion in the face of inflammation of the pancreas worsen the prognosis?

Goodgame and Fischer[200] have compared the results of patients with acute pancreatitis treated with TPN, with historical controls from the pre-TPN era. TPN clearly maintains nutritional status. The survival rate of severely ill patients treated with TPN was 80 per cent, whereas in an earlier report of severely ill patients managed with surgery and jejunostomy feeds the survival rate was 74 per cent, not a significant difference. TPN led to an 80 per cent survival rate in a subset of patients with a gastrointestinal tract that was nonfunctioning for more than one month, emphasizing its role in preventing nutritional decompensation. The incidence of, and mortality rates from, pancreatitis-associated renal failure and respiratory failure were not substantially different from pre-TPN studies. It is obviously difficult to draw conclusions from retrospective studies separated by many years, especially since pancreatitis encompasses a number of pathophysiologic processes, but there appears to be no clear-cut advantage to bowel rest per se in the patient with acute pancreatitis unless there is bowel ileus. In patients with a functioning gastrointestinal tract TPN seems an unnecessarily sophisticated and expensive means of nutritional support.

Elemental diets have been proposed as a means of providing enteral nutrition without stimulating pancreatic secretion. Rivilis et al.[84] concluded in dog studies that an elemental diet induces less gastric acid secretion than does dog food. Ragins et al.[201] infused boluses of Vivonex, amino acids, or glucose into the stomach, duodenum, or a 45-cm Thiry-Vella jejunal fistula. Each nutrient solution evoked increases in pancreatic volume and secretion of bicarbonate and protein when infused into the stomach, but not when infused into the duodenum or Thiry-Vella loop. Koretz and Meyer[202] have pointed out that since boluses of nutrients injected directly into the duodenum or into Thiry-Vella fistulas are rapidly absorbed, the duration of the stimulus for secretion will be less than when food is slowly emptied from the stomach into the duodenum.

Kelly and Nahrwold[197] perfused an elemental diet for 90 minutes into the duodenum of dogs with chronic pancreatic fistulas. A second group of dogs received the same total amount of elemental diet in the form of an oral bolus. Both diets stimulated pancreatic protein outputs to a similar degree. The oral diet, however, stimulated a greater volume and greater bicarbonate output than the perfused diet. The authors concluded that the additional bicarbonate and volume outputs were caused by increased gastric secretions in the orally fed animals. Other studies comparing the effects on pancreatic secretion of an elemental diet versus whole food have produced results that are hard to evaluate. In one study Flexical, a fat-containing peptide diet, produced greater pancreatic volume and secretion of bicarbonate and protein than blenderized food,[203] whereas in another dog study Flexical induced less secretion than standard dog chow.[204] Since these diets were not always isonitrogenous,[151] and the route of administration was not always specified, no conclusions can be reached.

The major stimulus for pancreatic enzyme secretion appears to be the presence of the amino acids phenylalanine and tryptophan, and possibly also valine, in the gastrointestinal tract,[205, 206] either in free form or as peptides. Absorption is not required to produce this secretory effect, and these amino acids are active at any site in the small bowel. Other amino acids singly or in combination do not cause pancreatic secretion. Undigested, whole protein infused intrajejunally does not stimulate pancreatic secretion, implying that free amino acids or peptides must be present. Intraduodenal fat has less of a stimulatory effect than phenylalanine or tryptophan,[206] whereas isotonic dextrose does not stimulate pancreatic secretions at all. Several clinical studies have corroborated these findings.[207-209]

Three uncontrolled studies have examined the usefulness of an elemental diet in the treatment of pancreatitis.[210-212] Vivonex was infused intragastrically into three patients with chronic pancreatitis and T-tube pancreatic drainage and resulted in diminished pancreatic output and enzyme secretion compared with whole food taken by mouth.[210] The differing routes of administration make it impossible to draw very clear conclusions. Voitk et al.[211] fed Flexical to six patients with complicated pancreatitis and pseudocyst formation. Up to 5 L/day of enteral diet was tolerated without exacerbation of pancreatitis. Blackburn et al.[212] used a combination of TPN and elemental diet in treating 13 patients with severe pancreatitis. Eleven patients did well on this combined nutritional support. The heterogeneity of patient populations make it difficult to compare these studies.

In summary, there is currently little evidence to conclude that prolonged bowel rest in the patient with pancreatitis and a functioning gastrointestinal tract is beneficial. The volume of pancreatic secretion will be diminished by infusing nutrients into the stomach and bypassing the cephalic phase of gastric secretion, and decreased even further by infusing directly into the small bowel and eliminating gastric secretion almost completely. Pancreatic enzyme output, on the other hand, is determined by the protein and fat content of the diet, and is unaffected by the route of administration. Elemental diets appear to be well tolerated by most patients with pancreatitis, perhaps because of their low protein content, but further studies are needed to determine whether polymeric diets with higher protein contents are equally efficacious.

Gastrointestinal Fistulas. The importance of nutrition in the management of gastrointestinal fistulas is well established. The optimal method of providing nutrition is still in question, however. TPN and bowel rest have been used recently in the hopes that this will lead to a decrease in fistula output and greater healing. Soeters et al.[213] in a recent retrospective study reviewed the Massachusetts General Hospital experience of 73 patients with gastrointestinal fistulas treated with bowel rest and TPN compared with 119 historical, pre-TPN controls. They concluded that the major improvement in survival of patients with fistulas occurred in the pre-TPN era when the impact of sepsis and malnutrition as important factors in mortality were recognized. TPN may have contributed to a decrease in mortality in esophageal, gastric, and duodenal fistulas. The published mortality rate in uncontrolled series of patients treated with TPN and bowel rest is approximately 14 per cent,[213–217] which does not differ from the 12 to 15 per cent mortality rate in the studies done when nutritional support was used but before TPN became available.[213, 218] It would seem that studies with very low mortality rates in TPN-treated patients have tended to involve a larger proportion of patients whose fistu-

las were in a favorable location for spontaneous closure.[214]

The effect of TPN and bowel rest on fistula output and spontaneous closure rate is also important. Although the presence of food in the gastrointestinal tract certainly stimulates secretion of enzymes, fluid, electrolytes, and bile, the use of TPN often causes only a very modest reduction in fistula output. Reber et al.[219] noted no decrease in fistula output in four patients with high output fistulas treated with TPN. Most authors find no correlation between fistula output and spontaneous closure rate. In a number of published series, the likelihood of spontaneous closure in enterally or parenterally nourished patients varies from 30 to 80 per cent.[213, 214, 217, 219–222] Spontaneous closure is more likely to occur in patients less than 65 years old whose fistulas are not caused by cancer, irradiation, or Crohn's disease,[219, 222] and whose fistulas are not complicated by sepsis, distal obstruction, or preexistent malnutrition. Although most fistulas that close spontaneously do so within one month, Byrne et al.[223] described 12 patients with complicated gastrointestinal fistulas not responding after one to two months of in-hospital TPN, but in 8 of the 12 patients the fistulas closed after a period of prolonged home TPN. TPN does appear to shorten the time in which spontaneous closure occurs. MacFadyen et al.[214] noted a decrease in average closure time from 59 days in pre-TPN patients to 35 days in TPN-treated patients. Other investigators have published similar clinical impressions.[217]

Wolfe et al.[224] showed that diet certainly alters bowel losses, since ileostomy outputs in dogs fed isocaloric diets of dog food, elemental diet, or TPN resulted in ostomy drainage of 1137, 220, and 80 ml/day, respectively. Several uncontrolled studies have reported on the management of gastrointestinal fistulas with elemental diets.[225–227] Some of the patients in these series also received TPN for variable periods of time. Spontaneous closure of the fistula occurred in 50 to 75 per cent of patients. Mortality rates with elemental feeding were comparable to those in published reports of patients treated with TPN and bowel rest.

Deitel[217] concluded that total bowel rest afforded superior results, and described several patients whose fistulas reopened when given an elemental diet. Rocchio and colleagues[226] noted a decrease in fistula output in 29 of 35 patients with high output fistulas (greater than 200 ml/day) treated with an elemental diet. There was a 50 per cent rate of spontaneous closure with upper or mid bowel fistulas. Clearly, nutrients must be absorbed to be effective, and thus must be infused at a location where the most absorption will occur before the fistula is reached. Alternatively, successful results of infusing an elemental diet distal to an upper small bowel fistula have been reported.[228]

In summary, prevention of malnutrition has played a major role in the reduction of mortality in patients with gastrointestinal fistulas. The cause and location of the fistula, control of sepsis, and presence of distal obstruction appear to be more important determinants of mortality and rate of spontaneous closure than the method of nutritional support. Total parenteral nutrition and bowel rest may promote more rapid healing of fistulas than enteral diets, although this does not appear to be related to fistula output. Enteral diets can be used in patients with fistulas, so long as the nutrients are not significantly expelled through the fistula. Compared with polymeric diets, elemental diets may decrease fistula output, but the importance of this observation awaits the results of controlled clinical trials.

REFERENCES

1. Rijke, R. P. C., Plaisier, H. M., deRuiter, H., and Galjaard, H.: Influence of experimental bypass on cellular kinetics and maturation of small intestinal epithelium in the rat. Gastroenterology, 72:896–901, 1977.
2. Dowling, R. H., and Booth, C. C.: Structural and functional changes following small intestinal resection in the rat. Clin. Sci., 32:139–149, 1967.
3. Obertop, H., Nundy, S., Malamud, D., and Malt, R. A.: Onset of cell proliferation in the shortened gut: Rapid hyperplasia after jejunal resection. Gastroenterology, 72:267–270, 1977.
4. Young, E. A., and Weser, E.: Nutritional adaptation after small bowel resection in rats. J. Nutr., 104:994–1001, 1974.
5. Weser, E., and Hernandez, M. H.: Studies of small bowel adaptation after intestinal resection in the rat. Gastroenterology, 60:69–75, 1971.
6. Hanson, W. R., Osborne, J. W., and Sharp, J. G.: Compensation by the residual intestine after intestinal resection in the rat. I. Influence of amount of tissue removed. Gastroenterology, 72:692–700, 1977.
7. Garrido, A. B., Jr., Freeman, H. J., Chung, Y. C., and Kim, Y. S.: Amino acid and peptide transport absorption after proximal small intestinal resection in the rat. Gut, 20:114–120, 1979.
8. Weinstein, L. D., Shoemaker, C. P., Hersh, T., and Wright, H. K.: Enhanced intestinal absorption after small bowel resection in man. Arch. Surg., 99:560–562, 1969.
9. Urban, E., and Pena, M.: In vivo calcium transport by rat small intestine after massive small bowel resection. Am. J. Physiol., 226:1304–1308, 1974.
10. Mackinnon, H. M.: Intestinal adaptation of vitamin B_{12} absorption [Abstract 9]. Clin. Sci., 42:29P, 1972.
11. Dowling, R. H.: The influence of luminal nutrition on intestinal adaptation after small bowel resection and bypass. In Dowling, R. H., and Riecken, E. D. (eds.): Intestinal Adaptation. Stuttgart, Schauttauer, 1974, pp. 35–46.
12. McCarthy, D. M., and Kim, Y. S.: Changes in sucrase, enterokinase and peptide hydrolase after intestinal resection. J. Clin. Invest., 52:942–951, 1973.
13. Williamson, R. C. N., Buchholtz, T. W., and Malt, R. A.: Humoral stimulation of cell proliferation in small bowel after transection and resection in rats. Gastroenterology, 75:249–254, 1978.
14. Bochenek, W. J., Narczewska, B., and Grzebieluch, M.: Effect of massive proximal small bowel resection on intestinal sucrase and lactase activity in the rat. Digestion, 9:224–230, 1973.
15. Freeman, H. U., Etzler, M. E., Garrido, A. B., Kim, Y. S.: Alterations in cell surface membrane components of adapting rat small intestinal epithelium: Studies with lectins after massive proximal jejunoileal resection and jejunoileal transposition. Gastroenterology, 75:1066–1072, 1978.
16. Adibi, S. A., and Allen, E. R.: Impaired jejunal absorption rates of essential amino acids induced by either dietary caloric or protein deprivation in man. Gastroenterology, 59:404–413, 1970.
17. Keren, D. F., Elliott, H. L., Brown, G. D., and Yardley, J. H.: Atrophy of villi with hypertrophy and hyperplasia of Paneth cells in isolated (Thiry-Vella) ileal loops in rabbits. Gastroenterology, 68:83–93, 1975.
18. Hanson, W. R., Rijke, R. P. C., Plaisier, H. M., Van Ewijk, W., and Osborne, J. W.: The effect of intestinal resection on Thiry-Vella fistulae of jejunal and ileal origin in the rat. Evidence for a systemic control mechanism of cell renewal. Cell Tissue Kinet., 10:543–555, 1977.
19. Levine, G. M., Deren, J. J., Steiger, E., et al.: Role of oral intake in maintenance of gut mass and disaccharidase activity. Gastroenterology, 67:975–982, 1974.
20. Eastwood, G. L.: Small bowel morphology and epithelial proliferation in intravenously alimented rabbits. Surgery, 82:613–620, 1977.
21. Assad, R. T., and Eastwood, G. L.: Relation between villus height and epithelial renewal in rats on intravenous, oral liquid, or oral solid feeding [Abstract]. Gastroenterology, 74:1004, 1978.
22. Morin, C. L., Ling, V., and Bourassa, D.: Small intestinal and colonic changes induced by a chemically defined diet. Dig. Dis. Sci., 25:123–128, 1980.
23. Young, E. A., Cioletti, L. A., Winborn, W. B., Traylor, J. B., and Weser, E.: Comparative study of nutritional adaptation to defined formula diets in rats. Am. J. Clin. Nutr., 33:2106–2118, 1980.
24. Buts, J. P., Morin, C. L., Bourassa, D., and Ling, V.: Influence of diet components on small bowel

adaptation after resection [Abstract]. Gastroenterology, 72:1035, 1977.

25. Castro, G. A., Copeland, E. M., Dudrick, S. J., and Johnson, L. R.: Intestinal disaccharidase and peroxidase activities in parenterally nourished rats. J. Nutr., 105:776–781, 1975.

26. Morin, C. L., Ling, V., and Van Caillie, M.: Role of oral intake on intestinal adaptation after small bowel resection in growing rats. Pediatr. Res., 12:268–271, 1978.

27. Alpers, D. H.: Protein synthesis in intestinal mucosa: The effect of route of administration of precursor amino acids. J. Clin. Invest., 51:167–173, 1972.

28. Sim, A. J. W., Wolfe, B. M., Young, V. R., Clarke, D., and Moore, F. D.: Glucose promotes whole-body protein synthesis from infused amino acids in fasting man: Isotopic demonstration. Lancet, 1:68–72, 1979.

29. Wilmore, D. W., Dudrick, S. J., Daly, J. M., and Vars, H. M.: The role of nutrition in the adaptation of the small intestine after massive resection. Surg. Gynecol. Obstet., 132:673–680, 1971.

30. Christie, D. L., and Ament, M. E.: Dilute elemental diet and continuous infusion technique for management of short bowel syndrome. J. Pediatr., 87:705–708, 1975.

31. Tepas, J. J., III, MacLean, W. C., Jr., Kolbach, S., and Shermeta, D. W.: Total management of short gut secondary to midgut volvulus without prolonged total parenteral alimentation. J. Pediatr. Surg., 13:622–625, 1978.

32. Weinberger, M., and Rowe, M. I.: Experience with an elemental diet in neonatal surgery. J. Pediatr. Surg., 8:175–184, 1973.

33. Bohane, T. D., Haka-Ikse, K., Biggar, W. D., Hamilton, J. R., and Gall, D. G.: A clinical study of young infants after small intestinal resection. J. Pediatr., 94:552–558, 1979.

34. Levine, G. M., Deren, J. J., and Yezdimir, E.: Small bowel resection: Oral intake is the stimulus for hyperplasia. Am. J. Dig. Dis., 21:542–546, 1976.

35. Feldman, E. J., Dowling, R. H., McNaughton, J., and Peters, T. J.: Effects of oral versus intravenous nutrition on intestinal adaptation after small bowel resection in the dog. Gastroenterology, 70:712–719, 1976.

36. Voitk, A. J., and Crispin, J. S.: The ability of an elemental diet to support nutrition and adaptation in the short gut syndrome. Ann. Surg., 181:220–225, 1975.

37. Tilson, M. D., and Wright, H. K.: Villus hyperplasia in parabiotic rats [Abstract]. Clin. Res., 19:405, 1971.

38. Dworkin, L. D., Levine, G. M., Farber, N. J., and Spector, M. H.: Small intestinal mass of the rat is partially determined by indirect effects of intraluminal nutrition. Gastroenterology, 71:626–630, 1976.

39. Fenyö, G., and Hallberg, D.: The influence of a chemical diet on the intestinal mucosa after jejuno-ileal bypass in the rat. Acta Chir. Scand., 142:270–274, 1976.

40. Fenyö, G., Hallberg, D., Soda, M., and Roosk, A.: Morphologic changes in the small intestine following jejuno-ileal shunt in parenterally fed rats. Scand. J. Gastroenterol., 11:635–640, 1976.

41. Gleeson, M. H., Cullen, J., and Dowling, R. H.: Intestinal structure and function after small bowel by-pass in the rat. Clin. Sci., 43:731–742, 1972.

42. Grenier, J. F., Dauchel, J., Marescaux, J., Eloy, M. R., and Schang, J. C.: Intestinal changes after jejuno-ileal shunt in obesity: A report of 2 cases. Br. J. Surg., 64:96–99, 1977.

43. Spector, M. H., Levine, G. M., and Deren, J. J.: Direct and indirect effects of dextrose and amino acids on gut mass. Gastroenterology, 72:706–710, 1977.

44. Sum, P. T., and Preshaw, R. M.: Intraduodenal glucose infusion and pancreatic secretion in man. Lancet, 2:340–341, 1967.

45. Johnson, L. R., and Chandler, A. M.: RNA and DNA of gastric and duodenal mucosa in antrectomized and gastrin-treated rats. Am. J. Physiol., 224:937–940, 1973.

46. Gregory, R. A., Grossman, M. I., Tracy, H. J., and Bentley, P. H.: Nature of the gastric secretagogue in Zollinger-Ellison tumours. Lancet, 2:543–546, 1967.

47. Landor, J. H., Behringer, B. R., and Wild, R. A.: Postenterectomy gastric hypersecretion in dogs: The relative importance of proximal versus distal resection. J. Surg. Res., 11:238–242, 1971.

48. Wickbom, G., Landor, J. H., Bushkin, F. L., and McGuigan, J. E.: Changes in canine gastric acid output and serum gastrin levels following massive small intestinal resection. Gastroenterology, 69:448–452, 1975.

49. Straus, E., Gerson, C. D., and Yalow, R. S.: Hypersecretion of gastrin associated with the short bowel syndrome. Gastroenterology, 66:175–180, 1974.

50. Junghanns, K., Kaess, H., Dörner, M., and Encke, A.: The influence of resection of the small intestine on gastrin levels. Surg. Gynecol. Obstet., 140:27–29, 1975.

51. Mak, K. M., and Chang, W. W. L.: Pentagastrin stimulates epithelial cell proliferation in duodenum and colonic crypts in fasted rats. Gastroenterology, 71:1117–1120, 1976.

52. Johnson, L. R., and Guthrie, P. D.: Mucosal DNA synthesis: A short term index of the trophic action of gastrin. Gastroenterology, 67:453–459, 1974.

53. Johnson, L. R., Lichtenberger, L. M., Copeland, E. M., Dudrick, S. J., and Castro, G. A.: Action of gastrin on gastrointestinal structure and function. Gastroenterology, 68:1184–1192, 1975.

54. Johnson, L. R., Copeland, E. M., Dudrick, S. J., Lichtenberger, L. M., and Castro, G. A.: Structural and hormonal alterations in the gastrointestinal tract of parenterally fed rats. Gastroenterology, 68:1177–1183, 1975.

55. Morin, C. L., and Ling, V.: Effect of pentagastrin on the rat small intestine after resection. Gastroenterology, 75:225–229, 1978.

56. Lichtenberger, L., Welsh, J. D., and Johnson, L. R.: Relationship between the changes in gastrin levels and intestinal properties in the starved rat. Am. J. Dig. Dis., 21:33–38, 1976.

57. Hughes, W., Tawil, T., and Weser, E.: Effect of antrectomy on ileal hyperplasia after jejunectomy in the rat. Clin. Res., 24:286A, 1976.

58. Sircar, B., Johnson, L. R., and Lichtenberger, L. M.: Effect of chemically defined diets on antral and serum gastrin levels in rats. Am. J. Physiol., 238:G376–G383, 1980.

59. Oscarson, J. E. A., Veen, H. F., Williamson, R. C. N., Ross, J. S., and Malt, R. A.: Compensatory postresectional hyperplasia and starvation atrophy in small bowel: Dissociation from endogenous gastrin levels. Gastroenterology, 72:890–895, 1977.

60. Tilson, M. D., and Axtmayer, A.: Antral exlcusion enhances compensatory hypertrophy of the gut after partial enterectomy. J. Surg. Res., 20:275–279, 1976.

61. Johnson, L. R., Guthrie, P. D., and Dudrick, S. J.: Effects of intraluminal gastrin on the growth of rat intestinal mucosa. Gastroenterology, 81:71–77, 1981.

62. Johnson, L. R., and Guthrie, P.: Effect of cholecystokinin and 16,16-dimethyl prostaglandin E$_2$ on RNA and DNA of gastric and duodenal mucosa. Gastroenterology, 70:59–65, 1976.

63. Hughes, C. A., Bates, T., and Dowling, R. H.: Cholecystokinin and secretin prevent the intestinal mucosal hypoplasia of total parenteral nutrition in the dog. Gastroenterology, 75:34–41, 1978.

64. Weser, E., Bell, D., and Tawil, T.: Effects of octapeptide-cholecystokinin, secretin, and glucagon on intestinal mucosal growth in parenterally nourished rats. Dig. Dis. Sci., 26:409–416, 1981.

65. Johnson, L. R., and Guthrie, P. D.: Secretin inhibition of gastrin-stimulated DNA synthesis. Gastroenterology, 67:601–606, 1974.

66. Gleeson, M. H., Bloom, S. R., Polak, J. M., Henry, K., and Dowling, R. H.: Endocrine tumour in kidney affecting small bowel structure, motility, and absorptive function. Gut, 12:773–782, 1971.

67. Bloom, S. R., Sagor, G. R., Al-Mukhtur, M. Y. T., Ghatei, M. A., and Wright, N. A.: Enteroglucagon and intestinal adaptation [Abstract]. Gastroenterology, 80:1113, 1981.

68. Liavag, I., and Vaage, S.: The effect of vagotomy and pyloroplasty on the gastrointestinal mucosa of the rat. Scand. J. Gastroenterol., 7:23–28, 1972.

69. Ballinger, W. F., Iida, J., Aponte, G. E., Wirts, C. W., and Goldstein, F.: Structure and function of the canine small intestine following total abdominal vagotomy. Surg. Gynecol. Obstet., 118:1305–1311, 1964.

70. Touloukian, R. J., and Spencer, R. P.: Ileal blood flow preceding compensatory intestinal hypertrophy. Ann. Surg., 175:320–325, 1972.

71. Altmann, G. G., and Leblond, C. P.: Factors influencing villus size in the small intestine of adult rats as revealed by transposition of intestinal segments. Am. J. Anat., 127:15–36, 1970.

72. Grönqvist, B., Engström, B., and Grimelius, L.: Morphological studies of the rat small intestine after jejuno-ileal transposition. Acta Chir. Scand., 141:208–217, 1975.

73. Altmann, G. G.: Influence of bile and pancreatic secretions on the size of the intestinal villi in the rat. Am. J. Anat., 132:167–178, 1971.

74. Weser, E., Heller, R., and Tawil, T.: Stimulation of mucosal growth in the rat ileum by bile and pancreatic secretions after jejunal resection. Gastroenterology, 73:524–529, 1977.

75. Roy, C. C., Laurendau, G., Doyon, G., Chartrand, L., and Rivest, M. R.: The effect of bile and of sodium taurocholate on the epithelial cell dynamics of the rat small intestine. Proc. Soc. Exp. Biol. Med., 149:1000–1004, 1975.

76. Shellito, P. C., Dahl, F. P., Terpstra, O. T., and Malt, R. A.: Postresectional hyperplasia of the small intestine without bile and pancreatic juice. Proc. Soc. Exp. Biol. Med., 158:101–104, 1978.

77. Bury, K.: Carbohydrate digestion and absorption after massive resection of small intestine. Surg. Gynecol. Obstet., 135:177–187, 1972.

78. Rosenszweig, N. S., and Herman, R. H.: Control of jejunal sucrase and maltase activity by dietary sucrose or fructose in man: A model for the study of enzyme regulation in man. J. Clin. Invest., 47:2253–2262, 1968.

79. Menge, H., Werner, H., Lorenz-Meyer, H., and Riecken, E. O.: The nutritive effect of glucose on the structure and function of jejunal self-emptying blind loops in the rat. Gut, 16:462–467, 1975.

80. Rodgers, J. B., Jr., and Bochenek, W.: Localization of lipid reesterifying enzymes of the rat small intestine. Effects of jejunal removal on ileal enzyme activities. Biochim. Biophys. Acta, 202:426–435, 1970.

81. Balint, J. A., Fried, M. B., and Imai, C.: Ileal uptake of oleic acid: Evidence for adaptive response to high fat feeding. Am. J. Clin. Nutr., 33:2276–2280, 1980.

82. Leleiko, N. S., Bronstein, A., and Munro, H. N.: Purine salvage in the small intestine, colon, and liver: Further evidence that enterally supplied nutrients are essential for optimal small intestinal mucosal cell turnover [Abstract]. Gastroenterology, 78:1205, 1980.

83. Ecknauer, R., Sircar, B., and Johnson, L. R.: Effect of dietary bulk on small intestinal morphology and cell renewal in the rat. Gastroenterology, 81:781–786, 1981.

84. Rivilis, J. A., McArdle, A. H., Wlodek, G. K., and Gurd, F. N.: Effect of an elemental diet on gastric secretion. Ann. Surg., 179:226–229, 1974.

85. Malagelada, J. R., Go, V. L. W., and Summerskill, W. H. J.: Different gastric, pancreatic, and biliary responses to solid-liquid or homogenized meals. Dig. Dis. Sci., 24:101–110, 1979.

86. Tompkins, R. K., Waisman, J., Watt, C. M.-H., Corlin, R., and Keith, R.: Absence of mucosal atrophy in human small intestine after prolonged isolation. Gastroenterology, 73:1406–1409, 1977.

87. Lifshitz, F., Coello-Ramirez, P., Gutierrez-Topete, G., and Cornado-Cornet, M. C.: Carbohydrate intolerance in infants with diarrhea. J. Pediatr., 79:760–767, 1971.

88. Lloyd-Still, J.: Gastroenteritis with secondary disaccharide intolerance: An outbreak in a premature unit. Acta Paediatr. Scand., 58:147–150, 1969.

89. Jeffries, G. H., Chapman, A., and Sleisenger, M. H.: Low-fat diet in intestinal lymphangiectasia: Its effect on albumin metabolism. N. Engl. J. Med., 270:761–766, 1964.

90. McGuigan, J. E., Purkerson, M. L., Trudeau, W. L., and Peterson, M. L.: Studies of the immunologic defects associated with intestinal lymphangiectasia. Ann. Intern. Med., 68:398–404, 1968.

91. Holt, P. R.: Dietary treatment of protein loss in intestinal lymphangiectasia: The effect of eliminating long chain triglycerides on albumin metabolism in this condition. Pediatrics, 34:629–635, 1964.

92. Berg, N. O., and Lindberg, T.: Incidence of coeliac disease and transient gluten intolerance in children in a Swedish urban community. Acta Paediatr. Scand., *68*:397–400, 1979.
93. Walker-Smith, J.: Transient gluten intolerance. Arch. Dis. Child., *45*:523–526, 1970.
94. Eastham, E. J., and Walker, W. A.: Adverse effects of milk formula ingestion on the gastrointestinal tract: An update. Gastroenterology, *76*:365–374, 1979.
95. Fischer, J. E., Yoshimura, N., Aguirre, A., James, J. H., Cummings, M. G., Abel, R. M., and Deindoerfer, F.: Plasma amino acids in patients with hepatic encephalopathy: Effects of amino acid infusions. Am. J. Surg., *127*:40–47, 1974.
96. Smith, A. R., Rossi-Fanelli, F., Ziparo, V., James, J. H., Perelle, B. A., and Fischer, J. E.: Alterations in plasma and CSF amino acids, amines, and metabolites in hepatic coma. Ann. Surg., *187*:343–350, 1978.
97. James, J. H., Hodgman, J. M., Funovics, J. M., Yoshimura, N., and Fischer, J. E.: Brain tryptophan, plasma free tryptophan and distribution of plasma neutral amino acids. Metabolism, *25*:471–476, 1976.
98. James, J. H., Escourroy, J., and Fischer, J. E.: Blood-brain neutral amino acid transport activity is increased after portacaval anastomosis. Science, *200*:1395–1397, 1978.
99. Fischer, J. E., Rosen, H. M., Ebeid, A. M., James, J. H., Keane, J. M., and Soeters, P. B.: The effect of normalization of plasma amino acids on hepatic encephalopathy in man. Surgery, *80*:77–91, 1976.
100. Gimmon, Z., James, J. H., and Fischer, J. E.: Effects of branched chain amino acids infusion on clearing of brain aromatic amino acids in hyperammonemic rats [Abstract]. Gastroenterology, *80*:1333, 1981.
101. Maddrey, W. C., Weber, F. L., Jr., Coulter, A. W., Chura, C. M., Chapanis, N. P., and Walser, M.: Effects of keto analogues of essential amino acids in portal-septemic encephalopathy. Gastroenterology, *71*:190–195, 1976.
102. Freund, H., Yoshimura, N., and Fischer, J. E.: Chronic hepatic encephalopathy: Long term therapy with a branched-chain amino-acid-enriched elemental diet. J.A.M.A., *242*:347–349, 1979.
103. Herlong, H. F., Maddrey, W. C., and Walser, M.: The use of ornithine salts of branched-chain ketoacids in portal-systemic encephalopathy. Ann. Intern. Med., *93*:545–550, 1980.
104. Michel, H., Pomier-Layrargues, G., Duhamel, O., Lacombe, B., Cuilleret, G., and Bellet, H.: Intravenous infusion of ordinary and modified amino-acid solutions in the management of hepatic encephalopathy [Abstract]. Gastroenterology, *79*:1038, 1981.
105. Ladefoged, K., Nicolaidou, P., and Jarnum, S.: Calcium, phosphorus, magnesium, zinc, and nitrogen balances in patients with severe short bowel syndrome. Am. J. Clin. Nutr., *33*:2137–2144, 1980.
106. Hylander, E., Ladefoged, K., and Madsen, S.: Calcium balance and bone mineral content following small intestinal resection. Scand. J. Gastroenterol., *16*:167–176, 1981.
107. Ammon, H. V., and Phillips, S. F.: Inhibition of ileal water absorption by intraluminal fatty acids: Influence of chain length, hydroxylation, and conjugation of fatty acids. J. Clin. Invest., *53*:205–210, 1974.
108. Crane, C. W., and Neuberger, A.: The digestion and absorption of protein by normal man. Biochem. J., *74*:313–323, 1960.
109. Borgström, B., Dahlqvist, A., Lundh, G., and Sjövall, J.: Studies of intestinal digestion and absorption in the human. J. Clin. Invest., *36*:1521–1536, 1957.
110. Gupta, J. D., Dakroury, A. M., and Harper, A. E.: Observations on protein digestion in vivo: Rate of disappearance of ingested protein from the gastrointestinal tract. J. Nutr., *64*:447–456, 1958.
111. Adibi, S. A., and Mercer, D. W.: Protein digestion in human intestine as reflected in luminal, mucosal, and plasma amino acid concentrations after meals. J. Clin. Invest., *52*:1586–1594, 1973.
112. Chung, Y. C., Kim, Y. S., Shadchehr, A., Garrido, A., MacGregor, I. L., and Sleisenger, M. H.: Protein digestion and absorption in human small intestine. Gastroenterology, *76*:1415–1421, 1979.
113. Adibi, S. A.: Intestinal transport of dipeptides in man: Relative importance of hydrolysis and intact absorption. J. Clin. Invest., *50*:2266–2275, 1971.
114. Silk, D. B. A.: Peptide transport. Clin. Sci., *60*:607–615, 1981.
115. Matthews, D. M., and Adibi, S. A.: Peptide absorption. Gastroenterology, *71*:151–161, 1976.
116. Meyer, J. H., Thomson, J. B., Cohen, M. B., Shadchehr, A., and Mandiola, S. A.: Sieving of solid food by the canine stomach and sieving after ulcer surgery. Gastroenterology, *76*:804–813, 1979.
117. Adibi, S. A., Gray, S. J., and Menden, E.: The kinetics of amino acid absorption and alteration of plasma composition of free amino acids after intestinal perfusion of amino acid mixtures. Am. J. Clin. Nutr., *20*:24–33, 1967.
118. Silk, D. B. A., Fairclough, P. D., Clark, M. L., Hegarty, J. E., Marrs, T. C., Addison, J. M., Burston, D., Clegg, K. M., and Matthews, D. M.: Use of a peptide rather than free amino acid nitrogen source in chemically defined "elemental" diets. J.P.E.N., *4*:548–553, 1980.
119. Hecketsweiler, P., Vidon, N., Emonts, P., and Bernier, J. J.: Absorption of elemental and complex nutritional solutions during a continuous jejunal perfusion in man. Digestion, *19*:213–217, 1979.
120. Ruppin, H., Bar-Meir, S., Soergel, K. H., and Wood, C. M.: Effect of liquid formula diets on proximal gastrointestinal function. Dig. Dis. Sci., *26*:202–207, 1981.
121. Binder, H. J., Filburn, C., and Volpe, B. T.: Bile salt alteration of colonic electrolyte transport: Role of cyclic adenosine monophosphate. Gastroenterology, *68*:503–508, 1975.
122. Krag, E., and Phillipps, S. F.: Effect of free and conjugated bile acids on net water, electrolyte, and glucose movement in the perfused human ileum. J. Lab. Clin. Med., *83*:947–956, 1974.
123. Bochenek, W., Rodgers, J. B., Jr., and Balint, J. A.: Effects of changes in dietary lipids on intestinal fluid loss in the short bowel syndrome. Ann. Intern. Med., *72*:205–213, 1970.
124. Simko, V., McCarroll, A. M., Goodman, S., Weesner, R. E., and Kelley, R. E.: High-fat diet in a

short bowel syndrome: Intestinal absorption and gastroenteropancreatic hormone responses. Dig. Dis. Sci., 25:333–339, 1980.

125. Ovesen, L., Chu, R., and Howard, L.: The effects of meals with different fat content on ostomy output of extreme short bowel patients. Accepted for publication. ASPEN meeting, Spring 1982.

126. Hogben, C. A. M.: Symposium on fat absorption. Fat absorption: A transport problem. Gastroenterology, 50:51–55, 1966.

127. Simko, V., and Linscheer, W. G.: Absorption of different elemental diets in short bowel syndrome lasting 15 years. Dig. Dis., 21:419–425, 1976.

128. Stephens, R. V., and Randall, H. T.: Use of a concentrated, balanced, liquid elemental diet for nutritional management of catabolic states. Ann. Surg., 170:642–665, 1969.

129. Bell, M. J., Martin, L. W., Schubert, W. K., Partin, J., and Burke, J.: Massive small-bowel resection in an infant: Long-term management and intestinal adaptation. J. Pediatr. Surg., 8:197–204, 1973.

130. Voitk, A. J., Echave, V., Brown, R. A., and Gurd, F. N.: Use of elemental diet during the adaptive stage of short gut syndrome. Gastroenterology, 65:419–426, 1973.

131. Thompson, W. R., Stephens, R. V., Randall, H. T., and Bowen, J. R.: Use of the "space diet" in the management of a patient with extreme short bowel syndrome. Am. J. Surg., 117:449–459, 1969.

132. Queen, P. M., Sutphen, J. L., and Tepper, D.: Nitrogen and mineral retention during feedings of defined formula diets in short small bowel. Accepted for publication, ASPEN meeting, Spring 1982.

133. Bury, K. D., and Jambunathan, G.: Effects of elemental diets on gastric emptying and gastric secretion in man. Am. J. Surg., 127:59–64, 1974.

134. Howard, L., Bigaouett, J., Chu, R., et al.: Water soluble vitamin requirements in home parenteral nutrition patients. Submitted for publication.

135. Bounous, G., Hugon, J., and Gentile, J. M.: Elemental diet in the management of the intestinal lesion produced by 5-fluorouracil in the rat. Can. J. Surg., 14:298–311, 1971.

136. Bounous, G., Gentile, J. M., and Hugon, J.: Elemental diet in the management of the intestinal lesion produced by 5-fluorouracil in man. Can. J. Surg., 14:312–324, 1971.

137. Bounous, G., and Maestracci, D.: Use of an elemental diet in animals during treatment with 5-flurouracil. Cancer Treat. Rep., 60:17–22, 1976.

138. Stanford, J. R., Carey, L. C., King, D. R., and Anderson, G. W.: Adverse effects of elemental diets on tolerance for 5-fluorouracil toxicity in rats. Surg. Forum, 27:42–43, 1976.

139. Donaldson, S. S., Jundt, S., Ricour, C., Sarrazin, D., Lenerle, J., and Schweisguth, O.: Radiation enteritis in children: A retrospective review, clinicopathologic correlation, and dietary management. Cancer, 35:1167–1178, 1975.

140. Morgenstern, L., and Hiatt, N.: Injurious effect of pancreatic secretions on postradiation enteropathy. Gastroenterology, 53:923–929, 1967.

141. Hugon, J. S., and Bounous, G.: Elemental diet in the management of the intestinal lesions produced by radiation in the mouse. Can. J. Surg., 15:18–26, 1972.

142. Pageau, R., and Bounous, G.: Systemic protection against radiation: Increased intestinal radioresistance in rats fed a formula-defined diet. Radiat. Res., 71:622–629, 1977.

143. McCardle, A. H.: The use of an elemental diet as prophylaxis in radiation enteropathy. Abstract presented at the Twelfth International Congress of Nutrition.

144. Homer, D. R., Grand, R. J., and Colodny, A. H.: Growth, course and prognosis after surgery for Crohn's disease in childhood and adolescents. Pediatrics, 59:717–725, 1977.

145. Kelts, D. G., Grand, R. J., Shen, G., Watkins, J. B., Werlin, S. L., and Boehme, C.: Nutritional basis of growth failure in children and adolescents with Crohn's disease. Gastroenterology, 76:720–727, 1979.

146. Morin, C. L., Roulet, M., Roy, C. C., and Weber, A.: Continuous elemental enteral alimentation in children with Crohn's disease and growth failure. Gastroenterology, 79:1205–1210, 1980.

147. Kirschner, B. S., Klich, J. R., Kalman, S. S., et al.: Reversal of growth retardation in Crohn's disease with therapy emphasizing oral nutritional restitution. Gastroenterology, 80:10–15, 1981.

148. Simmons, J. M., Wilson, C. J., Potter, D. E., and Holliday, M. A.: Relation of calorie deficiency to growth failure in children on hemodialysis and the growth response to calorie supplementation. N. Engl. J. Med., 285:653–656, 1971.

149. Barot, L. R., Rombeau, J. L., Steinberg, J. J., Crosby, L. O., Feurer, I. D., and Mullen, J. L.: Energy expenditure in patients with inflammatory bowel disease. Arch. Surg., 116:460–462, 1981.

150. Grand, R. J., Kelts, D. G., Shen, G., and Boehme, C.: Energy and nitrogen balance in children with Crohn's disease and growth failure before and during parenteral nutrition [Abstract]. Gastroenterology, 80:1162, 1981.

151. Motil, K. J., Grand, R. J., Young, V. R., Matthews, D. E., and Bier, D. M.: The effect of dietary protein and energy supplementation on whole body protein and nitrogen metabolism in children with Crohn's disease and growth failure [Abstract]. Gastroenterology, 80:1235, 1981.

152. Kirschner, B. S.: Somatomedin deficiency: A possible cause of growth failure in children with chronic inflammatory bowel disease [Abstract]. Gastroenterology, 80:1192, 1981.

153. Segal, A. W., Levi, A. J., and Loewi, G.: Levamisole in the treatment of Crohn's disease. Lancet 2:382–384, 1977.

154. Axelsson, C. K., and Justesen, T.: Studies of the duodenal and fecal flora in gastrointestinal disorders during treatment with an elemental diet. Gastroenterology, 72:397–401, 1977.

155. Calam, J., Crooks, P. E., and Walker R. J.: Elemental diets in the management of Crohn's perianal fistulae. J.P.E.N., 4:4–8, 1980.

156. Giorgini, G. L., Stephens, R. V., and Thayer, W. R.: The use of "medical by-pass" in the therapy of Crohn's disease: Report of a case. Am. J. Dig. Dis., 18:153–157, 1973.

157. Bury, K. D., Turnier, E., and Randall, H. T.: Nutritional management of granulomatous colitis with perianal ulceration. Can. J. Surg., 15:108–113, 1972.

158. Banwell, J. G., and Sherr, H.: Effect of bacterial enterotoxins on the gastrointestinal tract. Gastroenterology, 65:467–497, 1973.

159. Sack, D. A., Islam, S., Brown, K. H., Islam, A., Kabir, A. K. M., Chowdhury, A. M. A. K., and Ali, M. A.: Oral therapy in children with cholera: A comparison of sucrose and glucose electrolyte solutions. J. Pediatr., 96:20–25, 1980.

160. Kent, T. H., and Lindenbaum, J.: Correlation of jejunal function and morphology in patients with acute and chronic diarrhea in East Pakistan. Gastroenterology, 52:972–984, 1967.

161. Agus, S. G., Dolin, R., Wyatt, R. G., Tousimis, A. J., and Northrup, R. S.: Acute infectious nonbacterial gastroenteritis: Intestinal histopathology. Histologic and enzymatic alterations during illness produced by the Norwalk agent in man. Ann. Intern. Med., 79:18–25, 1973.

162. Torres-Pinedo, R., Rivera, C. L., and Fernandez, S.: Studies on infant diarrhea: Absorption of glucose and net fluxes of water and sodium chloride in a segment of the jejunum. J. Clin. Invest., 45:1916–1922, 1966.

163. Billich, C., Bray, G. A., Gallagher, T. F. Jr., Hoffbrand, A. V., and Levitan, R.: Absorptive capacity of the jejunum of obese and lean subjects: Effect of fasting. Arch. Intern. Med., 130:377–380, 1972.

164. Pergolizzi, R., Lifshitz, F., Teichberg, S., and Wapnir, R. A.: Interaction between dietary carbohydrates and intestinal disaccharidases in experimental diarrhea. Am. J. Clin. Nutr., 30:482–489, 1977.

165. Davidson, G. P., Gall, D. G., Petric, M., Butler, D. G., and Hamilton, J. R.: Human rotavirus enteritis induced in conventional piglets: Intestinal structure and transport. J. Clin. Invest., 60:1402–1409, 1977.

166. Rodriguez, W. J., Kim, H. W., Arrobio, J. O., Brandt, C. D., Chanock, R. M., Kapikian, A. Z., Wyatt, R. G., and Parrott, R. H.: Clinical features of acute gastroenteritis associated with human reovirus-like agent in infants and young children. J. Pediatr., 91:188–193, 1977.

167. Sack, D. A., Chowdhury, A. M. A. K., Ensof, A., Ali, M. A., Merson, M. H., Islam, S., Black, R. E., and Brown, K. H.: Oral hydration in rotavirus diarrhea: A double blind comparison of sucrose with glucose electrolyte solution. Lancet, 2:280–283, 1978.

168. Nalin, D. R., Cash, R. A., Rahman, M., and Yunus, M. D.: Effect of glycine and glucose on sodium and water absorption in patients with cholera. Gut, 11:768–772, 1970.

169. Chung, A. W., and Viščorová, B.: The effect of early oral feedings versus early oral starvation on the course of infantile diarrhea. J. Pediatr., 33:14–22, 1948.

170. Iyngkaran, N., Abdin, Z., Davis, K., Boey, C. G., Prathap, K., Yadav, M., Lam, S. K., and Puthucheary, S. D.: Acquired carbohydrate intolerance and cow milk protein sensitive enteropathy in young infants. J. Pediatr., 95:373–378, 1979.

171. Avery, G. B., Villavicencio, O., Lilly, J. R., and Randolph, J. G.: Intractable diarrhea in early infancy. Pediatrics, 41:712–722, 1968.

172. Hyman, C. J., Reiter, J., Rodman, J., and Drash, A. L.: Parenteral and oral alimentation in the treatment of the nonspecific protracted diarrheal syndrome of infancy. J. Pediatr., 78:17–29, 1971.

173. Lloyd-Still, J. D., Schwachman, H., and Filler, R. M.: Protracted diarrhea of infancy treated by intravenous alimentation: Clinical study of 16 infants. J. Dis. Child., 125:358–368, 1973.

174. Sherman, J. O., Hamly, C. A., and Khachadurian, A. K.: Use of an oral elemental diet in infants with severe intractable diarrhea. J. Pediatr., 86:518–523, 1975.

175. Greene, H. L., McCabe, D. R., and Merenstein, G. B.: Protracted diarrhea and malnutrition in infancy: Changes in intestinal morphology and disaccharidase activities during treatment with total intravenous nutrition or oral elemental diets. J. Pediatr., 87:695–704, 1975.

176. Rossi, T. M., Lebenthal, E., Nord, K. S., and Fazili, R. R.: Extent and duration of small intestinal mucosal injury in intractable diarrhea of infancy. Pediatrics, 66:730–735, 1980.

177. Aufses, A. H., Jr., and Kreel, I.: Ileostomy for granulomatous ileocolitis. Ann. Surg., 173:91–96, 1971.

178. Strobel, C. T., Byrne, W. J., and Ament, M. E.: Home parenteral nutrition in children with Crohn's disease: An effective management alternative. Gastroenterology, 77:272–279, 1979.

179. Greenberg, G. R., Haber, G. B., and Jeejeebhoy, K. N.: Total parenteral nutrition and bowel rest in the management of Crohn's disease. Gut, 17:828, 1976.

180. Elson, C. O., Layden, T. J., Nemchausky, B. A., Rosenberg, J. L., and Rosenberg, I. H.: An evaluation of total parenteral nutrition in the management of inflammatory bowel disease. Dig. Dis. Sci., 25:42–48, 1980.

181. Reilly, J., Ryan, J. A., Strole, W., and Fischer, J. E.: Hyperalimentation in inflammatory bowel disease. Am. J. Surg., 131:192–200, 1976.

182. Vogel, C. M., Corwin, T. R., and Baue, A. E.: Intravenous hyperalimentation in the treatment of inflammatory diseases of the bowel. Arch. Surg., 108:460–467, 1974.

183. Anderson, D. L., and Boyce, H. W., Jr.: Use of parenteral nutrition in treatment of advanced regional enteritis. Am. J. Dig. Dis., 18:633–640, 1973.

184. Dickinson, R. J., Ashton, M. G., Axon, A. T. R., Smith, R. C., Yeung, C. K., and Hill, G. L.: Controlled trial of intravenous hyperalimentation and total bowel rest as an adjunct to the routine treatment of acute colitis. Gastroenterology, 79:1199–1204, 1980.

185. Voitk, A. J., Echave, B., Feller, J. H., Brown, R. A., and Gurd, F. N.: Experience with elemental diet in the treatment of inflammatory bowel disease: Is this primary therapy? Arch. Surg., 107:329–333, 1973.

186. Rocchio, M. A., Mo Cha, C.-J., Haas, K. F., and Randall, H. T.: Use of chemically defined diets in the management of patients with acute inflammatory bowel disease. Am. J. Surg., 127:469–475, 1974.

187. Axelsson, C., and Jarnum, S.: Assessment of the therapeutic value of an elemental diet in chronic inflammatory bowel disease. Scand. J. Gastroenterol., 12:89–95, 1977.

188. O'Morain, C., Segal, A. W., and Levi, A. J.: Elemental diets in treatment of acute Crohn's disease. Br. Med. J., 281:1173–1175, 1980.

189. Goode, A., Feggetter, J. G. W., Hawkins, T., and Johnston, I. D. A.: Use of an elemental diet for long-term nutritional support in Crohn's disease. Lancet, 1:122–124, 1976.

190. Logan, R. F. A., Gillon, J., Ferrington, C., and Ferguson, A.: Reduction of gastrointestinal protein loss by elemental diet in Crohn's disease of the small bowel. Gut, 22:383–387, 1981.

191. Morin, C. L., Roulet, M., Weber, A., Roy, C. C., and Lapointe, N.: Nasogastric infusion of elemental diet as primary therapy in Crohn's disease [Abstract 478]. Pediatr. Res., 13:405, 1979.

192. Andresen, A. F. R.: Ulcerative colitis: An allergic phenomenon. Am. J. Dig. Dis., 9(O.S.):91–98, 1942.

193. Binder, H. J., Gryboski, J. D., Thayer, W. R., Jr., and Spiro, H. M.: Intolerance to milk in ulcerative colitis. Am. J. Dig. Dis., 11:858–864, 1966.

194. Gudnand-Høyer, E., and Jarnum, S.: Incidence and clinical significance of lactose malabsorption in ulcerative colitis and Crohn's disease. Gut, 11:338–343, 1970.

195. Kirschner, B. S., DeFavaro, M. V., and Jensen, W.: Lactose malabsorption in children and adolescents with inflammatory bowel disease. Gastroenterology, 81:829–832, 1981.

196. Isenberg, J. I., and Maxwell, V.: Intravenous infusion of amino acids stimulates gastric acid secretion in man. N. Engl. J. Med., 298:27–29, 1978.

197. Kelly, G. A., and Nahrwold, D. L.: Pancreatic secretion in response to an elemental diet and intravenous hyperalimentation. Surg. Gynecol. Obstet., 143:87–91, 1976.

198. Adler, M., Pieroni, P. L., Takeshima, T., Nacchiero, M., Dreiling, D. A., and Rudick, J.: Effects of parenteral hyperalimentation on pancreatic and biliary secretions. Surg. Forum, 26:445–446, 1975.

199. Johnson, L. R., Schanbacher, L. M., Dudrick, S. J., and Copeland, E. M.: Effect of long-term parenteral feeding on pancreatic secretion and serum secretin. Am. J. Physiol., 233:E524–E529, 1977.

200. Goodgame, J. T., and Fischer, J. E.: Parenteral nutrition in the treatment of acute pancreatitis. Ann. Surg., 186:651–658, 1977.

201. Ragins, H., Levenson, S. M., Signer, R., Stamford, W., and Seifter, E.: Intrajejunal administration of an elemental diet at neutral pH avoids pancreatic stimulation: Studies in dog and man. Am. J. Surg., 126:606–614, 1973.

202. Koretz, R. L., and Meyer, J. H.: Elemental diets—Facts and fantasies. Gastroenterology, 78:393–410, 1980.

203. Lewis, J. W., and Freeman, J. B.: Canine pancreatic exocrine secretion in response to low and high fat elemental diet [Abstract]. Gastroenterology, 70:907, 1976.

204. McArdle, A. H., Echave, W., Brown, R. A., and Thompson, A. G.: Effect of elemental diet on pancreatic secretion. Am. J. Surg., 128:690–692, 1974.

205. Meyer, J. H., Kelly, G. A., Spingola, L. J., and Jones, R. S.: Canine gut receptors mediating pancreatic responses to luminal L-amino acids. Am. J. Physiol., 231:669–677, 1976.

206. Go, V. L. W., Hofmann, A. F., and Summerskill, W. F. J.: Pancreozymin assay in man based on pancreatic enzyme secretion: Potency of specific amino acids and other digestive products. J. Clin. Invest., 49:1558–1564, 1970.

207. Vidon, N., Hecketsweiler, P., Butel, J., and Bernier, J. J.: Effect of continuous jejunal perfusion of elemental and complex nutritional solutions on pancreatic enzyme secretion in human subjects. Gut, 19:194–198, 1978.

208. Wolfe, B. M., Keltner, R. M., and Kaminski, D. L.: The effect of an intraduodenal elemental diet on pancreatic secretion. Surg. Gynecol. Obstet., 140:241–245, 1975.

209. Cassim, M. M., and Allardyce, D. B.: Pancreatic secretion in response to jejunal feeding of elemental diet. Ann. Surg., 180:228–231, 1974.

210. Keith, R. G.: Effect of a low fat elemental diet on pancreatic secretion during pancreatitis. Surg. Gynecol. Obstet., 151:337–343, 1980.

211. Voitk, A., Brown, R. A., Echave, V., McArdle, A. H., Gurd, F. N., and Thompson, A. G.: Use of an elemental diet in the treatment of complicated pancreatitis. Am. J. Surg., 125:223–227, 1973.

212. Blackburn, G. L., Williams, L. F., Bistrian, B. R., Stone, M. S., Phillips, E., Hirsch, E., Clowes, G. H. A., Jr., and Gregg, J.: New approaches to the management of severe acute pancreatitis. Am. J. Surg., 131:114–124, 1976.

213. Soeters, P. B., Ebeid, A. M., and Fischer, J. E.: Review of 404 patients with gastrointestinal fistulas: Impact of parenteral nutrition. Ann. Surg., 190:189–202, 1979.

214. MacFadyen, B. V. J., Dudrick, S. J., and Ruberg, R. L.: Management of gastrointestinal fistulas with parenteral hyperalimentation. Surgery, 74:100–105, 1973.

215. Freund, H., Anner, C., and Saltz, N. J.: Management of gastrointestinal fistulas with total parenteral nutrition. Int. Surg., 61:273–275, 1976.

216. Blackett, R. L., and Hill, G. L.: Postoperative external small bowel fistulas: A study of a consecutive series of patients treated with intravenous hyperalimentation. Br. J. Surg., 65:775–778, 1978.

217. Deitel, M.: Nutritional management of external gastrointestinal fistulas. Can. J. Surg., 19:505–511, 1976.

218. Sheldon, G. F., Gardiner, B. N., Way, L. W., and Dunphy, J. E.: Management of gastrointestinal fistulas. Surg. Gynecol. Obstet., 133:385–389, 1971.

219. Reber, H. A., Roberts, C., Way, L. W., and Dunphy, J. E.: Management of external gastrointestinal fistulas. Ann. Surg., 188:460–467, 1978.

220. Bury, K. D.: Elemental diets. In Fischer, J. E. (ed.): Total Parenteral Nutrition. Boston, Little, Brown and Co., 1976, pp. 395–411.

221. Fischer, J. E.: Hyperalimentation. Adv. Surg., 11:1–69, 1977.

222. Thomas, R. J. S.: The response of patients with fistulas of the gastrointestinal tract to parenteral nutrition. Surg. Gynecol. Obstet., 153:77–80, 1981.

223. Byrne, W. J., Burke, M., Fonkalsrud, E. W., and Ament, M. E.: Home parenteral nutrition: An alternative approach to the management of complicated gastrointestinal fistulas not responding to conventional medical or surgical therapy. J. P. E. N., 3:355–359, 1979.

224. Wolfe, B. M., Keltner, R. M., and Willman, V. L.: Intestinal fistula output in regular, elemental, and intravenous alimentation. Am. J. Surg., 124:803–806, 1972.

225. Voitk, A. J., Echave, V., Brown, R. A., McArdle,

A. H., and Gurd, F. N.: Elemental diet in the treatment of fistulas of the alimentary tract. Surg. Gynecol. Obstet., *137*:68–72, 1973.

226. Rocchio, M. A., Mo Cha, C.-J., Haas, K. F., and Randall, H. T.: Use of chemically defined diets in the management of patients with high output gastrointestinal cutaneous fistulas. Am. J. Surg., *127*:148–156, 1974.

227. Bury, K. D., Stephens, R. V., and Randall, H. T.: Use of a chemically defined, liquid, elemental diet for nutritional management of fistulas of the alimentary tract. Am. J. Surg., *121*:174–183, 1971.

228. Tanski, E. V., and Weismann, R. E.: Management of upper gastrointestinal fistula with a double lumen tube. Am. J. Surg., *121*:426–431, 1971.

CHAPTER 21

Enteral Nutrition and Renal Disease

WILLIAM P. STEFFEE
CARL F. ANDERSON

The advent of techniques to intervene nutritionally has provided the clinician with a considerable advantage when treating the patient with impaired renal function. This is particularly true for enteral hyperalimentation, which has the ability to meet the patient's nutrient and metabolic demands by use of controlled delivery of solutions to the intestinal tract. This chapter will address issues relative to this method of therapy and not necessarily relate to broader dietary aspects or the use of total parenteral nutrition.

The hospitalized patient with renal disease who requires nutritional support nearly always has additional problems that frequently include malnutrition, trauma, surgical intervention, and infection. Care depends on evaluation of the degree of acute or chronic renal disease, whether or not dialysis therapy is necessary, as well as the nutritional state and the degree of stress to which the patient is exposed.

Acute renal failure is characterized by increasing levels of serum urea, creatinine, uric acid, hydrogen ions, potassium, and phosphorus, while levels of serum sodium, bicarbonate, and calcium fall. Acute renal failure may be classified as oliguric (less than 500 ml of urine/day) or nonoliguric (more than 500 ml of urine/day, often 1500 ml). When oliguric renal failure is present, nutritional treatment is severely limited by fluid restriction and in most cases will require dialysis. Nonoliguric acute renal failure, often preceded by aminoglycoside therapy or less prolonged renal ischemia, is probably much more common in hospital-

ized patients.[1] The serum creatinine and urea levels tend to increase at slower rates and the urine sodium losses are often fixed between 50 and 75 mEq/L.[2] In general, nutritional therapy can be more easily implemented without the necessity for dialysis therapy.

From the perspective of nutritional intervention, chronic renal failure may be divided into three categories depending upon residual renal function.

Renal function greater than 50 per cent of normal. The serum creatinine levels are usually between 2 and 3 mg/dl. The blood pH is normal. The hematocrit level is within normal range as is the level of serum phosphorus. Protein delivery is generally well tolerated and, as a rule, little modification is needed apart from closer attention to water and sodium intake.[3]

Renal function between 20 and 50 per cent of normal. These patients represent a group whose well-being is greatly dependent on nutritional treatment. If the nutritional therapy is carefully chosen, dialysis can often be avoided. Renal adaptation is less complete, especially at the lower level in this category. The serum creatinine may be 5 mg/dl or more, the blood pH 7.35, the hematocrit low, and the level of serum phosphorus elevated. Water excess, hyperkalemia, sodium excess or, less commonly, depletion, and hypermagnesemia are all common unless close attention is paid to intakes and losses. Total nitrogen intake depends not only on the level of renal function but also on the presence or absence of uremic signs and symptoms.

Renal function less than 20 per cent of normal. Serum creatinine levels are nearly always greater than 5 mg/dl and blood urea nitrogen levels are above 100 mg/dl. Renal regulatory capacity is severely tested. Acidemia, hyperphosphatemia, and anemia are invariably present. Whereas strict adherence to a dietary prescription may allow some degree of stability, when trauma, major surgery, or infection are added, intake modification alone is usually inadequate. Hemodialysis or peritoneal dialysis is often necessary.

Other renal diseases or states of malfunction may also affect nutritional therapy. Massive proteinuria is almost invariably associated with a decreased ceiling of sodium excretion that requires moderate to marked sodium restriction.[4] Renal tubular acidosis may require additional bicarbonate therapy.

Hyperglycemia[5, 6] after a carbohydrate load and hypertriglyceridemia[7] are both frequently noted in patients with chronic renal failure. Although one might be tempted to alter nutritional therapy if one or both are found, to do so is usually counterproductive. Insulin may be necessary if hyperglycemia is a problem. Insulin should be administered in quantities sufficient to maintain an optimal blood glucose level at times of optimal caloric delivery. Hypertriglyceridemia alone in these patients has not been convincingly shown to be a cardiovascular risk factor.

With the belief that the majority of hospitalized patients requiring major nutrient modification due to renal failure have renal function in the range of 20 to 50 per cent of normal, considerable effort will be devoted to this group with nonoliguric renal failure. In addition, it is commonly true that patients with acute oliguric renal failure often experience multi-organ dysfunction. This often makes use of the gastrointestinal tract marginally successful at best, with total parenteral nutrition then being the more realistic approach to nutritional therapy.

THE FAILING KIDNEY

When considering the pathophysiology of renal failure, it is important to remember that the failure of renal function is primarily a failure of regulation. Whereas the patient with healthy kidneys can perform wonders to maintain the internal milieu in face of oftentimes extreme variations of intake, the patient with renal failure demands that the delivery of nutrients, water, and electrolytes be adjusted to the relatively fixed ability of the kidneys to excrete or retain elements.

We are normally endowed with approximately two million intact nephrons. As the number decreases, either due to disease or the aging process, those that remain are thought to hypertrophy as adaptation occurs. As nephron loss progresses, the urine volume that is produced reflects primarily a solute diuresis with the total solute load excreted daily being near normal. It is the ability to manipulate the load presented for excretion that becomes impaired, that is, a failure of regulatory capacity. Efforts to treat the patient must be directed toward defining this regulatory capacity and altering the burden requiring excretion either by direct modification of intake or by influence of endogenous metabolic pathways by nutritional therapy.

What would happen without renal adaptation? With an unchanged intake and a decrease in the number of functioning nephrons, there would be an obligatory increase in the body content of substances that depend on renal excretion. Without adaptation, the body's content of water, sodium, potassium, and magnesium would quickly increase to lethal levels. The kidney adapts by increasing excretion of each of these substances per hypertrophied nephron. Renal regulation of excretion of phosphate, urates, and ammonia is less complete and the excretion of phosphorus results in a "trade-off" phenomenon. There seems to be little if any renal adaptation to increased levels of urea, although the liver can utilize the nitrogen from the urea-generated ammonia to aminate some carbon compounds.[8] Tubular secretion of creatinine seems to increase[9] and some of the creatinine can be metabolized in the gastrointestinal tract.[10]

Renal excretion equals the excretion per nephron times the number of functioning nephrons. Since the number of functioning nephrons is less, there must be increased excretion per nephron. In general, the adaptation seems relatively solute-specific and the price for adaptation (trade-off) may include some of the findings observed in these patients. This adaptation is best understood for phosphate. Assuming a constant intake of phosphorus, the serum level of ionized calcium falls as nephron loss occurs. This happens before any fall in serum levels of 1,25 dihydroxycholecalciferol becomes apparent. The serum level of parathyroid hormone increases, urine phosphate increases, urinary calcium falls, and the serum levels of phosphate and ionized calcium return to normal. However, the serum level of parathyroid hormone remains elevated. The trade-off for maintaining normal levels of serum phosphate and ionized calcium includes the extrarenal effects of parathyroid hormone. Increased levels of parathyroid hormone may be important in producing the osteitis fibrosa cystica component of renal osteodystrophy, pruritus, prolonged nerve conduction, and carbohydrate and lipoprotein abnormalities.[11-13] If intake of phosphorus is decreased concomitant with nephron loss in animal studies, there is less excretion of phosphate per nephron, lower serum parathyroid levels, and less bone disease.[14]

PROTEIN AND ENERGY CONSIDERATIONS

Biochemical considerations of the metabolic syndrome associated with renal failure have long held that products of nitrogen metabolism are intimately related to the clinical expression of the disease state. Since kidneys are major excretory organs, and since the uremic syndrome resembles so closely that of an intoxication, it has been the fashion to assume a simple cause and effect relationship between the failure of excretory function, the accumulation of "toxic" nitrogenous waste products, and the clinical syndrome. In 1822, Prévost and Dumas found elevated blood urea levels in nephrectomized animals, a finding that has become a biochemical hallmark of the human disease.[15] Since that time, many efforts have been made to substantiate or disprove the possible toxicity of urea in the disease syndrome. At present, most clinicians would agree that urea plays a relatively minor role, mainly because there appears to be little consistent or strong correlation between elevated blood urea levels and other parameters of the disease state.[16] It is quite uncertain, however, whether changes in blood metabolite levels, particularly those of nitrogenous origin, are the direct results of a failure in excretory function, or whether these changes are in part reflective of an ill-defined and poorly understood disturbance in the pathways of body protein metabolism, or a combination of both disturbances.

It is not often appreciated that, in the adult human, total nitrogen turnover and rates of protein anabolism and catabolism are from two to three times greater than the normal dietary protein consumption and perhaps even eight to ten times higher than current estimates of the minimal amount of dietary nitrogen required to maintain nitrogen balance in health.[17] It is unknown whether these quantitative relationships apply to the patient with renal failure, but it is conceivable that alterations in anabolic or catabolic rates of total body protein may be an important abnormality in the uremic syndrome. If such is the case, it follows that clinical efforts to control these endogenous rates are perhaps of greater importance than the actual delivery of exogenous dietary protein.

Case Study

The following case study, in which these parameters were evaluated under controlled conditions in a patient with severe renal failure before and after the initiation of high dose steroid therapy, seems to add insight into the relative importance of dietary protein intake and endogenous protein turnover.

The patient, a 55-year-old woman with a height of 150 cm and a weight of 49 kg, was admitted to the Clinical Research Center (CRC) of the Mayo Clinic as a participant in a study designed to assess parameters of endogenous protein turnover in adults. She had a history of chronic renal failure and a renal biopsy had revealed interstitial nephritis. Systemic lupus erythematosus was subsequently diagnosed but at this point the diagnosis had not been firmly established. She was moderately hypertensive. Renal osteodystrophy was present.

Initial renal evaluation revealed a blood urea concentration of 219 mg/dl (blood urea = BUN × 2.14), plasma creatinine 5.6 mg/dl, and bilaterally small kidneys. Insulin and para-aminohippuric acid clearances were 8 and 30 ml/min/1.73 m² respectively. The patient was given a 40-gm high biologic protein, high caloric, 40 mEq sodium diet. One year later, her blood urea had dropped to 69 mg/dl and her plasma creatinine to 3.5 mg/dl. She remained relatively stable during the year prior to study with her blood urea slowly increasing to 93 mg/dl and plasma creatinine to 6.3 mg/dl at the time the study began. She was never dialyzed.

The study protocol called for the provision of a rotating-pair diet containing 0.38 gm of egg protein/kg/day and 45 kcal/kg/day primarily in the form of carbohydrate. The patient was instructed in this diet two weeks prior to entering the CRC. As was anticipated, this initial period of prehospitalization dietary therapy resulted in a reduction of both blood urea and creatinine concentrations (Fig. 21–1). However, once on the study, a divergent pattern emerged. Blood urea fell and was maintained at a stable level between 55 and 60 mg/dl. Creatinine, contrary to our experience, began to rise from an admission level of 4.0 mg/dl to a peak of 7.8 mg/dl 18 days after initiation of the protocol. At this point, the patient complained of severe headaches followed by the abrupt onset of a right hemiparesis.

A diagnosis of a brainstem lesion secondary to vasculitis of acute lupus erythematosus was made and therapy was initiated with prednisone, 20 mg three times a day. Optimal nutrition was not maintained during the first few days; however, the patient responded rapidly to therapy and was able to resume eating. An effort was made to maintain an intake similar to that provided in the CRC, and approximately two weeks later the patient was returned to the CRC for reevaluation of parameters of endogenous protein turnover. The previous study had been performed on days 9 to 12 of the protocol prior to steroid therapy. Of interest is the marked increase in blood urea levels to approximately 250 mg/dl and a concurrent return of plasma creatinine to 4.2 mg/dl. This divergent pattern was interpreted to represent the catabolic effects of steroids on muscle metabolism and the improvement of presumed coincident glomerulonephritis.

Rates of total body nitrogen flux and protein anabolism and breakdown were obtained using the constant infusion model described by Picou and Taylor-Roberts[15] in malnourished children and applied with modifications to normal adults.[19] Daily 24-hour urine collections were obtained for analysis of total nitrogen, urea, creatinine, and 3-methylhistidine.

Compared to values for normal adults on a similar diet, the single study in this uremic subject prior to steroid therapy reveals an acceleration of protein turnover and rates of protein anabolism and catabolism (Table 21–1). In this instance, the amount of protein being synthesized was slightly greater than that being degraded, a pattern similar to that found in the normal subjects on a high protein diet.[19] However, the patient's plasma albumin was found to be subnormal prior to study (2.5 gm/dl) and the enhanced rate of synthesis compared to breakdown may reflect an ongoing repair of a body protein deficit.

After steroid therapy, total body turnover was enhanced 77 per cent above normal, protein anabolic rates increased slightly, and those of catabolism increased quite markedly. The net difference between rates of synthesis and catabolism was reversed, and the patient became "catabolic."

Support for these findings can be found in blood and urine urea and 3-methylhistidine levels (Fig. 21–2). Presteroid blood urea values were stable in face of apparently deteriorating renal function (rising creatinine). In this period of time the efficiency of total body protein turnover remained relatively stable with no change in the net amount of nitrogen requiring excretion as urea. On the other hand, the creatinine levels increased, suggesting decreased glomerular perfusion. Levels of plasma 3-methylhistidine were measurable, this not being the case in nonuremic subjects.[20] Twenty-four hour urine 3-methylhistidine levels were maintained within limits defined as normal for the control subjects on a similar diet.

As a consequence of steroid therapy, not only did blood urea levels rise from 50 to 250 mg/dl, but urine urea excretion increased nearly five-fold, supporting a marked disproportion between rates of synthesis and catabolism. Likewise, both plasma and urine 3-methylhistidine increased. This amino acid is methylated only after incorporation into actin and myosin moieties of muscle.[20] Once released by protein breakdown, the 3-methylhistidine is not reincorporated but

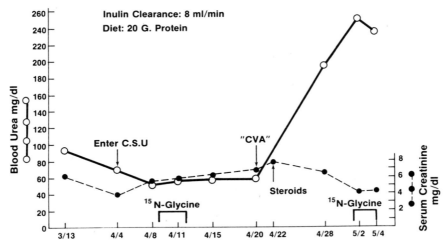

Figure 21–1. The clinical course of a uremic patient who underwent controlled study of parameters of endogenous protein turnover before and after steroid therapy.

Table 21–1 COMPARISON OF TOTAL BODY "PROTEIN" (NITROGEN) TURNOVER AND PROTEIN ANABOLISM AND CATABOLISM IN NORMAL ADULTS AND A UREMIC PATIENT*

	NORMAL	UREMIC	PER CENT CHANGE FROM NORMAL	UREMIC WITH STEROID THERAPY	PER CENT CHANGE FROM NORMAL
Total "protein" turnover	188.9	286.7	+52	334.4	+77
Protein anabolism	170.5	277.8	+63	290.3	+70
Net difference (anabolism-catabolism)	−0.8	+10.3		−25.0	
Percentage of total protein entering amino acid "pool" from diet	9.8	6.5	−33.7	5.6	−42.9

*Studies were done before and after steroid therapy while patient was consuming dietary protein of 18.6 gm/day. Values are expressed as gm of protein/day.

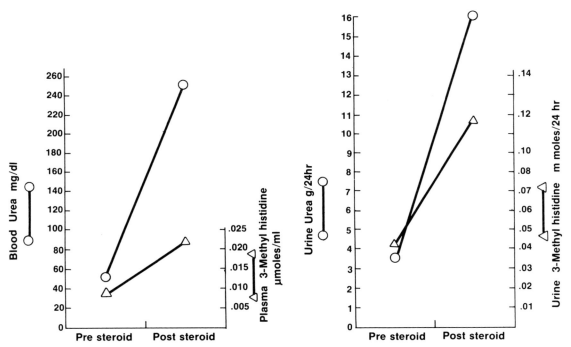

Figure 21–2. Changes in blood and urine urea and 3-methylhistidine in a uremic patient before and after steroid therapy. Note that urea levels are approximately twice those of urea nitrogen.

excreted. In view of its unique metabolism, it has been proposed that 3-methylhistidine be used as an indicator of muscle breakdown.[21] Its rise in this instance suggests that much of the protein being degraded was derived from skeletal muscle. In spite of this, urine creatinine did not rise significantly and plasma values fell to presteroid levels, again suggesting that the glomerulitis was favorably affected by steroids leading to an improved glomerular filtration rate. The contribution of dietary protein to the overall turnover of protein was only 9.8 per cent in healthy adults, decreased by one third to only 6.5 per cent in uremia, and even further, in comparison, once steroids were added to the regimen. Clearly for the stressed patient, intensive efforts should relate to those factors that have the potential to moderate endogenous turnover rather than to an uncritical manipulation of dietary protein intake to lowest levels. The administration of optimal energy substrates to reduce catabolism and of amino acids in quantities necessary to support enhanced endogenous protein synthetic demands must be accomplished.

TREATMENT CONSIDERATIONS

Energy Substrates. Energy requirements are dependent upon the basal energy expenditure and the degree of stress to which the patient is exposed. It is well established that amino acids are diverted for use as energy substrates, particularly for conversion to glucose, in the stress state. It is also accepted that the delivery of exogenous energy can blunt this response. Perhaps more than any other advantage, our ability to deliver nutrients regardless of the patient's clinical state has allowed us the reasonable assurance that the protein delivered is being used for synthetic purposes rather than being diverted in unknown quantities to meet fuel requirements. This assurance rests, of course, on our ability to define and meet the energy requirements of the individual patient.

One approach to defining this requirement, using the computer, is presented elsewhere in this book. In general, however, a level 1½ to 2 times the patient's basal energy expenditure is a reasonable starting point, with adjustments made dependent upon clinical response. The total amount may range from less than 2000 calories for an elderly patient to levels approaching 5000 calories for a young man with multiple injuries.

The ratio of carbohydrates and fat administered as non-protein calories is probably not of importance relative to renal function, per se. The preferred fuel of the renal cortex is fatty acids, and the cells of the renal medulla appear to be glucose dependent. Medium-chain triglycerides (octanoic acid) can be utilized by the kidney as well as by other body tissues. Therefore, clinical decisions relative to the commercial formula of choice rest more upon other factors such as the need for an elemental diet, the impact of fat on gastric emptying, and pancreatic exocrine functional capacity—factors that influence delivery rather than metabolic utilization.

Protein and Amino Acids. Protein should be delivered in sufficient quantity and quality to support optimal endogenous protein synthetic demands. With the full realization that complications of uremia, such as pericarditis and gastrointestinal bleeding, appear more commonly when levels of blood urea nitrogen exceed 100 mg/dl, it is not necessarily the goal of nutritional support to maintain blood urea levels as low as possible at the expense of impaired protein synthesis. Provided that the patient with renal failure is not malnourished, the stress is minimal, and adequate non-protein calories can be supplied to minimize diversion of amino acid for use as energy substrates, the protein intake can be controlled to match renal function. In patients with renal function greater than 50 per cent of normal, a protein intake of 0.8 to 1.0 gm/kg/day is commonly advised. If more protein is needed for synthesis, an even larger intake is possible. In patients with renal function between 20 and 50 per cent of normal, 0.6 gm of protein/kg/day seems adequate for protein synthesis. In addition, for both groups at least one 24-hour urine protein determination should be made, and that amount of protein added to the daily intake. Generalizations concerning patients with renal function less than 20 per cent of normal and for those with acute renal failure are more difficult because marked stress and concomitant malnutrition are much more common. Even with minimal stress and without marked proteinuria, the daily protein intake should be no lower than 0.45 gm/kg/day. If hemodialysis becomes necessary, the daily protein intake should be increased to 1 to 1.5 gm/kg/day to replace amino acid loss during dialysis.

The precise protein requirements for stressed patients are not known; however, some investigators suggest that amounts approaching 2 gm/kg of body weight/day are necessary to support both the healing process and the repair of tissues depleted secondary to malnutrition. Is there any reason to think that renal failure substantially reduces this requirement? In fact, the case study reported earlier in this chapter would suggest that the reverse can be true: that renal failure further enhances the protein demands for synthetic purposes. It is therefore reasonable to suggest that these demands be met and, if need be, blood urea nitrogen levels reduced to less than 100 mg/dl by dialysis. Most importantly, protein restriction should not be prescribed solely for the purpose of delaying or preventing dialysis. In fact, the reverse should be the case. One of the principal indications for dialysis should be its use to allow the optimal delivery of nutrients for the stressed patient.

There is also a need for enteral solutions with minimal protein and amino acid content. They are indicated for those individuals for whom the renal shutdown is only temporary—with expected return of function in two or three days—or in the instance in which dialysis must be delayed for technical reasons such as access difficulties. Their long-term use is to be deplored.

The amino acid content should reflect the metabolic demands of the patient. This may be the inherent content of the complex protein used in the formula, or perhaps an amino acid mix with added branched-chain amino acids either for the treatment of hepatic encephalopathy or to meet the specific demands of the stress response itself. It should, at a minimum, meet the requirements as currently understood for the essential amino acids.

The studies of Rose during the 1940s and 1950s that defined the eight essential amino acid requirements for healthy young males are useful[22] but are not necessarily applicable to the stressed, ill patient, particularly one with renal failure.

Recent work has suggested that even the designation of these amino acids be changed: that essential be called "indispensable," the unessential "dispensable," and a new category be called the "conditionally indispensable" (Table 21–2). Such a change is perhaps most useful for the consideration of renal failure. In addition to the original eight essential amino acids, histidine has been

Table 21–2 AMINO ACIDS IN CLINICAL NUTRITION*

DISPENSABLE	INDISPENSABLE	CONDITIONALLY INDISPENSABLE
Glutamic acid	Leucine	Histidine
Glutamine	Isoleucine	Arginine
Alanine	Valine	Tyrosine (?)
Serine	Tryptophan	Others (?)
Proline	Methionine	
Hydroxyproline	Threonine	
Cystine	Phenylalanine	
Cysteine	Lysine	
Aspartic acid		

*Amino acids are perhaps better grouped as dispensable (unessential), indispensable (essential), and conditionally indispensable, depending upon age, degree of stress, clinical state, etc.

demonstrated to be essential for adult patients with impaired renal function.[23] More recently, it has been suggested that inadequacies of arginine in nutritional solutions result in impaired Krebs-Henseleit urea cycle activity and lower blood urea levels, but create a rise in blood ammonia concentrations.[24]

One has to consider if there are also sufficient amounts of tyrosine (despite "adequate" phenylalanine delivery) to allow optimal neurotransmitter synthesis. Other amino acids, while recognized as dispensable in healthy young adults, may be indispensable under the conditions of renal failure, sepsis, surgery, and other forms of stress to which the hospitalized patient is exposed. It would seem most reasonable to give the patient the benefit of the doubt and provide him with amounts adequate to meet needs, rather than eliminating them to arbitrarily lower blood urea levels. Again, should dialysis be required, it should not be withheld.

Actually, dialysis is required more often to repair fluid and electrolyte problems than to reduce urea levels. More often than not, the clinical challenge is to nourish an individual whose limited fluid excretory capacity is already exceeded by the delivery of intravenous antibiotics, pressor agents, or other life-saving drugs. In such cases, nutritional efforts may be relegated to a lesser priority due to "fluid restrictions." Such an individual should be dialyzed to allow nutritional support regardless of blood urea levels.

Once dialysis is initiated, the requirement for amino acid delivery is enhanced by the additional losses imposed by the procedure itself (Table 21–3). During hemodialysis, small molecules such as amino acids

Table 21–3 PROTEIN LOSS WITH DIALYSIS*

	AMINO ACIDS	PEPTIDES	ALBUMIN
Hemodialysis	8–10	3–4	—
Peritoneal dialysis	+15	?	10–40

*Protein losses can be considered as a result of the dialysis process. Estimates are in grams per dialysis and represent average losses. Albumin and other whole protein losses with peritoneal dialysis are dependent upon the degree of peritoneal inflammation present.

and short peptides are lost indiscriminately across the membrane in amounts dependent upon nonphysiologic factors such as membrane area, membrane pore size, and the duration of dialysis. These losses are greater if peritoneal dialysis is used and, particularly if peritoneal irritation is present, considerable amounts of whole proteins such as albumin can be lost. These should be replaced by solutions containing a more liberal amino acid formulation.

Some clinicians recommend the delivery of amino acids to the patient at the conclusion of a dialysis procedure. In most instances, 500 ml of a 7 to 10 per cent solution is administered intravenously via the dialysis return (venous) line, or left in the peritoneal cavity at the termination of peritoneal dialysis. It would seem easier simply to administer enteral feeding in adequate amounts to cover such losses.

Fluid and Electrolyte Requirements. Our ability to define and meet requirements imposed by a lack of renal regulatory function perhaps is better for fluid and electrolytes. Reference to Table 21–4 will demonstrate the range and usual limits imposed by a functional capacity of 20 to 30 per cent of normal.

Fluid Requirements. The patient with normal kidneys can reduce urine volume to as low as 350 ml with enhancement up to 22 L daily should intake so demand. The usual daily volume is approximately 1.5 L. Contrary to popular opinion, the patient with renal dysfunction actually excretes more urine than do normal subjects. Most importantly, the range is contracted, being from 1 to 4 L overall. Confirmatory evidence relates to concentrating ability. The normal individual can create a urine with a concentration as low as 30 and as high as 1500 mOsm/L with a usual value of 1200. The patient with renal failure loses the ability to concentrate, perhaps because of a disruption of medullary countercurrent capacities. Likewise, optimal dilution is also restricted. What often results is a solute-dependent diuresis; that is, the amount of water lost is more dependent upon the solute submitted for excretion. This relatively fixed osmolality is the basis for several observations.

In the past, patients with azotemic renal failure were often advised to increase their fluid intake to "flush out their kidneys." Since the clearance of urea is related to the square root of urine volume when the urine output is less than 2 ml/min, the urine volume increased and the serum urea level decreased. The physician noted a lower serum urea value and perhaps felt better, but the patient with a lower ceiling for water excretion often became hyponatremic and felt nauseated.

With decreased water intake, normal

Table 21–4 REGULATION FAILURE IN RENAL DISEASE*

	NORMAL		RENAL FAILURE	
	Usual	*Range*	*Usual*	*Range*
Fluid (L)	1	0.35–22	2	1–4
Concentration (mOsm)	1200	30–1500	300	250–300
Sodium (mEq)	Dependent upon intake	1–160	40–50	10–500
Potassium (mEq)	Dependent upon intake	10–125	30	20–50
Acid-Base (mEq)	60–80	−300–+500	30–60	30–60

*A comparison of regulatory capacities of the normal patient with one with moderate failure of renal function (glomerular filtration rate of 20 to 30 per cent of normal) clearly reveals the inability to respond to wide variations of nutrient intake.

subjects can conserve water normally and decrease urine volume. Because patients with renal failure cannot conserve water normally, their urine volume does not decrease at night when water intake is less and nocturia ensues.

Any marked sudden fall in urine output in patients with chronic renal failure is cause for alarm. Since they have a very limited ability to concentrate urine, a sudden marked fall in urine output is seldom caused by a variation in water intake. Instead, after ruling out the possibility of bladder dysfunction, consider a decrease in glomerular filtration rate as resulting from sodium depletion or hemorrhage.

These limitations must be understood for the uncomplicated delivery of enteral hyperalimentation. The routine use of super-concentrated solutions with the belief that all patients have difficulties excreting water can quickly lead to dehydration and the development of a hyperosmolar state. Dehydration, if severe, can lead to prerenal failure due to poor renal perfusion, an acceleration of biochemical abnormalities of the uremic syndrome, followed by dialysis or death.

On the other hand, too much fluid can create the syndrome of water intoxication which is expressed by nausea, vomiting, and mental obtundation, a clinical syndrome very similar to uremia. The obvious answer lies in an initial thoughtful consideration of fluid regulatory capacity and sufficient daily monitoring of serum electrolytes and body weight to detect and allow correction of abnormalities.

Sodium Requirements. The normal individual has an astounding capacity to reduce sodium excretion to as low as 1 mEq/day. If one considers the amount of sodium filtered by the glomeruli on a daily basis, this is indeed an accomplishment. The highest excretory rates are likewise broad but limited, the amount being dependent upon intake. As might be expected, this range is markedly narrowed by renal failure in 90 per cent of instances. The usual sodium excretion at this functional level is between 30 and 50 mEq/day. Therefore, a restriction of sodium intake is generally required. However, it must be recognized that approximately 10 per cent of patients with renal failure have a salt-losing nephropathy. In these instances, sodium excretion can rise to 500 mEq/day no matter what the intake.

In the adapted kidney, each remaining nephron has enhanced its individual capacities for sodium excretion. Factors that might explain increased sodium excretion per nephron include aldosterone secretion, changes in single nephron glomerular filtration rate, redistribution of blood flow between deep and superficial nephrons, other changes in intrarenal hemodynamics, changes in physical factors, and a natriuretic hormone.

Aldosterone secretion is neither consistently increased nor decreased in these patients. Differences in single nephron glomerular filtration rates between experimental glomerular and interstitial renal disease have been demonstrated. Bricker[25] is a staunch supporter of the natriuretic hormone concept. A natriuretic substance has been isolated from the urine and plasma of sodium-fed uremic humans and from a nonuremic man undergoing water emersion natriuresis.[26] Sodium excretion per nephron can be decreased in patients with chronic renal disease by very slowly and carefully decreasing sodium intake.[27] If such a natriuretic hormone is present, might it also influence sodium handling at other membranes in the body? Might some of the other incompletely explained findings in uremia such as serositis be a result of this trade-off to increase renal sodium excretion?

It should be obvious that a normal sodium intake of 3 to 4 gm daily will cause salt and water overload in most individuals with renal failure, and in 1 out of 10, severe salt and water depletion, dehydration, and acceleration of the uremic syndrome. The best clinical approach would be to monitor sodium excretion during a defined intake and make appropriate changes in prescription according to output.

Potassium. Like sodium excretion, potassium excretion in the healthy adult is largely dependent upon intake and ranges from near zero to as great as 125 mEq/day. The patient with limited function exhibits a contracted capability to deal with the potassium load delivered to the kidney.

Actually, the kidney maintains the potassium secretory capacity of the distal tubule until quite late in the evolution of chronic renal failure. In the absence of acute oliguric failure, hyperkalemia is not a common event in the hospitalized setting unless this excretory capacity is exceeded by exogenous potassium delivery. Hypokalemia may be even more troublesome, particularly if gastrointestinal suction or fistula losses are large.

The potassium burden can be generated in large part from endogenous perturbations resulting from the stress state. Potassium is one of the principal intracellular ions that can be released into body fluids as cells are contracted secondary to malnutrition, or disrupted for whatever reason—trauma, abscess, or blood in the intestinal tract. In addition to a definition of the excretory capacity and appropriate modification of intake, the clinician must also be alert to potential endogenous sources and make every attempt to eliminate them. From a nutritional perspective, the primary goals of nutritional intervention must be attained. Fuel requirements must be defined and met to aid in the prevention of potassium release due to cellular destruction secondary to malnutrition. Other factors leading to real or apparent hyperkalemia may include (1) hemolysis of red blood cells in the blood sample; (2) an increase in exogenous potassium load such as food or potassium-containing medications; (3) the use of diuretics that interfere with potassium excretion in the distal nephron; and (4) hyporeninemic hypoaldosteronism, usually found in older patients with only mild renal insufficiency. Interstitial renal disease or diabetes mellitus is often present. Hyperchloremic rather than uremic acidosis is also often documented.[28, 29]

Blood potassium levels do not always reflect total body potassium levels. Extracellular potassium is highly dependent upon hydrogen ion concentrations rising 0.5 mEq/dl for every 0.1 pH unit fall, and vice versa. For example, if a patient is first evaluated while acidotic, perhaps during a ketotic state secondary to either starvation or uncontrolled diabetes mellitus, potassium levels may be high initially but plummet once sufficient base is delivered to correct the acid-base imbalance.

Another clinical state in which blood potassium levels fall abruptly is well known to nutritionists. As glucose is administered to patients in need, intracellular potassium is quickly replenished with a resultant fall in extracellular concentrations. Actually, what we often accomplish in the course of nutritional intervention, particularly with total parenteral nutrition, is one of the therapeutic modalities for the treatment of hyperkalemia, the administration of concentrated glucose along with insulin.

Acid-Base Requirements. The normal patient can excrete either hydrogen ions or bicarbonate as the kidney interacts with endogenous buffer systems to maintain the internal milieu at the appropriate pH. The patient with renal dysfunction is again limited in this capacity, being confined to a relatively narrow range of ± 30 mEq of hydrogen ion per day.

Since states of stress and starvation entail considerable hydrogen ion production, it is important that the clinician use the techniques of enteral hyperalimentation available to minimize the excretory demands for hydrogen ion excretion. As cells contract and are destroyed by malnutrition, the release of phosphate, sulfate, and other intracellular ions contribute to the burden. Their release can be minimized by preventing the cellular effects of malnutrition. Likewise, a considerable portion of the fuel requirements is met by the release of fatty acids from endogenous triglycerides, a process that can be inhibited by appropriate nutritional intervention.

Other Micronutrients. We do not have a clear understanding of the requirements for vitamins and trace elements in the stress state. Nearly all commercially available solutions contain these micronutrients (with exceptions noted below) in amounts understood for the healthy individual. One must hope that such is also the case for the patient with renal failure. If hemodialysis therapy is undertaken, one multiple vitamin plus 1.0 mg of folate should be given at the end of each dialysis to replace losses, even in face of otherwise "normal" micronutrient delivery.

Nutritional Intervention. All solutions should be delivered by the continuous infusion method which offers a reasonable chance that nutrient requirements can be met and complications of the delivery process itself by minimized. The details of such a controlled delivery system are outside of the context of this chapter and the reader is referred to the appropriate chapter in this text.

Nearly all commercial formulas, if prepared or delivered as recommended, have some drawbacks for the patient with renal failure. Those formulas with a caloric density of one calorie per milliliter will most often result in excessive delivery of fluid, sodium, potassium, and/or protein if the primary intent, as always, is to meet the patient's caloric requirements. The most common limiting factors are the salt and water content. Those more calorically dense solutions available commercially are, in most cases, also high in electrolytes and protein.

The availability of powdered, nonelectrolyte-containing caloric sources provides the clinician with the option of creating a "partial modular" solution by adding these products to a standard commercial formula of choice. Table 21–5 lists a selected number of "base" solutions to which caloric substrates have been added to a level of 2 kcal/ml. In order to deliver 3000 kcal/day in 1.5 L of solution, a base solution would be selected that best met the constraints as defined by the clinical state. From the few examples given, daily protein delivery ranges from 38 to 66 gm, sodium from 33 to 65 mEq, potassium from 27 to 49 mEq, and phosphorus from approximately 500 to 800 mg. It should be obvious that a more precise prescription could be developed by close attention to detail and extensive knowledge of the formula content. Herein lies one of the potential uses of the computer in nutritional support (see Chapter 8).

Most useful would be the ability to develop a completely "modular" approach, whereby a precise solution could be compounded to meet the individual requirements for fluid, protein, electrolytes, and micronutrients. Such systems are commercially available; however, the commitment and dedication of a nutrition support team must be present, particularly if the definition, preparation, and delivery of solutions are to be accomplished for patients with rapidly changing clinical disease states. In such instances, patient monitoring must be continuous and precise if the clinician wishes to affect patient outcome in a meaningful way.

Should the special renal formulas be used? The answer is definitely yes, but only for short periods of time that may be required to allow the clinical course to become manifest. The renal insult may be brief with rapid correction anticipated. Problems with vascular access may require a few days' wait before hemodialysis can be initiated. These solutions can provide for optimal calorie administration with absolute minimal nitrogen and electrolyte load. Their intentional use to delay or prevent dialysis for prolonged periods is unacceptable. Most hospitals have access to dialysis facilities, the procedure having been developed to a degree that complications are a minor consideration. Once dialysis is initiated, the losses of amino acids, peptides, and whole protein resulting from the procedure itself require a return to more protein dense solutions to cover both those losses and meet the requirements of enhanced endogenous protein synthetic demands.

Newer solutions may prove to be more useful. "Stress formulas" are emerging in the marketplace which have the indispensable amino acids enhanced to a degree that with caloric augmentation, a general reduction in total amino acid amount can be accomplished, and some degree of confidence maintained that at least meets Rose's minimal recommendations for health (Table 21–6). Such confidence is not always present when reduced amounts of usual high biologic value proteins are administered.

The patient with renal failure produces a significant challenge to the clinical nutritionist. A thorough knowledge of all formulas, a commitment to close monitoring of multiple clinical parameters, a dedication to detail, and an ability to change formulations to meet rapidly evolving clinical demands result in the type of clinical care that brings credibility and plaudits to the discipline of Clinical Nutrition.

Table 21–5 AUGMENTATION OF SELECTED COMMERCIAL FORMULAS TO MEET VARIED NUTRIENT REQUIREMENTS IN RENAL FAILURE*

BASE SOLUTION	FLUID (L)	PROTEIN (gm)	SODIUM (mEq)	POTASSIUM (mEQ)	PHOSPHORUS (mg)
Criticare HN	1.5	54	39	48	750
Ensure	1.5	56	48	48	750
Isocal	1.5	51	33	49	750
Precision PN	1.5	66	65	35	500
Travasorb Whole Protein	1.5	52	48	49	790
Vipep	1.5	38	49	33	750
High Nitrogen Vivonex	1.5	63	51	27	495

*If the caloric density of commercial formulas is augmented by the addition of a powdered, nonelectrolyte caloric source to a density of 2 kcal/ml, the resultant mix will often serve to meet the requirements of most patients with renal failure.

Table 21-6 AMINO ACID CONTENT OF SELECTED FORMULAS DESIGNED TO TREAT PATIENTS
WITH RENAL FAILURE

AMINO ACIDS	AMIN AID	TRAVASORB RENAL	"STRESS FORMULA"*	ROSE REQUIREMENTS†
Indispensable				
Leucine	1.62	1.58	11.02	1.10
Isoleucine	1.03	1.33	5.50	0.70
Valine	1.18	1.97	5.50	0.80
Tryptophan	0.37	0.43	0.85	0.25
Threonine	0.74	0.99	1.66	0.50
Lysine	1.18	1.18	3.29	0.80
Methionine	1.62	1.50	2.14	1.10
Phenylalanine	1.62	1.29	3.31	1.10
Conditionally Indispensable				
Histidine	0.37	1.11	1.73	—
Arginine	—	1.37	5.08	—
Tyrosine	—	0.13	0.59	—
Dispensable				
Alanine	—	1.46	2.44	—
Aspartic acid	—	—	3.68	—
Glutamine	—	—	8.55	—
Glycine	—	—	6.09	—
Proline	—	0.99	3.25	—
Serine	—	0.92	1.95	—
Cystine	—	—	0.11	—

*The "stress formula" in a commercial solution became available in early 1983.
†Based on an assumption of 2000 kcal/day of energy intake and "safe" intake of amino acids.

REFERENCES

1. Anderson, R. J., Linas, S. L., Berns, A. S., Henrich, W. L., Miller T. R., Gabow, P. A., and Schrier, R. W.: Nonoliguric acute renal failure. N. Engl. J. Med., 296:1134–1138, 1977.
2. Finn, W. F.; Acute renal failure. *In* Earley, L. E., and Gottschalk, C. W. (eds.): Strauss and Welt's Diseases of the Kidney, Vol. I. Edition 3. Boston, Little, Brown and Co., 1979, pp. 167–210.
3. Anderson, C. F., Nelson, R. A., Margie, J. D., Johnson, W. J., and Hunt, J. C.: Nutritional therapy for adults with renal disease. J.A.M.A., 223:68–72, 1973.
4. Hutt, M. P., and Glassock, R. J.: Proteinuria and the nephrotic syndrome. *In* Schrier, R. W. (ed.): Renal and Electrolyte Disorders. Edition 2. Boston, Little, Brown and Co., 1980, pp. 501–520.
5. Pierides, A. M.: Chronic renal failure. *In* Spittel, J. A., Jr. (ed.): Clinical Medicine, Vol. 7. Philadelphia, Harper and Row, 1981, p. 6.
6. Knochel, J. P., and Seldin, D. W.: The pathophysiology of uremia. *In* Brenner, B. M., and Rector, F. C., Jr. (eds.): The Kidney. Edition 2. Philadelphia, W. B. Saunders Co., 1981, pp. 2156–2167.
7. Wochos, D. N., Anderson, C. F., and Mitchell, J. C., III.: Serum lipids in chronic renal failure. Mayo Clin. Proc., 51:660–664, 1976.
8. Giordano, C.: Use of exogenous and endogenous urea for protein synthesis in normal and uremic subjects. J. Lab. Clin. Med., 62:231–246, 1963.
9. Anderson, C. F., Jaecks, D. M., Ballon, H. S., DePalma, J. R., and Cuttler, R. E.: Renal handling of creatinine in nephrotic and non-nephrotic patients. Clin. Sci., 38:555–562, 1970.
10. Jones, J. D., and Burnett, P. C.: Creatinine metabolism and toxicity. Kidney Int., 7:S94–S98, 1975.
11. Guisado, R., Arieff, A. I., Massry, S. G., Lazarowitz, V., and Kerian, A.: Changes in the electroencephalogram in acute uremia: Effects of parathyroid hormone and brain electrolytes. J. Clin. Invest., 55:738–745, 1975.
12. Hampers, C. L., Katz, A. I., Wilson, R. E., and Merrill, J. P.: Disappearance of "uremic" itching after subtotal parathyroidectomy. N. Engl. J. Med., 279:695–697, 1968.
13. Massry S. G., Popovtzer, M. M., Coburn, J. W., Makoff, D. L., Maxwell, M. H., and Kleeman, C. R.: Intractable pruritus as a manifestation of secondary hyperparathyroidism in uremia: Disappearance of itching after subtotal parathyroidectomy. N. Engl. J. Med., 279:697–700, 1968.
14. Rutherford, W. E., Border, P., Marie, P., et al.: Phosphate control and 25-hydroxycholecalciferol administration in preventing experimental renal osteodystrophy in the dog. J. Clin. Invest., 60:332–341, 1977.
15. Prévost, J. L., and Dumas, J. A.: Examen du sand de son action das les divers phénomènes de la vie. Ann de Chimie et de Physique (2me série), 23:90–104, 1821.
16. Johnson, W. J., Hagge, W. W., Wagoner, R. D., Dinapoli, R. P., and Rosevear, J. W.: Effects of urea loading in patients with far-advanced renal failure. Mayo Clin. Proc., 47:21–29, 1972.
17. Joint FAO/WHO Ad Hoc Expert Committee on En-

ergy and Protein Requirements: Energy and Protein Requirements. Rome, Food and Agriculture Organization of the United Nations. World Health Organization Technical Report Series, No. 522, 1973.

18. Picou, D., and Taylor-Roberts, T.: The measurement of total protein synthesis and catabolism and nitrogen turnover in infants in different nutritional states and receiving different amounts of dietary protein. Clin. Sci., 36:283–296, 1969.

19. Steffee, W. P., Goldsmith, R. S., Pencharz, P. B., Scrimshaw, N. S., and Young, V. R.: Dietary protein intake and dynamic aspects of whole body nitrogen metabolism in adult humans. Metabolism, 25:281–297, 1976.

20. Young, V. R., Alexis, S. D., Baliga, B. S., and Munro, H. N.: Fate of administered 3-methylhistidine. Lack of muscle transfer ribonucleic acid charging and quantitative excretion as 3-methylhistidine and its N-acetyl derivative. J. Biol. Chem., 247:3592–3600, 1972.

21. Young, V. R.: The role of skeletal and cardiac muscle in the regulation of protein metabolism. In Munro, H. N. (ed.): Mammalian Protein Metabolism, Vol. IV, New York, Academic Press, 1970, pp. 585–674.

22. Rose, W. C.: Amino acid requirements of man. Fed. Proc., 8:546–552, 1949.

23. Kopple, J. D., and Swendseid, M. E.: Evidence that histidine is an essential amino acid in normal and chronically uremic man. J. Clin. Invest., 55:881–891, 1975.

24. Rapp, R. P., Bivins, B. A., and McRoberts, W. R.: Hyperammonemic encephalopathy occurring in a patient receiving essential amino acid/dextrose parenteral nutrition. Clin. Pharmacol., in press.

25. Bricker, N. S., and Fine, L. G.: The renal response to progressive nephron loss. In Brenner, B. M., and Rector, F. C., Jr. (eds.): The Kidney. Edition 2. Philadelphia, W. B. Saunders Co., 1981, pp. 1056–1090.

26. Epstein, M., Bricker, N. S., and Bourgoignie, J. J.: Presence of a natriuretic factor in urine of normal men undergoing water immersion. Kidney Int., 13:152–158, 1978.

27. Danovitch, G. M., Bourgoignie, J. J., and Bricker, N. S.: Reversibility of the "salt-losing" tendency in chronic renal failure. N. Engl. J. Med., 296:14–19, 1977.

28. Perez, G. O., Oster, J. R., and Vaamonde, C. A.: Renal acidosis and renal potassium handling in selective hypoaldosteronism. Am. J. Med., 57:809–816, 1974.

29. Williams, G. H.: Aldosterone, potassium, and acidosis [Editorial]. N. Engl. J. Med., 294:392–393, 1976.

CHAPTER 22

Enteral Nutrition and Liver Disease

DANNY O. JACOBS
MARCIA C. BORAAS
JOHN L. ROMBEAU

"The goals in nutritional support of patients with hepatic failure should include the maintenance of adequate nutrition, enhancement of liver regeneration or recovery, and prevention and/or amelioration of hepatic encephalopathy."

—JOSEF E. FISCHER

The liver is a unique and highly specialized organ, receiving up to 40 per cent of the total cardiac output and continuously performing a wide range of essential metabolic functions. It has the capacity for storage, activation, degradation, and excretion of both endogenous and exogenous substances, and is critically involved in the regulation of carbohydrate, protein, and fat metabolism. The liver synthesizes albumin, coagulation factors, and other plasma proteins, and plays a central role in the storage and activation of vitamins, as well as in the inactivation and excretion of toxic wastes.

Nutritional abnormalities attributable to poor dietary intake or induced by alterations in nutrient absorption, substrate requirements, or hepatic nutrient metabolism are often found in association with primary liver disease. Chronic fibrosing processes (alcoholic or primary biliary cirrhosis), infections (viral hepatitis), and hereditary metabolic diseases (hemochromatosis and Wilson's disease) may be associated with malnutrition and cause specific alterations such as glucose, vitamin, and protein metabolism. Conversely, it is also true that primary nutritional diseases (kwashiorkor) may have marked effects on hepatic morphology and function.

Among the average hospitalized population in the United States, the most widespread and significant liver problem is alcohol-related liver disease, which ranges from reversible fatty infiltration to acute alcoholic hepatitis and cirrhosis. Chronic ingestion of ethanol is not invariably followed by clinically evident hepatic disease, but there is some evidence for a direct relationship between the amount of ethanol consumed and the risk of cirrhosis.[1]

Histologically, cirrhosis is often preceded by inflammatory changes in the hepatic parenchyma, but the exact cause is often unknown. Alcoholic, or Laennec's cirrhosis, probably results from a direct toxic effect of alcohol on the liver. Protein, calorie, and vitamin deficiencies are frequently associated with acute and chronic alcohol intake and may contribute to liver injury. Once hepatic fibrosis is established, the clinical course is generally one of progressive deterioration with the development of portal hypertension and its sequelae, encephalopathy and progressive hepatic failure.

This chapter will review the hepatic aspects of carbohydrate, protein, and fat metabolism, the role of the liver in the regulation of other vital substances, alcohol-induced liver diseases, and their nutritional effects. The contribution of nutrient deficiencies to liver injury and common alterations in nutrient metabolism, water and electrolyte balance, and red blood cell homeostasis will be discussed. Finally, the principles that guide the alimentation of patients with end-stage liver disease will be examined.

LIVER AS A NUTRITIONAL ORGAN

Within the body's complex system of homeostatic mechanisms, the liver serves as a focal point for regulation and metabolism of both endogenous and exogenous substrates. In addition, it is a major site of protein synthesis, of detoxification and excretion of drugs and toxic substances, and is important in the storage and activation of many vitamins. Although the liver is composed of several cell types, the intense metabolic activity occurs primarily within the hepatocyte. The hepatocyte forms the bulk of hepatic parenchyma, and is regulated both by complex hormone signals and direct enzymatic feedback controls. Under physiologic conditions, exogenous substrates are absorbed across the intestinal epithelium and into the portal circulation where they are modified by the liver prior to reaching the systemic circulation. Because the intestinal mucosa actively modifies the ingested protein, carbohydrates, and fats, these substances reach the portal blood in the form of free amino acids, monosaccharides, and short- or medium-chain fatty acids. Long-chain dietary fatty acids are not carried to the liver but form chylomicrons and are taken up by the lymphatics. In addition to these dietary sources, the liver receives endogenously generated substrates including free fatty acids released from adipose tissue stores, and amino acids and lactate derived from tissue catabolism. The metabolism of all these substances is closely interrelated with the liver as the central regulatory site.

Normal Carbohydrate Metabolism

Dietary carbohydrates are generally absorbed in the form of hexose polymers, including galactose, fructose, and glucose. Although pathways for breakdown of other hexose molecules exist, the major source of energy and the major circulating sugar in the body is glucose. All active cells contain a nonspecific hexokinase enzyme for the breakdown of sugar, but the liver has a unique role in carbohydrate metabolism and regulates the circulating level of glucose in the blood (Fig. 22–1). Because of its anatomic position, exogenous carbohydrates traverse the liver prior to reaching the systemic circulation. Simultaneously, through the portal circulation, the liver is exposed to higher concentrations of insulin than are the peripheral tissues. Hepatocytes contain a unique glucokinase which, unlike tissue hexokinase, is specific for the glucose molecule, and is induced by high levels of insulin. With the exception of the kidney, the liver is also the only organ which contains glucose-6-phosphatase, an enzyme that reverses the hexokinase-glucokinase reaction and allows regeneration of free glucose molecules for use by the rest of the body.

Fifty-five to sixty per cent of an oral glu-

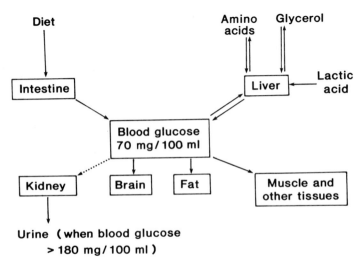

Figure 22–1. Blood glucose homeostasis, illustrating the glucostatic function of the liver.

cose load is taken up by the liver, 25 per cent is used to meet the energy needs of the brain and noninsulin-dependent tissues, and 15 per cent is used by muscle adipose tissue in the periphery.[2, 3] Glucose molecules reaching the liver are either polymerized and stored as glycogen (glycogenesis) or catabolized (glycolysis) by one of two main pathways (Fig. 22–2). The hexose-monophosphate shunt, which requires the presence of oxygen, generates large amounts of high energy bonds in the form of nicotinamide adenine dinucleotide phosphate (NADPH) which can enter the mitochondria to generate adenosine triphophosphate (ATP) by oxidative phosphorylation. The hexose-monophosphate shunt also forms pentoses, which are used in the synthesis of nucleotides. An alternative route of glucose catabolism is anaerobic glycolysis via the Embden-Meyerhof pathway, which results in the formation of pyruvate and lactate. Pyruvate can then enter the citric acid cycle (Fig. 22–3) to generate additional energy as ATP, can be converted to acetyl coenzyme A (Co-A) for formation of ketone bodies or fatty acids, or can be metabolized to alanine and subsequently enter pathways of protein metabolism. There is some autoregulation of these processes in the hepatocyte. However, the relative plasma concentrations of glucagon and insulin have regulatory importance. High insulin: glucagon ratios, which follow enteral glucose loading, enhance glycogen synthesis and glycolysis.

In contrast, when the body's requirement for glucose exceeds that supplied by the exogenous sources, the liver is capable of reversing these processes to supply glucose to other body tissues. Under the influence of low insulin levels and elevated plasma glucagon, glucose catabolism is slowed and glucose synthesis and output by the liver increase. Lactate and amino acids, primarily alanine, derived from muscle catabolism, enter the blood from peripheral tissues and can be converted by the liver to pyruvate and then to glucose by gluconeogenesis. During a short fast, however, the body's initial energy needs are met through breakdown of stored glycogen rather than by gluconeogenesis (Fig. 22–4). When exogenous glucose supplies are abundant, glycogen is formed in the liver by polymerization of glucose molecules. This requires conversion of glucose to glucose-6-phosphate by glucokinase (hexokinase) (Fig. 22–5). The average adult liver in the "fed" state contains approximately 75 gm of glycogen which can be degraded to provide 70 to 75 per cent of the required hepatic glucose output during an overnight fast.[3] This requires glucose-6-phosphatase, which is found primarily in the liver but also in the kidney. Skeletal muscle also contains the enzymes necessary to form glycogen and is the other major storage site of glycogen. Muscle, however, lacks glucose-6-phosphatase and cannot form free glucose molecules from glycogen. Muscle glycogen is therefore metabolized directly to pyruvate and lactate via the Embden-Meyerhof pathway. These end prod-

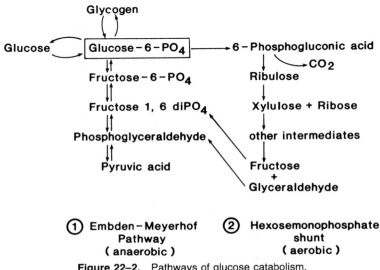

Figure 22–2. Pathways of glucose catabolism.

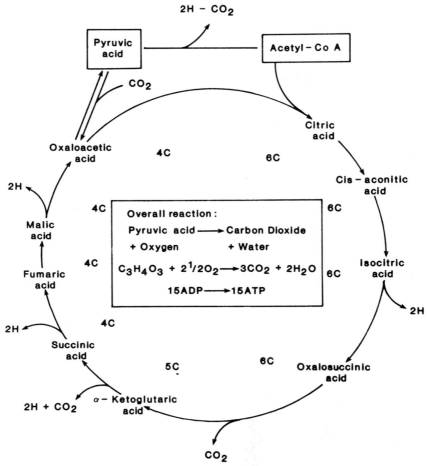

Figure 22–3. Citric acid cycle.

ucts, however, can then be returned to the liver and used for gluconeogenesis, or enter the other metabolic pathways previously described.

Normal Protein Metabolism

Like the substrates involved in carbohydrate metabolism, free amino acids reach the liver from either endogenous or dietary sources. Although a healthy adult synthesizes a total of 300 to 400 gm of body protein per day, the average Western diet supplies only 90 to 100 gm daily.[4] Endogenous proteins are therefore undergoing a continuous process of hydrolysis and resynthesis at variable rates depending on specific tissue characteristics (high rates in the intestinal mu-

cosa, low in collagen). In addition to active protein turnover, there is also a constant interchange by transamination, amination, and deamination reactions between amino acids and the non-protein products of carbohydrate and fat metabolism, the "common metabolic pool" (Fig. 22–6). The enzymatic transamination of amino acids to the corresponding keto acids (Fig. 22–7) provides a variety of substrates for incorporation into energy producing pathways. In addition, through oxidative deamination (Fig. 22–8), nitrogen can be removed from amino acids directly to form ammonia. In the liver ammonia is converted to urea by the urea cycle (Fig. 22–9) and can subsequently be excreted into the urine. The deaminated carbon skeletons are then used as gluconeogenic substrates or in the formation of acetyl Co-A

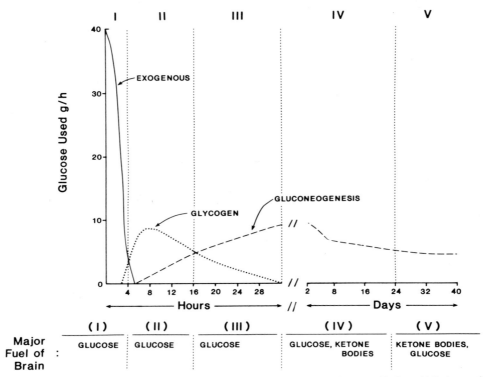

Figure 22–4. Sources of glucose production in normal subjects. (*From* Wurtman, R. J. and Wurtman, J. J. (eds.): Disorders of Eating and Nutrients in Treatment of Brain Diseases. Nutrition and the Brain, Volume 3, New York, Raven Press, 1979, with permission.)

and ketone bodies. They may also directly enter the citric acid cycle and be used to generate ATP (Figs. 22–10 and 22–11).

The rate of hepatic turnover and catabolism of amino acids varies with the availability of the substrate, and is affected by the hormonal milieu. Following enteral administration of a protein load, portal vein amino acid levels rise. Elwyn showed in dogs that 57 per cent of ingested amino acids were converted by the liver to urea and 20 per cent were incorporated into either plasma or hepatic proteins.[5] Only 23 per cent entered the plasma amino acid pool, reflecting the immediate capacity of the liver to respond to an acute substrate load. Hormonal changes, including an elevation in plasma insulin, can also influence amino acid metabolism by increasing the uptake of branched-chain amino acids into muscle and adipose tissue. A fall in insulin concentration and a rise in plasma glucagon concentration, characteristic of the catabolic state, however, will result in increased circulating levels of amino acids. The amino acids can then be used by the liver for protein synthesis or catabolized by transamination and oxidative pathways.

Normal Fat Metabolism

The liver is important in the metabolism of endogenous and dietary lipids, including triglycerides and phospholipids. These fatty substances circulate in the blood bound to hepatically synthesized proteins and sterols. Medium- and short-chain fatty acids from dietary sources reach the liver via the portal vein, and, together with free fatty acids derived from adipose tissue triglyceride stores, can be converted in the liver to acetyl Co-A and thus enter the citric acid cycle. Glycerol, which remains after fatty acids are cleared from triglycerides, can be converted in the liver to glucose, although this is a quantitatively unimportant pathway of gluconeogenesis. Prolonged starvation, accompanied by low levels of plasma insulin and elevation in serum glucagon concentrations, increases the mobilization of free fatty acids from adi-

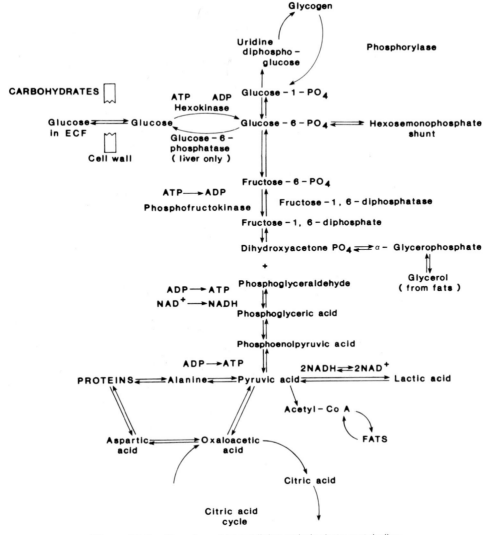

Figure 22–5. Overview of intracellular carbohydrate metabolism.

pose tissue and fat oxidation, and decreases fat synthesis. Although fatty acids can be directly metabolized by tissues including skeletal muscle, the increased formation of acetyl Co-A from fatty acids is followed in the liver by condensation of acetyl Co-A units to form ketone bodies—acetoacetate, β-hydroxybutyrate, and acetone (Fig. 22–12). Body tissues including the brain (see Fig. 22–4) can metabolize ketones in lieu of glucose. This mechanism decreases the need for gluconeogenesis in the liver and therefore decreases the demand for gluconeogenic precursors derived from the breakdown of muscle protein stores.

Other Hepatic Functions

In addition to serving as a focal point in the complex regulation of carbohydrate, fat, and protein metabolism, the liver also synthesizes many essential substances such as albumin, coagulation factors (prothrombin, V, VII, IX, and X), alpha and beta globulins, haptoglobin, and transferrin. Apoproteins and lipoproteins are also synthesized as well as cholesterol—the precursor of steroid hormones, bile acids, and some vitamins.

The liver is also the major storage organ for both water-soluble and fat-soluble vitamins, and is the site of conversion of many

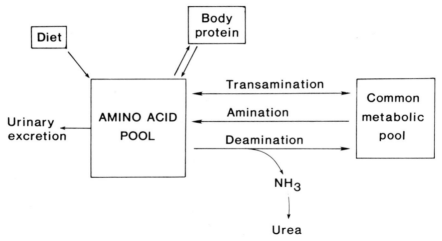

Figure 22–6. Amino acid metabolism.

vitamins to their metabolically active forms. In some cases, the liver is also the source of vitamin transport proteins, including retinol-binding protein and prealbumin, which serve as carriers for vitamin A.

Diseases affecting the liver parenchyma are therefore capable of interrupting both the well coordinated intricacies of substrate metabolism and the myriad of vital synthetic and enzymatic processes that occur within the hepatocyte. The nature and degree of injury, as well as the underlying reserve of hepatic parenchyma, will dictate the ultimate degree of hepatic dysfunction. However, once irreversible damage has occurred, the metabolic consequences may be rapid and are frequently fatal.

THE LIVER AND ITS RESPONSE TO INJURY

The classification of liver disease is difficult because the etiology and pathogenesis are often obscure.[6] Therefore classification is commonly based on morphology. Cirrhosis then accounts for the majority of recognized cases of liver disease.

There is no universally accepted defini-tion of cirrhosis. The word is derived from the Greek "kirrhos," and translated literally means tawny. It was originally used to describe one form of cirrhosis associated with alcohol abuse in which the liver was indeed tawny in color.[6]

Morphologically, the cirrhotic liver is characterized by fibrosis, which represents an actual or relative increase in connective tissue, and cell necrosis, which is associated with nodular regeneration of liver cells.[6] Many liver diseases can cause these injuries and the patterns may sometimes be characteristic of particular disease states. However, morphologic patterns may overlap, especially in end-stage liver disease. Clinically the liver's response to severe injury is fairly stereotypical. Jaundice occurs secondary to deranged bilirubin metabolism, liver function is impaired, and varying degrees of liver failure or insufficiency develop.

In urban areas in the United States, 90 per cent of the fatal cases of liver cirrhosis are secondary to alcoholism.[7] In 1975, cirrhosis of the liver was the seventh leading cause of death in the United States with an incidence of 15 deaths per 100,000 population.[7] Thus, the impact of alcoholism on liver disease and the importance of cirrhosis in

$$
\begin{array}{ccccccc}
CH_3 & & CH_2-CH_2-COOH & & CH_3 & & CH_2-CH_2-COOH \\
| & & | & \longrightarrow & | & & | \\
CH-COOH & + & O=C-COOH & \longleftarrow & C=O & + & CH-COOH \\
| & & & & | & & | \\
NH_2 & & & & COOH & & NH_2 \\
\end{array}
$$

Alanine a–Ketoglutaric acid   Pyruvic acid   Glutamic acid

Figure 22–7. Transamination.

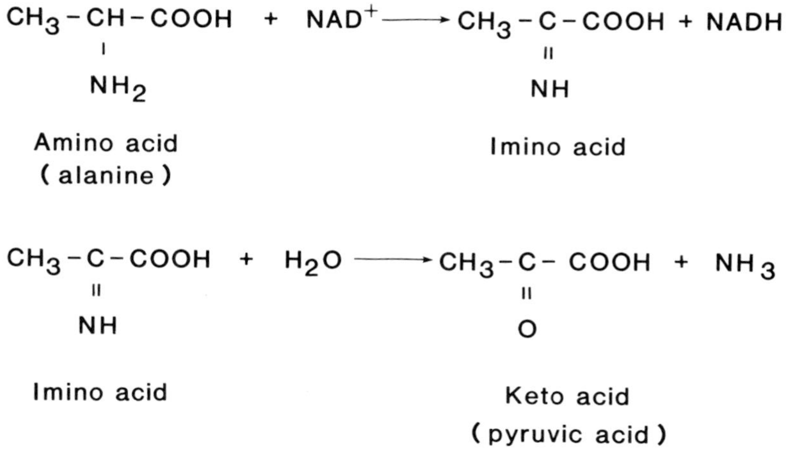
CH3 - CH - COOH + NAD+ → CH3 - C - COOH + NADH
NH2
NH
Amino acid
(alanine)
Imino acid
CH3 - C - COOH + H2O → CH3 - C - COOH + NH3
NH
O
Imino acid
Keto acid
(pyruvic acid)

Figure 22–8. Oxidative deamination.

the pathogenesis of liver insufficiency and liver failure are obvious.

The liver is probably the only human organ which retains the propensity for secondary regeneration. In some circumstance, the liver can regenerate 80 per cent of its pre-injury mass.[8] In other instances, it seems that liver regeneration is limited by an overgrowth of fibrous tissue.[8] Fischer states that therapy in liver disease is a "play for time to allow the liver to regenerate." Furthermore he notes that of all the factors that are known to influence liver regeneration (growth hormone, triiodothyronine, adrenal hydrocortisone, ileal factor, insulin, and glucagon), physicians are currently best able to manipulate nutrition.[9]

ALCOHOLIC LIVER INJURY

Three histologic types of alcoholic liver injury are well recognized: fatty metamorphosis, hepatitis, and cirrhosis.

Exactly how alcohol causes alcoholic hepatitis and cirrhosis has not been determined. Whereas the cirrhotic, alcoholic patient commonly has a reduced nutrient intake and primary malnutrition, this does not implicate malnutrition as the sole etiologic factor in alcoholic cirrhosis.[10–14] Lieber et al. demonstrated adverse effects of alcohol that occurred despite a nutritious diet.[14]

The major pathways of ethanol metabolism in the liver can be seen in Fig. 22–13. Alcohol dehydrogenase oxidizes ethanol to acetaldehyde. The oxidation of ethanol transfers hydrogen to nicotinamide adenine dinucleotide and hence increases NADH:NAD ratios. This alteration in redox state changes the ratios of those metabolites that are reduced by NADH-NAD exchanges and is thought to be responsible for the major metabolic changes associated with alcohol abuse including: (1) hyperlactacidemia (increased lactate to pyruvate ratios); (2) secondary hyperuricemia; (3) impaired gluconeogenesis; (4) increased alpha-glycerophosphate con-

Flow of amino groups into the urea cycle in ureotelic organisms

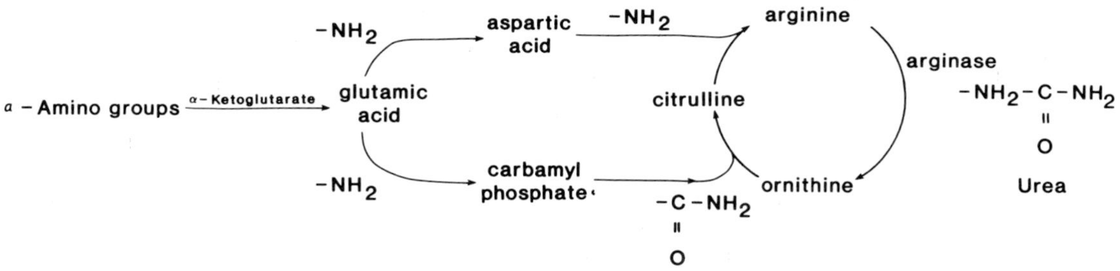
-NH2
aspartic acid
-NH2
arginine
arginase
α - Amino groups
α - Ketoglutarate
glutamic acid
citrulline
-NH2 - C - NH2
O
-NH2
carbamyl phosphate
ornithine
Urea
-C - NH2
O

Figure 22–9. The urea cycle.

Glycogenic

Ala	His
Arg	Met
Asp	Pro
Asn	Ser
Cys	Thr
Glu	Trp
Gln	Val
Gly	

Ketogenic

Leu

Glycogenic and ketogenic

He
Lys
Phe
Tyr

Figure 22–10. Fate of amino acids.

hepatic oxaloacetate concentrations). (Ultimately mitochondria use hydrogen equivalents which originate from ethanol, rather than from the oxidation of two carbon fragments from fatty acids) and (6) an alteration in redox state at the hepatocyte which can reduce protein synthesis but this effect is attenuated with chronic alcohol exposure.[14]

Acetaldehyde, which is produced by the oxidation of alcohol, may be responsible for some of the complications of alcoholism. The metabolism of acetaldehyde by aldehyde dehydrogenase generates NADH. Hence, some of the effects of acetaldehyde may be mediated by altered redox states as described previously. Acetaldehyde may also have direct toxic effects including: (1) neurologic damage; (2) decreased activity of mitochondrial shuttles which transport reducing equivalents between compounds; (3) inhibition of oxidative phosphorylation; and (4) decreased mitochondrial fatty acid oxidation; and (5) decreased glutathione levels, a compound that aids in free radical detoxification. This favors peroxidative membrane damage and may precipitate liver injury[14] and cirrhosis.[15]

In Lieber's opinion, depressed fatty acid

centrations, which may predispose the liver to triglyceride accumulation; (5) a decrease in overall metabolic activity including major changes in the citric acid cycle (altered alpha-ketoglutarate oxidation and decreased

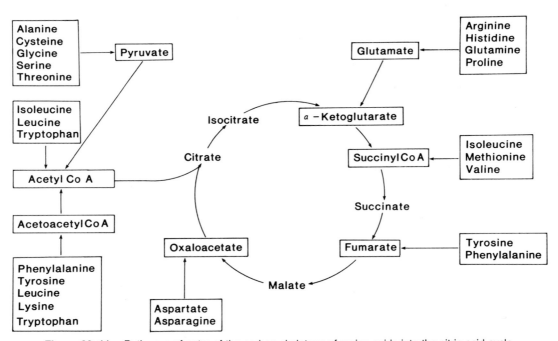

Figure 22–11. Pathways of entry of the carbon skeletons of amino acids into the citric acid cycle.

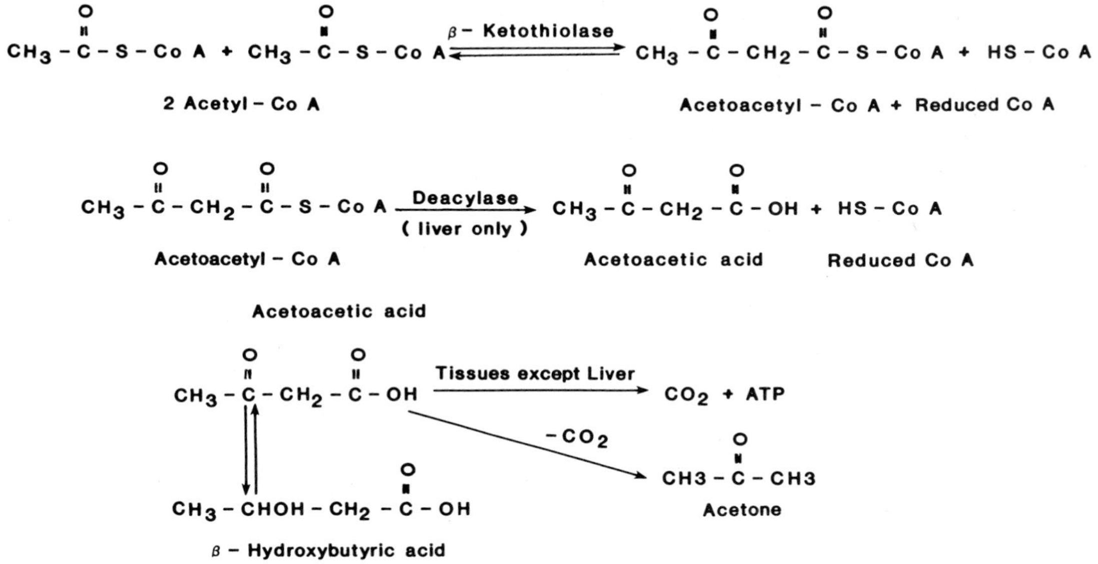

$$CH_3 - \overset{\overset{O}{\parallel}}{C} - S - Co\,A + CH_3 - \overset{\overset{O}{\parallel}}{C} - S - Co\,A \underset{\beta - Ketothiolase}{\rightleftharpoons} CH_3 - \overset{\overset{O}{\parallel}}{C} - CH_2 - \overset{\overset{O}{\parallel}}{C} - S - Co\,A + HS - Co\,A$$

2 Acetyl – Co A   Acetoacetyl – Co A + Reduced Co A

$$CH_3 - \overset{\overset{O}{\parallel}}{C} - CH_2 - \overset{\overset{O}{\parallel}}{C} - S - Co\,A \xrightarrow[\text{(liver only)}]{\text{Deacylase}} CH_3 - \overset{\overset{O}{\parallel}}{C} - CH_2 - \overset{\overset{O}{\parallel}}{C} - OH + HS - Co\,A$$

Acetoacetyl – Co A   Acetoacetic acid   Reduced Co A

Acetoacetic acid

$$CH_3 - \overset{\overset{O}{\parallel}}{C} - CH_2 - \overset{\overset{O}{\parallel}}{C} - OH \xrightarrow{\text{Tissues except Liver}} CO_2 + ATP$$

$$-CO_2 \quad CH3 - \overset{\overset{O}{\parallel}}{C} - CH3$$

Acetone

$$CH_3 - CHOH - CH_2 - \overset{\overset{O}{\parallel}}{C} - OH$$

β – Hydroxybutyric acid

Figure 22–12. Formation and metabolism of ketone bodies.

oxidation plays a major role in the development of alcoholic fatty liver, which may be the first stage of alcoholic liver injury.[16] As he notes, the effects of a potential alteration of redox state are attenuated with chronic alcohol ingestion and thus the progression of liver disease beyond fatty infiltration must be attributed to other mechanisms. Fatty liver occurs very commonly in alcoholics and is a relatively benign condition since it is completely reversed after several weeks of normal, alcohol-free diet.[14, 17] Exactly what causes the hepatocellular damage in alcoholic liver injury is unknown. Two basic

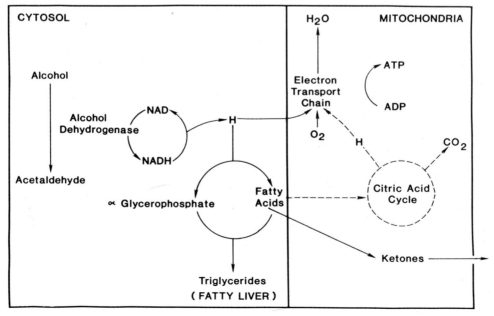

Figure 22–13. Degradation of alcohol and its metabolic effects. Broken lines indicate inhibition. (*From* Mezey, E.: Alcoholic liver disease: Roles of alcohol and malnutrition. Am. J. Clin. Nutr., *33*:2709–2718, 1980, with permission.)

mechanisms are proposed: central hypoxia and hepatocyte hypertrophy.[11] Hepatomegaly is known to occur after chronic ingestion of ethanol and is probably caused by an increase in fat and protein content. Approximately one-half of the increase in the dry weight of the liver is accounted for by lipids, the other half by protein.[18] These effects may be mediated by the effects of ethanol and its metabolic by-products as described previously. The end result of the protein, fat, amino acids, and concomitant water and electrolyte accumulation is a twofold to threefold increase in the diameter, and a fourfold increase in the volume, of some hepatocytes.[14] This so-called "ballooning" has a number of potentially adverse effects including an increase in intrahepatic pressure, which may correlate with collagen deposition,[11] and chronic cellular disorganization, which may promote liver injury. The latter mechanism is supported by observations of patients with alpha-antitrypsin deficiencies in whom protein accumulates in the liver. Morphologic studies have demonstrated sclerosis and collagen deposition in association with fatty liver infiltration but the collagen deposition is variable.[14] Uncomplicated fatty liver may have collagen detectable by chemical means only. Patients in whom pericentral sclerosis and cirrhosis develop may or may not have alcoholic fatty liver infiltration or hepatitis.[13] Neither the duration of drinking nor the amount of alcohol consumed accurately predicts the severity of the histologic lesions seen in alcoholic liver disease.[13]

Whereas it is unclear whether fatty liver is a precursor of alcoholic cirrhosis, it is generally believed that alcoholic cirrhosis may develop from alcoholic hepatitis (Fig. 22–14).[11, 13, 14] The hepatocytic ballooning, extensive necrosis, and polymorphonuclear inflammation seen in alcoholic hepatitis may progress to sclerosis and cirrhosis. Morphologic studies of patients with acute alcoholic hepatitis have demonstrated centrilobular fibrosis which progressively extends to the portal tract—so-called bridging. Bridging is believed to be a precursor of cirrhosis.[13] Baboons fed alcohol develop fatty livers and "ballooned" hepatocytes, and one third of the animals develop cirrhosis.[14, 18] Different morphologic types of cellular infiltration occur under the influence of alcohol.[18] Some patient populations develop cirrhosis without intermediate stages of severe or flagrant alcoholic hepatitis.[11] Thus "simple" fatty liver does not necessarily progress to alcoholic hepatitis or cirrhosis, and alcoholic hepatitis is not necessarily a precursor of alcoholic cirrhosis.

Alcoholic liver injuries are unusual in that they may progress despite discontinuation of alcohol consumption. This suggests an immunologic role in the genesis of alcoholic liver disease. Indeed, cell-mediated and other immunologic abnormalities are common in patients with alcoholic liver disease. A decreased lymphocyte response to mitogens, sequestration of T lymphocytes, an increased incidence of histocompatibility antigen HLA-B8 in patients with biopsy-proven fatty liver, and hyaline antibody and antigen interactions which can alter chemotaxis and cause cell necrosis, have been described in patients with alcoholic liver injury.[14] Although many immunologic alter-

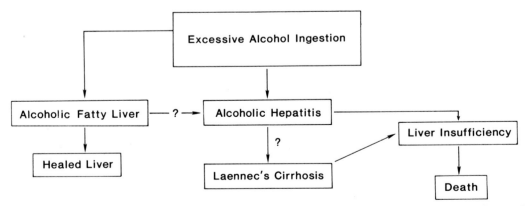

Figure 22–14. Schematic diagram depicting the spectrum of alcoholic liver disease. (*From* Greenberger, N. J., and Winship, D. H.: Liver in Gastrointestinal Disorders: A Pathophysiologic Approach. Chicago, Year Book Medical Publishers Inc., 1976, pp. 253–339, with permission.)

ations are documented in patients with alcoholic liver disease, especially in patients with alcoholic hepatitis, a direct causal relationship between cell-mediated immunologic events and ethanol-induced liver injury has not be established.[19] The exact timing of immunologic events is not clear.[19]

Finally, it appears certain that the development of liver injury is influenced by diet. Protein, vitamin, and other nutrient deficiencies probably potentiate the effects of alcohol on the liver.[11] Fibrosis develops in children with kwashiorkor, and fatty infiltration of the liver and cirrhosis are more common in some malnourished populations.[11] Centrilobular collagen deposition and liver cell necrosis occur, although rarely, in obese patients, and in patients after jejunoileal bypass.[20, 21] Although malnutrition may promote these changes in liver morphology, the fatty infiltration seen in kwashiorkor and in protein-deficient Rhesus monkeys does not necessarily progress to cirrhosis.[11]

In humans, nutrient deficiencies and excessive ethanol intake may combine to produce liver disease.[11] Limited financial resources, disorganized life styles, and gastritis contribute to the histories of inadequate dietary intakes found in two thirds of hospitalized alcoholic patients.[10] Decreased caloric intakes, altered storage and absorptive mechanisms, metabolic abnormalities, and increased nutrient losses further predispose the alcoholic person to nutritional deficiences and subsequent liver injury.[10, 11, 14]

CARBOHYDRATE METABOLISM AND LIVER DISEASE

Liver injury commonly alters carbohydrate metabolism. Abnormal glucose tolerance curves are most common but hypoglycemia also occurs. Both have been well described.[22]

Hypoglycemia may complicate fulminant viral hepatitis and has also been described in patients with severe hepatic damage, primary hepatic carcinoma, and cholangitis.[22] Two mechanisms probably protect patients with liver injury from significant hypoglycemia.[22] First, hepatocytes have a significant reserve; normal homeostasis can be maintained with as little as 20 per cent of the total liver mass. Second, the kidneys also have a significant capacity for gluconeogenesis which may be operative in patients with chronic liver disease.

The proposed explanations for hypoglycemia seen in liver disease are many. In general, hypoglycemia may be associated with impaired glycogen synthesis or breakdown, or impaired gluconeogenesis.[22]

As Johnston and Alberti imply, direct and indirect evidence suggests that gluconeogenesis is impaired in patients with liver disease.[22] The fasting blood levels of gluconeogenic precursors such as lactate tend to increase. An increase in nonesterified fatty acid concentration combined with an inhibition of pyruvate oxidation may elevate lactate levels. Studies of animal models of hepatitis have documented elevated lactate levels, decreased gluconeogenesis, and decreased uptake of all the major gluconeogenic precursors,[22] possibly owing to decreased phosphoenolpyruvate activity.[23] Alcohol inhibits gluconeogenesis and can cause hypoglycemia when the hepatic glycogen content is reduced as occurs in fasting. Histologic studies in patients with viral hepatitis have demonstrated decreased glycogen stores but their diets were not controlled.[22]

Hypoglycemia is also thought to be due to either enhanced or normal production of insulin in the presence of decreased degradation of insulin by the liver.[22] There may also be an abnormal response to glucagon in some patients with cirrhosis. This may reflect abnormal glucagon shunting prohibiting normal action, true hypersection, decreased glucagon metabolism by the diseased liver, or damaged or altered glucagon receptors in patients with significant liver injury.[22]

Hypoglycemia may also occur in patients with cryptogenic cirrhosis, which is cirrhosis that occurs after portal systemic bypasses are created surgically. Theoretically, these shunts cause pancreatic insulin to enter the systemic venous system directly, bypassing the liver. High blood levels of insulin would be expected and are found in these patients.[24]

Patients with chronic liver disease and cirrhosis generally have normal or elevated fasting blood glucose levels.[25] Indeed, impaired glucose tolerance is common in the cirrhotic patient. Patients with cryptogenic cirrhosis commonly have decreased or normal lactate responses to intravenous glucose.[26] Variable changes are associated with other liver diseases[22] and the interpretation of these findings is controversial.

Although fasting blood glucose levels are normal or slightly elevated, plasma insulin levels, although initially normal, slowly rise to supranormal levels in most patients.[24] Elevated insulin levels are generally attributed to hypersecretion, portal diversion, or decreased hepatic clearance.[22] Various studies have shown that the rates of disappearance of injected insulin from the circulation are normal.[27] Studies with C-peptide assays by Johnston et al. have demonstrated decreased insulin degradation.[22]

In any case, glucose intolerance in the presence of elevated insulin levels implies insulin resistance. As Johnston notes, several mechanisms can account for this effect; (1) the total number of parenchymal cells may be decreased and thus insulin would have decreased substrate with which to bind; (2) the number of insulin receptors may be reduced; or (3) insulin may be shunted away from the liver.[22] Extrahepatic factors may also influence insulin resistance.[22] Growth hormone, glucagon, corticosteroids, sex hormones, and other end organ abnormalities such as pancreatitis may precipitate a diabetogenic state. Potassium deficiency has also been shown to impair glucose tolerance.[22]

Although glucose metabolism is most commonly altered, other carbohydrate abnormalities occur but are less well studied. Galactose intolerance may occur secondary to decreased galactose-1-phosphate uridyl transferase levels in some patients. Galactose-1-phosphate uridyl transferase is thought to decrease because of an altered redox state at the hepatocyte.[22] The accumulation of galactose-1-phosphate inhibits galactokinase, and galactose utilization is consequently impaired.[22]

Anderson's disease and hereditary fructose intolerance are caused by specific enzyme deficiencies which alter carbohydrate metabolism and can apparently cause cirrhosis.[28] Idiopathic hemochromatosis, characterized by abnormal iron deposition in the pancreas and liver, can also cause diabetes and cirrhosis.[28]

FAT METABOLISM AND MALABSORPTION IN LIVER DISEASE

As has been reviewed, there are many mechanisms by which fatty liver infiltration may occur; some are peculiar to ethanol-induced liver injury: (1) fatty infiltration may occur secondary to the effects of certain drugs such as ethanol which mobilize lipids from adipose tissue; (2) liver fatty acid levels may increase because of enhanced synthesis or (3) decreased fatty acid oxidation. (4) As noted, ethanol may increase the concentration of alpha-glycerophosphate, a compound that is used for fatty acid esterification. (5) Triglyceride release requires lipoprotein formation; hence lipids may accumulate because of decreased apoprotein synthesis. This mechanism is primarily responsible for the lipid accumulation caused by toxins such as CCl_4 and phosphorus. (6) Impaired lipoprotein synthesis or (7) impaired lipoprotein secretion from the liver may occur and produce fatty metamorphosis.[24]

Cholesterol is synthesized by the liver and by the small intestine to a lesser degree. A decrease in plasma cholesterol ester concentration may reflect hepatic damage. Severe liver injuries may be associated with a decrease in total serum cholesterol levels owing to decreased synthesis of cholesterol and cholesterol esters and/or a decreased synthesis of apolipoproteins.[25]

Steatorrhea is the most common manifestation of malabsorption in patients with cirrhosis,[10] and fat malabsorption may contribute to malnutrition in many cirrhotic patients. One third to two thirds of patients with cirrhosis will have fat malabsorption.[29] However, only 10 per cent of patients will have severe steatorrhea, that is, greater than 30 gm/day of fat in their stools.[10] The etiology of fat malabsorption in cirrhosis is not clear. Alcohol intake may contribute to mild steatorrhea by direct effects on the intestine, but cirrhotic patients deprived of alcohol may still have steatorrhea.[30] An altered pancreatic response to secretin and pancreozymin has been noted in some patients, but this does not necessarily correlate with fat content in stools.[10] Empirical treatment of cirrhotic patients with pancreatic enzyme preparations sometimes decreases fecal fat content.[30, 31] Bile salt abnormalities may contribute to the steatorrhea seen in patients with cirrhosis.[10] Decreased synthesis and premature deconjugation of traurocholic and glycocholic acids have been noted in some cases. Cholestyramine and neomycin, used to treat patients with liver disease, may also aggravate fat malabsorption.[10]

Treatment with medium-chain triglycerides decreases fat excretion in stools in some cirrhotic patients with steatorrhea.[30]

VITAMINS AND LIVER INJURY

Vitamin deficiencies are common in patients with chronic liver disease. Several mechanisms contribute to hypovitaminosis: (1) an increased need for vitamins in the face of inadequate intake; (2) intestinal malabsorption; and (3) a reduced hepatic storage capacity.[10, 32] Clinical stigmata of vitamin deficiency may also occur in the presence of normal stores when liver dysfunction prevents conversion of vitamins into useful forms.[32] Russell notes that patients with liver disease can have a "function malnutrition."[33] According to this model, a nutrient is present in sufficient quantities but cannot be normally metabolized or transported to its end organ, and thus a deficiency state results.

Most vitamins are distributed on plasma proteins in the alpha and beta globulin fractions. Hence abnormalities in red blood cell and protein metabolism may alter circulating vitamin levels. Indeed, circulating vitamin levels are commonly altered in liver disease.[32] Studies by Leevy et al. noted that all of 40 patients with Laennec's cirrhosis, 8 of 10 patients with chronic viral hepatitis, and 9 of 12 patients with biliary cirrhosis, had levels of two or more vitamins that were 20 per cent or less of the range established for healthy subjects.[32] Folic acid was most commonly altered, followed by vitamin B_6 and thiamine. In this study vitamin deficiencies were not necessarily correlated with dietary intake, as in some cases hypovitaminosis occurred despite oral vitamin supplementation.

Conversion of folate to its principal circulating form, 5-methyl tetrahydrofolic acid, occurs primarily in the liver.[33] Similarly, thiamine deficiency in patients with liver disease may result from inadequate conversion of thiamine to its active form.[10]

Decreased vitamin B complex levels commonly occur in hepatocellular disease, as its release from necrotic cells increases its losses.[32] There is also increased demand for this complex, which is needed for nucleic acid synthesis and liver regeneration.[32]

Hypervitaminemia may be seen in the acute phases of viral or CCl_4-induced hepatitis.[32] Vitamin levels generally return to normal within one to two weeks except for vitamin B_{12}, which follows a slower time course.

Hospitalized alcoholic patients in whom acute fatty livers develop may have elevated serum panthothenic acid concentrations despite low levels of folic acid, thiamine, and vitamin B_6.[32] As the fatty changes disappear with nutritional therapy so do the elevated levels of panthothenic acid levels. The cause of elevation of levels of pantothenic acid is unknown.

Catheterization studies of hepatic and umbilical veins demonstrate that orally administered, water-soluble vitamins are absorbed from the intestine into the portal circulation.[32] Vitamin A is absorbed equally by the liver and lymphatics. Vitamin E absorption occurs primarily via the lymphatics.[32] Patients with biliary obstruction, chronic hepatocellular disease, or steatorrhea have reduced uptakes of vitamins A and E. Adaptation to darkness is impaired in some patients with cirrhosis,[10, 33] which may be attributed to the decreased synthesis of retinol-binding protein and prealbumin. These substances are necessary for normal transport of vitamin A.

The metabolism and absorption of vitamin D may be altered in alcoholic patients with significant liver disease, but especially in patients with primary biliary cirrhosis who malabsorb fat-soluble vitamins. 25-hydroxylation of cholecalciferol is reduced in alcoholic liver injury.[34] Furthermore, enhanced mixed function oxidases may speed the degradation of vitamin D. As noted by Korstein and Lieber, abnormal activation of vitamin D may contribute to the increased incidence of fractures and osteonecrosis seen in alcoholic populations.[34]

Patients with alcoholic liver disease have decreased absorption of thiamine and folic acid. Ethanol intake, even in the absence of significant liver disease, adversely affects the metabolism of folic acid, thiamine, pyridoxine, and other vitamins.[12, 35, 36] The effects of ethanol on pyridoxine metabolism are probably mediated by acetaldehyde, which accelerates the degradation of pyridoxal-5-phosphate, the active form of pyridoxine.[11] Acetaldehyde may mediate this effect by displacing pyridoxal-5-phosphate from its cytosolic binding protein.[11] Plasma levels of pyridoxal-5-phosphate are decreased in patients with alcoholic cirrhosis.[11]

Malabsorption may contribute to abnormal vitamin homeostasis. Chronic liver disease is associated with malabsorption caused by alterations in bile salt metabolism and other imprecisely defined mechanisms as discussed earlier. Alcohol may act directly on the liver, pancreas, and intestines to further disturb absorption. Many cirrhotic patients without "significant" liver disease malabsorb D-xylose and vitamins.[11] Vitamin deficiencies may potentiate and perpetuate malabsorption. Folic acid, for example, is known to influence intestinal absorption.[7, 11]

Vitamin storage is altered in patients with significant hepatocellular disease. Total levels of nicotinic acid, vitamins B_{12} and B_6, thiamine, and folate in the liver are decreased in patients with cirrhosis.[32] The liver is a principal storage site for thiamine.[35] Thiamine in the liver may be decreased as a result of decreased uptake, altered binding, or decreased cellular affinity.[32, 35]

TRACE ELEMENTS

The liver is involved in the digestion, absorption, storage, and metabolism of most essential micronutrients. Significant liver disease can be associated with changes in the level of activity of these elements. Both decreased dietary intake of elements and anorexia contribute to the mineral deficiencies seen in patients with liver disease, but the former is probably more important.

Serum zinc levels may be increased or decreased in cirrhosis of the liver.[37] Cirrhosis impairs zinc metabolism and hyperzincuria is observed in many cirrhotic patients.[33] Red blood cells and hair from patients with portal cirrhosis have reduced zinc contents as compared with normal controls.[37] Zinc is normally bound to serum albumin. The decreased serum zinc levels and hyperzincuria seen in many cirrhotic patients may be related to decreased levels of serum albumin.[33] Studies by Hankin and Smith have demonstrated that the amount of zinc excreted in the urine varies with the amount of micromolecular liganded zinc, that is, the amount of zinc bound to amino acids.[38] Cirrhosis, which alters amino acid levels, could theoretically decrease serum zinc levels by increasing glomerular filtration of this compound. Acute ethanol intake is also associated with increased urinary zinc loss through mechanisms that are incompletely described.[33]

Some patients with viral hepatitis have elevated serum zinc levels and excrete abnormally large amounts of zinc in the urine.

This is thought to result from the release of zinc-containing enzymes from damaged hepatic cells.[37]

Copper metabolism is also altered in patients with chronic liver disease. Hemachromatosis and portal and biliary cirrhosis are associated with increased serum copper levels.[37] In these conditions, the copper content of the liver is increased. Wilson's disease, or hepatolenticular degeneration, is associated with abnormal copper metabolism. In Wilson's disease, urinary excretion of copper is high and serum copper levels are low. Excess copper appears in various organs including the liver.[37] The exact pathophysiologic abnormality is unknown but various mechanisms have been proposed, including deranged tissue and carrier protein synthesis which could bind copper abnormally.[25, 37]

The manganese content of the liver may be decreased in some forms of liver disease including portal cirrhosis.[37] Similar changes in levels of molybdenum, cadmium, and selenium have been described.[37] The clinical and nutritional importance of these changes are not known and warrant further study.

WATER AND ELECTROLYTES

Fluid retention is commonly seen in patients with end-stage liver disease and is well described.[25] Patients with ascites have greatly increased total body water and total body exchangeable sodium because of alterations in hydrostatic equilibrium and other endocrine, renal, and biochemical abnormalities. For instance, secondary hyperaldosteronism commonly develops in cirrhotic patients. Dilutional hyponatremia represents water overload in excess of sodium retention. Total body exchangeable potassium levels are usually low. This abnormality may reflect dietary inadequacies, muscle wasting, diuretic therapy, secondary hyperaldosteronism, and renal tubular acidoses which may be present singly or in combinations.[39] Potassium deficiency may contribute to the alkalosis, hyperammonemia, hepatic coma, and renal tubular dysfunction seen in some patients with cirrhosis.

Hyperkalemia may develop in cirrhotic patients secondary to use of diuretics such as spironolactone or if oliguric renal failure develops in end-stage liver disease. Hypochloremia, which is rarely important clinically, is occasionally seen and most often occurs in patients receiving diuretics.[39]

Respiratory alkaloses develop in some patients with hepatic coma. This may represent central neurogenic effects of their liver insufficiency.[39]

ANEMIAS

The cause of anemia in patients with liver disease is generally multifactorial. As alluded to earlier, nutrient deficiencies may predispose these patients to various anemias. However, just the presence of significant liver disease may alter red blood cell mechanics. Cooper recently reviewed the distinct hematologic syndromes that occur in liver disease:[40] (1) spherocytosis may develop in cirrhotic patients from secondary splenomegaly which erodes or "conditions" red blood cell membranes and ultimately leads to destruction of red blood cells in the spleen; (2) acute portal hypertension and splenic congestion, which may occur in patients with acute fatty livers, may be associated with mild hemolysis; and (3) spur cell formation, secondary to membrane structural abnormalities, may occur in alcoholic cirrhosis. These cells are destroyed by the spleen which recognizes them as abnormal. Spur cells are thought to develop secondary to the selective transfer of cholesterol from lipoproteins to red cell membranes, and this adversely affects membrane fluidity. As Cooper notes, alcohol is the most commonly implicated etiologic agent in acute and chronic liver disease and may decrease red blood cell production. If cirrhotic patients have deficiencies of vitamins such as B_{12} and folate, or iron, red blood cell homeostasis may be further disturbed. Iron deficiency anemia is common in patients with chronic liver disease secondary to inadequate intake and/or blood loss.

PROTEIN METABOLISM AND ENCEPHALOPATHY IN LIVER INSUFFICIENCY

Protein metabolism is commonly altered in severe liver disease. The central problem for the nutritionist is how to provide adequate calories and protein to the patient with liver insufficiency without precipitating or exacerbating hepatic encephalopathy.

Two basic hypotheses of hepatic encephalopathy exist. Hepatic encephalopathy may occur as a result of the accumulation of specific "neurotoxins" or the physiologic changes that occur in liver failure may alter "normal" neurotransmitter function and hence mental status. The possibility that the liver fails to excrete or synthesize some protective substance has not been fully examined.[41]

Early research suggested that ammonia might be the specific neurotoxin that accumulates in hepatic encephalopathy. According to this theory, ammonia, which originates from the actions of gut bacteria, amino acid deamination, and protein catabolism, is not detoxified by the liver, but accumulates and damages the central nervous system. The ammonia theory is unsatisfactory for many reasons. Perhaps the most damaging criticism is that the subtle changes of hepatic encephalopathy cannot be explained on the basis of this toxic hypothesis.[42]

The correlation between blood ammonia and the severity of hepatic encephalopathy is poor. Methionine sulfoximine increases the concentration of ammonia in the central nervous system but decreases toxicity.[43] Monoamine oxidase inhibitors, which decrease blood ammonia levels, increase the severity of hepatic encephalopathy.[44] These findings make it unlikely that ammonia is the sole etiologic factor.

Other researchers have suggested that ammonia inhibits cerebral energy production by an alteration in the malate-aspartate shuttle and in cytoplasmic to mitochondrial NADH:NAD ratios.[41] Walker suggested that ammonia might inhibit acetylcholine synthesis.[45] Goetchus and Webster proposed that elevated ammonia levels could cause the inhibitory neurotransmitter gamma-aminobutyric acid to accumulate.[46] Ammonia may affect neuronal cell membranes by inhibiting ATP-ase activity activated by sodium and potassium ions.[47]

Short-chain fatty acids have also been implicated in encephalopathy.[48] Zieve proposed that mercaptans and methanetioles could act synergistically with short-chain fatty acids and ammonia to produce encephalopathy.[48] Others have proposed that fatty acids cause encephalopathy by interfering with ammonia detoxification.[41]

Recent studies suggest that the aminergic system may play a neuromodulator, co-transmitter, or regulatory role in determining the overall level of consciousness.[42] Aminergic terminals comprise only 5 per cent of the total number in the central nervous system.[42] Anatomic studies have shown that the synapses of the catecholaminergic and serotonergic system diffuse freely throughout the glial substance of the central nervous system, rather than terminating on end-plates.[42] Thus small changes in the balance of serotonergic and catecholaminergic modulating systems could theoretically cause the neurologic changes seen in hepatic encephalopathy.[42] Fischer's hypothesis is that the central nervous system neurotransmitters norepinephrine and dopamine are replaced by co-transmitters or false neurotransmitters such as octopamine and other beta-hydroxyphenylethanolamines. The concentration of serotonin, a putative transmitter of the indoleamine system, is also altered.[9]

As Fischer notes, neurotransmitter function is altered by a complex metabolic process beginning with a "deranged hormonal milieu."[9] Hepatic failure is characterized by a glucagon and insulin imbalance. Steroid and epinephrine levels increase because of inadequate liver metabolism. Hyperglucagonemia in the presence of elevated steroid and epinephrine levels forces gluconeogenesis.[9] The liver fails to maintain energy output and its production of glucose and ketone bodies decrease, which in turn increases catabolism. Branched-chain amino acids, which are not released in normal amounts, are consumed locally by muscle and fat.[9] The plasma concentrations of aromatic amino acids, which are normally catabolized by the liver, are altered. Thus, the plasma aminogram changes in hepatic failure. Typically the aromatic amino acids (phenylalanine, tyrosine, tryptophan, and methionine) increase and the branched-chain amino acids (valine, leucine, and isoleucine) decrease. Levels of monoamine precursors and aromatic amino acids also increase in the brain.[49, 50] Potential false neurotransmitter amines effectively bypass metabolism because of inadequate liver function and physiologic or surgical shunting of blood.

Evidence against the false neurotransmitter theory is accumulating, as elucidated by Schenker et al. and Zieve in recent reviews.[41, 48] Massive amounts of octopamine fail to induce coma when administered directly into rat brains even though octopamine levels much greater than normal are produced.[48] Eighty-five to ninety per cent reductions in whole brain, norepinephrine, and dopamine levels in rats given octopamine or gamma hydroxydopamine failed to alter consciousness.[41] Controlled trials have not demonstrated any beneficial effects of

L-dopa in patients with portal systemic encephalopathy, and levels of regional brain norepinephrine and dopamine are not altered in these patients.[47]

It is difficult to account for the observed concentrations of various neutral amino acids in the brain on the basis of plasma competition even in the presence of an altered blood brain barrier.[51] James et al. noted that patients with encephalopathy had elevated levels of glutamine in the brain.[51] He proposed that glutamine could accumulate in the brain secondary to elevated plasma levels of ammonia. According to this theory, ammonia entering the brain is rapidly detoxified or combined with glutamate to form glutamine. The brain, in its efforts to normalize neutral amino acid levels, rapidly exports glutamine by the same mechanism responsible for the influx of neutral amino acids. In support of this hypothesis, James et al. found an excellent correlation between the observed and predicted concentrations of various aromatic amino acids and glutamine.[51] Thus, ammonia may contribute to amino acid imbalances in the brain and aggravate hepatic encephalopathy by its metabolic by-product glutamine. The beauty of this theory is that it incorporates multiple factors in the pathogenesis of hepatic encephalopathy; it explains the contribution of ammonia and correlates this with the observed aminergic neurotransmitter imbalances. It also explains the excellent correlation between encephalopathy grade and glutamine concentration in cerebrospinal fluid.

Schenker has summarized the current hypotheses of etiology of hepatic encephalopathy as follows. All encephalopathies may not have the same pathogenesis, and the etiology of hepatic encephalopathy is most likely multifactorial: Different factors may summate or synergize to produce the changes seen in encephalopathy. The precise mechanisms that induce coma are still uncertain.[41] Futher research will help to elucidate these mechanisms.

TREATMENT

Not just alcoholic cirrhosis results in clinically significant hepatic decompensation. Many other diseases of the liver, which are nutritionally important, disturb detoxification and metabolic systems.[9] Specific nutritional intervention is generally required only when liver insufficiency results. End-stage liver disease, regardless of etiology, is characterized by abnormalities that sometimes have specific clinical manifestations. These abnormalities are perhaps best defined in studies of alcohol and its effects on organ systems. Indeed, it is often difficult to separate the biochemical changes caused by alcohol from those changes that occur in end-stage liver diseases owing to alcoholism. In some cases, alcoholic cirrhosis may not be a valid model of end-stage liver disease, and other times not. The nutritional aberrations of liver failure and liver insufficiency, however, are generally not disease specific. We, as nutritionists, are most often involved with the clinical sequelae of the disease rather than the etiology. Therapy is therefore guided by certain basic principles. These goals are, as Fischer notes, "the maintenance of adequate nutrition, enhancement of liver regeneration, and the recovery and prevention, or amelioration of hepatic encephalopathy."[9]

Principles of Treatment

The nutritional therapy of patients with liver disease is guided by several basic principles. Generally, therapeutic intervention is directed at improving liver function and at avoiding exacerbation of disease. Whether this is accomplished by avoiding the unnecessary use of sedatives, tranquilizers, alcohol, and anesthetics, by preventing metabolic abnormalities, constipation, uremia, infections, or gastrointestinal hemorrhage or by providing aggressive nutritional support, all manipulations are directed toward these goals.

Fluid restriction may be necessary in patients with diffuse liver disease in order to avoid or ameliorate ascites formation. Restriction of dietary sodium is often mandatory. Many patients with ascites will excrete less than 30 mg/day of sodium urine, feces, and sweat, and will need low sodium diets to minimize sodium retention. Similarly, patients with ascites may need to limit daily fluid intake to 1000 to 1500 ml. Sufficient protein and calories must be provided to help maintain nitrogen balance and facilitate liver healing. Since a large proportion of patients with cirrhosis (especially Laennec's cirrhosis) may have deficiencies of vitamins such as folic acid, B_6, and thiamine (with or without clinical manifestations), intensive

replacement therapy may be needed. Failure to adequately correct vitamin deficiencies can have major consequences. For example, it is well known that the administration of glucose, without giving thiamine, to patients with preexisting thiamine deficiencies may precipitate Wernicke's encephalopathy.[41]

Attempts to severely restrict dietary protein in patients with diffuse liver disease in order to avoid precipitating hepatic encephalopathy are misguided. Studies of protein turnover in acute and chronic liver disease indicate that protein restrictions will not significantly affect hepatic or serum amino acid levels.[52] The effect of severe protein restriction in patients with hepatic encephalopathy has been to worsen rather than to improve their nutritional status.[53, 54]

Patients with minor hepatic insufficiency may tolerate modest amounts of protein in the diet, and may require only minimal alterations in fat, sodium, and water contents. These patients may not need special dietary formulations other than those commonly used in most hospitals. Frequently these patients can be nourished at home.

Although some patients with diffuse liver disease who may have mild encephalopathy are able to nourish themselves orally, a significant percentage of these patients are anorexic. Even mild hepatic encephalopathy may prohibit substantive caloric intake. These patients may need to be fed by nasoenteric tube.[56]

Some patients with liver disease require special enteral formulas. When standard formulas are excessive in water, sodium and/or protein contents, modular feedings are particularly well suited for these patients.[56, 57] There is little evidence that nutritional therapy improves outcome in patients with liver disease. Adequate nutrition appears important for recovery but excess calories do not improve survival or rate of healing.[9, 59] Glucose and amino acid therapy may affect the rate of hepatic regeneration.

The intravenous administration of glucose, amino acids (75 to 85 gm/day), minerals, and vitamins, coupled with ad libitum caloric and protein intake (generally 1400 to 1500 kcal/day and 40 to 60 gm/day of protein) in hospitalized patients with alcoholic hepatitis and cirrhosis, was shown to reduce mortality and improve liver function and nutritional indices as compared to diet alone.[59]

Smith et al. used enteral techniques to try and achieve the same goals.[60] Their preliminary results indicated a great potential for this method. By using a low sodium, high caloric density, high protein (70 gm/L) or low protein (40 gm/L) formula, they were able to successfully aliment ascitic cirrhotic patients. This was evidenced by improvements in serum albumin, creatinine: height ratios, and mid-arm muscle and fat indices. Thus while there is as yet no hard evidence to suggest that nutritional therapy significantly alters outcome, aggressive nutritional support of patients with liver disease is warranted.

The principal obstacle to the successful nutritional support of patients with hepatic failure is encephalopathy. The administration of sufficient protein to patients with liver disease will decrease gluconeogenesis, spare catabolism, and encourage overall protein synthesis.[61] Patients with severe or minimal disease who do not tolerate commercial formula, may benefit from solutions with increased ratios of branched-chain amino acids (BCAA) to aromatic amino acids (AAA).

Although at this time no controlled studies have demonstrated that treatment with BCAA influences the outcome of patients with cirrhosis and encephalopathy, there are two potential benefits to using formulas enriched with BCAA:[61] (1) BCAA in combination with other amino acids and hypertonic glucose may be used to prevent or ameliorate encephalopathy and support nutrition; and (2) oral preparations of BCAA may be used for the long-term nutritional support of some cirrhotic patients.

The use of parenteral formula containing high concentrations of BCAA in combination with hypertonic glucose has been shown to be therapeutically effective in producing nitrogen equilibrium and improving encephalopathy.[62, 63] The use of these parenteral formulas will be discussed in volume II of this book.

Oral, defined formula diets, enriched in BCAA (such as Hepaticaid) are now commercially available and are being evaluated in clinical trials. These enterally administered BCAA formulas may prove as effective as parenteral BCAA formulas in ameliorating encephalopathy.[64–67]

Recent work by Maddrey et al.[68] and Herlong et al.[69] has suggested that ornithine salts of BCAA ketoanalogs may be superior to BCAA alone, and to the calcium salts of the BCAA ketoanalogs, in improving the symptoms of hepatic encephalopathy. Their preliminary data demonstrated stabilized or improved liver function and decreased blood ammonia and free tryptophan levels in patients treated with this regimen. More studies are needed to document this phenomenon.

It should be noted that the beneficial effects of BCAA in ameliorating or preventing encephalopathy might not be the result of changes in BCAA concentration. Rather, the effects may be from the marked reductions in the content of ammonia-generating amino acids such as glycine or increases in the levels of arginine, which aid in processing of ammonia. As Zieve notes, the only work that convincingly associates changes in amino acid ratios with the production of encephalopathy is work by Fahey et al. published in the 1950's.[70] In Fahey's studies, infusions of pure amino acid mixtures, lacking arginine, precipitated encephalopathy by generating excess ammonia which the liver could not metabolize to urea.[71] Controlled studies that address these variables independently will help to establish which changes are responsible for the observed therapeutic effects.

APPROACH TO THE PATIENT WITH LIVER DISEASE

As is true with any patient who might require nutritional therapy, patients with liver disease need a thorough nutritional assessment (see Chapter 7). This of course begins with the history and physical examination. One is especially interested in a history of alcoholism, pancreatitis, or coexistent renal or cardiovascular disease. Also, one should determine if there is a history of cirrhosis and how this was documented. The physical examination will provide evidence of cirrhosis, peripheral edema, ascites, and encephalopathy, and should enable the physician to determine the severity of the patient's disease. One should note whether the patient has had previous episodes requiring admission (such as encephalopathy) and whether he or she has had portal systemic shunts created surgically. A key issue is whether the patient will be able to adequately nourish himself orally. Whereas an initial screen may suffice to answer this question, long-term follow-up with calorie counts and serial examinations may be necessary. Nutritional indices and skilled examinations will determine if the patient is malnourished. The basic questions that the nutritionist must then answer are the following. Can the gastrointestinal tract be used safely or will parenteral techniques be necessary? Will the patient require salt and fluid restriction? Is protein restriction necessary? Will special dietary formulations be necessary because of concurrent disease? Will the patient who is unable to take adequate calories orally tolerate nasoenteric tube feeding?

High protein intakes are usually not needed to achieve positive nitrogen balance in most patients with liver disease.[72, 73] From 0.5 to 0.7 gm of protein per kg of body weight will allow nitrogen equilibrium or positive nitrogen balance in most cirrhotic patients.[72, 73] Portal systemic shunting, either iatrogenic or naturally occurring, does not appear to alter nitrogen balance in stable conditions.[72, 73]

Preliminary work suggests that vegetable protein may be superior to animal protein in patients with liver disease and encephalopathy.[74] Other evidence has suggested that milk protein may be superior to animal protein formulas.[75, 76] The tolerance to different proteins may be related to their amino acid contents.[74] The administration of diets high in vegetable proteins is limited by their bulk and palatibility.

Although some cirrhotic patients will have abnormal glucose tolerance curves, treatment with insulin or oral hypoglycemic agents is rarely needed. (Patients with preexisting diabetes mellitus or hemochromatosis may be exceptions to this rule.) As a corollary, high calorie feedings are not contraindicated.

Low fat diets are not needed by most patients with liver disease.[77] Indeed, most will tolerate 150 to 200 gm of dietary fat per day without adverse consequences. Patients with severe jaundice and decreased bile excretion may need dietary fat restriction for short periods[72] until enterohepatic circulation returns to normal. Patients with severe steatorrhea may benefit from trials of medium-chain triglycerides, although diarrhea, decreased protein tolerance, and abdominal discomfort may result.[72] The sodium content of some medium-chain triglyceride formulas may also be excessive.

Patients with nonalcoholic acute liver injury whose intakes are suboptimal for short periods of time generally do not require vitamin supplementation. Patients with liver injury who may not be alcoholic may have specific (vitamin) deficiencies that require replacement therapy. Oral vitamin supplements may also be needed by patients with hepatic encephalopathy who may have decreased intake of B-complex vitamins. Patients with biliary cirrhosis may need fat-soluble vitamin supplementation.

After this initial assessment, the potential route for nutrient administration can be identified. Patients who are severely ill and malnourished and whose gastrointestinal tracts cannot be used safely are best served by total parenteral nutrition.

From a therapeutic standpoint, patients can then be grouped into three basic categories: (1) those with stable liver disease; (2) those with acute fulminant liver injury; and (3) those with decompensated chronic cirrhosis.

Most patients with chronic stable liver disease whose intake is not limited by anorexia, vomiting, or diarrhea can be managed with oral diets. Fluid and/or sodium intakes are restricted as needed for patients who have ascites and edema. These patients are commonly managed by their primary physicians and usually do not require special enteral feedings.

Peripheral intravenous feedings may be used to supplement oral intakes in patients who cannot receive central parenteral nutrition (for example, because of a refractory coagulopathy prohibiting safe subclavian vein puncture) or who are not yet ready to support themselves with oral feedings.

Patients with acute fulminant hepatitis most often are not able to nourish themselves orally. Although their gastrointestinal tracts may be functional, the severity of their disease is such that tube feedings are rarely used. In general, parenteral nutrition is used in these patients because caloric goals may be more readily achieved. Furthermore, these patients may require highly individualized therapy because of varying fluid and electrolyte requirements. At present these patients are more easily managed with parenteral techniques, which allow fluid and electrolyte changes more rapidly and easily. Nutritional therapy for these patients is thus more readily individualized. Modular feeding techniques, which are currently being developed, may allow the same flexibility to be attained with enteral feeding.

Special Considerations

Patients who require artificial feeding and who are not candidates for parenteral or modular techniques are candidates for fixed formula diets. Most of these patients have decompensated chronic cirrhosis.

The nutritional assessment should provide an estimate of the minimum caloric requirement. A critical issue will be whether fluid restriction is required. Standard fixed formula diets generally provide 1.0 kcal/ml of solution. Furthermore, these formulas may have prohibitively high sodium contents (35 to 45 mEg/1000 kcal of sodium). If adequate calories cannot be provided within the limits of fluid restriction, a high caloric density formula may be needed (2 kcal/ml).

Table 22–1 provides a partial listing of high caloric density formulas. In addition to their relatively low sodium and water contents, these formulas have the advantage of being nutritionally complete. Whole proteins provide the protein source in most high caloric density formulas. Carbohydrate is provided as complex oligosaccharides and starches in combination with monosaccharides such as glucose. Certain formulas such as Travasorb (Travenol Laboratories, Deerfield, Il.) provide fat as the easily absorbed medium-chain triglycerides.

Most patients with minimal or absent encephalopathy, and with mild or moderate ascites or edema, can be managed initially with standard fixed formulas. These formulas provide 350 to 500 mg of sodium and 20 to 40 gm of protein per liter. Sixty per cent of patients with liver disease will tolerate 40 to 60 gm of protein per day.[9]

Those patients with severe ascites and edema may require more severe sodium restriction. Similarly some patients who are protein intolerant or who have significant encephalopathy may require special enteral formulas. In these patients we start with 250 mg of sodium and 50 gm of protein per day and increase this according to patient tolerance. As tolerance is ascertained, protein is increased by 10 to 15 gm per day and caloric intake by 200 to 300 calories per day until the nutritional requirements are reached.

Patients with severe steatorrhea can be managed with a formula based on medium chain triglycerides and partially hydrolyzed protein (such as Vital) (Ross Laboratories, Columbus, Ohio). These formulas require minimal digestion and can be absorbed directly. Patients with coexistent pancreatic insufficiency may benefit from a trial with pancreatic enzyme preparations. Linoleic acid supplementations at 4 to 7 gm/day may be needed when medium chain triglycerides are the sole fat source for extended time periods.

When diabetes and glucose intolerance complicate the care of patients with liver disease, formulas based on complex, long-chain sugars may reduce hyperglycemia and glucosuria.[78]

Renal insufficiency may further complicate the care of patients with liver disease. These renal patients may require low sodium, high caloric density, low potassium formulas. In addition, increased calorie to nitrogen ratios and total free water restriction may be needed. If severe hepatic encephalopathy is present, these patients may be especially difficult to manage. At this point modular feedings of formulas which are enriched with BCAA should be considered.

Specific vitamin deficiencies are treated when they are recognized. For example, patients with prolonged prothrombin times (such as patients with biliary cirrhosis) may benefit from parenteral vitamin K therapy.

Table 22–1. SELECTED HIGH CALORIC DENSITY FORMULAS

FORMULA	CALORIES (per ml)	VOLUME (ml/1000 kcal)	OSMOLALITY (mOsm/kg)	PROTEIN (gm/1000 kcal)	CARBO-HYDRATE (gm/1000 kcal)	FAT (gm/1000 kcal)	NA (mg/1000 kcal)	K (mg/1000 kcal)
Magnacal (Organon)	2.0	1000	520	35	125	40	500	625
Ensure Plus (Ross)	1.5	666	600	36.6	133	36	704	1268
Isocal HCN (Mead-Johnson)	2.0	1000	650	75	225	91	800	1400

Patients with macrocytic anemias who have B_{12} or folate deficiencies may need to have these vitamins replaced. We recommend that vitamin supplements be administered to all patients with liver disease, particularly thiamine to alcoholic patients.

When electrolyte deficiencies are encountered they are treated specifically. At times these are best managed by parenteral supplementation. Other electrolytes, such as potassium, can be easily and safely repleted orally. Electrolyte excesses are not as easily treated with fixed enteral formulas. Often other exogenous sources of the particular electrolyte can be identified. The content or amount of these sources can be decreased, thus diminishing the intake of the offending electrolyte. This may be the case in patients in whom potassium excesses develop. While the potassium content of the fixed formula cannot be decreased, the amount of potassium in intravenous fluids can be reduced. Discontinuing oral potassium supplements or changing potassium-based medications may further decrease potassium intake.

Trace element and other micronutrient deficiencies or excesses are handled in a similar fashion and in general most patients will present with vitamin and mineral deficiencies. Once again, deficiencies are more easily treated. As mentioned previously, a modular formula is ideally suited to match the patient's individual requirements. Magnesium, calcium, iron, and other micronutrient deficiencies are treated when they are present by supplementing the formula. Excesses are rare and usually iatrogenic. These micronutrient excesses may develop when patients are given inappropriate amounts in improperly mixed modular formulas, especially when the body's homeostasis is altered, such as in renal disease, when magnesium excretion is impaired. Excesses can also result from inappropriate replacement therapy.

Finally, those patients with severe hepatic encephalopathy or who are protein intolerant should be given BCAA formulas, as tolerated. These formulas may improve nutritional indices, protein tolerance, and decrease encephalopathy as discussed. We should point out that these formulas are currently being examined in carefully controlled, clinical trials to fully document their beneficial effects.

Continual assessment of the patient is mandatory for several reasons. One must ensure that nutritional goals are attained and met on a perpetual basis. Caloric requirements are subject to change according to the patient's condition, including the presence of infection, surgery, and other catabolic stresses. Similarly, protein, fluid, and electrolyte requirements are subject to change. Careful monitoring is necessary to recognize these changes and to treat them appropriately.

Patient Examples

This section will illustrate the principles of enteral alimentation of patients with liver disease followed at the Philadelphia Veterans Administration Medical Center.

Example 1. The Nutritional Support Service is called to evaluate a 42-year-old man admitted to the medical service with a diagnosis of alcoholic hepatitis. His oral intake is significantly limited by nausea and anorexia. Dietary history reveals a chronically inadequate intake of all nutrients. There is no history of ascites or encephalopathy.

> *Physical Examination*—Height: 5'8";
>   weight: 55 kg (IBW = 63. kg); minimal
>   to absent ascites; grade 0 encephalopathy
> *Laboratory Studies*—Albumin 3.2 gm/dl;
>   transferrin 180 mg/dl
> *Caloric Requirement*—2400 kcal/day
>   (see Chapter 11)
> *Sodium/Fluid Restriction*—None
> *Nutritional Assessment*—Moderately
>   malnourished
> *Enteral Prescription*
>   Route: Nasogastric tube
>   Method: Intermittent
>   Formula: Standard fixed formula
>   (such as Isocal)
>   Rate:

Day	Volume (ml)	Strength	Frequency	Time for Delivery
1	150	Full	Q4⁰	20–30 min
2	250	Full	Q4⁰	20–30 min
3	400	Full	Q4⁰	20–30 min

Comments. There are no contraindications to using the gastrointestinal tract in this patient. His oral intake is limited only by the symptoms of his disease, and tube feedings can be used safely. No disease process, sign, or symptom would suggest that this patient is at increased risk for aspiration. Nasogastric feedings are commonly used for patients who require tube feedings, and they are the preferred feedings for patients without increased risk for aspiration. The stomach has a tremendous reservoir capacity that allows full-strength formula to be used immediately. Bolus feedings are easily administered and require less nursing time and effort.

By day 3 of this prescription, the patient will receive 2400 kcal, 78 gm of protein, and 53 mEq of sodium per day in 2400 ml. Greater than 100 per cent of the recommended dietary allowance for vitamins and trace elements are provided in 2400 ml of this fixed formula diet. We would normally supplement the diet with an oral multivitamin preparation (such as 1 capsule/day or Theragram-M), as patients with liver disease may need additional vitamin supplementation. Parenteral thiamine is also administered as needed. The exact requirements for vitamins in the stressed and sick patient are unknown.

The patient must be monitored for signs of protein intolerance such as the development of encephalopathy. Clinical examination for asterixis, confusion, loss of coordination, and other objective tests (such as trail tests, venous ammonia levels) are used for this purpose. The patient may tolerate 80 gm/day of protein as there is no prior history of encephalopathy.

Similarly, the patient will probably tolerate 1200 mg/day of sodium (which is less than the average daily intake for most adults in this country) and no sodium restriction is required.

Example 2. The same patient returns five years later. He has continued to drink and is admitted with another episode of alcoholic hepatitis. A liver biopsy performed during the intervening five-year period demonstrated alcoholic cirrhosis. He has significant ascites and peripheral edema which has been treated with sodium restriction (2 gm) and diuretics. Oral intake is insufficient.

Physical Examination—Mild to moderate ascites; grade 0–1 encephalopathy
Laboratory Studies—Albumin 3.0 gm/dl; transferrin 140 mg/dl
Caloric Requirements—2400 kcal/day
Fluid Limit—1500 ml/day
Nutritional Assessment—Moderately malnourished

Enteral Prescription
   Route: Nasoduodenal tube
   Method: Continuous
   Formula: High caloric density fixed formula (such as Magnacal)
   Rate:

Day	Volume (ml)	Strength	Frequency	Delivery
1	50	½	hourly	Continuous pump
2	50	¾	hourly	Continuous pump
3	50	full	hourly	Continuous pump

Comments. This patient with mild encephalopathy is a candidate for nasoduodenal feeding, which is thought to decrease the incidence of aspiration. Once again there is no contraindication to using the gastrointestinal tract. Our assessment has indicated that this patient needs nutritional maintenance primarily and not repletion.

Using this prescription, 2400 kcal and 77 gm of protein are given in 1200 ml of fluid daily. A restricted sodium intake of 1200 mg/day is given in this volume. This diet provides 100 per cent of the recommended dietary allowance of vitamins and trace elements, but vitamin intake would again be supplemented.

The fixed formula diets are limited as to the number of calories that can be administered without risking significant protein intolerance. This regimen could conceivably worsen the patients's encephalopathy. If this occurs, the patient would be treated empirically with lactulose and neomycin. If this treatment fails, protein intake will have to be decreased.

Another option in this patient would be to use modular feedings. Modular feedings (when available) adjust nutrient intakes more readily to patients needs (see Chapter 11). For example, our patient could also be managed with a formula consisting of:

   750 cc (2kcal/cc) Magnacal
      (Organon, West Orange, New Jersey)
   250 cc (2 kcal/cc) Polycose
      (Ross Laboratories, Columbus, Ohio)
   60 cc (8.3 kcal/cc) MCT Oil
      (Mead Johnson, Evansville, Indiana)
                or
   110 cc (4.5 kcal/cc) Microlipid
      (Organon, West Orange, New Jersey)
                and
   1 Multivitamin capsule daily.

This formula would provide 2500 kcal/day, 1060 mg/day of sodium and 54 gm/day of protein. As many calories are provided as in the original fixed formula diet but with far less sodium, protein, and total volume. This prescription may be more easily tolerated by the protein-intolerant patient. By decreasing the amount of the fixed formula and adjusting the ratios of the other components even smaller amounts of protein may be administered. If medium chain triglycerides constitute the only fat source for an extended time, patients may develop essential fatty acid deficiencies. Furthermore one must be aware of their potential to exacerbate encephalopathy.

Example 3.   The patient again recovers and is discharged only to return two years later with an other episode of alcoholic hepatitis. He appears to be malnourished. Anorexia and encephalopathy prevent significant oral intake.

> *Physical Examination*—Significant ascites; 2–3+ peripheral edema; grade 2 encephalopathy
> *Laboratory Studies*—Serum albumin 3.0 gm/dl; serum transferrin 150 mg/dl
> *Caloric Requirement*—2500 kcal/day
> *Fluid Limit*—1500 ml/day
> *Sodium Restriction*—<1 gm/day
> *Nutritional Assessment*—Moderately malnourished
> *Enteral Prescription*
> Route: Nasoduodenal tube
> Method: Continuous
> Formula: Branched chain amino acid enriched (such as Hepatic-Aid)
> Rate:

Day	Volume (ml/hr)	Strength
1	50	¼
2	63	½
3	63	½
4	63	½
5	63	¾
6	63	¾
7	63	Full

Comments.   We would start feedings in the duodenum at one-quarter strength and increase the rate as determined by patient tolerance. Volume is increased before concentration, as the duodenum has a smaller reservoir capacity as compared to the stom-ach. A formula with BCAA may ameliorate or prevent encephalopathy.

Hepatic-Aid, 1500 ml, provides 2500 kcal and 65 gm of protein per day. The sodium content of this formula is negligible if distilled water is used in reconstitution. If 60 gm of protein are not tolerated, smaller volumes of Hepatic-Aid may be administered and additional calories provided by an intravenous or enteral modular source.

Other options are available. For example, essential amino acids may be used: 1775 ml of Aminaid will provide 2500 kcal, 22.5 gm of protein, and 7.5 mEq of sodium per day. This formula does not provide the increased BCAA ratios thought to be effective in ameliorating encephalopathy. Furthermore, vitamins and trace elements must be added to this diet to make it nutritionally complete.

SUMMARY

The liver serves as the focal point for regulation and metabolism of both endogenous and exogenous compounds. It is a major site of protein synthesis, drug and toxin detoxification and excretion.

The classification of liver disease is difficult; however, the histologic result in many cases is cirrhosis. Cirrhosis is very common and is a leading cause of death in the United States. Alcoholic cirrhosis accounts for most of the fatal cases of cirrhosis in urban areas in this country.

The pathophysiologic effects of alcohol on the liver and the role of alcohol in the genesis of cirrhosis and liver failure has been extensively studied. Three histologic types of alcoholic liver injury are well recognized: fatty metamorphosis, hepatitis, and cirrhosis.

Exactly how alcohol causes cirrhosis and alcoholic hepatitis has not been determined. Alcoholic hepatitis is not necessarily a precursor of alcoholic cirrhosis. Alcohol may cause cirrhosis by directly altering enzyme systems and redox states or by the effects of metabolic by-products such as acetaldehyde at the microsomal level. Cell-mediated immunologic abnormalities, genetic factors, and nutrient deficiencies may potentiate the development of cirrhosis.

Carbohydrate metabolism is commonly altered in end-stage liver disease. Both hyperglycemia and hypoglycemia occur but the former is more common. Glucose intolerance is thought to occur because of relative insulin resistance. Other carbohydrate abnormalities may occur but are less well studied.

Altered fat metabolism and steatorrhea may be seen. An increased need for vitamins, deficient dietary intake, intestinal malabsorption, and reduced hepatic storage capacities contribute to the vitamin deficiencies seen in most patients with liver disease.

Trace element deficiencies are also common. The liver is intimately involved in the digestion, absorption, and metabolism of most micronutrients. Zinc and copper deficiencies and their pathophysiologic and clinical consequences are well described. Deranged water, electrolyte, and red blood cell homeostasis also occur with severe liver injury.

Abnormalities in protein metabolism cause significant morbidity and are thought to be primarily responsible for the signs and symptoms of hepatic encephalopathy, although the exact pathophysiological mechanisms are unclear.

Specific nutritional intervention is only required when liver insufficiency or decompensation occurs. The nutrient-metabolic requirements and intolerances of liver failure or insufficiency are probably not disease specific. Nutritional therapy is often directed at the clinical manifestations of the disease rather than the etiology. As noted by Fischer, the goals of nutritional therapy are to maintain adequate nutrition, to facilitate regeneration and recovery, and to prevent or ameliorate hepatic encephalopathy where possible.[9] Sufficient protein and calories must be provided to help maintain nitrogen balance. Sodium, water, and protein restriction are usually necessary. Severe protein restriction, however, is not always necessary and may be harmful. Most patients with grade 0 to 1 encephalopathy will tolerate modest amounts (40 to 60 gm/day) of protein in their diets. Patients who are protein intolerant and develop encephalopathy may benefit from diets enriched with branched-chain amino acids which are now available for enteral use. High caloric density formulas, which are low in sodium, are useful for those patients in need of sodium and water restriction and who require enteral alimentation. Modular feedings may be ideal for alimenting patients with liver disease who do not tolerate standard fixed formula diets.

REFERENCES

1. Lelbach, W. K.: Cirrhosis in the alcoholic and its relation to the volume of alcohol abuse. Ann. N.Y. Acad. Sci., 252:85–105, 1975.
2. Felig, P., Wahren, J., and Hendler, R.: Influence of oral glucose ingestion on splanchnic glucose and gluconeogenic substrate metabolis in man. Diabetes, 24:468–475, 1975.
3. Wahren, J.: Carbohydrate homeostasis and the liver. Acta Med. Scand. [Suppl.], 639:37–41, 1980.
4. Munro, H.: Parenteral nutrition: Metabolic consequences of bypassing the gut and liver. In Green, Holiday, and Munro (eds.): Clinical Nutrition Update: Amino Acids. Chicago, American Medical Association, 1977, pp. 141–146.
5. Elwyn, D. H.: The role of the liver in the regulation of amino acid and protein metabolism. In Munro, H. N. (ed.): Mammalian Protein Metabolism, Vol. IV. New York, Academic Press, 1970, pp. 523–571.
6. Robbins, S. L.: The liver and biliary tract. In Robbins, S. L., and Cotran, S. (eds.): Pathologic Basis of Disease. Philadelphia, W.B. Saunders Co., 1974, pp. 985–1055.
7. Halsted, C. H.: Alcoholism and Malnutrition: Introduction to the symposium. Am. J. Clin. Nutr., 33:2705–2708, 1980.
8. Schwartz, S. I.: Liver. In Schwartz, S. I. Lillehei, R. C., Shires, G. T., et al. (eds.): Principles of Surgery. Edition 3. New York, McGraw-Hill, 1979, pp. 1177–1220.
9. Fischer, J. E., and Bower, R. H.: Nutritional support in liver disease. Surg. Clin. North Am., 61:653–660, 1981.
10. Mezey, E.: Liver disease and nutrition. Gastroenterology, 74:770–783, 1978.
11. Mezey, E.: Alcoholic liver disease: Roles of alcohol and malnutrition. Am. J. Clin. Nutr., 33:2709–2718, 1980.
12. Patek, A. J.: Alcohol, malnutrition, and alcoholic cirrhosis. Am. J. Clin. Nutr., 32:1304–1312, 1979.
13. Van Thiel, D. H., Lipsitz, H. D., Porter, L. E., Schade, R. R., Gottlieb, G. P., and Graham, T. O.: Gastrointestinal and hepatic manifestations of chronic alcoholism. Gastroenterology, 81:594–615, 1981.
14. Lieber, C. S.: Metabolism and metabolic effects of alcohol. Semin. Hematol., 17:85–99, 1980.
15. Lewis, K. O., and Paton, A.: Could superoxide cause cirrhosis? Lancet, 2:188–189, 1982.
16. Lieber, C. S.: Metabolism of ethanol. In Medical Disorders of Alcoholism: Pathogenesis and Treatment. Philadelphia, W. B. Saunders Co., 1982.
17. Baraona, E., and Lieber, C. S.: Effects of chronic ethanol feeding on serum lipoprotein metabolism in the rat, J. Clin. Invest., 49:769–778, 1970.
18. Lieber, C. S., DeCarli, L. M., and Rubin, E.: Sequential production of fatty liver, hepatitis, and cirrhosis in sub-human primates fed ethanol with adequate diets. Proc. Nat. Acad. Sci., 72:437–441, 1975.
19. Zetterman, R. K., and Sorrell, M. F.: Immunologic aspects of alcoholic liver disease. Gastroenterology, 81:616–624, 1981.
20. Shibata, H. R., Mackenzie, J. R., and Huang, S.: Morphologic changes of the liver following small intestinal bypass for obesity. Arch. Surg., 103:229–237, 1971.

21. Ackerman, N. B.: Protein supplementation in the management of degenerating liver function after jejunoileal bypass. Surg. Gynecol. Obstet., *149*:8–14, 1979.

22. Johnston, D. C., and Alberti, K. G. M. M.: Carbohydrate metabolism in liver disease. Clin. Endocrinol. Metabol., *5*:675–702, 1976.

23. Record, C. O., Alberti, K. G. M. M., and Williamson, D. H.: Metabolic studies in experimental liver disease resulting from D(+)-galactosamine administration. Biochem. J., *130*:37–44, 1972.

24. Megyesi, C., Samols, E., and Marks, V.: Glucose tolerance and diabetes in chronic liver disease. Lancet, 2:1051–1055, 1967.

25. Shafritz, D. A., Yap, S. H., and Isselbacher, K. J.: Derangements of hepatic metabolism. *In* Isselbacher, K. J., Adams, R. D., Braunwald, E., Petersdorf, R. G., and Wilson, J. D. (eds.): Harrison's Principles of Internal Medicine. Edition 9. New York, McGraw-Hill, 1980, pp. 1445–1449.

26. Alberti, K. G. M. M.: Some metabolic aspects of liver disease. *In* Truelove, S. C., and Trowell, J. (eds.): Topics in Gastroenterology, Oxford, Blackwell, 1974, pp. 341–359.

27. Collins, J. R., Lacy, W. W., Stiel, J. N., and Crofford, O. B.: Glucose intolerance and insulin resistance in patients with liver disease. II. A study of etiological factors and evaluation of insulin actions. Arch. Intern. Med., *126*:608–614, 1970.

28. Sherlock, S.: The iron storage diseases. *In* Sherlock, S. (Ed.): Diseases of the Liver and Biliary System. Edition 4. Philadelphia, F. A. Davis, 1968, pp. 437–455.

29. Baraona, E., Orrego, H., Fernandez, O., Amenabar, E., Maldonado, E.: Tag, F., and Salina, A.: Absorptive function of the small intestine in liver cirrhosis. Am. J. Dig. Dis., 7:318–330, 1962.

30. Linscheer, W. G.: Malabsorption in cirrhosis. Am. J. Clin. Nutr., 23:488–492, 1970.

31. Sun, D. C. H., Albacete, R. A., and Chen, J. K.: Malabsorption studies in cirrhosis of the liver. Arch. Intern. Med., *119*:567–572, 1967.

32. Leevy, C. M., Thompson, A., and Baker, H.: Vitamins and liver injury. Am. J. Clin. Nutr., 23:493–499, 1970.

33. Russell, R. M.: Vitamin and mineral supplements in the management of liver disease. Med. Clin. North Am., *63*:537–544, 1979.

34. Korsten, M. A., and Lieber, C. S.: Nutrition in the alcoholic. Med. Clin. North Am., *63*:963–972, 1979.

35. Hoyumpa, A. M.: Mechanisms of thiamine deficiency in chronic alcoholism. Am. J. Clin. Nutr., 33:2750–2761, 1980.

36. Lindenbaum, J., and Roman, M. J.: Nutritional anemia in alcoholism. Am. J. Clin. Nutr., 33:2727–2735, 1980.

37. Prasad, A. S., Oberleas, D., and Rasjasekaran, G.: Essential micronutrient elements. Biochemistry and changes in liver disorders. Am. J. Clin. Nutr., 23:581–591, 1970.

38. Henkin, R. I., and Smith, F. R.: Zinc and copper metabolism in acute viral hepatitis. Am. J. Med. Sci., 264:401–409, 1972.

39. Summerskill, W. H. J., Barnardo, D. E., and Baldus, W. P.: Disorders of water and electrolyte metabolism in liver disease. Am. J. Clin. Nutr., 23:499–507, 1970.

40. Cooper, R. A.: Hemolytic syndromes and red cell membrane abnormalities in liver disease. Semin. Hematol., 17:103–112, 1980.

41. Schenker, S., Henderson, G. I., Hoyumpa, A. M., and McCandless, D. W.: Hepatic and Wernicke's encephalopathies: Current concepts of pathogenesis. Am. J. Clin. Nutr., 33:2719–2726, 1980.

42. Freund, H. R., and Fischer, J. E.: Hepatic failure. *In* Hill, G. L. (ed.): Nutrition and the Surgical Patient, Vol. 2, Clinical Surgery International. New York, Churchill Livingstone, 1981, pp. 201–218.

43. Warren, K. S., and Schenker, S.: Effect of an inhibitor of glutamine synthesis (methionine and sulfoximine) on ammonia toxicity and metabolism. J. Lab. Clin. Med., 64:442–449, 1964.

44. Dawson, A. M., and Sherlock, S.: Effect of an amine-oxidase inhibitor on arterial ammonium levels in liver disease. Lancet, 1:1332–1333, 1957.

45. Walker, C. O., Speeg, K. V., Levinson, J. D., and Schenker, S.: Cerebral acetylcholine, serotonin, and norepinephrine in acute ammonia intoxication. Proc. Soc. Exper. Biol. Med., 136:668–671, 1971.

46. Goetcheus, J. S., and Webster, L. T.: α-Amino-butyrate and hepatic coma. J. Lab. Clin. Med., 65:257–267, 1965.

47. Schenker, S. D., McCandless, D. W., Brophy, E., and Lewis, M. S.: Studies on the intracerebral toxicity of ammonia. J. Clin. Invest., 46:838–848, 1967.

48. Zieve, L.: Hepatic encephalopathy: Summary of present knowledge with an elaboration on recent developments. *In* Popper, H., and Schaffer, F. (eds.): Progress in Liver Diseases, Vol. VI. New York, Grune and Stratton, 1979, pp. 327–342.

49. Rosen, H. M., Yoshimura, N., Hodgman, J. M., and Fischer, J. E.: Plasma amino acid patterns in hepatic encephalopathy of differing etiology. Gastroenterology, 72:483–487, 1977.

50. Soeters, P. B., and Fischer, J. E.: Insulin, glucagon, aminoacid imbalance, and hepatic encephalopathy. Lancet, 2:880–882, 1976.

51. James, J. H., Jeppsson, B., Ziparo, V., and Fischer, J. E.: Hyperammonaemia, plasma aminoacid imbalance, and blood-brain aminoacid transport: A unified theory of portal-systemic encephalopathy. Lancet, 2:772–774, 1979.

52. O'Keefe, S. J. D., Abraham, R. R., Davis, R., and Williams, R.: Protein turnover in acute and chronic liver disease. Acta Chir. Scand. [Suppl.], *507*:91–101, 1981.

53. Silk, D. B. A.: Malnutrition in liver disease and its relationship to hepatic encephalopathy. Acta Chir. Scand. [Suppl.], *507*:106–111, 1981.

54. Fischer, J. E.: The etiology of hepatic encephalopathy—nutritional implications. Acta Chir. Scand. [Suppl.], *507*:50–68, 1981.

55. Bethel, R. A., Jansen, R. D., Heymsfield, S. B., Ansley, J. D., Hersh, T., and Rudman, D.: Nasogastric hyperalimentation through a polyethylene catheter: An alternative to central venous hyperalimentation. Am. J. Clin. Nutr., 32:1112–1120, 1979.

56. Heymsfield, S. B., Horowitz, J., and Lawson, D. H.: Enteral hyperalimentation. *In* Berk, J. E. (ed.): Developments in Digestive Diseases. Philadelphia, Lea and Febiger, 1980, pp. 59–83.

57. Freed, B. A., Hsia, B., Smith, J. P., and Kaminiski, M. V.: Enteral nutrition: Frequency of formula modification. J.P.E.N., 5:40–45, 1981.

58. Galambos, J. T., Hersh, T., Fulenwider, J. T., Ansley, J. D., and Rudman, D.: Hyperalimentation in alcoholic hepatitis. Am. J. Gastroenterol., 72:535–541, 1979.

59. Nasrallah, J. M., and Galambos, J. T.: Aminoacid therapy of alcoholic hepatitis. Lancet, 2:1276–1277, 1980.

60. Smith, J., Horowitz, J., Henderson, M., and Heymsfield, S.: Enteral hyperalimentation in undernourished patients with cirrhosis and ascites. Am. J. Clin. Nutr., 35:56–72, 1982.

61. Fischer, J. E., and Fishman, A. P.: Panel report on nutritional support of patients with liver, renal, and cardiopulmonary diseases. Am. J. Clin. Nutr., 34:1235–1245, 1981.

62. Fischer, J. E., Rosen, H. M., Ebeid, A. M., James, J. H., Keane, J. M., and Soeters, P. B.: The effect of normalization of plasma amino acids on hepatic encephalopathy in man. Surgery, 80:77–91, 1976.

63. Okada, A., Ikeda, Y., Itakura, T., Kim, C. W., Kamata, S., and Kawashima, Y.: Treatment of hepatic encephalopathy with a new parenteral amino acid mixture. J.P.E.N., 2:218, 1978.

64. Freund, H., Yoshimura, N., and Fischer, J. E.: Chronic hepatic encephalopathy: Long-term therapy with a branched-chain amino-acid-enriched elemental diet. J.A.M.A., 242:347–349, 1979.

65. Horst, D., Grace, N., Conn, H. O., Schiff, E., Schenker, S., Viteri, A., Law, D., and Atterbury, C. E.: A double-blind randomized comparison of dietary protein and an oral branched-chain amino acid (BCAA) supplement in cirrhotic patients with chronic portal systemic encephalopathy (PSE). Hepatology, 2:184, 1982.

66. Keohane, P. P., Attrill, H., Grimble, C., Spiller, R., and Silk, D. B. A.: Nutritional support of malnourished encephalopathic cirrhotic patients using a specially formulated enteral diet. Gastroenterology, 82:1098, 1982.

67. Simko, V.: Long-term tolerance and nutritional value of oral branched chain amino acids (Hepatic-aid) in patients with liver disease and history of encephalopathy. Gastroenterology, 82:1244, 1982.

68. Maddrey, W. C., Weber, F. L., Coulter, A. W., Chura, C. M., Chapanis, N. P., and Walser, M.: Effects of ketoanalogues of essential amino acids in portal-systemic encephalopathy. Gastroenterology, 71:190–195, 1976.

69. Herlong, H. B., Maddrey, W. C., and Walser, M.: The use of ornithine salts of branched-chain ketoacids in portal-systemic encephalopathy. Ann. Intern. Med., 93:545–550, 1980.

70. Zieve, L.: Amino acids in liver failure. Gastroenterology, 76:219–221, 1979.

71. Fahey, J. L., Perry, R. S., and McCoy, P. F.: Blood ammonia elevation and toxicity from intravenous L-amino and administration to dogs: The protective role of L-arginine. Am. J. Physiol., 192:311–317, 1958.

72. Gabuzada, C. J.: Nutrition and liver disease. Med. Clin. North Am., 54:1455–1472, 1970.

73. Rogers, A. I.: Therapeutic considerations in selected forms of acute and chronic liver disease. Med. Clin. North Am., 55:373–390, 1971.

74. Morgan, M. Y.: Enteral nutrition in chronic liver disease. Acta Chir. Scand. [Suppl.], 507:81–90, 1981.

75. Fenton, J. C. B., Knight, E. J., and Humpherson, P. L.: Milk-and-cheese diet in portal-systemic encephalopathy. Lancet, 1:164–166, 1966.

76. Condon, R. E.: Effect of dietary protein on symptoms and survival in dogs with an Eck fistula. Am. J. Surg., 121:107–114, 1971.

77. Crews, R. H., and Faloon, W. W.: The fallacy of a low-fat diet in liver disease. J.A.M.A., 181:754–759, 1962.

78. Heymsfield, S. B., Smith, J., Redd, S., and Whitworth, H. B., Jr.: Nutritional support in cardiac failure. Surg. Clin. North Am., 61:635–652, 1981.

CHAPTER 23

Enteral Nutrition and Sepsis

VAL SELIVANOV
GEORGE F. SHELDON

The current clinical consensus that sick patients who are fed do better than those not fed has evolved in part by inference from the historical association of famine and pestilence, and by a formidable array of clinical observations linking malnutrition with altered response to infection.[1] A consistently beneficial role specific for enteral nutrition in sepsis has not been unequivocally substantiated with controlled data. Nevertheless, multiple relationships between nutrition and infection can be identified: (a) important infections in human populations are rendered more serious by presence of malnutrition;[1] (b) many infections precipitate nutritional disturbances;[1] and (c) some infections surprisingly appear less severe when associated with nutritional deficiency.[2]

The metabolic consequences of infection are well described, and this review will focus on the effects of infection. Also, we shall cite data in support of enteral alimentation as adjunctive supportive treatment of sepsis.

Historically, there have been divergent views for the role of alimentation in stressed, infected patients. "Starve a fever" is an old adage paraphrasing the underlying concept that anorexia of infection may have some protective role. Proponents of this concept are not limited to earlier centuries. Interesting but anecdotal observations are presented by Murray[2] on the apparent paradox of suppression of infections by famine (illustrating the relationship (c) listed above). Murray[3] also attempts to provide a controlled study documenting decreased survival in force-fed mice challenged with *Lysteria monocytogenes*.

Though such observations are of interest, they presumably reflect untreated infection, and serve to reinforce the principle that nutritional manipulation alone is not the primary treatment of sepsis. Primary therapy is still the treatment of the microorganisms whose foreign proteins and/or antigenic substances have initiated the septic insult. Usually, this entails surgical intervention as well as appropriate antimicrobial agents. The current role of enteral nutrition is supportive and is affected by modifying relationships (a) and (b) as noted above.

Concepts of the role of oral alimentation in hospitalized patients stem from the recognition that inanition compounds the effects of the primary disease. Graves is credited with suggesting relationships between sepsis and nutrition, and noted that "want of a sufficiency or food of an unwholesome or an improper character predisposes the human frame to disease by its debilitating effect on the system."[4] Graves advocated a diet of sugar water, meat broth, and toast and jelly for patients with sepsis and thyrotoxicosis.[5, 6]

Fever and infection themselves exert a nutritional toll, as demonstrated by the calorimetric studies of typhoid fever patients in 1915 by Coleman and Dubois, who summarized: "protein, fat, and carbohydrate are oxidized to the same or approximately same end products as in health and in their oxidation give off the standard amounts of heat . . . the basal heat production rises and falls in a curve roughly parallel with the temperature. At the height of the fever it averages about 40% above the normal, but in some cases rises to more than 50% above the normal."[7] These authors concluded: "There is a toxic destruction of protein in typhoid

Supported in part by National Institutes of Health Grants Nos. GMO 7032 and NIGMO 18470.

fever."[7] Thus, since 1915, there has been evidence for an increased metabolic rate and an increased protein requirement in infection.

DEFINITION OF SEPSIS

Although sepsis may be defined as an invasive infection documented by positive blood culture and evidence of an infective focus,[8] it is more useful to further characterize sepsis as a metabolic and physiologic response to foreign protein and other antigenic substances of invading microorganisms, possibly mediated by release of kinin and bradykinin which induces deranged intermediary metabolism and subsequent physiologic compensation.[9] Sepsis is an underlying metabolic process with specific physiologic manifestations.[9]

Clinical indices that summarize the physiologic manifestation of the underlying process of sepsis are: (1) increased cardiac index, possibly followed by decrease as state deteriorates; (2) decreased peripheral resistance; (3) decreased venous capacitance; (4) decreased blood volume; (5) increased core temperature until terminal decrease; (6) decreased oxygen extraction (narrow arteriovenous difference); (7) metabolic acidosis; and (8) increased capillary muscle blood flow (warm shock).[10]

The metabolic characterization of sepsis is quite distinct from that of simple starvation (Table 23–1). Whereas simple starvation shows adaptation within a few days and decrease in resting metabolic rate (RME), which reaches a plateau by 30 days, sepsis of peritonitis has a marked increase in RME[11] and remains elevated until resolution of sepsis. The consensus of most authorities is that sepsis unassociated with major burns is responsible for an increase in resting or basal metabolic rates of 30 to 60 per cent.[12, 13]

Besides increased metabolic rate, the altered intermediary metabolism consists of a peripheral energy deficit in skeletal muscle with obligate proteolysis and subsequent stimulation of hepatic (central) gluconeogenesis.[8, 14–16] These changes are mediated by an altered hormonal milieu as described below.[8, 15]

↑ *Catecholamines*
↑ ↓ *Insulin* (function of glucose) insulin resistance at muscle;
   insulin sensitive at adipocyte causing lipolysis.
↑ *Glucagon*-enhancing hepatic gluconeogenesis
↑ *Glucocorticoids*
↓ *Growth hormone*
   Insulin:glucagon ratio favors gluconeogenesis

GLUCONEOGENESIS AND METABOLISM IN SEPSIS

The hepatic glucose synthesis is in part a function of increased loads of alanine, pyruvate, and lactate, which are available from proteolysis and hydrolysis of leucine and other branched-chain amino acids (BCAA) in (periphery) skeletal muscle.[15] Glucagon has an effect on enhancing gluconeogenesis by increasing hepatocellular accumulation of cyclic adenosine monophosphate. Epinephrine also induces gluconeogenesis but is not as potent a stimulator as glucagon. A low ratio of insulin to glucagon is a predictor of active hepatic gluconeogenesis.

Ureagenesis from the increased utilization of alanine and other amino acids providing increased amino nitrogen is cycled through the liver.[15] The liver plays a key role in regulating ketone body production in sepsis.

Long[11] and Wannemacher[17] et al. suggest conversion of glucose carbon to fat was increased in septic patients. There is progressive increase in lipid content and rate of incorporation of labeled oleic acid in livers from fasted infected rats in the face of decreased plasma free fatty acids.[17] Increased synthesis of triglycerides in the liver is thought to be the explanation for both the fatty metamorphosis seen in hepatocytes during sepsis and for the lack of ketosis in sepsis.[16]

Events in the skeletal muscle are thought to reflect an energy deficit state induced intracellularly by the septic insult. This leads to irreversible combustion BCAA which skeletal muscle is able to oxidize for

---

Table 23–1 CHARACTERISTICS OF METABOLISM IN SEPSIS*

Increased release of alanine and other amino acids from muscle.
Increased gluconeogenesis (liver) (renal).
Increased ureagenesis and nitrogen excretion (negative nitrogen balance).
Decreased ketogenesis.

*These responses may be altered in the pre-moribund state or if sepsis develops in a severely malnourished host.

energy,[15, 18] and makes available other amino acids for release which cannot be formed into protein because of insufficient BCAA. Leucine is a BCAA which is linked in this manner to muscle protein synthesis.[15]

The septic metabolic response may be characterized as peripheral energy deficit associated with oxidation of BCAA and increased peripheral release of alanine[19] and other amino acids that are utilized in the liver for gluconeogenesis under the stimulation of glucagon, thus increasing ureagenesis. Simultaneously, the gluconeogenesis and proteolysis are accompanied by decreased plasma ketone bodies and decreased free fatty acids (FFA), which prevent the energy starved muscle from utilizing these for oxidation energy and further forces BCAA combustion. The liver may trap FFA and synthesize triglycerides during this process explaining the lack of ketosis.[15–19]

ENERGY AND PROTEIN NEEDS

From the known alterations of metabolism in sepsis, rational guidelines for nutritional support may be formulated. Septic metabolism is hypermetabolic, frequently 20 to 60 per cent above normal resting rates. This represents an increased caloric expense from about 34 kcal/kg/day to 43 kcal/kg/day in the adult.[11] Because sepsis is also proteolytic, an absolute requirement is for additional calories and protein or amino acids, as well as cofactors of protein synthesis—potassium, phosphorus, ascorbic acid, and vitamin A—if negative nitrogen balance is to be avoided.

The prime rationale for protein nutritional support rests upon the observed negative nitrogen balance and the following concept: "an inadequate supply of any one of the full complement of amino acids necessary for the synthesis of a protein molecule will result in the termination of the synthetic process and hydrolysis of the nascent peptide fragment."[15]

This is a plausible explanation for the generation of gluconeogenic precursors (such as alanine) from skeletal muscle that is undergoing proteolysis. BCAA, especially leucine, have a role in regulating muscle nitrogen balance in a dose dependent manner.[20] Irreversible combustion of leucine is accelerated with 72 hours in fasted septic rabbits[15] and in humans; BCAA tend to fall

with sepsis.[18] Loss of this amino acid places the remaining amino acids of the budding nascent peptide available for release from the muscle for hepatic gluconeogenesis and ureagenesis.

The above concepts have led to the postulation that increasing BCAA oxidation may be a specific septic process and that BCAA may serve as a specific protein-nitrogen source for skeletal muscle during sepsis. Therapeutic addition of BCAA may correct a theoretical intracellular BCAA deficit and thus allow protein synthesis to proceed. In vivo influence of BCAA on muscle catabolism in rats has shown improved nitrogen balance and body weight.[21] Patients surviving sepsis had higher levels of BCAA than non-survivors, and infusion of amino acid mixtures rich in BCAA have been advocated.[18, 21]

For sepsis without hepatic or renal failure, protein and energy requirements are met with essential amino acids and calories, supplied in 1 gm nitrogen to 150 non-nitrogen calories, so that total calories provided range anywhere from 20 to 60 per cent above an estimate resting caloric energy expenditure.

Measurements of human energy expenditure have been performed by direct calorimetry which requires methodology impractical for routine clinical use. Indirect calorimetry based on oxygen consumption and carbon dioxide expiration analysis correlate well with direct measurements at resting levels and less so if the subject is active.[22] All current methods of measuring human energy changes have assumptions or technical drawbacks that make them difficult to apply to acutely ill patients.

For practical purposes, we use an estimated "basal" normal energy expenditure (BEE) in kcal/day calculated by the Harris-Benedict equations:

Female
$$BEE = 655 + 9.6W + 1.8H - 4.7A$$

Male
$$BEE = 66 + 13.7W + 5H - 6.8A$$

Where W is weight in kg, H is height in cm, and A is age in years.

A starved, unstressed patient would be provided 0.8 to 1.0 BEE in non-nitrogen calories per day. We consider resting in the hospital to require 1.2 BEE for non-nitrogen calories, and we add to, or multiply 1.2 BEE by a subjective stress factor to estimate energy needs of various stressed patients, such that a patient with burns of greater than 50 per cent of total body area may require 2.0 BEE, whereas a septic or severely traumatized patient with multiple fractures and muscle injury may require 1.6 BEE non-nitrogen calories/day.

Protein needs are estimated as 1 gm/kg/day for unstressed patients, 1.5 to 2.5 gm/kg/day for moderately stressed patients, and 3 gm/kg/day for maximally catabolic patients. We do not include the caloric content of protein as part of the total energy needs, in part because of the theoretic concept that all protein provided is incorporated into functional body cell mass and none is oxidized for energy use.

The nitrogen:calorie ratio should remain in the 1:100 to 1:170 range for optimal utilization in sepsis.

Any number of nutrition supplements or chemically defined diets may be selected (Table 23–2). Though the non-protein calories may be carbohydrate or fat in variable mixture, the proportion of carbohydrate to fat has some significance in affecting lipogenesis and respiratory physiology of the patient. High carbohydrate loads and diets with high ratios of carbohydrate to fat increase production of carbon dioxide and therefore minute ventilation, placing a stress on patients with suspected pulmonary reserve.[12]

TRACE ELEMENTS, MINERALS, AND VITAMINS

Trace elements, minerals, and vitamins are needed as cofactors in enzyme reactions for protein synthesis. Zinc, copper, chromium, iron, and manganese have been identified as important in maintaining nutritional homeostasis. Cobalt, selenium, iodine, fluorine, and molybdenum are also known to have essential roles. Mechanisms of their action are poorly understood and may vary. Chromium is thought to combine with insulin to form a ternary complex which acts on cell membrane receptors and in this way may exert its effect in creating the abnormal glucose tolerance known to occur with chromium deficiency.[23] Chromium levels are depressed with infection,[24] but the glucose intolerance of sepsis is not considered to be due exclusively to a lack of chromium.

Infection also induces alterations in zinc, copper, and iron metabolism. Zinc and iron are sequestered in the reticuloendothelial system, and thus plasma levels are lowered. Copper and its ceruloplasmin levels are increased.[24] Zinc levels, normally 12 to 18 mm/L of plasma, fall with infection. Zinc is mainly albumin bound, though some is bound to alpha$_2$-macroglobulins and some to amino acids. These are fair suggestions that zinc is involved in the efficiency of protein synthesis.[25]

The need for mineral supplements in enteral feedings must not be overlooked. Mineral content of the various formulas is variable, though most meet recommended dietary allowances. An increased need for all minerals is not consistently demonstrated in sepsis, but Ca^{++}, Fe^{++}, PO_4^{--}, Mg^{++}, K^+ should all be monitored to determine need (Table 23–3).

The crucial role of vitamins has been understood for years. A 1939 study by Robertson and Tisdall[4] demonstrated clearly the roles of vitamin A and B deficiency, along with low mineral diet, in worsening survival in rats stressed with salmonella infection. Survival was 40 per cent for vitamin A deficient rats compared with 79 per cent for controls; survival was 20 per cent in vitamin B deficient rats compared with 72 per cent for

Table 23–2 COMPARISONS OF CONTENT OF COMMERCIALLY AVAILABLE NUTRITIONAL SUPPLEMENTS

	CAL/CC	PROTEIN (gm/250 cc)	N/CAL*	PER CENT FAT†	PER CENT CHO†
Compleat B	1.0	9.6	1:131	36	48
Compleat Mod.	1.0	10.7	1:131	31	53
Ensure	1.06	8.7	1:155	31.5	54.5
Isocal	1.05	8.1	1:169	38.5	49.6
Precision HN	1.0	10.4	1:125	.42	82.9
Travasorb Std.	1.0	7.5	1:202	12.0	76
Travasorb HN	1.0	11.3	1:126	12.0	70
Vivonex HN	1.0	10.8	1:127	.78	84.1

*Non-nitrogen calories.
†Per cent of calories.

Table 23–3   FORMULA COMPARISONS*

	CA (MG)	PO₄ (MG)	MG (MG)	FE (MG)	MN (MG)
Ensure (Ross) 2400 cc	1300	1300	500	22.5	5
Ensure Plus 2400 cc	1500	1500	750	33.8	5
Osmolite 2400 cc	1300	1300	500	22	5
Isocal (Mead Johnson) 2400 cc	1500	1250	500	22.5	6
Vivonex (Eaton Lab.) 300 cc	1333	1332.7	533.3	24	3.74
Vivonex HN 300 cc	800	800	319	14.4	2.25
Precision LR (Doyle) 300 cc	1360	1360	536	24	5.33
Precision HN 300 cc	800	800	320	14.4	3.19
Precision Isotonic 300 cc	1360	1360	536	24	5.36
Vital (Ross) 300 cc	1600	1600	640	28.8	3.2
Compleat-B (Doyle) 240 cc	1600	3200	640	30	6.7
Compleat-Modified 240 cc	1600	2240	640	30	6.39

*Courtesy, Department of Nutrition and Dietetics, San Francisco General Hospital.

controls; and survival was 54 per cent in mineral deficient rats compared with 00 per cent in controls. It is safe to conclude that the effects of vitamin and mineral deficiency are detrimental, but that the mechanisms of these effects are only understood in part.

The crucial roles of vitamins C and A are well appreciated in protein synthesis. Hydroxylation of proline and lysine, essential for collagen synthesis, requires alpha₂-ketoglutarate and ascorbic acid.[26] Vitamin A requirements may be increased by the corticosteroids of infection, since increased cortisol levels have been shown to deplete vitamin A from the liver and kidney of rats.[27] Local host resistance factors may depend upon tissue levels of vitamin A, since its deficiency causes epithelium lining the urinary tract, eyes, hair folicles, and respiratory tract to undergo changes, causing replacement of secretory cells by cells unable to produce mucus, IgA, or lysozymes. Also, infections that develop in vitamin A deficiency usually involve the epithelial surfaces.[28]

Overwhelming sepsis may increase all vitamin requirements because of hypermetabolism and because of competition for available vitamins between host and invading organisms.[29] Data quantitating the percentage of increase in specific vitamins from sepsis are not available, but recommended dietary allowances as summarized by Munro[30] should be adhered to, keeping in mind that fat soluble vitamins (A,D,E, and K) can be stored, whereas water-soluble vitamins (C, thiamine, riboflavin, niacin, and B₆) cannot be stored as readily by the body.

HOST DEFENSE

Sepsis is a function of host defense, which in turn is partially dependent upon nutrition. The mechanisms relating nutrition and defense remain incompletely understood. Studies showing a significant correlation between an immune parameter and a metabolic one are rare. There remains the issue of which causes which. Sepsis can induce malnutrition and accelerate deterioration of host defense; conversely, failing defenses accelerate establishment and severity of sepsis.

The immune system is comprised of local and systemic factors involving (1) thymic (T) derived or influenced lymphocytes; (2)

marrow or "bursa" (B) derived lymphocytes; (3) A cells, which are macrophages, monocytes, and neutrophils; (4) reticuloendothelial cells; (5) intestinal and pulmonary secretory epithelial cells; and (6) the various molecular products or stimulants of these cells, such as immunoglobulins, kinins, bradykinins, opsonic proteins, lymphokines, and complement.

The classic separation of cell-mediated and humoral-mediated phenomena of a few years ago, with its assignment of T cells as exclusive effectors for cell-mediated immunity and B cells as specific effectors for humoral-mediated immunity, is no longer considered valid. In vitro measurements of lymphocyte blastogenesis, mitogen response, antibody formation, and cell-mediated cytotoxicity are considered to require interaction of B, T, and A cells.[31, 32] The further identification of subpopulations of T lymphocytes in helper cells, suppressor cells, and effector cells has compounded the difficulty in assigning specific mechanisms for failing host defenses in sepsis and malnutrition.

A recent review by Kahan[33] discussing nutrition and host defense concludes that T lymphocytes are most frequently depressed in malnutrition and show impaired T helper cell function in antibody production. He also concludes that septic neutrophils show altered chemotaxis response and that altered bactericidal and fungicidal neutrophil function is the most consistently demonstrated defect in protein-calorie malnutrition in children. Impairment of neutrophil function correlates with, and has been shown to precede bacteremic episodes.[34]

The crucial role of neutrophils is reinforced by the study by Alexander et al.,[35] a rare study that correlates improved neutrophil bactericidal indices and opsonic indices with a metabolic intermediate, such as elevated serum asparagine. They also showed strong evidence that a high protein diet gave better survival (100 per cent) than a lower protein content diet (56 per cent) in severely burned children.

Another study correlating immune parameters with a metabolic intermediary by Jose and Good[36] showed the leucine deficiency depressed cytotoxicity of T cells in mice.

The role of serum immunoglobulins in sepsis relates to their function as opsonins. However, opsonin requirements vary considerably for various bacteria,[37] and most serum immunoglobulins do not fall in protein-calorie malnutrition. However, secretory antibodies IgA and IgE[28] are reduced in malnutrition, and this may predispose to decreased local resistance in gut mucosa and respiratory tract.

Finally, a hypothesis relating host defense to the altered metabolism of sepsis is that the peripheral proteolysis is a mechanism by which "non-crucial" proteins of muscle are diverted as amino acids to the liver, not only for gluconeogenesis but for visceral protein synthesis. The ability of the liver to maintain its protein content during the catabolism of sepsis supports such a view.[38]

The peripheral translocation of substrate to support visceral protein synthesis in sepsis is effected by altered intermediary metabolism, which may affect neutrophil functions and T helper cells, leading to decreased host defense, thus furthering a septic stimulus to altered metabolism and increasing the severity of sepsis.

EFFECT OF SEPSIS ON THE GASTROINTESTINAL TRACT

The effects of sepsis on the gastrointestinal tract are variable and reflect the underlying causes or sources of sepsis as well as how far the natural course has progressed. There is increased hepatic flow and hepatic oxygen consumption concomitant with a 7 per cent increase in splanchnic blood flow, which was one-half of the increase in cardiac output caused by fever from intraperitoneal infection.[39]

Anorexia of disease, including infection and sepsis, is poorly understood and remains unclear. Various theories implicate the ventromeidal nucleus and the lateral area of the hypothalamus as satiety and feeding centers that may be sensitive to peripheral arteriovenous glucose difference.[40] Other theories favor afferent nervous stimulation of some central nervous system locus as in the anorexia associated with acute appendicitis. Anorexia may be triggered by catecholamines[40] or by alteration in plasma owing to bacterial toxic peptides, amino acid imbalances, or virus-induced proteins.[41]

Antibiotics used in the treatment of sepsis may have a profound effect on gastrointestinal mucosa and on the hepatocytes. Almost 20 per cent of patients on ampicillin, and nearly 30 per cent on clindamycin, will experience diarrhea.[42] Similarly, pseudomembranous colitis associated with antibiotics and antibiotic-associated enterocolitis have severe effects on the mucosa and may themselves lead to septic shock.[43]

Although it is routine to advise enteral feeding for patients considered to require nutritional support, conditions of specific exclusion of this route are rarely clearly stated. An estimation of the degree of inflammation of either the serosa or mucosa of the small intestine becomes the deciding clinical factor. Peritonitis sufficient to cause ileus and regional enteritis are two examples for which enteral nutrition is not advised, whereas an enterocutaneous fistula represents a localized inflammatory process, and even though it may threaten sepsis, it is not a contraindication for elemental diets, if such substrate is delivered to an appropriate location vis à vis the fistula.

A major effect of sepsis on the gut is the result of lack of luminal substrate and nutrients. Their absence may result from anorexia or may be iatrogenic. In either case there is a loss of the normal interplay of neurohumoral reflexes stimulated by the physical and chemical properties of orally ingested food. Many studies compare enteral and intravenous nutrition on a large array of gut parameters.[44–47] Absence of intraluminal nutrients causes the following changes in morphology and function: (1) proximal gut mass decreases;[44, 45] (2) loss of DNA from the small bowel;[45] (3) mucosa undergoes loss of villus height;[44, 46] (4) intestinal disaccharidase activities decrease;[44] (5) serum glucagon immunoreactivity is higher in intravenously fed animals;[47] and (6) antral gastrin is decreased in the absence of enteral nutrients.[45] Collectively, these data suggest that absence of nutrients within the lumen of the small intestine induces hypoplasia of structure and atrophy of some functions. Moreover, enteral nutrients seem to be trophic to the gut.

The presence of luminal nutrients and their natural processing by portal and hepatic routes is extremely important for survival in experimental peritonitis. Kudsk et al. have demonstrated that refeeding of protein-calorie depleted rats by regular diet and by oral D_{25}-4.25 per cent amino acids restored survival in hemoglobin E. coli peritonitis, but intravenous repletion with the same solution gave the same poor survival as uncorrected protein-calorie malnourished controls.[48, 49]

Studies in humans comparing enteral to parenteral feeding have shown that parenteral administration of D_{25}-3.5 per cent amino acid solution revealed increased levels of insulin, cortisol, and glucose in the parenteral group, with concomitant decrease in serum free fatty acids in the intravenous group compared to the enteral group.[50] Nitrogen balance has been achieved with nasogastric tube and jejunal tube delivery in patients with life-threatening sepsis characterized by pyrexia, leukocytosis, tachycardia, and having intraperitoneal abscesses and fistulas;[51] such studies suggest that delivery of the necessary calories and nitrogen may be more readily achieved by enteral rather than parenteral routes.[50, 51]

In summary, the effects of sepsis on the gut are variable and are in part due to inflammation and absence of luminal nutrients. Absence of enteral nutrients induces a form of disuse atrophy of the small intestine and absence of enteral substrate, even in the presence of TPN sufficient to maintain positive nitrogen balance, and correlates with decreased survival to septic challenge in an experimental model.[49]

The effect of enteral nutrition on function of gut lymphocytic tissue (such as Peyer's patches) and on the reticuloendothelial system remains to be investigated, as do the possible antigenic and immunostimulatory differences the divergent routes of administration of nutrients cause.

SYNOPSIS

Uncorrected sepsis and malnutrition have become linked in current thinking as a final, common pathway leading to multiple organ failure and death in surgical patients. Sepsis may be viewed as a powerful stimulus to alteration of protein metabolism, and this change in intermediary metabolism may adversely affect host immune response and cause loss of structural and physiologic integrity of the organism.

The role of enteral nutrition in supporting the organism during sepsis is vital and encompasses not only provision of substrate to meet the needs of the altered metabolism, but also the maintenance of a positive, trophic influence on gastrointestinal mucosa and gut lymphocytic tissue. Nevertheless, it must be kept in mind that the primary cause of sepsis is exposure of the organism to foreign protein of microorganisms, and any therapy must be based on the elimination of this cause while providing adequate substrate for metabolism as well as appropriate hemodynamic support.

REFERENCES

1. Scrimshaw, N. S., Taylor, C. E., and Gordon, J. E.: Interactions of nutrition and infection. Am. J. Med. Sci., 237:367–404, 1959.
2. Murray, J., and Murray, A.: Suppression of infection by famine and its activation by refeeding—A paradox? Perspec. Biol. Med., 20:471–483, 1977.
3. Murray, M. J., and Murray, A. B.: Anorexia of infection as a mechanism of host defense. Am. J. Clin. Nutr., 32:593–596, 1979.
4. Robertson, E. C., and Tisdall, F. F.: Nutrition and resistance to disease. Can. Med. Assoc. J., 40:282–284, 1939.
5. Rombeau, J. L., and Barot, L. R.: Enteral nutritional therapy. Surg. Clin. North Am., 61:605–620, 1981.
6. Graves, R. J.: Lectures on the practice of medicine. New Syndenham Society. 1884.
7. Coleman, W., and Dubois, E. F.: Calorimetric observations on the metabolism of typhoid patients with and without food. Arch. Intern. Med., 15:887–938, 1915.
8. McLean, A. P. H., and Meakins, J. L.: Nutritional support in sepsis. Surg. Clin. North Am., 61:681–690, 1981.
9. Seigel, J. H., Cerra, F. B., Coleman, B. et al.: Physiological and metabolic correlations in human sepsis. Surgery, 86:163–193, 1979.
10. Sheldon, G. F.: Blood and fluid replacement in shock. In Walt, A. J. (ed.): American College of Surgeons' Early Care of the Injured Patient. Edition 2. Philadelphia, W.B. Saunders Co., 1981.
11. Long, C. L.: Energy balance and carbohydrate metabolism in infection and sepsis. Am. J. Clin. Nutr., 30:1301–1310, 1977.
12. Elwyn, D. H.: Nutritional requirements of adult surgical patients. Crit. Care Med., 8:9–20, 1980.
13. Blackburn, G. L., and Bistrian, B. R.: Nutritional care of the injured and/or septic patient. Surg. Clin. North Am., 56:1195–1224, 1976.
14. Clowes, G. H. A., Jr., O'Donnell, T. F., Blackburn, G. L., and Maki, T. N.: Energy metabolism and proteolysis in traumatized and septic man. Surg. Clin. North Am., 56:1169–1184, 1976.
15. Ryan, N. T.: Metabolic adaptations for energy production during trauma and sepsis. Surg. Clin. North Am., 56:1073–1090, 1976.
16. Beisel, W. R., and Wannemacher, R. W., Jr.: Gluconeogenesis , ureagenesis, and ketogenesis during sepsis. J.P.E.N., 4:277–285, 1979.
17. Wannemacher, R. W., Jr., Page, J. G., Beall, F. A., et al.: Role of the liver in regulation of ketone body production during sepsis. J. Clin. Invest., 64:1565–1572, 1979.
18. Freund, H. R., Ryan, J. A., Jr., and Fischer, J. E.: Amino acid derangements in patients with sepsis: Treatment with branched chain amino acid rich infusions. Ann. Surg., 188:423–429, 1978.
19. Clowes, G. H. A., Jr., Heideman, M., Lindberg, B., et al.: Effects of parenteral alimentation on amino acid metabolism in septic patients. Surgery, 88:531–540, 1980.
20. Buse, M. G., and Reid, S. S.: Leucine: A possible regulator of protein turnover in muscle. J. Clin. Invest., 56:1250–1261, 1975.
21. Freund, H. R., Yoshimura, N., Lunetta, L., and Fischer, J. E.: The role of the branched-chain amino acids in decreasing muscle catabolism in vivo. Surgery, 83:611–618, 1978.
22. Elwyn, D. H., and Kinney, J. M.: A unique approach to measuring total energy expenditure by indirect calorimetry. In Assessment of Energy Metabolism in Health and Disease. Report of the First Ross Conference on Med Res. Columbus, Ohio, Ross Laboratories, 1980.
23. Mertz, W.: Chromium and its relation to carbohydrate metabolism. Med. Clin. North Am., 60:739–744, 1976.
24. Mills, C. B., and Kaminski, M. V.: Trace element requirements. In Deitel, M. (ed.): Nutrition in Clinical Surgery. Baltimore, Williams and Wilkins, 1980, pp. 113–122.
25. Fell, G. S., and Burns, R. R.: The importance of zinc and other essential elements after injury. In Wilkinson, A. W., and Cuthbertson, D. (eds.): Metabolism and the Response to Injury. Chicago, Year Book Medical Publishers, 1976.
26. Levenson, S. M., et al.: Influence of injury on vitamin metabolism. In Wilkinson, A. W., and Cuthbertson, D. (eds.): Metabolism and the Response to Injury. Chicago, Year Book Medical Publishers, 1976.
27. Clark, I., and Coburn, R. W.: Relationship between vitamin A metabolism and cortisone. Endocrinology, 56:232–238, 1955.
28. Dreizen, S.: Nutrition and the immune response—a review. Int. J. Vitam. Nutr. Res., 49:220–228, 1979.
29. Gann, D. S., and Robinson, H. B., Jr.: Salt, water, and vitamins. In Ballinger, W. F., Collins, J. A., Drucker, W. R., et al. (eds.): American College of Surgeons' Manual of Surgical Nutrition. W.B. Saunders Co., 1975, pp. 73–90.
30. Munro, M. N.: Nutritional requirements in health. Crit. Care Med., 8:2–8, 1980.
31. Miller, C. L.: Immunological assays as measurements of nutritional status: A review. J.P.E.N., 2:554–566, 1978.
32. Golub, E. S.: The Cellular Basis of the Immune Response: An Approach to Immunobiology. Edition 2. Sunderland, Massachusetts, Sinauer Assoc., 1981, pp. 25–40.
33. Kahan, B. D.: Nutrition and host defense mechanisms. Surg. Clin. North Am., 61:557–570, 1981.
34. Alexander, J. W., Stinnett, J. D., Ogle, C. K., et al.: A comparison of immunologic profiles and their influence on bacteremia in surgical patients with a high risk of infection. Surgery, 86:94–104, 1979.
35. Alexander, J. W., MacMillan, B. G., Stinnett, J. D., et al.: Beneficial effects of aggressive protein feeding in severely burned children. Ann. Surg., 192:505–517, 1980.
36. Jose, D. G., and Good, R. A.: Quantitative effects of nutritional essential amino acid deficiency upon immune responses to tumors in mice. J. Exper. Med., 137:1–9, 1973.
37. Alexander, J. W.: Host defense mechanisms against

infection. Surg. Clin. North Am., *52*:1367–1378, 1972.

38. Reiss, E.: Protein metabolism in infection. I. Changes in certain visceral proteins studied with glycine-N[15]. Metabolism, *8*:151–159, 1959.
39. Gump, F. E., Price, J. B., Jr., and Kinney, J. M.: Whole body and splanchnic blood flow and oxygen consumption measurements in patients with intraperitoneal infection. Ann. Surg., *171*:321–328, 1970.
40. Weser, E., and Kim, Y.: Nutrition and the gastrointestinal tract. *In* Sleisenger, M. H., and Fordtran, J. S. (eds.): Gastrointestinal Disease: Pathophysiology, Diagnosis, Management. Philadelphia, W.B. Saunders Co., 1978, pp. 21–52.
41. Theologides, A.: Anorexia-producing intermediary metabolites. Am. J. Clin. Nutr., *29*:552–558, 1978.
42. Calderwood, S. B., and Moellering, R. C., Jr.: Common adverse effects of antibacterial agents on major organ systems. Surg. Clin. North Am., *60*:65–81, 1980.
43. Gorbach, S. L., and Bartlett, J. G.: The role of clindamycin in anaerobic bacterial infections. A symposium. J. Infect. Dis., *135*:51–133, 1977.
44. Levine, G. M., Deren, J. J., Steiger, E., and Zinno, R.: Role of oral intake in maintenance of gut mass and disaccharide activity. Gastroenterology, *67*:975–982, 1974.
45. Johnson, L. R., Copeland, E. M., Dudrick, S. J., et al.: Structural and hormonal alterations in the gastrointestinal tract of parenterally fed rats. Gastroenterology, *68*:1177–1183, 1975.
46. Feldman, E. J., Dowling, R. H., McNaughton, J., and Peters, T. J.: Effects of oral versus intravenous nutrition on intestinal adaptation after small bowel resection in the dog. Gastroenterology, *70*:712–719, 1976.
47. Lickley, H. L. A., Track, N. S., Vranic, M., and Bury, K. D.: Metabolic responses to enteral and parenteral nutrition. Am. J. Surg., *135*:172–176, 1978.
48. Kudsk, K. A., Carpenter, G., and Sheldon, G. F.: Effect of route of nutrient administration on survival with hemoglobin-*E. coli* adjuvant peritonitis in normal rats. Surg. Forum, *32*:102–104, 1981.
49. Petersen, S. R., Kudsk, K. A., Carpenter, G., and Sheldon, G. F.: Malnutrition and immunocompetence: Increased mortality following an infectious challenge during hyperalimentation. J. Trauma, *21*:528–533, 1981.
50. McArdle, A. H., Palmason, C., Morency, I., and Brown, R. A.: A rationale for enteral feeding as the preferable route for hyperalimentation. Surgery, *90*:616–623, 1981.
51. Allardyce, D. B., and Groves, A. C.: A comparison of nutritional gains resulting from intravenous and enteral feeding. Surg. Gynecol. Obstet., *139*:179–184, 1974.

CHAPTER 24

Enteral Nutrition in Patients with Burns or Trauma

JOSEPH A. MOLNAR
STACEY J. BELL
RICHARD D. GOODENOUGH
JOHN F. BURKE

In the last decade, much of the literature on the nutritional support of the surgical patient has emphasized the use of total parenteral nutrition. However, because of the variety of complications associated with this mode of therapy, it has become apparent that enteral nutrition is preferable when feasible. This is especially important in patients with burns or trauma since these individuals usually have normal gastrointestinal tracts at the time of injury such that enteral nutrition is frequently a viable alternative. Unfortunately, much of our knowledge of the nutrient requirements of the trauma patient is derived from studies of parenteral nutrition. Assuming that such information may be precisely applied to enteral nutrition is likely to be erroneous. However, such investigations must suffice until further knowledge is gained on enteral nutrition in burns and trauma.

The stress of thermal injury provides an excellent model for examining the metabolic response to trauma since a major burn induces a response that is typically of greater magnitude and duration while qualitatively similar to other forms of trauma. As a result, when determining the nutrient requirements of patients with non-burn trauma, one can usually assume that they are less than or equal to those of patients with burns.

Although meeting the nutritional requirements of the trauma patient is essential, avoiding nutrient excess may be just as important. Nutritional substrates, much like drugs, have a therapeutic range of administration. Even apparently innocuous nutrients may have adverse effects when supplied in overabundance to the critically ill. Providing adequate nutrients to the patient with burns or trauma with an enteral diet, while avoiding excess, is the topic of this chapter.

PHYSIOLOGIC RESPONSE TO INJURY

The metabolic response to injury, as described by Cuthbertson,[1] may be divided into two phases. The initial response is one of hypometabolism known as traumatic shock or the "ebb" phase. This period is relatively brief, lasting hours with minor trauma and a few days in the burn patient. While previously a period of extremely high mortality, the improved knowledge in fluid resuscitation and critical care medicine of this century has greatly increased survival so that most patients proceed to the "flow" phase of injury. The flow phase is a period of hypermetabolism that may last days to months depending upon the etiology of the traumatic insult. While the value of nutritional support during the ebb phase is uncertain, nutritional support during the flow phase is less controversial. It is the metabolic response and nutritional requirements during this hypermetabolic phase of injury that form the basis of this discussion.

Metabolic Rate and Caloric Requirement

One of the universal responses to injury is an increase in metabolic rate. However, the magnitude of the increase is highly dependent upon the type of traumatic insult. Burn patients manifest the greatest degree of hypermetabolism while lesser responses are found in patients with other major injuries such as multiple trauma.[2, 3] Increases in metabolic rate of 100 to 150 per cent above basal have been reported for burn patients,[2, 4–6] although in our experience elevations greater than 100 per cent above basal are rare (Fig. 24–1).[7] Uncomplicated elective surgical cases will demonstrate only mild and transient increases in basal energy expenditure, which may actually remain within normal limits.[2]

Numerous variables, including treatment and pre-injury physical state of the patient, may influence the degree of metabolic response. In general, young, healthy persons have a quantitatively greater response than elderly or debilitated patients. Psychic stress may have significant metabolic effects,[8] and Danielsson has demonstrated that excitement may increase metabolic rate transiently in burn patients.[9] Thus, providing a restful environment and adequate pain relief may be helpful to minimize energy consumption.

Activity is an important variable in determining metabolic rate. Even the increase in energy expenditure associated with burns is overshadowed by moderate physical exercise (Fig. 24–2). Moving a patient from a bed to a chair may increase metabolic expenditure 10 to 20 per cent and ambulation may produce two- to three-fold increases.[3] In the patient with severe burns or multiple trauma, bedrest is likely to be obligatory, making metabolic rate more constant throughout the day. However, in the patient with relatively minor injury or during convalescence for a severe injury, the level of activity must be considered in estimations of caloric expenditure. Frequently, the increase in energy expenditure with activity during convalescence will offset and surpass the decrease caused by recovery from the original injury. By the time the patient is fully ambulatory, caloric requirements are more likely to approximate pre-injury intakes.

The amount of nutritional intake will itself alter energy expenditure. It is well described that energy consumption decreases with starvation or malnutrition.[3, 10] Similarly, feeding has been demonstrated to increase metabolic rate in a manner that cannot simply be explained as the specific dynamic action of the food.[11–13] It is possible that this effect may account for some of the extremely high metabolic rates observed in patients receiving the excessive substrate intakes by "hyper" alimentation.[11, 14]

A significant factor in determination of metabolic rate is maintenance of thermoneutrality. Burn and trauma patients, much like normal individuals, are subject to heat loss from such mechanisms as radiation, conduction, convection, and evaporation. However, in the area of the burn wound, normal skin thermoregulatory mechanisms are impaired such that the loss of body surface heat may assume greater importance. A number of investigations have examined the

Figure 24–1. The average increase in metabolic rate in burn patients treated with early excision and grafting and occlusive dressings rarely exceeds 100 per cent. (*From* Royle, G. T., Wolfe, R. R., and Burke, J. F.: Metabolic expenditure in severely burned children and adults treated with early excision and closure of wounds. Submitted for publication.)

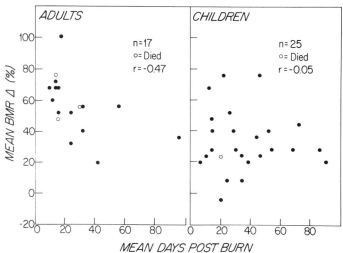

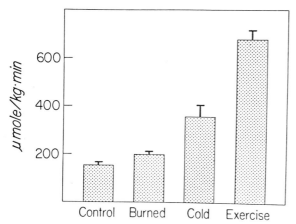

Figure 24–2. Oxygen consumption increases significantly with exercise and can overshadow the increase observed in burn patients. Patient activity must be considered in estimation of caloric requirements. (Courtesy of R. R. Wolfe, Ph.D.)

burn victim with occlusive dressings may offer a metabolic advantage over topical antibacterials with open dressings.[21]

Ambient temperature may also modify the metabolic response to injury by its effect on radiation and conductive heat loss. Oxygen consumption decreases in burn patients when the environmental temperature is raised from 21° C to 33° C (Fig. 24–3).[6] Similar reductions in the metabolic response to trauma of the lower extremity has been demonstrated in humans and animals treated at higher ambient temperatures.[22, 23] These observations suggest that maintenance of a warm environment will minimize the metabolic requirements of the trauma patient.

It has been suggested that burn size is a critical factor in determining the metabolic response of the burn patient.[6, 24] Surely, the burn must be a certain minimal size to evoke a significant metabolic response. However, in a review of patients with burns of 30 to 95 per cent of body surface area treated with early excision and grafting, metabolic rate, although related to area of the open wound at the time of measurement, increased minimally despite substantial increases in initial burn size.[7] Thus, it appears that it is the extent of open wound at the time of metabolic assessment, and not the initial burn size, that determines metabolic rate. It is evident that the method of management of the burn wound may explain some of this discrepancy. It is possible that wound closure with early excision and grafting results in a more rapid lessening of metabolic rate than other methods of management of burn wounds. In any case, it would appear that estimation of caloric requirements for the burn patient

role of evaporative water loss from the wound in determining the metabolic rate of the burn patient. Evaporation of 1 ml of water consumes 0.576 kcal of heat.[5] If the burn victim loses 2.5 to 4.0 L of water from the wound daily and all of the energy supplying the heat of evaporation came from the patient, then 1440 to 2300 kcal would need to be generated to maintain thermal equilibrium.[15] It appears, however, that a substantial portion of this energy comes from environmental heat, reducing the patient's energy contribution. While this topic remains controversial, several investigations suggest that evaporative wound losses are at least a contributor to the hypermetabolism of burns.[5, 16–20] As a result, treatment of the

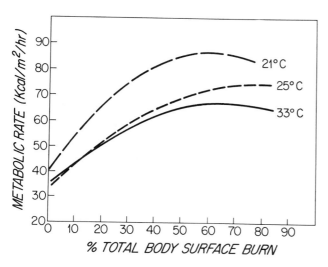

Figure 24–3. Metabolic rate in the burn patient may vary with ambient temperature. (*From* Wilmore, D. W., Long, J. M., Mason, A. D., Jr., Skreen, R. W., and Pruitt, B. A., Jr.: Catecholamines: Mediator of the hypermetabolic response to thermal injury. Ann. Surg., *180*:653–668, 1974; reproduced with permission.)

need not be adjusted for the size of the initial burn wound.

Since the trauma patient is hypermetabolic, the clinician's temptation is to provide a surfeit of calories to insure that caloric requirements are met. However, caloric excess must also be avoided, since it may increase metabolic rate and induce the problems of specific nutrient excess such as fatty liver and increased pulmonary demands. As a result, it is essential that some method be employed to more closely approximate caloric requirements. Ideally, one might measure the energy expenditure by indirect calorimetry. This method has proved effective in the nutritional management of postoperative, trauma, and burn patients.[4, 25] Unfortunately, the necessary equipment for these measurements is not universally available.

As a result, a variety of methods to mathematically estimate caloric requirements for the burn and trauma patient have been devised.[26-29] One approach is to provide the patient with calories based on some multiple of the basal metabolic rate based on the Harris-Benedict equation (Fig. 24–4, Table 24–1). In this manner, one automatically accounts for the variables of age, sex, height, and weight. Certain advantages are gained by substituting ideal body weight for actual body weight in this formula. Accurate weight measurements are difficult to obtain in patients with burns or severe trauma because of fluid shifts, bulky dressings, cases, and other attached supportive paraphernalia. In addition, using the ideal body weight tends to minimize caloric intake for the obese individual while maximizing intake for underweight patients. Nonetheless, this must be tempered with clinical judgment. For example, the caloric requirement of the mesomorph is more likely to be approximated by using actual weight in the formula. Based on this method, the caloric requirements of the burn patient may be met by providing calories at twice the predicted basal metabolic rate. Severely traumatized patients who are

nonambulatory may be given calories at 50 to 75 per cent above the basal metabolic rate (see Table 24–1). However, once the patient becomes ambulatory, consumed calories should more closely approximate pre-injury intake.

Carbohydrate Metabolism

The fundamental change in carbohydrate metabolism found in patients with burns, trauma, and sepsis is increased gluconeogenesis.[30-36] While blood glucose concentrations may be elevated in these conditions, frequently a concomitant rise in glucose clearance may result in euglycemia. Isotopic studies examining the fate of this glucose demonstrate that, although thermal injury is associated with increased cellular glucose uptake, there is no corresponding increase in oxidation of this substrate to carbon dioxide.[33-35] While some of this glucose carbon skeleton may be used for glycogen, triglyceride, or amino acid synthesis, much of the increased glucose turnover is due to recycling through lactate and alanine (Fig. 24–5).[33-35, 37]

Given this basic pattern of response of carbohydrate metabolism in trauma, one must determine how this may be modified by nutritional support to the advantage of the patient. From Figure 24–5, it may be inferred that the beneficial effects of carbohydrate on protein metabolism may be either from direct utilization as an energy source or from suppression of gluconeogenesis. Thus, carbohydrate minimizes the degradation of amino acids that would be oxidized for energy or to provide gluconeogenic precursors. Although it may be tempting to provide large quantities of carbohydrate to ensure adequate intake, it must be recognized that excess carbohydrate may have adverse side effects. Carbohydrate excess has been implicated as a cause of impaired liver function,[38-40] and fatty metamorphosis of the liver has been described in postmortem examination of burn patients receiving high rates of parenterally administered carbohydrate (Table 24–2).[40] The mechanism proposed to account for these hepatic abnormalities is that the chronic hyperinsulinemia of continuously infused glucose interferes with lipid mobilization in adipose tissue and the liver. It is possible that this is a less important problem with enteral feeding since

$$\text{Male}$$
$$\text{BMR (kcal)} = 66 + (13.7 \times W) + (5 \times H) - (6.8 \times A)$$
$$\text{Female}$$
$$\text{BMR (kcal)} = 665 + (9.6 \times W) + (1.7 \times H) - (4.7 \times A)$$

Figure 24–4. Harris-Benedict equation for estimation of basal metabolic rate (BMR). W, weight in kg; H, height in cm; and A, age in years. (*From* Harris, J. A., and Benedict, F. G.: Biometric Study of Basal Metabolism in Man. Carnegie Institute, 1919.)

Table 24–1   SUGGESTED MACRONUTRIENTS FOR PATIENTS WITH BURNS OR TRAUMA*

	TOTAL CALORIES (MULTIPLE OF BMR)	CARBOHYDRATE (MG/KG/MIN)	PROTEIN (GM/KG/DAY)	FAT
BURNS	2	5	2.5	Fat Calories = Total kcal
TRAUMA	1.5–2	5	1.5	(carbohydrate kcal + protein kcal)

*To be delivered at an average rate over 24 hours. See text.

the insulin response may be less to carbohydrate provided in this manner.[41] Nonetheless, biochemical essential fatty acid deficiency, which is also postulated to result from chronic hyperinsulinemia, has been induced by continuous enteral feedings of carbohydrate and amino acids.[42] This would suggest that some of the toxic effects of carbohydrate excess may be independent of route of administration.

Excess carbohydrate may also have adverse effects on pulmonary function. First, the physical effect of an enlarged, fatty liver may interfere with diaphragmatic excursion. Second, excess carbohydrate may increase demands upon the respiratory system. Provision of glucose at a rate equivalent to the oxidation rate would maximize use of carbohydrate as an energy source and result in production of carbon dioxide equal to oxygen consumed (Fig. 24–6A). However, at higher rates of glucose intake, triglyceride will be synthesized resulting in an increased production of carbon dioxide, and energy will be consumed in the synthetic process (Fig. 24–6B). The carbon dioxide thus produced must be removed by increased minute ventilation. This in turn will also increase energy expenditure and may require ventilatory assistance or may result in respiratory failure in patients with ongoing pulmonary compromise.[43–45] Finally, excess carbohydrate may hinder pulmonary surfactant synthesis by inhibition of lipolysis and, thus, interfere with the availability of palmitic acid.[46]

Several studies give some indication of the ideal carbohydrate intake by which one may maximize the beneficial effects brought about by carbohydrate oxidation and suppression of gluconeogenesis, while avoiding excess production of fat and carbon dioxide. Maximal glucose oxidation rates in burn patients were found with infusion rates of approximately 5 mg/kg/min (Fig. 24–7).[40] Investigations in normal and postoperative patients demonstrate maximal suppression of gluconeogenesis with intravenous glucose infusion rates of 4 mg/kg/min.[47, 48] Maximal glucose oxidation in postoperative patients occurred at 7 mg/kg/min. With higher infusion rates, there was elevated glucose clear-

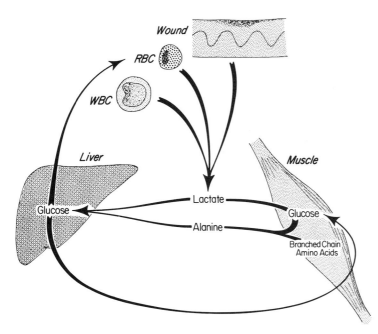

Figure 24–5. The glucose-alanine cycle. (*From* Molnar, J. A., Wolfe, R. R., and Burke, J. F.: Metabolism and nutritional therapy in thermal injury. *In* Schneider, H. A., Anderson, C. E., and Coursin, D. B. (eds.): Nutritional Support of Medical Practice. Edition 2. New York, Harper & Row, in press; reproduced with permission.)

Table 24–2 AUTOPSY FINDINGS IN PATIENTS TREATED WITH VERY HIGH GLUCOSE INFUSIONS

PATIENT	SEX	AGE	PER CENT BSA BURNED*	MUSCLE ATROPHY	HYPERCAL FOR 3 WEEKS BEFORE DEATH	RATE OF IV GLUCOSE (MG/KG/MIN)	LIVER WEIGHT AT AUTOPSY (PER CENT ABOVE NORMAL)
1	M	11	80	0	yes	13.5	254
2	F	14	66	0	yes	14.8	246
3	F	10	86	0	yes	9.3	164
4	M	13	54	0	yes	10.8	309
5	F	16 mo.	47	0	yes	17	291
6	M	10 mo.	39	0	yes	17	324
7	M	3	85	0	yes	13.1	440
8	F	4	70	0	yes	14.3	331

*BSA = body surface area.

ance but a plateau in glucose oxidation rates (Fig. 24–8). Since the respiratory quotient at these higher infusion rates was greater than one, it may be inferred that the increased cellular glucose uptake was used for fatty acid synthesis. In burn patients, infusion rates of 4.7 to 6.8 mg/kg/min also allowed maximal whole body protein synthetic rates (Table 24–3), but with higher infusion rates production of carbon dioxide increased rapidly, suggesting increased fatty acid synthesis (Fig. 24–9).

From these studies, it would appear that in postoperative and burn patients there is an optimal rate of glucose infusion (approximately 5 mg/kg/min) to maximize protein sparing while minimizing adverse side effects. At present, no controlled studies have investigated whether these parameters are identical in the enterally nourished patient. However, in view of the potential "toxicity" of carbohydrate excess, it would be prudent to use restraint in administration of carbohydrate regardless of the route.

There is considerable controversy regarding the role of exogenous insulin in the provision of carbohydrate and its effect upon protein metabolism. It has been suggested from in vitro muscle studies,[2, 49] and from investigations in burns and other trauma[50] that administration of insulin has beneficial effects on protein metabolism independent of its effect on carbohydrate metabolism. However, when this was investigated in burn patients receiving glucose at approximately 6 mg/kg/min, administration of insulin resulted in a slight but not significant increase in protein synthesis and increased glucose clearance without a concomitant increase in glucose oxidation.[40] From this, one may conclude that while the direct anabolic effects of exogenous insulin may exert positive effects on protein metabolism, provision of insulin to "cover" administration of carbohydrate in excess of needs is likely to result only in increased production of fat. As a result, the preferred treatment of hyperglycemia with nutritional support is decreasing carbohydrate intake rather than providing more insulin.

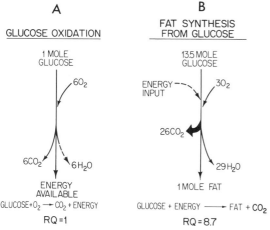

Figure 24–6. *A*, The oxidation of glucose makes energy available, and CO_2 produced is equivalent to oxygen consumed, resulting in an RQ of 1. *B*, However, synthesis of fat from glucose requires energy and releases much more CO_2 than O_2 consumed, resulting in an elevated RQ. (*From* Wolfe, R. R., O'Donnell, T. F., Jr., Stone, M. D., Richmond, D. A., and Burke, J. F.: Investigation of factors determining the optimal glucose infusion rate in total parenteral nutrition. Metabolism, 29:892–900, 1980; reproduced with permission.)

Protein Metabolism

The early investigations of Cuthbertson demonstrated that trauma was associated with a tendency toward negative nitrogen

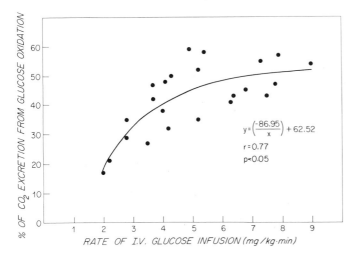

Figure 24–7. As glucose infusion rates in burn patients receiving total parenteral nutrition increased above 5 to 6 mg/kg/min, the per cent of CO_2 from glucose oxidation reached a plateau. (*From* Burke, J. F., Wolfe, R. R., Mullany, C. J., Mathews, D. E., and Bier, D. M.: Glucose requirements following burn injury: Parameters of optimal glucose infusion and possible hepatic and respiratory abnormalities following excessive glucose intake. Ann. Surg., *190:* 274–283, 1979; reproduced with permission.)

balance disproportionate to local tissue damage.[1, 51] The major loss of this nitrogen is by increased urinary urea excretion reflecting increased degradation of amino acid.[29, 52] Whole body protein turnover studies have demonstrated net catabolism of protein with trauma, although net catabolism may be accomplished by different mechanisms under different stress conditions. For example, after elective surgery whole body synthetic rates decrease while catabolic rates remain constant.[53–55] However, similar kinetic studies performed in sepsis,[56,] burns,[57] and skeletal trauma[58] suggest that both synthetic and catabolic rates are increased but that a larger absolute increase in the latter results in net catabolism.

Cuthbertson noted that the increased urinary urea nitrogen was associated with increased losses of sulfur, potassium, phosphorus, and creatinine and postulated that the increased urinary nitrogen loss was primarily the result of increased muscle catabolism,[51, 59, 60] "to meet both the exigencies of repair and maintenance."[51] Recent studies examining urinary N$^\tau$-methylhistidine excretion confirm that muscle catabolism is increased in burns, trauma, and sepsis.[61–63] From such investigations has derived the concept of a peripheral to visceral redistribution of protein and other nutrients during periods of metabolic stress.[64–66] Under this paradigm, the carcass undergoes net catabolism to support activities of more essential tissues such as visceral organs and reparative tissue.

From investigations of the metabolism of starvation, one may infer that the transfer of nitrogen from carcass to viscera is primarily by alanine and glutamine.[67–69] Alanine ap-

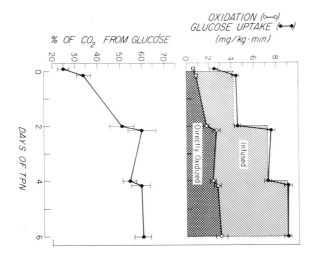

Figure 24–8. Increasing glucose infusion rate from 4 mg/kg/min to 7 mg/kg/min resulted in increased glucose uptake and oxidation in patients receiving total parenteral nutrition. However, while infusion rates above 7 mg/kg/min resulted in even greater uptake, oxidation was not significantly changed, suggesting use in other pathways such as fat synthesis and glycogen production. (*From* Wolfe, R. R., O'Donnell, T. F., Jr., Stone, M. D., Richmond, D. A., and Burke, J. F.: Investigation of factors determining the optimal glucose infusion rate in total parenteral nutrition. Metabolism, *29:*892–900, 1980; reproduced with permission.)

Table 24–3 WHOLE BODY PROTEIN SYNTHETIC RATES IN BURN PATIENTS AS A FUNCTION OF INTRAVENOUS GLUCOSE INFUSION RATE

RATE OF GLUCOSE INFUSION (MG/KG/MIN)	WHOLE BODY PROTEIN SYNTHESIS (GM/KG/DAY)
1.4–4.5	4.3 ± 0.54
4.7–6.8	5.2 ± 0.28
7.03–9.31	5.05 ± 0.183

pears to be synthesized in the muscle with branched chain amino acids as the major nitrogen donor.[67, 68, 70] Upon transfer to the liver, alanine and glutamine may be transaminated to synthesize non-essential amino acids, and the carbon skeletons thus produced may be used as gluconeogenic precursors (see Fig. 24–5). This glucose may then be consumed by leukocytes, erythrocytes, and reparative tissue, which solely utilize carbohydrate as an energy source. The resultant glycolysis may provide more three-carbon moieties for gluconeogenesis or amino acid synthesis.

While the general mechanisms of the alterations in protein metabolism in response to trauma have been delineated, translation of this information to determination of the protein requirements of patients with burns or trauma is difficult. This is not surprising in light of problems in determining protein requirements for normal health.[71–74] However, it is apparent that the question of adequate protein intake cannot be entirely dissociated from other nutrient intake. If adequate non-nitrogenous calories are supplied, protein may be catabolized as an energy source (see Fig. 24–5). Furthermore, other nutrients such as potassium, phosphorus, and sodium must be available for optimal utilization of exogenously administered amino acids.[26, 75]

Given that other nutrient intake is sufficient, one still has the difficulty of arriving at appropriate criteria for measuring the adequacy of protein intake in the trauma patient. Sutherland has reported positive nitrogen balance in burned children with intakes of protein similar to those of healthy individuals.[76] Yet, nitrogen balance studies are fraught with pitfalls and one is never certain whether a greater positive balance would be beneficial.[74] Markley et al.[77] examined the effect of protein intake on mortality in burned mice and demonstrated no advantage to protein intakes at twice normal. However, in humans one would also wish to consider the effects of dietary intake on morbidity. Alexander et al.[78] attempted to examine the effects of protein intakes of 105 and 134 gm/m²/day on support of immune function in burn patients. While they concluded that the higher protein intake was advantageous, their groups were not strictly comparable. Shizgal and Forse investigated the effect of 1.3 and 2.4 gm/kg/day protein intake on body composition in a variety of surgical patients including those with trauma.[79] They concluded that there was no advantage to the higher protein intake. Wolfe et al.[80] examined the effect of diets of 1.5 and 2.5 gm/kg/day protein intakes on whole body protein kinetics in burn patients. While the higher protein intake resulted in increased

Figure 24–9. As glucose infusion rates in burn patients receiving total parenteral nutrition increased above 5 to 6 mg/kg/min, the respiratory quotient increased rapidly, suggesting increased fat production. (*From* Burke, J. F., Wolfe, R. R., Mullany, C. J., Mathews, D. E., and Bier, D. M.: Glucose requirements following burn injury: Parameters of optimal glucose infusion and possible hepatic and respiratory abnormalities following excessive glucose intake. Ann. Surg., *190*:274–283, 1979; reproduced with permission.)

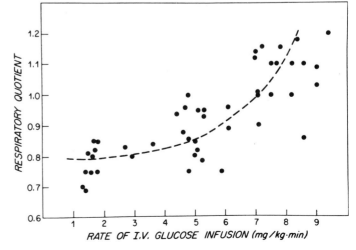

rates of protein synthesis, catabolic rates also increased such that net synthesis was similar in the two groups. Unfortunately, such studies of whole body turnover of protein provide no information on the distribution of protein synthesis. Hence, one cannot be certain that the higher protein intake may not aid synthesis of certain essential proteins.

While the results are somewhat conflicting, these investigations would suggest that protein intakes as low as 1.5 gm/kg/day may be adequate for patients with burns or trauma. Nonetheless, we presently recommend provision of protein at 2.5 gm/kg/day to the critically ill burn patient as added insurance of meeting metabolic requirements (see Table 24–1). While it may be tempting to provide even greater quantities of protein, it would be at the price of increased metabolic rate and hypoxic ventilatory response[11] and increased urinary calcium excretion.[81, 82]

Fat Metabolism

Fats are the body's major energy source in fasting and exercise,[83] and the evidence suggests this also to be true in burns, trauma, and sepsis.[14, 40, 84, 85] Even with high carbohydrate infusions, nearly one-fourth of the CO_2 production results from fat oxidation.[47] In general, serum free-fatty acid concentrations are elevated with trauma and burns,[18, 86–88] suggesting increased lipolysis which is supported by the observed increased glycerol turnover in injury.[89] While serum triglyceride levels tend to remain normal with uncomplicated trauma,[90] they may be elevated in burns[86, 87] and infection.[90] Nonetheless, it would appear that trauma is associated with an enhanced capacity to clear circulating triglyceride,[91, 92] although conflicting results have been found in sepsis.[90, 91] While changes in lipoprotein lipase activity may account for some of the observed differences in triglyceride clearance, alterations in tissue perfusion may also play a role.[90]

Relevant to the issue of fat metabolism in trauma is the importance of ketone bodies. The observed elevation of serum ketone bodies with uncomplicated trauma appears to be of adaptive value by a peripheral protein sparing effect.[85, 93–95] However, ketone bodies are not always elevated in burns,[96] and infection inhibits ketogenesis.[97]

There are two main reasons to include fat in the diet of the trauma or burn patient. The first is to provide calories and thus minimize catabolism of endogenous proteins by meeting energy requirements. Despite the fact that fats may be a preferential fuel source in the trauma patient, isocaloric substitution of fat for carbohydrate may not result in equivalent protein sparing. It would appear that carbohydrate has unique effects on protein metabolism not shared by fat such that a minimal amount of carbohydrate should be included in all diets.[39, 98–100] Above this minimal level, isocaloric substitution of fat for carbohydrate is likely to be effective.[101, 102]

The second major reason to include fat in the diet is to avoid essential fatty acid deficiency. In adults undergoing starvation, essential fatty acid deficiency is unlikely to occur because of the mobilization of essential fatty acids from significant endogenous fat stores. This is also likely to be true in patients with burns or trauma who are not receiving any source of caloric intake. However, when carbohydrate or amino acids are continuously provided, the secondary insulin response inhibits lipolysis, and mobilization of endogenous stores of essential fatty acids is curtailed. As a result, under such circumstances, essential fatty acids must be provided exogenously. Biochemical evidence of this deficiency has been described in patients with burns or trauma.[103–105] While primarily a complication of parenteral nutrition that lacks lipids,[106] it has also been observed in individuals receiving continuously infused enteral diets of only carbohydrate and amino acid.[42]

At present, it is not clear precisely how much essential fatty acid needs to be supplied to the burn and trauma patients to avoid deficiency. However, because of the importance of this nutrient to cellular integrity, hepatic lipid metabolism, and wound repair, it should be included in the diet of every patient. It has been suggested that 1 to 2 per cent of the total caloric intake be provided as essential fatty acid to patients receiving TPN. However, with enteral nutrition this is less of a problem since most enteral formulas contain fat. Presently, we simply administer fat to meet total caloric requirements after providing protein and carbohydrate, regardless of the route of alimentation (see Table 24–1).

Micronutrients

Although precise macronutrient requirements are poorly defined for burn or trauma patients, even less is known about micronutrient requirements. This is partially because the physiologic significance of biochemical assays for many of these nutrients is unknown. Even if one can make recommendations for an intake that will assure a "normal value" for a biochemical parameter, one is frequently uncertain of the clinical relevance of this normal value. In the case of the trace elements, multiple indices must be measured to have confidence in the overall status of the element.

Despite these frustrations, micronutrients cannot be overlooked, for deficiencies have far-reaching effects on cellular activities and macronutrient utilization. Vitamin B[12], folate, and zinc, for example, are essential for normal nucleic acid metabolism. Deficiencies of chromium and manganese alter carbohydrate utilization, while carbohydrate intake helps to determine thiamine requirements. Pyridoxine is essential for normal protein metabolism, and vitamin C, iron, and copper are all necessary for collagen synthesis.

Vitamins. Ascorbic acid has received the attention of surgeons because of its role in collagen synthesis and thus an obvious relationship to wound repair. Lund[108] noted decreased plasma levels and urinary excretion of vitamin C in burn patients that paralleled the severity of the burn, and described alterations of nitrogen metabolism. Crandon[109] observed increased wound dehiscence in postoperative patients with low blood levels of ascorbate. Subsequent investigators have also found decreased leukocyte or urinary ascorbate in surgical patients, the clinical significance of which is unknown.[110, 111] Nonetheless, it is reasonable to administer supplements of 250 to 1000 mg of vitamin C daily to burn or trauma patients. However, extremely large doses should be avoided since even ascorbate may have adverse side effects.[112]

A variety of studies have suggested increased requirements for nicotinic acid, biotin, pyridoxine, thiamine, and folate in the burned patient.[108, 113–117] While this may in part be due to losses from the burn wound itself, it is likely that the metabolic response to trauma is the major reason for increased requirements of the nutrients.

Some vitamins are less likely to be deficient in the patient with trauma. B[12], for example is extensively stored in the liver as is vitamin A. Similarly, fat-soluble vitamins will be stored in adipose tissue. In addition, vitamin K will continue to be produced by colonic bacteria unless oral antibiotics suppress normal gastrointestinal flora. Whether utilization of these stores of micronutrients is impaired in the patient with trauma is unknown.

Trace Elements. Among the trace elements, zinc has received the most attention by surgeons owing to its proposed importance in wound repair and protein metabolism.[23, 118–120] Approximately 20 per cent of the body store of zinc is in the skin so that cutaneous thermal injury would of necessity decrease total body zinc.[121] Urinary losses of zinc increase and blood and hair levels decrease with burn injury.[23, 121–123] In addition, animal studies have suggested increased requirements for zinc to minimize nitrogen loss after fracture of the femur.[124] Some investigators have recommended administration of large amounts of zinc to improve wound repair,[118, 120] but this remains controversial.[121, 125] Also, oral zinc has been implicated in producing gastritis and will interfere with absorption of other trace elements such that excessive use is not without complications. At present, we recommend administration of zinc to patients with burns or major trauma at two to three times the Recommended Dietary Allowance for normal individuals.

Requirements of other trace elements in the patients with burns or trauma are largely unknown. Magnesium deficiency attributable to wound and urinary losses has been reported in burns,[126, 127] and copper and manganese intake to maintain nitrogen equilibrium is increased in animals with fracture of the femur.[124] While deficiencies of zinc, magnesium, copper, chromium, and selenium have been reported with TPN,[128–130] the enteral utilization of these nutrients in trauma remains unknown.

It is likely that requirements for all micronutrients are increased with burns or trauma, but there is no solid evidence for megadose therapy with any of these nutrients. In addition, each has its potential toxicity such that their administration should be optimized. Clinical deficiencies are probably uncommon in the patient receiving standard enteral formulas owing to the ubiquity of many of these nutrients in normal foodstuffs. However, greater care in supplementation is necessary in patients receiving TPN, defined formula, or elemental diets.

Gastrointestinal Changes with Trauma

One of the most frustrating problems in attempting to employ enteral nutrition in the patient with burns or trauma is paralytic ileus. While perhaps most severe after direct injury to the peritoneal cavity by the initial trauma or surgical intervention, it also accompanies injury distant to the abdomen, including burns.[131–133] The etiology is likely multifactorial, but alpha-adrenergic hyperactivity associated with stress has been implicated as an important mediator.[134–138]

The various segments of the gastrointestinal tract are not equally susceptible to paralytic ileus. Studies observing the passage of radiologic contrast material[131, 139, 140] and more direct measures of motility[141–143] suggest that the small bowel is relatively resistant to the development of postoperative or traumatic ileus, and activity usually returns within the first few hours following the insult. However, colonic motility may not return for 24 hours after extra-abdominal procedures,[132] and may require 72 hours or more after intra-abdominal manipulations.[131, 132, 139, 140, 142] Similarly, return of gastric motility may be delayed 24 to 96 hours,[131, 139, 140] although this has been questioned.[142]

The therapeutic implication of this differential gastrointestinal activity is that even if the stomach and colon may not readily tolerate enteral feeding in the first few days after traumatic stress, the small bowel may. Since the major gastrointestinal absorption and digestion occur in the small bowel, if special measures were taken to bypass the stomach, earlier enteral nutrition might be possible. Indeed, Glucksman et al. have demonstrated normal glucose and sodium absorption in the early postoperative period.[144] This has prompted therapeutic trials of early postoperative feeding via the small bowel.[145–147]

While the evidence suggests that such measures are beneficial in postoperative patients,[145, 146] recent studies by Carter et al.[147] would suggest that such may not be true for patients with burns. When rats were subjected to a 40 per cent burn, transport of calcium, 3-0 methylglucose, and cycloleucine in gut sacs were significantly decreased compared to controls at 18 hours post-burn. In addition, in vivo fat absorption was dramatically decreased. From this, one may conclude that even if motility returns to normal in this early post-burn period, absorption may be decreased such that enterally supplied nutrients may be poorly utilized.

One of the most common gastrointestinal complications of trauma and burns is stress ulceration.[133] Frequently, such lesions are associated with ongoing sepsis. While the etiology is uncertain, alterations in gastric acid secretion,[148, 149] mucosal blood flow,[150–153] and gastric mucosal barrier and mucosubstances have been implicated.[152, 154–157] However, nutritional status may also be a factor. The hypoproteinemia of malnutrition has been suggested to predispose to gastric mucosal injury in burns,[150] and energy and nitrogen balance may also play a role.[158] In addition, vitamin A alone may be important since it is known to be deficient in stressed patients[159, 160] and to be involved in maintaining the integrity of the mucus-secreting cells of the gastrointestinal tract.[161, 162] It has been suggested that the observed decrease in stress ulceration with nutritional supplementation may be secondary to direct enteral effects such as buffering of gastric pH or direct utilization of nutrients.[163, 164] However, the observed minimization of stress ulceration with parenteral alimentation implies that the support of systemic nutritional balance may be the dominant factor.[158, 165–167]

Unfortunately, relatively little is known about the effects of traumatic stress on the rest of the gastrointestinal tract. Hepatic oxygen consumption is increased,[168] and histologic changes in the liver[169] and potential circulating hepatotoxins[170] have been described in burns. The effect of such alterations in hepatic function upon the utilization of splanchnic nutrients from enteral nutrition is uncertain. Similarly, acalculous cholecystitis,[171–174] pancreatitis,[133] and superior mesenteric artery syndrome[175] are entities associated with burns and trauma lacking precise etiologies and therapeutic implications. Carter et al[176] have demonstrated decreased mucosal weight and DNA synthesis in the small bowel of rats within the first 24 hours after burn injury. Whether this may be ameliorated with early nutritional support remains to be seen.

Summary and Nutritional Recommendations

The metabolic response to injury may be conveniently divided into a hypometabolic "ebb" phase followed by a hypermetabolic "flow" phase. It is in the flow phase that nutritional demands are greatest and that nutritional support is of greatest value. The increase in metabolic rate of a given patient depends upon numerous variables including general physical status, activity, pain, psychic stress, nutritional intake, environmental temperature, evaporative water loss, and, in some cases, method of treatment. While it is essential to provide adequate calories to the burn or trauma patient, caloric excess should be avoided. At present we recommend that burn patients receive approximately twice the basal metabolic rate and that patients with major trauma receive 1.5 to 1.75 times the basal metabolic rate as calculated by the Harris-Benedict equation.

Not only must adequate calories be supplied to the burn or trauma patient, but those calories must have the proper nutrient composition. Carbohydrate must be supplied so that the body's nitrogen may be spared by direct utilization of carbohydrate as an energy source and by suppression of gluconeogenesis. However, carbohydrate excess must be avoided because of the potential problems of fatty liver and pulmonary compromise secondary to increased production of carbon dioxide. It would appear that the optimal rate of administration of carbohydrate is approximately 5 mg/kg/min. While it would appear that protein requirements are elevated in the burn or trauma patient, with presently available methodology it is difficult to accurately estimate ideal protein intake. Presently, we provide burn patients with 2.5 gm/kg day of protein and trauma patients with a 1.5 gm/kg/day. After providing a minimal carbohydrate intake, fat may be substituted for carbohydrate as a caloric source. In addition, provision of fat in the diet may be helpful to avoid essential fatty acid deficiency in the face of continuously administered carbohydrate.

Even less is known regarding the micronutrients. However, it would appear that injury increases the requirements of nearly all micronutrients. Nonetheless, one must avoid excessive administration since some micronutrients have significant toxicity.

MODULAR FORMULA

Rationale

Given the above nutritional guidelines for the patients with burns or trauma (see Table 24–1), one must determine how these nutrients may be provided without deficiency or excess. Unfortunately, owing to the relatively high carbohydrate content of prepared tube feeding formulas, it is difficult to use them in patients with burns or trauma without carbohydrate and caloric excess, or protein deficiency.

There are several solutions to this problem and the best solution at a given institution is somewhat dependent upon available facilities and personnel. For example, one alternative is simply to add protein to a standard tube feeding formula. While reasonably convenient to prepare, such diets are relatively expensive, have a high osmolality, and one has little control over total volume or amount of micronutrients. We have found it more efficient to employ a modular formula. In this manner, one has precise control over all nutrients allowing maximum flexibility. By utilizing powdered materials, total fluid intake and osmolality can be optimized to meet patient needs. In addition, this formula can be prepared at a cost that is actually less than normal kitchen diets. All necessary components of this diet are discussed below and described in Table 24–4.

Macronutrient Sources

Protein. The major protein source for our enteral formula is whole egg powder (United Egg Producers, Decatur, Georgia). Based on FAO-WHO recommendations,[177] this is the highest quality protein source for normal man, and assuming no special amino acid requirements or alterations in protein utilization, it should also be the ideal source

Table 24–4 MODULAR TUBE FEEDING FOR BURN PATIENTS

NUTRIENT	SOURCE	DAILY QUANTITY	
		Adult (70 kg)	*Child (15 kg)*
Calories		3400 kcal	1500 kcal
Protein			79 gm
	Whole egg	220 gm	0 gm
	Egg white	89 gm	114 gm
Carbohydrate	Polycose*	501 gm	
Fat	Corn oil	None—adequate fat in whole egg	75 ml
Vitamins			
Water soluble	Whole egg solids	2 ml Berrocca-C†	1 Capsule
Fat soluble	plus	500 mg Ascorbic acid	B-Complex with C‡
	supplements	1 mg Folate	0.5 mg folate
		No additions	Pediatric
			Multivitamin§
			three times per week
Minerals	Whole egg solids plus following supplements:		
Sodium	Sodium chloride	Additions	14 mEq
Potassium	Potassium chloride	as needed	11 mEq
Calcium	Calcium gluconate	per laboratory	40 mEq
Phosphorus	Phospho-Soda	monitoring	26 mM
Magnesium	Mangesium sulfate		13 mEq
Zinc	Zinc sulfate	440 mg	220 mg

*Ross Laboratories, Columbus, Ohio.
†Roche Laboratories, Nutley, New Jersey.
‡Squibb, Princeton, New Jersey.
§Miles Laboratory, Elkhart, Indiana.

for patients with burns or trauma. In addition, it is inexpensive and provides other nutrients including fat, carbohydrate, vitamins, and minerals (Table 24–5). Other high quality protein sources such as egg white powder, lactalbulin, and casein are available and may be used to minimize the lipid and cholesterol intake of the whole egg powder. For example, we use egg white powder in our adult tube feeding to avoid excessive administration of fat (see Table 24–4). However, it has been shown that even a diet of 35 eggs per day in the burn patient has no demonstrable adverse effects.[178] Furthermore, due to the additional non-protein nutrients in whole egg powder, the total diet is less expensive using this protein source.

Carbohydrate. While glucose or sucrose would appear to be appropriate carbohydrate sources because of their ease of digestion and absorption, they unfortunately make an enteral feeding of high osmolality. As a result, it is preferable to provide carbohydrate in the modular diet as a polysaccharide. Polycose (Ross Laboratories, Columbus, Ohio), Sumacal (Organon Nutritional Products, West Orange, New Jersey), and Controlyte (Doyle Pharmaceutical Co., Minneapolis, Minnesota) are glucose poly-

mers that are readily digestible but will minimally contribute to the osmolality and cost of the feeding.

Fat. The source of fat chosen for a modular formula should be inexpensive, readily available, and high in essential fatty acids. While sunflower, safflower, and corn oil all contain adequate essential fatty acids, corn oil is the least expensive.

Micronutrient Sources

Mineral and Trace Elements. Whole egg powder contains a variety of micronutrients (see Table 24–5). However, most are inadequate quantities for patients with burns or trauma and must be supplemented when using this protein source with Polycose and corn oil as a tube feeding formula. For example, this diet will be deficient in sodium, potassium, and magnesium and have a low calcium to phosphorus ratio. These minerals may be supplemented at the time the tube feeding is prepared or administered by the feeding tube by the nursing staff. Exact amounts administered will depend on the amount of egg protein provided and the patient's needs. Such parameters may readily

Table 24–5　COMPOSITION OF WHOLE EGG SOLIDS*

Macronutrients		
	per 100 gm	
Protein	47.4	gm
Fat	43.1	gm
Carbohydrate	0	gm
Calories	577.5	kcal
Micronutrients		
Minerals	mg/100 gm	
Calcium	209	
Chlorine	691	
Copper	0.24	
Iodine	0.19	
Iron	7.8	
Mangesium	45	
Manganese	0.15	
Phosphorus	798	
Potassium	533	
Sodium	510	
Sulfur	648	
Zinc	5.1	
Vitamins	per 100 gm	
Vitamin A	1896	IU
Vitamin B$_{12}$	3.5	μg
Biotin	79	μg
Choline	1.70	gm
Vitamin D	198	IU
Vitamin E	6.7	mg
Folic Acid	0.24	mg
Niacin	0.32	mg
Pantothenic acid	6	mg
Pyridoxine	0.47	mg
Riboflavin	1.30	mg
Thiamine	0.36	mg

*Adapted from Cotterill, O. J., and Glauret, J. L.: Nutrient values for shell, liquid/frozen, and dehydrated egg derived by linear regression analysis and conversion factors. Poultry Science, 58:131, 1979.

be monitored by serum chemistry and treated appropriately. For the reasons discussed above, zinc is added to the tube feedings in the form of zinc sulfate, 220 mg a day for children, and 220 mg twice a day for adults.

Vitamins. Vitamins must also be supplemented with this modular formula. When using whole egg as a protein source, reasonable amounts of fat soluble vitamins are present and need not be supplemented in adults. As a result, only 2 ml of Berocca C (Roche Laboratories, Nutley, New Jersey) and 500 mg of ascorbic acid are added daily. Since the egg powder approximates the child's vitamin requirements to a smaller degree, a multivitamin preparation that includes fat-soluble vitamins is added three times a week and B-complex on the other days to the pediatric formula. Other approaches to vitamin supplementation may

be preferable at other institutions. Nonetheless, one should provide all vitamins at equal to or greater than normal recommended dietary allowances (RDA),[177] while avoiding toxicity, especially with fat-soluble vitamins.

Implementation

It is imperative that nutritional support of the patient with burns or trauma be implemented expeditiously once it is clear that the patient will not be eating for a period of more than a few days. In general, the trauma patient is well nourished at the time of injury. Procrastination in regard to nutritional support while awaiting adequate oral intake will only complicate treatment of the injury with superimposed malnutrition. However, it is not clear that it is advantageous to begin nutritional support during the "shock phase" of injury. In addition, because of problems of post-traumatic ileus and fluid and electrolyte balance, it is difficult to provide nutrients enterally or parenterally immediately after injury. As a result, it is frequently necessary to wait as much as three to five days after burns and major trauma to begin nutritional support. If the gastrointestinal tract is functional at this time, nutrients should be provided enterally. However, if the patient is unable to tolerate an enteral diet, it is essential that TPN be initiated until gastrointestinal function returns (Fig. 24–10). Proper administration of tube feeding is discussed elsewhere in this volume, but use of a soft, small-bore feeding tube and continuous infusion are preferable.

Once administration of the tube feeding is begun, it is essential to have "feedback" to assess the success at reaching the prescribed dietary goal and to determine if this goal is appropriate for the patient. Attainment of the dietary goal may be monitored by dietary staff using a table such as that in Figure 24–11. Nutritional assessment determines if the goal is appropriate. Laboratory monitoring is helpful in this regard (Table 24–6). In addition, anthropometric measurements and skin anergy testing may be advantageous in the trauma patient. However, routine nutritional assessment is extremely difficult in the burn patient. For example, serum indices, such as albumin and transferrin, may vary as a result of transfusional therapy. Anthropometrics such as triceps

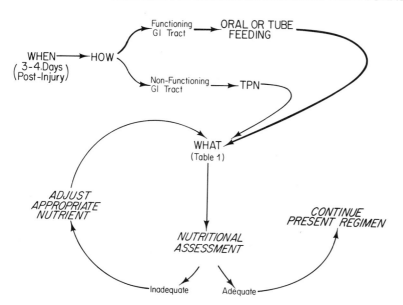

Figure 24–10. Nutritional support in the burn or trauma patient should begin 3 to 4 days after injury, preferably via the enteral route. However, with gastrointestinal conditions such as a prolonged ileus, parenteral nutritional support must be initiated. In either case, the proper nutrients must be supplied and nutritional assessment employed to determine efficacy of treatment. (*From* Molnar, J. A., Wolfe, R. R., and Burke, J. F.: Metabolism and nutritional therapy in thermal injury. *In* Schneider, H. A., Anderson, C. E., and Coursin, D. B. (eds.): Nutritional Support of Medical Practice. Edition 2. New York, Harper & Row, in press; reproduced with permission.)

skinfold and arm circumference are unreliable because of the edema and inapplicability to burned extremities. Weight measurements may be erroneous secondary to the variability in fluid balance, support paraphernalia and dressings, and the weight loss of excisional therapy. Skin testing has been employed in burns with some success,[179] although one would prefer not to jeopardize potential donor sites. Nonetheless, it is important to employ all feasible methods of clinical assessment, as well as good clinical judgment, to optimize the nutritional support for each patient (Fig. 24–11).

OTHER ENTERAL FORMULAS

While the modular formula is usually the ideal enteral formula for patients with burns or trauma in our experience, on occasion other enteral formulas may be useful. For example, patients beginning an oral intake may consume inadequate quantities to meet the total daily nutrient requirements. Under these circumstances, a standard formula, either as an oral supplement or as a tube feeding at night, may be helpful. Rarely will an elemental diet be required in burn patients since typically they have a normal gastrointestinal tract that may readily accommodate complex foodstuffs. However, specific indications include the patient with preexisting gastrointestinal disease or associated abdominal trauma. In addition, the patient requiring prolonged parenteral

nutrition may develop atrophic gut changes such that an elemental diet may be an appropriate initial tube feeding because of its relative ease of digestion.

COMBINED ENTERAL AND PARENTERAL NUTRITION

Combined enteral and parenteral nutrition is often ignored in discussions of nutritional support but may actually be an important means by which to meet the complete dietary requirements of a patient. It is not infrequent that only a portion of the desired intake may be provided enterally because of such complications as diarrhea or abdominal discomfort. Under these circumstances, enteral intake may be supplemented parenterally. Several alternatives are available depending upon the specific dietary problem. Frequently, it is preferable to provide some

Table 24–6 RECOMMENDED ROUTINE LABORATORY MONITORING FOR PATIENTS ON MODULAR TUBE FEEDING

DAILY	WEEKLY
Na, K, Cl, CO_2	Triglycerides
BUN, creatinine	Cholesterol
Blood sugar	Total protein, albumin
Calcium	
Phosphorus	
Magnesium	Patient weight
Sugar and acetone (urine) each 8 hours	

Name _____ Age _____ Sex _____

Per Cent Body Surface Area Burn _____

Actual Admission   Ideal Body   Weight by
Weight (kg) _____ Weight _____ History _____

Height (cm) _____ Basal Metabolic Rate _____

Surface Area (M^2) _____ Estimated Caloric Requirement _____

24-HOUR INTAKE -- WEEK OF

	Clinical Ideal	Mon.	Tues.	Wed.	Thurs.	Fri.	Sat.	Sun.
Body Weight								
% Weight Loss	< 10%							
% Open Wound								
Caloric Intake/Day								
Carbohydrate Intake mg/kg/min/Daily total	5							
Carbohydrate calories/day								
Protein Intake gm/kg/day/Daily total	1.5 – 2.5							
Protein calories/day								
Fat Intake gm/kg/day/Daily total								
Fat calories/day								
Nitrogen Balance Nitrogen Intake								
Nitrogen Excretion								
Balance	> 0							

Figure 24–11. Daily nutritional assessment sheet to monitor intake of a seriously ill patient. Ideal body weight is obtained from standard tables. Basal metabolic rate is calculated with the Harris-Benedict equation. (*From* Molnar, J. A., Wolfe, R. R., and Burke, J. F.: Metabolism and nutritional therapy in thermal injury. *In* Schneider, H. A., Anderson, C. E., and Coursin, D. B. (eds.): Nutritional Support of Medical Practice. Edition 2. New York, Harper & Row, in press; reproduced with permission.)

fraction of all nutrients parenterally. Under these circumstances, a TPN solution may be infused via a central line while enteral tube feedings are simultaneously administered. This situation frequently arises when a patient receiving TPN begins to receive an enteral diet but prolonged gut rest demands careful advancement of the rate of infusion of tube feeding. While enteral nutrition is being increased, parenteral nutrition may be decreased until it is discontinued after a few days. Under other circumstances, specific nutrients such as a 3 per cent amino acid solution, lipid emulsion, or specific micronutrients may be infused peripherally to supplement an inadequate enteral diet.

FUTURE DIRECTION

While this chapter attempts to review and make recommendations for nutrient requirements in burns and trauma, it is apparent that these recommendations are frequently based on a paucity of knowledge. Injury initiates a number of well-described metabolic alterations. In many cases, it is not known how this response to injury may be manipulated by administration of exogenous nutrients to the benefit of the patient. At present, the guidelines for administration of calories and carbohydrate would seem to be fairly appropriate for optimal patient benefit. However, much less is known regarding the provision of ideal quantities of protein, fat, and micronutrients in trauma. While more investigation is necessary in all areas of nutrient metabolism in trauma, emphasis should be placed on examining functional parameters that relate to morbidity and mortality, and on elaboration of the adverse effects of specific nutrient excess. Furthermore, in order that we may more accurately meet the requirements of each patient, reliable and inexpensive methods for assessment of specific nutrient status must be developed for burn patients.

Further investigation of the physiologic response of the gastrointestinal tract to trauma is needed. Understanding of the neural and hormonal mechanisms involved in post-traumatic ileus may allow pharmacologic manipulation to minimize this impediment to enteral nutrition. Not only must motility be examined, but knowledge of nutrient absorption and utilization from the gastrointestinal tract is essential to place enteral nutrition in patients with burns or trauma on a more solid scientific basis.

Acknowledgments

The authors with to express their appreciation for the contributions of Beverly T. Nuss, Kathleen A. Gilleran, and Andrea M. Frank in the preparation of this manuscript.

REFERENCES

1. Cuthbertson, D. P.: Observations on the disturbance of metabolism produced by injury to the limbs. Quart. J. Med., 1:233–246, 1932.
2. Long, C. L.: Energy balance and carbohydrate metabolism in infection and sepsis. Am. J. Clin. Nutr., 30:1301–1310, 1977.
3. Gump, F. E., Martin, P., and Kinney, J. M.: Oxygen consumption and caloric expenditure in surgical patients. Surg. Gynecol. Obstet., 137:499–513, 1973.
4. Bartlett, R. H., Allyn, P. A., Medley, T., and Wetmore, N.: Nutritional therapy based on positive caloric balance in burn patients. Arch. Surg., 112:974–980, 1977.
5. Roe, C. F., Kinney, J. M., and Blair, C.: Water and heat exchange in third-degree burns. Surgery, 56:212–220, 1964.
6. Wilmore, D. W., Long, J. M., Mason, A. D., Jr., Skreen, R. W., and Pruitt, B. A., Jr.: Catecholamines: Mediator of the hypermetabolic response to thermal injury. Ann. Surg., 180:653–668, 1974.
7. Royle, G. T., Wolfe, R. R., and Burke, J. F.: Metabolic expenditure in severely burned children and adults treated with early excision and closure of wounds. Submitted for publication.
8. Scrimshaw, N. S., Habicht, J. P., Piché, M. L., Cholakos, B., and Arroyave, G.: Protein metabolism of young men during university examinations. Am. J. Clin. Nutr., 18:321–324, 1966.
9. Danielsson, U., Arturson, G., and Wennberg, L.: Variations of metabolic rate in burned patients as a result of the injury and the care. Burns, 5:169–173, 1978.
10. Brooke, O. G., Cocks, T., and March, Y.: Resting metabolic rate in malnourished babies in relation to total body potassium. Acta Paediatr. Scand., 63:817–825, 1974.
11. Zwillich, C. W., Sahn, S., and Weil, J. V.: Effects of hypermetabolism on ventilation and chemosensitivity. J. Clin. Invest., 60:900–906, 1977.
12. Wolfe, R. R., Durkot, M. J., Clarke, C. C., Bode, H. H., and Burke, J. F.: Effect of food intake on hypermetabolic response to burn injury in guinea pigs. J. Nutr., 110:1310–1312, 1980.
13. Garrow, J. S.: Energy Balance and Obesity in Man. Amsterdam, Elsevier/North Holland Biomedical Press, 1978.
14. Askanazi, J., Carpentier, Y. A., Elwyn, D. H., Nordenström, H., Jeevanandam, M., Rosenbaum, S. H., Gump, F. E., and Kinney, J. M.: Influence of total parenteral nutrition on fuel utilization in injury and sepsis. Ann. Surg., 191:40–46, 1980.
15. Gump, F. E., and Kinney, J. M.: Caloric and fluid losses through the burn wound. Surg. Clin. North Am., 50:1235–1248, 1970.
16. Neely, W. A., Petro, A. B., Holloman, G. H., Rushton, F. W., Turner, M. D., and Hardy, J. D.: Researches on the cause of burn hypermetabolism. Ann. Surg., 179:291–294, 1974.
17. Zawacki, B. E., Spitzer, K. W., Mason, A. D., Jr., and Johns, L. A.: Does increased evaporative water loss cause hypermetabolism in burned patients? Ann. Surg., 171:236–240, 1970.
18. Birke, G., Carlson, L. A., von Euler, U. S., Liljedahl, S. O., and Plantin, L. O.: Lipid metabolism, catecholamine excretion, basal metabolic rate, and water loss during treatment of burns with warm dry air. Acta Chir. Scan., 138:321–333, 1972.
19. Caldwell, F. T., Jr.: Energy metabolism following thermal burns. Arch. Surg. 111:181–185, 1976.
20. Harrison, H. N., Moncrief, J. A., Duckett, J. W., Jr., and Mason, A. D., Jr.: The relationship between energy metabolism and water loss from vaporization in severely burned patients. Surgery, 56:203–211, 1964.

21. Caldwell, F. T., Jr., Bowser, B. H., and Crabtree, J. H.: The effect of occlusive dressings on the energy metabolism of severely burned children. Ann. Surg., *193*:579–590, 1981.

22. Crowley, L. V., Seifter, E., Kriss, P., Rettura, G., Nakao, K., and Levenson, S. M.: Effects of environmental temperature and femoral fracture on wound healing in rats. J. Trauma, *17*:436–445, 1977.

23. Cuthbertson, D. P., Fell, G. S., Smith, C. M., and Tilstone, W. J.: Metabolism after injury. I. Effects of severity, nutrition, and environmental temperature on protein, potassium, zinc, and creatinine. Br. J. Surg., *59*:925–931, 1972.

24. Shires, G. T., and Black, E. A. (eds.): Second conference on supportive therapy in burn care: Proceedings of a conference held at NIH 9–10 October 1980. J. Trauma, *21*(Suppl.):665–750, 1981.

25. Gazzaniga, A. B., Polachek, J. R., Wilson, A. F., and Day, A. T.: Indirect calorimetry as a guide to caloric replacement during total parenteral nutrition. Am. J. Surg., *136*:128–133, 1978.

26. Elwyn, D. H.: Nutritional requirements of adult surgical patients. Crit. Care Med., *8*:9–20, 1980.

27. Molnar, J. A., Wolfe, R. R., and Burke, J. F.: Metabolism and nutritional therapy in thermal injury. *In* Schneider, H. A., Anderson, C. E., and Coursin, D. B. (eds.): Nutritional Support of Medical Practice. Edition 2. Hagerstown, Maryland, Harper and Row, in press.

28. Rutten, P., Blackburn, G. L., Flatt, J. P., Hallowell, E., and Cochran, D.: Determination of optimal hyperalimentation infusion rate. J. Surg. Res., *18*:477–483, 1975.

29. Wilmore, D. W.: Nutrition and metabolism following thermal injury. Clin. Plast. Surg., *1*:603–619, 1974.

30. Ryan, N. T.: Metabolic adaptations for energy production during trauma and sepsis. Surg. Clin. North Am., *56*:1073–1090, 1976.

31. Long, C. L., Kinney, J. M., and Geiger, J. W.: Nonsupressibility of gluconeogenesis by glucose in septic patients. Metabolism, *25*:193–201, 1976.

32. Long, C. L., Spencer, J. L., Kinney, J. M., and Geiger, J. W.: Carbohydrate metabolism in man: Effect of elective operations and major injury. J. Appl. Physiol., *31*:110–116, 1971.

33. Wolfe, R. R., Miller, H. I., Elahi, D., and Spitzer, J. J.: Effect of burn injury on glucose turnover in guinea pigs. Surg. Gynecol. Obstet., *144*:359–364, 1977.

34. Wolfe, R. R., Durkot, M. J., Allsop, J. R., and Burke, J. F.: Glucose metabolism in severely burned patients. Metabolism, *28*:1031–1039, 1979.

35. Wolfe, R. R., and Burke, J. F.: Effect of burn trauma on glucose turnover, oxidation, and recycling in guinea pigs. Am. J. Physiol., *233*:E80–85, 1977.

36. Wilmore, D. W., Mason, A. D., and Pruitt, B. A., Jr.: Alterations in glucose kinetics following thermal injury. Surg. Forum, *26*:81–83, 1975.

37. Wilmore, D. W., Aulick, L. H., Mason, A. D., Jr., and Pruitt, B. A., Jr.: Influence of the burn wound on local and systemic responses to injury. Ann. Surg., *186*:444–456, 1977.

38. Sheldon, G. F., Peterson, S. R., and Sanders, R.: Hepatic dysfunction during hyperalimentation. Arch. Surg., *113*:504–508, 1978.

39. Long, J. M., III, Wilmore, D. W., Mason, A. D., Jr. Pruitt, B. A., Jr.: Effect of carbohydrate and fat intake on nitrogen excretion during total intravenous feeding. Ann. Surg., *185*:417–422, 1977.

40. Burke, J. F., Wolfe, R. R., Mullany, C. J., Mathews, D. E., and Bier, D. M.: Glucose requirements following burn injury: Parameters of optimal glucose infusion and possible hepatic and respiratory abnormalites following excessive glucose intake. Ann. Surg., *190*:274–283, 1979.

41. McArdle, A. H., Palmason, C., Morency, I., and Brown, R. A.: A rationale for enteral feeding as the preferable route for hyperalimentation. Surgery, *90*:616–622, 1981.

42. Wene, J. D., Connor, W. E., and DenBesten, L.: The development of essential fatty acid deficiency in healthy men fed fat-free diets intravenously and orally. J. Clin. Invest., *56*:127–134, 1975.

43. Askanazi, J., Rosenbaum, S. H., Hyman, A. I., Silverberg, P. A., Milic-Emili, J., and Kinney, J. M.: Respiratory changes induced by the large glucose loads of total parenteral nutrition. J.A.M.A., *243*:1444–1447, 1980.

44. Askanazi, J., Elwyn, D. H., Silverberg, P. A., Rosenbaum, S. H., and Kinney, J. M.: Respiratory distress secondary to a high carbohydrate load: A case report. Surgery, *87*:596–598, 1980.

45. Askanazi, J., Rosenbaum, S. H., Hyman, A. I., Foster, R. J., Milic-Emili, J., and Kinney, J. M.: Effects of total parenteral nutrition on gas exchange and breathing patterns [Abstract]. Crit. Care Med., *7*:125, 1979.

46. Wolfe, R. R., Snowden, J. M., and Burke, J. F.: Influence of insulin and palmitic acid concentration on pulmonary surfactant synthesis. J. Surg. Res., *27*:262–267, 1979.

47. Wolfe, R. R., O'Donnell, T. F., Jr., Stone, M. D., Richmond, D. A., and Burke, J. F.: Investigation of factors determining the optimal glucose infusion rate in total parenteral nutrition. Metabolism, *29*:892–900, 1980.

48. Wolfe, R. R., Allsop, J. R., and Burke, J. F.: Glucose metabolism in man: Responses to intravenous glucose infusion. Metabolism, *28*:210–220, 1979.

49. Pozefsky, T., Felig, P., Tobin, J. D., Soeldner, J. S., Cahill, G. F., Jr.: Amino acid balance across tissues of the forearm in postabsorptive man. Effects of insulin at two dose levels. J. Clin. Invest., *48*:2273–2282, 1969.

50. Woolfson, A. M. J., Heatley, R. V., and Allison, S. P.: Insulin to inhibit protein catabolism after injury. N. Engl. J. Med., *300*:14–17, 1979.

51. Cuthbertson, D. P.: The disturbance of metabolism produced by bone and non-bony injury, with notes on certain abnormal conditions of bone. Biochem. J., *24*:1244–1263, 1930.

52. Nardi, G. L.: "Essential" and "nonessential" amino acids in the urine of severely burned patients. J. Clin. Invest., *33*:847–854, 1954.

53. Hoover-Plow, J. L., and Clifford, A. J.: The effect of surgical trauma on muscle protein turnover in rats. Biochem. J., *176*:137–142, 1978.

54. Kien, C. L., Young, V. R., Rohrbaugh, D. K., and Burke, J. F.: Whole-body protein synthesis and breakdown rates in children before and after reconstructive surgery of the skin. Metabolism, *27*:27–34, 1978.

55. Waterlow, J. C., Golden, M., and Picou, D.: The measurement of rates of protein turnover, synthesis, and breakdown in man and the effects of

nutritional status and surgical injury. Am. J. Clin. Nutr., 30:1333–1339, 1977.

56. Long, C. L., Jeevanandam, M., Kim, B. M., and Kinney, J. M.: Whole body protein synthesis and catabolism in septic man. Am. J. Clin. Nutr., 30:1340–1344, 1977.

57. Kien, C. L., Young, V. R., Rohrbaugh, D. K., and Burke, J. F.: Increased rates of whole body protein synthesis and breakdown in children recovering from burns. Ann. Surg., 187:383–391, 1978.

58. Birkhahn, R. H., Long, C. L., Fitkin, P., Geiger, J. W., and Blakemore, W. S.: Effects of major skeletal trauma on whole body protein turnover in man measured by L-[1,^{14}C]-leucine. Surgery, 88:294–299, 1980.

59. Cuthbertson, D. P.: Physical injury and its effects on protein metabolism. In Munro, H. N., and Allison, J. B. (eds.): Mammalian Protein Metabolism, Vol. II. New York, Academic Press, 1964, pp. 373–414.

60. Cuthbertson, D. P., and Tilstone, W. J.: Nutrition of the injured. Am. J. Clin. Nutr., 21:911–922, 1968.

61. Threlfall, C. J., Stoner, H. B., and Galasko, C. S. B.: Patterns in the excretion of muscle markers after trauma and orthopedic surgery. J. Trauma, 21:140–147, 1981.

62. Munro, H. N., and Young, V. R.: Urinary excretion of N$^{\tau}$-methylhistidine (3-methylhistidine): A tool to study metabolic responses in relation to nutrient and hormonal status in health and disease of man. Am. J. Clin. Nutr., 31:1608–1614, 1978.

63. Bilmazes, C., Kien, C. L., Rohrbaugh, D. K., Uauy, R., Burke, J. F., Munro, H. N., and Young, V. R.: Quantitative contribution by skeletal muscle to elevated rates of whole-body protein breakdown in burned children as measured by N$^{\tau}$-methylhistidine output. Metabolism, 27:671–676, 1978.

64. Beisel, W. R.: Interrelated changes in host metabolism during generalized infectious illness. Am. J. Clin. Nutr., 25:1254–1260, 1972.

65. Powanda, M. C.: Changes in body balances of nitrogen and other key nutrients. Description and underlying mechanisms. Am. J. Clin. Nutr., 30:1254–1268, 1977.

66. Wannemacher, R. W., Jr.: Key role of various individual amino acids in host response to infection. Am. J. Clin. Nutr., 30:1269–1280, 1977.

67. Goldberg, A. L., and Chang, T. W.: Regulation and significance of amino acid metabolism in skeletal muscle. Fed. Proc., 37:2301–2307, 1978.

68. Felig, P.: The glucose-alanine cycle. Metabolism, 22:179–207, 1973.

69. Cahill, G. F., Jr.: Starvation in man. N. Engl. J. Med., 282:668–675, 1970.

70. Imamura, M., Clowes, G. H. A., Jr., Blackburn, G. L., O'Donnell, T. F., Jr., Trerice, M., Bhimjee, T., and Ryan, N. T.: Liver metabolism and glucogenesis in trauma and sepsis. Surgery, 77:868–880, 1975.

71. Young, V. R., and Scrimshaw, N. S.: Nutritional evaluation of proteins and protein requirements. In Milner, M., Scrimshaw, N. S., Wang, D. I. C. (eds.): Protein Resources and Technology. Westport, Connecticut, AVI Publishing, 1978, pp. 136–173.

72. Rand, W. M., Scrimshaw, N. S., and Young, V. R.: Determination of protein allowances in human adults from nitrogen balance data. Am. J. Clin. Nutr., 30:1129–1134, 1977.

73. Bodwell, C. E., Schuster, E. M., Kyle, E., Brooks, B., Womack, M., Steele, P., and Ahrens, R.: Obligatory urinary and fecal nitrogen losses in young women, older men, and young men and the factorial estimation of adult human protein requirements. Am. J. Clin. Nutr., 32:2450–2459, 1979.

74. Hegsted, D. M.: Assessment of nitrogen requirements. Am. J. Clin. Nutr., 31:1669–1677, 1978.

75. Rudman, D. Millikan, W. J., Richardson, T. J., Bixler, T. J. II, Stackhouse, W. J., and McGarrity, W. C.: Elemental balances during intravenous hyperalimentation of underweight adult subjects. J. Clin. Invest., 55:94–104, 1975.

76. Sutherland, A. B., and Batchelor, A. D. R.: Nitrogen balance in burned children. Ann. N.Y. Acad. Sci., 150:700–710, 1968.

77. Markley, K., Smallman, E., and Thornton, S. W.: The effect of diet protein on late burn mortality. Proc. Soc. Exp. Biol. Med., 135:94–98, 1970.

78. Alexander, J. W., MacMillan, B. G., Stinnett, J. D., Ogle, C., Bozian, R. C., Fischer, J. E., Oakes, J. B., Morris, M. J., and Krummel, R.: Beneficial effects of aggressive protein feeding in severely burned children. Ann. Surg., 192:505–516, 1980.

79. Shizgal, H. M., and Forse, R. A.: Protein and calorie requirements with total parenteral nutrition. Ann. Surg., 192:562–568, 1980.

80. Wolfe, R. R., Goodenough, R. D., Wolfe, M. H., and Burke, J. F.: Isotopic study of protein metabolism in burn patients given isocaloric diets with differing protein content [Abstract]. American Burn Association, 1982.

81. Schuette, S. A., Zemel, M. B., and Linkswiler, H. M.: Studies on the mechanism of protein-induced hypercalcuria. J. Nutr., 110:305–315, 1980.

82. Worthington, G. S., III, and Moylan, J. A.: Hypercalciuresis in trauma patients in high-nitrogen enteral and parenteral diets. J. Trauma, 19:227–233, 1979.

83. Bergström, J., and Hultman, E.: Nutrition for maximal sports performance. J.A.M.A., 221:999–1005, 1972.

84. Al Shamma, G. A., Goll, C. C., Baird, T. B., Broom, J., Nicholas, G. A., and Richards, J. R.: Changes in body composition after thermal injury in the rat. Br. J. Nutr., 42:367–375, 1979.

85. Birkhahn, R. H., Calvin, L. L., Fitkin, D. L., Busnardo, A. C., Geiger, J. W., and Blakemore, W. S.: A comparison of the effects of skeletal trauma and surgery on the ketosis of starvation in man. J. Trauma, 21:513–519, 1981.

86. Allison, S. P., Hinton, P., and Chamberlain, M. J.: Intravneous glucose-tolerance, insulin, and free-fatty-acid levels in burned patients. Lancet, 2(7578):1113–1116, 1968.

87. Schumer, W.: Supportive therapy in burn care. Consensus summary on metabolism. J. Trauma, 19(11 Suppl.): 910–911, 1979.

88. Kitchell, B. B., Rauckman, E. J., Rosen, G. M., Lazar, J. D., and Moylan, J. A.: Changes in plasma free fatty acids and hepatic enzymes following traumatic injury in the rat. Biochem. Pharmacol., 30:537–539, 1981.

89. Carpentier, Y. A., Askanazi, J., Elwyn, D. H., Jeevanandam, M., Gump, F. E., Hyman, A. I., Burr, R., and Kinney, J. M.: Effect of hypercaloric glucose infusion on lipid metabolism in injury and sepsis. J. Trauma, 19:649–653, 1979.

90. Robin, A. P., Askanazi, J., Greenwood, M. R. C., Carpentier, Y. A., Gump, F. E., Kinney, J. M.: Lipoprotein lipase activity in surgical patients: Influence of trauma and infection. Surgery, 90:401–407, 1981.

91. Robin, A. P., Nordenström, J., Askanazi, J., Elwyn, D. H., Carpentier, Y. A., and Kinney, J. M.: Plasma clearance of fat emulsion in trauma and sepsis: Use of a three-stage lipid clearance test. J.P.E.N., 4:505–510, 1980.

92. Hallberg, D.: Studies on the elimination of exogenous lipids from the blood stream. Acta Physiol. Scan., 65:153–163, 1965.

93. Smith, R., Fuller, D. J., Wedge, J. H., Williamson, D. H., and Alberti, K. G. G. M.: Initial effect of injury on ketone bodies and other blood metabolites. Lancet, 1(7897):1–3, 1975.

94. Williamson, D. H., Farrell, R., Kerr, A., and Smith, R.: Muscle-protein catabolism after injury in man, as measured by urinary excretion of 3-methylhistidine. Clin. Sci. Mol. Med., 52:527–533, 1977.

95. Sherwin, R. S., Hendler, R. G., and Felig, P.: Effect of ketone infusions on amino acids and nitrogen metabolism in man. J. Clin. Invest., 55:1382–1390, 1975.

96. Long, C.: Energy expenditure of major burns. J. Trauma., 19:904–905, 1979.

97. Neufeld, H. A., Kaminski, M. V., Jr., and Wannemacher, R. W., Jr.: Effect of inflammatory and noninflammatory stress on ketone bodies and free fatty acids in rats. Am. J. Clin. Nutr., 30:1357–1358, 1977.

98. Richardson, D. P., Wayler, A. H., Scrimshaw, N. S., and Young, V. R.: Quantitative effect of an isoenergetic exchange of fat for carbohydrate on dietary protein utilization in healthy young men. Am. J. Clin. Nutr., 32:2217–2226, 1979.

99. Munro, H. N.: Carbohydrate and fat as factors in protein utilization and metabolism. Physiol. Rev., 31:449–488, 1951.

100. Freund, H., Yoshimura, N., and Fischer, J. E.: Does intravenous fat spare nitrogen in the injured rat? Am. J. Surg., 140:377–383, 1980.

101. Kirkpatrick, J. R., Dahn, M., and Wis, L.: Selective versus standard hyperalimentation. Am. J. Surg., 141:116–121, 1981.

102. Kirkpatrick, J. R., Dahn, M., Hynes, M. J., and Williams, D.: The therapeutic advantages of a balanced nutritional support system. Surgery, 89:370–374, 1981.

103. Tempel, G., Lohninger, A., Jelen, S., Riedl, W., and Blümel, G.: Changes in essential fatty acids in plasma lipid fractions of polytraumatized patients with different parenteral nutrition. Resuscitation, 6:107–113, 1977.

104. Helmkamp, G. M., Jr., Wilmore, D. W., Johnson, A. A., and Pruitt, B. A., Jr.: Essential fatty acid deficiency in red cells after thermal injury: Correction with intravenous fat therapy. Am. J. Clin. Nutr., 26:1331–1338, 1973.

105. McCarthy, M. C., Cottam, G. L., and W. W. Turner, Jr.: Essential fatty acid deficiency in critically ill surgical patients. Am. J. Surg., 142:747–751, 1981.

106. Collins, F. D., Sinclair, A. J., Royle, J. P., Coats, D. A., Maynard, A. T., and Leonard, R. F.: Plasma lipids in human linoleic acid deficiency. Nutr. Metab., 13:150–167, 1971.

107. Goodgame, J. T., Lowry, S. F., and Brennan, M. F.: Essential fatty acid deficiency in total parenteral nutrition: Time course of development and suggestions for therapy. Surgery, 84:271–277, 1978.

108. Lund, C. C., Levenson, S. M., Green, R. W., et al.: Ascorbic acid, thiamine, riboflavin and nicotinic acid in relation to acute burns in man. Arch. Surg., 55:557–583, 1947.

109. Crandon, J. H., Lennihan, R., Jr., Mikal, S., and Reif, A. E.: Ascorbic acid economy in surgical patients. Ann. N.Y. Acad. Sci., 92:246–267, 1961.

110. Irvin, T. T., Chattopadhyay, D. K., and Smythe, A.: Ascorbic acid requirements in postoperative patients. Surg. Gynecol. Obstet., 147:49–55, 1978.

111. Mason, M., Matyk, P. W., and Doolan, S. A.: Urinary ascorbic acid excretion in post-operative patients. Am. J. Surg., 122:808–811, 1971.

112. Hodges, R. E.: Ascorbic acid. In Goodhart, R. S., and Shils, M. E. (eds.): Modern Nutrition in Health and Disease. Edition 6. Philadelphia, Lea and Febiger, 1980, pp. 259–273.

113. Barlow, G. B.: The effects of burns on blood folate levels in children. In Mašek, J., Ošancová, K., and Cuthbertson, D. P. (eds.): Nutrition: Proceedings of the Eighth International Congress, Prague, September 1969. Amsterdam, Excerpta Medica, 1970, pp. 506–508.

114. Barlow, G. B., Dickerson, J. A., and Wilkinson, A. W.: Plasma biotin levels in children with burns and scalds. J. Clin. Pathol., 29:58–59, 1976.

115. Barlow, G. B., Sutton, J. L., and Wilkinson, A. W.: Metabolism of nicotinic acid in children with burns and scalds. Clin. Chim. Acta, 75:337–342, 1977.

116. Barlow, G. B., and Wilkinson, A. W.: 4-Amino-imidazole-5-carboxamide excretion and folate status with burns and scalds. Clin. Chim. Acta, 29:355–359, 1970.

117. Barlow, G. B., and Wilkinson, A. W.: Plasma pyridoxal phosphate levels and tryptophan metabolism in children with burns and scalds. Clin. Chim. Acta, 64:79–82, 1975.

118. Pories, W. J., Henzel, J. H., Rob, C. G., and Strain, W. H.: Acceleration of wound healing in man with zinc sulfate given by mouth. Lancet, 1(7482):121–124, 1967.

119. Hsu, J. M., and Anthony, W. L.: Effect of zinc deficiency on urinary excretion of nitrogenous compounds and liver amino acid-catabolizing enzymes in rats. J. Nutr., 105:26–31, 1975.

120. Brodribb, A. J. M., and Ricketts, C. R.: The effect of zinc in the healing of burns. Injury 3:25–29, 1971.

121. Solomons, N. W.: Zinc and copper in human nutrition. In Karcioglu, Z. A., and Sarper, R. M. (eds.): Zinc and Copper in Medicine. Springfield, Illinois, Charles C Thomas, 1980, pp. 224–275.

122. Larson, D. L., Maxwell, R., Abston, S., and Dobrkovsky, M.: Zinc deficiency in burned children. Plast. Reconstr. Surg., 46:13–21, 1970.

123. Fell, G. S., Cuthbertson, D. P., Morrison, C., Fleck, A., Queen, K., Bissent, R. S., and Husain, S. L.: Urinary zinc levels as an indication of muscle catabolism. Lancet, 1(7798):280–282, 1973.

124. Thompson, H. J., Griminger, P., and Evans, J. L.: Effect of dietary copper, manganese, and zinc on nitrogen equilibrium and mineral distribution subsequent to trauma in mature rats. J. Nutr., 106:1421–1428, 1976.

125. Wacker, W. E. C.: Biochemistry of zinc—Role in wound healing. In Hambridge, K. M., and Ni-

chols, B. L. (eds.): Zinc and Copper in Clinical Medicine. Jamaica, New York, SP Scientific and Medical Books, 1978, pp. 15–24.

126. Broughton, A., Anderson, I. R. M., and Bowden, C. H.: Magnesium-deficiency syndrome in burns. Lancet, 2(7579):1156–1158, 1968.

127. Domres, B., Heller, W., Koslowski, L., and Schmidt, K.: Das Verhalten der Serumspiegel von Magnesium und Zink nach einem kontrollierten Verbrennungstrauma der Ratte. [Serum levels of magnesium and zinc after a controlled thermal trauma of the rat.] Langenbecks Arch. Chir., 343:107–112, 1977.

128. Kay, R. G., Tasman-Jones, C., Pybus, J., Whiting, R., and Black, H.: A syndrome of acute zinc deficiency during total parenteral alimentation in man. Ann. Surg., 183:331–340, 1976.

129. van Rij, A. M., Thomson, C. D., McKenzie, J. M., and Robinson, M. F.: Selenium deficiency in total parenteral nutrition. Am. J. Clin. Nutr., 32:2076–2085, 1979.

130. Freeman, J. B., and Wittine, M. F.: Magnesium requirements are increased during total parenteral nutrition. Surg. Forum, 28:61–62, 1977.

131. Nachlas, M. M., Younis, M. T., Roda, C. P., and Wityk, J. J.: Gastrointestinal motility studies as a guide to postoperative management. Ann. Surg., 175:510–522, 1972.

132. Wilson, J. P.: Postoperative motility of the large intestines in man. Gut, 16:689–92, 1975.

133. Kirksey, T. D., Moncrief, J. A., Pruitt, B. A., Jr., and O'Neill, J. A., Jr.: Gastrointestinal complications in burns. Am. J. Surg., 116:627–633, 1968.

134. Catchpole, B. N.: Ileus: Use of sympathetic blocking agents in its treatment. Surgery, 66:811–820, 1969.

135. Smith, J., Kelly, K. A., and Weinshilboum, R. M.: Pathophysiology of postoperative ileus. Arch. Surg., 112:203–209, 1977.

136. Dubois, A., Weise, V. K., and Kopin, I. J.: Postoperative ileus in the rat: Physiopathology, etiology and treatment. Ann. Surg., 178:781–786, 1973.

137. Dubois, A., Kopin, I. J., Pettigrew, K. D., and Jacobowitz, D. M.: Chemical and histochemical studies of postoperative sympathetic activity in the digestive tract in rats. Gastroenterology, 66:403–407, 1974.

138. Dubois, A., Watanabe, A. M., and Kopin, I. J.: Postoperative gastric ileus. Am. J. Dig. Dis., 18:39–42, 1973.

139. Wells, C., Rawlinson, K., Tinckler, L., Jones, H., and Saunders, J.: Ileus and postoperative intestinal motility: Preliminary communication. Lancet, 2:136–137, 1961.

140. Rothnie, N. G., Harper, R. A. K., and Catchpole, B. N.: Early postoperative gastrointestinal activity. Lancet, 2(7298):64–67, 1963.

141. Tinckler, L. F.: Surgery and intestinal motility. Br. J. Surg., 52:140–150, 1965.

142. Woods, J. H., Erickson, L. W., Condon, R. E., Schulte, W. J., and Sillin, L. F.: Postoperative ileus: A colonic problem? Surgery, 84:527–532, 1978.

143. Mishra, N. K., Appert, H. E., and Howard, J. M.: Studies of paralytic ileus. Effects of intraperitoneal injury on motility of the canine small intestine. Am. J. Surg., 129:559–563, 1975.

144. Glucksman, D. L., Kalser, M. H., and Warren, W.

D.: Small intestinal absorption in the immediate postoperative period. Surgery, 60:1020–1025, 1966.

145. Moss, G.: Early enteral feeding after abdominal surgery. In Deitel, (ed.): Nutrition in Clinical Surgery. Baltimore, Williams and Wilkins, 1980, p. 161.

146. Page, C. P., Carlton, P. K., Andrassy, R. J., Feldtman, R. W., and Shield, C. F., III: Safe, cost-effective postoperative nutrition: Defined formula diet via needle-catheter jejunostomy. Am. J. Surg., 138:939–945, 1979.

147. Carter, E. A., Udall, J., and Walker, W. A.: The effect of acute burn trauma on rat small intestine. Submitted for publication.

148. Rosenthal, A., Czaja, A. J., and Pruitt, B. A.: Gastrin levels and gastric acidity in the pathogenesis of acute gastroduodenal disease after burns. Surg. Gynecol. Obstet., 144:232–234, 1977.

149. Robbins, R., Idjadi, F., Stahl, W. M., and Essiet, G.: Studies of gastric secretion in stressed patients. Ann. Surg., 175:555–562, 1972.

150. Czaja, A. J., McAlhany, J. C., Jr., Andes, W. A., and Pruitt, B. A., Jr.: Acute gastric disease after cutaneous thermal injury. Arch. Surg., 110:600–605, 1975.

151. Czaja, A. J., McAlhany, J. C., and Pruitt, B. A., Jr.: Acute gastroduodenal disease after thermal injury: An endoscopic evaluation of incidence and natural history. N. Engl. J. Med., 291:925–929, 1974.

152. O'Neill, J. A., Jr., Ritchey, C. R., Mason, A. D., and Villarreal, Y.: Effect of thermal burns on gastric mucous production. Surg. Gynecol. Obstet., 131:29–33, 1970.

153. Friesen, S. R.: The genesis of gastroduodenal ulcer following burns. Surgery, 28:123–158, 1956.

154. Skillman, J. J., and Silen, W.: Stress ulcers. Lancet, 2(7790):1303–1306, 1972.

155. Kitajima, M., Allsop, J. R., Trelstad, R. L., and Burke, J. F.: Experimental studies on stress ulcer of the stomach following thermal injury with special reference to H^+ back diffusion and microcirculation. Gastroenterol. Jpn., 13:175–183, 1978.

156. Lucas, C. E., Sugawa, G., Friend, W., and Walt, A. J.: Therapeutic implications of disturbed gastric physiology in patients with stress ulcerations. Am. J. Surg., 123:25–34, 1972.

157. Skillman, J. J., Gould, S. A., Chung, R. S. K., and Silen, W.: The gastric mucosal barrier: Clinical and experimental studies in critically ill and normal man, and in the rabbit. Ann. Surg., 172:564–582, 1970.

158. Carrasquilla, C., Weaver, A., Amarasinghe, D. C., Rota, A., Walt, A. J., and Park, A.: Gastroesophageal erosions and ulcerations. Arch. Surg., 107:447–451, 1973.

159. Chernov, M. S., Hale, H. W., Jr., and Woods, M.: Prevention of stress ulcers. Am. J. Surg., 122:674–677, 1971.

160. Rai, K., and Courtemanche, A. D.: Vitamin A assay in burned patients. J. Trauma, 15:419–424, 1975.

161. De Luca, L., and Wolf, G.: Vitamin A and protein synthesis in mucous membranes. Am. J. Clin. Nutr., 22:1059–1062, 1969.

162. De Luca, L., Little, E. P., and Wolf, G.: Vitamin A and protein synthesis by rat intestinal mucosa. J. Bio. Chem., 244:701–708, 1969.

163. Choctaw, W. T., Fujita, C., and Zaracki, B. E.: Prevention of upper gastrointestinal bleeding in

burn patients: A role for elemental diet. Arch. Surg., *115*:1073–1076, 1980.

164. Solem, L. D., Strate, R. G., and Fischer, R. P.: Antacid therapy and nutritional supplementation in the prevention of Curling's ulcer. Surg. Gynecol. Obstet., *148*:367–370, 1979.

165. Hobbs, C. L., Mullen, J. L., Buzby, G. P., Morrison, B., and Rosato, E. F.: The effects of nutrition on aspirin-induced mucosal ulceration in primates. Surgery, *86*:49–54, 1979.

166. Deysine, M., Katzka, D., and Rosario, E.: Stress gastric bleeding. Prevention of experimental lesions by intravenous hyperalimentation. Am. J. Gastroenterol., *67*:152–156, 1977.

167. Hunt, T. K.: Injury and repair in acute gastroduodenal ulceration. Am. J. Surg., *125*:12–17, 1973.

168. Wilmore, D. W., Goodwin, C. W., Aulick, L. H., Powanda, M. C., Mason, A. D., Jr., and Pruitt, B. A., Jr.: Effect of injury and infection on visceral metabolism and circulation. Ann. Surg., *192*:491–502, 1980.

169. Langlinais, P. C., and Panke, T. W.: Intrasinusoidal bodies in the livers of thermally injured patients. Arch. Pathol. Lab. Med., *103*:499–504, 1979.

170. Scholmerich, J., Kremer, B., Richter, I. E., Schmidt, K., Setyadharma, H., and Schoenenberger, G. A.: Effect of cutaneous human or mouse burn toxin on the metabolic function of isolated liver cells. Scand. J. Plast. Reconstr. Surg., *13*:223–230, 1979.

171. Lindberg, E. F., Grinnan, G. L. B., and Smith, L.: Acalculous cholecystitis in Viet Nam casualties. Ann. Surg., *171*:152–157, 1970.

172. Munster, A. M., Goodwin, M. N., and Pruitt, B. A., Jr.: Acalculous cholecystitis in burned patients. Am. J. Surg., *122*:591–593, 1971.

173. Weeder, R. S., Bashant, G. H., and Muir, R. W.: Acute noncalculous cholecystitis associated with severe injury. Am. J. Surg., *119*:729–732, 1970.

174. Rice, J., Williams, H. C., Flint, L. M., and Richardson, J. D.: Posttraumatic acalculous cholecystitis. South. Med. J., *73*:14–17, 1980.

175. Lescher, I. J. Sirinek, K. R., and Pruitt, B. A., Jr.: Superior mesenteric artery syndrome in thermally injured patients. J. Trauma, *19*:567–571, 1979.

176. Carter, E. A., and Walker, W. A.: Stress induced by acute burn trauma and cold inhibits DNA synthesis in regenerating rat liver. Submitted for publication.

177. Recommended Dietary Allowances. Edition 9. National Research Council, Food and Nutrition Board, Washington, D.C., National Academy Press, 1980.

178. Hirshowitz, B., Brook, J. G., Kaufman, T., Titelman, U., and Mahler, D.: 35 eggs per day in the treatment of severe burns. Br. J. Plast. Surg., *28*:185–188, 1975.

179. Hiebert, J. M., McGough, M., Rodeheaver, G., Tobiason, J., Edgerton, M. T., and Edlich, R. F.: The influence of catabolism on immunocompetence in burned patients. Surgery, *86*:242–246, 1979.

CHAPTER 25

Pediatric Enteral Nutrition

CHRISTINE KENNEDY-CALDWELL
MICHAEL D. CALDWELL

HISTORICAL PERSPECTIVE

As early as 1792 Danz suggested that fetal salivary glands might function in utero.[1] In 1855, Chievitz reportedly demonstrated salivary buds from the buccal epithelium of a two-month-old fetus. Subsequently, in 1908 Ibrahim[2] reported ptyalin (salivary amylase) activity in fetuses older than five months. Schiffer[3] in 1872 and Keating[4] in 1883 reported the salivary digestion of starch by term infants suggesting the presence of amylase in their saliva. During this same period, morphologic development of the small intestine had been studied carefully by Barry.[5] He reported absence of villi in a 1.7 cm, seven-week-old fetus; villi confined to the duodenum in an eight- to nine-week-old fetus; and villi along the length of the entire small intestine by 12 weeks of gestational age. The beginning of the modern era of research in the development of human gastrointestinal function can be attributed to the observations of such workers as Hess,[6] Johnson,[7] Keane,[8] Hewer,[9] and Tachibana[9–14] during the period of the 1920s through the 1930s. The reader is referred to an extensive review of this subject, "Development of the Human Gastrointestinal Tract," by Grande, Watkins, and Torti.[15]

Other chapters discuss normal human digestion and absorption and the alterations of digestion and absorption with disease. The purpose of this chapter is to point out special considerations of gastrointestinal physiology in infants and children and to discuss the resultant alterations required in enteral formulae for feeding sick children (Table 25–1).

DEVELOPMENTAL CONSIDERATIONS

The function of the gastrointestinal tract of the fetus is not as well defined as that of the neonate. The nutritive significance of fetal gastrointestinal absorption relates primarily to maturational events in readiness for birth and separation from the constant placental supply of substrates. At birth several small intestinal absorptive functions are marginal and barely able to complete digestion and facilitate absorption of nutrients. If gestation is interrupted by premature delivery, the margin of adequacy is further decreased. Furthermore, anoxia or sepsis will affect the adaptive response to the extrauterine environment.[16]

Three generalized patterns can be seen within the development of gastrointestinal function. In early gestation, specific morphologic characteristics of organs develop. By mid to late gestation, functioning components (such as hormones and enzymes) are present. At birth and during the early neonatal period, integrated gastrointestinal function (for example, the relationship between enterokinase and pancreatic digestive enzyme activation) is seen.[17] From the few reported attempts to study motility in utero, it is apparent that gastrointestinal peristalsis can only be demonstrated in the later stages of gestation.[17] Despite its importance to the care of newborn infants, our knowledge of integrated gastrointestinal function during the perinatal period is limited.

During gestation, most nutrients are provided to the fetus via the placenta. The fetus is able to swallow amniotic fluid at 16

Table 25–1   NORMAL DEVELOPMENTAL NUTRITION PROFILES*

THE PREMATURE INFANT

- ≦28 weeks' gestation (1–2 lb) sucking and swallowing reflexes weak or absent
- ≧32 weeks' gestation (3–4 lb) sucking and swallowing reflex present, not adequate to maintain nutrition
- not interested in feeding
- appetite no guide to nutritional requirements

FULL-TERM NEONATE

- peristalsis and swallowing unstable
- hiccups after ''burping''
- vigorous sucking elicited only when hungry, preceded by rooting movements; may stop sucking, rest, and even sleep for brief periods during a feeding
- definitely feels hunger and satiation
- indicates desire for food by crying and rooting movement
- notice: steady weight gain after first 4 to 5 days
- danger signals which may be organic or reactional to adult tensions are referable chiefly to GI tract: i.e., anorexia, failure to suck, vomiting, diarrhea

INFANT AT ONE MONTH

- gain of 1 lb over birthweight
- sucking when hungry still preceded by rooting movements; it now remains vigorous until hunger is appeased and is no longer interrupted by short catnaps
- sucking desire present when not hungry; will accept pacifier
- hunger constitutes powerful demand for attention
- periodicity of need for food becoming regularized
- enjoys sensation of warmth and body contact while eating

THREE MONTHS OLD

- gain in weight rapid
- peristalsis is usually in right direction and a little slower than earlier (less ''spitting up,'' stools less frequent and slightly firmer)
- sucking is strong and vigorous and is no longer preceded by rooting movements
- sucks and ''mouths'' fingers and anything held in hands
- shows excitement at sight of food
- enjoys spoon-fed food, though with considerable spluttering
- wants to be held when sucking milk

SEVEN MONTHS OLD

- weight gain in infant's own channel of growth
- vigorous sucking, enjoys sucking milk but also sucks fingers and anything baby can carry to mouth
- chews on everything, drools constantly
- has taste preferences and will spit out food not liked
- wants to feed self
- pats bottle
- may dive into bowl of food with both hands
- may take few sips of water or juice from cup
- chews food put into mouth with fingers, but may object to lumps in spoon-fed food

NINE MONTHS OLD

- weight gain in own channel of growth
- vigorous sucking
- holds own bottle; some prefer to lie on back and hold own bottle; others insist on being held to take bottle
- wants to feed self with hands
- interested in chewing
- interested in cup for water or juice

THE YEARLING

- tripled birthweight
- sucking is fading
- anticipation on sight of food; many also associate sounds with food
- has definite food preferences
- eats spoon-fed food well
- wants to feed self with fingers
- chews soft lumps in food
- enjoys sucking and may insist on holding own bottle
- prefers water or juice from cup and takes some swallows of milk from cup

Table continued on following page

Table 25–1   NORMAL DEVELOPMENTAL NUTRITION PROFILES* *(Continued)*

FIFTEEN MONTHS OLD

- growth has slowed down
- sucking is fading
- wants to feed self, except when unusually tired
- drinks water and juice from cup
- drinks some milk from cup, but may want bottle, especially when sleepy
- chews soft lumps in food
- amount of food consumed has decreased

THE TODDLER

- gain in weight is slow but steady
- sphincter control developing
- abandons bottle (large variation in age; this occurs spanning from late infancy to 2 years old)
- feeds self and resents any help except when unusually tired
- dining pleasures consist of getting food into mouth; conversation and companionship at meals more often a distraction
- table manners rudimentary; frequently uses fingers instead of conventional tools
- food consumption small

PRESCHOOLER

- weight gain slow and steady
- has mastered art of getting food into mouth
- drinks completely from cup or glass
- chews easily; eats what family eats
- table manners reasonably acceptable
- interested in companionship at mealtime
- actual food consumption small

SCHOOL-AGE CHILD

- growth is steady
- usually accepts family food patterns
- desires companionship at dining
- desires after-school snacks

PUBERTY—EARLY ADOLESCENCE

- rapid growth, males gain more weight and height than females
- constantly hungry
- companionship desired with meals

LATE ADOLESCENCE

- growth has subsided
- full stature almost attained
- food requirements approaching adult level
- companionship desired with meals

Adapted from: Sutterly, D. C., and Donnelly, G. F.: Perspective in Human Development. Philadelphia, J. B. Lippincott Co., 1973.

to 17 weeks of gestation. At term, fetal swallowing accounts for nearly half of the total amniotic fluid per day. This process can supply up to 0.6 gm/kg/day of protein as a nutrient source. Despite this ability to swallow amniotic fluid in early gestation, sucking mechanisms are not efficient until 33 to 35 weeks of gestation.[18]

Premature Infants

Appropriate for Gestational Age Infants

The premature infant has a defined gestational age of less than 38 weeks, usually weighs less than 2.5 kg, and is between the tenth and ninetieth percentiles of acceptable norms for intrauterine growth.[19]

In recent years, there has been renewed interest in the provision of optimal nutrition to high-risk neonates. This interest has been stimulated by the availability of more small premature infants (less than 1500 gm) because of their increased survival in modern neonatal intensive care units. In addition, it has been shown that malnutrition produces adverse effects on many organs and physiologic functions. The well-publicized studies of the pediatric population from Third World nations have documented impaired organ growth, specifically the human brain, caused by malnutrition.[20, 21] As might be expected, the organs most severely affected were the ones in an active phase of growth at the time the malnutrition occurred.

The myriad of problems associated with prematurity complicates the provision of adequate nutrition. First, the premature infant's energy stores are small; the fetal body contains only 3.5 per cent fat at a weight of 1.5 kg and 11 per cent at term, while glycogen stores are virtually nonexistent. The fat deposits are small because most of the fat deposition in the fetus takes place in the last six weeks of pregnancy. Thus, early provision of adequate calories is essential to minimize body composition losses and to reduce the incidence of hypoglycemia. Second, the premature infant has relatively higher energy needs than the term infant owing to a higher metabolic rate per unit body weight. This is a result of greater heat losses caused by the lack of subcutaneous fat insulation and a relatively greater surface area.[22]

Based on resting metabolic requirements of 40 to 55 cal/kg/day, Hierd and associates[23] estimated that without being fed, a neonate weighing 1 kg could theoretically live for four days, a 2-kg neonate for 12 days, and the full-term neonate for 31 days. The caloric requirements upon which these figures are based do not allow for growth, biochemical maturation, activity, or responses to stresses such as hypothermia or respiratory distress syndrome. This caloric intake only allows for survival. Third, the premature infant of less than 32 to 34 weeks' gestation has an immature sucking and swallowing reflex; thus regurgitation and aspiration are common. This is further complicated in the smallest preterms by absence of a cough reflex and weakened respiratory muscles. For the infants of less than 34 weeks' gestation, the imparied ability to coordinate suck and swallow usually mandates tube feeding. Frequent bolus or continuous feedings by nasogastric or nasojejunal routes are used.

Other factors affecting the immature neonate to limit nutrient intake are an incompetent esophageal sphincter leading to gastroesophageal reflux, delayed gastric emptying, and decreased intestinal peristalsis.[18] In addition several studies recently have been reported that suggest a delay in the maturation of anal-rectal continence in premature and newborn infants.[17] Although gastrointestinal motility is present in the newborn period, it is incompletely developed and is subject to suppression by prenatal complications. Further extrauterine motility studies are needed to determine if infants can respond to medications that facilitate peristalsis. The anatomic distribution of ganglion cells, even within the normal rectal and anal canal, is sparse in premature infants. This fact might account for delay in normal contractions and tone. Work by Boston and Scott,[16] who measured contractility of the anorectal sphincter in premature infants, demonstrated that contractions were generally apparent by 34 weeks of gestation but could be depressed for long periods with such complications as sepsis, hypoxia, or hypothermia.

The gastrointestinal digestive system is also immature. Sucrase and maltase enzymes do not attain maximal activity until the eighth month of gestational age. Lactase activity is present at approximately nine months of gestational age.[19] Thus, preterm infants are particularly predisposed to impaired lactose tolerance during the first weeks of life.

Another factor contributing to enhanced intestinal maturation and function is the presence of an adequate, mature intestinal surface for the final stages of digestion and absorption of nutrients into the circulation. Several studies have reported that the weight of the jejunum and the ileal villus:crypt ratio are decreased during the period of late gestation. Some observers suggest that an immature intestinal surface exists at birth and that the rate of cell differentiation is considerably less than that of the mature intestines.[24, 25] Other observers have suggested that accelerated maturation of the small intestines occurs when enteric feeding is instituted.[26]

Compared with adults, premature infants have decreased concentration and different composition of bile salts, which possibly account for their decreased ability to digest fats. Even fats more readily digested by term infants, such as those contained in human milk, are not as well assimilated by the preterm infant. Medium-chain fatty acids, however, are readily absorbed by the premature infant and thus are frequently used in formulas for these infants. No differences of practical significance in protein digestion have been demonstrated between full-term and premature infants, although difficulties with utilization of amino acids, as in the tyrosinemia of prematurity, have been described.

Small for Gestational Age Infants

Another subgroup of low birth weight infants includes those either small for gestational age (SGA) who may be at term (38 to 40 weeks of gestation) but weigh less than 2.5 kg, or premature infants who are less than 38 weeks of gestation but who are below the tenth percentile for normal group. These infants have lower nutrient stores because of limited transplacental acquisition.

Enteral feedings are preferable from a physiologic standpoint and should be the first choice if the SGA neonate demonstrates adequate function of the gastrointestinal tract. In addition to the biologic advantages achieved by the utilization of normal metabolic processes, it has been shown that intestinal mucosal integrity and function are better maintained if small amounts of nutrients are given continuously into the bowel.[26]

Early provision of calories may be even more crucial here than for the premature infant of the same gestational age who did not suffer from intrauterine malnutrition. Thermoregulation is often precarious in the SGA infant and hypothermia can lead to hypoglycemia, acidosis, vasoconstriction, and bradycardia. Higher caloric intakes are necessary for adequate growth, apparently owing to inefficient formula utilization resulting from the premature gastrointestinal tract and the increased metabolic demands. All low birth weight neonates (especially those who are small for gestational age) should be given nutritional support as soon as possible, and no later than the first eight hours following birth. Sick neonates in whom enteral feedings are precluded by virtue of their clinical picture should be started on parenteral feedings until toleration of enteral feedings is possible.

Term Infants and Children

The term infant and the child differ considerably from adults in regard to sufficient reservoir capacity for absorption of nutrients and adaptation to alterations in diet. The intestinal tract of a full-term newborn infant is approximately 240 to 300 cm in length. In studies by Requium[27] and Seaburg,[28] an average intestinal length of about 270 cm was found in neonates. The length of the small intestine from the ligament of Treitz to the ileocecal valve was measured in 183 infants and children ranging up to 15 years of age. Elongation of the intestine was rapid until crown–heel length was 60 cm and remained constant from 100 to 140 cm of body length. The small intestine continues to grow throughout the early years of life and doubles in length by the beginning of adolescence. The liver, which has developed to approximately 5 per cent of body weight at birth, represents only about 2.5 per cent of the weight of the adult. The gallbladder grows rapidly during the first two years.

"Anatomic" gastric capacity at birth does not necessarily reflect the functional capacity of the infant's stomach and thus provide a guideline for feeding of infants. Little objective information is available on the proper volume to administer to infants during initial introduction to feeding. Scammon and Dole[29] found the mean nursing intake of infants weighing between 2000 and 2500 gm to be 2, 4, 10, and 16 ml/kg of feeding on the first four days of life with a corresponding maximum intake being 3, 8, 15, and 24 ml/kg of feeding. This contrasts with the postmortem anatomic capacity of only 13 ml/kg in newborn infants weighing between 1500 and 2500 gm at birth. Thus, the functional capacity is far less than the anatomic capacity at birth, but rises rapidly to surpass the anatomic capacity by four days of age.

A general rule of thumb is that, at birth, an infant's stomach is approximately the same size as its fist. It continues to expand and by the tenth day it will hold approximately 3 per cent of the infant's weight; the 3 per cent rule holds during the first six months of life. Physiologically, the capacity may triple in the first two weeks of life for a normal newborn infant and is estimated to be 90 to 150 ml at one month, 210 to 360 ml by one year, 500 ml at two years, and up to 900 ml in later preadolescence.

The stomach empties fastest when the infant is in the right lateral position. The prone position also produces rapid gastric emptying. The stomach empties much more slowly when the infant is placed supine or in the left lateral position.[30]

The emphasis on infants should not suggest that the older hospitalized child is exempt from nutritional problems. Surveys among various children's hospitals show that malnutrition is evident in a high percentage of the population seeking primary care there. Especially in critical care and intensive care units for older children, the percentage of the population that is malnourished upon entry into the hospital is much higher than the general population of children in the United States.[31-33]

NUTRIENT REQUIREMENTS

The recommended dietary allowances (RDA) are the levels of intake of essential nutrients considered, in the judgment of the Food and Nutrition Board on the basis of available scientific knowledge, to be adequate to meet the known nutritional needs of practically all healthy children (Table 25–2). It is particularly important to note the following:

1. Since the requirements of many nutrients for children have not been established, and the essentiality of several nutrients has only recently been established, it is generally suggested that the RDA should be provided from as varied a selection of foods as practical to guarantee that possibly unrecognized nutritional needs are met.

2. The RDA are recommendations of the amounts of nutrients that should be consumed daily; they do not take into consideration losses of nutrients that occur during the processing and preparation of foods.

3. The RDA should not be confused with requirements, because the RDA (except for energy) are estimated to exceed the requirements of most children and thereby guarantee that the needs of nearly all are met.

4. The RDA do not cover therapeutic needs (they give intakes that meet needs of healthy children only) and consequently may not meet requirements as affected by disease states or medication.

5. The RDA are expressed for term infants and children with normal growth and development; they do not provide guidelines for premature infants.

The problems encountered in using RDA to determine nutrient intake include the lack of sufficient data in children regarding nutrient requirements, the difficulty in assessing when the requirement has been met, and the difficulty in assessing absorption in vivo. The attempted solution has been to err on the positive side to avoid producing deficits. Conditions that frequently require adjustment in dietary allowances include alteration in physiologic state, physical activity and climate, and illness and rehabilitation. With all of the previously mentioned shortcomings duly considered,

the RDA still provide the principal guidelines for enteral nutrient intake for children in the continental United States.[34]

Water

The normal rate of water turnover approaches 6 per cent of body content per day in an adolescent and 15 per cent per day in a young infant. The obligatory urine volume depends on the solute load to be excreted. In general this load is composed of urea, sodium, potassium, and chloride with other nitrogenous material and minerals as a minor fraction. The fluid requirement for a 24-hour period for newborn infants is generally 85 ml/kg, for infants under three months 140 to 160 ml/kg, and for children over three months approximately 120 ml/kg until two years of age. The infant has a relatively more liquid diet than an adult and more rapid water turnover, and hence is especially subject to dehydration. The infant is particularly susceptible to lack of water intake because his obligatory urine and insensible water losses are considerably greater than those of the adult. In addition he is far more subject to pathologic processes causing water loss, specifically vomiting and diarrhea. Symptoms of dehydration appear rapidly and have serious consequence. Premature infants, particularly those in intensive care units, have variable insensible water loss, dependent on their environment. In a study by Baumgart,[35] insensible water loss for infants nursed either in a wall-chambered Isolette or under a thin plastic blanket was significantly decreased in comparison with a controlled environment of an open bed. In addition, insensible water loss was significantly less for infants nursed under the plastic blanket compared with the wall chamber (1.55 ± 0.47 versus 2.45 ± 0.67 ml/kg/hr). In the controlled open bed environment, insensible water loss was 3.38 ± 0.69 ml/kg/hr.

Water balance must be considered a primary factor in these infants because frequently fluid intake is low, extrarenal losses of fluid can be very great (especially with diarrhea or during phototherapy), renal concentrating ability is low, and the diet generally yields a high renal solute load. Protein and mineral content of the formula is related to the overall renal solute load. In the more concentrated formulas fed to premature infants, the renal solute load is increased. In

Table 25–2 RECOMMENDED DIETARY ALLOWANCES, REVISED 1980*

	AGE (yr)	WEIGHT (kg)	WEIGHT (lb)	VITAMIN A (IU)	VITAMIN D (IU)	VITAMIN E (IU)	VITAMIN C (mg)	FOLACIN (µg)	B_3 (mg)	B_2 (mg)	B_1 (mg)	B_6 (mg)	B_{12} (µg)	CALCIUM (mg)	PHOSPHORUS (mg)	IODINE (µg)	IRON (mg)	MAGNESIUM (mg)	ZINC (mg)
Infants	0.0–0.5	6	13	2100	400	4	35	30	6	0.4	0.3	0.3	0.5	360	240	40	10	50	3
	0.5–1.0	9	20	2000	400	6	35	45	8	0.6	0.5	0.6	1.5	540	360	50	15	70	5
Children	1–3	13	29	2000	400	7	45	100	9	0.8	0.7	0.9	2.0	800	800	70	15	150	10
	4–6	20	44	2500	400	9	45	200	11	1.0	0.9	1.3	2.5	800	800	90	10	200	10
	7–10	28	62	3500	400	10	45	300	16	1.4	1.2	1.6	3.0	800	800	120	10	250	10

*Adapted from *Recommended Dietary Allowances*, 9th ed., with the permission of the National Academy of Sciences, Washington, D.C., 1980.

addition, if the formula is very concentrated, sufficient water may not be supplied to compensate for the impaired renal concentrating ability of the premature infant. Infants consuming less than a normal volume of formula are particularly vulnerable because, under constant conditions of extrarenal loss, the lower the formula intake, the greater the proportion of water required for renal excretion of the solute load. Infants whose water balance is threatened (by heat, phototherapy, cold stress, infection, or diarrhea) should have formulas of low renal load and should not be fed formulas of caloric density greater than 24 cal/oz.[36, 37]

Also related to fluid requirements in enteral feeding of children is the osmotic concentration or osmolality. For a detailed explanation of this crucial factor, see Chapter 10. The ideal osmolality of an oral feeding for children is the same as either human milk (approximately 277 to 303 mOsm/kg of water) or normal blood serum (approximately 275 to 325/kg of water).[36] Feedings greatly exceeding these values may cause osmotically induced diarrhea. As a consequence, the Committee on Nutrition of the American Academy of Pediatrics has recommended that formulas for normal infants that have concentrations greater than 400 mOsm/L should be labeled with a warning statement concerning potential side effects.

A number of factors may influence the osmolality of the formula: caloric concentration, formula composition, method of preparation, and variations in products within and between manufacturers' lots. Formulas containing supplemental iron do not significantly change the osmolality of the formula. There is no important difference in the osmolality of powdered formulas before or after terminal heat sterilization.[36]

Protein

At birth, roughly 2 per cent of the body consists of nitrogen as contrasted with slightly over 3 per cent for the adult. Most of this change occurs during the first year. As infancy advances, the curve of protein requirement falls off sharply, more sharply than the curve for caloric requirement. The reason for this is that activity is now the major function for which calories are required, and activity, unlike growth and maintenance, does not require a comparable expenditure of nitrogen. For the infant, about 35 per cent of the

dietary protein allowance of 2 gm/kg/day should be provided as indispensable (essential) amino acids. It must be remembered that the demand for energy takes first priority in metabolism and, as a consequence, if nonprotein caloric sources are not consumed in sufficient amounts, some of the amino acids—even from a diet inadequate in protein—will be used as a source of energy and will not be available for protein synthesis. The recommendations for protein intake for infants and children in Table 25–2 are based on ingestion of milk protein in infancy and a mixed diet that provides protein with an efficiency of utilization of 75 per cent in older children.

During periods of catch-up growth, protein requirements increase. Intakes of 3.2 gm/kg of milk protein when energy intakes are adequate have been suggested.[38] Foman has suggested that during infancy it would be more meaningful to express amino acid requirements per unit of calories consumed. Since this method would reflect both size and rate of growth, it should prove more useful than expressions of requirements on the basis of body weight alone. On this basis an estimate of protein requirements would be 1.6 gm/100 cal for children one to four months of age, and 1.4 gm/100 cal for children 8 to 12 months of age.[39] The American Academy of Pediatrics has set minimum standards for infant formula of 1.8 gm/100 cal with a protein efficiency ratio equal to that of casein. The protein requirement for any child will depend on the rate of growth and the quality of protein in the diet.

Protein is more efficiently utilized when carbohydrate and/or fats are consumed at the same time or soon after. It has been suggested that a safe ratio of protein to energy in the diets of children two to three years of age is close to 5 per cent.[39]

Energy

The energy expended by any child is determined primarily by body size and composition, physical activity, and the rate of growth. Energy costs of growth have been estimated to approximate 4.4 to 5.7 cal/gm of tissue gained. Decreasing rates of growth result in decreasing requirements for energy per unit of size (cal/kg). In other words, as children grow older they need a greater number of calories because of larger body size, but their need for energy per unit of size decreases. The caloric requirements of newborn infants are two to three times as great as those of the adult in terms of body weight. It should be pointed out that what is commonly referred to as basal metabolism—metabolism under conditions of rest—is actually not basal in the growing child, but represents the requirement for growth as well as maintenance. Energy required for growth is greatest in the newborn period, decreasing rapidly during the first year and more gradually up to the time of puberty when a spurt in growth occurs. The requirement for activity is surprisingly great, particularly in small infants; crying has been shown to double the metabolic rate.[40] There is considerable variation in the caloric requirements of individual children, chiefly because of differences in activity. The recommended daily dietary allowances established by the Food and Nutrition Board (see Table 25–2) assume that 50 per cent of the calories will be expended for maintenance, 25 per cent for activity, and 25 per cent for growth during infancy. Two sources generally provide energy in childhood: fats and carbohydrates.

Carbohydrates. Carbohydrates should generally supply between 40 and 50 per cent of the energy consumed by most infants and children. The Food and Nutrition Board of the National Research Council suggests minimum intakes of 50 to 100 gm/day of carbohydrate for children. In the infant over 50 per cent of ingested carbohydrate and in the adolescent over 80 per cent is eventually hydrolyzed to glucose. If intakes of carbohydrates are low, amino acids and fats are metabolized for energy. When this happens, there is a risk of ketosis from the breakdown of fat. Urea formed from the breakdown of protein will obligate additional water for excretion. Symptoms include dehydration, ketosis, loss of body protein, fatigue, and loss of energy intake. Excessive intakes of carbohydrate may load the enzyme system at least temporarily, and diarrhea may result.

Fat. The other main source of meeting the caloric requirements of children is through the substrate nutrient, fat. Fat, the most calorically concentrated nutrient, supplies between 40 and 50 per cent of the energy consumed in infancy and approximately 40 per cent of the energy consumed by children thereafter. A greater percentage of fat is absorbed in later life than in infancy. Approximately 95 per cent of ingested fat is ab-

sorbed by adolescents. Newborn infants absorb approximately 85 to 90 per cent of the fat provided by human milk. Many infants absorb less than 70 per cent of calf milk fat. Absorption of fat begins to reach adult levels between the ages of six and nine months. Mixtures of vegetable oils in infant formulas are generally absorbed well, although the degree of absorption is variable in disease states. The concentrated source of energy provided by fats per unit of volume is an asset during periods of rapid growth and illness when the volume that an infant or child can consume is limited.

Fat in the form of essential fatty acids provides components for cellular membranes and is a precursor for the synthesis of prostaglandins. Biochemical evidence of essential fatty acid deficiency appears when linoleic acid is fed at less than 1 per cent of the total calories. On this basis, the minimal requirements for linoleic acid for children are considered to be approximately 1 per cent of the calories consumed, and an optimal intake is thought to be 4 to 5 per cent of the calories consumed. Approximately 4 per cent of the total calories in human milk and 1 per cent of the calories in cow's milk are provided by linoleic acid. Commercially available infant formulas contain blends of vegetable oils and contribute greater amounts of linoleic acid. The Committee on Nutrition of the American Academy of Pediatrics has recommended that infant formulas contain a minimum of 300 mg of 18:2 fatty acids/100 calories (1.7 per cent of the energy content).[37] Human milk, cow's milk, and commercial infant formulas provide approximately 50 per cent of their calories as fat. No recommendation for intakes of fat has been made. However, if less than 30 per cent of energy intakes are derived from fat, a dry and unpalatable diet may result.

Vitamins

For premature infants on enteral feedings, formulas frequently do not meet the needs for certain vitamins and minerals. Thus it is recommended that the following additional supplements be provided until the premature infant is taking in an adequate amount of formula to meet his needs (Table 25–3): a multivitamin solution without iron and an aqueous vitamin E preparation (in infants less than 36 weeks of gesta-

Table 25–3 VITAMIN SUPPLEMENTS*

	A (IU)	D (IU)	E (IU)	B₁ (mg)	B₂ (mg)	B₃ (mg)	B₅ (mg)	B₆ (mg)	B₁₂ (µg)	C (mg)	FA (mg)	Fe (mg)	Fl (mg)	ADDITIONAL INFORMATION
Multivitamins (Content given per capsule, tablet, 1 ml injection or 0.6 ml drops, except as noted.)														
Adabee Tablets† (Robins)	10,000			15	10	50		5		250				Alcohol-free
Abedec Drops† (Parke-Davis)	5000	400		1	1.2	10	5	1		50				
Novacebrin Drops‡‡ (Lilly)	2500	400		1	1	10		0.8		60				30 µg d-biotin
Vi-Penta Multivitamin Drops‡‡ (Roche)	5000	400	2	1	1	10	10	1		50				
Polysorbin Drops† (Reid-Provident)	3000	400	5	1	1.2	8	3	1		60				Per 1 ml
Multivitamins with B₁₂ (Content given per capsule or tablet, or as noted.)														
Chew-Vite Chewable Tablets† (North American)	5000	400		3	2.5	20		1	1	50				
Vita-Tot Chewable Tablets† (Century Pharm.)	5000	400		3	2.5	20		1	1	50				
Poly-Vi-Sol Drops‡‡ (Mead Johnson)	1500	400	5	0.5	0.6	8		0.4	2	35				Per 1 ml
Vi-Daylin Drops‡‡ (Ross)	1500	400	5	0.5	0.6	8		0.4	1.5	35				Less than 0.5% alcohol; content per 1 ml
Bon-A-Day, Improved Tablets† (Spencer-Mead) Bugs Bunny Tablets† (Miles) Chocks Tablets† (Miles) Flintstones Tablets† (Miles) Multi-Chewz, Improved Tablets† (Spencer-Mead) One Tablet Daily† (Rexall) Spider-Man Vitamin Tablets† (Hudson) Unicap Capsules† (Upjohn) Unicap Tablets† (Upjohn) Unicap Chewable Tablets† (Upjohn) Vi-Magna Capsules† (Lederle)	5000	400	15	1.5	1.7	20		2	6	60	0.4			
Poly-Vi-Sol Chewable Tablets† (Mead Johnson)	2500	400	15	1.05	1.2	13.5		1.05	4.5	60	0.3			

Table continued on following page

Table 25-3 VITAMIN SUPPLEMENTS* (Continued)

	A (IU)	D (IU)	E (IU)	B₁ (mg)	B₂ (mg)	B₃ (mg)	B₅ (mg)	B₆ (mg)	B₁₂ (μg)	C (mg)	FA (mg)	Fe (mg)	Fl (mg)	ADDITIONAL INFORMATION
Vi-Daylin Chewable Tablets† (Ross) ⎱ Vigran Chewable Tablets† (Squibb) ⎰	2500	400	10	0.7	0.8	9		0.7	3	40	0.2			
Multivitamins with Minerals (Content given per capsule, tablet, or 5 ml.)														
Clusivol Syrup† (Ayerst)	2500	400		1	1	5	3	0.6	2	15				Mg, Mn, Zn
Nuclomin Tablets† (Miller)	2500	200	12.5	1.125	1.125	12.5	7.5	1.5	3	25				10 mg Fe, Cu, I, Mg, Mn, Zn, biotin, folinic acid
Mitey Vites Tablets† (Spencer-Mead)	2000	200	5	1.6	1.5	0.9	1.6	1.6	5	30				1 mg Fe, Cu, I, Mg, Mn
Cardenz Tablets† (Miller)	2000	100	5			20		1.5	1	25				I, K, Mg, inositol, PABA
Lemivite Tablets† (Lemmon)	1666	66	0.4	1	1	8	1.6	0.166	1	16				3 mg Fe, Ca, Cu, K, Mg, Mn, P, Zn
Stuart Formula Liquid† (Stuart)	3333	333	0.1	1.33	1.33	10	1.43	0.067						5 mg Fe, Mn
Ominal Tablets† (Kenwood)	3333	133		10	10	100	20	5	5	200				Cu, Mg, Mn, Zn
Multivitamins with Iron (Content given per tablet or 1 ml.)														
Tri-Vi-Sol with Iron Drops†† (Mead Johnson) ⎱ Vi-Daylin Plus Iron ADC Drops†† (Ross) ⎰	1500	400								35		10		
Taystron Tablets† (Vale				3					4	20		15		
Ferric B Jr. Tablets† (Jenkins)				2					5	30		10		
Feostim Tablets† (O'Neal)				3				1	5	20		18		Biotin
Abdol with Minerals Capsules† (Parke-Davis)	5000	400		2.5	2.5	20	2.5	0.5	1	50	0.1	15		Ca, Cu, I, K, Mg, Mn, P, Zn
Bugs Bunny Plus Iron Tablets† (Miles) ⎱ Chocks Plus Iron Tablets† (Miles) Flintstones Plus Iron Tablets† (Miles) ⎰	2500	400	15	1.05	1.2	13.5		1.05	4.5	60	0.3	15		
Multi-Chewz w/Iron, Improved Tablets† (Spencer-Mead)														

Table 25–3 VITAMIN SUPPLEMENTS* (Continued)

	A (IU)	D (IU)	E (IU)	B_1 (mg)	B_2 (mg)	B_3 (mg)	B_5 (mg)	B_6 (mg)	B_{12} (µg)	C (mg)	FA (mg)	Fe (mg)	Fl (mg)	ADDITIONAL INFORMATION
Pals Plus Iron Tablets† (Bristol-Myers)	3500	400		0.8	1.3	14	5	1	2.5	60	0.05	12		
Poly-Vi-Sol with Iron Tablets† (Mead Johnson)	2500	400	15	1.05	1.2	13.5		1.05	4.5	60	0.3	12		
Vi-Daylin Plus Iron Tablets† (Ross)	2500	400	10	0.7	0.8	9		0.7	3	40	0.2	10		
Monster with Iron Tablets† (Bristol-Myers)	3500	400		1.1	1.2	15	5	1.2	5	40	0.1	10		
Poly-Vi-Sol with Iron Drops†† (Mead Johnson)	1500	400	5	0.5	0.6	8		0.4		35		10		
Vi-Daylin Plus Iron Drops†† (Ross)	1500	400	5	0.5	0.6	6		0.4	1.5	35		10		
Multivitamins with Fluoride (Content given per tablet)														
Poly-Vi-Flor Chewable Tablets§ (Mead Johnson)	2500	400	15	1.05	1.2	13.5		1.05	4.5	60	0.3		1	
Standard F Chewable Tablets§ (Spencer-Mead)	2500	400	15	1.02	1.2	13.4		1.28	4.5	60	0.2		1	
Vi-Daylin w/ Fluoride Chewable Tablets§ (Ross)	2500	400	15	1.05	1.2	13.5		1.05	4.5	60	0.3		1	
Poly-Vi-Flor with Iron Chewable Tablets§ (Mead Johnson)												12	1	
Tri-Vi-Flor Tablets§ (Mead Johnson)	2500	400								60			1	
Cari-Tab Softab Tablets§ (Stuart)	2000	200					3			75			0.5	
Dentavite Chewable Tablets§ (Reid-Provident)	3000	400		1	1.2	8		1		60			1	
(Content given per 1 ml or as noted.)														
Florvite Pediatric Drops§ (Everett Labs)														
Poly-Vi-Flor 0.5 mg Drops†§ (Mead Johnson)	1500	400	5	0.5	0.6	8		0.4	2	35			0.5	
Vi-Daylin/F Drops†§ (Ross)	1500	400	5	0.5	0.6	8		0.4		35			0.25	
Poly-Vi-Flor 0.25 mg Drops†§ (Mead Johnson)	1500	400	5	0.5	0.6	8		0.4	2	35			0.25	

Table continued on following page

Table 25–3 VITAMIN SUPPLEMENTS* (Continued)

	A (IU)	D (IU)	E (IU)	B_1 (mg)	B_2 (mg)	B_3 (mg)	B_5 (mg)	B_6 (mg)	B_{12} (μg)	C (mg)	FA (mg)	Fe (mg)	Fl (mg)	ADDITIONAL INFORMATION
Florvite + Iron Pediatric Drops§ (Everett Labs)	1500	400	5	0.5	0.6	8		0.4		35	10		0.5	
ViDaylin/F + Iron Drops§ (Ross)	1500	400	5	0.5	0.6	8		0.4		35	10		0.25	
Ad-Cebrin c̄ Fluoride Drops†§ (Lilly)	2500	400								60			0.5	Per 0.6 ml
Baby Mins Drops§ (Spencer-Mead)	1500	400												
Tri-Vi-Flor 0.5 mg Drops†§ (Mead Johnson)										35			0.5	
Tri-Vi-Flor 0.25 mg Drops†§ (Mead Johnson)	1500	400								35			0.25	
Vi-Daylin/F ADC Drops†§ (Ross)														
Vi-Penta F Infant Drops†§ (Roche)	5000	400	2							50			0.5	Per 0.6 ml
Trisorbin F Drops§ (Reid-Prov.)	3000	400		1				1		60			0.5	
Adeflor Drops§ (Upjohn)	2000	400		1				1		50			0.5	Per 0.6 ml
Initia with Fluoride Drops§ (Parke-Davis)	1500	200		1				1		50			0.5	Per 0.6 ml
Vi-Daylin/F ADC + Iron Drops§ (Ross)	1500	400	5							35	10		0.25	
Abdec with Fluoride Baby Vitamin Drops§ (Parke-Davis)	5000	400		1	1.2	10	5.5	1		50			0.5	Per 0.6 ml
Novocebrin c̄ Fluoride Drops†§ (Lilly)	4000	400		1	1	10		1		60			0.5	Per 0.6 ml
Dentavite Drops§ (Reid-Prov.)	3000	400		1	1.2	8	3	1		60			0.5	
Vi-Penta F Multivitamin Drops§ (Roche)	5000	400	2	1	1	10	10	1		50			0.5	Per 0.6 ml
Polysorbin F Drops§ (Reid-Provident)	3000	400	5	1	1.2	8	3	1		60			0.5	
Fluoride Vitamin Drops§ (Spencer-Mead)	2000	400	5	0.6	0.6	8	4	0.6	1	60			0.25	

*Adapted from Facts and Comparisons, June 1980.
†Over-the-counter preparation.
‡Sugar-free preparation.
§By prescription only.

tion—50 IU daily until 40 weeks of gestation; minimally 1 IU of vitamin E/1 gm of polyunsaturated fatty acid (PUFA) in the formula). The age at which iron should be supplemented and in what amounts is still controversial. Many believe it should be given from two weeks on (or as soon as enteral feedings are established) in a dose of 2 to 3 mg/kg of body weight. Others feel that particularly premature infants do not need therapeutic iron and that this may inhibit absorption of vitamin E and increase hemolysis, and thus suggest iron be withheld until two to three months of age.[37] Folic acid should be supplemented to provide 50 μg/day until formula intake is meeting the RDA. Also a calcium source supplementation should be used to provide 50 mg/kg/day of elemental calcium until a weight of 2.25 kg is reached. Some premature infants discharged on breast milk may also need supplemental calcium.[22]

The breast-fed term infant should receive supplements of iron (7 mg daily from ferrous sulfate or other preparation of high bioavailability), vitamin D (400 IU daily), and on occasion fluoride if the infant lives in a deficient region (0.25 mg daily). Infants fed commercially prepared, iron-fortified formulas require no supplements, with the exception of fluoride, depending on fluoride content of local drinking water.

Vitamin supplementation of diets of toddlers and older children should be recommended only after careful evaluation of the child's actual food intake. Diets of children who restrict their intake of milk because of real or imagined allergies, lactose intolerance, or for hospitalization reasons should be monitored for calcium, riboflavin, and vitamin D status. Diets of infants and children receiving goat's milk should be carefully monitored for food sources of folacin. Diets of children who consume limited amounts of fruits and vegetables should be checked for sources of vitamins A and C. Medication intake should also be ascertained in order to extrapolate the role of any drug-nutrient interactions (Table 25–4).

Few satisfactory data are available for establishing vitamin requirements in the adolescent. Although most needs are met by usual foods, mild vitamin deficiencies are not uncommon in this age group, resulting both from a poorly chosen diet and the in-

Table 25–4   PEDIATRIC DRUG:NUTRIENT INTERACTION*

DRUG	EFFECT ON NUTRIENTS	RECOMMENDATION
Analgesics		
Aspirin	↓ absorption of vitamin C and folic acid, intake > 12 tabs a day significantly ↓ platelet aggregation and plasma ascorbic acid level	↑ use of food high in vitamin C
Morphine	↓ gastric and pancreatic secretions and appetite	supplement with vitamin and mineral capsule to meet RDA
Antacids		
Aluminum hydroxide	destroys thiamine; phosphate depletion if dietary intake is low	supplement; check dietary balance
Aluminum carbonate gel	in conjunction with restriction of dietary calcium and phosphorus may produce persistently lowered serum phosphate and mildly ↑ alkaline phosphatase	monitor with long-term therapy
Maalox	↓ absorption of iron if gastric content is not kept acidic	iron supplementation therapy if > 2 weeks
Anticonvulsants		
Carbamazepine	can lead to aplastic anemia	monitor
Phenobarbital	↓ absorption of folic acid, B_{12}, B_6, vitamin D, vitamin K; ↓ taste sensitivity	supplement; counsel patient and family
Primidone	↓ folic acid	supplement
Valpronle	affects gastrointestinal tract → cramps, nausea, vomiting, diarrhea, or constipation	monitor intake and output

Table continued on following page

Table 25–4   PEDIATRIC DRUG: NUTRIENT INTERACTION* *(Continued)*

DRUG	EFFECT ON NUTRIENTS	RECOMMENDATION
Anti-inflammatory Corticosteroids	↑ protein catabolism and sodium retention, ↓ glucose tolerance, ↑ urinary loss of zinc, calcium and potassium; causes fat mobilization and redistribution, especially in truncal area; ↑ metabolic need for vitamins B_6, C, and D	counsel patient and family; ↓ dietary sodium (2–4 gm), ↑ protein; restrict simple sugars, vitamin and mineral supplements
Antimitotics Methotrexate	inhibits folic acid utilization; ↓ B_{12} absorption; ↑ excreting nucleic acid metabolites	folic acid level should be 0.1–0.5 mg daily as excessive amounts alter response to methotrexate supplement with vitamin mineral capsule to meet RDA
Cardiac Glycoside Digoxin	↑ serum calcium level	monitor
Diuretics Furosemide	↑ urinary excretion of vitamin C, calcium, potassium, magnesium, and sodium	supplement
Hypocholesterolemics Cholestyramine	↓ absorption of vitamins A, D, K, B_{12}, carotene, and folic acid, fat, MCT, sugar, iron and calcium	supplement with fat-soluble vitamins and B_{12}
Laxatives Milk of Magnesia	↓ absorption of calcium and potassium, causes steatorrhea	supplement Ca and K
Mineral oil	↓ absorption of carotene, vitamins A, D, and K	counsel patient and family; do not use with food or at meal times
Minerals Ferrous compounds	with milk iron complexes and interferes with iron absorption	counsel patient and family; do not drink milk 1–2 hours before or after ingestion of iron
Neurologic Methylphenidate	suppression of growth, inhibits metabolism of anticonvulsants, ↑ loss of appetite, abdominal pain and weight loss	monitor anthropometric status and concurrent use of other drug therapy
Vitamins Fat-soluble preparations	toxicity with megadoses	monitor supplementation and counsel on OTC usage

*References: Molleson, A. L., and Gallagher-Allred, C. R.: Nutrient and Drug Interactions. Nutrition and Primary Care Series. Columbus, Ohio State University, 1980; Physicians' Desk Reference.

creased metabolic requirements during the growth spurt. As with other nutrients, vitamin requirements are best correlated not with age but with growth demands. Of additional special concern within the adolescent age group is calcium, iron, and zinc status. In the pregnant adolescent, studies indicate that inadequate amounts of iron, calcium, calories, and vitamin A are ingested.

COMPENDIUM OF ENTERAL FORMULATIONS

Tables 25–5 and 25–6 make up a compendium of pediatric commercially available enteral diets. There are two major subdivisions, the first being formulations appropriate for children over one year of age, the second for children under one year of age.

The first section includes indications for commercial tube feedings and supplements including a breakdown of the composition with specific factors of concern in the childhood population. The composition values are listed per 100 ml, and include preferred administrative routes and specific indications for use. This section includes: (1) tube feedings without lactose; (2) tube feedings and oral supplements without lactose; (3) elemental (predigested) diet without lactose; (4) modular formulas or components; and (5) oral supplements without lactose. The second section for children of under one year of age includes: (1) formulas appropriate for the full-term infant; (2) formulas specially designed for premature infants with an immature gastrointestinal tract; (3) formulations with low renal solute load; (4) formulas with manipulations of carbohydrate source secondary to allergy or disaccharidase deficiency; (5) hypoallergenic protein hydrolysate for easy protein digestion; (6) fat sources modified for use in significant steatorrhea; (7) oral electrolyte solutions for replacement of water and electrolyte losses; (8) carbohydrate-induced diarrhea; (9) feedings for inborn errors of metabolism; and (10) modular components for infant formulas.

METHODS OF FEEDINGS

The methods of enteral feeding for infants and children are similar to those for adults. Some of the common problems and their causes are addressed in this book in other chapters (see Chapter 13). However, in many instances the patient's condition and indications for different routes and feedings vary in children from the adult population. Common feeding routes are indwelling nasogastric tube feeding, transpyloric intubation, intermittent feeding by gastric tube, and continuous feeding by gastric and transpyloric tube. Also used in a pediatric patient, especially after surgery, is the feeding gastrostomy.

Common indications for nasogastric and oral gastric tube feedings are prematurity of generally less than 34 weeks of gestational age, short-term coma, need for constant drip feedings after severe diarrhea, major burns and hypermetabolic states, refusal to eat (such as anorexia nervosa), and nocturnal feedings. Contraindications include gastroesophageal reflux and intractable vomiting. Complications with these feeding methods include risk of aspiration, occlusion of airway in premature infants, intestinal perforation, lactobezoar, and nasal colonization.[41–45]

Transpyloric jejunal tubes in feedings have been used since the early 1970s in infants and children.[42] The indications for use include congenital gastrointestinal anomalies, inadequate gastric motility, and after upper gastrointestinal surgery. Jejunal feedings have not proved to be more efficacious than intermittent gastric gavage feedings in low birth weight infants. This route is generally not advocated for the routine feeding of low birth weight infants.[43, 46] For larger infants with bowel disease such as protracted diarrhea or surgically created short bowel syndrome and children at home with chronic disease, continuous and intermittent feedings into the jejunum have been found to be beneficial for maintenance and improvement of nutritional status.[47, 48] Complications involved in jejunal tube feeding have included bowel perforation, bacterial overgrowth, and malabsorption.

Gastrostomy tube feedings should be considered in those critically ill children who require extensive prolonged tube feeding, who have had undesirable side effects of intermittent tube feeding, or who have had an upper gastrointestinal tract anatomic abnormality. Other common indications include inability to suck or swallow as in developmentally delayed children; congenital anomalies such as esophageal atresia, tracheoesophageal fistula, and some types of cleft palate; esophageal injury with obstruction after ingestion of caustic chemicals; long-term coma; hypermetabolic states as in cardiac disease and severe respiratory disease; and home feeding management when parents are unable to follow nasogastric feeding regimens.

Gastrostomy tube feedings are generally contraindicated in children who have severe gastroesophageal reflux, intractable vomiting, or inadequate gastric emptying. Precautions must be taken that the tube does not obstruct the pyloric outlet and is secure enough to prevent removal by the patient.

Two developmental characteristics of children and infants must be taken into consideration when tube feedings will be given for prolonged periods of time. It has been demonstrated that premature infants who are supplied with nonnutritive sucking (such

Table 25–5 INDICATIONS FOR COMMERCIAL TUBE FEEDINGS AND SUPPLEMENTS*
(for children over 1 yr of age)

	ROUTE OF ADMINISTRATION	INDICATIONS AND COMMENTS

COMPLETE DIETS WITHOUT LACTOSE

Appropriate for patients with normal gut function or slight dysfunction of the gastrointestinal tract. These diets contain normal nutrient distribution with an optimal nonprotein kcal:N ratio of 150–200:1 and are available in a ready-to-use form. Used in hypermetabolic states, head and neck injuries (for example, radiation to these areas or wired jaws), coma, burns, protein-calorie malnutrition, inflammatory bowel disease, celiac disease, and mild pancreatic insufficiency. These formulas contain intact nutrients that require normal digestion and are not suitable in the presence of severe pancreatic insufficiency, a short or damaged intestine, or when the patient needs bowel rest (that is, during treatment of intestinal fistulas). All require additional free water secondary to solute load. Unless otherwise indicated all products are unpalatable when taken orally, contain no lactose, gluten or oxalate, and are very low in purine, cholesterol, and residue content. Most provide 1 kcal/cc. Certain formulas indicate NJ or J as an acceptable, well-tolerated route of administration and as such should usually be given as continuous infusions.

TUBE FEEDINGS WITHOUT LACTOSE

Complete B Modified	NG, G, bolus	To be used when a home-blenderized diet is anticipated. Contains moderate amounts of fruit and plant fiber. Lactose-containing version is still available (with dry skim milk) and may be beneficial when a higher residue diet is needed. Contains purines.
Isocal	NG, G, NJ or J bolus	Contains intact sources of nutrients (protein isolates) with exception of fat. Of 37%, 30% is soy oil and 7% MCT oil. It has been successfully used as an NJ or J feed. Can be used as a home-blenderized diet and is isotonic.
Osmolite	NG, G, NJ or J bolus	Is very similar in composition to Isocal except a greater per cent of kcal come from MCT oil (16%) and therefore may be helpful in the management of patients with fat malabsorption. Also isotonic.
Portagen	NG, G, NJ or J	Unique in that 34% of total kcal come from MCT oil. Product should be used when fat absorption is impaired such as may occur in the following clinical conditions: pancreatic insufficiency, bile acid deficiency, some intestinal resections, and lymphatic anomalies. Needs to be ordered as 1 kcal/ml because it is also available as an infant formula. Requires mixing.

TUBE FEEDINGS/ORAL SUPPLEMENTS WITHOUT LACTOSE

Precision	P.O., NG, G bolus	Slightly lower fat content at 28%. This well accepted oral supplement has been well tolerated, particularly with inflammatory bowel diseases. Orange and vanilla flavors available. Isotonic. Requires mixing.
Ensure	P.O., NG, G bolus	Because it is slightly hypertonic it should be sipped slowly to avoid diarrhea and is not suggested as a transpyloric feeding. Multi-flavored: vanilla, chocolate, and strawberry. All but chocolate are purine-free.
Ensure Plus (1.5 kcal/cc)	P.O., continuous NG, or G	Contains less than optimal nonprotein kcal-to-nitrogen ratio, but is actually more palatable than Ensure 1 kcal/cc. It is particularly important to sip slowly (600 mOsm H_2O) and is not recommended as a transpyloric feeding. Flavors as above.
Magnacal (2 kcal/cc)	P.O., continuous, NG, or G	Particularly useful in fluid restrictions or when patient is unable to ingest adequate volumes of food (as oncology patients). Transpyloric feedings are not recommended. Available in bland vanilla so a variety of flavors can be added. As product is a concentrated source of nutrients, fluid balance must be closely monitored.

ELEMENTAL (PREDIGESTED) DIET WITHOUT LACTOSE

Vital	Continuous NG, G	Indicated when significant gastrointestinal dysfunction is present, such as that found in steatorrhea secondary to severe pancreatic insufficiency, radiation therapy to the bowel, and short-gut syndrome. Also indicated for treatment of intractable diarrhea, exudative enteropathy, bowel rest, and lower intestinal fistulas. Because it is absorbed proximally and has a low-residue content, it is appropriate as a bowel preparation. Note that it contains an adequate per cent of linoleic kcal to prevent fatty acid deficiency. Not suggested as a transpyloric feeding secondary to its high osmolality.
	P.O. when flavored	

Table 25–5　INDICATIONS FOR COMMERCIAL TUBE FEEDING AND SUPPLEMENTS*
(for children over 1 yr of age) *(Continued)*

				COMPOSITION PER 100 ML							
kcal/ml	CARBO-HYDRATE	PROTEIN	FAT	mOsm/kg H$_2$O	N:NPK	% kcal Linoleic	gm PRO-TEIN	Vit. D (IU)	mg CA/mg P	mg Fe	mEq Na/mEq K
1	53% (hydro-lyzed cereal, solids, fruit, vegetables, and orange juice)	16% (beef puree)	31% (corn oil; mono- and diglycerides)	300	1:131	11%	4.2	26.6	67/93	1.2	2.9/3.6
1	50% (glucose, oligosaccha-rides)	13% (Ca and Na caseinate soy protein isolate)	37% (soy oil, 80%; MCT oil, 20%)	300	1:167	16%	3.4	21	63/53	1	2.3/3.4
1	55% (corn syrup solids)	14% (Na and Ca caseinate soy protein isolate, 12%)	31% (MCT oil, 50%; corn oil, 40%; soy oil, 10%)	300	1:153	10%	3.5	21	54/54	.92	2.4/2.2
1	45% (corn syrup solids, 73%; sucrose, 25%; lactose, 2%)	14% (sodium caseinate)	40% (MCT oil, 86%; corn oil 14%)	348	1:161	4%	3.5	78	94/70	1.9	2.0/3.2
1	60% (glucose oligosaccha-rides, 75%; su-crose, 25%)	12% (egg white solids, sodium caseinate)	28% (soy oil, and mono- and diglycerides)	300	1:183	—	3.1	27	68/68	1.2	3.5/2.6
1	54% (corn syrup solids, 74%; sucrose, 26%)	14% (Na and Ca caseinate, 88%; soy protein iso-late, 12%)	32% (corn oil)	450	1:153	17%	3.7	21	54/54	.94	3.3/3.2
1.5	53% (corn syrup solids, 74%; sucrose, 26%)	15% (Na and Ca caseinate, 88%; soy protein iso-late, 12%)	32% (corn oil)	600	1:140	17%	5.4	21	62/62	1.4	4.5/4.8
2	50% (malto-dextrin sucrose)	14% (Ca and Na caseinates)	36% (soy oil)	590	1:154	13%	7	40	100/100	1.8	4.3/3.2
1	74% (glucose oligopolysac-charides, 83%; sucrose, 17%	17% (di- and tripeptides; whey and soy meat protein, 87%; free amino acids, 13%)	9% (MCT oil, 45%; safflower oil, 55%)	460	1:124	4%	4.2	27	67/67	1.2	1.7/3.0

Table continued on following page

Table 25–5 INDICATIONS FOR COMMERCIAL TUBE FEEDING AND SUPPLEMENTS*
(for children over 1 yr of age) (Continued)

	ROUTE OF ADMINISTRATION	INDICATIONS AND COMMENTS
MODULAR FORMULAS/COMPONENTS		

The following modular formulas/components are not designed as complete feedings. They can be added alone or in combination to increase calories, thereby changing the caloric distribution of that tube feeding or formula. Each component listed mixes well in beverages, formulas, or tube feedings. For infants under 1 yr of age, increasing the caloric concentration, and thus maintaining the caloric distribution, is more desirable than initially adding modular components.

	ROUTE OF ADMINISTRATION	INDICATIONS AND COMMENTS
Citrotein (.67 kcal/cc)	P.O.	Very well-accepted high-protein (24%) supplement with a flavor resembling Kool-Aid, with some vitamins and minerals added. It is also cholesterol-, gluten-, purine-, lactose-, and oxalate-free.
Polycose Liquid (2 kcal/cc)	Add to beverages, supplements and formulas	Liquid source of carbohydrate calories for protein- or electrolyte-restricted diets. Contributes minimally to taste. Caution is advised regarding amounts added to formulas or tube feedings, as the osmolality will be increased.
Controlyte Powder	Add to beverages, supplements and formulas	Concentrated source of calories for restricted protein and electrolyte diets, such as for renal disease.
MCT Oil (7.6 kcal/cc)	Add to beverages, supplements and formulas	Unlike LCFA, undergoes very rapid intestinal lipolysis. Does not require micellar solubilization for digestion and absorption and therefore is not dependent on bile acid availability. MCTs are absorbed adequately via the portal vein even when intestinal area is reduced. MCT oil appears to enhance absorption of LCFA. MCTs do not contribute to osmolality or contain essential fatty acids.
Vegetable Oil (9 kcal/cc)	To be added in formulas	This is more desirable to add to infant formulas when fat absorption is not impaired, as it provides slightly increased calories.
ORAL SUPPLEMENTS WITH LACTOSE		
Sustacal Pudding	P.O. only	An acceptable high-protein supplement with an optimal nonprotein kcal-to-nitrogen ratio, with vitamins and minerals added. Available in vanilla, chocolate, and butterscotch.
Delmark Milkshakes	P.O. only	Very palatable. Available in vanilla, chocolate, and strawberry.
Special Milk	P.O. only	Well-accepted supplement containing WCM plus dry skim milk powder (which does not alter taste of milk). It can also be flavored as desired and still retains milk-like consistency. Provides 16 mEq K per cup.
High-Protein High-kcal CHOP Milkshakes	P.O. only	Flavors available: chocolate, strawberry, banana, and vanilla.

G, gastrostomy; NG, nasogastric; J, jejunostomy; NJ, nasojejunum; WCM, whole cow's milk; LCFA, long-chain fatty acids; MCT, medium-chain triglycerides; kcal, kilocalories; N:NPK, gm N to nonprotein kilocalories; NA, not applicable
*Zitarlli, M. B., Healy, M., Lechner, D., Parker, L.: Children's Hospital of Philadelphia, Philadelphia, PA, with permission, 1982.

as a pacifier during gavage feedings) experience shortened time for completion of initial, and transition to total, nipple feeding. Findings suggest an increased weight gain in premature infants given pacifiers that may be due to an influence of lingual lipase on nutrient absorption.[48] Later, generally at six to seven months of age, infants who are developmentally ready for solids are at risk for developing rumination or other adverse side effects if not exposed to feedings during this critical sensitive period. It has been shown that children not exposed to feedings at this sensitive period later have difficulty taking normal feedings, failing to chew, refusing solids, or vomiting. Programs of oral stimulation and gratification should be designed to coexist when tube feedings are the sole source of nourishment during this first year of infancy.

Table 25–5 INDICATIONS FOR COMMERCIAL TUBE FEEDING AND SUPPLEMENTS*
(for children over 1 yr of age) (Continued)

				COMPOSITION PER 100 ML								
$\frac{kcal}{ml}$	CARBO-HYDRATE	PROTEIN	FAT	mOsm/ kg H$_2$O	N:NPK	% kcal Linoleic	gm PRO-TEIN	Vit. D (IU)	$\frac{mg\ CA}{mg\ P}$	mg Fe	$\frac{mEq\ Na}{mEq\ K}$
.66	73% (sucrose, maltodextrin)	24% (egg white solids)	2% (mono- and diglycer-ides partially hydrogenated soy oil)	496	1:78	—	4	42	104/104	3.75	2.9/1.7
2	100% (glucose polymers from hydrolysis of cornstarch)	NA	NA	850	NA	NA	NA	NA	30/6	NA	2.5/0.5
2	57% (polysaccha-rides)	NA	43% (partially hydrogenated soybean oil)	598	NA	—	NA	NA	1.6/3.2	NA	.17/.04
7.7	NA	NA	100% (frac-tionated coco-nut oil)	300	NA	0%	NA	NA	NA	NA	NA
9.0	NA	NA	100% (saf-flower oil)	300	NA	80%	NA	NA	NA	NA	NA
1.7	53% (sucrose, modified food starch, lactose)	11% (nonfat milk)	36% (partially hydrogenated soy oil)	—	1:211	13%	4.5	40	147/147	1.8	3.5/4.9
.95	51% (lactose, sucrose)	15% (cow's milk)	35% (cow's milk)	480	1:149	—	3.4	40	117/94	.061	2.8/3.7
.90	37% (lactose)	26% (whole and nonfat milk)	37% (whole cow's milk)	490	1:75	—	5.6	10	202/158	.083	3.6/6.7
2.8	28% (lactose, sucrose)	6% (whole and nonfat milk)	66% (cow's milk)	612	1:389	—	4.3	49	152/122	.06	3.3/5.0

MONITORING NUTRITIONAL STATUS

Sound, clinical judgment aided by factual data is necessary to monitor children with conditions that interfere with normal growth and place them at nutritional risk. The real value of measurements of physical growth and laboratory data depends on their accuracy and interpretation, and on implementation of appropriate follow-up efforts after identification of abnormality. There is little point in measuring physical growth anthropometrics if it is not done accurately or if the finding of an abnormal value does not trigger specific nutritional intervention procedures and treatments as indicated.

The goal of assessment of nutritional status in an office or clinical practice/hospitalized setting is to detect not only a malnourished child but also the child who is at risk for undernutrition or overnutrition. Early intervention will hopefully prevent full-blown nutritional disease and identify individuals

Text continued on page 458

Table 25–6   INDICATIONS FOR COMMERCIAL INFANT FORMULAS
(for infants under 1 yr of age)

FORMULAS APPROPRIATE FOR THE FULL-TERM INFANT
   Products listed are suitable for the full-term infant when a cow's milk formula of normal dilution or a calorically concentrated formula is desired. Nutrient distribution is essentially the same as human milk and there is no difference in composition among these products.

A. *Normal Dilution* (20 kcal/oz)

Enfamil, without iron	Available as ready-to-feed, concentrate or powder.
Enfamil, with iron	Available as ready-to-feed, concentrate or powder.
Similac, without iron	Available as ready-to-feed, concentrate or powder.
Similac, with iron	Available as ready-to-feed, concentrate or powder.

B. *Concentrated Caloric Density*

Enfamil, with iron only (24 kcal/oz)	Available as ready-to-feed; can be made from powder or concentrate by adjusting amount of water added.
Similac, without iron (24 kcal/oz)	Available as ready-to-feed; can be made from powder or concentrate by adjusting amount of water added.
Similac, with iron (24 kcal/oz)	Available as ready-to-feed; can be made from powder or concentrate by adjusting amount of water added.
Similac, without iron only (27 kcal/oz)	Available as ready-to-feed; can be made from powder or concentrate by adjusting amount of water added.

FORMULAS SPECIALLY DESIGNED FOR PREMATURE INFANTS WITH AN IMMATURE GASTROINTESTINAL TRACT
   Formulas designed for the premature infant necessitate manipulation of all three major nutrients. Lactose is found in human milk and may therefore have special significance; however, the LBW infant's lactase activity does not reach that of the full-term infant until the ninth month of gestation. Therefore, in these formulas only 40 to 50 per cent of the carbohydrate is available as lactose. This mixture of carbohydrates facilitates utilization because multiple digestive and absorptive pathways are involved. The whey-to-casein ratio (60:40) of human milk is incorporated in these formulas because (1) whey forms smaller, more digestible curds, avoiding lactobezoar formation; (2) offers a more appropriate amino acid composition which is higher in cystine (may be essential to the LBW infant), and lower in tyrosine, an amino acid which a LBW infant may not have the metabolic pathways to handle. LBW infants frequently are unable to digest long-chain saturated fats which form insoluble calcium–fatty-acid complexes, resulting in impaired absorption of fats, calcium, and other minerals. This poor digestion is thought to be related to low bile acid pools and poor reabsorption of the bile acids; thus MCT oil has been utilized. None of these formulas are fortified with iron, nor are they available outside the hospital. The LBW infant still requires supplementation with a multivitamin preparation with these products.

Similac Special Care 20 kcal/oz	Requires approximately 8–10 oz/day to meet calcium needs.
Similac Special Care 24 kcal/oz	Requires approximately 8–10 oz/day to meet calcium needs.
Premature Enfamil 20 kcal/oz	Requires approximately 12–14 oz/day to meet calcium needs.
Premature Enfamil 24 kcal/oz	Requires approximately 12–14 oz/day to meet calcium needs.
"Preemie" SMA	Requires approximately 16–18 oz/day to meet calcium needs.

Table 25–6 INDICATIONS FOR COMMERCIAL INFANT FORMULAS
(for infants under 1 yr of age) *(Continued)*

kcal/oz	CARBO-HYDRATE	PROTEIN	FAT	gm PRO-TEIN	Vit. D (I.U.)	mg Ca / mg PO₄	Folic Acid (µg)	mg Fe / mg Zn	Vit. E (I.U.)	Na mg/ mEq	K mg/ mEq	mOsm kg H₂O
20	41% (lactose)	9% (cow's milk)	50% (soy oil, 80%; coconut oil, 20%)	1.5	42	52/44	11	.2/.4	1.3	23/1.0	67/1.7	290
20	41% (lactose)	9% (cow's milk)	50% (soy oil, 80%; coconut oil, 20%)	1.5	42	52/44	11	1.3/.4	1.3	23/1.0	67/1.7	290
20	43% (lactose)	10% (cow's milk)	47% (coconut oil, 60%; soy oil, 40%)	1.6	40	51/39	10	.2/.5	1.7	25/1.0	78/2	290
20	43% (lactose)	10% (cow's milk)	47% (coconut oil, 60%; soy oil, 40%)	1.6	40	51/39	10	1.2/.5	1.7	25/1.0	78/2	290
24	42% (lactose)	9% (cow's milk)	49% (soy oil, 80%; coconut oil, 20%)	1.8	50	66/55	13	1.5/.5	1.5	34/1.5	83/2	355
24	42% (lactose)	11% (cow's milk)	47% (coconut oil, 60%; soy oil, 40%)	2.2	48	73/56	12	.2/.6	1.8	33/1.4	107/2.7	360
24	42% (lactose)	11% (cow's milk)	47% (coconut oil, 60%; soy oil, 40%)	2.2	48	73/56	12	1.5/.6	1.8	33/1.4	107/2.7	360
27	42% (lactose)	11% (cow's milk)	47% (coconut oil, 60%; soy oil, 40%)	2.4	54	81/62	14	.2/.6	2	38/1.7	125/3.2	420
20	42% (lactose, 50%; corn solids, 50%)	11% (lactalbumin and lactoglobulin, 60%; casein, 40%)	47% (MCT oil, 50%; corn oil, 30%; coconut oil, 20%)	1.8	100	120/60	25	.25/1.0	2.5	29/1.3	83/2.1	220
24	42% (lactose, 50%; corn solids, 50%)	11% (lactalbumin and lactoglobulin, 60%; casein, 40%)	47% (MCT oil, 50%; corn oil, 30%; coconut oil, 20%)	2.2	120	144/72	30	.3/1.2	3.0	35/1.5	100/2.6	300
20	44% (corn syrup solids, 60%; lactose, 40%)	12% (lactalbumin, 60%; casein, 40%)	44% (MCT oil, 40%; corn oil, 40%; coconut oil, 20%)	2.0	42	78/39	20	.11/.67	1.3	26/1.1	74/1.9	244
24	44% (corn syrup solids, 60%; lactose, 40%)	12% (lactalbumin, 60%; casein, 40%)	44% (MCT oil, 40%; corn oil, 40%; coconut oil, 20%)	2.4	50	94/49	24	.13/.80	1.56	31/1.3	89/2.3	300
24	43% (lactose, 50%; maltodextrins, 50%)	10% (lactalbumin, 60%; casein, 40%)	47% (MCT oil, 13%)	2.0	51	75/40	10	.3/.5	1.5	32/1.4	75/1.9	268

Table continued on following page

Table 25–6   INDICATIONS FOR COMMERCIAL INFANT FORMULAS
(for infants under 1 yr of age) *(Continued)*

FORMULATIONS WITH LOW RENAL SOLUTE LOAD

These formulas are often used when the infant's status requires a low sodium intake (contains approximately half the sodium of other infant formulas). Both formulas have often been used with the premature infant secondary to their whey-to-casein ratio (60:40) and have been well tolerated. However, less than optimal features for the premature infant include (1) carbohydrate content as 100 per cent lactose and (2) inadequate levels of folic acid, calcium, and vitamin E.

SMA 20 kcal/oz, with iron	
SMA 24 kcal/oz, with iron	Available in ready-to-feed, concentrate liquid and powder form; can be easily diluted to 20, 24, 27, and 30 kcal/oz formula.
SMA 27 kcal/oz, with iron	
PM 60/40 20 kcal/oz	Not iron-fortified. Only 20 kcal/oz available as ready-to-feed. Other dilutions can be easily mixed from concentrate liquid or powder form.

FORMULAS WITH MANIPULATIONS OF CARBOHYDRATE SOURCE SECONDARY TO ALLERGY OR DISACCHARIDASE DEFICIENCY

All formulas are designed for the full-term infant and are iron-fortified.

Soy Protein Base and Lactose-Free Isomil 20 kcal/oz	Hypoallergenic soy protein isolate to be used when cow's milk allergy is diagnosed. Lactose-free for the management of lactose intolerance due to diarrhea, primary lactose intolerance, and galactosemia. 20 kcal/oz available as ready-to-feed. Concentrate liquid and powder form can be easily mixed to increase kcal concentration. Will be substituted for Soyalac. Use in the premature infant can induce phosphorus-deficiency rickets.
Soy Protein Base, Lactose- and Sucrose-Free Prosobee 20 kcal/oz	Indications listed above also applicable. In addition, it is appropriate when a chronic or transient diarrhea also causes a sucrase deficiency and can be used in gluten sensitivity. Available in ready-to-feed and liquid concentrate which can be diluted to 20, 24, 27, and 30 kcal/oz.
Soy Protein Base, Lactose- and Corn-Free Nursoy 20 kcal/oz	For use when corn allergy is diagnosed; available in ready-to-feed and liquid concentrate.

HYPOALLERGENIC PROTEIN HYDROLYSATE FOR EASY PROTEIN DIGESTION

Nutramigen 20 kcal/oz	Indicated primarily in cow's milk allergy or other protein allergic sensitivity, severe or multiple food allergies, severe or persistent diarrhea, or other gastrointestinal disturbances. Also used as maintenance diet during elimination diet testing and in galactosemia. Iron-fortified. Available ready-to-feed and as powder that can easily be calorically concentrated.
Pregestimil 20 kcal/oz	Appropriate for idiopathic defects in digestion or absorption, intestinal resection, intractable diarrhea, cystic fibrosis, steatorrhea, and also food allergies. Contains 40% of fat kcal as MCT oil. Iron-fortified. Available as ready-to-feed and powder that can easily be calorically concentrated. It is an ideal elemental formula for infants.

Table 25–6 INDICATIONS FOR COMMERCIAL INFANT FORMULAS
(for infants under 1 yr of age) *(Continued)*

				COMPOSITION per 100 ml								
$\frac{kcal}{oz}$	CARBO-HYDRATE	PROTEIN	FAT	gm PRO-TEIN	Vit. D (I.U.)	$\frac{mg\ Ca}{mg\ PO_4}$	Folic Acid (µg)	$\frac{mg\ Fe}{mg\ Zn}$	Vit. E (I.U.)	Na mg/ mEq	K mg/ mEq	mOsm kg H_2O
20	43% (lactose)	9% (lactalbumin, 60%; casein, 40%)	48% (oleo, 33%; oleic, 25%; coconut oil, 27%; soy oil, 15%)	1.5	42	44/32.5	5	1.3/.4	.94	15/.7	55/1.41	300
24	43% (lactose)	9% (lactalbumin, 60%; casein, 40%)	48% (oleo, 33%; oleic, 25%; coconut oil, 27%; soy oil, 15%)	1.8	50	53/39	6	1.5/.4	1.13	18/.8	66/1.69	364
27	43% (lactose)	9% (lactalbumin, 60%; casein, 40%)	48% (oleo, 33%; oleic, 25%; coconut oil, 27%; soy oil, 15%)	2.0	56	59/44	7	1.7/.5	1.27	20/.9	75/1.91	416
20	41% (lactose)	9% (lactalbumin, 60%; casein, 40%)	50% (coconut oil, 60%; corn oil, 40%)	1.6	40	40/20	5	.26/.4	20	16/.7	50/1.5	260
20	42% (corn syrup, sucrose)	12% (soy protein isolate)	46% (coconut oil, 60%; soy oil, 40%)	2.0	40	70/50	10	1.2/.5	1.7	30/1.3	71/1.8	250
20	42% (corn syrup solids)	12% (soy protein isolate)	46% (soy oil, 80%; coconut oil, 20%)	2.0	42	63/49	11	1.2/.5	1	29/1.3	81/2	160
20	42% (sucrose)	12% (soy protein isolate)	46% (oleo, soy oil, coconut oil, safflower oil)	2.1	40	60/42	5	1.2/.3	.9	20/.9	73/1.8	244
20	52% (sucrose, 72%; modified tapioca starch, 28%)	13% (casein hydrolysate)	35% (corn oil)	2.2	42	63/49	10	1.3/.42	1.04	31/1.4	68/1.7	479
20	54% (corn syrup solids, 85%; modified tapioca starch, 15%)	11% (casein hydrolysate)	35% (corn oil, 60%; MCT oil, 40%)	1.9	42	63/42	10	1.3/.42	1.6	31/1.4	73/1.9	348

Table continued on following page

Table 25–6   INDICATIONS FOR COMMERCIAL INFANT FORMULAS
(for infants under 1 yr of age) *(Continued)*

FAT SOURCE MODIFIED FOR USE IN SIGNIFICANT STEATORRHEA

Portagen
20 kcal/oz

> Should be used when significant steatorrhea occurs in the following conditions: cystic fibrosis, intestinal resections, pancreatic insufficiency, lymphatic anomalies (intestinal lymphangiectasia, etc.) celiac disease, and biliary atresia. Available only in powder form. Iron-fortified. Contains 86% of fat kcal as MCT oil.

ORAL ELECTROLYTE SOLUTIONS FOR REPLACEMENT OF WATER AND ELECTROLYTE LOSSES

For maintenance of fluid and electrolyte balance during mild to moderate diarrhea and in recovery from diarrhea; contains balanced formulation including electrolytes, calories, and water in proportions needed to prevent metabolic deficits.

Pedialyte

Lytren

FOR INFANTS WITH CARBOHYDRATE-INDUCED DIARRHEA

RCF
20 kcal/oz

> For dietary management of infants or children unable to tolerate disaccharides or other carbohydrates found in commercial formulas. Specific indications include intractable diarrhea and glycogen storage disease. The concentrate does not provide a completely balanced formula unless diluted with table sugar, dextrose, polycose (glucose polymers), or corn syrup. Allows the physician to prescribe type and amount of carbohydrate that can be tolerated. Also contains soy protein to avoid symptoms of cow's milk allergy or sensitivity. Available only as 24 kcal/oz concentrate. Iron-fortified.

MANAGEMENT OF INFANTS WITH LEUCINE-SENSITIVE HYPOGLYCEMIA

S-14
20 kcal/oz

> S-14 by virtue of its low protein content, has a reduced leucine content. The formula supplies low, though adequate, quantities of leucine and other essential amino acids as judged by published estimates of requirements as amounts supplied by human milk.

FOR THE MANAGEMENT OF BRANCHED-CHAIN KETOACIDEMIA

MSUD
20 kcal/oz

> An amino acid mixture free of the branched-chain amino acids that also contains the fat, carbohydrate, vitamins, and minerals essential for the infant. It can be used as the sole diet until plasma level of leucine, isoleucine, and valine return to normal range. Supplementation with an infant formula or milk to provide sufficient branched-chain amino acids to meet minimal requirements is necessary as soon as plasma levels of each return to normal.

FOR THE MANAGEMENT OF INFANTS WITH PHENYLKETONURIA

Lofenalac

> Contains 11 mg phenylalanine per 100 ml, which is not adequate to meet the total daily requirement of the growing infant. Sufficient phenylalanine from other sources such as infant formula, breast milk, or cow's milk must be added to Lofenalac to meet the patient's minimum requirements for growth and development.

MODULAR COMPONENTS FOR INFANT FORMULAS
(Refer to Section III under Tube Feedings).

who may be in need of counseling and careful follow-up. The presence of chronic underlying disease or disability seriously interferes with adequate nutrition. As previously mentioned, nutritional assessment of the hospitalized pediatric population reveals that 20 to 50 per cent have nutritional deficits.[31-33] Nutritional assessment should begin as soon as the child is admitted to the hospital or in the pre-admission work-up in the office in nonacute admissions. The assessment should include anthropometric measurements, biochemical, laboratory, and x-ray studies, assessment of dietary intake, and basic physical examination.

Anthropometry, the measurement of

Table 25–6 INDICATIONS FOR COMMERCIAL INFANT FORMULAS
(for infants under 1 yr of age) *(Continued)*

				COMPOSITION per 100 ml								
kcal/oz	CARBO-HYDRATE	PROTEIN	FAT	gm PRO-TEIN	Vit. D (I.U.)	mg Ca / mg PO_4	Folic Acid (µg)	mg Fe / mg Zn	Vit. E (I.U.)	Na mg/mEq	K mg/mEq	mOsm kg H_2O
20	45% (corn syrup solids, 73%; sucrose, 25%; lactose, 2%)	14% (sodium caseinate)	40% (MCT oil, 86%; corn oil, 14%)	2.4	52	63/47	10	1.3/.63	2.1	31/1.4	83/2.1	158
6			3 mEq Na / 3 mEq Na	2 mEq K / 2.5 mEq K	3 mEq Cl / 2.5 mEq Cl							
20	40% (added carbohydrates)	12% (soy protein isolate)	48% (soy oil, 50%; coconut oil, 50%)	2.0	40	70/50	10	.15/.5	1.7	30/1.3	71/1.8	
								RCF with added sucrose				305
								RCF with added polycose				158
								RCF with added corn syrup				241
								RCF with added dextrose				520
20	61% (lactose)	9% (cow's milk)	30% (oleo, coconut oil, safflower oil, soybean oil)	1.1	42	42/31	5.2	1.25/.36	.93	16/.7	46/1.2	276
20	54%	7% (crystalline amino acids)	39%	1.2	42	69/38	10.4	1.25/.41	1.04	31/1.4	46/1.2	—
20	52% (corn syrup solids, 84%; tapioca, 16%)	13% (casein hydrolysate)	35% (corn oil)	2.2	42	63/47	10.4	1.25/.41	1.04	31/1.4	68/1.7	356

body size, weight, and proportions, is one of the most frequently performed child health and nutrition screening procedures. Reliability and accuracy cannot be stressed enough in the measurement and recording of growth parameters. To illustrate the impact of errors, for example, an error of 0.5 kg (1 lb) of body weight can displace an infant from above the tenth percentile to below the fifth percentile. An error of 2 cm (1 in) of body length can result in a similar displacement. Such errors can lead to incorrect conclusions regarding nutritional intervention and therapy.

To obtain an accurate weight measurement, a balance beam scale with nondetachable weights should be used. Infants and young children are weighed while lying down. A pan-type pediatric scale, accurate to within 10 gm ($\frac{1}{3}$ oz) is required. For older children, the standard platform beam scale, sensitive to within 100 gm ($\frac{1}{4}$ lb), is suitable. The accuracy of scales should be checked with a set of standard weights by a local dealer or inspector of weights and measurements at least two to three times a year.

Recumbent length is measured for children younger than 24 months or for children between 24 and 36 months of age who cannot stand unassisted. Two people are required for measuring an infant's length accurately. If at all possible, a length footboard should be used for accuracy. Length should be recorded to the nearest 0.1 cm ($\frac{1}{8}$ in). With premature infants in intensive care settings who are supported by critical care equipment (respirators and intravenous lines), length can be measured while daily weight is being obtained on the pan scale by taping a paper tape measure to the inside border of the metal scale. Stature should be used for children two years and older if cooperation can be obtained. It is essential to note whether length or stature was measured because length is greater than stature by up to 2 cm (nearly 1 in).

Head circumference should be measured routinely in infants and children until they are 36 months of age by a flexible, nonstretchable measuring tape. The tape should be pulled snugly to compress the hair because the objective is to measure maximal head circumference. The measurement should be read and recorded to the nearest 0.1 cm ($\frac{1}{8}$ in). Expected head circumference during infancy can be estimated by remembering that the average full-term infant will show the following increments in head growth: first four months, 2 cm a month; fourth to sixth months, 1 cm growth a month; and sixth to twelfth months, $\frac{1}{3}$ cm a month growth, for a total of a 12 cm of growth during the first year. In sick premature infants the head circumference increases at a slower rate. Patterns of head growth in premature infants seem to be a function of gestational age as well as of the infant's health. Intrauterine growth of head circumference in weeks 28 to 32 of gestation averages approximately 0.9 cm a week. The healthy premature infant of 30 to 33 weeks' gestational age averages, during the first 8 weeks of life, an increment of 1.1 cm per week, and during

weeks 9 to 16 of life an increment of 0.5 cm per week; thus total growth during the first 16 weeks of life is 12.8 cm. The older premature infant's (34 to 37 weeks) total increment during the first 16 weeks of life is 9.6 cm, with 0.8 cm a week during the first 8 weeks average, and 0.4 cm a week during the next 8 weeks of life. The sick premature averages only 0.25 cm a week during the whole first 16 weeks of life. Sick premature infants are defined as those requiring artificial ventilation or intravenous feedings for a period of greater than two weeks or longer (Figs. 25–1 to 25–3).[30, 49, 50]

Apparently, abnormality of growth is a nonspecific sign. Many conditions retard growth; some accelerate it. In addition, birth can be normal in the presence of disease, and growth can appear abnormal in the absence of disease (short children of short parents). Adjustments for parental stature can be made to the infant's measured length.[51] Interpretation and utilization of indices and standards vary from setting to setting. Different populations are better monitored by standards established for the population in question. At present there are not enough standardized data to monitor arm circumference and triceps skinfolds in premature infants. Head circumference, length, and weight are the only available standardized indices. An intrauterine growth chart reflecting growth based on actual gestational age is recommended for charting the increments for any infant less than 40 weeks of gestation. For infants and children of normal term delivery there are a number of standards available for comparison.[39] These include the weight for height for age index by McClaren and Reed published in 1972; the weight for height index by Waterlow published in 1972 and 1976; the height for age designed by Kanawati and McClaren published in 1970; the National Center for Health Statistics (NCHS) weight for height percentiles published in 1976; and Zerfas' weight for height classification published in 1977.

Although the nutritional assessment factors for children reflect the present adult assessment parameters, the future should bring us indices that represent specific variations within the pediatric population. Work on retinol-binding protein, prealbumin, 3-methylhistidine, somatomedin, and constituents of hair offers possible avenues for more specific nutritional assessment and

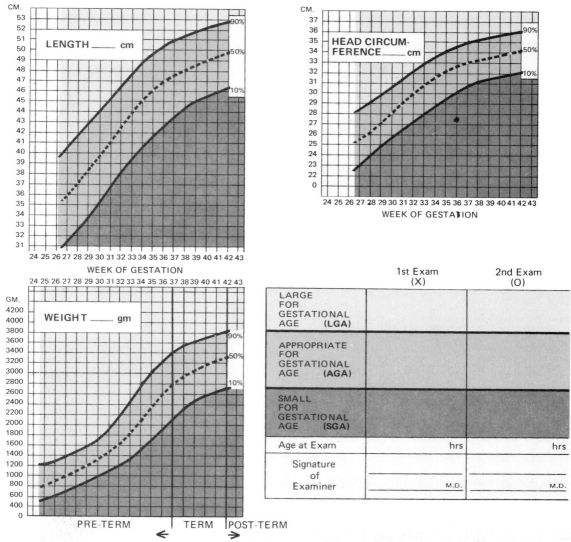

Figure 25–1. Classification of newborns, based on maturity and intrauterine growth. (*Adapted from* Lubchenko, L. C., Hansman, C., and Boyd, E.: Pediatrics, *37*:403, 1966; Battaglia, F. C., and Lubchenko, L. C.: J. Pediatr., *71*:159, 1967.)

monitoring. Systemic daily nutritional monitoring has led to a one week earlier discharge with greater improvements in length and serum protein levels at certain pediatric institutions.[22] See Figure 25–4 for recommended enteral parameters to be monitored.

NUTRITIONAL IMPLICATION OF PEDIATRIC DISORDERS

Nutritional therapy for children frequently follows the same channel of principles outlined for the adult; however, attention is directed to the need of additional calories and protein so that the child can meet the requirement for growth and development as well as the increase in basal metabolic rate. The following section is provided to briefly highlight the nutritional aspects in treatment of selected pediatric disorders which differ from the adult management. The reader is referred to other chapters in this text for comprehensive discussion of nutritional principles involved in management of conditions that are similar for both the child and adult.

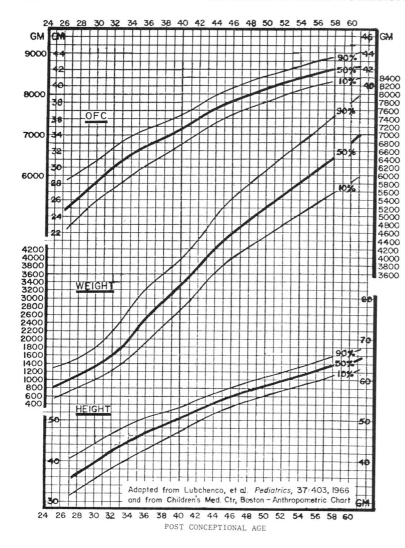

Figure 25–2. Combined intrauterine-neonatal growth chart for height, weight, and occipitofrontal circumference. (*Adapted from* Lubchenko, L. C., Hansman, C., and Boyd, E.: Pediatrics, *37*:403, 1966, and from Children's Medical Center, Boston, Anthropometric chart; *reproduced from* Stahler-Miller, K.: Neonatal and Pediatric Critical Care Nursing. New York, Churchill Livingstone, 1982.)

POST CONCEPTIONAL AGE

Bronchopulmonary Dysplasia (BPD). BPD is a well-recognized complication of hyaline membrane disease and its treatment. Recovery is often slow and prolonged, the therapy being largely supportive. Affected infants have been noted to grow more slowly and remain at a lower percentile during the first four months of age.[52] The reason for slower growth is probably a combination of several factors. In one study it was demonstrated that these children had a 25 per cent higher resting metabolic rate by measurements of oxygen consumption. This finding that resting VO_2 is higher in infants with BPD, and that as a consequence, resting caloric needs are greater, is of significant importance in the care of these infants. Caloric density of enteral formulations through both the fat and carbohydrate components must be increased to meet the needs of these children. Since these infants frequently are tachypneic, tube feedings or frequent oral nipple feedings are usually required.

Congenital Heart Disease. Congenital anomalies of the heart make up 12 per cent of all infant anomalies. Approximately 95 per cent of babies who require hospitalization for heart disease in the first month of life are term infants. Although most of these babies are appropriately grown at birth, they suffer from early growth failure from multiple factors. Inadequate caloric intake from decreased volume of intake due to rapid fatigue and labored respirations interfere with their ability to meet the increased metabolic requirements. Inefficient gastrointestinal absorption further prevents meeting their needs.

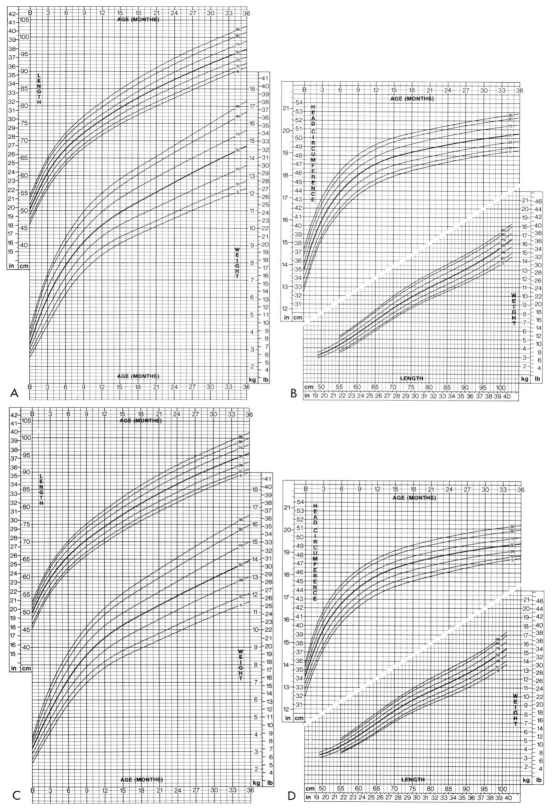

Figure 25–3. NCHS percentiles. *A,* For length and weight for age, boys, birth to 36 months. *B,* For weight and length, boys, less than 4 years, and for head circumference, boys, birth to 36 months. *C,* For length and weight for age, girls, birth to 36 months. *D,* For weight and length, girls, less than 4 years, and for head circumference, girls, birth to 36 months.

Illustration continued on following page

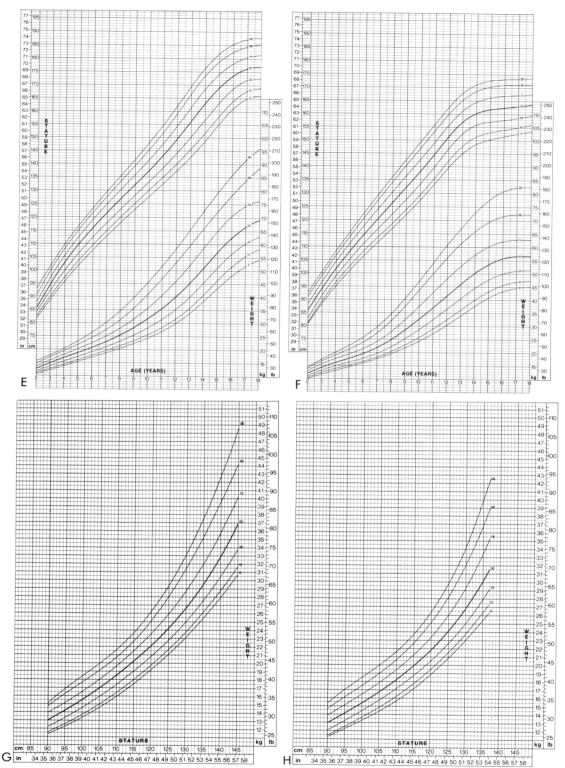

Figure 25–3 *(Continued).* *E,* For stature and weight for age, boys, 2 to 18 years. *F,* For stature and weight for age, girls, 2 to 18 years. *G,* For weight and stature, prepubescent boys. *H,* For weight and stature, prepubescent girls. From: Hamill P. V. V., Drizd T. A., Johnson C. L., Reed R. B., Roche A. F., Moore W. M.: Physical growth: National Center for Health Statistics percentiles. Am J Clin Nutr, *32:*607–629, 1979. Data from the Fels Research Institute, Wright State University School of Medicine, Yellow Springs, Ohio, with permission.

CHILDREN'S HOSPITAL OF PHILADELPHIA
NEONATOLOGY DIVISION
Enteral Nutrition Flow Sheet

Name: Problems:

Date of Birth: Birth Weight: gm Present Length cm Present Gestational Age: wk
Gestational Age: wk Birth Length: cm Ideal Weight: gm Head Circumference: cm

Date	Age (days)	Weight (grams)	Variation gm/day	Type of Feedings Ordered	Total Volume (ml)	ml/kg/day	Calories/day	Cal/kg/day	Protein/day	Pro/kg/day	Vit./Min. Supplements	Vitamin E	Folic Acid (ug)	Vit D (IU)	Calcium (mg) / mg/kg	Iron (mg) / mg/kg	Residuals/ Vomited (ml)	Stool/day	COMMENTS: RECOMMENDATIONS LABS
Weekly Average																			
Goal																			______ R.D. Nutrition Support

Figure 25–4. Enteral nutrition flow sheet. (Courtesy of Children's Hospital of Philadelphia.)

Growth failure is also affected by chronic hypoxia, acidosis, pulmonary hypertension, and repeated infections. Despite the fact that the weights of many of these infants equal or exceed average weight as newborn infants, the majority fall below the fifth percentile before they reach the ninth month. A clinical picture of failure to thrive frequently presents early in their management. Congestive heart failure is a complicating factor in children suffering from congenital heart disease, and they have been shown to have increased evaporated losses and a greater oxygen consumption exaggerating nutritional and fluid problems. Because of the ability to take only small volumes, formulas and foods with high caloric density must often be utilized. Clinically we have found it useful to add carbohydrate and fat to a standard 24 cal/oz commercial formula to increase the total calories to a 30 cal/oz solution, thus providing 100 cal/100 ml. Skillful and careful dietary management and monitoring are important so that manipulations of the protein and calorie sources do not lead to protein dilution, especially when the child is started on semisoft foods. When formulas are concentrated by adding less water to the commercial product, the renal solute load must be carefully considered. Sodium balance is of particular concern since an excess may precipitate congestive heart failure or jeopardize water balance because of high renal solute load. Sodium intake of 7 mEq/kg/day is advised for adequate growth, although the estimated requirement is 2.1 to 2.6 mEq/kg/day.[37] Fruits are frequently offered because of their ready digestibility and acceptability to young infants. Later when cereal is started, home-prepared unsalted vegetables may also be added. Supplements of vitamins, calcium, and iron should be given because of the decreased intake. An increased prevalence of biochemical riboflavin deficiency and folic acid deficiency has been documented in this population (see Table 25–4 for details). In older infants and children, meat may be given if the renal solute load is not considered to be a problem, otherwise meat should be limited to less than 1 oz/day or omitted completely.

Oncology. Children at particular risk for nutrient deficits are those with cancer involving the gastrointestinal tract, those with rapidly growing tumors, those undergoing major surgery, those with serious infections, radiation-treated children, and those on drugs that adversely affect nutrient absorption and metabolism. Children with cancer frequently suffer from both the disease and its treatment. Nausea and vomiting, changes in taste sensations, diarrhea, water retention, constipation, heartburn, bloating, and dryness and soreness of the mouth leading to swallowing difficulties are all incurred in this population. Generally, there is a need for increased protein and calories in a smaller volume than usually is taken in by children of the same age. There are relatively few studies of energy balance in patients with cancer and no detailed studies of energy balance in children with cancer. It appears, however, that there is evidence that increased energy requirements may be a variable along with insufficient food composition and alterations in metabolic status that lead to the rampant cancer cachexia seen in children. Estimation of energy requirements for children with cancer vary considerably. The unknown factor is how many calories should be allocated as a stress allowance by virtue of tumor growth. The work by DeWys on the pathophysiology of cancer cachexia suggests a 20 per cent addition to a basal metabolic requirement of 1270 cal/m^2/24 hr. To this was added a growth requirement of 0.4 to 1.1 cal/kg and in addition an activity allowance of 50 per cent to individualize the caloric requirements. Total protein requirements were estimated to be approximately 1.5 gm/kg/day utilizing nitrogen balance studies for this determination. Children with intestinal graft versus host disease may benefit by a specific nutritional enteral transition as employed by those at the Fred Hutchinson Cancer Research Center in Seattle.[53] Children with advanced cancer who are hospitalized frequently must rely on total parenteral nutrition because of inability to maintain enteral feedings alone. There are only a few cancer chemotherapeutic agents in common use in pediatric oncology today which are not associated with nausea and vomiting. The reader is referred elsewhere[54] for a comprehensive review of many nutri-

tional aspects of oncologic management and treatment.

Celiac Disease. This is a genetically transmitted disease with an age of onset varying between four months and sixteen years. The majority of cases occur between the first and the third years of life. Children with the disease frequently present as weak, underweight, and malnourished with retarded growth, a bulging distended abdomen, and excessive irritability. They suffer from a sensitivity to the gluten fraction in wheat, oats, barley, rye, flours, or cereals. The response is diarrhea and steatorrhea, with multiple vitamin and mineral deficiencies. Usually the child requires additional calories, protein, fat in the form of medium-chain triglycerides, and supplemental administration of vitamins A and D (in water-soluble form) and iron. Some children also require calcium and vitamin B$_{12}$ and folate to treat macrocytic anemia. The response to gluten restriction in the diet is not immediate and frequently requires two to six weeks of treatment before improvement becomes evident. A severely dehydrated child in a state of crisis should be started on intravenous therapy. If a child presents who is questionable, a formula such as Pregestimil, Nutramigen, or Portagen is safe to give until the diagnosis is established. At that point a gluten-free, high-protein, low-fat diet is usually started, after which the child is switched to a high-calorie diet excluding gluten as indicated (see Appendix for more recommendations).

Cerebral Palsy. This chronic disease frequently causes difficulty in sucking and swallowing, thus causing feeding problems. The subsequent inanition and fatigue experienced by these children leads to difficult problems with malnutrition. It is helpful with patients who tend to drool or expectorate to have them hyperextend their necks when being fed. Chewing is frequently a problem, and dental caries appears to be more prevalent than in the normal child. Drooling is frequently exaggerated by citrus fruits and, if these are avoided, a vitamin C supplement must be provided. A program of oral motor stimulation and physical therapy should be enlisted for these children during hospitalization.[55]

Cystic Fibrosis. Eighty to ninety per cent of these children have gastrointestinal involvement. They suffer from a decrease in the secretion of trypsin amylase and lipase into the duodenum. Therefore, they frequently suffer from poorly absorbed fat-soluble vitamins from intermittent intestinal obstruction from the thick mucoid secretions, anemia, and rectal prolapse. Fluid intake is kept relatively high to keep sputum thin and thus increase expectorations. A high-carbohydrate, high-protein, and low-fat diet is used to allow adequate caloric intake and increase weight gain. Frequently, medium-chain triglycerides are added to increase caloric density. Pancreatic enzymes are added with meals. Vitamins are given in two times the RDA in split doses to help improve the absorption of fat-soluble vitamins and iron. Alteration in the increasing amounts of pancreatic enzyme administered leads to altered stool pattern. Thus, changes should not occur more frequently than every other day. Caloric and fluid requirements for patients with cystic fibrosis are approximately double the average recommendation. For small infants the caloric intake should be 200 cal/kg/24 hr; for older children 100 cal/kg/24 hr. Protein should be supplied in the amount of at least 2.5 gm/kg the first year of life. Feeding should be frequent, every two to three hours, because these patients generally have voracious appetites.

Diabetes Mellitus. The diet for a diabetic child follows the same general pattern as that suggested for a diabetic adult; however, a child's calorie and protein requirements per kilogram of body weight are higher to allow for growth and development. Protein requirements range from 1 to 2 gm/kg, depending on the age of the child. Mineral and vitamin requirements are also increased. The diet is usually adjusted to provide 15 to 20 per cent of the calories from protein, 35 per cent from fat, and 50 to 55 per cent from carbohydrates (see Appendix 25–1 for a breakdown of different levels of diabetic diets).

Chronic Diarrhea. Diarrhea is considered chronic if formless stools are passed for 14 days or more. Some patients will have intermittent chronic diarrhea—a few days per week of diarrhea alternating with normal stool. Periods of poor weight gain may result from malabsorption or lack of caloric intake. Frequently, lack of growth is due to the feeding of dilute hypocaloric formulas or clear liquids in an effort to reduce diarrhea as opposed to actual malabsorption. Nutritional treatment of diarrhea depends on the diagnosis and the age of the child. From birth to four months the causes are generally formula protein intolerance, absorptive defects, cystic fibrosis, short bowel syndrome, transport defects, and disaccharidase deficiencies. In infants from four months to three years, the causes are somewhat different: a chronic nonspecific diarrhea of infancy, milk or protein sensitivity, celiac disease, giardiasis, and congenital sucrase-isomaltase deficiency. Chronic diarrhea is less likely to be a pediatric complaint in children from three to eighteen years of age. But within this group it may be a presenting symptom in Crohn's disease and ulcerative colitis. Enteral nutritional regimens will vary depending on the diagnosis.

Duodenal Atresia. Oral feedings are usually possible two to three days after corrective surgery. TPN may be required if functional obstruction of the anastomosis complicates the case.

Failure to Thrive. Failure to thrive is usually considered when a child presents with a weight of less than the third percentile, a weight for height ratio less than the tenth percentile, and skinfold thicknesses less than the tenth percentile with no other organic cause of growth failure. The poor growth pattern is accompanied or masked by a variety of physical symptoms such as vomiting and diarrhea, and there are usually significant developmental delays or aberrations in development. Nutritional treatment should include meeting protein and caloric needs determined according to ideal weight beginning with three- to five-day calorie counts, daily weighings, and observation of the mother-child feeding interactions, and, if caloric intake is inadequate for growth, tube feedings may be necessary. If the child is severely malnourished with low total proteins and edema, parenteral nutrition is generally advised first. At particular risk are premature infants in the ambulatory setting.

Gastroesophageal Reflux. Gastroesophageal reflux is a nonspecific term to describe any episode in which gastric contents are returned to the esophagus. The presence of this condition may be either physiologic or pathologic. Reflux may present as chronic vomiting and regurgitation, rumination, cyanosis, poor weight gain and malnutrition, chronic wheezing and cough, recurrent aspiration, dysphasia, or chest or abdominal pain. Sequelae of gastroesophageal reflux are esophagitis, failure to thrive, recurrent pneumonia, apneic or cyanotic episodes, iron deficiency anemia, chronic asthma, esophageal stricture, and Sandifer syndrome. During the diagnostic evaluation and differential testing, many contributing factors can be delineated. It is important to elucidate the cause, but during the evaluation the child may still be able to be enterally fed. Upright positioning and thickening of feedings will not change the physiologic abnormalities. This may, however, diminish the overt amount of reflux and in the cases of less severe reflux postpone further invasive therapy until a later date. The upright position must be maintained for at least two hours following every meal and it may be necessary to change to nearly continuous upright position. In some children the problem improves with age. Others with significant sequelae, particularly severe failure to thrive, cyanosis, pneumonia, or gross esophagitis, require surgical intervention. Hiatus hernia with gastroesophageal reflux is treated similarly with small thickened feedings and nursing in the upright position. Parenteral nutrition is necessary if significant esophageal stricture or severe aspiration pneumonia develops.

Myelomeningocele. Myelomeningocele occurs in 1 of every 200 births. There is an 80 per cent incidence of hydrocephalus, along with muscle weakness and paralysis of the lower extremities, and loss of bladder and bowel innervation. Because of the relative inactivity imposed upon these infants by paralysis and leg deformities, they are predisposed to obesity from the time of birth. Obesity is a significant problem in these children and is usually present after the first 24 months of life. A decrease in muscle tissue and increase in fat in the lower extremities are readily apparent when surgery is performed on the paralyzed limbs. Thus, standard normal growth is absent and there may be a risk for disordered nutritional status when followed on a standard weight for height growth chart. There is very little information on nutritional considerations in the first three years of life. Excessive bottle feeding, early introduction of solids, and genetic influences, along with overprotective parental influence, lead to a teenage population with 90 per cent being overweight. The main goal, then, is to design a nutritional regimen that maintains stable weight while providing sufficient calories for continued linear growth.[56]

Necrotizing Enterocolitis–Short Bowel Syndrome. There is considerable evidence that early enteral feedings are involved in predisposing premature, high-risk infants to this disorder.[57] Evidence suggests that a 48-hour delay in the initiation of feeding in the high-risk infant, while not totally effective in eliminating necrotizing enterocolitis, might reduce the incidence. Although animal studies have demonstrated a protective influence of breast milk on the newborn rat, clinical studies in the human neonate have not totally substantiated this relationship.[57, 58] The children who survive necrotizing enterocolitis (if spared from short bowel syndrome) generally do not suffer significant late gastrointestinal problems. Other children who survive but require extensive intestinal resection frequently have to be supported on TPN for extensive periods before the remaining small intestine adapts to absorb adequate nutrients. Factors thought to regulate intestinal adaptation include: (1) exposure of the residual bowel to nutrients; (2) stimulation of the mucosa by biliary and pancreatic secretions; and (3) enteric and other hormones. Depending on the section of the bowel resected, additional or different routes of supplying vitamin and mineral nutrients must be provided.[59]

Renal Disease. Nephrotic syndrome is a general metabolic disturbance resulting in continuing large losses of protein mainly in the urine. This relatively uncommon pediatric syndrome generally occurs in the two- to four-year-old age group, and 80 per cent of the cases occur in children under 15 years of age. Nutritional care involves increasing the protein in the diet to 1.5 gm/kg of body weight or 60 to 100 gm/day in an attempt to maintain positive nitrogen balance. Sodium intake is restricted to limit edema formation. The intake is usually restricted to 500 mg/day, depending on a child's 24-hour excretion of sodium. Supplemental protein nourishments are listed in Table 25–5 for the child requiring these. Children with chronic renal disease frequently show a decrease in growth velocity and significant malnutrition. The energy requirements per kilogram of body weight are higher than in adults because of the differences in body composition and activity levels. The major cause of energy deficit in these patients with uremia is inadequate appetite or anorexia. Drug therapy frequently depresses appetite. Dietary manipulation by increasing carbohydrate intake with the use of carbohydrate polymers must be balanced with the frequent hypertriglyceremia seen in uremic children. Children with renal insufficiency and on dialysis have sodium restrictions to at least 50 mg/kg/day (2 to 3 mEq/kg/day) if hypertension, edema, or excessive interdialysis weight gain is present. Restrictions of dietary potassium and administration of potassium-binding agents is recommended when there is decreased renal function. It is generally recommended that these children receive additional folacin, 1 mg after dialysis, 50 to 100 mg/day of vitamin C, and possibly additional B_6 (1.2 to 5.0 mg/day may be given safely). Iron, zinc, and copper are also frequently low in children with renal insufficiency.[60]

Tracheoesophageal Fistula. Frequently, tracheoesophageal fistula repair is carried out as a primary procedure. However, if a child receives a staged procedure, many surgeons will also advocate a temporary gastrostomy. Feedings can proceed with the standard formula. It is important to provide sufficient water when feeding by this route. Oral feedings are usually started four to seven days after the definitive repair is done. Obstruction or leakage from the anastomosis might require a change to parenteral nutrition for these children.

REFERENCES

1. Feldman, W. M.: The Principles of Ante-Natal and Post-Natal Child Physiology Pure and Applied. London, Longmans, Green and Co., 1920.
2. Ibrahim, J.: Neure Forschungen uber die Verdauungs physiologie des Sauglingssalters. Verh Ges Deutsch Naturforsch Aerzte, 80:316, 1908.
3. Schiffer, J.: Uber die saccarificirenden Eigenschaften des kindlichen speichels. Arch. Anat. Physiol. Wissensch. Med., 72:469–473, 1872.
4. Keating, J. M.: Some observations on the salivary digestion of starch by infants. Med. Surg. Rep. (Phila.), 49:357–376, 1883.
5. Berry, J. M.: On the development of the villi of the human intestine. Anat. Anz., 17:242–249, 1900.
6. Hess, A. F.: The gastric secretion of infants at birth. Am. J. Dis. Child., 6:264–284, 1913.
7. Johnson, F. B.: The development of the mucuous membrane of the esophagus, stomach and small intestine of the human embryo. Am. J. Anat., 10:522–561, 1910.
8. Keene, M. F. L., Hewer, E. E.: Digestive enzymes of the human fetus. Lancet, 1:767–769, 1929.
9. Tachibana, T.: Physiological investigation of the fetus. I. On the trypsinogen in the pancreas. Jpn. J. Obstet. Gynecol., 10:27–32, 1927.
10. Tachibana, T.: Physiological investigation of the fetus. II. Peptone decomposing ferment in intestinal canal. Jpn. J. Obstet. Gynecol., 10:40–46, 1927.
11. Tachibana, T.: Physiological investigation of fetus. IV. Lipase in pancreas. Jpn. J. Obstet. Gynecol., 11:92–99, 1928.
12. Tachibana, T.: Physiological investigation of fetus. VIII. Invertase in intestinal canal. Jpn. J. Obstet. Gynecol., 12:40–49, 1929.
13. Tachibana, T.: Physiological investigation of the fetus. VII. Maltese in intestines and pancreas. Jpn. J. Obstet. Gynecol., 12:21–32, 1929.
14. Tachibana, T.: Physiological investigation of fetus. IX. Lactase in intestinal canal. Jpn. J. Obstet. Gynecol., 12:100–110, 1929.
15. Grand, R. J., Watkins, J. B., and Torti, F. M.: Development of the human gastrointestinal tract—a review. Gastroenterology, 70:790–810, 1976.
16. Boston, V. E., and Scott, J. E.: Anorectal monometry as a diagnosis method in the neonatal period. J. Pediatr. Surg., 11:9, 1976.
17. Walker, W. A.: Development of gastrointestinal function and selected dysfunctions. In Selected Aspects of Perinatal Gastroenterology. Mead Johnson Symposium, No. 11, 1977.
18. Fitzgerald, J. F.: Development of gut function: Motility, digestion, enzymes, absorption, microflora and sucking response. In Sunshine, P. (ed.): Feeding the Neonate Weighing Less than 1,500 Grams—Nutrition and Beyond. Ross Conference on Pediatric Research, No. 79, Columbus, Ohio, Ross Laboratories, 1980.
19. Rickard, K., and Gresham, E.: Nutritional considerations for the newborn requiring intensive care. J. Am. Diet. Assoc., 66:592, 1975.
20. Dickerson, J. W. T.: Nutrition, brain growth and development. Clin. Dev. Med., no. 77/78, 1981.
21. Dobbing, J.: The later development of the brain and its vulnerability. Scientific Foundations of Pediatrics.
22. Avery, G. B., and Fletcher, A. B.: Nutrition. In Avery, G. (ed.): Neonatology. Edition 2. Philadelphia, J. B. Lippincott, 1981.
23. Nutritional care for the low-birth-weight and high-risk neonate. p. 736–754.
24. Sunshine, P.: Absorption and malabsorption of carbohydrates. In Selected Aspects of Perinatal Gastroenterology, Mead Johnson Symposium, No. 11, 1977.
25. Sunshine, P.: Digestion and absorption of proteins. In Selected Aspects of Perinatal Gastroenterology, Mead Johnson Symposium, No. 11, 1977.
26. Reimer, S. L., Michener, W. M., and Steiger, E.: Nutritional support of the critically ill child. Pediatr. Clin. North Am., 27:647, 1980.
27. Reiquium, C. W., Allen, R. P., and Akers, D. R.: Normal and abnormal small bowel lengths. Am. J. Dis. Child., 109:447, 1965.
28. Siebert, J. R.: Small intestinal length in infants and children. Am. J. Dis. Child., 134:593, 1980.
29. Scammon, R. E., and Doyle, L.O.: Am. J. Dis. Child., 20:516–538, 1920.
30. McMillan, J. A., Stockman, J. A., and Oski, F. A.: The Whole Pediatrician Catalog, Volume 2, Philadelphia, W. B. Saunders Co., 1979.
31. Merrit, R. J., and Suskind, R. M.: Nutritional survey of hospitalized pediatric patients. Am. J. Clin. Nutr., 32:1320, 1979.
32. Parsons, H. B., Fiancoeur, T. E., et al.: The nutritional status of hospitalized children. Am. J. Clin. Nutr., 33:1140, 1980.
33. Cooper, A., Jacobowski, D., et al.: Nutritional assessment: An integral part of the preoperative surgical evaluation. J. Pediatr. Surg., 16:554, 1981.
34. Caldwell, M. D., and Kennedy-Caldwell, C.: Normal nutritional requirements. Surg. Clin. North Am., 61:489, 1981.

35. Baumgart, S., Engle, W. D., Fox, W. W., et al.: Effect of heat shielding on convective and evaporative heat losses and on radiant heat transfer in the premature infant. J. Pediatr., 99:948, 1981.
36. Zenk, K. E., and Huxtable, P. F.: Osmolarity of infant formulas, tube feeding, and total parenteral nutrition solutions. Hosp. Formulary, 577, 1978.
37. Pediatric Nutrition Handbook. American Academy of Pediatrics Committee on Nutrition, Evanston, Illinois, 1979.
38. Fomon, S. J., et al.: Requirements for protein and essential amino acids in early infancy. Acta Pediatr. Scand., 62:33, 1973.
39. Pipes, P. L.: Nutrition in Infancy and Childhood. St. Louis, C. V. Mosby, 1981.
40. Snydeman, S. E.: Nutrition in infancy and adolescence. In Goodhart, R. S., and Shils, M. E. (eds.): Modern Nutrition in Health and Disease. Edition 6. Philadelphia, Lea and Febiger, 1980.
41. Robbins, S., Thorp, J., and Wadsworth, C.: Tube feeding of infants and children. ASPEN Monograph, A.S.P.E.N. Washington D.C., 1982.
42. Ehrenkranz, R. A.: Continuous and bolus techniques for alimentation of the low-birth-weight infant. In Sunshine, P. (ed.): Feeding the Neonate Weighing Less than 1,500 grams—Nutrition and Beyond. Ross Conference on Pediatric Research, No. 79, Columbus, Ohio, Ross Laboratories, 1980.
43. Pereira, G. R., and Lemons, J. A.: Controlled study of transpyloric and intermittent gavage feeding in the small preterm infant. Pediatrics, 67:68, 1980.
44. Personal communication. Children's Hospital National Medical Center, Washington, D.C., February, 1979.
45. Merten, D. F., Mumford, L., Filston, H., et al.: Radiological observations during transpyloric tube feeding in infants of low birth weight. Pediatr. Radiol., 136:67, 1980.
46. Drew, J. H., Johnston, R., Finocchiaso, C., et al.: A comparison of nasojejunal with nasogastric feedings in low birth weight infants. Aust. Paediatr. J., 15:98, 1979.
47. Parker, P., Stroop, S., and Greene, H.: A controlled comparison of continuous versus intermittent feeding in the treatment of infants with intestinal disease. J. Pediatr., 99:360, 1981.
48. Bernbaum, J., Pereira, G. R., Watkins, J. B., et al.: Enhanced growth and gastrointestinal function in premature infants given non-nutritive sucking (abstract). In Proceedings of Society for Pediatric Research, San Francisco, April 1980.
49. Mark, K. H., Maisels, M. J., Moore, E., et al.: Head growth in sick premature infants—A longitudinal study. J. Pediatr., 94:282, 1979.
50. Dine, M. S., Gartside, P. S., Glueck, C. J., et al.: Relationship of head circumference to length in the first 400 days of life: A mnemonic. Pediatrics, 67:506, 1981.
51. Himes, J. H., Roche, A. F., et al.: Parent-specific adjustments for assessment of recumbent length and stature. Monographs in Pediatrics, Vol. 13, Switzerland, S. Karger. 1981.
52. Weinstein, M. R., and Oh, W.: Oxygen consumption in infants with bronchopulmonary dysplasia. J. Pediatr., 99:958, 1981.
53. Graurreau, J. M., Lenssen, P., Cheney, C. L., et al.: Nutritional management of patients with intestinal graft-versus host disease. J. Am. Diet. Assoc., 79:673–677, 1981.
54. DeWys, et al: Cancer Res., 42:721–726, 1982.

BIBLIOGRAPHY

Alfin-Slater, R. B., and Jelliffe, D. B.: Nutritional requirements with special reference to infancy. Pediatr. Clin. North Am., 24:3–16, 1977.

American Academy of Pediatrics—Committee on Nutrition. Vitamin and mineral supplement needs in normal children in the United States. Pediatrics, 66:1015, 1980.

Andrassy, R. J., Page, C. P., Feldtman, R. W. et al.: Continual catheter administration of an elemental diet in infants and children. Surg. Nutr. 82:205–210, 1977.

Andrassy, R. J., and Wooley, M. M.: Progress in the use of elemental diets in infants and children. Surg. Gynecol. Obstet., 147:701–704, November, 1978.

Atkinson, S. A., Bryan, M. H., and Anderson, G. H.: Human milk feeding in premature infants: Protein, fat and carbohydrate balances in the first two weeks of life. J. Pediatr., 99:617–624, 1981.

Aynsley-Green, A., Lucas, A., and Bloom, S. R.: The control of the adaptation of the human neonate to postnatal nutrition. Acta Chir. Scand. Suppl. 507, 1980.

Babson, S. G., Benson, R. C., Pernoll, M. L., and Benda, G. I.: Management of High-Risk Pregnancy and intensive Care of the Neonate. Edition 3. St. Louis, C.V. Mosby Co., 1975.

Baens, G. S., Lundeen, E., and Cornblath, M.: Studies of carbohydrate metabolism in the newborn infant. VI. Levels of glucosin blood in premature infants. Pediatrics, 31:580–589, April, 1963.

Casolaro, M. B.: Nutrition and the sick child. Department of Clinical Nutrition. Children's Hospital of Philadelphia, January, 1982 (personal communication).

Chessex, P., Reichman, B. L., Verellen, G. J. E., et al.: Influences of postnatal age, energy intake and weight gain on energy metabolism in the very low-birth-weight infant. J. Pediatr., 99:761–766.

Christie, D. L., and Ament, M. E.: Dilute elemental diet and continuous infusion technique for management of short bowel syndrome. J. Pediatrics, 87:705–708, 1975.

Congden, P. J., Bruce, G., Rothburn, M. M., et al.: Vitamin status in treatment of patients with cystic fibrosis. Arch. Dis. Child., 56:708, 1981.

Cornblath, M., Wybreqt, S. H., and Baens, G. S.: Studies of carbohydrate metabolism in the newborn infant. VII. Tests of carbohydrate tolerance in premature infants. Pediatrics, 32:1007–1024, 1963.

Cox, J. H., and Gallagher-Allred, C. R.: Normal diet: Age of dependency, No. 4 in Nutrition in Primary Care Series, Ohio State University, Columbus, Ohio, 1980.

Daries, D. P., and Evans, T. J.: Nutrition and early growth of preterm infants. Early Hum. Dev., 2:383, 1978.

Enzi, G., Zanardo, V., Carett, F., et al.: Intrauterine growth and adipose tissue development. Am. J. Clin. Nutr., 34:1785–1790, September 1981.

Fomon, S. J., Filer, L. J., Anderson, T. A., et al.: Recommendations for feeding normal infants. Pediatrics, 63:52–59, 1979.

Glorieaux, F. H., Salle, B. L., Delvin, E. E., et al.: Vitamin D metabolism in preterm infants: Serum calcitriol values during the first five days of life. J. Pediatr., 99:640, 1981.

Greene, H. L.: Gastrointestinal development. In Johnson, T. R., Move, W. M., and Jeffries, J. E. (eds.): Children are Different: Developmental Physiology,

2nd Edition 2. Columbus, Ohio, Ross Laboratories, 1978.

Hartline, J. V.: Continuous intragastric infusion of elemental diet. Clin. Pediatr., 16:1105–1109, 1977.

Heittamper, M., Hansen, R., and Hansen, B. C.: Effects of rate and volume of tube feeding in normal human subjects. In Baily, M. V. (ed.): Communicating Nursing Research. Boulder, WICHE, 1973.

Illingworth, R. S., and Lister, J.: The critical or sensitive period, with special reference to certain feeding problems in infants and children. J. Pediatr., 65:839, 1964.

Jelliffe, E. F. P.: Infant feeding practices: Associate iatrogenic and commerciogenic diseases. Pediatr. Clin. North Am., 24:49, 1977.

Kagawa-Busby, K. S., Heitkemper, M. D., Hansen, B. C., et al.: Effects of diet temperature on tolerance of enteral feedings. Nurs. Res., 29:276–280, 1980.

Klish, W. J., Potts, E., Ferry, G. D., et al.: Modular formula: An approach to management of infants with specific or complex food intolerances. J. Pediatr., 88:948, 1976.

Krauss, A. N., and Auld, P. A.: Metabolic requirements of low birth weight infants. J. Pediatr., 75:952, 1969.

Larter, N.: Cystic fibrosis. Am. J. Nursing, 81:527, 1981.

LeLeiko, N. S., Murray, C., and Munro, H. N.: Enteral support of the hospitalized child. In Suskind, R. (ed.): Textbook of Pediatric Nutrition. New York, Raven Press, 1981, pp. 357–374.

MacKeith, R., and Wood, C.: Infant Feeding and Feeding Difficulties. Churchill Livingstone, London, 1977, p. 28, 31 (Figures 14 and 15).

McSherry, E. M.: Disorders of acid-base equilibrium. Pediatr. Ann., 10:44–58, 1981.

McWilliams, M.: Nutrition for the Growing Years. Edition 2. New York, John Wiley and Sons, 1980.

Merrit, R. J.: Neonatal nutritional support. Clinical Consults, 1:5, 1981.

Parker, L.: Glycogen storage disease. Department of Clinical Nutrition. Children's Hospital of Philadelphia, January, 1982 (personal communication).

Recommendation for infant feeding practice-Child Health and Disability Prevention Branch. Maternal and Child Health Branch, California, Department of Health Services, August, 1979.

Richmond, J. B., Eddy, E., and Green, M.: Rumination: A psychosomatic syndrome of infancy. Pediatrics, 21:49, 1958.

Roy, C. C., Sainte-Marie, M., Chartrand, L., et al.: Correction of the malabsorption of the preterm infant with a medium-chain triglyceride formula. J. Pediatr. 86:446–450, 1975.

Schreiner, R. L., Eitzen, H., Gfell, M. A., et al.: Environmental contamination of continuous drip feedings. Pediatrics, 63:232, 1979.

Shils, M. E., Bloch, A. S., and Chernoff, R.: Liquid Formulas for Oral and Tube Feeding. Edition 2, New York, Memorial Sloan-Kettering Cancer Center, 1979.

Sinclair, J. C., Saigal, S., and Yeung, C. Y.: Early postnatal consequences of fetal malnutrition. In Winick, M. (ed.): Nutrition and Fetal Development. New York, John Wiley and Sons, 1972.

Smith, D. W.: Basis and standards, approach and classifications, growth deficiency disorders, growth excess disorders, obesity. In Growth and Its Disorders. Philadelphia, W.B. Saunders, Co., 1977.

Stothers, J. K., and Warner, R. M.: Effect of feeding on oxygen consumption. Arch. Dis. Child., 54:415–420, 1979.

Sutterly, D. C., and Donnelly, G. F.: Perspectives in Human Development. Philadelphia, J. B. Lippincott Co., 1973.

Tuckermanty, E., and Gallagher-Allred, C. R.: Normal diets in adolescence, No. 6 in Nutrition in Primary Care Series, Columbus, Ohio State University, 1980.

Tuckermanty, E., and Gallagher-Allred, C. R.: Normal diets: Age of dependency, No. 4 in Nutrition in Primary Care Series, Columbus, Ohio State University, 1980.

Williams, H. H.: Differences between cow's and human milk. J.A.M.A., 175:104–107, 1961.

Williams, R. C.: Intestinal adaptation (Part I—Structural, functional and cytokinetic changes, pp. 1393–1444; and Part II—Mechanisms of control, pp. 1444–1449). N. Engl. J. Med., 298:22, 1978.

Worthington, P.: Infant nutrition and feeding techniques. Pediatr. Nurs., Jan–Feb 1977.

Zerfas, A. J., Shorr, I. J. et al.: Office assessment of nutritional status. Pediatr. Clin. North Am., 24:253, 1977.

APPENDIX 25–1
PEDIATRIC CONSIDERATIONS IN MODIFIED DIETS

The following is a collection of selected pediatric considerations in modified hospital and home diets. It is adapted from the work of the pediatric nutritionists of the Clinical Nutrition group, Children's Hospital of Philadelphia.

Diet for Diarrhea
(Brat Diet)

Purpose: The pediatric diet for diarrhea is used to eliminate or decrease the frequency and looseness of stools. Fluids are increased to avoid dehydration.

Use: It is used to introduce foods that are easily absorbed with limited digestive capacity. It is designed for children with symptoms associated with diarrhea not caused by lactose or gluten intolerance.

Adequacy: This diet is inadequate in all nutrients according to the National Research Council's Recommended Daily Dietary Allowances and should be used for a short period of time only.

Recommended Foods:

*Ripe banana	Rice	*Buttermilk
*Banana flakes	Toast	*Skim milk
Grated apple	*Crackers	Jell-O
Applesauce	Jelly	Sherbet
Cream of rice	*Cottage cheese	Popsicle
Farina	*American cheese	*Beef broth
Rice cereal	*Vanilla pudding	Weak tea

Foods should be served often and in small amounts. Other foods can be added gradually until the child can tolerate a general diet.

Note: This diet, though not supported by extensive controlled research studies, has been found to be effective treatment for pediatric diarrhea. The pectin in apples and the particular configuration of cellulose in bananas have a documented binding effect.

---

*These foods help to replace the sodium and potassium lost in diarrhea.

Tonsillectomy and Adenoidectomy Diet
(T and A)

Principle: The Tonsillectomy and Adenoidectomy Diet provides foods that will not irritate a sore throat. The foods listed for the first postoperative day may be ordered for any child with an acute sore throat.

Indications: The Tonsillectomy and Adenoidectomy Diet for the day of operation consists of cold, nonirritating foods. On the second day some solid and hot foods are added.

Adequacy: The diet is nutritionally inadequate until the child is able to eat the complete soft diet including citrus fruits and sources of ascorbic acid.

Recommended Foods:
Day of Operation
  Ice, water, carbonated beverages as tolerated
  Milk, ice cream, popsicle at supper
First Postoperative Day (Small Meals)
  Weak tea
  Milk, milkshakes
  No bread
  Cooked, refined cereal
  Plain ice cream, puddings, popsicles, plain gelatin
  Soft cooked, poached, or scrambled eggs
  Cottage cheese
  Canned peaches or pears, or their juices, banana

Recommended
  Mashed potato, strained vegetables
  Strained cream soups, except tomato

Gluten-Free Diet
(The Wheat-, Rye-, Oat-Free Diet)

Principle: Gluten is removed from the diet by eliminating all foods prepared with wheat, rye, oats, barley, and buckwheat. The diet is not restricted in fat or fiber.

Indications: Those glutens found in wheat, rye, oats, and barley interfere with the absorption of food in patients with celiac diseases which may also be called gluten-induced enteropathy, nontropical sprue, or idiopathic steatorrhea. LABELS MUST BE READ CAREFULLY TO DETERMINE PRODUCTS.

Adequacy: The gluten-restricted diet is nutritionally adequate according to the Recommended Daily Dietary Allowances of the National Research Council.

Galactose-Free Diet

Principal Use: This diet is used in infants who have a deficiency in the enzyme Gal-1-P uridyl transferase. This diet is effective in halting the progression of hepatic, ophthalmic, renal, and central nervous system involvement of the disease.

Nutritional Adequacy: Galactose is most commonly present in the diet in the form of lactose (glucose + galactose), the disaccharide found in milk. It is difficult to produce a diet that is entirely free of galactose. Hydrolyzed casein and soybean protein are standard sources of protein in the diet of the galactosemic child. However, the casein is prepared from milk, and a day's supply of the hydrolyzed product could contain from a fraction of a gram to 3 to 4 gm of galactose. Soybean products also contain some galactose in the form of oligosaccharides, but galactose in this form does not appear to be readily digested.

Until two years of age the diet will need vitamin and trace element supplementation. There is no evidence that dietary restriction of galactose may be harmful.

Sucrose- and Fructose-Free Diet

Principal Use: The causes of secondary disaccharide intolerance in infancy and childhood are many: gastrointestinal infections, nonspecific diarrheas, prematurity, intestinal operations in small infants, infective hepatitis, and so

Nutritional Adequacy:
forth. This diet is ordered to relieve the patient while other therapy (drugs, surgery) is investigated.
This diet is very restrictive. Sugar must be eliminated from the diet and also from drugs and medicines. Many tablets contain sugar, even mineral supplements.

Fructose- (Sucrose-), Galactose- (Lactose-) Restricted Diet

Description:
The content of monosaccharides fructose and galactose (therefore, including the disaccharides, sucrose, and lactose) is severely reduced or eliminated from this diet. These hexoses are avoided because they may exacerbate lactic acidosis.

This diet provides energy-protein needs for a child of comparable age. Approximately 2/5 to 1/2 of daily kcalorie needs are given as nocturnal infusions. The remaining kcalories are divided into equal-portioned meals to be eaten at 3- to 4-hour intervals during the day.

Composition of this diet is approximately 60 to 70% carbohydrate [almost exclusively starch (95%), with the remaining 5% as simple sugar], 10 to 15% protein, and the remaining 20 to 30% as fat. The major goal of this diet is to maintain blood glucose levels at 70 to 150 mg/dl.

Indications:
This diet is suggested for patients with type I glycogen storage disease (von Gierke's disease).

Adequacy:
This diet is sufficient in all nutrients to support growth (altered growth pattern is secondary to disease course) in children as long as the patient is consuming approximately 1 L of a special therapeutic formula per day along with adequate kcalorie intake.

However, one patient has been reported to have experienced an increased growth velocity in which the calcium intake of this diet was insufficient to meet his needs for normal ossification.

Low-Protein Diet

"Zero"-gram protein. This diet is inadequate in all nutrients, except possibly calories, according to National Research Committee's Recommended Daily Allowances and should be used only for a short period of time. It is recommended that multiple vitamin supplements be used with this diet.

Renal Diets

Principle:
Protein: Protein not used for growth is broken down by the body to urea and excreted by the kidneys. In renal failure the kidneys cannot adequately remove urea and therefore the blood urea concentration rises. To lessen the build-up of urea and other protein end-products, the kind and amount of protein in the diet must be carefully controlled.

Diet Calculations for Diabetic Children (1981)*

Calorie Level	1000	1100	1200	1300	1400	1500	1600	1700	1800	1900	2000	2100	2200	2300	2400	2500	2600	2700	2800	2900	3000
Protein (gm)	50	55	60	65	70	75	80	85	90	95	100	105	110	115	120	125	130	135	140	145	150
Fat (gm)	33	37	40	43	47	50	53	57	60	63	67	70	73	77	80	83	87	90	93	97	100
Carbohydrate																					
Total (gm)	125	136	150	163	175	188	200	213	225	238	250	263	275	288	300	313	325	338	350	363	375
Simple sugars (gm)	42	42	42	42	52	52	52	62	68	68	68	68	78	78	78	88	88	88	98	98	98
Starch (gm)	82	97	112	127	127	127	127	157	163	163	178	193	193	208	223	223	238	253	253	268	283
Total food/group																					
Milk	2	2	2	2	2	2	2	2	3	3	3	3	3	3	3	3	3	3	3	3	3
Protein	3	4	4	4	5	6	7	7	6	7	8	8	9	9	10	10	10	11	12	12	13
Starch	4	5	6	7	7	7	8	9	9	9	10	11	11	12	13	13	14	15	15	16	17
Vegetables	2	2	2	2	2	2	2	2	2	2	2	2	2	2	2	2	2	2	2	2	2
Fat	3	3	4	4	4	4	4	4	6	6	5	6	6	6	6	7	7	7	7	7	7
Fruit	3	3	3	3	4	4	4	5	5	5	5	5	6	6	6	7	7	7	8	8	8

*Protein, 20%; fat, 30%; carbohydrate, 50% (simple sugar, 30%; starch, 70%).

Sample Meal Patterns for Diabetic Children

Calorie Level	1000	1100	1200	1300	1400	1500	1600	1700	1800	1900	2000	2100	2200	2300	2400	2500	2600	2700	2800	2900	3000
Breakfast																					
Fruit Exchange	1	1	1	1	1	1	1	1	1	1	1	1	2	2	2	2	2	2	2	2	2
Meat Exchange	1	1	1	1	1	2	2	2	2	2	2	2	2	2	2	2	3	3	3	3	3
Bread Exchange	½	1	2	2	2	2	2½	2½	2½	2½	3	3½	3½	3½	4	4	4	4	4	5	5
Fat Exchange	1	1	1	1	1	1	1	1	2	2	2	2	2	2	2	3	3	3	3	3	3
Milk Exchange	1	1	1	1	1	1	1	1	1	1	1	1	1	1	1	1	1	1	1	1	1
Lunch																					
Fruit Exchange	1	1	1	1	—	—	—	1	1	1	1	1	1	1	1	1	1	1	2	2	2
Meat Exchange	1	1	1	1	2	2	2	2	2	2	2	2	2	2	3	3	3	3	3	3	3
Bread Exchange	½	1	1	1½	1½	1½	1½	1½	1½	1½	2	2	2	2	2	2	2	3	3	3	3
Vegetable Exchange	1	1	1	1	1	1	1	1	1	1	1	1	1	1	1	1	1	1	1	1	1
Fat Exchange	1	1	1	1	1	1	1	1	1	1	1	2	2	2	2	2	2	2	2	2	2
Milk Exchange	—	—	—	—	—	—	—	—	½	½	½	½	½	½	½	½	½	½	½	½	½
Afternoon Snack																					
Fruit Exchange	—	—	—	—	1	1	1	1	1	1	1	1	1	1	1	1	1	1	1	1	1
Meat Exchange	—	—	—	—	—	—	—	—	—	—	1	1	1	1	1	1	1	1	1	1	1
Bread Exchange	1	1	1	1	1	1	1	1½	1½	1½	1	1	1	1½	1½	1½	1½	2	2	2	2
Milk Exchange	½	½	½	½	½	½	½	½	½	½	½	½	½	½	½	½	½	½	½	½	½
Dinner																					
Fruit Exchange	1	1	1	1	1	1	1	1	1	1	1	1	1	1	1	2	2	2	2	2	2
Meat Exchange	1	2	2	2	2	2	3	3	2	3	2	2	3	3	3	3	3	3	4	4	5
Bread Exchange	1	1	1	1½	1½	1½	2	2	2	2	3	3½	3½	3½	4	4	4	4	4	4	5
Vegetable Exchange	1	1	1	1	1	1	1	1	1	1	1	1	1	1	1	1	1	1	1	1	1
Fat Exchange	1	1	2	2	2	2	2	2	3	3	2	2	2	2	2	2	2	2	2	2	2
Milk Exchange	—	—	—	—	—	—	—	—	½	½	½	½	½	½	½	½	½	½	½	½	½
Evening Snack																					
Fruit Exchange	—	—	—	—	1	1	1	1	1	1	1	1	1	1	1	1	1	1	1	1	1
Meat Exchange	—	—	—	—	—	—	—	—	—	—	1	1	1	1	1	1	1	1	1	1	1
Bread Exchange	1	1	1	1	1	1	1	1½	1½	1½	1	1	1	1½	1½	1½	1½	2	2	2	2

Sodium: A sodium restriction may be necessary to control hypertension and/or fluid retention. A specific level of sodium should be ordered according to patient needs.

Potassium: A potassium restriction may be necessary to control bradycardia.

$$39 \text{ mg K} = 1 \text{ mEq K}$$
$$74 \text{ mg KCl} = 1 \text{ mEq K}$$

Fluid: A fluid restriction is often essential in treatment of renal and/or hepatic disease. The restriction will vary with patient's urinary output. All foods that liquefy at room temperature will be counted as fluid.

Phosphorus: To prevent hyperphosphotemia, most patients with chronic renal disease have phosphate-binding gels prescribed. When these medications are not used, dietary phosphorus may have to be restricted. With all its limitations, a renal diet is usually already low in phosphorus. To limit phosphorus further, milk, milk products, eggs, and dried peas and beans may have to be further limited.

Indications:

A protein-controlled diet may be ordered for acute renal insufficiency, acute glomerulonephritis, and hepatic failure.

Commonly used levels of protein are "zero," 20, 40, and 60 gm.

Nutritional Adequacy:

Protein-restricted diets (up to 60 gm of protein) are inadequate in all nutrients except vitamins A and C.

Caloric intake must be sufficient to maximize the sparing of endogenous protein breakdown.

PROTEIN

	20 gm	*40 gm*	*60 gm*
Calories	1092	1391	1860
Fat (gm)	40	55	80
Carbohydrate (gm)	162	183	225

Sodium-Restricted Diets

Principal Use:	Intake of sodium has been implicated in disorders of the cardiac and renal system. An increase in blood levels of sodium (as can occur in renal failure) may lead to edema and result in congestive heart failure.
Indications for Use:	The following are some common indications for a sodium-restricted diet:

a) diseases of the kidney in which edema or high blood pressure occurs, such as acute nephritis, nephrotic syndrome, and chronic renal failure;
b) congestive heart failure with edema;
c) severe cirrhosis of the liver.

Nutritional Adequacy: A normal diet contains about 3000 to 6000 mg of Na. Average sodium intake is 4 to 10 gm per day in the U.S. When sodium is restricted, other sources of iodine should be prescribed, especially for children and pregnant females. A severe sodium restriction also reduces the intake of vitamin A owing to restriction of dark-green leafy vegetables.

Conversion Table:

$$23 \text{ mg Na} = 1 \text{ mEq Na}$$
$$58 \text{ mg NaCl} = 1 \text{ mEq Na}$$

Potassium-Restricted Diet

Principle:

Potassium excess (hyperpotassemia or hyperkalemia) is a frequent complication in renal failure in severe dehydration, following too rapid parenteral administration of potassium and in adrenal insufficiency. Hyperkalemia is corrected by using a low-potassium, low-protein, liberal-carbohydrate diet.

Nutritional Adequacy:

Because potassium is so widely distributed in foods in large amounts, diets restricted in potassium will be low in protein and inadequate in calcium, iron, and most vitamins, particularly ascorbic acid. On a low-protein diet a more generous potassium intake is helpful to allow bulk from fruit, vegetables, and potato.

Low-Fat Diet

Principles: 1. The fat content of this diet may be reduced by:
   a) using skimmed milk
   b) omitting butter, margarine, and other visible fats
   c) selecting lean meats such as poultry (with skin removed), and fish, and using them in restricted amounts
2. A higher protein content may be increased by using:
   a) skimmed milk
   b) cottage cheese made from skimmed milk
3. To increase calories the following foods are encouraged:
   a) cereal
   b) sweetened fruits
   c) fruit juice
   d) sugar and other sweets

Indications for Use: A low-fat diet may be used in the treatment of disease of the gallbladder, liver, or pancreas; atherosclerosis; and coronary heart disease.

Some fruits and vegetables that cause an increase in stomach juices may be restricted.

Nutritional Adequacy: If a diet has less than 50 gm of fat a day, there may be a need for a vitamin A supplement. Commonly used levels of fat are 30, 40, and 50 gm.

FAT

	30 gm*	40 gm
Calories	1400	1600
Protein (gm)	60	80
Carbohydrate (gm)	225	220

*Less than 15% of the total calories of this diet comes from fat.

Low-Calcium, Low-Phosphorus Diet

Principal Use: This diet is used for children with parathyroid tumors and orthopedic problems associated with hypercalcemia. It may also be used for the treatment and prevention of recurrent renal calculi composed largely of phosphates and may be used after an acute stage of lead poisoning.

Nutritional Adequacy: This diet meets the Recommended Dietary Allowances for all essential nutrients except iron, thiamine, and riboflavin. This should be supplemented by physician order if diet is used long-term.

Calories	2150
Protein (gm)	90 (360 calories)
Fat (gm)	90 (810 calories)
Carbohydrate (gm)	245 (980 calories)

SELECTED BIBLIOGRAPHY: MODIFIED PEDIATRIC DIETS

General

Manual of Clinical Dietetics. Chicago Dietetic Association.

Galactose-Free Diet

"Parents' Guide to The Galactose Restricted Diet," Bureau of Public Health Nutrition, California State Department of Public Health, 2151 Berkeley Way, Berkeley, CA 94740, 1968.
McLaren, D. S., and Burman, D.: Textbook of Paediatric Nutrition. "Galactosaemia" Disorders of Carbohydrate Metabolism, pg. 245, Churchill Livingstone, New York, 1976.

Sucrose- and Fructose-Free Diet

Krause, M. V., and Hunscher, M. A.: Food Nutrition and Diet Therapy, Fifth Edition. "Metabolic Disorders Related to Nutrition," pp. 397 and 415, W. B. Saunders Company, Philadelphia, 1972.
McLaren, D. S., and Burman, D.: Textbook of Paediatric Nutrition. "Sucrose-Free Regimen" Disorders of Carbohydrate Metabolism, pg. 319, Churchill Livingstone, New York, 1976.

Juvenile Diabetes Mellitus

Renewed Interest in Diet Therapy for the Diabetic Patient. Nutrition and the M.D., Vol. IV, No. 5, March, 1978. Publisher PM, Inc., Van Nuys, CA 91405.
Marble, Alexander, et al.: Joslin's Diabetes Mellitus, Eleventh Edition, pg. 346, Lea & Febiger, Philadelphia, 1971.
Fajans, S. S., and Sussman, K. E.: Diabetes Mellitus: Diagnosis and Treatment, Vol. 11. The American Diabetes Association, 1971. "The Adolescent Diabetic Patient," pg. 338.
Read, C. H.: What is Diabetes Mellitus? Copyright 1976. Department of Pediatrics, University Hospitals, University of Iowa, Iowa City, Iowa 52242.
Casewell, J.: Constant Carbohydrate Diet Management for Diabetes Mellitus. Copyright 1977. Department of Pediatrics, University Hospitals, University of Iowa, Iowa City, IA 52242.
Davidson, J. K.: Controlling Diabetes Mellitus with Diet Therapy. Postgraduate Medicine, *59*(1): 114–122, 1976.

CHAPTER 26

Enteral Nutrition for Older Persons

DONALD M. WATKIN
DAVID A. LIPSCHITZ

A chapter on the management of older persons in a book devoted to enteral nutrition serves two purposes: it provides the reader with some insight into what transpires in the aging process in mature adults; and it sets some logical limits for what can and cannot be accomplished by nutrition enterally administered.

DEFINITIONS

Essential to an understanding of this chapter are definitions of terms used in the discussion.

Aging in Mature Adults. The process of biologic aging begins no later than conception and ends at death. For purposes of this chapter, only aging in the latter half of the technical life span of human beings (TLS[h]) will be considered. The technical life span of a given species is the oldest age to which a member of that species is *documented* to have survived. Since the TLS[h] is 115 years,[1] this chapter will deal with persons whose chronologic ages are 58 and older.

Since major improvements in environmental sanitation, quality of the water supply, food safety, the control of infectious diseases, and, in the past two decades, decrements in the mortality rates for major killer diseases have led to marked increases in life expectancy and in the average age at death, more genetically elite persons endowed with inherited longevity are alive at ages 58 and older than ever before. Hence, some additional definitions are justified. Just as persons between birth and maturity cannot be considered as a uniform monolith, neither can persons 58 and older be viewed as separate but equal. A convenient infra-

structure upon which to build considerations of aging in mature adults is based on the TLS[h]. From 58 through 68, persons continue to be classified as *middle-aged*. On entering the 69th year, the beginning of the final two-fifths of the TLS[h], they may be classified as *aging* (used here as a collective noun to distinguish particular cohorts undergoing the aging process). On entering the 77th year, the beginning of the final one-third of the TLS[h], they may be classified as *elderly*. On entering the 86th year, the threshhold of the last quarter of the TLS[h], they may be classified as *aged*.

These definitions make sense economically but also from the standpoint of health. The diseases afflicting those 58 and older differ greatly with the age of the cohort. In addition, nutritional requirements among healthy persons have been studied to some extent through age 85, but virtually no information is available in regard to the nutritional needs of persons 86 and older. Finally, there is considerable doubt that so-called preventive nutrition plays any role in persons 58 and older for the simple reason that it is difficult to prevent pathology already in situ. However, of great importance to considerations of enteral nutrition, the nutritional care of older persons is essential to their recovery and rehabilitation when they are victims of acute infectious diseases and of the life-threatening complications of chronic ailments, of accidents, and of the stresses imposed by major surgery.

ORIENTATION

Indications for enteral nutrition as it is now utilized among older persons are both consumer- and provider-oriented. When the level of provider care is high, the indications are consumer-oriented, or based on specific consumer needs. In situations in which the level of provider care is low, either because the professionals in charge are poorly trained or because they are too few in number even though they have excellent training, the indications are provider-oriented. Under these circumstances, the indications may be specific (that is, the consumer could not survive without enteral nutrition) or nonspecific (that is, the management of the consumer's nutrient intake is simplified by the use of enteral nutrition). Obviously, consumer-oriented indications are preferable. Nonetheless, in view of the incredibly low staffing ratios in many health care settings today, provider-oriented indications are widely used and certainly cannot be ignored.

PRECAUTIONS WITH COMPONENTS

Enteral nutrition is not an innocuous mode of alimentation. Precautions with several components must be taken to assure preservation of or attainment of optimal health status by the recipients.

Water. The water content of enteral regimens for older persons must be planned with great care. A major complication of enteral nutrition among older persons is hypernatremia. This may result from inadequate hydration of recipients during enteral alimentation.

If the enteral formula is high in protein and salt, the resulting load of urea and salt that must be excreted increases the obligatory renal water loss sufficiently to create an imbalance between water intake and water loss, which in turn produces hypernatremia. Consequently, careful attention must be given to water requirements of enterally nourished recipients, especially if they are obtunded, comatose, or for some reason unable to respond to the sensation of thirst.

Should hypernatremia occur, the appropriate treatment is administration of water sufficient to add 4 per cent of the body weight in kilograms for each 10 mEq/L increase in serum sodium above normal. If sufficient water cannot be included in the enteral mixture, water should be supplied by other routes, such as intravenously as a 5 per cent glucose solution. Considerable caution should be exercised in the correction of hypernatremia, since too rapid replacement of water may lead to cerebral edema. A prudent course would entail replacing half of the fluid deficit in the first 24 hours. This usually can be accomplished by increasing the water content of the enterally administered nutrient and monitoring the slow reduction in serum sodium over an interval of 48 hours.

Carbohydrate. For older recipients, ample carbohydrate, preferably in complex rather than simple form, should be incorporated in the enteral formula. Complex carbohydrates produce lower osmotic loads than do simple sugars. Constant carbohydrate ingestion, as is possible through the use of enteral nutrition, reduces insulin requirements in elderly diabetic persons, reduces serum cholesterol concentrations, and induces greater nitrogen retention.

Fat. The fat content of enterally administered mixtures should be tailored to meet the needs of the recipient. Fat, the most concentrated source of food energy, 9 cal/gm, enables an enteral regimen to meet energy deficits while at the same time not adding to the osmotic load. This is especially significant among elderly and aged recipients in whom energy deficits in dietaries are very prevalent and being underweight is extremely common. When energy is required, fat, up to the point of inducing undesirable signs and symptoms, is an indicated ingredient. In recipients intolerant to conventional triglycerides, medium-chain triglycerides provide an energy source that is absorbed directly into the portal circulation without requiring bile salts or pancreatic enzymes for preliminary digestion. Medium-chain triglycerides are valuable in managing older persons with malabsorption syndromes as a result of surgical removal of portions of, radiation to, or chemotherapy affecting the small bowel.

Protein. The protein content of a daily regimen of enteral nutrition should be prescribed after a careful clinical evaluation of the recipient, including evaluation of prior and present protein intake, estimated lean body mass, desirable lean body mass, and present renal function. As noted above, the higher the protein content of the regimen, the more water must be incorporated into the formula. Little if any information is available on protein requirements of the aged. Available information of protein requirements of the aging and the elderly suggests that the health status of the individual is a far more important determinant of protein intake than is chronologic age. Since most older persons requiring enteral nutrition manifest poor health status, the protein intake must be adjusted to meet the particular needs of the individual. Among those requiring additional protein are persons with acute febrile illnesses, serious burns, extensive trauma, and hypermetabolism from endocrine and neoplastic diseases.

Among persons not falling into the categories mentioned immediately above, a protein intake—with two major exceptions—of at least 1 gm/kg of body weight per day is indicated.

One major exception is the person with severely compromised renal function in whom the protein intake must be quantitatively restricted and qualitatively adjusted to provide protein of the highest possible biologic value. Successful enteral therapy with regimens containing 30 to 40 gm daily of protein and the amino acid proportions of whole egg or of the Protein Quality Reference Standard* will reduce laboratory parameters of azotemia and usually will induce clinically evident improvement in the health of the recipient.

The second major exception is the person with hepatic encephalopathy from severely impaired liver function or the person with a portocaval shunt (or hyperammonemia from any cause capable of manifesting itself in mature adults). In such persons, the protein should be reduced quantitatively and its biologic value increased so that the smallest amount compatible with the maintenance of nutritional status may be used. If reduction in protein intake alone fails to relieve the encephalopathy, lactulose or neomycin or both should be added to the enteral regimen.

Chemically defined or so-called elemental diets whose "protein" comprises free amino acids or small peptides have specific indications, few of which are found in older persons. These include such conditions as inflammatory bowel disease, chronic pancreatitis, gastrointestinal fistulas, radiation or chemotherapeutic enteropathy, the short gut syndrome, states of malabsorption and maldigestion, and situations in which a low

residue diet is required. They also may be utilized in preoperative preparation of the bowel. Unless there is a very specific indication for their use, compounds of this type are too costly for routine use in enteral regimens for older persons.

Minerals and Trace Elements. *Calcium and Phosphorus.* Unless specifically contraindicated, the calcium:phosphorus ratio should be maintained at 1 or higher. Such ratios are unusual among technically advanced societies for two principal reasons: (1) the popularity of red meat, high in phosphorus and low in calcium; and (2) the quantities of soft drinks imbibed by persons of all ages, beverages that are high in phosphorus and negligible in calcium. Diets high in phosphorus should be used with caution by older persons whose reduced renal function, especially when complemented by renal disease, places them at risk for hyperphosphatemia. If high-carbohydrate, low-protein, low-phosphorus enteral regimens are unattainable or cannot be prepared, aluminum hydroxide compounds which bind and make unabsorbable phosphorus in ingested foods and gastrointestinal fluids may be added to the enteral alimentation. If used, this technique for preventing hyperphosphatemia must be accompanied by scheduled laboratory and clinical evaluation of recipients, since such compounds are virtually the only cause of the true phosphorus deficiency syndrome in older persons who are free from advanced liver disease.

In terms of the pathogenesis of osteopenia in older persons, the only finding suggesting an etiologic role for phosphorus is the inverse relation between concentrations of serum phosphate and 1,25-dihydroxyvitamin D.[2] While bone metabolism involves at least 10 factors other than calcium and phosphorus in dietary regimens, present consensus among investigators suggests that older persons should ingest daily at least the recommended dietary allowance (RDA) of 800 mg of calcium and that the calcium:phosphorus ratio should be at least 1. Dairy products as sources of calcium should not be avoided in enteral regimens unless proof positive is obtained indicating individual idiosyncrasy or a very high level of lactose intolerance, neither of which is found frequently among older persons.

Magnesium. Magnesium is an important component of enteral regimens and should be consumed in the amount of 300 to

---

*Published by the Food and Nutrition Board, National Research Council–National Academy of Sciences: Recommended Dietary Allowances, Edition 9, 1980.

400 mg daily. Among older persons, factors contributing to magnesium deficiency include parenteral alimentation, certain diuretics, certain antibiotics, excessive enemas, abuse of alcohol, malabsorption syndromes and the syndrome of inappropriate secretion of antidiuretic hormone (SIADH). The common manifestations of magnesium deficiency are hypocalcemia and hypokalemia. Since the prevalence rates for diseases and their treatments among older persons correlate well with the prevalence of magnesium deficiency, the importance of magnesium in enteral regimens is apparent. Less apparent but vital to older persons is the proper diagnosis of magnesium deficiency and its prompt treatment by parenterally administered solutions of magnesium salts.

Potassium. Potassium sufficient to maintain serum potassium concentrations in the normal range is mandatory. Potassium is especially important in the enteral feeding of persons who may be on potassium-losing diuretics or who have suffered serious fluid losses from the gastrointestinal tract. In persons whose renal tubules fail to secrete enough potassium, hyperkalemia may result, requiring a reduction in potassium intake. Both hypokalemia and hyperkalemia in advanced stages produce characteristic changes in electrocardiograms; however, these changes should never be used as indices of the adequacy of potassium nutrition.

Sodium. Sodium, with particular reference to hypernatremia, has been discussed previously. Computing the ideal sodium content of enteral regimens used in the alimentation of older persons requires careful estimation of total body water as well as the serum sodium concentration. In older persons who are ill, low serum sodium concentrations are usually ominous signs. Such persons frequently have excessive total body water and have new homeostatic sets for their serum sodium concentrations. In fact, they usually have an excess total body sodium if one examines the product of the serum concentration and the total body water. Under such circumstances, increasing sodium intake in the absence of fluid restriction will lead only to an increase in total body water. The only way to correct this electrolyte abnormality in the short term is to restrict water intake, a process that is unpleasant for the recipient of enteral nutrition (if conscious) and usually of little consequence per se in improving the health status

of the person involved. Correction, if possible, of the pathology underlying the electrolyte abnormality is the only measure that will in the long run improve health status.

Chloride. Enteral regimens deficient in chloride are rarities. However, hypochloremia usually associated with alkalosis is found among older persons, particularly those whose maintenance of health status has required gastric suction or who have suffered from long-term diarrhea or fluid losses from intestinal fistulas. The resolution of the hypochloremia lies not in augmenting the chloride intake but in filling the underlying potassium deficit which, when eliminated, will be accompanied by resolution of the hypochloremia. Hyperchloremia and particularly hyperchloremic acidosis is encountered in older persons with a variety of clinical conditions. It may be found in persons whose ureters have been implanted in their large intestines and then serve as substitutes for urinary bladders that have been surgically removed, usually for cancer. This form of hyperchloremia may also present in situations involving parenteral alimentation with synthetic amino acid mixtures. The excess of cationic amino acids (arginine, histidine, and lysine) contributes hydrogen and chloride to body fluids as they are converted to urea or converted into peptides, producing a hyperchloremic metabolic acidosis. This may be prevented by adding sodium bicarbonate rather than sodium chloride to the regimen when synthetic amino acid mixtures are administered.

Iron. Iron is supplied in most commercially available enteral regimens. If noncommercial enteral mixtures are prepared, the iron content should approximate the RDA of 1980, 10 mg daily, even when pathologic blood loss is excluded in the older person. Since many older persons with anemias do have pathologic causes of iron depletion, and since many also have gastric achlorhydria, which alone can decrease the absorption of ferric iron by 50 per cent, a strong case may be developed for an iron intake daily higher than the RDA for older persons.

Chromium. The major function of chromium, that of potentiating the peripheral action of insulin, may be of importance in enteral alimentation of older persons because of their well-documented carbohydrate intolerance, whether or not they are diabetic. Chromium is thought to be effective only when it is a component of substances having the generic term glucose tolerance factor. In foods, glucose tolerance factor is most abundant in brewer's yeast and is also found in non-fish animal protein and in foods made from whole grain, all of which may be used as components of enteral feeding mixtures. While meaningful recommendations for a chromium RDA are still lacking, a minimum daily requirement for man of approximately 10 μg is frequently mentioned.

Copper. Copper, widely distributed in foodstuffs, is essential for the proper functioning of enzymes in virtually every organ system. Under normal dietary practices, copper deficiency in healthy adults is highly unlikely to occur. However, when enteral alimentation is used to supply nutrients, dietary copper should be maintained in the range of 2 to 5 mg daily, with the exception of persons with Wilson's disease in whom a low copper diet is indicated.

Fluoride. Fluoride has been used in older persons in conjunction with calcium and vitamin D in the management of senile osteoporosis. The principal vehicle, sodium fluoride, may be used in amounts as high as 50 mg daily, but, since it may produce toxic manifestations such as anorexia, epigastric pain, ectopic calcification, optic neuritis, and retinal damage, its use as a component of enteral regimens must be monitored with great care and used only when the indication is highly specific.

Iodine. Iodine, whose RDA is 150 μg daily, was once so deficient in the diets of persons living in inland North America that goiter was endemic. However, data collected during the 1968 to 1970 Ten State Nutrition Survey showed no relationship between the prevalence of goiter and the iodine intake of the persons studied. The reason lies primarily in the fact that in recent years the use of iodine in animal feeds and medications and as a component of bactericidal agents used in processing food and dairy products has introduced exogenous iodine into the food chain to the extent that the mean amount ingested daily per person is well in excess of the RDA. This is an important consideration in designing enteral regimens, many of which are based on dairy products.

Selenium. Selenium is an essential component of the enzyme glutathione peroxidase, which utilizes glutathione as an electron donor for the reduction of peroxides, thereby helping to stabilize the lipid-containing biologic membranes of subcellular components such as mitochondria, microsomes, and lyosomes. Selenium therefore joins other dietary factors responsible for the integrity of cell membranes, essential in the prevention of cell death and therefore of the aging process per se. In animals, diets containing 0.1 μg/gm have prevented selenium deficiency. This concentration is present in the average mixed American diet. However, selenium deficiency has been reported in persons with alcoholic cirrhosis[3] and among those receiving prolonged parenteral alimentation.[4] Hence, in persons receiving enteral feedings, especially chemically defined or elemental diets, consideration should be given to the selenium content, especially in older persons, whom studies from New Zealand[5] have shown to have lower selenium and glutathione peroxidase concentrations in blood than younger subjects serving as controls.

Vanadium. Vanadium, although present in abundance virtually everywhere, has been implicated as a deficient element in human diets primarily because of its extremely low concentrations in milk, liver, meat, fish, and highly refined foods. The implication seems unjustified even in considerations of enteral nutrition, since most components of enteral regimens are prepared in contact with some vanadium-containing metal or compound.

Zinc. In contrast to other trace elements, zinc has received wide attention and has been incorporated in 1974 and 1980 into the widely disseminated tables of RDA, in which its quantity for older persons has been set at 15 mg daily. Overt zinc deficiency is virtually never seen in North America, but marginal zinc deficiency has been inferred frequently from improved wound healing and improved taste acuity observed in adult humans when zinc intake was deliberately increased. In addition, conditioned zinc deficiencies are numerous among older persons. Since only 10 to 15 per cent of ingested zinc is absorbed under the ideal circumstances afforded by diets high in animal protein, dietary components, medications, and pathologic factors may reduce the effective zinc intake well below that needed for optimal functioning of zinc-dependent metallo-enzymes. Hypotheses are one thing, but proving that marginal zinc deficiencies exist is extremely difficult. The best compromise lies in assuring that enteral regimens contain at least the RDA. Few if any reliable data are available indicating that zinc supplements far in excess of the RDA have any benefit, whereas they do pose serious risks of zinc toxicity.

Summary. Many factors are involved in considerations of minerals and trace elements in enteral nutrition. Each must be related to other nutrients in the diet. Each must be related to the genetic, toxic, traumatic, and disease factors that influence the nutrient requirements of each person. Each must be considered with respect to the vehicle, compound, or format through which it will be ingested and metabolized by the older person.

The experience of the Nutrition Program for Older Americans (NPOA) in evaluating the acceptability of Limited Use Supplemental Food (LUSF), a nonfat, dry milk–based product to which vitamins, trace minerals, and a small quantity of corn syrup solids had been added, a product that would provide excellent enteral alimentation, revealed the impossibility of evaluating the effectiveness of a dietary supplement or an enteral regimen without objective measures at the disposal of investigators. The number and variety of health-related events, 96 per cent favorable, following consumption of LUSF by 6000 older persons reporting subjectively could only be viewed as classic examples of the Hawthorne phenomenon.[6, 7]

Vitamins. Many investigators have sought to prove that older persons as a class are vitamin deficient. With the possible exception of the aged, for whom no reliable data are available, this hypothesis remains unsupported. However, factors associated with diseases, medications, insufficient education, and deplorable socioeconomic conditions are far more prevalent and potentially more remediable causes of vitamin deficiency syndromes.

Enteral alimentation provides a convenient means of rectifying vitamin deficiency states from any cause. Clinical signs and symptoms combined with available biochemical parameters are useful in identifying specific deficiency states. However, in older persons vitamin deficiencies when present tend to be generalized. Furthermore, most commercial enteral regimens contain at least the RDA for all water- and fat-soluble vitamins. When noncommercial regimens are being prepared, multivitamin preparations are available that may be added to the mixture. These preparations should be examined carefully, since some lack folate and others contain sufficiently high concentrations of fat-soluble vitamins to create potential hazards if carelessly used over long intervals. If liquid preparations are not accessible, multivitamin tablets may be used by first crushing them and then mixing them with other components of the regimen.

Perhaps the most important consideration involving vitamins in enteral nutrition is their potential for being eliminated from the body or altered disadvantageously in the course of their metabolism by medications being administered concurrently. In the realm of fat-soluble vitamins, mineral oil given for the management of chronic constipation may make unavailable for absorption sufficient fat-soluble vitamins to induce clinical deficiency states. Cholestyramine in doses ranging from 12 to 36 gm daily increases fecal fat excretion to quantities comparable to those found in persons with active sprue. By interfering with normal fat absorption, cholestyramine diminishes the availability of all fat-soluble vitamins.

The availability and metabolism of water-soluble vitamins are also influenced by medications. Antibiotics alter the flora of the small intestine, diminishing the microbial production of biotin, riboflavin, and possibly folacin (as well as fat-soluble vitamin K). Other drugs widely used in the management of health problems in older persons adversely affect absorption and metabolism of folacin. These include methotrexate, aminopterin, pyrimethamine, trimethoprim, phenytoin, primadone, barbiturates, cholestyramine, polydexide, and even aspirin.[8]

In addition to medications, various diseases and conditions in older persons may lead to deficiencies of one or more vitamins. A few of these include addisonian pernicious anemia, gluten-induced enteropathy, regional ileitis, Crohn's disease, intestinal resections, and inadequate exocrine pancreatic secretions.

Finally, food faddists, especially strict vegetarians, may have vitamin deficiency signs and symptoms or may not, as in the case of those with extremely low serum concentrations of vitamin B_{12} but no other evidence of B_{12} deficiency.

Caution is needed in regulating the doses of fat-soluble vitamins A and D and of water-soluble C, all of which may produce toxic syndromes if administered in large multiples of the RDA.

Calories. Derived from fat, carbohydrate, and protein, energy has been found by many investigators to be a major deficiency in the diets of older persons. This is particularly pertinent in view of recent information suggesting that the 1959 Metropolitan Life Insurance Company data in tables giving desirable weights for sex and heights and the even leaner desirable weights promulgated in the 1980 edition of *Recommended Dietary Allowances* are associated with higher mortality rates at any age than weights approximately 15 per cent higher.[9] These findings suggest that energy should be given top priority in designing enteral regimens for older persons.

Enteral regimens high enough in energy content to provide the calories needed for weight gain or even for weight maintenance in older persons whose conditions clearly indicate such alimentation must contain relatively large quantities of fat, the nutrient of highest energy density. Such regimens should contain no less than 35 per cent calories from fat. If tolerated—no evidence of sprue-like syndromes or complaints of upper abdominal or chest pain (in persons who are both conscious and communicative)—the fat content may be raised to as high as 50 per cent of total calories. For those older persons who demonstrate intolerance to 14-carbon and longer fatty acids, the chain length may be shortened by the use of medium-chain triglycerides derived from coconut oil and having their triglycerides composed primarily of C_8 and C_{10} saturated fatty acids.

The fatty acid composition of these regimens (whether high or low in saturated or unsaturated triglycerides) should be of little concern, since evidence is lacking that altering the lipid composition of the serum in older persons has any impact on morbidity or mortality from cardiovascular diseases (with the possible exception of high-density lipoprotein [HDL] fractions). This is true[10] even if the lipid hypothesis, which has yet to be confirmed, is valid or not.[11]

In managing indicated enteral regimens in older persons, energy needs deserve a very high priority,[12] and, in fulfilling those needs, fat plays a crucial role.

DESIGN

Commercial Formulas. A broad spectrum of commercial formulas are available and are referred to elsewhere in this book. The suppliers make available to providers information on proximate analyses, macro-

nutrient and micronutrient composition, energy content, and amino acid and lipid analyses of their various products. They also provide detailed instructions on the preparation of the enteral regimens and suggested indications for uses of the various formulas. Less detailed information is available in standard references[13, 14] and in other chapters of this book. When such commercial formulas are used, they may be modified by the addition of other ingredients at the discretion of the providers.

Special Formulas. Those providers interested in less costly enteral nutrition who have access to blenders or food processors may produce their own enteral regimens. In these, liquified conventional foods may be used with the daily dietaries planned in conventional manners. The viscosities and textures of the regimens may be regulated by adjusting the times used in blending or processing and the fluid contents of the mixtures. Enteral regimens so prepared have a feature important to many older persons not usually present in commercial mixtures: they may contain the same quantities of fiber found in conventional diets.

Enteral Nutrition Combined with Parenteral Nutrition. As already noted, enteral nutrition may be and often must be combined with parenteral nutrition to meet adequately the nutritional requirements of older persons. If enteral nutrition is feasible, its use may avoid the need to resort to TPN and its requirements for catheter placement and its attendant complications. The parenteral component should complement the enteral to provide a satisfactory total daily nutrient and water regimen.

Enteral Combined with Nutrition by Mouth. Whenever feasible, oral alimentation should be used in conjunction with enteral in older persons. Taking food by mouth not only keeps mastication and deglutition in practice but also reassures older persons that they are functionally normal in that they are able to eat as do other healthy persons. In weaning older persons from enteral regimens, careful records of nutrients and water taken orally should be kept and the quantities of the enteral regimens administered reduced accordingly.

MONITORING

In older recipients who are conscious and communicative, symptoms reported by them deserve scrupulous attention. Their own impressions of the clarity of their sensoria should be evaluated to determine the reliability of their reports of other symptoms, including sensations of thirst, regurgitation, shortness of breath, abdominal pain, diarrhea, and constipation.

In all older recipients of enteral nutrition, monitoring of physical signs is critical. These include the state of oral hygiene, odor of the breath, presence of pulmonary congestion or edema, presence of abdominal ascites and of dependent edema, clarity of the sensorium, color of the tongue, body weight, fluid intake and output, nutrient intake, frequency and consistency of bowel movements, presence of diarrhea and of constipation, bowel sounds, and size of the urinary bladder.

When quantification of blood constituents and chemistries is accessible, their monitoring is desirable. Particularly important are measurements of sodium, chloride, potassium, total osmolality, and pH. Calcium, phosphorus, magnesium, glucose, total protein, albumin, creatinine, and hematology are important in the initial work-up and periodically thereafter in monitoring the success of the enteral regimen in achieving and maintaining normal parameters. Quantification of levels of vitamins and trace elements is important in clinical investigations but, in view of the fact that enteral regimens are designed to provide at least the RDA, such quantification is rarely essential in the clinical management of older persons. The exception would be in those older persons with absorption deficiencies or medication regimens that could interfere with absorption and metabolism of micronutrients, in which instances it would become important to know the specific micronutrients affected so that replacements by parenteral administration or by increasing their concentrations in the enteral mixture could be undertaken.

Physiotherapy

When older persons are sustained by enteral nutrition, active or passive physiotherapy should be an integral part of their daily routines. If trained therapists are not available, other staff members in institutional settings or family and friends in home settings must make certain that joints are flexed and extended and that muscles retain tone and strength. Ambulation by enterally fed older persons themselves is very desirable and can be achieved either by discontinuing alimentation during periods of ambulation or by devising methods whereby the enteral regimens may be transported by or with the older recipient.

Good Nursing Care

In institutional settings, the ultimate determinant of the success of enteral alimentation in older persons is the quantity and quality of nursing care. Even with the most highly skilled and imaginative professional staffs, good care cannot be provided if the staff-to-patient ratio is too low. Experience in nursing homes run by the Federal government suggests that, with seriously ill and disabled persons, ratios of 2.0 are required. Needless to say, many institutions function with ratios ranging from 0.5 to as low as 0.1. When a low staffing ratio is present, serious consideration should be given to moving older persons for whom enteral alimentation is indicated to other better-staffed institutions or to the care of family and friends in a home setting.

Very frequently in providing enteral alimentation many compromises with ideal conditions are required. For innumerable reasons, staffing ratios rarely reach those desirable. Under such circumstances, one knowledgeable professional should be on call at all times to make critical decisions. These may include avoiding enteral alimentation, transferring older persons to other institutions or sending them to their homes, or modifying the total regimens to minimize the risk of complications. If enteral nutrition is being conducted in a home setting, monitoring by a home care team or by knowledgeable visiting nurses is mandatory. When such are not available, arrangements should be developed under which health industry representatives are accessible at all times to render advice or activate emergency assistance, as indicated.

WHEN TO STOP ENTERAL NUTRITION

The enteral alimentation of older persons should be discontinued when they are sufficiently recovered from the indications for enteral nutrition to consume voluntarily by mouth the dietary regimens deemed appropriate. Usually this would imply dietaries containing the RDA appropriate for age and sex. Occasionally, supplemental vitamins, minerals, or even mixtures such as LUSF may be indicated to assure appropriate nutrition after discontinuation of enteral alimentation.

In some cases, when brain death has occurred or when jurisdictional law permits, families may request discontinuation of all life support mechanisms, including enteral nutrition. Usually such requests should be honored only after thorough consultation with the family, other health professionals, institutional administrators, the families' spiritual advisers, and legal counsel.

Finally, enteral nutrition should be stopped (or never initiated) in older persons in whom the risk far exceeds the possible benefit.

PROTEIN-ENERGY MALNUTRITION

The prevalence rate of protein-energy malnutrition in general has been discussed in detail elsewhere in this book. The prevalence in older persons remains unknown. Such persons do compose the majority of hospitalized patients. In the experience of one of the authors (D.A.L.), the prevalence for malnutrition is highest in this group. Malnutrition is sometimes overlooked or completely ignored while attention is focused on the primary reason for hospitalization. The clinical features of protein-energy malnutrition in older persons, the problems associated with its diagnosis, and, once diagnosed, the relative ease with which it may be eliminated by appropriate nutritional management are discussed below.

Etiology and Significance. Protein-energy malnutrition in the hospitalized older patient, as in any other age group, is most frequently secondary to a primary disease requiring hospitalization. Primary diseases include neoplasia, chronic heart failure, chronic lung disease, renal failure, and hepatic disease, to mention a few examples. Protein-energy malnutrition reduces the malnourished older person's resistance to infections. In regard to these, the effects of protein-energy malnutrition on the immune and the hematopoietic systems have been examined. Cell-mediated immunity is impaired. T cells are reduced with a relative increase in T-suppressor and a reduction of T-helper cells. In contrast, B-cell function is unaffected. Reduction in the neutrophil response to infection is also found. A defect

appears to be a decreased ability of hematopoietic stem cells to proliferate. This contributes to anemia, which is one of the earliest manifestations of protein-energy malnutrition. Deficiencies of other nutrients such as iron, pyridoxine, and folate may also contribute to the anemia, as may shortened red cell survival and a relative reduction of erythropoietin secretion by the kidney. These sequelae of protein-energy malnutrition are important in differential diagnosis, since alterations in the immune and hematopoietic system which result from the aging process per se closely mimic those caused by protein-energy malnutrition.[15-19] Decreased cell-mediated immunity, alterations in number and function of T cells, and changes in hematopoiesis caused by aging are similar to those described above for protein-energy malnutrition. In a population of older persons in whom host defenses already may be compromised, the effects of protein-energy malnutrition may be severe, and mortality and morbidity correspondingly high. For these reasons, the diagnosis of protein-energy malnutrition and the implementation of appropriate nutritional intervention are especially important in older persons.

Clinical Presentation. As indicated above, chronic diseases are usually the indicators for hospitalization. Protein-energy malnutrition may already be present on admission or may develop during the course of a complicated hospital stay. Patients presenting with acute infections may on further evaluation be found to have protein-energy malnutrition. Such patients are usually over 70, indigent, and in marginal social circumstances. When available, dietary histories reveal grossly inadequate food intake. Histories of being unable or unwilling to cook for themselves are common. Severe endogenous depressions from deaths of spouses or close relatives and friends frequently contribute to poor nutrient intakes. Patients transferred from other long-term care institutions may also manifest protein-energy malnutrition. Frequently they have required prolonged enteral feeding because of cerebrovascular accidents or other organic brain syndromes. Protein-energy malnutrition is particularly common in older persons who have been discharged a short time before from both acute care and long-term care institutions.

The most frequent symptom of protein-energy malnutrition is confusion or a history of recent alterations in mental status. These may be already present on admission or may develop during hospitalization. The symptoms in older persons are extremely nonspecific and may be the initial manifestations of other diseases. In patients who have been hospitalized for some time, careful examinations of their records reveal significant weight losses since admission. Such losses are particularly common in older persons recovering from recent major surgical procedures.

Fifteen such patients have recently been evaluated by one of us (D.A.L.) for the presence of protein-energy malnutrition. Of these, the majority (11 patients) had required emergency surgery including aneurysm repair, appendectomy, and a variety of orthopedic procedures. Their initial postoperative courses were usually uneventful, but, after periods ranging from 14 to 30 days, these patients were more and more confused and increasingly bedfast. Reviews of their hospital charts revealed weight losses ranging from 6 to 15 per cent of their weights on admission. In 12 of the 15, acute infections unrelated to the surgical procedures developed and in two wound sepses occurred. Infections included pneumonia, those of the urinary tract, and, in one patient, septicemia of unknown origin. Clues suggesting the presence of malnutrition may be found occasionally by physical examinations. Flaky paint dermatitis may be seen, and glossitis is common. The usual manifestations of kwashiorkor or marasmus are very unusual. In some patients, dehydration may be obvious, whereas in others edema may be present.

Diagnosis. The nutritional evaluation of hospitalized patients has been reviewed extensively elsewhere and recommendations regarding the most appropriate way to assess nutritional status are available. As noted above, many changes which occur as a result of aging per se are frequently found in protein-energy malnutrition. This problem has been examined by comparing nutritional parameters in groups of young and of older healthy males and females and in groups of young and older patients with protein-energy malnutrition.[20]

One of the most impressive features of advancing age is the marked agewise reduction in lean body mass.[21] In the Arkansas studies, 30 to 50 per cent of healthy older persons had mid-arm muscle circumferences and urinary creatinine excretions in the moderately to severely deficient ranges.

The usefulness of serum transferrin as a predictor of nutritional status in older persons is diminished when compared with its usefulness in the young. In addition to being affected by nutrient intake, circulating transferrin also varies inversely with tissue iron stores. Studies have shown that iron stores in older persons are significantly greater than in young persons, the difference being most pronounced in females. For this reason, many older persons with high tissue iron stores have reductions in circulating transferrin not related to altered nutritional status. The value of anemia, anergy, and lymphocytopenia as parameters for the nutritional assessment of older persons remains to be determined. Although invariably found in malnourished older persons, these abnormalities are detected not infrequently in healthy older persons. Also demonstrated by studies in Arkansas, many older persons with severe protein-energy malnutrition were overweight, emphasizing that malnutrition may occur among those who appear to be obese.

The only parameter of nutritional assessment not affected by the aging process in persons in Arkansas was serum albumin. Irrespective of age or sex, healthy persons rarely have serum albumin concentrations below 4 gm/dl. By contrast, a concentration greater than 3.5 gm/dl is extremely unusual in older persons with protein-energy malnutrition. Naturally, many factors affect serum albumin concentrations. Albumin behaves as an acute phase reactant with modest reductions occurring in a wide variety of acute disease processes. In addition, before hypoalbuminemia can be attributed to protein-energy malnutrition, hepatic dysfunction and renal and gastrointestinal losses of protein must be excluded.

Based upon the above discussion, the following methods for diagnosing protein-energy malnutrition are recommended: (1) careful histories and physical examinations; (2) a history of recent weight loss together with a serum albumin of less than 3.5 gm/dl not attributable to hepatic failure or renal disease; and (3) anemia, lymphocytopenia, and anergy. Currently other anthropometric measures including urinary excretion of creatinine have been found to be of little value.

Management. Once a diagnosis of protein-energy malnutrition has been made, clinical judgment is extremely important in deciding the appropriate time to commence nutritional support. In the acutely ill patient, attention should first be directed at correcting major diseases and physiologic abnormalities. Thus management of infections, control of blood pressure, and the restoration of metabolic, electrolyte, and fluid homeostasis should receive priority. During this period, fluid and nutrient intake should be recorded to assist in estimating future needs. Once the acute processes have stabilized, daily calorie counts should be performed. Patients should be encouraged to consume voluntarily as much food as possible. If fluid overload is not a major concern, the use of liquified commercially available dietary supplements between meals and in the late evening should be considered. The objective should be to obtain a caloric intake of approximately 35 cal/kg based on ideal rather than actual body weight. In Arkansas, by encouragement alone, only 10 per cent of older patients with protein-energy malnutrition consumed sufficient food voluntarily to correct their nutritional deficiencies. Most required more aggressive nutritional intervention. Except in patients with abnormal gastrointestinal tracts, the most appropriate method of nutritional intervention was enteral hyperalimentation through a small-bore nasogastric polyethylene catheter. Interventions were begun with undiluted liquified commercially available dietary supplements at continuous rates of 25 ml/hr. The supplements contained no more than 1 cal/ml. Fluids too viscous to pass through the tubing with ease were avoided. Delivery rates were gradually increased until after 48 hours the daily protein and calorie requirements of the patients were fulfilled by enteral alimentation alone.

Enteral hyperalimentation had side effects particularly bothersome in older persons. The most commonly encountered of these was excessive fluid retention. Invariably when nutritional support commenced weight gain was noticed within the first two to three days. This reflected fluid retention, since weight gains were associated with significant reductions in concentrations of serum albumin and hemoglobin. The average increase in weight during this time was 1.3 kg, while the mean concentration of serum albumin fell from 2.8 gm/dl prior to nutritional support to 2.3 gm/dl by day three. Occasionally, and particularly in older patients with inadequate renal function, excessive fluid retention resulted in peripheral edema or even heart failure. When this occurred, diuretic therapy or calorically dense supplements were used to correct the underlying problems.

Major alterations in circulating electrolytes have been described. Hyponatremia and hypocalcemia occur frequently. In addition, hypophosphatemia and decreased concentrations of serum magnesium may be found, often associated with worsening confusion and delirium on the part of the older patients. Occasionally, hyperglycemia and glycosuria are noted. Frank diabetic coma may develop. Severe diarrhea may occur; its risk can be minimized if enteral supplements are infused slowly. Bolus administration of dietary supplements through nasogastric tubes increases the risk of diarrhea and, particularly in older persons, increases the possibility of vomiting and aspiration pneumonia.

In Arkansas, a large number of older patients with severe protein-energy malnutrition have been supported nutritionally by means of enteral hyperalimentation. In them, dramatic clinical improvement has usually been demonstrated. This was particularly apparent in patients with primary protein-energy malnutrition or those with a disease process that was improved or corrected by appropriate medical management. The Arkansas experience in nine such persons has been reported recently.[22] Moreover, in a period of 18 months following that report, 35 additional patients have been managed by similar means. When first diagnosed, these patients invariably were confined to their beds. After 21 days of enteral hyperalimentation, 33 of the 35 were observed to be markedly less confused. They were more mobile and could transfer from their beds to chairs without assistance. When the underlying medical problems were correctable, 80 per cent of the patients improved sufficiently to return to their homes. In addition, objective improvements of nutritional parameters were documented. After the initial prompt weight gain seen in the first three days, a more gradual increase averaging 7.1 kg occurred over 21 days (Fig. 26–1). In addition, highly significant increases in plasma protein measurements were noted. In the nine subjects shown in Figure 26–1, the mean serum albumin increased from a nadir of 2.3 gm/ml to a mean of 3.5 gm/ml at day 21. The total iron-binding capacity (TIBC) in-

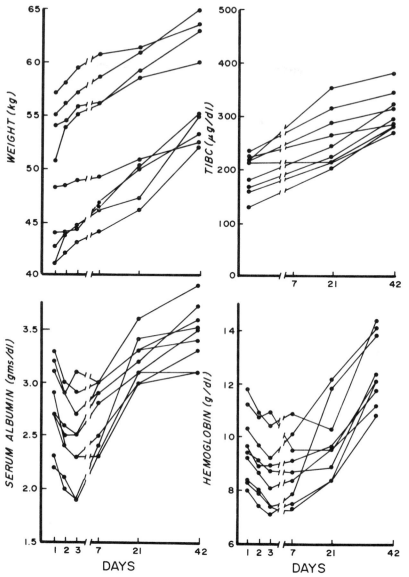

Figure 26–1. Changes in weight, serum albumin, hemoglobin, and total iron-binding capacity (TIBC) in nine elderly patients with severe protein energy malnutrition who received intensive nutritional support. For the first 21 days, the nutritional supplement was given by nasogastric tubes. The tubes were then removed and the patients followed for another 21 days during which time liquefied commercially available dietary supplements were given between meals. The initial falls in albumin and hemoglobin reflect fluid retention. Significant increases in weight, serum albumin, and TIBC occurred by 21 days and were even greater by day 42. This is not surprising, since hemoglobin is the last nutritional parameter to return to normal.

creased from a mean of 215 µg/dl to a mean of 290 µg/ml.

When nutritional supplements were given through a nasogastric tube, satiety did not occur. In most subjects, some voluntary consumption of food continued even though delivery of nutrients by infusion was adequate to meet their nutritional needs. After one week of enteral support and, presumably, as anorexia decreased, a large number of patients consumed all their meals voluntarily, and the average caloric intake frequently exceeded 4000 cal/day. An example of such a patient receiving enteral hyperalimentation and voluntarily eating a meal is shown in Figure 26–2. After three weeks of

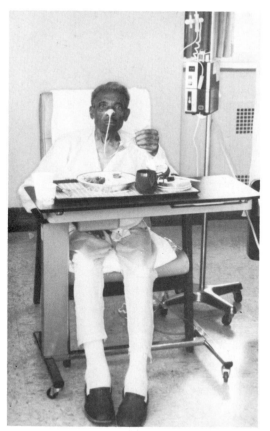

Figure 26–2. An 89-year-old patient with severe protein energy malnutrition receiving enteral hyperalimentation by slow continuous infusion through a nasogastric tube. The patient was initially confused and confined to bed. This picture was taken 14 days after nutritional therapy was begun, at which time the patient was relatively mobile and could transfer from his bed to a chair with assistance. Enteral hyperalimentation given by slow infusion did not cause satiety, so this patient consumed all his meals daily.

counts were less than 1.6×10^3 cells/μl. After 21 days of nutritional support, significant increases in lymphocyte counts were noted in virtually all patients studied. In addition, after 21 days, 80 per cent of patients were no longer anergic, developing significant induration (greater than 10 mm in 2 planes at 24 or 48 hours) to at least three of the five antigens that were reapplied intradermally. In addition to frequently correcting these immune abnormalities, substantial improvement in hematologic functions was demonstrated. As noted above, hemoglobin values improved markedly after six weeks. In addition, in measurements of the hematopoietic myeloid stem cell (CFU-C) in older patients with severe protein-energy malnutrition, the CFU-C values were markedly reduced prior to nutritional support, averaging 0.23×10^7 cell/kg compared with a normal value of 0.84×10^7 cell/kg. After three weeks of nutritional support, CFU-C had invariably increased to a mean value of 0.65×10^7 cell/kg. The importance of these observations lies in the fact that they highlight a possible role for nutrition-impaired host defense in older patients. They also emphasize the need for a careful nutritional assessment prior to ascribing all immune and hematopoietic abnormalities to the aging process per se.

SUMMARY

Older persons have needs that vary depending on the cohort to which they belong: middle-aged, aging, elderly, or aged. Their needs for enteral nutrition should be consumer-oriented but frequently are provider-oriented. The determinants of enteral nutrition are specific and should be used in estimating the quantitative and the qualitative aspects of the regimens selected. Precautions must be taken in designing the nutrient and water contents of the mixtures. Commercial formulas are available, varied, and easily prepared. They are expensive, however, and may be replaced by mixtures of regular foods and beverages liquified in blenders and food processors. Monitoring by knowledgeable people—not necessarily professionally trained—is a requisite. Physiotherapy, good nursing care, and knowledgeable nutritional advice are essential. Considerations of food safety must be entertained by all providers. Team rounds pro-

nutritional support, voluntary caloric intakes were such that the nasogastric tubes were removed. The patients continued to consume food voluntarily and, over the three subsequent weeks, further increases in weight, serum albumin, and TIBC were documented. In addition, hemoglobin, which had not increased after 21 days of nutritional support, had risen markedly by day 42.

Some additional points deserve special comment. As indicated above, both protein-energy malnutrition and the aging process cause major alterations in hematopoietic and immune functions. The Arkansas patients with severe protein-energy malnutrition were invariably anergic, and their lymphocyte vide an excellent method of assuring coordination of the activities of all involved providers. When compromises must be made, a single knowledgeable person should have authority to make decisions. Enteral nutrition in older persons should be discontinued when it is no longer indicated and when the risks entailed in its use exceed possible benefits.

REFERENCES

1. McWhirter, N.: Guinness Book of World Records. 1981 Annual Edition. New York, Bantam Books, Inc., 1981, pp. 25–29.
2. Gray, R. W., Wilz, D. R., Caldas, A. E., and Lemann, J., Jr.: The importance of phosphate in regulating 1,25(OH)$_2$-vitamin D levels in humans: Studies in healthy subjects, in calcium-stone formers, and in patients with primary hyperparathyroidism. J. Clin. Endocrinol. Metab., 45:299–306, 1977.
3. Aaseth, J., Thomassen, Y., Alexander, J., and Norheim, G.: Decreased serum selenium in alcoholic cirrhosis. N. Engl. J. Med., 303:944–945, 1980.
4. Johnson, R. A., Baker, S. S., Fallon, J. T., Maynard, E. P., III, Ruskin, J. H., Wen, Z., Ge, K., and Cohen, H. J.: An Occidental case of cardiomyopathy and selenium deficiency. N. Engl. J. Med., 304:1210–1212, 1981.
5. Thompson, C. D., Rea, H. M., Robinson, M. F., and Chapman, O. W.: Low blood selenium concentrations and glutathione peroxidase activities in elderly people. Proc. Univ. Otago. Med. Schl., 55:18–19, 1977.
6. Watkin, D. M.: Modern nutrition for those who are already old: The challenges of the eighties. Aging, Sept.–Oct., Nos. 311–312, 1980, pp. 21–28.
7. Watkin, D. M.: Aging and the food service industry: Effects upon consumers, employees and executives. In Proceedings of the 36th Conference: The Food Service Industry in the 1980s—A More Complex Environment, San Antonio, Texas, November 6–8, 1980. Fort Wayne, Indiana, The Society for the Advancement of Food Service Research, 1981, pp. 31–40.
8. Roe, D. A.: Drug-Induced Nutritional Deficiencies. Westport, Connecticut, AVI Publishing Company, Inc., 1976. pp. 1–272.
9. Andres, R.: Influence of obesity on longevity in the aged. In Borek, C. (ed.): Aging, Cancer, and Cell Membranes, Vol. III, Advances in Cancer Biology Series. New York, Stratton Intercontinental Medical Book Corporation, 1980, pp. 238–246.
10. Hazzard, W. R.: Aging and atherosclerosis: Interactions with diet, heredity, and associated risk factors. In Rockstein, M., and Sussman, M. L. (eds.): Nutrition, Longevity, and Aging. New York, Academic Press, 1976, pp. 143–195.
11. Rifkin, B. M.: The coronary primary prevention trial: Design and implementation. The lipid research clinics program. J. Chron. Dis., 32:609–631, 1979.
12. Schaefer, A. E.: Nutrition policies for the elderly. In Kamath, S., and Kohrs, M. B. (eds.): Proceedings of a Symposium on Nutrition and Aging, Chicago, July 23–24, 1981. Am. J. Clin. Nutr., 36:819–822, 1982.
13. Bloch, A. S., and Shils, M. E.: Appendix. In Modern Nutrition in Health and Disease. Edition 6. Philadelphia, Lea and Febiger, 1980, pp. 1312–1330.
14. Wilmore, D. W.: Enteral and parenteral nutrition in hospital In Rubenstein, E., and Federman, D. D. (eds.): Scientific American Medicine. New York, Scientific American, Inc., 1981, pp. 4:XIV 1–16.
15. Chandra, R. K.: Lymphocyte subpopulations in human malnutrition: cytotoxic and suppressor cells. Pediatrics, 59:423–427, 1977.
16. Adams, E. B.: Anemia associated with protein deficiency. Semin. Hematol., 7:55–66, 1970.
17. Reissman, K. R., and Udupa, K. B.: Effect of inflammation on erythroid precursors (BFU-E and CFU-E) in bone marrow and spleen of mice. J. Lab. Clin. Med., 92:22–29, 1978.
18. Weksler, M. E., and Hütteroth, T. M.: Impaired lymphocyte function in aged humans. J. Clin. Invest., 53:99–104, 1974.
19. Gupta, S., and Good, R. A.: Subpopulations of human T lymphocytes. X. Alterations in T, B, third population cells and T cells with receptors for immunoglobulin M (Tμ) or G (Tγ) in aging humans. J. Immunol., 122:1214–1219, 1979.
20. Mitchell, C. O., and Lipschitz, D. A.: The effect of age and sex on the routinely employed measurements used to assess the nutritional status of hospitalized patients. Am. J. Clin. Nutr., 36:340–349, 1982.
21. Forbes, G. B., and Reina, J. C.: Adult lean body mass declines with age: Some longitudinal observations. Metabolism, 19:653–663, 1970.
22. Lipschitz, D. A., and Mitchell, C. O.: The correctability of the nutritional, immune, and hematopoietic manifestations of protein-calorie malnutrition in the elderly. J.P.E.N., 4:621, 1982.

CHAPTER 27

Enteral Tube Feeding at Home

CATHERINE H. BASTIAN
RICHARD H. DRISCOLL

In recent years health care professionals have begun to place appropriate emphasis on the treatment of chronic disease. The important concept in this trend is the return of the affected patient to the home environment as a viable and functioning member of the family unit. "Self-care" of the patient, with or without family assistance, is the cornerstone of this philosophy. That the physician for too long has been unable or unwilling to relinquish this responsibility has ultimately resulted in prolonged or repeated hospitalizations and has compounded the already present emotional and economic burdens. An excellent example of this situation is the patient who is unable to maintain adequate oral nutrition.

Enteral tube feeding and total parenteral nutrition (TPN) are readily used in appropriate hospitalized patients who are incapable of voluntarily consuming adequate calories and protein. However, when the primary disease is rendered stable, the patient is usually discharged regardless of his or her nutritional status. The physician's decision may have been reached without sufficient consideration of the adequacy of the patient's oral intake, or may have been based on the prohibitive cost of a hospital bed to be used solely for providing prolonged nutritional support. Unfortunately, many patients are unable to sustain an appropriate dietary intake at home. Malnutrition often persists, despite intensive dietary counseling and encouragement from medical personnel and family, and results in hospitalization.[1] Conversely, the physician who is concerned about the nutritional status of the patient may hospitalize the patient for prolonged tube feeding until adequate oral intake is achieved or until nutritional sufficiency allows medical or surgical therapy.

Three issues may arise, and the options clearly need to be addressed. Specifically, is the patient's nutritional status in jeopardy? If so, is the patient a candidate for enteral tube feeding, and could this program be managed at home effectively and safely? Generally, the goal of such treatment is to provide either complete or supplemental tube feedings sufficient to promote positive energy-protein balance and weight gain. The patient may consume whatever foods are tolerated. The duration of time for enteral tube feeding depends on the desired end point—the patient's ability to resume adequate oral intake, or to achieve acceptable nutritional balance, or both. When the desire to eat begins to return or nutritional parameters have improved to adequate levels, enteral tube feeding may be tapered or discontinued.

Tremendous attention has been focused on the importance of nutrition in the comprehensive management of disease processes. Protein-calorie malnutrition frequently accompanies many disorders. It may affect the overall prognosis and well-being of any given patient.[2, 3] Therefore, it is important to identify those persons who, because of their underlying disorders, may be subject to chronic progressive malnutrition and debility. Clearly, patients who cannot eat, will not eat, or should not eat are at obvious risk and need specific attention focused on maintenance or repletion of normal nutritional balance. If such is the case, can enteral tube feeding at home sustain or improve proper energy-protein balance and weight for prolonged periods in patients with an accessible and functioning gastrointestinal tract? If so, what are the cost and safety of such an approach, and should other options be considered?

Enteral tube feeding at home is not a new concept or practice, but it has been underutilized because its potential benefits have not been appreciated. It has also been misdirected because often only the terminally ill or institutionalized patient is committed to such an endeavor. The practice of enteral tube feeding at home needs to be examined so that patients with a variety of disorders can be successfully introduced to this technique to ensure the already established benefits. Positive nitrogen balance, progressive weight gain, and restoration of lean body tissue can be achieved while the medical or surgical disease is being corrected or controlled at home.[1, 4, 5]

Through the use of various access routes, a variety of blenderized or defined formula diets, and intermittent or continuous infusion, enteral tube feeding at home has been demonstrated to provide adequate nutrition in patients with a wide spectrum of disorders.[6, 7] Enteral feedings may be administered for various time periods, depending on the short-term or long-term needs of the patient. In addition, improvement in the primary disease may occur directly or indirectly from nutritional therapy in certain patients.[1, 5] If oral restitution cannot be attained, then enteral tube feeding seems to be a viable alternative for long-term nutritional maintenance, either as a complete or as a supplemental feeding. Though clinical experiences seem to support this concept, clear documentation in the literature is lacking for significant numbers of patients treated longer than 18 to 24 months. Certainly, long-term studies are needed.

The major alternative to enteral tube feeding in patients unable to achieve adequate oral intake is home TPN. The remarkable progress made in home TPN since its advent 10 years ago has been substantial.[8, 9] Home TPN has enabled patients with intestinal failure and short-bowel syndrome to return to nearly normal living while sustaining normal nutritional and fluid balance.[10, 11] The great excitement in parenteral nutrition has relegated enteral tube feeding to the background. As clinical experience has accumulated, the indications for home TPN, primarily for acute or chronic gastrointestinal dysfunction or failure, have been realized. Wide application has been inhibited somewhat by the unknowns of long-term parenteral feeding and by the time commitment, cost, and potential complications. Recently, physicians have been realizing the potential benefit and broad application that enteral tube feeding possesses for patients with acceptable gastrointestinal function. Home enteral tube feeding may not be applicable to all patients, but when used in appropriate clinical situations, it provides a more physiologic, safer, less time-consuming, and less expensive method of nutritional support.

Clinical studies comparing nutritional gains resulting from intravenous and enteral feeding have been limited and somewhat conflicting.[5, 12, 13, 14] Studies of this type are difficult because many variables exist. There is increasing evidence that short-term nutritional repletion may be achieved more rapidly with TPN.[13] However, this may depend on the specific disease process and the effect of that disease on gastrointestinal function (mechanical, digestive, and absorptive capacity), which could adversely affect enteral tube feeding. It has been demonstrated that home enteral tube feeding compares favorably with home TPN (regardless of underlying disease process) with respect to weight gain, improved anthropometric measures, physical fitness, and quality of life over a 2- to 15-month period. Both techniques eliminated the need for prolonged hospitalization. Complications in the TPN group were significantly greater and potentially life-threatening.[5] Unfortunately, the number of patients was small, and the groups were not clearly comparable. Further studies are warranted.

Enteral feeding of nutrients appears to possess physiologic benefits that may be lacking in long-term intravenous administration. Luminal nutrition appears important in maintaining the functional and structural integrity of the gastrointestinal mucosa.[15, 16] The observed effects may be attributed not only to the exclusion of luminal nutrients, but also to alteration in gastrointestinal hormonal function.[16] The clinical significance of these observations in patients who have had prolonged bowel rest needs documentation. The insulin response to enteral glucose is greater than the response to parenteral glucose, which apparently results from complex gut–hormone interactions.[17, 18] To what extent hormonal balance and function are altered, and what role these changes play in nutrient metabolism after prolonged parenteral nutrition are unknown. Although bypassing the normal enterohepatic axis may not affect overall energy and nitrogen balance, what effect does parenteral nutrition have on hepatic nutrient processing (such as specific amino acid, lipoprotein, and vitamin metabolism)? Recommended daily allowances of essential nutrients are derived from enteral nutrition and are not known for parenteral nutrition. Nutrient needs and excess can often be regulated by the enterohepatic axis, but are similar controlling mechanisms operational with parenteral delivery? Severe metabolic bone disease has been well documented in patients on long-term TPN.[19, 20] The exact mechanism of this disorder has not been clearly established; however, it appears that TPN adversely affects vitamin D bone metabolism in certain individuals.[21] Whether other clinically significant metabolic alteration will occur in patients on home TPN remains to be described.

The time constraints placed on the patient on home enteral tube feeding appear to be much less than those of the patient on home TPN. The enterally fed patient does not have the time-consuming task of preparation of parenteral solutions. Administration of the enteral formula is accomplished more quickly and safely. Infusion time may be comparable, but enteral feeding allows the patient greater flexibility that may shorten the adjustment period and allow the patient to return to a more normal life-style.[5] Enteral tube feeding is, for the most part, simple for the patient to learn. Care of the feeding tube and administration set is easy, and there is no fear of dislodged, thrombotic, or septic catheters.[5]

With careful selection of patients, a knowledgeable staff, thoroughly educated patients, hospital trials to simulate at-home feeding conditions, and frequent monitoring, home enteral tube feeding can be relatively safe. Under similar circumstances, home TPN can be conducted with an acceptable low rate of complications.[10, 11] However, catheter-related complications do occur and may be potentially life-threatening. Large series detailing complications associated with tube feeding at home have not been reported. The clinical experience to date would indicate that this procedure is far safer for long-term nutritional therapy.[1, 4, 5]

Finally, in times when cost considera-tions must be an important priority, hospital versus home economics certainly favors home enteral tube feeding. Though costs may vary considerably, depending on the products and the volume, the yearly expense for home enteral tube feeding averages between $4,000 and $15,000 ($10 to $40 per day).[4, 5] Home TPN in a comparable patient would cost between $25,000 and $90,000 per year ($70 to $250 per day), a sizeable cost differential.[5, 9] The comparison of home enteral tube feeding with home TPN is not meant to condemn the latter, but to place the two techniques into proper perspective. Each has an important role when used appropriately. Enteral tube feeding at home is beneficial, safe, cost effective, and adaptable to diverse disease processes in patients with adequate gastrointestinal function.

CLINICAL APPLICATION

Disease Considerations

Any disease process that adversely affects oral consumption will lead to nutritional deprivation of varying degree, depending on: (1) the severity of the disease and associated complications; (2) the duration of disease activity; and (3) the balance of nutritional supply versus the demands of body metabolism. A variety of diseases and disorders, though different in their pathophysiologic manifestations, may adversely affect appetite or interfere with the patient's capacity to consume or assimilate adequate nutrients. The consequences of nutritional depletion associated with inadequate oral intake are well described.[2, 3] If gastrointestinal function is preserved, these problems can virtually be overcome by various modes of enteral tube feeding. Adequate nutritional supply can be maintained until proper medical or surgical therapy cures or palliates the disease and normal oral intake resumes. If a successful end point cannot be achieved, then enteral tube feeding may be used indefinitely. In many situations in which enteral tube feeding is indicated for three to four weeks or longer, and continued hospitalization is otherwise unwarranted, the patient may be a candidate for home enteral tube feeding. The skyrocketing costs of hospitalization should compel the physician to consider strongly the role of home enteral tube feeding or other options for nutritional maintenance. The ultimate role of home enteral tube feeding has yet to be realized since its use has been restricted primarily to the terminally ill or institutionalized patient. Though its use in these situations is entirely appropriate, attention must be extended to patients with treatable or controllable disorders who are capable of some form of natural life-style.

This chapter considers the broad applications of enteral tube feeding in the overall management of a wide variety of disorders. Table 27–1 outlines the various disorders in which home enteral tube feeding may be po-

Table 27–1 DISEASES IN WHICH HOME ENTERAL TUBE FEEDING IS POTENTIALLY APPROPRIATE

DISEASES OR DISORDERS	REFERENCES
Metabolic	
Glycogen storage disease, type I (glucose-6-phosphatase deficiency)	1,22–27
Gastrointestinal	
Inflammatory bowel disease	
Intestinal manifestations	1,2,5,30–41
Fistula(s)	30,33,35,36,38,41,45–48,50
Growth retardation	51–55
Short-bowel syndrome	1,30,31,33,34,36,37,42–44
Abdominal fistula(s) (non-Crohn's)	34,45–50
Radiation enteropathy	34,35,47,56
Other	—
Cancer	
Obstructing disease	
Head and neck	5,58–67,70–76
Esophagus	5,68–76
Stomach	5,70–76
Abnormalities of deglutition following surgical intervention	
Head and neck	5,58–65, 70–76
Esophagus	5,68–76
Gastrointestinal side effects of cancer (or chemotherapy and/or radiotherapy)	1,2,5,34,70–83
Terminal supportive care	2,5,70–76
Neurologic	79–86
Comatose patient	
Cerebrovascular accident	
Head injury	
Encephalopathy	
Dysphagia	
Cranial nerve dysfunction (IX,X,XI)	
Basal ganglion disease (Parkinson's)	
Myasthenia gravis	
Muscular dystrophies, polymyositis	
Geriatric patient with cerebral dysfunction	
Mental retardation	
Psychologic	
Anorexia nervosa	87
Major affective disorders (depression)	—
Schizophrenia (catatonia)	—
Phobic anxiety states	—
Other Systemic Disorders	
Chronic renal disease (hemodialysis and peritoneal dialysis)	1
Chronic cardiac disease	1,2
Chronic pulmonary disease	—
Chronic liver disease	2

tentially useful—chronic disorders for which long-term nutritional maintenance may be necessary.

Glycogen storage disease, type I, is a rare metabolic disorder in which the liver cannot maintain adequate glucose homeostasis because of glucose-6-phosphatase deficiency. The long-term management of the metabolic and clinical problems of this disorder depends on home enteral tube feeding. With the use of frequent, high-starch meals during the day and continuous intragastric feedings at night, hypoglycemia and acidosis, which contribute to catabolism and anorexia, can be suppressed.[22] Similarly, other manifestations of the disease can be effectively controlled. Continuous intragastric feeding at night has promoted anabolism and caloric intake, which accounts for the catch-up growth seen in many pediatric patients with associated growth retardation.[23] A number of reports have confirmed these observations, and follow-up has been as long as five years.[22-27] Nasogastric feeding tubes are inserted nightly, and may be removed each morning to allow the child a normal life-style during the day. Since complications have been minimal to absent, and patient tolerance has been remarkably acceptable, experience to date has found it unnecessary to perform gastrostomy. As patients with this disorder age, they are better able to extend periods between feedings and may only occasionally require nocturnal tube feeding.[22] The role of home enteral tube feeding in this disorder is somewhat unique. It provides (supplements) necessary calories, primarily in the form of glucose, and thus satisfies the nutritional needs of the patient and controls the clinical manifestations of the disease. In addition, enteral tube feeding can be undertaken with safety and acceptable compliance in a young age group.

Nutritional depletion is common in many gastrointestinal disorders, and the physician must recognize this association to deal effectively with the special problems encountered in these disorders. The typical patient has some element of malabsorption or excessive gastrointestinal nutrient loss and is unable to satisfy increased nutritional needs through oral consumption, which is often limited by appetite, symptoms, or prescription.[28] Although the frequency and diversity of nutritional derangements in patients with gastrointestinal disease have been clearly documented,[29] what should be the practical approach to their management? The answer lies in the physician's ability to recognize the development of specific nutritional abnormalities and then to correct them. A logical sequence of dietary manipulation is as follows: (1) alterations in the normal diet content and meal frequency to meet the patient's appetite and desires; (2) selective additions to correct specific deficits (such as iron, folic acid, supplemental protein, and total calories); (3) isolated deletions or diminutions of specific nutrients (such as fiber, lactose, or fat) in response to pathophysiologic changes associated with the disease; and (4) consideration of the use of special enteral or parenteral formulas when indicated.[30] Attention to this sequence of therapy will minimize complications, cost, and hospitalization.[30] Defined formula diets are valuable in situations requiring maintenance of nutritional balance, and in many instances are effective in controlling symptoms of gastrointestinal disease. Extensive experience with such diets, primarily through oral administration, has been reported.[31-45] If one considers the degree of anorexia, the adverse symptoms associated with oral consumption of food, and the unpalatability of many defined formula diets, enteral tube feeding would appear to be a beneficial and viable option for providing adequate nutritional intake. However, relatively few reports have been published concerning its use in patients with gastrointestinal disease requiring long-term nutritional maintenance.[1, 5, 31, 32] The clinical applications of enteral tube feeding in patients with such disorders appear to have great potential and are worthy of discussion. Table 27–2 summarizes gastrointestinal disorders in which home enteral tube feeding could be used to supply a complete or supplemental diet.

The acute gastrointestinal disorders refer to short-term or temporary (four to eight weeks) nutritional deprivation that persists until medical and/or surgical intervention can either cure or palliate the disease and normal oral intake can be resumed. Many such patients exist and should be considered as candidates for home enteral tube feeding. Adequate current experience is clearly lacking and is worthy of future investigation.

The chronic gastrointestinal disorders serve as a prototype for use of home enteral tube feeding. By virtue of their nature, they are long-standing chronic diseases (months to years) characterized by periods of remis-

Table 27–2 GASTROINTESTINAL DISORDERS IN WHICH HOME ENTERAL TUBE FEEDING COULD BE POTENTIALLY BENEFICIAL FOR SUPPLYING A COMPLETE OR SUPPLEMENTAL DEFINED FORMULA DIET

	OBJECTIVES	SUGGESTED APPROACH
Acute Disorders (4 to 8 Weeks) Obstructive disease (acid-peptic disease of upper gastrointestinal tract, gastrointestinal cancer of the esophagus or stomach)	To replete nutritional status prior to (or during) major medical, surgical, and/or radiotherapy intervention and to maintain same until therapy for the underlying disease allows for adequate oral intake.	Tube feeding delivered distal to obstruction; complete or supplemental feeding; administered as 24-hour continuous or intermittent infusion during the day and/or night.
Inflammatory disorders (acute radiation injury) Postsurgical anorexia (prolonged anorexia following major abdominal surgery)	To provide short-term nutritional support until anorexia or other interfering symptoms abate, allowing for resumption of normal or modified diet.	Nasogastric infusion to supplement oral intake; may only require intermittent or nocturnal infusion.
Chronic Disorders (Months to Years) Postgastrectomy malnutrition Inflammatory bowel disease with fistula(s) or with growth retardation Short-bowel syndrome Radiation enteropathy Abdominal fistula (non-Crohn's)	To provide long-term nutritional support to maintain or promote weight gain and/or linear growth; additional benefits may result in improved intestinal symptoms and fistula closure; when remission occurs, oral intake can be resumed.	Depending on oral intake, tube feeding can provide complete or supplemental calories and protein; delivery by nasogastric route as 24-hour continuous drip, intermittent infusions during day, or nocturnal infusion.

sions and exacerbations and often require either continuous or intermittent nutritional therapy. This patient population is certainly one for which home management should be advocated. A number of published reports verify the usefulness of defined formula diets administered orally or by feeding tube within the hospital, primarily in patients with inflammatory bowel disease [30–41] or short-bowel syndrome. [30, 31, 33, 34, 36, 37, 42–44] The experience with oral, defined formula diets at home also has been gratifying. Such diets have demonstrated value in sustaining positive nitrogen balance, relieving symptoms of bowel obstruction, aiding in fistula closure [45–48, 50] and symptomatic management of choleraic diarrhea, [33] and initiating linear growth in children whose growth has been retarded. [51–55] The use of home enteral tube feeding in these disorders has received little attention in the literature. [1, 5, 32] Although the number of cases reported has been small, the overall results and safety compare favorably with those achieved within the hospital. At the same time, the cost savings is tremendous. The majority of these patients use tube feedings to supplement their oral intake. This is accomplished by continuous or intermittent nasogastric infusion during the day or overnight, using a defined formula diet designed to achieve optimal assimilation and cost containment. As home enteral tube feeding becomes more widely accepted and practiced, and as adequate experience is gained, it should offer an excellent alternative for long-term nutritional support in patients with chronic gastrointestinal disease. These patients are otherwise destined to chronic debility and repeated hospitalizations, or, alternatively, are candidates for long-term home TPN. [57]

For the other disorders reviewed in Table 27–1, home enteral tube feeding may also have potential benefits. These have been discussed in previous chapters, and appropriate references that provide additional details are listed in Table 27–1. Future prospective studies should provide the data needed to adequately define the proper role of long-term enteral tube feeding in these disorders.

Patient Selection

If one recognizes that long-term enteral tube feeding can maintain nutritional balance and preserve the well-being of patients, then which patients should use this technique at home? Figure 27–1 depicts var-

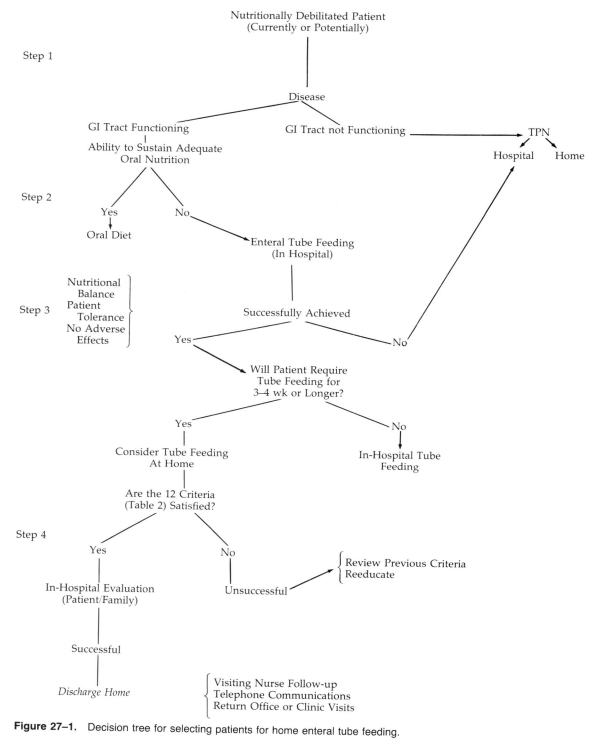

Figure 27–1. Decision tree for selecting patients for home enteral tube feeding.

ious steps involved in the decision-making process.

The first consideration (step 1) concerns whether the patient is at nutritional risk by virtue of the underlying disease process, and/or as a result of medical or surgical intervention. Once nutritional risk has been determined, step 2 evaluates the adequacy of gastrointestinal function and the ability of the patient to consume sufficient nutrients by the oral route.

Table 27–3 lists situations in which oral intake may be compromised, and optional modes of feeding need careful consideration. Every attempt should be made to allow the patient to consume food as naturally as possible before other methods are undertaken. Proper selection of diet and encouragement by family and professional staff are essential. If, after a sufficient trial, oral intake is inadequate and the gastrointestinal tract is functional, then enteral tube feeding in the hospital would be indicated. At this juncture, it would be appropriate to consider whether long-term enteral tube feeding may be necessary. If the patient is destined for tube feeding for three to four weeks or more, then home administration is a logical alternative. The other important considerations at this time would be as follows: (1) Is the patient's underlying disease process stable so that continued hospitalization is no longer warranted and home management could be undertaken without difficulty or complicating problems? (2) What would be the most appropriate route for delivering the enteral tube feeding (nasogastric tube, gastrostomy)? (3) Can enteral tube feeding be used successfully to supply nutritional needs with acceptable patient tolerance and without adverse effects? A period of time in the hospital will be necessary to formulate a tube feeding program and to determine its potential success (step 3).

Once tube feeding is successfully conducted in the hospital and prolonged administration is deemed likely, then home enteral tube feeding should be strongly considered (step 4). Table 27–4 lists the minimum criteria for selecting such patients. The time period of three to four weeks has been chosen somewhat arbitrarily. However, the allotment of seven to ten days to formulate and administer a successful enteral tube feeding program and to adequately train the patient and family to use it would leave at least 10 to 14 days for tube feeding at home. Shorter periods of home enteral tube feeding are probably not cost effective when the time involved by multiple health care professionals is considered.

Patient selection is critical for successful management and outcome. All patients requiring long-term enteral tube feeding are not candidates for automatic discharge to the home. A social worker should be involved in the planning for all potential candidates for home enteral tube feeding. The physical, psychological, and socioeconomic status of each patient and the patient's family must be thoroughly assessed before home training is undertaken within the hospital. If such patients or families are deemed unconcerned and fraught with risk, long-term tube feeding should be conducted within the hospital or a chronic care facility where appropriate attention can be directed to techniques and potential side effects.

REVIEW OF TECHNIQUES

Once the patient is deemed a candidate for home enteral tube feeding, the most appropriate access route must be achieved, and discharge planning for the patient should be set in motion. Careful coordination and individual attention requires the expertise of

Table 27–3 CLINICAL SITUATIONS IN WHICH ENTERAL TUBE FEEDING (SHORT- OR LONG-TERM) SHOULD BE CONSIDERED

CLINICAL SITUATION	ETIOLOGIC FACTOR
Anorexia (patient will not eat)	Active disease process, treatment of disease, psychologic state
Inability to eat (patient cannot eat)	Coma, cerebrovascular disease, mental retardation, dysphagia
Contraindicated (patient should not eat)	Obstruction, abnormal digestive and/or absorptive process, fistula(s)
Other	Metabolic instability

Table 27–4 CRITERIA FOR SELECTING PATIENTS TO RECEIVE HOME ENTERAL TUBE FEEDING

1. Inability to consume nutritional requirements orally when nutritional status is in jeopardy
2. Underlying disease process appears stable and continued hospitalization is no longer warranted
3. Continued tube feeding will be necessary for 3 to 4 weeks or longer
4. Most appropriate delivery route used for enteral tube feeding
5. Successful hospital experience documenting nutritional adequacy, patient acceptance, and lack of adverse effects
6. Willingness and cooperation of patient and/or family to continue tube feeding at home in suitable emotional and physical environment
7. Home enteral tube feeding must achieve advantages to the patient that could not be obtained in the hospital (such as psychological, mobility, and cost)
8. Predetermined goals and objectives of home tube feeding formulated and discussed between health care team and patient and family
9. Comprehensive education given to patient and family by knowledgeable health care professional(s)
10. Financial arrangements (cost reimbursement) reviewed, discussed, and accepted by patient and family
11. Proper support and follow-up must be available to patient and family at all times
12. Successful in-hospital trial (two days) achieved by patient and family

Table 27–5 CONSIDERATIONS FOR DETERMINING ACCESS ROUTE FOR HOME ENTERAL TUBE FEEDING

Duration of illness
Disease pathology
Patient considerations
   Age
   State of consciousness
   General overall health
   Comfort and tolerance
   Ability to perform necessary tube care
Aspiration potential and risk
   State of consciousness
   Cranial nerve dysfunction (IX, X, XI)
   Abnormal cough reflex
   Dysphagia
   Gastric retention
   Underlying pulmonary disease
In-hospital evaluation
   Patient tolerance
   Observed complications
   Unacceptable gastric residual
Surgical considerations
   Surgical & anesthetic risk
   Surgical experience and preferred procedure(s)

the physician, clinical dietitian, nurse specialist, social worker, and home health service. Consideration of the patient's and family's needs with respect to his or her medical condition, emotional and psychological outlook, and social and economic situation will determine the effectiveness of the home feeding program.[88]

Determining the Access Route for Feeding Tube Delivery

Strong consideration needs to be given to the most appropriate access route for delivery, which usually is either a nasopharyngeal tube or tube enterostomy. The specifics of these currently available techniques are discussed in detail in Chapters 16 and 17. This chapter discusses the determination of optimal sites for enteral tube feeding for prospective home patients.

The obvious and major consideration is what is best for the patient. The choices vary greatly and should be individualized for each patient (Table 27–5). The first consideration is the duration of illness. If the underlying illness is chronic and/or progressive, then some form of tube enterostomy would be appropriate.[85, 89–91] However, if such a patient requires long-term intermittent feeding to supplement oral intake, a nasogastric feeding tube for nocturnal infusions may be preferred. With short-term feedings (four to eight weeks), some form of nasopharyngeal tube or temporary enterostomy should be used.

The underlying disease process often dictates what type of delivery site should be used. Tube feeding, which is always delivered distal to the obstructive process, may often dictate an enterostomy, though often nasopharyngeal tubes may pass through obstructive lesions of the esophagus or stomach.[68] A conservative approach may be most appropriate in patients of increased age, of decreased state of consciousness, and with poor underlying health.[91] High morbidity and mortality have been associated with certain types of gastrostomy and jejunostomy in this patient population.[90, 91] The pediatric population appears to be at risk for development of complications after gastrostomy, and probably another approach should be used.[89]

The possibility of aspiration, which is

the major, life-threatening complication associated with tube feeding, needs to be assessed prior to discharging the patient from the hospital. Any patient with an altered state of consciousness or dysfunction of the cranial nerves (IX to XI) should be considered a candidate for either a gastrostomy or jejunostomy.[85] The risk of aspiration from nasogastric tube feeding is unacceptably high in this patient population.[81] If the above illnesses are judged to be temporary, a nasoduodenal feeding tube is an option. However, it is still not clear whether this truly reduces the risk of aspiration, since these tubes may dislodge proximally into the stomach or esophagus. Similarly, in patients with problems of deglutition after head and neck surgery with cervical esophagostomy, the risk of aspiration is significant. A small nasogastric tube or other type of tube enterostomy may be more appropriate. This remains to be determined. If abnormal deglutition is deemed a long-term problem, then either a gastrostomy or jejunostomy may be the most logical choice. Since aspiration may be particularly serious in patients with pulmonary disease (and this appears to be a very common problem in patients with head or neck cancer), similar procedures should be strongly considered.

Advocating an aggressive approach to the surgical construction of gastrostomy or jejunostomy depends on the risks of surgery and anesthesia and the experience and expertise of the surgeon. Gastrostomy and jejunostomy can be performed under local anesthesia with good results.[89] If the risk of surgical laparotomy is too high, a percutaneous endoscopic gastrostomy should be considered. The initial results of this technique are encouraging.[92–94] Gastrostomy and jejunostomy are underutilized procedures, and potentially offer greater benefits and safety for the patient.[89–91, 95] Studies are clearly needed to compare these and other feeding tube techniques in specific patient populations to determine the most advantageous approach.

The ultimate decision for the optimal method of tube delivery should result from the postprocedural assessment. The patient's tolerance, reaction, and attitudes to the selected procedure should be carefully observed. The patient's compliance and eventual outcome at home depend on favorable acceptance. The choice of the most appropriate access route for home enteral tube feeding cannot be overemphasized and clearly needs to be individualized for each patient. The overall success and longevity of the home program are extremely dependent on this decision.

Aspiration is a major complication.[81, 96] For this reason, checking gastric residual and evaluating the patient for subjective symptoms of gastric retention (such as abdominal distention or fullness, nausea, and bloated feeling) are appropriate. Evaluating secretions around the site of tracheostomy, pharyngostomy, or esophagostomy is most important. The development of respiratory distress, fever, or pulmonary infiltrates on chest x-ray film should be considered evidence of clinical aspiration until proved otherwise. Though gastric retention almost certainly predisposes to aspiration in a variety of disorders, it remains to be demonstrated what volume of gastric residual is clinically significant. Current literature recommends that gastric residuals be checked every eight hours with continuous feeding (pump-assisted) and before each feeding with the intermittent gravity method. Feedings should be withheld if the residual is greater than 150 ml.[97] For the present time these guidelines seem to be appropriate, but clinical documentation remains to be defined.

Selecting the Proper Enteral Formula Diet

A clinical dietitian should be responsible for evaluating the nutritional status of the patient, calculating nutritional requirements, and considering the most effective feeding modality and administration schedule to meet the patient's overall needs.[88] The nutritional adequacy of the enteral feeding program needs careful consideration to satisfy the patient's needs for a prolonged or indefinite period. This includes requirements for energy, protein, electrolytes, minerals, essential fatty acids, vitamins, trace elements, and water. The choice of the enteral dietary formulation will depend on complete nutritional adequacy, tube size and location, patient tolerance, formula availability, and cost.

A great variety of enteral products are available, including defined formula diets (polymeric, monomeric, and modular) and home- or commercially-blenderized diets.[2]

Standard use of home-blenderized products is not recommended primarily because: (1) the more commonly used access routes (nasogastric, nasoduodenal, and jejunostomy) do not usually permit their infusion; (2) bolus feeding is often not appropriate and needs to be discouraged as general practice; (3) nutritional adequacy may often be questioned; and (4) time of preparation, inadequate kitchen facilities, and the patient's unwillingness or inability to prepare the formula may jeopardize its success. Factors that favor use of home-blenderized diets may be economical and psychological. Patients may feel they are receiving "better nutrition" from commonly accepted food products and may feel more involved in family dynamics if they receive blenderized portions of food that other family members are consuming at mealtime.[88] Because of rising food costs and proposed changes in food stamp legislation that may restrict their availability, the cost advantages of home-blenderized diets are unclear. However, many health insurance plans and government programs (Medicare) are providing cost reimbursement for commercial formula diets.

Many aspects of selection of enteral formulas are detailed in previous chapters.[2] One aspect of the nutritional care plan that needs emphasis is the determination of the patient's requirement for water. This is rarely a problem in the patient who is capable of consuming water orally to satisfy thirst. However, in the unconscious or extremely debilitated patient, hyperosmolarity and dehydration are potentially life-threatening.[98–103] Water requirements will vary from patient to patient and will depend on normal metabolic fluid loss (insensible water loss, loss in stool and urine) and medical problems that may alter fluid balance (fever, diarrhea, renal disease, and fistula).[104]

Randall utilizes the guidelines in Table 27–6 to determine water requirements for each patient.[104] It is best to use ideal body weight for the obese and actual weight for others when calculating total water requirements. Once water requirements are calculated, how should they be satisfied? It is fallacious to assume that enteral formula volume is equal to free water content. The total free water content for each defined formula or blenderized diet varies: Compleat-B (Doyle) contains approximately 84 per cent free water (840 ml of water per 1000 ml of formula); Ensure-plus (Ross) contains approximately 78 per cent free water (780 ml of water per 1000 ml of formula); and Magnacal (Organon) contains approximately 58 per cent free water (577 ml of water per 1000 ml of formula). Since total free water content may vary with each enteral formula, the commercial industry needs to provide this information for each product. It is best to assume that for enteral formulas with caloric densities of 1.5 cal/ml or less, 80 per cent of the product volume is free water. For products with caloric densities of greater than 1.5 cal/ml, 60 per cent of the volume is free water. With this in mind, an adequate amount of water can be administered to achieve the necessary requirements. In patients unable to relate thirst and to achieve voluntary water intake, formulas with 1 cal/ml should be used if possible. If additional

Table 27–6 BASELINE FLUID REQUIREMENTS IN TEMPERATE CLIMATE*

	AGE (YR)	AVERAGE WATER REQUIREMENTS (ML/KG/DAY)
Adults, based on "ideal" weight for height and age		
Average adults	25–55	35
Young active adults	16–30	40
Older patients	55–65	30
Elderly	>65	25
Children over 5 kg body weight to age 18		
First 10 kg	—	100
Second 10 kg	—	50
Weight >20 kg	—	25

*From Randall, H.T. Fluid, electrolyte, and acid-base balance. Surg. Clin. North Am., *56*:1636, 1976, with permission.

water volume is required above the amount supplied in the administered formula, the formula can be diluted or water can be added directly through the feeding tube (as a wash) after the formula is delivered.[88, 97]

If the patient's fluid status is considered tenuous, the water generated through body metabolism may need consideration. This parameter is estimated by calculating 10 per cent of total administered calories as that volume (in milliliters) of water produced endogenously. This value can then be subtracted from the patient's total water requirement.[104]

Regardless of how perfect or imperfect these calculations for water requirements may be, caution should be taken and fluid balance should be watched carefully. All patients should be carefully monitored within the hospital and after discharge. Studies to evaluate acceptable hydration would involve measuring weight, serum sodium content, serum and urine osmolality, and blood urea nitrogen.

Choosing the Optimal Schedule for Administration of Formula

In determining the best schedule for formula delivery, two objectives clearly need to balance: which schedule will allow the patient the most free time, mobility, and ease of actual administration; and which system will best deliver the required tube feeding to provide adequate assimilation and avoid adverse effects and complications. The considerations for determining the schedule are listed in Table 27–7. There are currently three methods for administering tube feedings: bolus feeding, intermittent gravity drip, and continuous pump infusion.[96, 97] The characteristics of each have been described in Chapter 16. The choice of method depends on the various considerations listed in Table 27–7 that need to be individualized for each patient. Although bolus feedings are convenient for home use, intermittent gravity feeding is preferable for stomach infusions. Contrary to popular beliefs, if performed properly, both techniques require comparable time for administration of formula. A frequent tendency is for bolus feedings to be administered too quickly, which may lead to adverse effects.

Intermittent gravity feedings are well tolerated by most patients, though the volume and rate need to be individualized. Normal individuals can tolerate feedings of 250 to 750 ml administered at 30 ml/min without distress.[105] However, this schedule certainly does not apply to the majority of

Table 27–7 CONSIDERATIONS FOR DETERMINING ADMINISTRATION SCHEDULE FOR HOME ENTERAL TUBE FEEDING

MAJOR CONSIDERATIONS	SITUATION	SUGGESTIONS
Feeding tube access site	Nasogastric, esophagostomy or gastrostomy	Bolus, int.* gravity or continuous pump
	Nasoduodenal, jejunostomy	Continuous pump
Volume required to achieve nutritional needs	Nasogastric, esophagostomy, or gastrostomy	Bolus or int. gravity for <2000 ml; Int. gravity or continuous pump for >2000 ml[109]
Specific formula utilized	Blenderized (home)	Bolus
	Blenderized (commercial)	Bolus or int. pump
	Defined formula diets	Int. gravity or continuous pump
Gastric emptying capacity (predisposition to aspiration)	Abnormal (or potentially)	Continuous or int. pump
	Normal	Bolus, int. gravity
Underlying gastrointestinal disease	Inflammatory bowel disease	Continuous pump
	Short bowel syndrome	Continuous pump
Patient ease (time factors)	Nasogastric, esophagostomy or gastrectomy	Bolus or int. gravity (or pump)
Patient tolerance (presence of side effects)	Multiple situations	Depends on situation
Additional personnel/family required to administer feeding	Nasogastric, esophagostomy or gastrostomy	Bolus or int. gravity (or pump)
	Nasoduodenal, jejunostomy	Continuous pump

*Int., intermittent.

patients who are candidates for home enteral tube feeding. The usual volume and rate prescribed is 250 to 500 ml administered during a 30 to 40 minute period (10 to 15 ml/min).[88, 96, 97] The exact volume and frequency of administration will depend on the nutritional needs and the schedule best suited for the patient. Some patients prefer intermittent gravity administration only during waking hours, whereas others may prefer to have more free time during the day and to infuse a certain amount of their formula by continuous nocturnal pump infusion. The experience to date would indicate that nocturnal feeding is not associated with increased risk in properly selected individuals.[1]

Continuous infusion with pump assistance is the preferred technique when gastrointestinal access is achieved by a nasoduodenal tube or jejunostomy and when gastric emptying is inadequate and aspiration is possible.[96, 97] Many patients with gastrointestinal disorders (see Table 27–2) are often best managed with continuous infusion. Studies comparing continuous tube feedings with intermittent oral feedings or with intermittent tube feedings have been reported. The results indicate that continuous infusions provide improved enteral balance of major nutrients in infants with underlying gastrointestinal disease[106] and significantly less stool frequency and time required to achieve nutritional goals in adult burn patients.[107] A recent study preliminarily reported by Rombeau compared the caloric intake, time required to achieve full caloric requirements, and complication rates in patients receiving total enteral nutrition by tube.[97] Continuous jejunal infusion of a protein isolate was comparable with both intermittent and continuous gastric nutrient delivery as to the percentage of kilocalories delivered and days required to meet full caloric intake. Intermittent jejunal infusion appeared to be inferior to the other routes, primarily because of poor patient tolerance.

Clearly, continuous infusion is an acceptable technique with certain important advantages in specific patients. The feeding schedule for continuous infusion is usually planned during an 8- to 24-hour period, depending on the volume and rate required to achieve nutritional needs and adequate patient acceptance. The major disadvantage would be the restraints of long infusion times on active ambulatory patients. If continuous infusion is to be used, it is probably in the best interest of the patient to use a pump to ensure a steady rate of formula delivery to allow the patient uninterrupted time without the aggravation of constantly checking and adjusting the rate of drip.[108, 109]

DISCHARGE PLANNING

At the time the specific diet and administration schedule are being designed, other aspects of discharge planning should begin. The nurse specialist coordinates the administration schedule, monitors the tube feeding for potential complications and side effects, and develops the teaching program with the patient, family, or other responsible party.[88] Patient education needs to be complete, yet simple and understandable to all involved participants. Patient education is best performed by a nurse specialist or other health care professional who is trained in education techniques and has knowledge of home tube feeding. Teaching materials are extremely useful and should include: (1) an audiovisual program reviewing the importance of good nutrition and the reason for tube feeding, demonstrating the fundamentals of formula preparation, administration, and proper use of equipment, and discussing the potential complications and necessary precautions; and (2) an individualized written instruction manual detailing a step-by-step home tube feeding program. In addition, the nurse and clinical dietitian should demonstrate to the patient or responsible individual the various procedures and protocol as part of the training program. The patient should then be allowed to perform the entire program on his own with supervision as to proper technique for a 48-hour period or until that time when all techniques are performed properly. During this period, close monitoring should be performed to assess patient tolerance and adverse effects and to determine whether nutritional requirements are being satisfied. Patient and family reaction to the procedures needs to be observed. The necessary equipment for home tube feeding should be assembled (Table 27–8) and used as part of the patient's in-hospital teaching program.[88] Certain aspects concerning storage, administration, and cleaning of equipment need to

Table 27–8　EQUIPMENT REQUIRED FOR HOME ENTERAL TUBE FEEDING*

EQUIPMENT	METHOD		
	Continuous	Intermittent	Bolus
Feeding tubes (stylets)	±[1]	±[1]	−
Administration set (Feeding bag or bottle with tubing)	+	+	−
Infusion pump (pump tubing)	+	±[2]	−
Intravenous pole	+	+	−
Roller clamp (tubing)[3]	+	+	
Feeding tube clamp or plug[4]	+	+	+
Syringes (10 cc and 50 cc)[5]	+	+	+
Measuring cup	+	+	+
Formula preparation container (1 quart)	+	+	+
Tape (adhesive or other)	+	+	+
Lubricating jelly	±	±	−
Blender or mixer[6]	−	−	+
Sieve[6]	−	−	+

*Adapted from Bayer, L., et al. Coordinating a discharge program for the tube-fed patient. Personal communication.[88]
[1]Optional if patient prefers reintubation for intermittent or continuous infusion.
[2]May be used for intermittent feedings depending on infusion time or patient tolerance.
[3]Usually included on most administration sets.
[4]Required for tube enterostomies.
[5]Fifty-cc syringes required for bolus feedings and water administration; 50-cc or 10-cc syringe may be used for stomach aspiration.
[6]Used for home-blenderized diets.

be stressed and individualized for each patient (Table 27–9).

The social worker evaluates the patient's emotional status, home environment, and economic situation prior to discharge from the hospital. Tube feeding may represent a significant adjustment in role function and interdependence relationships.[110] For the patient, tube feeding represents a drastic change in physical conditions of food and food intake.[111] Tube feeding reduces eating to its barest essential, that of providing nourishment to the patient.[112] It drastically limits the sensory pleasures that normally accompany eating and contributes to dissocialization. In a recent study discussing patient reaction to tube feeding, Padilla et al. found that the most common and distressing experiences associated with tube feeding were "feeling thirsty," "being deprived of tasting food," and "having an unsatisfied appetite for certain foods."[112] These psychosensory disturbances are potential problems that need to be discussed with the patient and family prior to discharge and on subsequent clinic visits. The patient needs emotional support and practical advice to deal with these percep-

tions. If oral food consumption is allowed, the patient should be encouraged to consume favorite foods and beverages as tolerated in an attempt to satisfy appetite and taste preferences. Patients should be encouraged to participate in family mealtime whenever possible so that social aspects of meals can be maintained.[112]

Mobility needs to be encouraged for both emotional and physical equilibrium. The feeding program should be designed to allow the patient time to maintain normal activities. Many patients will be concerned about the appearance of a continuous indwelling nasopharyngeal tube. Every effort should be made to allow the patient freedom from such a tube by using self-intubation for intermittent or continuous infusions. Patients who will require long-term tube feeding should be equipped with some unexposed form of tube enterostomy to alleviate embarrassment or self-consciousness.[88]

A home enteral tube feeding program may be an overwhelming financial burden for the patient and family. In most instances cost reimbursement will be essential. In recent years many health insurance plans and

Table 27–9   SUGGESTIONS CONCERNING CERTAIN ASPECTS OF HOME ENTERAL TUBE
FEEDING

	SUGGESTIONS	COMMENTS
Formula Diets		
Storage	Room temperature	Any opened and unused liquid should be refrigerated (not longer than 24 hr).*
Form	Powder	Powder is preferred because of cost, storage space, no need for refrigeration, and least waste.
Preparation	24-hr supply	24-hr supply should be prepared daily and refrigerated; formulas should be allowed to come to room temperature before administration.
Formula spoilage	4 to 12 hr*	Most manufacturers recommend formula be discarded if it remains 4 to 8 hr at room temperature.*
Cleaning and Reuse of Equipment		
Administration set and bag	Clean after every use and discard every 24 hr	Liquid soap and hot water are probably sufficient; air dry; manufacturers recommend discarding after each use.*
Feeding tube	Clean after each infusion	If feeding tube is to remain in place, then flushing tube with sufficient water is adequate; if feeding tube is removed intermittently, then the same practices apply as with administration set and bag; most nasopharyngeal tubes can be reused indefinitely.
Pump	Proper cleansing and maintenance	Depending upon how pump is purchased or rented, some regular maintenance schedule should be arranged with clinical engineering department; pump replacement should be possible within 24 hr.

*Manufacturer recommendations only. Documentation of recommendation lacks sufficient data.

government programs (Medicare) have realized the medical importance and cost-saving benefits derived from home tube feeding.

Commercial health care plans are beginning to accept consignment for home enteral tube feeding if such a program is proved to be a medical necessity and if one can demonstrate considerable cost savings through the use of home enteral tube feeding instead of prolonged and repeated hospitalizations or home TPN.

Medicare has recently accepted coverage for home enteral tube feeding only as a prosthetic device (Section 3110.4).[113] Medicare recognizes "enteral nutrition to be a reasonable and necessary alternative to parenteral nutrition for a patient with a functioning gastrointestinal tract but for whom regular oral feeding is impossible."[113] The underlying diseases or disorders listed by Medicare that indicate this approach are similar to those listed in Table 27–1. However, home enteral tube feeding will be reimbursed only if accompanied by a prosthetic device, more specifically, a feeding pump. "Payment will be made for necessary supplies, adjustments, repairs and replacements that are necessary for the effective use of the prosthetic device."[113] Therefore, Medicare will cover the cost of the enteral formula, administration set and bag, infusion pump (rental or purchase fee and necessary maintenance), and other necessary equipment listed in Table 27–8.

Thorough investigation of the patient's eligibility for cost reimbursement is required and should be undertaken early by the social worker or financial counselor. Other financial benefits to be evaluated include possible income tax deductions and/or use of food stamps.

REFERENCES

1. Greene, H. L., Helinek, G. L., Folk, C. C., Courtney, M., Thompson, S., MacDonell, R. C., Jr., and Lukens, J. N.: Nasogastric tube feeding at home: A method for adjunctive nutritional support of malnourished patients. Am. J. Clin. Nutr., 34:1131–1138, 1981.
2. Heymsfield, S. B., Horowitz, J., and Lawson, D. H.: Enteral hyperalimentation. In Berk, J. E. (ed.): Developments in Digestive Diseases. Philadelphia, Lea and Febiger, 1980, Vol. 3, pp. 59–83.
3. Butterworth, C. E., Jr., and Weinsier, R. L.: Malnutrition in hospital patients: Assessment and treatment. In Goodhart, R. S., and Shils, M. E. (eds.): Modern Nutrition in Health and Disease. Edition 6. Philadelphia, Lea and Febiger, 1980, pp. 667–684.
4. Newmark, S. R., Simpson, S., Beskitt, P., Black, J., and Suhlett, D.: Home tube feeding for long-term nutritional support. J.P.E.N., 5:76–79, 1981.
5. Chrysomilides, S. A., and Kaminski, M. V., Jr.: Home enteral and parenteral nutrition support. Am. J. Clin. Nutr., 34:2271–2275, 1981.
6. Gormican, A., Liddy, E., Thrush, L. B., Jr.: Nutritional status of patients after extended tube feeding. J. Am. Diet. Assoc., 63:247–253, 1973.
7. Woolfson, A. M. J., Saour, J. N., Ricketts, C. R., Hardy, S. M., et al.: Prolonged nasogastric tube feeding in critically ill and surgical patients. Postgrad. Med. J., 52:678–682, 1976.
8. Wretlind, A.: Parenteral nutrition. Nutr. Rev., 39:257–265, 1981.
9. Goodgame, J. T., Jr.: A critical assessment of the indications for total parenteral nutrition. Surg. Gynecol. Obstet., 151:433–441, 1980.
10. Fleming, C. R., Beart, R. W., Jr., Berkner, S., McGill, D. B., and Gaffron, R.: Home parenteral nutrition for management of the severely malnourished adult patient. Gastroenterology, 79:11–18, 1980.
11. Miller, D. G., Ivey, M., and Young, J.: Home parenteral nutrition in treatment of severe radiation enteritis. Ann. Intern. Med., 91:858–860, 1979.
12. Allardyce, D. B., and Groves, A. C.: A comparison of nutritional gains resulting from intravenous and enteral feeding. Surg. Gynecol. Obstet., 139:179–184, 1974.
13. Lim, S. T. K., Choa, R. G., Lam, K. H., Wong, J., and Ong, G. B.: Total parenteral nutrition versus gastrostomy in the preoperative preparation of patients with carcinoma of the esophagus. Br. J. Surg., 68:69–72, 1981.
14. McArdle, A. H., Palmason, C., Morency, I., and Brown, R. A.: A rationale for enteral feeding as

the preferable route for hyperalimentation. Surgery, 90:616–623, 1981.
15. Levine, G. M., Deren, J. J., Steiger, E., and Zinno, R.: Role of oral intake in maintenance of gut mass and disaccharidase activity. Gastroenterology, 67:975–982, 1974.
16. Williamson, R. C. N., and Chir, M.: Intestinal adaptation. N. Engl. J. Med., 298:1393–1402, 1444–1450, 1978.
17. McIntyre, N., Holdsworth, C. D., and Turner, D. S.: Intestinal factors in the control of insulin secretion. J. Clin. Endocrinol. Metab., 25:1317–1324, 1965.
18. Lickley, H. L. A., Track, N. S., Vranic, M., and Bury, K. D.: Metabolic responses to enteral and parenteral nutrition. Am. J. Surg., 135:172–176, 1978.
19. Shike, M., Harrison, J. E., Sturtridge, W. C., Tam, C. S., Bobechko, P. E., Jones, G., Murray, T. M., and Jeejeebhoy, K. N.: Metabolic bone disease in patients receiving long-term total parenteral nutrition. Ann. Intern. Med., 92:343–350, 1980.
20. Klein, G. L., Targoff, C. M., Ament, M. E., Sherrand, D. J., Bluestone, R., Young, J. H., Norman, A. W., and Coburn, J. W.: Bone disease associated with total parenteral nutrition. Lancet, 2:1041–1044, 1980.
21. Shike, M., Sturtridge, W. C., Tam, C. S., Harrison, J. E., Jones, G., Murray, T. M., Husdan, H., Whitwell, J., Wilson, D. R., and Jeejeebhoy, K. N.: A possible role of vitamin D in the genesis of parenteral-nutrition-induced metabolic bone disease. Ann. Intern. Med., 95:560–568, 1981.
22. Greene, H. L., Slonim, A. E., Burr, I. M., and Moran, J. R.: Type I glycogen storage disease: Five years of management with nocturnal intragastric feeding. J. Pediatr., 96:590–595, 1980.
23. Fernandes, J., Jansen, H., and Jansen, T. C.: Nocturnal gastric drip feeding in glucose-6-phosphatase deficient children. Pediatr. Res., 13:225–229, 1979.
24. Davidson, A. G. F., Wong, L. T. K., Kirby, L., Tze, W. J., Rigg, J. M., and Applegarth, D. A.: Glycogen storage disease Type I: Effect of continuous nocturnal nasogastric feeding. Monogr. Hum. Genet., 9:29–36, 1978.
25. Greene, H. L., Slonim, A. E., O'Neil, J. A., Jr., and Burr, I. M.: Continuous nocturnal intragastric feeding for management of Type I glycogen storage disease. N. Engl. J. Med., 294:423–425, 1976.
26. Perlman, M., Aker, M., and Slonim, A. E.: Successful treatment of severe Type I glycogen storage disease with neonatal presentation by nocturnal intragastric feeding. J. Pediatr., 94:772–774, 1979.
27. Slonim, A. E., Terry, A., Greene, H. L., Lacy, W. W., Burr, I. M.: Amino acid and hormonal response to long-term nocturnal nasogastric feeding therapy of glycogen storage disease Type I (GSD-I). Monogr. Hum. Genet., 9:37–41, 1978.
28. Driscoll, R. H., Jr., and Rosenberg, I. H.: Total parenteral nutrition in inflammatory bowel disease. Med. Clin. North Am., 62:185–201, 1978.
29. Driscoll, R. H., Jr., and Rosenberg, I. H.: The nutritional aspects of malabsorption. In Handbook of Nutrition and Food, Cleveland, CRC Press, Inc., 1981.

30. Law, D. H.: Use of elemental diet and parenteral nutrition in patients with inflammatory bowel disease. *In* Kirsner, J. B., and Shorter, R. G. (eds.): Inflammatory Bowel Disease. Philadelphia, Lea and Febiger, 1980, pp. 447–464.

31. Rocchio, M. A., Cha, C. M., Haas, K. F., and Randall, H. T.: Use of chemically defined diets in the management of patients with acute inflammatory bowel disease. Am. J. Surg., 127:469–475, 1974.

32. Main, A. N. H., Morgan, R. J., Hall, M. J., et al.: Home enteral tube feeding with a liquid diet in the long-term management of inflammatory bowel disease and intestinal failure. Scott. Med. J., 25:312–314, 1980.

33. Russell, R. I., and Hall, M. J.: Elemental diet therapy in the management of complicated Crohn's disease. Scott. Med. J., 24:291–295, 1979.

34. Bounous, G., Devroede, G., Haddad, H., Beaudry, R., Perey, B. J., and Lejeune, L-P.: Use of an elemental diet for intestinal disorders and for the critically ill. Dis. Colon Rectum, 17:157–166, 1974.

35. Voitk, A. J., Echave, V., Feller, J. H., Brown, R. A., and Gurd, F. N.: Experience with elemental diet in the treatment of inflammatory bowel disease. Arch. Surg., 107:329–333, 1973.

36. Axelsson, C., and Jarnum, S.: Assessment of the therapeutic value of an elemental diet in chronic inflammatory bowel disease. Scand. J. Gastroenterol., 12:89–95, 1977.

37. Simko, V., and Linscheer, W. G.: Absorption of different elemental diets in a short-bowel syndrome lasting 15 years. Am. J. Dig. Dis., 21:419–425, 1976.

38. Calam, J., Crooks, P. E., and Walker, R. J.: Elemental diets in the management of Crohn's perianal fistulae. J.P.E.N., 4:4–8, 1980.

39. Logan, R. F. A., Gillon, J., Ferrington, C., and Ferguson, A.: Reduction of gastrointestinal protein loss by elemental diet in Crohn's disease of the small bowel. Gut, 22:383–387, 1981.

40. O'Morain, C., Segal, A. W., and Levi, A. J.: Elemental diets in treatment of acute Crohn's disease. Br. Med. J., 281:1173–1175, 1980.

41. Goode, A., Feggetter, J. G. W., Hawkins, T., and Johnston, I. D. A.: Use of an elemental diet for long-term nutritional support in Crohn's disease. Lancet, 1(7951):122–124, 1976.

42. Voitk, A. J., Echave, V., Brown, R. A., and Gurd, F. N.: Use of elemental diet during the adaptive stage of short gut syndrome. Gastroenterology, 65:419–426, 1973.

43. Zurier, R. B., Campbell, R. G., Hashim, S. A., and Van Itallie, T. B.: Use of medium-chain triglyceride in management of patients with massive resection of the small intestine. N. Engl. J. Med., 274:490–493, 1966.

44. Winawer, S. J., Broitman, S. A., Wolochow, D. A., Osborne, M. P., and Zamcheck, N.: Successful management of massive small-bowel resection based on assessment of absorption defects and nutritional needs. N. Engl. J. Med., 274:72–78, 1966.

45. Holmes, J. T.: Nutritional support of fistulas. Br. J. Surg., 64:695–697, 1977.

46. Monod-Broca, P.: Treatment of intestinal fistulas. Br. J. Surg., 64:685–689, 1977.

47. Halasz, N. A.: Changing patterns in the management of small bowel fistulas. Am. J. Surg., 136:61–65, 1978.

48. Bury, K. D., Stephens, R. V., and Randall, H. T.: Use of a chemically defined, liquid, elemental diet for nutritional management of fistulas of the alimentary tract. Am. J. Surg., 121:174–183, 1971.

49. Voitk, A. J., Echave, V., Brown, R. A., McArdle, A. H., and Gurd, F. N.: Elemental diet in the treatment of fistulas of the alimentary tract. Surg. Gynecol. Obstet., 137:68–72, 1973.

50. Nutritional management of enterocutaneous fistulas [Editorial]. Lancet, 2(8141):507–508, 1979.

51. Kirschner, B. S., Voinchet, O., and Rosenberg, I. H.: Growth retardation in inflammatory bowel disease. Gastroenterology, 75:504–511, 1978.

52. Kirschner, B. S., Klich, J. R., Kalman, S. S., deFavaro, M. V., and Rosenberg, I. H.: Reversal of growth retardation in Crohn's disease with therapy emphasizing oral nutritional restitution. Gastroenterology, 80:10–15, 1981.

53. Kelts, D. G., Grand, R. J., Shen, G., Watkins, J. B., Werlin, S. L., and Boehme, C.: Nutritional basis of growth failure in children and adolescents with Crohn's disease. Gastroenterology, 76:720–727, 1979.

54. Grand, R. J.: Malnutrition and inflammatory bowel disease. Curr. Concepts Nutr., 9:125–140, 1980.

55. Morin, C. L., Roulet, M., Roy, C. C., and Weber, A.: Continuous elemental enteral alimentation in children with Crohn's disease and growth failure. Gastroenterology, 79:1205–1210, 1980.

56. Shils, M. E.: Enteral nutrition by tube. Cancer Res., 37:2432–2439, 1977.

57. Rosenberg, I. H.: Nutritional support in inflammatory bowel disease. Gastroenterology, 77:393–395, 1979.

58. Sessions, D. G., and Zill, R.: Deglutition after conservative surgery for cancer of the larynx and hypopharynx. Otolaryngol. Head Neck Surg., 87:779–796, 1979.

59. Copeland, E. M., III, Daly, J. M., and Dudrick, S. J.: Nutritional concepts in the treatment of head and neck malignancies. Head Neck Surg., 4:350–365, 1979.

60. Noone, R. B., and Graham, W. P., III: Nutritional care after head and neck surgery. Postgrad. Med., 53:80–86, 1973.

61. Fleming, S. M., Weaver, A. W., and Brown, J. M.: The patient with cancer affecting the head and neck: Problems in nutrition. J. Am. Diet. Assoc., 70:391–394, 1977.

62. Aguilar, N. V., Olson, M. L., and Shedd, D. P.: Rehabilitation of deglutition problems in patients with head and neck cancer. Am. J. Surg., 138:501–507, 1979.

63. Steffee, W. P., and Krey, S. H.: Enteral hyperalimentation for patients with head and neck cancer. Otolaryngol. Clin. North Am., 13:437–448, 1980.

64. Sobol, S. M., Conoyer, J. M., Zill, R., Thawley, S. E., and Ogura, J. H.: Nutritional concepts in the management of the head and neck cancer patient. II. Management concepts. Laryngoscope, 89:962–979, 1979.

65. Close, L. G.: Indications for hyperalimentation in the treatment of head and neck malignancies. Otolaryngol. Head Neck Surg., 88:700–706, 1980.

66. Welty, M. J., Graham, W. P., III, and Rosillo, R. H.: The patient with maxillofacial cancer. Nurs. Clin. North Am., *8*:137–151, 1973.

67. Dingman, D. L.: Postoperative management of the severe oral cripple. Plast. Reconstr. Surg., *45*:263–267, 1970.

68. Dobbie, R. P., and Butterick, O. D., Jr.: Continuous pump/tube enteric hyperalimentation—use in esophageal disease. J.P.E.N., *1*:100–104, 1977.

69. Butler, F. S.: Cancer of the esophagus: Modern method of maintaining nutrition. J. Am. Geriatr. Soc., *15*:462–469, 1967.

70. Shils, M. E.: Enteral nutritional management of the cancer patient. Cancer Bull., *30*:98–101, 1978.

71. Shils, M. E.: Enteral nutrition by tube. Cancer Res., *37*:2432–2439, 1977.

72. Soukop, M., and Calman, K. C.: Nutritional support in patients with malignant disease. J. Hum. Nutr., *33*:179–188, 1979.

73. Calman, K. C.: Nutritional support in malignant disease. Proc. Nutr. Soc., *37*:87–93, 1978.

74. Van Eys, J.: Nutritional therapy in children with cancer. Cancer Res., *37*:2457–2461, 1977.

75. Shils, M. E.: Enteral nutritional management of the cancer patient. Cancer J. Clin., *29*:78–83, 1979.

76. Shils, M. E.: Nutritional therapy of the cancer patient: Guidelines for enteral and parenteral feeding. Curr. Probl. Cancer, *4*:66–76, 1979.

77. Rickard, K. A., Kirksey, A., Baehner, R. L., Grosfeld, J. L., Provisor, A., Weetman, R. M., Boxer, L. A., and Ballantine, T. V. N.: Effectiveness of enteral and parenteral nutrition in the nutritional management of children with Wilms' tumors. Am. J. Clin. Nutr., *33*:2622–2629, 1980.

78. Welch, D.: Nutritional compromise in radiation therapy patients experiencing treatment-related emesis. J.P.E.N., *5*:57–60, 1980.

79. Sundaram, R., Megna, D., and Sibley, J.: Long-term tube feeding in the aged. N.Y. State J. Med., *79*:1226, 1979.

80. O'Hara, J. G., Kennedy, S., and Lizewski, W.: Effects of long-term elemental nasogastric feeding on elderly debilitated patients. Can. Med. Assoc. J., *108*:977–980, 1973.

81. Olivares, L., Segovia, A., and Revuelta, R.: Tube feeding and lethal aspiration in neurological patients: A review of 720 autopsy cases. Stroke, *5*:654–657, 1974.

82. Chernoff, R., and Young, E.: Clinical case presentation. J.P.E.N., *2*:41–42, 1978.

83. Day, S., and Buckell, M.: Feeding the unconscious patient. Proc. Nutr. Soc., *30*:184–190, 1971.

84. Jones, D. C., and Dickerson, J. W. T.: Decision making in the nutritional care of unconscious patients. J. Adv. Nurs., *1*:359–365, 1976.

85. Pomerantz, M. C., Salomon, J., and Dunn, R.: Permanent gastrostomy as a solution to some nutritional problems in the elderly. J. Am. Geriatr. Soc., *28*:104–117, 1980.

86. Heimbach, D. M.: Surgical feeding procedures in patients with neurologic disorders. Ann. Surg., *172*:311–314, 1970.

87. Halmi, K. A., Powers, P., and Cunningham, S.: Treatment of anorexia nervosa with behavior modification. Effectiveness of formula feeding and isolation. Arch. Gen. Psychiatry, *32*:93–96, 1975.

88. Bayer, L. M., Evans, D. K., and Ford, E. G.: Coordinating a discharge program for the tube fed patient. Personnel communication.

89. Torosian, M. H., and Rombeau, J. L.: Feeding by tube enterostomy. Surg. Gynecol. Obstet., *150*:918–927, 1980.

90. Meguid, M. M., and Williams, L. F.: The use of gastrostomy to correct malnutrition. Surg. Gynecol. Obstet., *149*:27–32, 1979.

91. Matino, J. J.: Feeding jejunostomy in patients with neurologic disorders. Arch. Surg., *116*:169–171, 1981.

92. Sacks, B. A., and Glotzer, D. J.: Percutaneous reestablishment of feeding gastrostomies. Surgery, *85*:575–576, 1979.

93. Preshaw, R. M.: A percutaneous method for inserting a feeding gastrostomy tube. Surg. Gynecol. Obstet., *152*:659–660, 1981.

94. Ponsky, J. L., and Gauderer, M. W. L.: Percutaneous endoscopic gastrostromy: A nonoperative technique for feeding gastrostomy. Gastrointest. Endosc., *27*:9–11, 1981.

95. Weinstein, E. C.: Gastrostomy. A neglected procedure. Geriatrics, *22*:157–161, 1967.

96. Rombeau, J. L., and Barot, L. R.: Enteral nutritional therapy. Surg. Clin. North Am., *61*:605–620, 1981.

97. Rombeau, J. L., and Miller, R. A.: Nasoenteric tube feeding. Practical aspects. Hedeco monograph, 1979.

98. Gault, M. H., Dixon, M. E., Doyle, M., and Cohen, W. M.: Hypernatremia, azotemia, and dehydration due to high-protein tube feeding. Ann. Intern. Med., *68*:778–791, 1968.

99. Walike, J. W.: Tube feeding syndrome in head and neck surgery. Arch. Otolaryngol., *89*:533–536, 1969.

100. Kubo, W., Grant, M., Walike, B., Bergstrom, N., Wong, H., Hanson, R., and Padilla, G.: Fluid and electrolyte problems of tube-fed patients. Am. J. Nurs., *76*:912–916, 1976.

101. Telfer, N., and Persoff, M.: The effect of tube feeding on the hydration of elderly patients. J. Gerontol., *20*:536–543, 1965.

102. Berenyi, M. Z., and Straus, B.: Hyperosmolar states in the chronically ill. J. Am. Geriatr. Soc., *17*:648–658, 1969.

103. Dehydration with high protein tube feeding [Editorial]. Nutr. Rev., *26*:271–273, 1968.

104. Randall, H. T.: Fluid, electrolyte and acid-base balance. Surg. Clin. North Am., *56*:1019, 1976.

105. Heitkemper, M. E., Martin, D. L., Hansen, B. C., Hanson, R., and Vanderburg, V.: Rate and volume of intermittent enteral feeding. J.P.E.N., *5*:125–129, 1981.

106. Parker, P., Stroop, S., and Greene, H.: A controlled comparison of continuous versus intermittent enteral feeding. J. Pediatr., *99*:360–364, 1981.

107. Hiebert, J. M., Brown, A., Anderson, R. G., Halfaire, S., Rodeheaver, G. T., and Edlich, R. F.: Comparison of continuous versus intermittent tube feedings in adult burn patients. J.P.E.N., *5*:73–75, 1981.

108. Jones, B. J. M., Payne, S., and Silk, D. B. A.: Indications for pump-assisted enteral feeding. Lancet, *1*(8177):1057–1058, 1980.

109. Gordon, A. M., Jr.: Enteral nutritional support. Guidelines for feeding tube selection and place-

ment. Postgrad. Med., *70*:155–162, 1981.

110. Rains, B. L.: The nonhospitalized tube-fed patient. Oncol. Nurs. Forum, *8*:8–13, 1981.

111. Hanson, R. L., Walike, B. C., Grant, M., et al.: Patient responses and problems associated with tube feeding. Wash. St. J. Nurs., 1975, pp. 9–13.

112. Padilla, G. V., Grant, M., Wong, H., Hanson, B. W., Hanson, R. L., Bergstrom, N., and Kubo, W. R.: Subjective distresses of nasogastric tube feeding. J.P.E.N., *3*:53–57, 1979.

113. Medicare Intermediary Manual. Part 3—Claims Process, July 1981.

CHAPTER 28

Pharmacologic Aspects of Enteral Nutrition

GEORGE MELNIK
KATHERINE WRIGHT

As the use of enteral nutrition increases in inpatient and outpatient settings, pharmacy involvement in this area of nutritional therapy will be greater. The pharmacist will take an active role in providing information on techniques of drug administration in tube-fed patients, in monitoring drug responses, in informing house staff of any actual or potential drug-nutrient interactions, and in compounding complicated enteral formulas. The purpose of this chapter is to discuss the pharmacologic aspects of enteral nutrition, including the administration of medications by enteral feeding tubes, commercial liquid medications, gastric emptying rate, drug therapy for diarrhea, and drug-nutrient interactions.

ADMINISTRATION OF MEDICATION BY ENTERAL FEEDING TUBES

The oral administration of medication may be thought of as a transitional process in which the drug is prepared by the stomach and delivered to the absorptive sites of the small intestine. When the entry route is altered by the placement of enteral feeding tubes, the pharmacologic agent and its mode of delivery are often modified. In this section we examine the process of drug dissolution in the stomach and the factors that must be considered when medication is delivered into the duodenum or jejunum.

The stomach responds similarly to oral dosage forms of drugs as it does to food. The primary event is the disintegration of large drug particles into smaller drug particles which are readily solubilized in the stomach. The dissolution of a drug in the stomach is the vital step in preparing the drug for absorption by the small intestine.[1] As the particle size of the drug decreases, the total surface area increases and absorption is enhanced. The administration of a drug with food can improve the dissolution process by increasing the time the drug remains in the stomach, ensuring that the medication goes into solution with the gastric contents. Only when the drug is dissolved can it be properly absorbed by the small intestine and produce a pharmacologic effect.

The concomitant administration of drugs with bolus enteral feedings delivered directly into the stomach by nasogastric or gastrostomy tubes enables the stomach to function in its normal capacity of preparing its contents for the rest of the gastrointestinal tract. Large-bore nasogastric or gastrostomy tubes permit the administration of large drug particles into the stomach. The placement of enteral tubes beyond the stomach will alter the method of drug delivery.

Jejunostomy, nasojejunal, or nasoduodenal feeding tubes bypass the stomach and its preparatory activity on food and drugs. When administering medication into the small intestine through these feeding tubes, one must use liquid drug preparation, taking into consideration: (1) internal tube diameter; (2) viscosity of drugs; and (3) enteral tube flushing. Before a drug can reach the absorptive sites in the small intestine (Fig. 28–1), it must pass through the small lumen of the enteral tube. Large drug particles cannot be accommodated, requiring the use of medication in liquid form. The drug's viscosity, however, may impede its passage into the small intestine. In such instances,

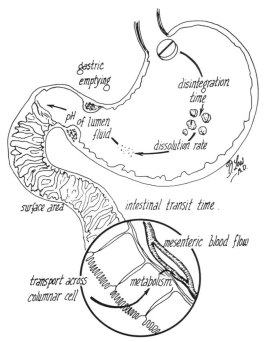

Figure 28–1. Examples of some factors affecting rate of absorption.

diluting the drug with 15 to 20 ml of luke-warm water will facilitate its delivery to the small bowel.[3] Flushing the enteral tube with 30 ml of warm water before and after administering the medication serves a triple purpose: it clears the tube for delivery of the medication; it aids in getting the drug into the intestine; and it indicates if the tube is clogged. Awareness of these technical points may aid in preventing complications with the tube.

When should medications be administered to tube-fed patients? Pharmacologic data indicate that many drugs are best absorbed in the "fasted" state as opposed to the fed condition. (This topic will be discussed in more detail in the section on gastric emptying rate and food.) Medications should, therefore, be administered one hour before or two hours after a meal. There is no hard evidence to suggest that drugs can be mixed in an enteral formula and administered in a continuous feeding over a long duration (eight hours) and still have a pharmacologic effect comparable to that of drugs administered in a bolus manner. At this time, therefore, medications should be administered in a bolus manner at the rec-

ommended dosage intervals. Patients who are fed continuously over a 24-hour period may have medication administered prior to the initiation of a new feeding volume, or may have their feeding interrupted. Patients who are given bolus intragastric feedings may receive medications at times that comply with the "one hour before or two hours after a meal" edict.

In summary, the stomach prepares medication for the remainder of the gastrointestinal tract by a process of dissolution; larger drug particles may be administered through large-bore gastric tubes; a drug delivered directly into the small bowel must be in solution; and until further research proves otherwise, medication should be given as a bolus one hour before or two hours after a feeding.

COMMERCIAL PREPARATIONS OF LIQUID MEDICATIONS

As the internal diameter of the enteric tube decreases, size of the drug particles must also decrease in order to traverse the tube successfully. This section discusses commercial preparations of liquid medication, extemporaneous preparation of liquid medications in a hospital pharmacy, and preparations of medications that should not be crushed.

To prepare a pharmaceutical liquid medication one must know the inherent physicochemical properties of drugs to be suspended in a liquid vehicle. Aqueous medications are available as four different entities: solution, a chemically and physically homogeneous mixture of two or more substances;[4] suspension, a coarse dispersion containing finely divided insoluble material suspended in a liquid medium;[5] elixir, a hydroalcoholic diluting agent suitable for drugs soluble in either water or diluted alcohol (approximately 25 per cent);[6] and emulsion, a dispersed system containing at least two immiscible liquid phases.[5]

Knowledge of the following three processes is essential in manufacturing pharmaceutically elegant and pharmacologically viable liquid products: interfacial phenomena, the properties of molecules situated at or very near the boundary between immiscible phases;[7] colloidal dispersion, the dispersion of very fine organic drug particles in a liquid medium;[8] and flocculation, the aggregation of small drug particles to form large clumps or floccules which rise or settle in an emulsion and represent an unstable product.[9] Commercially available preparations of liquid medications are a product of this scientific knowledge and manufacturing expertise. Liquid products available are listed in Appendix 28–1.

When a liquid product is not available, the pharmacy must prepare a solution or a suspension from solid oral dosage forms. The initial step is to pulverize the oral solid form by using a mortar and pestle.

Mortars and pestles currently used are made from Wedgwood ware, porcelain, or glass. Each type has a specific use. For example, glass mortars are primarily designed for preparing solutions and suspensions because they are characteristically nonporous and do not stain easily. This nonporous property of glass ensures that the drug will not adhere to the mortar or pestle during mixing. Glass cannot be used for comminuting hard solids (the mechanical process of reducing particle size). Wedgwood mortars and pestles are best suited for comminution of crystalline solids. However, they are porous and easily stained, and require meticulous washing to ensure that particles are not trapped on their surfaces. Porcelain mortars and pestles are similar to Wedgwood but their exterior surface is glazed, making them less porous. Mortars and pestles made of porcelain are best suited for mixing powders.[10] After choosing the proper mortar and pestle for preparing the liquid medication, one may begin the process of compounding.

The extemporaneous preparation of a liquid dosage form for tube feeding is as follows: (1) Establish the amount of drug per dose and the duration of therapy. (2) Using a Wedgwood mortar and pestle, pulverize an adequate amount of solid oral dosage form for the duration of the therapy. (3) Wash these utensils carefully with 5 to 10 ml of water to extract any residual drug. (4) Transfer the pulverized drug and washings, then (5) wet the suspending agent to defloccuate solids suspended in the liquid and to stabilize their dispersion. The agent used to wet the suspending agent should be a nonadsorbing liquid—alcohol, glycerine, or propylene glycol. A commonly used suspending agent is methylcellulose, which is soluble in cold water. Other suspending agents include carboxymethylcellulose, acacia, bentonite, and carbopol. The pulverized drug, washings, and wetted suspending agent are mixed together and the resulting suspension is transferred into a graduated cylinder. The mortar and pestle are rinsed with the liquid vehicle that will be added to the graduated cylinder. The product is then brought to the desired volume.[11]

Not all solid oral dosage forms are suitable for compounding into a liquid dosage form. Alternative liquid products should be considered for those drugs that are available as enteric-coated or slow-release compounds. Enteric-coated products are usually acid labile or gastric-irritating drugs. They are coated with a protective barrier that may or may not dissolve in the acidic stomach. The pharmacologic integrity of the drug, however, is maintained. Pulverizing an enteric-coated or slow-release compound may destroy the integrity of the drug if it is administered into the stomach.[12] The preparation of the slow-release product allows a small amount of drug to be released continuously so that absorption may occur over a longer time period as the drug traverses the intestinal tract. The solubilization and administration of a slow-release product into an enteral tube located in the jejunum will not result in an extended activity. The use of alternative liquid medications for these products entails more attention to titrating the drug to achieve the desired response. Drugs available as enteric-coated or slow-release products are listed in Appendix 28–2.

In the extemporaneous preparation of liquid medications, one must be concerned with interfacial phenomena, colloidal dispersion, flocculation, and enteric-coated and slow-release compounds. Otherwise problems such as nonuniformity of particle size, choice of an improper suspending agent, production of an unstable drug product, and improper use of a slow-release compound may occur. A commercial liquid medication should always be used when it is available. When a liquid medication must be compounded, however, all precautions should be taken to assure product stability and uniformity. Slow-release or enteric-coated compounds should not be used in extemporaneous liquid compounding, and equivalent generic solid dosage forms should be used when no liquid product is available.

Text continued on page 532

Appendix 28–1 ORAL LIQUID MEDICAL PREPARATIONS

MEDICATION	CONCENTRATION	TYPE	TRADE NAME
ANTIBIOTICS			
Amphotericin B USP, Tetracycline	25 mg/5 ml 125 mg/5 ml	Syrup	Mysteclin-F Syrup
Griseofulvin USP	125 mg/5 ml	Suspension	Grifulvin V
Nystatin USP	100,000 units/ml	Suspension	Nilstat
Nystatin, Demeclocycline HCl	125,000 units/ml 75 mg/5 ml	Suspension	Declostatin
Nystatin, Oxytetracycline, Glucosamine HCl	125,000 units/ml 125 mg/5 ml 138 mg/5 ml	Suspension	Terrastatin
Nystatin, Tetracycline	125,000 units/ml 125 mg/5 ml	Suspension	Achrostatin V, Tetrastatin
Cephalexin	100 mg/5 ml 125 mg/5 ml 250 mg/5 ml	Suspension	Keflex
Cephradine	125 mg/5 ml 250 mg/5 ml	Suspension	Anspor, Velosef
Chloramphenicol palmitate	150 mg/5 ml	Suspension	Chloromycetin Palmitate
Erythromycin ethylsuccinate	200 mg/5 ml	Suspension	E.E.S. 200 Liquid, Pediamycin Liquid
	400 mg/5 ml	Suspension	E.E.S. 400 Liquid, Pediamycin 400 Liquid
Amoxicillin (as trihydrate)	50 mg/ml 125 mg/5 ml 250 mg/5 ml	Suspension	Amoxil
Ampicillin	100 mg/ml 125 mg/5 ml 250 mg/5 ml 500 mg/5 ml	Suspension Suspension Suspension Suspension	Omnipen, Penbritin Omnipen, Penbritin Omnipen, Penbritin Omnipen

Appendix 28–1 ORAL LIQUID MEDICAL PREPARATIONS *(Continued)*

MEDICATION	CONCENTRATION	TYPE	TRADE NAME
Ampicillin trihydrate	100 mg/ml	Suspension	Amcill, Polycillin, SK-Ampicillin
	125 mg/5 ml	Suspension	Alpen, Amcill, Ampi-Co, Amplin, Pen-A, Pensyn, Polycillin, Principen, QID-amp, SK-Ampicillin, Supen, Tabocillin, Totacillin
	250 mg/5 ml	Suspension	Alpen, Amcill, Amplin, Pen-A, Pensyn, Polycillin, Principen, QID-amp, SK-Ampicillin, Supen, Tabocillin, Totacillin
	500 mg/5 ml	Suspension	Polycillin
Cloxacillin sodium	125 mg/5 ml	Solution	Tegopen
Dicloxacillin sodium	62.5 mg/5 ml	Suspension	Dynapen, Pathocil
Hetacillin	112.5 mg/5 ml	Suspension	Versapen Oral
Nafcillin sodium	250 mg/5 ml	Solution	Unipen
Oxacillin sodium	250 mg/5 ml	Solution	Prostaphlin
Penicillin G benzathine	150,000 units/5 ml	Suspension	Bicillin
	300,000 units/5 ml	Suspension	Bicillin
Penicillin G potassium	100,000 units/5 ml	Solution	Pen-Can Formula #1
	125,000 units/5 ml	Solution	Sugracillin 125M
	200,000 units/5 ml	Solution	Kesso-Pen, Pentids
	250,000 units/5 ml	Solution	Sugracillin 250M

Appendix 28–1 ORAL LIQUID MEDICAL PREPARATIONS *(Continued)*

MEDICATION	CONCENTRATION	TYPE	TRADE NAME
Penicillin G potassium	400,000 units/5 ml	Solution	G-Recillin, Kesso-Pen, Pentids "400," Pfizerpen G
Penicillin V USP	208 mg/ml	Suspension	V-Cillin Drops
Penicillin V benzathine	180 mg/5 ml	Suspension	Pen-Vee Suspension
Penicillin V hydrabamine	180 mg/5 ml	Suspension	Compocillin-V
Penicillin V potassium	125 mg/5 ml	Solution	Betapen-VK, Compocillin-VK, Kesso-Pen-VK, Ledercillin VK, Penapar VK, Pen-Vee, Pfizerpen VK, QID-pen VK, Repen-VK, Robocillin VK, Ro-Cillin VK, SK-Penicillin VK, Uticillin VK, V-Cillin K, Veetids "125"
	250 mg/5 ml	Solution	Betapen-VK, Compocillin-VK, Kesso-Pen-VK, Ledercillin VK, Ora-VK, Penapar-VK, Pen-Vee K, Pfizerpen VK, QIDpen VK, Repen VK, Robicillin VK, Ro-Cillin VK, SK-Penicillin VK, Uticillin VK, V-Cillin K, Veetids "250"

Appendix 28–1 ORAL LIQUID MEDICAL PREPARATIONS *(Continued)*

MEDICATION	CONCENTRATION	TYPE	TRADE NAME
Demeclocycline HCl	60 mg/ml 75 mg/5 ml	Suspension Suspension	Declomycin Declomycin
Doxycycline monohydrate	25 mg/5 ml	Suspension	Vibramycin Monohydrate
Methacycline HCl	75 mg/5 ml	Suspension	Rondomycin
Minocycline HCl	50 mg/5 ml	Suspension	Minocin Vectrin
Oxytetracycline calcium	125 mg/5 ml	Suspension	Terramycin Syrup
Tetracycline HCl	100 mg/ml	Suspension	Achromycin V, Panmycin, Premocycline, Tetrachel-S, Tetrex (phosphate complex)
	125 mg/5 ml	Suspension	Achromycin, Achromycin V, Panmycin, Panmycin KM, Premocycline, Retet-S, Robitet, SK-Tetracycline, Sumycin, T-125, Tetrachel-S, Tetracyn, Tetrex (phosphate complex)
	250 mg/5 ml	Suspension	Achromycin
Clindamycin palmitate HCl	75 mg/5 ml	Solution	Cleocin Pediatric
Lincomycin HCl	250 mg/5 ml	Syrup	Lincocin
Colistin sulfate	25 mg/5 ml	Suspension	Coly-Mycin S Oral Suspension
Neomycin	125 mg/5 ml	Solution	Mycifradin Sulfate

Appendix 28–1 ORAL LIQUID MEDICAL PREPARATIONS *(Continued)*

MEDICATION	CONCENTRATION	TYPE	TRADE NAME
Novobiocin calcium	125 mg/5 ml	Suspension	Cathomycin Calcium
Oleandomycin base	125 mg/5 ml	Suspension	TAO
Vancomycin HCl	500 mg/6 ml	Solution	Vancocin
Amantadine HCl	50 mg/5 ml	Syrup	Symmetrel
Sulfacetamide, Sulfadiazine, Sulfamerazine	162 mg/5 ml (each) 165 mg/5 ml (each)	Suspension Suspension	Sulford Liquid Buffonamide
Sulfadiazine, Sulfamerazine	250 mg/5 ml (each)	Suspension	Sufonamides Duplex, Aldiazol-M
Sulfadiazine, Sulfamerazine, Sulfamethazine	167 mg/5 ml (each)	Suspension	Sulfose
Trisulfapyrimidines, USP (sulfadiazine, sulfamerazine, sulfamethazine)		Suspension	Citrasulfas, Diazolac, Meride, Neotrizine, Syrasulfas, Terfonyl, Tri-Azo-Mul, Trisulfazine
Phthalylsulfathiazole, USP Succinylsulfathiazole	250 mg/5 ml 250 mg/5 ml	Elixir	Intestol
	1 gm/5 ml	Suspension	Cremothalidine
Sulfadiazine	500 mg/5 ml	Suspension	Coco-Diazine
Sulfamethizole	250 mg/5 ml	Suspension	Renasul, Thiosulfil
	500 mg/5 ml	Suspension	Sulfurine, Proklar
Sulfamethoxazole NF	500 mg/5 ml	Suspension	Gantanol

Appendix 28–1 ORAL LIQUID MEDICAL PREPARATIONS *(Continued)*

MEDICATION	CONCENTRATION	TYPE	TRADE NAME
Sulfamethoxazole, Trimethoprim (co-trimoxazole)	200 mg/5 ml 40 mg/5 ml	Suspension	Bactrim Septra
Sulfamethoxypyridazine acetyl	250 mg/5 ml	Suspension	Midicel Acetyl Suspension
Sulfaphenazole	500 mg/5 ml	Suspension	Orisul
Sulfisoxazole acetyl USP	500 mg/5 ml 1 gm/5 ml	Suspension Suspension, extended release	Gantrisin Pediatric Lipo-Gantrisin
Methenamine	100 mg/5 ml 300 mg/5 ml 400 mg/5 ml	Elixir Elixir	Uritone Compound Uritone
Methenamine mandelate	250 mg/5 ml 500 mg/5 ml	Suspension Suspension	Mandelamine Mandelamine Forte
Nitrofurantoin	25 mg/5 ml	Suspension	Furadantin
Furazolidone	16.7 mg/5 ml	Suspension	Furoxone
CARDIOVASCULAR DRUGS			
Digoxin	50 mcg/ml	Elixir	Lanoxin
Reserpine	250 mcg/ml	Solution	Serpasil Elixir
CENTRAL NERVOUS SYSTEM DRUGS—ANALGESICS			
Hydromorphone HCl NF	1 mg/5 ml	Syrup	Dilaudid HCl
Meperidine HCl USP	50 mg/5 ml	Syrup	Demerol HCl
Methadone HCl USP	1.7 mg/5 ml	Syrup	Dolophine
Acetaminophen NF	120 mg/5 ml 130 mg/5 ml 325 mg/5 ml	Elixir Elixir Suspension	various names Neopap Pyrapap

Appendix 28–1 ORAL LIQUID MEDICAL PREPARATIONS *(Continued)*

MEDICATION	CONCENTRATION	TYPE	TRADE NAME
Propoxyphene napsylate	50 mg/5 ml	Suspension	Darvon-N
Aspirin	324 mg	Tablet	Alka-Seltzer
Choline salicylate	870 mg/5 ml	Liquid	Actasal, Arthropan
Salicylates sodium salicylate, phenacetin, caffeine	500 mg/5 ml 100 mg/5 ml 20 mg/5 ml	Liquid	Sal-Ge-Sic
ANTICONVULSANTS			
Ethosuximide USP	250 mg/5 ml	Syrup	Zarontin
Paramethadione USP	300 mg/ml	Solution	Paradione
Phenobarbital USP	7.5 mg/5 ml 10 mg/5 ml 15 mg/5 ml 20 mg/5 ml 100 mg/5 ml	Solution Solution Solution Elixir Solution	Bar Elixir Henomint Infadorm Orpine Sedadrops
Phensuximide NF	300 mg/5 ml	Suspension	Milontin
Phenytoin USP	30 mg/5 ml 125 mg/5 ml	Suspension Suspension	Dilantin-30 Dilantin-125
Primidone USP	250 mg/5 ml	Suspension	Mysoline
Trimethadione USP	200 mg/5 ml	Solution	Tridione
Valproate	250 mg/5 ml	Solution	Depakene Syrup
PSYCHOTHERAPEUTIC AGENTS			
Doxepin HCl	10 mg/ml	Solution	Sinequan Concentrate
Nortriptyline HCl NF	10 mg/5 ml	Solution	Aventyl HCl

Appendix 28–1 ORAL LIQUID MEDICAL PREPARATIONS *(Continued)*

MEDICATION	CONCENTRATION	TYPE	TRADE NAME
Chlorpromazine HCl USP	30 mg/ml 100 mg/ml 10 mg/5 ml	Liquid Liquid Syrup	Thorazine Concentrate Thorazine Concentrate
Chlorprothixene	100 mg/5 ml	Liquid	Taractan
Fluphenazine HCl NF	500 µg/ml 5 mg/ml	Elixir Solution	Prolixin Permitil Oral Concentrate
Haloperidol NF	2 mg/ml	Solution	Haldol Concentrate
Hydroxyzine HCl NF	10 mg/5 ml	Syrup	Atarax
Perphenazine	4 mg/ml 2 mg/5 ml	Liquid Syrup	Trilafon Concentrate
Prochlorperazine edisylate USP	10 mg/ml 5 mg/5 ml	Liquid Syrup	Compazine Concentrate
Promazine HCl	30 mg/ml 100 mg/ml 10 mg/5 ml	Liquid Liquid Syrup	Sparine Concentrate Sparine Concentrate
Thiothixene HCl	5 mg/ml	Liquid	Navane Concentrate
Trifluoperazine	10 mg/ml	Liquid	Stelazine
Triflupromazine	50 mg/5 ml	Suspension	Vesprin
Dextroamphetamine sulfate	5 mg/5 ml	Elixir Elixir (w/amobarbital)	Dexedrine, Dexamyl
Methamphetamine HCl USP	3.3 mg/5 ml 5 mg/5 ml	Elixir Elixir	Desoxyn Syndrox
Nikethamide	1.25 gm/5 ml	Solution	Coramine
Pentylenetetrazol	100 mg/5 ml	Solution	Metrazol Liquidum, Nioric Elixir
Aprobarbital NF	40 mg/5 ml	Elixir	Alurate

Appendix 28–1   ORAL LIQUID MEDICAL PREPARATIONS *(Continued)*

MEDICATION	CONCENTRATION	TYPE	TRADE NAME
Butabarbital sodium NF	30 mg/5 ml 10 mg/5 ml	Elixir Solution	Buta-Kay, Butal, Butisol Sodium Ruck-Sed
Chloral hydrate	625 mg/5 ml 267 mg/5 ml 250 mg/5 ml 500 mg/5 ml	Solution Elixir Syrup Syrup	Fello-Sed Somnos —— Kessodrate, Noctec
Paraldehyde	——	Liquid	Paral
Pentobarbital NF Pentobarbital sodium USP	18.2 mg/5 ml 20 mg/5 ml	Elixir Elixir (w/Carbromal)	Nembutal Carbrital
Phenobarbital USP Phenobarbital sodium USP	7.5 mg/5 ml 10 mg/5 ml 15 mg/5 ml 20 mg/5 ml 40 mg/5 ml	Solution Elixir Elixir Elixir Elixir	—— —— —— Sherital ——
Promethazine HCl USP	6.25 mg/5 ml 12.5 mg/5 ml 25 mg/5 ml	Syrup Syrup Syrup	Phenergan ZiPAN Phenergan
Secobarbital USP	22 mg/5 ml	Elixir (w/methenamine)	Seconal
Triclofos	500 mg/5 ml	Liquid	Triclos
ELECTROLYTE SOLUTIONS			
Ammonium chloride USP	500 mg/5 ml	Syrup	——
Sodium bicarbonate USP	0.15%	Solution	Moyer's Solution
Sodium lactate	2 Molar	Syrup	——
Lactulose	3.33 gm/5 ml	Syrup	Cephulac
Calcium glubionate	115 mg Ca/5 ml	Solution	Neo-Calglucon Syrup

Appendix 28–1 ORAL LIQUID MEDICAL PREPARATIONS (*Continued*)

MEDICATION	CONCENTRATION	TYPE	TRADE NAME
Potassium chloride USP	3.3 mEq K$^+$/5 ml 5 mEq K$^+$/5 ml 6.7 mEq K$^+$/5 ml 10 & 13.3 mEq K$^+$/5 ml	Solution Solution Solution Solution	—— Kay-Pote Various names Various names
Potassium gluconate NF	6.7 mEq K$^+$/5 ml	Solution	KG, Kalinate, Kaon
Potassium acetate, Potassium bicarbonate, Potassium citrate	2.5 mEq K$^+$/5 ml 15 mEq K$^+$/5 ml	Liquid	Tri-K Potassium Triplex, Potassium Tri-Pli, Randall's Solution, Triple Potassium
Potassium chloride, Potassium bicarbonate	20 mEq K$^+$/tablet	Tablet	Various names
Potassium chloride, Potassium bicarbonate, Potassium citrate	20 mEq K$^+$/tablet	Tablet	Kaochlor-EFF
Potassium chloride, Potassium gluconate	6.7 mEq K$^+$/5 ml 20 mEq K$^+$/5 ml	Liquid Liquid	Kolyum Kolyum
Potassium gluconate, Potassium citrate	6.7 mEq K$^+$/5 ml	Liquid	Twin-K Elixir
Sodium chloride	0.3%	Solution	Moyer's Solution
Saccharin sodium	225 mg/ml	Solution	
Chlorothiazide	250 mg/5 ml	Suspension	Diuril
EXPECTORANTS			
Ammomium chloride USP	500 mg/5 ml	Syrup	
Calcium iodide	150 mg/5 ml 152 mg/5 ml	Syrup Syrup	Norisodrine Calcidrine
Carbetapentane	7.25 mg/5 ml	Syrup	Todase

Appendix 28–1 ORAL LIQUID MEDICAL PREPARATIONS *(Continued)*

MEDICATION	CONCENTRATION	TYPE	TRADE NAME
Chlophedianol HCl	15 mg/5 ml	Syrup	Acutuss, Ulominic
Codeine NF	8.4 mg/5 ml	Syrup	Calcidrine
Codeine phosphate USP	5 to 10 mg/5 ml	Elixir Liquid Syrup	Various names
Dextromethorphan	5, 10, & 15 mg/5 ml	Syrup	Various names
Glycerol guaiacolate	Various strengths	Elixir Suspension Syrup	Various names
Hydrocodone bitartrate	Various strengths	Liquid Suspension Syrup	Various names
Noscapine	10 mg/5 ml	Syrup	Conar, Noscomel
GASTROINTESTINAL DRUGS			
Aluminum carbonate		Suspension	Basaljel
Aluminum hydroxide		Suspension	Alkagel, Amphojel, Hydroxal
Aluminum phosphate		Suspension	Phosphaljel
Calcium carbonate		Suspension	Titralac
Magaldrate (Aluminum magnesium hydroxide)		Suspension	Riopan
Magnesium hydroxide		Suspension	Various names
Aluminum hydroxide, Magnesium hydroxide		Suspension	Various names
Aluminum hydroxide, Magnesium trisilicate		Suspension	A-M-T, Neutracomp, Trisogel

Appendix 28–1 ORAL LIQUID MEDICAL PREPARATIONS *(Continued)*

MEDICATION	CONCENTRATION	TYPE	TRADE NAME
Aluminum hydroxide, Calcium carbonate, Magnesium hydroxide		Suspension	Camalox
Aluminum hydroxide, Dihydroxyaluminum aminoacetate, Magnesium hydroxide		Suspension	Aluscop, Tralmag
Aluminum hydroxide, Magnesium hydroxide, Magnesium trisilicate		Suspension	Magnatril
Diphenoxylate hydrochloride, Atropine sulfate	2.5 mg/5 ml 25 μg/5 ml	Solution	Lomotil
Opium	Various	Suspension	Paregoric, USP
Simethicone	Various	Suspension	Cosil, Mylanta, Silain-Gel
Cascara sagrada fluidextract		Suspension	Cas-Evac Liquid
Danthron	37.5 mg/5 ml	Solution	Modane Liquid
Senna	325 mg/5 ml 350 mg/5 ml	Solution Solution	Fletcher's Castoria Dr. Caldwell's Senna Laxative
	400 mg/5 ml	Solution	Casafru
Senna Fruit Extract	7.5 mg/5 ml	Solution	Senokot Syrup, X-Prep Liquid
Senna Syrup	1 gm/5 ml	Solution	Black Draught Syrup
Malt Soup Extract	4 gm/5 ml	Solution	Maltsupex Liquid
Methylcellulose	450 mg/5 ml 985 mg/5 ml	Solution Solution	Cologel Liquid Hydrolose Syrup
Psyllium hydrophilic Mucilloid, Mineral oil	7.5 mg/5 ml 142 mg/5 ml		Petro-Syllium No. 1 Plain

Appendix 28–1 ORAL LIQUID MEDICAL PREPARATIONS *(Continued)*

MEDICATION	CONCENTRATION	TYPE	TRADE NAME
Castor oil	34% w/w 60% w/w 95% w/v	Suspension Suspension Suspension	Neoloid Liquid Alphamul G-W Emulsoil
Diphenylmethane Phenolphthalein, Mineral oil	15 mg & 3.25 ml/5 ml	Suspension	Petrogalar and Phenolphthalein
	49 mg & 2.75 ml/5 ml	Suspension	Kondremul with Phenolphthalein
	65 mg & 1.6 ml/5 ml	Suspension	Agoral, Agoral Raspberry
Glycerin	75%	Liquid	
Sorbitol	70%	Solution	
Mineral oil, heavy	55% w/w 1.6 ml/5 ml 2.75 ml/5 ml 3.25 ml/5 ml	Jelly Solution Solution Solution	Neo-cultol Agoral Plain Kondremul Plain Emulsion Petrogalar Plain
Mineral oil, Milk of Magnesia	1 ml & 4 ml/5 ml 1.25 ml & 3.75 ml/5 ml	Suspension Suspension	Various names Haley's M-O
Mineral oil, Phenolphthalein	1.6 ml & 65 mg/5 ml	Suspension	Agoral, Agoral Raspberry
Mineral oil, Cascara sagrada Phenolphthalein	2.75 ml & 220 mg/5 ml 2.75 ml & 49 mg/5 ml		Kondremul with Cascara Emulsion Kondremul with Phenolphthalein
Magnesium citrate	77–141 mEq	Solution	Various names
Magnesium hydroxide	82–164 mEq	Suspension	Various names
Sodium biphosphate, Sodium phosphate	2.4 gm & 900 mg/5 ml	Solution	Fleet Phospho-Soda
Dioctyl sodium sulfosuccinate (DSS)	16.7 mg/5 ml 20 mg/5 ml 50 mg/5 ml 250 mg/5 ml	Solution Solution Solution Solution	Various names Colace, Disonate Colace, Disonate Doxinate

Appendix 28–1 ORAL LIQUID MEDICAL PREPARATIONS *(Continued)*

MEDICATION	CONCENTRATION	TYPE	TRADE NAME
DSS, Casanthranol	20 mg 10 mg/5 ml	Solution	Peri-Colace Syrup
Ipecac syrup USP		Syrup	
Prochlorperazine edisylate USP	10 mg/ml 5 mg/5 ml	Liquid Syrup	Compazine Concentrate Compazine
SPASMOLYTIC AGENTS			
Aminophylline USP hydrous	Various strengths	Solution	Various names
Dyphylline	33 mg/5 ml 53 mg/5 ml	Solution Solution	Lufyllin Elixir, Airet Dlor Elixir, Neothylline Elixir
Theophylline USP anhydrous	Various strengths	Solution	Various names
VITAMINS			
Oleovitamin A & D	6490 IU of A 520 IU of D/5 ml	Liquid	Super D
Vitamin B Complex		Elixir	Various names
Vitamin C	500 mg/5 ml	Syrup	Vitamin C Syrup
Dihydrotachysterol	250 µg/ml	Solution	Hytakerol
Ergocalciferol	200 µg/ml	Solution	Drisdol
Vitamin E	50 IU/ml	Solution	Aquasol E
Multivitamin	Various strengths	Elixirs Liquids Solutions	Various names

Appendix 28–2 ORAL DOSAGE FORMS THAT SHOULD NOT BE CRUSHED*

DRUG	DOSAGE FORM	REASON
Aerolate SR, JR, III	Capsule	Slow release
Afrinol Repetabs	Tablet	Slow release
Aminodur Dura-Tabs 300 mg	Tablet	Slow release
Ananase	Tablet	Enteric coated
Artane Sequels	Capsule	Slow release
Azulfidine EN-tabs	Tablet	Enteric coated
Bellergal-S	Tablet	Slow release
Benzedrine Spansule	Capsule	Slow release
Bisacodyl	Tablet	Enteric coated
Bronchobid Duracap	Capsule	Slow release
Bronkodyl S-R 300 mg	Tablet	Slow release
Butibel-Zyme	Tablet	Slow release
Cartrax	Tablet	Slow release
Chexit	Tablet	Enteric coated
Chlorpheniramine Maleate TD	Capsule	Slow release
Chlor-Trimeton Repetabs	Tablet	Slow release
Chymoral 100,000 Units	Tablet	Interference with enzymatic activity
Clistin R-A	Tablet	Slow release
Combid Spansules	Capsule	Slow release
Compazine Spansule	Capsule	Slow release
Congess SR and JR TD	Capsule	Slow release
Contac Continuous Action Decongestant	Capsule	Slow release
Cotazym-S	Capsule	Enteric coated
Deconamine-SR	Capsule	Slow release
Demazin Repetabs	Tablet	Slow release
Depakene	Capsule	Irritating to mouth and throat
Diacin 200 mg	Capsule	Slow release
Diamox Sequels	Capsule	Slow release
Dimetane Extentabs	Tablet	Slow release
Dimetapp Extentabs	Tablet	Slow release
Dipav	Capsule	Slow release
Disophrol Chronotat	Tablet	Slow release
Donnatal Extentabs	Tablet	Slow release
Donnazyme	Tablet	Enteric coated
Drixoral Sustained Action	Tablet	Slow release
Dulcolax	Tablet	Enteric coated
Duotrate	Capsule	Slow release
Ecotrin	Tablet	Enteric coated
Elixophyllin SR	Capsule	Slow release
E-Mycin	Tablet	Enteric coated
Entozyme	Tablet	Enteric coated
Eskabarb Spansule	Capsule	Slow release
Extendryl	Capsule	Slow release
Feosol	Tablet	Enteric coated
Feosol Spansule	Capsule	Slow release
Fero-Grad-500 mg Filmtabs	Tablet	Slow release
Fero-Gradumet	Tablet	Slow release
Ferrobid Duracaps	Capsule	Slow release
Ferro-Sequels	Capsule	Slow release
Festal	Tablet	Enteric coated
Fortespan	Capsule	Slow release
Gaviscon Antacid	Tablet	Crushing may reduce foaming action
Geroniazol TT	Tablet	Slow release
Guaiahist TT	Tablet	Slow release
Hepicebrin	Tablet	Enteric coated
Histabid SR	Capsule	Slow release
Histatapp TD	Tablet	Slow release
Iberet	Tablet	Slow release
Ilotycin	Tablet	Enteric coated
Isoclor Timesule	Capsule	Slow release
Isordil Chewable 40 mg	Tablet	Partial absorption may not be obtained in mouth when crushed
Isordil Sublingual	Tablet	Tablets are made to disintegrate under the tongue
Isordil Tembid	Capsule	Slow release

Appendix 28–2   ORAL DOSAGE FORMS THAT SHOULD NOT BE CRUSHED* *(Continued)*

DRUG	DOSAGE FORM	REASON
Isuprel HC Glossets	Tablet	Tablets are made to disintegrate under the tongue
Kanulase	Tablet	Enteric coated
Kaon-Cl	Tablet	Slow release
K-Tab	Tablet	Slow release
KEFF 20 mEq	Tablet	Effervescent tablet must be dissolved in water
Klotrix 10 mEq	Tablet	Slow release
Laxadane Supules	Tablet	Enteric coated
Leder-BP Sequels	Capsule	Slow release
Leder-CC Sequels	Capsule	Slow release
Leder-CPI Sequels	Capsule	Slow release
Lithobid	Tablet	Slow release
Marblen	Tablet	Decreased duration of activity
Meprospan	Capsule	Slow release
Mestinon Timespan	Tablet	Slow release
Mi-Cebrin	Tablet	Enteric coated
Mi-Cebrin T	Tablet	Enteric coated
Modane	Capsule	Capsule contains a liquid
MSC Triaminic	Tablet	Enteric coated
Multicebrin	Tablet	Enteric coated
Naldecon	Tablet	Slow release
Napril	Capsule	Slow release
Nico 400	Capsule	Slow release
Nicobid	Capsule	Slow release
Nico-Span	Capsule	Slow release
Nitroglycerin TD	Capsule	Slow release
Nitroglyn	Tablet	Slow release
Novafed	Capsule	Slow release
Novafed A	Capsule	Slow release
Novahistine LP	Tablet	Slow release
Nu'Leven	Tablet	Enteric coated
Obestat	Capsule	Slow release
Ornade Spansule	Capsule	Slow release
Pabalate, Pabalate-SF	Tablet	Enteric coated
Pancrease	Capsule	Enteric coated
Papaverine HCL TR	Capsule	Slow release
Pathilon Sequels	Capsule	Slow release
Pavabid	Capsule	Slow release
Pavakey	Capsule	Slow release
PBZ-SR	Tablet	Slow release
Pentritol	Capsule	Slow release
Peritrate SA	Tablet	Slow release
Permitil Chronotab	Tablet	Slow release
Phazyme	Tablet	Slow release
Phazyme-95	Tablet	Slow release
Phazyme-PB	Tablet	Slow release
Phyllocontin	Tablet	Slow release
Polaramine Repetabs	Tablet	Slow release
Pretts	Tablet	Crushing reduces foam formation
Proternol	Tablet	Slow release
Quibron Bidcaps	Capsule	Slow release
Quinaglute Dura-Tabs	Tablet	Slow release
Quinidex Extentabs	Tablet	Slow release
Rhinex-D•Lay	Tablet	Slow release
Ro-Bile	Tablet	Enteric coated
Robimycin Robitabs	Tablet	Enteric coated
Roniacol Timespan	Tablet	Slow release
Singlet	Tablet	Slow release
SK-Bisacodyl	Tablet	Enteric coated
SK-Erythromycin	Tablet	Enteric coated
Sorbitrate SA	Tablet	Slow release
Sprx-105	Capsule	Slow release
Sudafed SA	Tablet	Slow release
Sustaire	Tablet	Slow release

Table continued on following page

Appendix 28–2   ORAL DOSAGE FORMS THAT SHOULD NOT BE CRUSHED* *(Continued)*

DRUG	DOSAGE FORM	REASON
Tedral SA	Tablet	Slow release
Teldrin Timed Release	Capsule	Slow release
Temaril Spansule	Capsule	Slow release
Theobid Jr. Duracap	Capsule	Slow release
Theo-Dur	Tablet	Slow release
Theophyl	Capsule	Slow release
Theovent Long-Acting	Capsule	Slow release
Thorazine Spansule	Capsule	Slow release
Triaminic	Tablet	Enteric coated
Triaminic Juvelets	Tablet	Enteric coated
Trilafon Repetabs	Tablet	Slow release
Triten	Tablet	Slow release
Tussagesic	Tablet	Enteric coated
Tussaminic	Tablet	Enteric coated
Tuss-Ornade Spansule	Capsule	Slow release
Wyamycin S	Tablet	Slow release

*From Mitchell and Liadis, Hosp. Pharm., *17*:148–156, 1982,[12] with permission.

GASTRIC EMPTYING RATE

The onset of absorption of food or drugs delivered into the stomach by oral, nasogastric, or gastrostomy feeding is determined by the gastric emptying rate (GER). The gastric emptying rate is the speed at which the stomach empties gastric contents into the small bowel. The GER directly influences the rate of drug absorption and onset of pharmacologic activity of oral agents. Hence, we shall address the physiologic control of GER, the extrinsic and intrinsic disease factors affecting GER, the effects of food and drugs on GER, and the surgical procedures that alter the GER.

Physiologic Control of Gastric Emptying.   Gastric distention is the only natural stimulus known to increase GER. Gastric slow waves, or the continuous electrical activity manifested in the stomach, represent electrical control activity. The rate of this electrical activity, three impulses per minute, may be associated with intermittent secondary electrical responses resulting in antral contraction. These contractions establish the frequency, velocity, and direction of peristalsis.[13] Local and distal nerve reflexes and hormones influence the rate of gastric slow waves and antral contractions. The exact mechanism, however, is not known. Acid, increased osmotic pressure, and amino acids in the duodenum delay gastric emptying. It is unclear whether the delay activated by these substances is mediated by neural, hor-

monal, or both receptors in the duodenum. Gastrin, secretin, and cholecystokinin all delay gastric emptying while glucagon inhibits gastric motility. It is doubtful, however, that these hormones have a physiologic role in the control of emptying. The pyloric sphincter, under the control of GER, relaxes with peristalsis, contracts in response to acid, fat, amino acids, and glucose, and also prevents duodenal reflux.

Effects of Disease on GER.   Diseases that affect GER are classified according to extrinsic and intrinsic factors. The current data on the effect of extrinsic factors on GER are anecdotal or hypothetical; only in a few instances has GER been measured in patients with these diseases. Generally any cause of peritoneal irritation is associated with a decrease in GER and diminished peristalsis. Gastric distention resulting from perforated peptic ulcer, appendicitis, pancreatitis, retroperitoneal hematoma, ruptured spleen, or subphrenic abscess, by inference, may delay GER. Other conditions that delay gastric emptying include severe trauma, laparotomy, head trauma, myocardial infarction, hepatic coma, hypercalcemia, diabetes mellitus, myxedema, and malnutrition.[13] Thus, the diseases that are alleged to inhibit GER are varied.

Intrinsic factors that are associated with delayed GER are atrophic gastritis in gastric carcinoma, pernicious anemia, pyloric stenosis, vagotomy, and diabetic autonomic neuropathy. The intrinsic and extrinsic influences affecting GER are thus multifactorial. When drug absorption is diminished as a consequence, alternative routes of drug administration must be considered (intravenous, intramuscular, or rectal) for adequate therapeutic response.

Effects of Drugs on GER. Drugs may alter the GER either by affecting the smooth muscle of the gastrointestinal tract or by influencing the release of intestinal hormones that modulate gastric activity. The following agents have been implicated in reducing GER: atropine, the antimuscarinic drug, scopolamine, and the belladonna alkaloids; propantheline when given intravenously; the phenothiazine class of drugs, which includes chlorpromazine and thioridazine; the antihistamines diphenhydramine and promethazine; the class of tricyclic antidepressant agents, such as amitriptyline and imipramine; the sympathomimetic drugs, which relax smooth muscle and inhibit propulsive contractions of the gastrointestinal tract; the antiparkinsonian drugs levodopa, trihexyphenidyl, and amantadine; antihypertensive agents; hypnotics; anesthetic agents; narcotic analgesics; and gastric antacids.[13-15]

Drugs increase GER by inhibiting dopamine receptors in the gastrointestinal tract (metoclopramide), by enhancing acetylcholine acitivity (anticholinesterases), or by stimulating gastric acid secretion (reserpine).

More pharmacologic agents decrease GER than enhance it (Table 28–1). An awareness of these agents and their inherent ac-

Table 28–1 FACTORS THAT INFLUENCE GASTRIC EMPTYING RATE (GER)*

	INCREASE GER	DECREASE GER
Physiologic Factors		
Liquids	+	
Solids		+
Acid		+
Fat		+
Increased osmotic pressure		+
Amino acids		+
Gastric distention	+	
Gastrin		+
Secretin		+
Cholecystokinin		+
Glucagon		+
Posture (prone or R side)	+	

Table 28–1 FACTORS THAT INFLUENCE GASTRIC EMPTYING RATE (GER)* *(Continued)*

	INCREASE GER	DECREASE GER
Pathologic Factors		
Acute abdomen		+
Chronic calculous cholecystitis	+	
Laparotomy		+
Trauma and pain		+
Labor		+
Myocardial infarction		+
Gastric ulcer		+
Duodenal ulcer	+	
Hepatic coma		+
Hypercalcemia		+
Diabetes mellitus		+
Myxedema		+
Malnutrition		+
Migraine		+
Raised intracranial pressure		+
Atrophic gastritis		
solids		+
liquids	+	
Pyloric stenosis		+
Gastric volvulus		+
Intestinal obstruction		+
Gastroenterostomy	+	
Pharmacologic Factors		
Anticholinergic drugs		
atropine		+
propantheline		+
tricyclics		+
trihexyphenidyl		+
Ganglion blocking drugs		
hexamethonium		+
Narcotic analgesics		
morphine		+
pentazocine		+
Isoniazid		+
Sodium nitrite		+
Chloroquine		+
Alcohol		+
Dioctyl sodium sulfosuccinate		+
Phenytoin		+
Metoclopramide	+	
Reserpine	+	
Anticholinesterases	+	
Sodium bicarbonate	+	
Aluminum hydroxide		+
Magnesium hydroxide		+

*From Nimmo, 1976.[13]

tivity on the gastrointestinal tract will minimize complications of enteral nutrition and delayed drug activity.

Effects of Food on GER. Food can have a positive or negative effect on GER, and this influence of food has a direct effect on drug absorption. The rate and amount of drug absorption are usually diminished when medications are taken with food. The ingested meal delays gastric emptying, and adsorption of the ingested drug by food constituents may occur. For example, serum levels of ampicillin, after being given with food, were shown to be half of the serum levels found when the drug was administered in the fasted state;[16] tetracycline absorption was diminished when taken with food;[17] and the hypnotic action of phenobarbital in rats was absent when the drug was given with food.[18]

Food has also had a positive effect on the absorption of some drugs. Studies have shown that the bioavailability of propranolol (Inderal) and metoprolol (Lopressor) was increased when administered with a meal to volunteers.[19] Griseofulvin absorption is greatly enhanced when given with a fatty meal.[20]

Since the pharmacologic activity of medications administered with food may either be enhanced or diminished, care should be taken to understand what will occur when drugs are given with food. Monitoring the clinical parameters of a drug that is delivered in this manner will optimize drug therapy.

Effects of Surgical Procedures on GER. In a study in dogs to determine the effect of surgically removing the distal antrum and pylorus, the results showed that after surgery there was increased gastric emptying of solids in comparison with gastric emptying in the intact stomach prior to surgery. There was no change in the GER of liquids after surgery. With respect to drug absorption, this indicates that large particles would be emptied faster into the small intestine and would not undergo the proper dissolution process, which ensures optimal drug absorption. Under such circumstances liquid dosage forms should be given to the patient to ensure maximal drug absorption and pharmacologic activity.[21]

Importance of GER in Drug Absorption. Gastrointestinal motility affects drug absorption. Absorption from the stomach is very slow, and therefore, GER is the rate-

limiting step in drug absorption. Administering a drug in solution, rather than in tablet form, will result in rapid absorption. Another factor that affects absorption is administering the drug in a large volume of fluid. This increases GER, whereas a concentrated drug solution in the stomach decreases GER.

In conclusion, GER may be affected by many factors, including diet, disease, and medications. Knowledge of the impact of the disease, of the enteral formulas, and of medications is vital to achieving a favorable response to both the drug therapy and enteral nutrition in tube-fed patients.

DRUG THERAPY FOR DIARRHEA IN TUBE-FED PATIENTS

Diarrhea is the most frequently encountered complication of enteral nutrition. In most medical institutions, whenever diarrhea occurs in tube-fed patients the tendency is to dilute the formula, decrease the rate, or discontinue enteral nutrition in order to alleviate the problem. The drug therapy for diarrhea is of special concern for enteral patients receiving concomitant drug therapy. As stated earlier the nutritional pharmacist is obliged to monitor drug-nutrient interactions and drug-drug interactions that may impede therapeutic goals. In this section we shall discuss the etiology of diarrhea and the drug therapy that is appropriate for a specific cause.

Diarrhea is defined as an increase in bowel frequency and/or fluid content of the stool. This problem is of special concern in patients on enteral nutrition because of nutrient losses that occur during the hypermotility of diarrhea. Diarrhea may result from a number of causative factors: bacterial or viral infection, hyperosmolar formula, lactose intolerance, antibiotic therapy, magnesium-containing antacids, the administration of abrasive drugs directly into the small intestine, and medications such as digoxin, guanethidine, methyldopa, propranolol, and quinidine.[22]

Drug theraphy for diarrhea depends on the cause. For example, if it is caused by magnesium-containing antacids, then alternating a magnesium-free antacid, such as aluminum hydroxide, with the magnesium-containing antacid throughout the day should eliminate the diarrhea. Diarrhea often develops in patients who are receiving oral antibiotic therapy as a result of the change in bacterial flora of the intestine. In this situation, the antidiarrheal agents diphenoxylate (Lomotil), loperamide (Imodium), camphorated opium (paregoric), and codeine should not be used. In patients with pseudomembranous colitis, use of diphenoxylate was actually shown to exacerbate diarrhea.[23] It is believed that diphenoxylate, with its constipating effects on the small intestine, enhances the absorption of *p*-cresol, the toxin of the *Clostridium difficile* pathogen, which in turn perpetuates the diarrhea. Cholestyramine has been used as an antidiarrheal agent secondary to clindamycin therapy in patients with diarrhea and pseudomembranous colitis. In this case, it is thought that the resin adsorbs the toxin.[24] Kaolin pectate may be used in uncomplicated diarrhea in patients who are receiving oral antibiotics. Diarrhea caused by digoxin (Lanoxin), guanethidine (Ismelin), propranolol (Inderal), methyldopa (Aldomet), and quinidine may be treated with diphenoxylate, loperamide, or paregoric. The adsorbing antidiarrheal agents may be detrimental in tube-fed patients taking these medications; for example, cholestyramine and kaolin pectate have been shown to bind digoxin when they are used chronically.

DRUG-NUTRIENT INTERACTIONS

Drug-nutrient interactions are of particular concern to nutritionists monitoring patient therapy in a hospital and home environment. Numerous parameters are known to affect the metabolic and nutritional status of the patient including sepsis, surgery, trauma, burns, malnutrition, and obesity. That drugs may also affect nutrient status received peripheral attention in the medical literature until Dr. Daphne Roe's work in this area was recognized. In this section, we will discuss the significant drug-nutrient interactions in hospitalized patients and patients on home enteral nutrition receiving concurrent drug therapy.

Fat-Soluble Vitamins

Vitamin A. Through various mechanisms, certain drugs have an impact on vitamin A absorption. Mineral oil decreases the absorption of vitamin A by acting as a solvent for the vitamin and causing its excretion in the feces.[25] Mineral oil may also impair micelle formation of the bile salts or may cause a physical barrier at the mucosal surface that inhibits absorption. Neomycin decreases vitamin A absorption by inhibiting pancreatic lipase, by inactivating bile salts, and by causing mucosal damage in the small intestine. Cholestyramine adsorbs bile salts, which causes steatorrhea and a reduction in vitamin absorption.[25, 26] Clofibrate may reduce absorption by precipitating bile salts in the common bile duct.[27] The basic interaction of drugs with vitamin A occurs by an inhibition of absorption by various mechanisms.

Vitamin K. The administration of a vitamin K–free oral diet in man has not produced a vitamin K deficiency. The assumption is that under normal circumstances the intestinal synthesis of vitamin K can supply the nutritional needs for adults and children. Administration of broad-spectrum antibiotics can decrease the synthesis of the vitamin, but no untoward effects are evident with an adequate dietary intake of the nutrient. Mineral oil and cholestyramine have been demonstrated to decrease the absorption of vitamin K. The warfarin anticoagulants are the most common group of drugs to cause vitamin K deficiency.[26]

Three case reports have been documented describing warfarin resistance in enteral nutrition patients. In all three instances the failure of warfarin therapy was attributed to the amounts of vitamin K contained in the prescribed enteral products (Table 28–2). In each case when the enteral formula was changed to products containing less vitamin K, prolongation of prothrombin time occurred.[28–30]

Vitamin D. Drugs may affect vitamin D status in various ways. Mineral oil decreases vitamin D absorption by inhibiting micelle formation of the bile salts, and may also impair vitamin D–dependent calcium transport at the brush border of the intestinal mucosa. Neomycin inactivates bile salts, thus decreasing the absorption of the vitamin.[33] The adsorbing activity of cholestyramine also reduces vitamin absorption. Excessive doses and chronic use of glucocorticoid steroids may interfere with the hepatic metabolism of the 25-hydroxycholecalciferol

Table 28–2 VITAMIN K CONTENT IN ENTERAL FEEDING FORMULAS*

PRODUCT	VITAMIN K (mg/1000 kcal)
Nutri-1000 LF	150
Vipep	75
Formula 2	NA
Compleat B (bottle)	NA
Compleat B (cans)	25
Meritene	NA
Precision LR	59
Precision Isotonic	64
Precision HN	35
Magnacal	NA
Renu	NA
Isocal	130
Flexical	125
Sustical (powder)	NA
Sustical (can)	40
Travasorb	1007
Travasorb STD	75
Travasorb HN	75
Travasorb Hepatic	46
Travasorb Renal	0
Travasorb MCT	950
Amin-Aid	0
Hepatic-Aid	0
Vivonex	37
Vivonex HN	22
Ensure	148
Ensure Plus	210
Vital	187
Osmolite	148

*Adapted from Lee et al., 1981;[28] Ross Laboratories, 1981;[31] and Travenol Laboratories, 1981.[32]

metabolite of the vitamin. Phenobarbital, phenytoin, primidone, and glutethimide all induce hepatic microsomal enzyme function, which results in an accelerated degradation of vitamin D_3 and 25-hydroxychole calciferol to inactive metabolites.[25] Diphosphones, which are used in the treatment of Paget's disease, block the metabolism of the physiologically active metabolite 1,25-dihydroxycholecalciferol in the kidney. Thus, mechanisms that affect vitamin D status decrease the absorption, block the normal metabolic pathway, or accelerate the degradation of the vitamin, all of which ultimately lead to an alteration of calcium status in the body.

Vitamin E. The only vitamin E moiety that is presently considered in dietary intake is alpha-tocopherol. Its absorption follows fat absorption, and therefore drugs have an impact on vitamin E through their effects on fat absorption (see the previous discussion on fat-soluble vitamins). Clofibrate, contra-ceptive steroids, and triiodothyronine cause a reduction in serum lipid concentration which results in a decrease in vitamin E concentration.[26]

Water-Soluble Vitamins

Ascorbic Acid. Depletion of ascorbic acid from tissue stores is caused by anorectic agents, anticonvulsants, oral contraceptives, and tetracycline. Aspirin is thought to cause depletion of vitamin C by increasing urinary excretion of the vitamin.[26] The diuretic furosemide (Lasix) also increases the urinary excretion of ascorbic acid.[27]

Thiamine. The enzymatic decarboxylation of pyruvic acid is a primary function of thiamine. Thus, blood pyruvate levels have been found to be elevated in severe thiamine deficiencies. Patients receiving digitalis alkaloids may have increased thiamine requirements. There have also been findings of elevated serum pyruvate levels in patients with digitalis intoxication.[34]

Riboflavin. Riboflavin absorption is increased by the presence of food in the intestine and decreased by the presence of any agent that causes hypermotility of the intestine. Metoclopramide may diminish riboflavin absorption by its ability to increase peristalsis. Antibiotics that cause diarrhea may likewise have a deleterious effect on riboflavin status, and diarrhea caused by magnesium-containing antacids similarly affects riboflavin absorption.[35]

Niacin. Drugs affecting niacin include the chemotherapeutic agents 5-fluorouracil and 6-mercaptopurine, which block the intracellular synthesis of the pyridine nucleotides (NAD and NADP). Niacin is a component of both pyridine nucleotides, which are vital in many metabolic functions through their role in electron transfer.

Folic Acid. Folic acid metabolism is affected by numerous drugs. Methotrexate and aminopterin are antineoplastic agents that inhibit the conversion of folate to tetrahydrofolate, the physiologically active metabolite, by blocking the converting enzyme dihydrofolate reductase (DHFR). Other drugs that inhibit the enzymatic activity of DHFR include pyrimethamine, an antimalarial agent; trimethoprim and pentamidine, antibiotics; and triamterene, a potassium-sparing diuretic. The anticonvulsants phenobarbital, phenytoin, and primidone interfere with the intestinal absorption of folate.[25, 26]

Pyridoxine. Drugs affecting pyridoxine are thought to act as antagonists to pyridoxine coenzymes. Hydralazine, isoniazid, and levodopa form hydrazones or Schiff bases with pyridoxal phosphate, the primary pyridoxine coenzyme, causing increased excretion of the coenzyme. Cycloserine and isoniazid inhibit pyridoxal kinase activity, which results in impaired synthesis of pyridoxal phosphate. Penicillamine directly competes with pyridoxal coenzymes for the apoenzyme surface and diminishes its activity.[35]

Vitamin B$_{12}$. Numerous drugs have affected the absorption of cyanocobalamin. The biguanides, metformin and phenformin, are oral antidiabetic agents that induce malabsorption either by competitive inhibition at the distal ileum absorption sites or by inactivation of the vitamin. Para-aminosalicylic acid is thought to decrease the absorption of vitamin B$_{12}$ by blocking a folate-dependent mucosal enzyme in the ileal wall. Cholestyramine, a bile acid adsorbent, prevents the formation of the cyanocobalamin–intrinsic factor complex by competitively binding with the intrinsic factor molecule. Potassium chloride inhibits B$_{12}$ absorption by lowering the pH at the ileal lumen absorptive site. Colchicine decreases cyanocobalamin absorption by producing histologic changes in the intestinal mucosa and may interfere with the cellular transporting mechanism of the vitamin.[26]

In contrast to the fat-soluble vitamins, the water-soluble vitamins interact with drugs primarily in the metabolic parameter. In the case of vitamin B$_{12}$ there are interactions that inhibit the absorption of the vitamin.

Minerals

Sodium. Episodes of hyponatremia have been attributed to diuretics used in hypertensive therapy, including chlorthalidone, furosemide, the thiazide derivatives, and ethacrynic acid. These agents block sodium uptake at specific regions in the renal tubule, from the descending nephron through the loop of Henle to the ascending nephron. Hyponatremia has occurred with conventional doses of these diuretics.[36]

Numerous pharmacologic agents have been reported to induce the syndrome of inappropriate secretion of antidiuretic hormone (SIADH): the oral hypoglycemic drugs chlorpropamide and tolbutamide; the antineoplastic and immunosuppressive drugs cyclophosphamide and vincristine; the psychoactive agents carbamazepine and amitriptyline; the hypolipemic drug clofibrate; the hormone oxytocin; and the thiazide and loop diuretics ethacrynic acid and furosemide.[36, 37] These drugs exert their antidiuretic effects either by stimulating an inappropriate secretion of antidiuretic hormone or by potentiating the tubular action of small amounts of antidiuretic hormone.[37]

Potassium. Hypokalemia has been caused by chronic use of laxatives; mineralocorticosteroids, which promote kaliuresis; diuretics (excluding the potassium-sparing diuretics spironolactone and triamterene), which may cause an exchange of sodium for potassium in the distal renal tubule; acetazolamide, which enhances potassium excretion; amphotericin B, which triggers potassium loss by causing numerous changes in the renal nephron; gentamicin in chronic doses greater than 10 gm cumulative, which causes hypokalemia; and carbenicillin, which behaves as a nonreabsorbable anion, creating an increase in the electronegativity of the distal nephron that enhances potassium and hydrogen excretion.[35, 38]

Calcium. Drugs also affect the status of calcium. Glucocorticosteroids reduce calcium absorption by antagonizing vitamin D activity. Anticonvulsant agents cause a malabsorption of calcium through the accelerated catabolism of vitamin D and its metabolites. The diphosphones suppress the formation of 1,25-dihydroxycholecalciferol, which reduces calcium absorption in the intestine. The diuretics furosemide, ethacrynic acid, and triamterene produce hypercalciuria. Digoxin augments the renal clearance of calcium in patients with congestive heart failure who are also receiving diuretic therapy. Gentamicin in cumulative doses greater than 10 gm has been shown to cause hypocalcemia.[36] Finally, laxatives also cause calcium depletion.[25]

Phosphates. Antacids are a common form of therapy for simple gastric distress and are used as phosphate binders in patients with renal failure. The mechanism by which aluminum-containing antacids bind phosphate in the gastrointestinal tract is illustrated in the following chemical equation:

$$Al(OH)_3 + 3HCl \rightarrow AlCl_3 + 3H_2O$$
$$AlCl_3 + PO_4 \rightarrow AlPO_4(insoluble) + 3Cl$$

Thirty milliliters given with or immediately following meals will bind dietary phosphates to produce insoluble complexes that are excreted in the stool. Although hypophosphatemia secondary to antacid therapy occurs with chronic use of antacids, one must also keep in mind the electrolyte shifts occurring during the anabolic refeeding period, which may also contribute to hypophosphatemia in patients with renal failure. Not all antacids have the same phosphate binding capacity, however (Table 28–3).

A depletion of phosphate by complexing with aluminum in the gut results in low serum inorganic phosphate levels. This inhibits red cell glycolysis and consequently the formation of adenosine triphosphate (ATP) and 2,3-diphosphoglycerate (2,3-DPG). Erythrocyte ATP and 2,3-DPG interact with hemoglobin to diminish its oxygen affinity.[41] Therefore, there is a linear relationship between red cell organic phosphate concentration and tissue oxygen saturation, but an inverse relationship between these phosphates and the affinity of hemoglobin for oxygen. Thus, during hypophosphatemia cell hypoxia may occur. Other consequences of hypophosphatemia are acute respiratory failure, neurologic abnormalities, hemolytic anemia, platelet dysfunction, diminished phagocytosis, and hemorrhage.[43] This clinical problem may be prevented by knowing the phosphate binding capacity of antacids, by providing adequate phosphate for absorption, and by monitoring blood phosphate on a weekly basis.

Magnesium. Medicinal agents also affect magnesium status. Digoxin in conjunction with diuretic therapy results in the hyperexcretion of magnesium. Gentamicin in a chronic cumulative dose of greater than 10 gm has caused hypomagnesemia. Neomycin, which precipitates bile salts and decreases pancreatic lipase activity, causes steatorrhea which results in fecal magnesium loss.[25]

Zinc. Zinc deficiency in humans has been attributed to D-penicillamine, which chelates zinc and is excreted in the urine. Corticosteroid therapy results in a renal loss of zinc as a result of catabolism of lean body tissue. Contraceptive steroids depress plasma zinc levels by altering transferrin and alpha$_2$-macroglobulin, which results in excretion of the element in the urine. Diuretics have been shown to increase zinc excretion.[25]

Iron. The inhibition of iron by pharmaceutical agents is accomplished by various means. Bicarbonate salts depress iron absorption by preventing oxidation of the element in the stomach. Cholestyramine binds heme and inorganic iron, and thereby blocks its absorption. There are two proposed mechanisms by which salicylates influence iron status: chronic aspirin intake causes intestinal bleeding that may be a prominent factor in iron deficiency anemia; and the antiplatelet activity of aspirin may potentiate the gastrointestinal effects that result in anemia.[25] The anticoagulant drugs coumadin and heparin may cause gastrointestinal hemorrhage during long-term therapy, which can initiate or exacerbate iron deficiency anemia.[43] Isoniazid impairs the uptake of iron into protoporphyrin, which may result in sideroblastic anemia.[25] Chloramphenicol, an antibiotic, suppresses the activity of ferrochelatase, the catalytic enzyme for hemoglobin synthesis within the mitochondria of erythroid cells. This effect occurs with normal or greater than normal levels of iron.[23]

Table 28–3 PHOSPHATE BINDING CAPACITY (PBC)*

PRODUCTS	CONTENTS	PBC
Basaljel	Aluminum carbonate	+4
Gelusil	Aluminum–magnesium hydroxide	+3
Maalox	Aluminum–magnesium hydroxide	+3
Amphojel	Aluminum hydroxide	+2
Mylanta	Aluminum–magnesium hydroxide	+2
Riopan	Aluminum–magnesium hydroxide	+1
Phosphaljel	Aluminum phosphate	0
Titralac	Calcium carbonate	0

*From Gambertoglio and Mangini, 1978.[40]

Copper. Copper is chelated by D-penicillamine. Manifestations of copper deficiency may appear as an iron deficiency anemia. More investigation of this mineral is needed.

Drugs affect mineral status primarily by enhancing their excretion. As a result, there is ineffective utilization of all of the substrates that compose a nutritional regimen.

Macronutrients

Protein. There are two mechanisms by which drugs affect protein status: inhibition of protein synthesis on the biochemical level and initiation of gluconeogenesis. Glucocorticosteroids in excessive doses induce the catabolism of body protein for the production of glucose for utilization by the central nervous system.[44] Tetracycline inhibits bacterial protein synthesis by binding to the 30S ribosome subunits and specifically inhibiting the enzyme-mediated binding of aminoacyl-tRNA to the adjacent ribosomal acceptor site. In high concentrations, tetracycline inhibits mammalian protein synthesis and may also affect protein status in postoperative patients receiving parenteral nutrition by inhibiting the utilization of amino acids for protein synthesis.[23]

Within the broad class of antineoplastic agents, individual drugs have exclusive mechanisms for protein synthesis suppression. Methotrexate, 6-mercaptopurine, and 6-thioguanine inhibit purine ring synthesis. Azaribine inhibits pyrimidine synthesis. Nucleotide interconversion reactions are inhibited by 6-mercaptopurine and 6-thioguanine. Hydroxyurea blocks the conversion of ribonucleotides to deoxyribonucleotides by inhibiting ribonucleotide reductase. Methotrexate and 5-fluorouracil inhibit thymidylate synthetase, blocking DNA synthesis. Cytarabine inhibits DNA polymerase and is also incorporated into both DNA and RNA to a limited extent. Bleomycin inhibits DNA synthesis and, to a lesser extent, RNA and protein synthesis. Dactinomycin, daunorubicin, and doxorubicin intercalate with the DNA helix and prevent the template activity of the nucleic acid. These agents are also thought to inhibit RNA synthesis. The alkylating agents mitomycin and cisplatin cross-link the DNA helix and thus prevent protein synthesis. L-Asparaginase deaminates aspar-agine and deprives malignant leukemic cells of this essential nutrient. The vinca alkaloids vinblastine and vincristine inhibit the function of microtubules, thus arresting cell division.[45] Protein status is therefore influenced by three classes of drugs—chemotherapeutic agents, antibiotics, and glucocorticosteroids—each of which has an effect on various nutrients.

Carbohydrates. Drugs that affect carbohydrate metabolism may cause either hypoglycemia or hyperglycemia. This discussion will review these drugs and the mechanisms by which these abnormalities are caused.

Numerous agents may cause hypoglycemia. When taken in large doses, acetaminophen is metabolized to a hepatotoxin. Its toxic effect on the liver has been associated with a decreased blood sugar. When glycogen stores have been depleted, ethanol may inhibit gluconeogenesis and may also increase insulin secretion. Anabolic steroids have been observed to decrease fasting blood sugar, reduce glycosuria, and reduce the amount of insulin required to transport glucose into the cell. These hormones may also, to some extent, inhibit the destruction of insulin. Fenfluramine has a synergistic effect on insulin by enhancing glucose uptake in the cell. Monoamine oxidase inhibitors potentiate insulin and sulfonylurea hypoglycemia by inhibiting the homeostatic response to hypoglycemia. Propranolol may block the glycogenolytic effects of the sympathomimetic amines in response to hypoglycemia and may, in addition, inhibit gluconeogenesis. Salicylates may increase the uptake of glucose, increase the glycolytic rate, and inhibit gluconeogenesis. Theophylline may augment the release of insulin.[46]

Hyperglycemia, or iatrogenic diabetes, has been caused by various drugs. Ethanol may suppress insulin release, increase glycogenolysis, stimulate glucocorticoid release, or inhibit the peripheral utilization of glucose. Arginine stimulates glucagon release from the alpha pancreatic islet, which in turn generates hepatic glycogenolysis. L-Asparaginase inhibits insulin synthesis or may destroy pancreatic tissue, and clonidine inhibits the secretion of insulin by alpha-adrenergic stimulation. Diazoxide has been implicated as the causative agent in hyperosmolar nonketotic coma in adult diabetic patients. It is believed that this agent blocks the secretion of insulin and decreases the postprandial plasma insulin levels in diabetic and nondiabetic patients. Diazoxide inhibits phosphodiesterase enzymes, which results in increased levels of 3',5'-cyclic adenosine monophosphate (AMP); phosphodiesterase promotes glycogenolysis and gluconeogenesis. Diuretics, including the thiazides, chlorthalidone, ethacrynic acid, furosemide, and triamterene, have all been noted to cause hyperglycemia in diabetic and nondiabetic patients. The proposed mechanism is similar to that of diazoxide; hypokalemia, secondary to diuretic therapy, may also be a contributing factor. Glucocorticoids stimulate gluconeogenesis, decrease peripheral glucose utilization by inhibiting phosphorylation of glucose, and may cause insulin resistance.[47] Levodopa increases plasma glucagon above basal levels, increases plasma glucose content, and increases growth hormone. Through a prostaglandin-mediated mechanism, nicotinic acid increases serum glucose. Phenothiazines have been noted to cause hyperglycemia in psychotic patients. Potassium administration in hypokalemia has been associated with hyperglycemia, which may result from decreased insulin and growth hormone output. Propranolol, a beta-blocking agent, impairs insulin secretion. Theophylline inhibits phosphodiesterase enzymes, causes an increase in the content of cyclic AMP, and may also increase the insulin response to glucose. The hyperglycemia that is resistant to insulin therapy may predominate, however, because of the glycogenolytic or gluconeogenic effects of the drug.[48]

Fats. Dietary linoleic acid is metabolized in a three-step sequence to arachidonic acid. This metabolite is then converted to prostaglandins of the two series by the activity of the enzyme cyclooxygenase. Nonsteroidal anti-inflammatory agents inhibit the activity of cyclooxygenase, and anti-inflammatory steroids reduce the availability of substrate fatty acids to this converting enzyme.[49–51] Agents that reduce the absorption of fat from the gastrointestinal tract are discussed in the section on fat-soluble vitamins.

CONCLUSION

There are four major principles of drug therapy in tube-fed patients. The administration of medication through these tubes should be in a liquid form. The gastric emptying rate can influence the absorption of nutrients and drugs. The drug treatment of diarrhea should be based on its etiology. The practitioner must be cognizant of drug-nutrient interactions that may affect nutrient utilization.

REFERENCES

1. Rowland, M.: Drug administration and regimens. In Melmon, K. L., and Morrelli, H. F. (eds.): Clinical Pharmacology: Basic Principles in Therapeutics. Edition 2. New York, MacMillan, 1978, pp. 25–70.
2. Barr, W. H.: Principles of biopharmaceutics. Am. J. Pharm. Educ., 52:958–981, 1968.
3. Rombeau, J. L., and Miller, R. A.: Nasoenteric Tube Feeding—Practical Aspects. Mountain View, California, HEDECO, 1979.
4. Sokoloski, T. D.: Solutions and phase equilibria. In Osol, A., et al. (eds.): Remington's Pharmaceutical Sciences. Edition 15. Easton, Pennsylvania, Mack, 1975, pp. 229–254.
5. Higuchi, W. I., Swarbrick, J., Ho, N. F. H., Simonelli, A. P., and Martin, A.: Particle phenomena and coarse dispersions. In Osol, A., et al. (eds.): Remington's Pharmaceutical Sciences. Edition 16. Easton, Pennsylvania, Mack, 1980, pp. 294–322.
6. Swinyard, E. A., and Lowenthal, W.: Pharmaceutical necessities. In Osol, A., et al. (eds.): Remington's Pharmaceutical Sciences. Edition 15. Easton, Pennsylvania, Mack, 1975, pp. 1221–1269.
7. Zografi, G.: Interfacial phenomena. In Osol, A., et al. (eds.): Remington's Pharmaceutical Sciences. Edition 15. Easton, Pennsylvania, Mack, 1975, pp. 285–298.
8. Schott, H.: Colloidal dispersions. In Osol, A., et al. (eds.): Remington's Pharmaceutical Sciences. Edition 16. Easton, Pennsylvania, Mack, 1980, pp. 266–293.
9. Swarbrick, J.: Coarse dispersions: Suspensions, emulsions, and lotions. In Dittert, L. W. (eds.): Sprowls' American Pharmacy. Edition 7. Philadelphia, J.B. Lippincott Co., 1974, pp. 175–232.
10. Felmeister, A.: Powders. In Osol, A., et al. (eds.): Remington's Pharmaceutical Sciences. Edition 15. Easton, Pennsylvania, Mack, 1975, pp. 1554–1575.
11. Swarbrick, J.: Coarse dispersions. In Osol, A., et al. (eds.): Remington's Pharmaceutical Sciences. Edition 15. Easton, Pennsylvania, Mack, 1975, pp. 322–339.
12. Mitchell, J. F., and Liadis, M.: Oral solid dosage forms that should not be crushed prior to administration. Hosp. Pharm., 17:148–156, 1982.
13. Nimmo, W. S.: Drugs, diseases, and altered gastric emptying. Clin. Pharmacokinet., 1:189–203, 1976.
14. Nimmo, W. S., Heading, R. C., Wilson, J., Tothill, P., and Prescott, L. F.: Inhibition of gastric emptying and drug absorption by narcotic analgesics. Br. J. Clin. Pharmacol., 2:509–513, 1975.
15. Prescott, L. F.: Gastric emptying and drug absorption. Br. J. Clin. Pharmacol., 1:189–190, 1974.
16. Fernandez, C. A., Menezes, J. P., and Ximenes, J.: The effect of food on the absorption of pivampi-

cillin and a comparison with the absorption of ampicillin potassium. J. Int. Med. Res., *1*:530–533, 1973.

17. Kirby, W. M. M., Roberts, C. E., and Burdick, R. E.: Comparison of two new tetracyclines with tetracycline and demethylchlortetracycline. Antimicrob. Agents Chemother., *1*:286–292, 1961.

18. Kojima, S., Smith, R. B., and Doluisio, J. T.: Drug absorption. V. Influence of food on oral absorption of phenobarbital in rats, J. Pharm. Sci., *60*:1639–41, 1971.

19. Melander, A., Danielson, K., Schersten, B., and Wahlin, E.: Enhancement of the bioavailability of propranolol and metoprolol by food. Clin. Pharmacol. Ther., *22*:108–112, 1977.

20. Crounse, R. G.: Human pharmacology of griseofulvin. The effect of fat intake on gastrointestinal absorption. J. Invest. Dermatol., *37*:529–533, 1961.

21. Dozois, R. R., Kelly, K. A., and Code, C. F.: Effect of distal antrectomy on gastric emptying of liquids and solids. Gastroenterology, *61*:675–681, 1971.

22. Hart, L. L.: General care: Constipation and diarrhea. *In* Koda-Kimble, M. A., Katcher, B. S., and Young, L. Y. (eds.): Applied Therapeutics for Clinical Pharmacists. Edition 2. San Francisco, Applied Therapeutics, 1978, pp. 115–128.

23. Kucers, A., and McK.Bennett, N.: The Use of Antibiotics: A Comprehensive Review with Clinical Emphasis. Edition 3. Philadelphia, J.B. Lippincott Co., 1979.

24. American Society of Hospital Pharmacists. Committee on Pharmacy and Pharmaceuticals. American Hospital Formulary Service. Washington, D.C., American Society of Hospital Pharmacists, 1981.

25. Roe, D. A.: Drug-Induced Nutritional Deficiencies. Westport, Connecticut, AVI Publishing, 1976.

26. Caldwell, M. D., and Kennedy-Caldwell, C.: Normal nutritional requirements. Surg. Clin. North Am., *61*:489–507, 1981.

27. Molleson, A. L., and Gallagher-Allred, C. R.: Nutrient and Drug Interactions. Columbus, Ohio State University Department of Family Medicine, 1980.

28. Lee M., Schwartz, R. N., and Sharifi, R.: Warfarin resistance and vitamin K. Ann. Intern. Med., *94*:140–141, 1981.

29. O'Reilly, R. A., and Rytand, D. A.: Resistance to warfarin due to unrecognized vitamin K supplementation. N. Engl. J. Med., *303*:160–161, 1980.

30. Lader, E., Yang, L., and Clarke, A.: Warfarin dosage and vitamin K in OSMOLITE, Ann. Intern. Med., *93*:373–374, 1980.

31. Ross Laboratories: Enteral Nutrition: Ready Reference. Chicago, Illinois, 1981.

32. Travenol Laboratories: Travasorb—Special Disease State—Diet Supplements. Deerfield, Illinois, 1981.

33. Hethcox, J. M., and Stanaszek, W. F.: Interactions of drugs and diet. Hosp. Pharm., *9*:373–378, 1974.

34. Zbinden, G.: Therapeutic use of vitamin B_1 in diseases other than beriberi. Ann. N.Y. Acad. Sci., *98*:550–561, 1962.

35. Cooper, J. W.: Food-drug interactions. U.S. Pharmacist, *1*(Nov-Dec):17–28, 1976.

36. Mangini, R. J., and Gambertoglio, J. G.: Diseases of the kidney. *In* Young, L. Y., and Kimble, M. A.

37. (eds.): Applied Therapeutics for Clinical Pharmacists. San Francisco, Applied Therapeutics, 1975, pp. 155–194.

37. Levinsky, N. G.: Fluids and electrolytes. *In* Isselbacher, K. J., Adams, R. D., Braunwald, E., et al. (eds.): Harrison's Principles of Internal Medicine. Edition 9. New York, McGraw-Hill, 1980, pp. 435–444.

38. Lipner, H. I., Ruzany, F., Dasgupta, M., Lief, P. D., and Bank, N.: The behavior of carbenicillin as a nonreabsorbable anion. J. Lab. Clin. Med., *86*:183–194, 1975.

39. Bailey, G. L.: Hemodialysis: Principles and Practice. New York, Academic Press, 1972, p. 119.

40. Gambertoglio, J. G., and Mangini, R. J.: Diseases of the kidney. *In* Koda-Kimble, M. A., Katcher, B. A., and Young, L. Y. (eds.): Applied Therapeutics for Clinical Pharmacists. Edition 2. San Francisco, Applied Therapeutics, 1978, pp. 347–409.

41. Sheldon, G. F., and Grzyb, S.: Phosphate depletion and repletion: Relation to parenteral nutrition and oxygen transport. Ann. Surg., *182*:683–689, 1975.

42. Lentz, R. D., Brown, D. M., and Kjellstrand, C. M.: Treatment of severe hypophosphatemia, Ann. Intern. Med., *89*:941–948, 1978.

43. Kayser, S. R.: Thrombosis. *In* Young, L. Y., and Kimble, M. A. (eds.): Applied Therapeutics for Clinical Pharmacists. San Francisco, Applied Therapeutics, 1975, pp. 106–119.

44. Haynes, R. C., Jr., and Larner, J.: Adrenocorticotropic hormone; adrenocortical steroids and their synthetic analogs; inhibitors of adrenocortical steroid biosynthesis. *In* Goodman, L. S., and Gilman, A. (eds.): The Pharmacological Basis of Therapeutics. Edition 5. New York, MacMillan, 1975, pp. 1472–1506.

45. Calabresi, P., and Parks, R. E., Jr.: Chemotherapy of neoplastic disease. *In* Gilman, A. S., Goodman, L. S., and Gilman, A. (eds.): The Pharmacological Basis of Therapeutics. Edition 6. New York, MacMillan, 1980, pp. 1249–1314.

46. Kimble, M. A.: Diabetes mellitus. *In* Young, L. Y., and Kimble, M. A. (eds.): Applied Therapeutics for Clinical Pharmacists. San Francisco, Applied Therapeutics, 1975, pp. 225–260.

47. Kishi, D. T.: Clinical use and toxicity of glucocorticoids. *In* Koda-Kimble, M. A., Katcher, B. S., and Young, L. Y. (eds.): Applied Therapeutics for Clinical Pharmacists. Edition 2. San Francisco, Applied Therapeutics, 1978, pp. 563–583.

48. Koda-Kimble, M. A.: Diabetes mellitus. *In* Koda-Kimble, M. A., Katcher, B. S., and Young, L. Y. (eds.): Applied Therapeutics for Clinical Pharmacists. Edition 2. San Francisco, Applied Therapeutics, 1978, pp. 449–493.

49. Flower, R. J.: Drugs which inhibit prostaglandin biosynthesis. Pharmacol. Rev., *26*:33–67, 1974.

50. Lands, W. E. M.: The biosynthesis and metabolism of prostaglandins. Ann. Rev. Physiol., *41*:633–652, 1979.

51. Van Itallie, T. B.: An overview of essential fatty acid deficiency: role of intravenous fat emulsions in prevention and treatment. *In* Barlow, L. (ed.): Liposyn Research Conference Proceedings, Abbott Laboratories, North Chicago, Illinois, 1979.

CHAPTER 29

Complications and Their Prevention

MARIE BERNARD
LORETTA FORLAW

There are relatively few clinically significant complications of enteral alimentation. Of those that are significant, most can be easily treated and prevented when patients are properly monitored. This chapter will describe the pathogenesis, diagnosis, and treatment of the gastrointestinal, metabolic, infectious, mechanical and psychological complications that result from enteral nutrition by tube (Fig. 29–1).

GASTROINTESTINAL COMPLICATIONS

Gastrointestinal abnormalities are among the most common complications of enteral feedings. Unfortunately, there are few series that carefully document the incidence of any of the complications of enteral alimentation. Table 29–1 summarizes the incidence of complications compiled from published series. The most common gastrointestinal complications are nausea and vomiting, and diarrhea.

Nausea and Vomiting. Nausea and vomiting are said to occur in as many as 10 to 20 per cent of patients who are tube fed.[1] The etiology of this complication may be multifactorial (Table 29–2). The smell of enteral formulas is often distressing to the patient and may cause nausea.[2] Formulas that are high in osmolality may lead to gastric retention,[3] nausea, and vomiting, particularly when formulas are infused very rapidly.[4] Nausea and vomiting may also be one of the many manifestations of lactose intolerance. With the increasing use of modular formulas, one must also be aware that an imbalance in the proportion of fat given a patient can promote nausea and vomiting, particularly in a patient with biliary tract disease. In view of these possible causes of nausea and vomiting, the need for preventive measures is evident. Flavorings can be added to formulas to increase their acceptance in terms of smell. This must be done cautiously, however, since large volumes of flavorings can significantly increase the osmolality of a solution. Nausea from gastric retention with hypertonic solutions is decreased by starting these solutions in diluted form, and gradually increasing their concentration over the course of several days to full strength. Heitkemper and associates[4] have shown that in normal volunteers, nausea and other forms

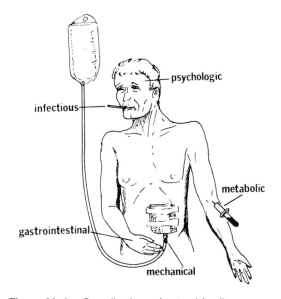

Figure 29–1. Complications of enteral feeding.

Table 29–1 INCIDENCE OF COMPLICATIONS IN TUBE FEEDING

	TOTAL PATIENTS	NAUSEA AND VOMITING	DISTENTION	DIARRHEA	ASPIRATION	HYPERGLYCEMIA	OVERHYDRATION	HYPERNATREMIC DEHYDRATION
Moore et al.[89]	30		3	4				
Roy et al.[92]	21		1					
Loo et al.[93]	17		1					
Chen and Wong[94]	13				3			
Cheek and Staub[90]	47				2			
Delany et al.[91]	19		+	+				
Winterbauer et al.[43]	20				6 clinically significant			
Heymsfield et al.[1]	150	10–15%		10–20%	<1%	10–15%	20–25%	5%
Andrassy et al.[82]	200	"many"			1		3	5
Mitty et al.[83]	13				0			
Bury et al.[84]	250	+		+				
Kaminski[8]	(160)					+		2
Stephens et al.[85]	16							
Levy et al.[86]	230	4		2	2			
Voitk et al.[21]	100				1			
Dobbie and Hoffmeister[87]	60			0	0			
Voitk et al.[88]	100		1-cramps					
Vanlandingham[32]	100			3	0			

Table 29–2 GASTROINTESTINAL COMPLICATIONS—NAUSEA AND VOMITING

CAUSE	DIAGNOSIS	THERAPY	PREVENTION
Offensive smell	Patient complains of smell of formula	Add flavorings to enteral formula	Use polymeric formulas whenever possible. Elemental formulas tend to have offensive odor
High osmolality leading to gastric retention	Gastric residual more than 100 ml 4 hours after bolus feeding or greater than 115% of vol/hour with continuous feeding	Dilute hyperosmolar formulas to isotonic strength, then slowly increase concentration over several days	Dilute hyperosmolar formulas to isotonic strength, then slowly increase concentration over several days
		Switch to isotonic formula	Use isotonic formulas when possible
Rapid rate of infusion	Nausea and vomiting develop within a short time after a change in infusion rate	Return infusion rate to previous level, and then advance by 25 ml/hr every 12 to 24 hr (if tolerated by patient)	Start gastric feedings at 40–50 ml/hr and jejunal and duodenal feedings at 20–25 ml/hr and advance at 25 ml/hr every 12–24 hr depending on clinical tolerance
Lactose intolerance	Review of past history to reveal lactose intolerance; lactose tolerance test; switch to lower lactose or non–lactose-containing formula with resolution of nausea and vomiting	Switch to lower lactose or non–lactose-containing formula	Use formulas with low lactose content (particularly in very ill patients with intestinal factors that predispose to relative lactose intolerance)
Excessive fat in diet	Review of past history to reveal fat intolerance or illness that predisposes to fat intolerance	Switch to lower fat diet	Maintain fat at no greater than 30–40% of total caloric intake

of gastrointestinal discomfort are minimized by giving bolus feedings at 30 ml/min. Nausea and vomiting from lactose intolerance or suspected lactose intolerance are best dealt with by switching to a lactose-free formula.

Diarrhea. Diarrhea is also a common gastrointestinal side effect of tube feeding (Table 29–3). Its incidence is reported at 10 to 20 per cent.[1] In order to deal with diarrhea effectively, one must have a clear understanding of the definition of diarrhea and its possible etiologies.

Diarrhea is usually defined as an increase in the frequency and/or volume of stool, or a decrease in the consistency of stool. Quantitatively, diarrhea is an increase in stool weight of more than 150 gm/24 hr, or an increase in stool water of more than 1500 ml/24 hr. Diarrhea occurs when the ab-

sorptive capacity of the colon is exceeded or altered. The small bowel usually has an absorptive capacity of approximately 12 L/day; the large bowel, of 4 to 6 L/day.[5, 6] The quantity of water that passes through the bowel is approximately 7 to 9 L in the small intestine, and 2 to 3 L in the large intestine. Water absorption in the bowel is passive, secondary to solute absorption; that is, water movement is caused by passive diffusion and relies upon the luminal-to-plasma osmotic gradient.[7] An increase in luminal osmolarity will slow water absorption. This can occur secondary either to nonabsorbed dietary solutes or to changes in intestinal mucosal transport processes. In addition, there is active secretion of some solutes by the large and small bowel, so that net solute movement is the sum of absorption versus

Table 29–3 GASTROINTESTINAL COMPLICATIONS—DIARRHEA

CAUSE	DIAGNOSIS	THERAPY	PREVENTION
Hyperosmolar solution	Osmolality of solution greater than 300 mOsm	Use isotonic solutions, or dilute hypertonic solutions to isotonic strength	Use isotonic solutions, or dilute hyperosmolar solutions to isotonic strength
Hyperosmolar solution	Increase in water content and frequency of stools without associated pain, blood, or pus in stool	Start at slow rate (40–50 ml/hr or less) and increase in 12–24 hr increments	Start at slow rate (40–50 ml/hr or less) and increase in 12–24 hr increments
		Increase caloric density with glucose polymers	Increase caloric density with glucose polymers
		Stop current formula for 12 hours—resume with isotonic formula at slow rate (40–50 ml per hour or less)	Stop current formula for 12 hr—resume with isotonic formula at slow rate of (40–50 ml/hr or less)
		Use Kaopectate or paregoric in appropriate dosage; Lomotil if necessary. Stop antidiarrheal medication at 2 days and monitor for impaction if required for longer	
Lactase deficiency	Review of past history to reveal lactose intolerance	Switch to lower lactose or non–lactose-containing formula	Use formulas with low lactose content (particularly in very ill patients, with small bowel factors that predispose to relative lactose intolerance)
	Lactose tolerance test Switch to lower lactose or non–lactose-containing formula with resolution of diarrhea		
Fat malabsorption	Review of past history to reveal diarrhea associated with fat ingestion or illness predisposing to fat malabsorption	Pancreatic enzyme supplements in patients with true pancreatic insufficiency	Use products with low fat content in patients with pancreatic insufficiency or other known illnesses that predispose to fat malabsorption
	72-hour fecal fat assessment	Switch to product with lower fat content	
Cold feedings	Tubing cold to touch	Discontinue feedings until formula has warmed to room temperature	Start recently refrigerated formulas at a slow infusion rate (40 ml/hr) to allow for warming to room temperature
Protein malnutrition	Albumin less than 3 gm/dl	Use isotonic solutions, or dilute hypertonic solutions to isotonic strength	Use isotonic solutions, or dilute hypertonic solutions to isotonic strength

Table continued on following page

Table 29–3 GASTROINTESTINAL COMPLICATIONS—DIARRHEA *(Continued)*

CAUSE	DIAGNOSIS	THERAPY	PREVENTION
		Start at slow rate, 20–25 ml/hr or less, and increase in 12–24 hr increments, depending on patient response	Start at slow rate, 20–25 ml/hr or less, and increase in 12–24 hr increments, depending on patient response
		Give parenteral nutrition concomitantly or prior to start of enteral feedings	Give parenteral nutrition concomitantly or prior to start of enteral feedings
		Use antidiarrheal agent for 48-hr period, if necessary	Use antidiarrheal agent for 48-hr period, if necessary
Factors independent of enteral formula	Careful review of patient history, physical examination, and medications	Reverse primary factor, e.g., discontinue antibiotics causing pseudomembranous enterocolitis or bacterial overgrowth; or treat infectious diarrheal agents	
Unidentifiable factors	Careful review of patient history, physical, and medications	Discontinue feedings for 48 hr, then resume at lower flow rate and utilize peripheral TPN in interim; or, decrease flow rate to 25–50 ml/hr for at least 24 hr then increase by 25–50 ml/hr every 24 hours; or, dilute formula and then slowly increase concentration over several days; or add an antidiarrheal agent; or add a bulk forming agent	

secretion. It is therefore possible for diarrhea to occur as a result of (1) a decrease in absorptive capacity, either generalized (celiac sprue) or selective (lactase deficiency); (2) an increase in active secretion of a solute owing to exogenous factors (cholera and other bacterial enterotoxins, commercial laxatives) or endogenous factors (vasoactive intestinal peptide, bile acids, fatty acids); or (3) a combination of abnormalities of absorption and secretion.

Formula Osmolality. Among a number of specific factors known to cause diarrhea in tube-fed patients is the osmolality of the solution. A hypertonic solution delivered directly into the small bowel has the potential to significantly retard the passive diffusion of water into the intestinal mucosa, and cause diarrhea. There can, in fact, be a net secretion of water to offset a very high luminal osmolality. If a hyperosmolar solution is delivered too rapidly directly into the jejunum, vascular collapse may result.[8] Hyperosmolar solutions are better tolerated delivered directly into the stomach and diluted by gastric juices, although, again, very rapid administration of a hyperosmolar solution into the stomach can lead to dumping of large volumes of the hyperosmolar solution into the small bowel, and subsequent diarrhea. This form of diarrhea is avoided or minimized by diluting all hyperosmolar solutions to an isosmotic (approximately 300 mOsm) concentration, and starting at a low flow rate. One can then slowly increase the concentration and flow rate until the patient's predicted nutritional needs are met. Table 29–3 provides therapeutic options when diarrhea develops with tube feeding.

Lactase Deficiency. Lactase deficiency,

or relative lactase deficiency, has also been demonstrated as a cause of diarrhea in tube-fed patients.[9, 10] In this condition, unhydrolyzed lactose causes diarrhea by increasing the colonic luminal osmolality and thereby decreasing the passive absorption of water from the bowel. The lactose is then fermented by bacteria into organic acids, causing the delivery of further water into the bowel and exacerbation of the diarrhea.[11]

True lactase deficiency occurs in as many as 60 per cent of black Americans and 6 to 20 per cent of white Americans. Walike and Walike[9, 10] reported that in approximately 87 per cent of patients given a large lactose load, such as that received in a typical blenderized formula, diarrhea developed. Only 14 per cent of these patients had true lactase deficiency as indicated by a lactose tolerance test. These results are commensurate with the variety of abnormalities in the small bowel that can reduce its lactase content.[12–14] For example, sprue, infectious diarrhea, intestinal resection, radiation enteritis, and malnutrition produce a range of lactose intolerance from partial to complete, depending upon the amount of bowel affected.[14] In addition, it appears that in a significant percentage of adults a natural decrease develops in the lactase content of their intestinal brush border, predisposing them to diarrhea when challenged by a large lactose load. As a result of the findings of Walike and Walike, the lactose content of many new products has been minimized.

Fat Malabsorption. There are a number of steps in the digestive process where fat absorption may be impaired, causing diarrhea in tube-fed patients. In pancreatic disease there may be insufficient lipase reaching the intestine to hydrolyze triglyceride. Gastric surgery may delay release of lipase or prevent adequate mixing of lipase with intestinal contents. Bile salts may not reach the intestinal lumen in adequate quantities in patients with biliary obstruction, ileectomy, or ileitis. All of these conditions will lead to decreased micellar solubilization of fats. Bacterial overgrowth, disordered mucosal phase of fat absorption associated with a wide range of intestinal diseases, and intestinal resection can all lead to different degrees of fat malabsorption. Paradoxically, in a few cases of documented fat malabsorption, medium-chain triglycerides, which are used to increase fat absorption, have caused increased diarrhea, flatulence, and abdominal pain because of intolerance to medium-chain triglycerides.[15]

The use of an enteral product with a lower fat content usually markedly decreases diarrhea related to fat malabsorption. Pancreatic enzyme supplements are generally required in patients with true pancreatic insufficiency and in whom a non-elemental diet is indicated. Patients with suspected intolerance to medium-chain triglycerides can on occasion be brought to greater tolerance with the addition of divided doses of medium-chain triglycerides to juices or solid foods (assuming that the patient is eating in addition to receiving tube feedings). Medium-chain triglycerides can also be used in cooking.

Diet Temperature. It is often felt that diarrhea and other gastrointestinal complaints (such as abdominal pain, nausea, vomiting, and flatulence) result from diet temperature. Kagawa-Busby and coworkers[16] have recently demonstrated that diets at room temperature or higher seem to have no clinical effect on tolerance for tube feeding. However, cold feedings (8 to 11°C) caused cramping and diarrhea in two of six patients in their study group. Thus cold feedings may increase the likelihood of gastrointestinal side effects in tube-fed patients.

Protein Malnutrition. Diarrhea may also occur as a consequence of marked protein malnutrition. Platt and coworkers[14] demonstrated that pigs fed diets markedly low in protein developed intestinal mucosal atrophy and consequent diarrhea with feedings. It has recently been demonstrated that serum albumin levels less than 3 gm/dl significantly correlated with the development of diarrhea at the initiation of feedings, while with albumin levels greater than 4 gm/dl there were generally no problems.[17] Diarrhea was particularly difficult when protein malnutrition was combined with sepsis. The initial diarrhea was generally alleviated by diluting the formulas, and very slowly advancing the flow rate and concentration.

Miscellaneous Factors. Finally, there are some patients who experience diarrhea during tube feedings for unknown or unidentifiable reasons. These are patients who may have subtle or transient fat or lactose malabsorption from any of the multiple factors listed previously. There may also be a cause of diarrhea in these patients which is unmasked by the tube feedings. A careful review of the patient's history is essential to be certain that the diarrhea did not antedate the start of tube feedings. Diarrhea associated with fever should raise the possibility of an infectious agent. The patient's medications should also be reviewed. Notorious among these are prolonged courses of antibiotics that alter the bacterial flora or cause pseudomembranous enterocolitis.

Diarrhea is a common side effect of the penicillin-like antibiotics, and efficacy of enteral feeding during their course must be individually evaluated. If diarrhea cannot be resolved with antidiarrheal medications, peripheral TPN may be appropriate if more calories can be delivered by this method than by the enteral route.

Lactulose therapy may also be an indication for peripheral TPN if nutritional needs cannot be met by the enteral route for a brief course of therapy.

Magnesium-based antacid therapy may also cause diarrhea in the tube-fed patient. Alternating magnesium-free antacid formulations may significantly reduce this problem.

Oral phosphate supplementation may be required initially in enteral feeding during intracellular anabolic shifts of phosphate. Small divided doses will generally decrease the incidence of diarrhea. Antidiarrheal medications may also be of assistance. Where there is no clearly identifiable cause of diarrhea, there are several options for therapy. Often a decrease in the flow rate alleviates diarrhea by permitting intestinal adaptation to the enteral formula, particularly in patients who have not been fed for a prolonged period, and who thus have relative malabsorption resulting from intestinal atrophy.[18, 19] The flow rate is then slowly increased to the desired level over the course of several days while the patient's clinical response is carefully monitored. If the diarrhea does not resolve with a decrease in flow rate, a decrease in the osmolality of the formula is often helpful. If diarrhea persists in spite of careful advancement of formula flow rate and concentration, many clinicians find that adding a small amount of paregoric or other antidiarrheal agent to the enteral solution will resolve the problem. This must be done with great caution, as at least one case of intestinal pseudo-obstruction which required surgery for diagnosis has been reported.[8] Another medication recently reported to be helpful in tube feeding associated diarrhea is Metamucil.[20] This bulk-increasing agent appears to absorb water, solidifying the stool and slowing the transit time. It is added to the enteral formula and titrated to the patient's needs. The average requirement at the University of San Diego was 7 gm per liter of formula. An area not yet investigated is the usefulness of bulk additives, such as bran, in controlling diarrhea associated with tube feedings.

Constipation. Constipation is another potential gastrointestinal complication of enteral feedings (Table 29–4). All of the formulas that are low in lactose may be expected to produce diminished fecal residue. Nonetheless, in a properly hydrated patient there should not be an absolute lack of feces. Patients complaining of constipation should be evaluated for nausea, vomiting, and distention, which may suggest concurrent obstruction. Rectal examination should always be performed to rule out fecal impaction. Extremely hard stools can be avoided by careful attention to the patient's free water balance.

METABOLIC COMPLICATIONS

Metabolic complications of enteral feeding are fairly frequent and are usually easily managed when patients are properly monitored (Fig. 29–2, Table 29–5).

Overhydration. Heymsfield and co-workers[1] report a 20 to 25 per cent incidence of overhydration in tube-fed patients. It is usually associated with the reintroduction of water and sodium to patients who have been deprived for long periods of adequate amounts of each and may be particularly pronounced in patients with any degree of cardiac, renal, or hepatic disease.[21, 22] Overhydration is treated by slowing the rate of enteral administration of fluid, and then slowly advancing it again, while carefully monitoring the patient's clinical response. Diuretics are rarely necessary unless the patient has prior significant cardiac, renal, or hepatic disease.

Dehydration. Hypertonic dehydration is a much more commonly discussed metabolic complication of enteral feedings. Its documented incidence appears to be from 5 to 10 per cent.[23-25] In the past it has been labeled the "tube feeding syndrome."[26] This

Table 29–4 GASTROINTESTINAL COMPLICATIONS—CONSTIPATION

CAUSE	DIAGNOSIS	THERAPY	PREVENTION
Dehydration	Intake less than output, dry skin and mucous membranes, orthostatic hypotension; BUN: creatinine ratio> 10:1	Supplemental fluids in enteral formula or by parenteral route	Careful watch of intake and output, giving supplements of free water when intake is not greater than output by 500–1000 ml (or more in febrile states)
Impaction	Rectal examination	Digital disimpaction	Careful watch of intake and output giving supplements of free water when intake is not greater than output by 500–1000 ml (or more in febrile states)
Obstruction	Nausea, vomiting, flat plate of abdomen showing dilated bowel with air fluid levels	Possible decompression by Miller-Abbott tube; generally requires surgery	

form of metabolic abnormality may develop when a formula of high osmolarity and high protein content is fed to patients unable to communicate their thirst, such as patients with tracheostomies, unconscious patients, very young patients, and debilitated elderly patients. The maximal renal concentrating ability of a healthy subject is thought to be

Metabolic Complications

Over-hydration

Dehydration

Hyperglycemia

Electrolyte and trace element imbalances

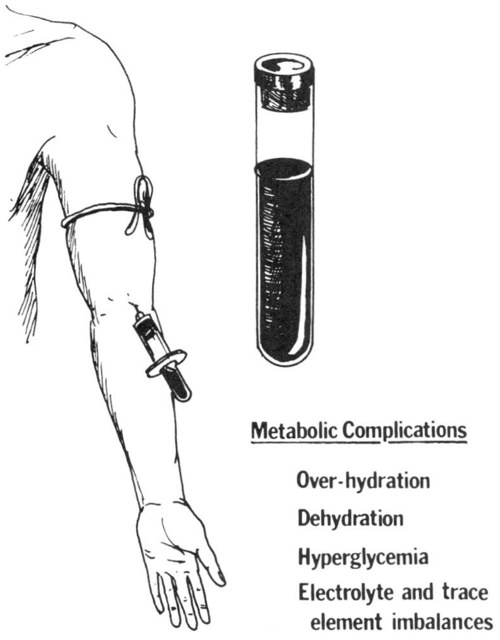

Figure 29–2. Metabolic complications of enteral feeding.

1300 mOsm/kg water.[27, 28] In many elderly subjects this concentrating ability is less than 1000 mOsm/kg of water. It should, therefore, be anticipated that with some enteral products supplementary water must be given if the patient is unable to respond voluntarily to his thirst mechanism. The necessary quantity of free water is best determined by knowing the amount of free water in the product being used, and by carefully following the patient for clinical signs of dehydration. The patient's intake, output, and serum electrolytes should be monitored.

Hyperglycemic Hyperosmolar Nonketosis. Another form of dehydration that may occur is associated with severe hyperglycemia. The syndrome of hyperglycemic hyperosmolar nonketosis occurs in less than 1 per cent of tube-fed patients.[29] It results from a relative insulin deficiency, usually in maturity onset diabetics or in previously borderline diabetics. The insulin reserves of these patients are adequate to prevent the development of true ketosis, but inadequate to control the serum glucose. The blood sugar, therefore, rises, leading to an osmotic diuresis and eventually marked dehydration. This complication fortunately is very uncommon because of the frequent use of protocols and careful metabolic monitoring of tube-fed patients. It is treated with small doses of intravenous or intramuscular insulin, and vigorous hydration.[30, 31]

Simple hyperglycemia occurs much more commonly, probably in 10 to 30 per cent of tube-fed patients.[1, 32] It is corrected by de-

Table 29–5 METABOLIC COMPLICATIONS

COMPLICATION	INCIDENCE (PER CENT)	CAUSE	THERAPY	PREVENTION
Overhydration	20–25	Severe malnutrition and refeeding	Decrease fluid flow rate	Careful monitoring of intake and output and clinical status
		Significant cardiac, renal, or hepatic disease	Occasional diuretics (particularly in patients with cardiac, renal, or hepatic disease)	
Hypertonic dehydration	5–10	Hypertonic formula given to a patient unable to communicate or respond to thirst	Supplemental water either in enteral formula or parenterally	Careful monitoring of intake and output and clinical status
HHNK	<1	Relative insulin lack	Discontinue feedings until blood sugar controlled, then restart at a slow rate, and slowly increase rate while titrating insulin	Careful monitoring of blood sugar on a daily basis as feedings are initiated; at least twice daily in patient with known diabetes
			Vigorous hydration	
			Small doses IV or IM insulin	
Hyperglycemia	10–30	Insulin lack	Slow enteral fluid administration rate initially; slow increase in flow rate	Give formulas with higher per cent fat; calories contributed by fat may require use of modular formula
			Insulin or an oral hypoglycemic	
Hypoglycemia	2	Sudden cessation of feedings in patients on medication for hyperglycemia	Taper feedings	Taper feedings
			Decrease fluid flow rate	Decrease fluid flow rate
Hyperkalemia	40	High potassium content of enteral formulas	Switch to formula with lower potassium content	Check electrolytes daily as flow rate is being increased; at least weekly once rate is established
		Renal insufficiency	Kayexalate; insulin and glucose	

Table 29–5 METABOLIC COMPLICATIONS *(Continued)*

COMPLICATION	INCIDENCE (PER CENT)	CAUSE	THERAPY	PREVENTION
		Acidosis		
Hypokalemia	8	Insulin administration	Potassium supplements in enteral formula or parenterally	Check electrolytes daily as flow rate is being increased; at least weekly once rate is established
		Diarrhea		
		Marked malnutrition		
Hypophosphatemia	30	Insulin administration	Phosphate supplements in enteral formula or parenterally	Check electrolytes daily as flow rate is being increased; at least weekly once rate is established
		Severe malnutrition		
Hyponatremia	31	See overhydration	Water restriction	Same as above
		Prolonged enteral therapy		
Hyperphosphatemia	14	Renal insufficiency	Switch to product with lower phosphate content	Same as above
Hypomagnesemia	3	Decreased carrier protein levels	Continued therapy	
Hypocupremia	3	Inadequate delivery	Supplement formula, as necessary	Check serum levels
Elevated transaminases	Unknown	Activation of hepatic enzymes	If progressively abnormal, discontinue formula, though there are reports of reversal of the abnormality in spite of continued enteral therapy	
Vitamin K deficiency	Unknown	Low vitamin K content of elemental formulas	Vitamin K replacement	Adequate provision of vitamin K
Essential fatty acid deficiency	Unknown	Low linoleic acid content of diet	Modular fat product added to enteral formula	Adequate provision of essential fatty acids
			Daily 5 ml of safflower oil orally	
			Parenteral fat administration	

creasing the flow rate of the enteral formula, and administering increasing doses of a rapid- or intermediate-acting insulin until the blood sugar is reduced to approximately 200 mg/dl. Some authors advocate the addition of an oral hypoglycemic drug to the enteral formula.[8] The flow rate may then be slowly advanced with continued titration of the insulin or oral hypoglycemic drug. Urine fractional measurements may be used as a guide to developing hyperglycemia, though treatment on the basis of these measurements alone can lead to adverse consequences in patients with a low urinary threshold for glucose.[33, 34]

Abnormalities of Electrolytes and Trace Elements. A number of abnormalities of electrolytes and trace elements may occur with enteral feedings. Vanlandingham and coworkers[32] reported a 2 per cent incidence of hypoglycemia, in each instance associated with sudden cessation of tube feedings in patients on insulin. There was a 40 per cent incidence of hyperkalemia (potassium greater than 5 mEq/L), although only 3 per cent of the potassium levels were greater than 6.0 mEq/L. Most cases of hyperkalemia were associated with metabolic acidosis combined with renal insufficiency. A recent report suggests that there is also an inappropriately high level of potassium in many enteral formulas, which may contribute to this observed incidence of hyperkalemia.[35]

Hypokalemia, as reported by Vanlandingham, occurred in 8 per cent of patients, usually in association with administration of insulin. Hypophosphatemia occurred in 30 per cent of patients and also was correlated with administration of insulin in a high percentage of cases. Hyponatremia occurred in 31 per cent of patients. One might anticipate some degree of hyponatremia after prolonged therapy, since most enteral formulas are equivalent to a 2-gm sodium diet. Hyperphosphatemia was seen in 14 per cent of patients, and was usually associated with renal failure.

There was a 3 per cent incidence of magnesium and copper deficiency as well as an 11 per cent incidence of zinc deficiency. Each of these deficits corrected spontaneously without special supplements, and was not associated with clinical signs of deficiency. The authors hypothesized that decreased carrier protein levels may have accounted for the decreased blood levels. True deficiency states should be expected in patients who chronically receive less than their predicted caloric needs in the form of enteral formula. Most formulas require an intake of 1500 to 2000 ml to meet all of the recommended daily allowances of vitamins and minerals.

Abnormalities of Liver Function. There has been at least one documented report of elevated transaminases associated with an elemental diet.[36] Areas of parenchymal necrosis with occasional acidophilic bodies in the biopsy of liver tissue in this case report suggested a toxic mechanism. Abnormalities resolved spontaneously with the cessation of tube feeding. The true incidence and pathogenesis of this abnormality are unknown. Two of 27 infants with diarrhea given elemental diets also had low-grade elevations of transaminase levels.[37] An unstated percentage of 28 patients in Kaminski's review had increased levels of alkaline phosphatase and transaminase. Rises in serum transaminase are nonspecific and are frequently seen in hospitalized patients. Transient rises in the transaminase have also been noted in patients receiving parenteral nutrition. In those patients the elevations have been ascribed to activation of hepatic enzymes by the new influx of large quantities of nutrients.[38] Though this problem has not been as carefully examined in patients receiving enteral nutrition, the mechanisms may be similar.

Deficiency States. Deficiency states may occasionally develop with enteral feedings despite the fact that the patient's predicted caloric needs have been met. Vitamin K deficiency has been reported[1, 39] with prolonged administration of formulas low in fat. Essential fatty acid deficiency may develop in patients fed long term with formulas low in linoleic acid.[40]

Formulas for Patients with Renal Failure. In patients with marked renal dysfunction, it is often preferable to limit intake of protein, potassium, phosphorus, magnesium, and other trace elements. This is best accomplished by giving enteral formulas especially designed for patients with renal failure. There are presently two commercially available formulas that are composed of essential amino acids as their protein sources. These formulas are based on the finding that essential amino acids given parenterally to patients with acute renal failure seem to increase the rate of recovery of renal function.[41]

Formulas for Patients with Hepatic Failure. In patients with hepatic failure, a low protein intake, primarily consisting of branched-chain amino acids (BCAA), may be desirable. There are some data to suggest that BCAA may help to reverse hepatic coma, and the presently available enteral formulas for hepatic failure have increased quantities of BCAA. Both the renal and hepatic formulas have virtually no electrolytes, vitamins, or minerals. These nutrients must therefore be added according to the patient's needs.

Formulas for Patients with Cardiac Failure. Patients with severe cardiac failure can generally tolerate the standard formulated enteral products, since they are usually equivalent to a 2-gm sodium diet. In cardiac patients who require severe fluid restriction, a more calorically dense formula may be preferable (2 cal/ml).

INFECTIOUS COMPLICATIONS

The two most common infectious complications are aspiration pneumonia and contamination of the formula (Fig. 29–3).

Aspiration Pneumonia. Aspiration pneumonia is a potential complication in all patients who receive tube feedings. The frequency of aspiration is difficult to determine because it is dependent upon one's definition of aspiration. Generally, aspiration pneumonia is defined as the sudden onset of respiratory distress or failure following an observed aspiration. Usually, chest x-ray films will show mottled densities in the lower lobes (or more diffusely). The patient produces frothy nonpurulent sputum. When defined in this manner, the incidence of aspiration associated with tube feedings is generally reported to be less than 1 per cent.

Unfortunately, aspiration of stomach contents can occur subtly, without overt evidence of vomiting, especially in patients with decreased mental status or decreased ability of glottic closure (tracheostomized patients, patients with an endotracheal tube). This form of aspiration is the result of regurgitation, a clinically silent event. Therefore, another definition of aspiration in tube feeding should be given: some combination of tachypnea, tachycardia, fever, hypoxemia, and a new infiltrate on chest x-ray film, with no obvious explanation of these findings, and a resolution of this syndrome with discontinuation of tube feedings. Using such a definition, the incidence of clinically significant aspiration has been reported to be as high as 30 per cent in a small group of pa-

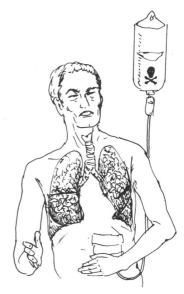

Figure 29–3. Infective complications of enteral feeding include aspiration and contamination of formula.

tients with tracheostomies or translaryngeal intubation.[43]

The consequences of aspiration are largely dependent upon pH and particle size of the aspirated material. After aspiration, gastric acid is rapidly distributed throughout the lungs, and damage occurs immediately. Isolated areas of atelectasis appear in the first several seconds, and the condition becomes extensive within minutes. Pathologic examination within the first few hours reveals epithelial degeneration of the bronchi, pulmonary edema, and hemorrhage.[44] During the next 24 to 36 hours, marked white blood cell infiltration occurs, and damage to the airways may cause mucosal sloughing.[45] Within 72 hours recovery has begun. It has been suggested by several authors that there is a critical pH of 2.5 in humans, below which these pathologic events occur.[46–50]

The pulmonary consequences of aspiration of gastric contents are also strongly related to the presence or absence of food particles.[51] Early pathologic studies have demonstrated that aspiration of neutral stomach contents containing small, nonobstructing particles of food cause a prolonged inflammatory response clinically similar to that caused by acid.[47, 52–55] The severity of the reaction is related to the size and the chemical composition of the particles. The composition of the particles is related to their ability to be phagocytosed, disintegrated, or removed from the lung. Hypertonic fluids can cause the same reaction, as can milk and formula.

The initial response to aspiration of foodstuff appears to be similar to that of aspiration of acid. But unlike in acid aspiration, at approximately 48 hours a widespread granulomatous reaction with numerous macrophages and giant cells develops. Within another 24 hours most of the reaction is mononuclear, and numerous granulomas are present. Within five days the macrophage infiltration is decreased, and focal granulomas are present.

One may then conclude that aspiration of blenderized diets may lead to a greater pulmonary consequence than elemental diets because of the presence of complex carbohydrates, fats, and proteins. In counterpoint, the high osmolality of elemental diets may be just as damaging to the tracheobronchial tree.

The patient's response to aspiration is determined by both the nature and quantity of the aspirate. If a large volume of enteral formula is aspirated, acute pulmonary edema may develop within minutes. Hypotension, tachypnea, dyspnea, and cyanosis ensue. Chest roentgenograms at six to eight hours may show diffuse, fluffy infiltrates, with a greater tendency for the infiltrates to occur in the lower lobes. The full extent of the pulmonary injury is usually not evident until 24 hours after the initial insult. In the following 24 to 48 hours, there may be progressive respiratory deterioration, and ultimate death with massive aspiration.

With very small volumes of aspiration, the initial event may go unrecognized. There may be such a small quantity of aspirate that there are no long-lasting pathologic or clinical changes. Alternatively, the patient may have fever and radiographic evidence of atelectasis or bronchopneumonia. Patients who are fed nasogastrically appear to have a higher likelihood of aspiration than patients fed by gastrostomy or jejunostomy.[56, 57] Likewise, patients with an endotracheal tube or a tracheostomy appear to have a high likelihood of aspiration.[58, 59] It has been claimed that nasojejunal feedings are associated with a lower likelihood of aspiration than nasogastric feedings. This theoretically is expected, since a tube positioned beyond the pylorus should allow for less refluxing into the oropharynx than a tube placed intragastrically. Good prospective studies to demonstrate this fact have yet to be reported,

though anecdotally many practitioners in nutritional support have observed this to be true.

A number of measures can be taken to decrease the likelihood of aspiration. First, maintaining elevation of the head of the bed at 30 degrees at all times will aid aboral progression of the feedings by simple gravitational pull, and decrease the likelihood of a significant amount of fluid being in the stomach at any one time. The higher the osmolality of the solution, the greater the likelihood of slow gastric emptying;[3] therefore, hypertonic fluids should be started in diluted form, and gradually built up to full strength. In addition, particularly in patients with any degree of depression of mental status, nasojejunal feedings appear to be preferable to nasogastric feedings. One must be careful to document that the feeding tube is in fact beyond the pylorus, both at the initiation of therapy and after vigorous coughing, vomiting, or any other maneuver that might dislodge the tube. Dislodgement of the tube renders a nasoduodenal tube equivalent to a nasogastric tube in terms of the risk of aspiration.

Frequent checks of the gastric residual should be made. In patients receiving bolus feedings, a gastric residual of more than 150 ml before initiation of feeding usually requires cessation of feedings until the residual is cleared. If residuals of this volume are found on two successive checks, enteral feedings should be discontinued. In patients receiving continuous feedings, a residual that is 10 to 20 per cent greater than the flow rate per hour should be considered significant, and the feedings should be stopped until the residual has cleared. Residuals of this volume on two successive checks mandates a cessation of feedings.

With the small-bore tubes that are commonly used for continuous feeding, it is often difficult to reliably check the gastric residual because the tube collapses with external suction. These patients should have abdominal girths checked serially, in addition to a check of gastric residuals. This is done by measuring the distance from one anterior superior iliac crest to the other. An increase in abdominal girth of 8 to 10 cm above baseline is thought to be significant, and to necessitate the temporary cessation of feeding. If a procedure requiring a recumbent position is anticipated, feedings should be stopped approximately 30 minutes to one hour prior to that procedure.

The diagnosis of aspiration is easy to make in the presence of a witnessed event; or, with the sudden onset of pulmonary edema, remains of the enteral feeding are identified with suction. In patients with silent, small volume aspiration, the diagnosis is often surmised when a fever develops, and chest x-ray infiltrate is unexplained on any other basis. The diagnosis can be aided in patients in whom there is direct access to the tracheobronchial tree by adding a small amount of Evans blue dye to the tongue every four hours,[59] or blue food dye to the enteral formula, and then checking the pulmonary secretions for the blue color. The diagnosis may also be made by testing pulmonary secretions for the presence of glucose via Clinistix.[43] One must be cautioned that this test for aspiration may not be applicable to all patients, since small amounts of blood in the respiratory secretions can make it falsely positive. This test in particular has yet to be tried in a prospective manner in patients without a tracheostomy or endotracheal tube.

The therapy of aspiration is easier than its diagnosis. In the case of a witnessed aspiration, immediate endotracheal suctioning should be undertaken. Though this may provide only a small volume of aspirate, it will stimulate continued coughing which helps to clear the trachea and major bronchi. It will also allow confirmation of the diagnosis. If solid particles are aspirated with the liquid formula (as is potentially the case in patients eating meals simultaneously with their tube feedings), immediate bronchoscopy should be performed to remove any residual food particles.

Depending upon the volume and pH of the aspirate, there may be rapid development of pulmonary edema which will require general supportive measures such as intravenous fluids with close monitoring with a central venous line or a Swan Ganz catheter for correction of hypotension; possible administration of albumin to help correct sequestration of fluids within the alveoli; and mechanical ventilation if fairly normal blood gases cannot be maintained by the usual means. Data from animal experiments suggest that early institution of positive pressure ventilation more rapidly reverses the physiologic changes induced by massive aspiration.[60] In some institutions, patients in whom massive aspiration is suspected are routinely placed on positive pressure ventilation for the first 12 hours after the event, and then rapidly weaned depending upon their clinical status.[61]

The role of steroids in massive aspiration is controversial. Although animal experiments suggest that steroids play a beneficial role,[62–66] this has not been successfully demonstrated in humans,[67–71] perhaps because in animal experiments steroids can be given within five minutes of the aspiration, whereas in humans the administration of the steroids relative to the aspiration is often delayed. It appears that unless steroids can be given concomitantly or within minutes of aspiration, their benefit is only theoretical.

Pulmonary infections often, but not invariably, follow aspiration. There appears to be no role for prophylactic antibiotics in patients with aspiration, but there is strong evidence that the damaged lung is more prone to superinfection. Patients should be carefully monitored, and at the first sign of purulent sputum, accompanied by fever and progressing pulmonary infiltrates, appropriate cultures should be taken and antibiotics begun. Since tube-fed patients will in the large majority of cases be in the hospital, they should receive antibiotic coverage for hospital contaminants as well as for the usual anaerobes residing in the oropharynx.[72–74] This usually requires a combination of an aminoglycoside and clindamycin; or an aminoglycoside, an antistaphylococcal drug, and an antianaerobic drug.

Contaminated Formulas and Feeding Equipment. Though aspiration pneumonia is the most frequently discussed potentially infectious complication of enteral alimentation, other infections associated with the feeding solution and tubing may occur. In 1976, Gutman and coworkers[75] reported four infants with staphylococcal enterocolitis associated with feeding catheters. In each patient, the feeding tube had been inserted through an area that was colonized with various strains of *Staphylococcus aureus*. All infants in whom this occurred developed disease or excreted *S. aureus* in their stools. Infants not fed by nasoduodenal or gastrostomy catheter or not colonized by *S. aureus* at the site of the feeding catheter did not acquire the disease. Reports from the 1950's[76] indicate the same mechanism can lead to infection in adults. This complication can be avoided by surveillance cultures in any area with a known high incidence of environmental contamination with staphylococci. This should be done prior to the placement of a nasoduodenal or gastrostomy tube in a high-risk patient, such as a low birth weight neonate.

A more generalized potential problem is direct contamination of the enteral formula. Unfortunately only a few studies address this problem.[77–80] Schreiner and coworkers[79] examined tube feeding contamination in 115 neonates in an intensive care unit. They found that 36 per cent of formula samples taken from drip chambers of gavage sets were contaminated. Attempts to induce contamination of the sets by retrograde infection were unsuccessful; however, follow-up cultures of nurses' hands showed a high incidence of bacteria similar to those found in the contaminated sets. They concluded that the primary cause of bacterial superinfection of enteral fluids was contamination by personnel when formula was placed in the delivery system.

White and colleagues[80] confirmed this finding in their study of the rate of contamination of 10 enteral solutions prepared in two different medical centers. They found that each of five bags of enteral formula prepared at one institution, without regard for sterile technique, grew bacteria at 48 hours from the time of feeding. The bacteria were avirulent, common skin contaminants. Only one of five bags grew bacteria at 48 hours in the center in which sterile technique was observed. Again, these bacteria were not enteric pathogens and were thought to be environmental contaminants. There was no significant bacterial growth in most enteral formulas hung as long as 12 hours at room temperature. Subsequently, they proposed that 12 hours was a safe hang time for enteral formulas. Schreiner and coworkers propose a 24-hour hang time for solutions. Neither group reported any clinically significant consequences of the bacterial contamination. However, there was at least one case report of septicemia probably arising from enteral fluid contamination.[81] In this patient, the contamination probably came from a kitchen detergent dispenser, since the formula was being prepared in the hospital.

One may conclude that with the observation of proper sterile techniques at each stage of the handling of enteral formulas, the likelihood of clinically significant bacterial contamination is low. Commercially prepared formulas are preferred over hospital prepared formulas in order to maintain a low incidence of contamination. Enteral formulas can probably be hung 8 to 12 hours at room temperature without clinically significant contamination. The complete delivery system, with the exception of the feeding tube itself, should be changed every 24 hours in the hospital setting. Patients at home can wash the enteral bags and reuse them every other day.

PSYCHOSENSORY COMPLICATIONS

It has been assumed by medical personnel that tube feeding is an unpleasant and distressing experience for the patient. This finding was only partially substantiated in a study by Padilla et al.,[95] who studied 30 adult subjects fed with either a rubber or plastic nasogastric tube (size 12, 14, or 16 French). They found that the most distressing experiences related to nasoenteric feeding were feelings of thirst, being deprived of tasting food, and having an unsatisfied taste for food. The most common physical complaint was that of a "sore nose or throat." In this study, however, it was difficult to assess whether this distress was caused by the patient's surgical procedure or by the presence of the nasogastric tube. The soft, small-bore feeding tubes were not used. Psychosensory discomforts that rated lower in level of distress included deprivation of liquids, chewing or swallowing of food, limited mobility, hearing sounds from the stomach, and exposure to regular food. Dry mouth, runny nose, breathing through the mouth, and breathing with a tube in the nose were additional complaints. The presence or absence of a tracheostomy did not significantly affect the distress associated with tube feedings.

Numerous measures may minimize psychosensory distresses. Assure hydration by adding additional water, if needed, to the feedings. When possible, allow the patient to drink additional water. Encourage the patient to breath through his nose. Provide the patient with water, mouthwash, a toothbrush, lubrication for the lips, lemon drops, and sugarless chewing gum. The benefit of gum must be assessed on an individual basis, as chewing may increase discomfort from swallowing additional saliva. Gargling with warm salt solution may be helpful for discomfort from a sore throat, if no open areas are in the throat or mouth. Soft, small-bore tubes may also be helpful in resolving this problem and in decreasing nasal discomfort. Proper taping of nasoenteric tubes to avoid pressure on the nasal alae is essential. Have patients state their meal preferences and allow them to have cool or warm feeding. Flavored formula may be preferable. Cinnamon or nutmeg may be used to "cover" formulas. Cooperative patients should be allowed to chew and spit out food if desired. Adjust the patients' feeding schedules so that they can be involved in other activities and/or provide privacy during feeding. Encourage patients to be active. Physical and occupational therapy should be provided. Mobile equipment should be utilized. Bedridden patients may be transported outside on a litter to the "solarium" if their medical condition permits.

Peteet et al.[96] have addressed the issue of artificial feedings in patients with cancer. They have found the patients' emotional responses to be influenced by both the diagnosis of cancer and their own personality characteristics, as well as those of their families. Three patterns of psychological response to artificial feeding were identified: (1) The demoralized or depressed patient often lost confidence in the ability to eat, as part of a more profound loss of confidence. Medical personnel must evaluate this type of patient closely, to avoid increasing dependency and fear of helplessness. Making decisions for them related to artificial feeding and other aspects of management promote their feelings of helplessness. (2) Patients with strongly independent personality traits may utilize control seeking. (3) Anxious patients express fears about dying by extreme preoccupation with their feeding regimen and their weight response to the regimen.

Peteet et al.[96] recommended the following principles to help the patient with cancer deal with the psychological implications of enteral feeding: recognize and understand the significance of eating and artificial feeding for the patient and his family; address obvious emotional issues directly, thus minimizing their effects upon eating and decisions about feeding regimens; address specific needs for dependency or control measures; allow patients to participate in their feeding, as well as in the decision to have feeding. These recommendations should also apply to noncancer patients.

Recognition of the psychological implications of enteral feeding is essential to promote the patient's acceptance of these feedings in both short- and long-term situations. Improvements in methods that promote physiological and psychological comfort require further investigation.

MECHANICAL COMPLICATIONS

Mechanical complications from feeding tubes are related to the size and position of the tube (Fig. 29–4). Complications of nasoenteric tubes, gastric tubes, and jejunal tubes will be described in the following sections (Table 29–6).

Nasoenteric Tubes. Mechanical complications from nasoenteric tubes are thought to be related primarily to size and pliability of the tube. The advantages of using fine-bore tubing with a mercury weight for nasoenteric feeding were described in the literature as early as the 1950's;[95] however, fine-bore tubes have been used routinely only since they became commercially available in the 1970's, with Silastic or silicone being advocated rather than polyvinylchloride.[98] The use of fine-bore, soft, mercury-weighted tubes should decrease, and, in fact, has decreased the incidence of mechanical complications according to reports of practitioners in nutritional support. Evidence to support this clinical observation is not found in the literature because complications, or the lack of them, are often viewed as part of the routine of tube feeding and because they can be corrected with little difficulty. A complication of the soft tubes that may be potentially fatal is inadvertent insertion of the tube into the trachea (Fig. 29–5). Aspiration of gastric contents or radiographic documentation of tube position will

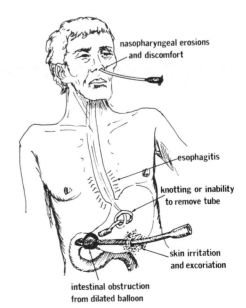

nasopharyngeal erosions and discomfort

esophagitis

knotting or inability to remove tube

skin irritation and excoriation

intestinal obstruction from dilated balloon

Figure 29–4. Mechanical complications of enteral feeding.

prevent inadvertent feeding by this route. Complications of large-bore, stiff tubing will be described since they are also potential problems with small-bore tubes, especially if appropriate care is not used.

Nasopharyngeal Discomfort. Nasopharyngeal discomfort can be caused by the absence of chewing, which is the normal stimulus to salivary secretions, and/or by mouth breathing, as a result of the nasoenteric tube being in place. Patients exhibit symptoms of sore throat, difficulty with swallowing, thirst, and dry mucous membranes. Measures which may decrease or eliminate the above symptoms include the use of soft, small bore tubes; lubrication of lips; gargling with warm water and a mouthwash solution, or physiologic saliva; and chewing sugarless gum. Analgesic or anesthetic lozenges may be required for severe discomfort. Anesthetic lozenges should be used cautiously because they may decrease swallowing or gag reflexes.

Nasal Erosions and Necrosis. Nasal erosions result from pressure on nasal alae from the nasoenteric tube (Fig. 29–6).[99] Erosions and necrosis can be severe enough to require reconstructive surgery. The patient will frequently complain of discomfort and/or feelings of pressure from the tube. Erythema occurs at the nasal alae with eventual ulceration. The nasoenteric tube should be taped so that pressure is not exerted against the nares. Tincture of benzoin should be applied to the bridge of the nose and allowed to dry. A piece of adhesive tape, 1 inch in diameter, can be cut longitudinally and applied to the bridge of the nose, with the cut pieces positioned so that they can be wrapped around the tube. An alternate method is to apply tincture of benzoin to the skin over the zygomatic process and to secure the tube at this point, making sure that the nasoenteric tube is not pulled taut against the side of the nares.

Abscess of the Nasal Septum. Pressure against the nasal cartilage from a nasoenteric tube, especially in the malnourished, dehydrated patient, can result in sloughing of nasal cartilage and the dropping of the dorsum of the nose. Prolonged use of the nasoenteric tube without treatment can result in retraction of columellar elements of the septum. The patient is described as having a "saddle nose." Reconstructive surgery may be required. If bacteria are present, an abscess may develop.

Acute Sinusitis. Acute sinusitis may occur when any of the sinus tracts are occluded by the nasoenteric tube. The symptoms are pain, nasal congestion with or without purulent discharge, malodorous breath in the absence of pharyngitis or dental decay, and mild fever. Acute suppurative drainage can occur if blockage persists without therapy. This is of particular concern if the frontal sinus is blocked and the potential for development of a brain abscess exists. Therapy and nursing measures include bedrest, analgesics, hot compresses to the face, and nonsurgical drainage. Removal of the nasoenteric tube is necessary. Soft, small-bore tubes should minimize the risk of development of this complication.

Otitis Media. The pressure of the nasoenteric tube at the eustachian tube opening can cause edema and pain. Severe, dull, throbbing ear pain, fever, chills, slight dizziness, nausea, and vomiting are suggestive of otitis media. Changing the nasoenteric tube to the other nostril may decrease the symptoms. If symptoms are not relieved by this, and enteral feeding is still required for a prolonged period, a gastrostomy, jejunal, or gastrojejunal tube may be required. Use of the soft, small-bore tube may prevent these symptoms.

Hoarseness. Hoarseness is a frequent complaint in patients fed with the large-bore tube. The mucous membranes of the larynx may become irritated by the tube. Use of a soft, small-bore tube, steam, or aerosol therapy may provide relief. Warm gargles or anesthetic lozenges may also be useful in treating hoarseness.

Intracranial Passage of Feeding Tube. A rare but potentially fatal complication of nasoenteric feeding is intracranial passage of the tube.[100, 101] This complication may occur in patients with severe head trauma. The risk of intracranial passage of the feeding tube may be reduced by the use of soft, pliable tubes and by very careful tube insertion (see Chapter 18).

Excessive Gagging. Excessive gagging is seen in anxious patients, in patients with a hypersensitive gag reflex, and when the tube is positioned in the back of the throat. Proper positioning of the tube as well as reassurance of the patient can reduce the frequency of gagging.

Laryngeal Ulceration and Stenosis. Development of this complication in the patient with a nasoenteric tube results from tube pressure against the mucosal surface of

Table 29-6 MECHANICAL COMPLICATIONS OF NASOENTERIC TUBES

COMPLICATION AND CAUSE	CLINICAL PRESENTATION	DIAGNOSIS	THERAPY	PREVENTION
Nasopharyngeal discomfort: Absence of chewing which is the normal stimulus to salivary secretions; mouth breathing as a result of the tube being in place	Sore throat, difficulty with swallowing, hoarseness, thirst, dry mucous membranes	Inspection	Lubrication of lips, chewing sugarless gum, gargling with warm water and a mouthwash solution, physiologic saliva or analgesic and/or anesthetic lozenges for severe discomfort (anaesthetic lozenges may decrease swallowing or gag reflexes)	Symptoms decreased to absent with use of soft, small-bore tubes; utilize therapeutic nursing measures
Nasal erosions and necrosis: Pressure on nasal ala from tube	Erosions of nasal ala	Inspection	Tape tube so that no pressure is exerted against nasal ala; apply tincture of benzoin to area where tape will be applied	Use of soft, small-bore tube; tape properly
Abscess—nasal septum: Pressure against the nasal cartilage especially in the malnourished, dehydrated patient with subsequent sloughing of nasal cartilage and dropping of the dorsum of the nose. If bacterial organisms are present, an abscess may develop	Complaints of continual pain and pressure from the tube; fever, chills	Symptomatic	Removal of tube; appropriate medical intervention if abscess is present	Soft, small bore tubing; proper taping of small or large bore tubing; evaluation of patient's nose size in relation to tube size
Acute Sinusitis: Sinus tract occluded by the nasoenteric tube	Pain; nasal congestion with or without purulent drainage; malodorous breath; mild fever	Symptomatic; culture of drainage	Removal of nasoenteric tube; Bedrest; analgesics; hot compresses to face; nonsurgical drainage	Soft, small-bore tubing; evaluation of patient's nose size in relation to tube size
Acute otitis media: Pressure at the eustachian tube opening from the nasoenteric tube, with entry of pathogenic bacteria into the middle ear	Severe, dull, throbbing ear pain, fever, chills, slight dizziness, nausea, and vomiting; the child may pull on affected ear	Symptomatic	Change nasoenteric tube to other nostril; antibiotic therapy if appropriate; myringotomy if severe	Use of soft, small-bore tubes

Table continued on following page

Table 29–6   MECHANICAL COMPLICATIONS OF NASOENTERIC TUBES *(Continued)*

COMPLICATION AND CAUSE	CLINICAL PRESENTATION	DIAGNOSIS	THERAPY	PREVENTION
Hoarseness: Irritation of mucous membranes of the larynx from presence of nasoenteric tube	Hoarseness	Symptomatic	Use of soft, small-bore tube, steam or aerosol therapy, warm gargle, anesthetic lozenges	Use of soft, small-bore tube, adequate hydration, mouth care
Intracranial passage of feeding tube: Passage of nasogastric tubes early on in patient with basal skull fracture	May be asymptomatic	X-ray of head	Removal of nasogastric tube; symptomatic	Careful passage of nasogastric tube; confirm placement in stomach
Excessive gagging: Anxious patient, or hypersensitive gag reflex	Excessive gagging; anxiety	Symptomatic	Reassurance	Careful explanation prior to placement of tube
Laryngeal ulceration stenosis: Pressure against the mucosal surface of the posterior pharynx from the limited mobility of both the tube and the anatomic structures in this area	Stenosis or ulceration of larynx on physical examination	Stenosis or ulceration of larynx on physical examination	Symptomatic; removal of tube	Use of soft, small-bore tube
Esophagitis: Predisposing factors: intestinal obstruction, persistent vomiting, poor nutritional status, supine position with an increase in acid reflux into the distal esophagus, large-bore tube obstructing the esophageal lumen	Heartburn; sour stomach; substernal and epigastric burning sensations with pain referred to the head, neck, and arms	Symptomatic; radiologic examination	Removal of tube	Use of soft, small-bore tubing; maintain elevation of the head of the bed; early recognition of patients at risk and those with symptoms of developing esophageal irritation
Esophageal ulceration and stenosis: Pressure against the mucosal surface of the esophagus particularly when esophagitis is present from persistent vomiting	Dysphagia prior to or after removal of nasoenteric tube	Symptomatic; radiologic examination; endoscopic examination	Removal of tube; esophagoscopy and dilation	Use of soft, small-bore tube; patients with persistent vomiting without removal of tube should be evaluated for jejunal tube
Tracheoesophageal fistula: Pressure necrosis with erosion occurring through the posterior wall of the tracheostomy and anterior wall of the esophagus	Presence of fistula on physical examination	Presence of fistula on physical examination	Symptomatic	Use of soft, small-bore tube; use of gastrostomy, jejeunal, or gastrojejunal tube

Table 29-6 MECHANICAL COMPLICATIONS OF NASOENTERIC TUBES *(Continued)*

COMPLICATION AND CAUSE	CLINICAL PRESENTATION	DIAGNOSIS	THERAPY	PREVENTION
Rupture of esophageal varices: Irritation and/or excessive pressure from stiff, large-bore tubes; esophagitis	Hematemesis melena	History of alcohol abuse; symptomatic; radiographic studies	Sedation and complete rest of the esophagus; other symptomatic measures as indicated by the patient's condition	Use of soft, small-bore tube. Use of parenteral feeding if other tubes (jejunal, gastrojejunal, or gastrostomy) are inappropriate
Gaseous distention of intestinal balloons: In unvented "balloons" the intestinal gases diffuse across the rubber membrane, producing an obstructing bolus in the intestinal tract	Nausea; abdominal distention; vomiting; abdominal cramping	Symptomatic; Radiologic studies	Deflation of balloon. Surgical intervention may be required	Placing a small needle hole in the finger cot or "balloon" or using commercially prepared mercury-weighted nasoenteric catheters
Knotting of the tube: Hyperactive peristalsis postulated	Unable to remove tube easily	Unable to remove tube easily	The tube may be removed by cutting it and allowing the lower portion to be evacuated per rectum. If the majority of the tube can be removed, a McGill forceps can be used to grab hold of the portion of the tube in the back of the throat, cut the tube outside the nares, and pull the rest of the tube out through the mouth.	None
Inability to withdraw the tube: Tube may be lodged within folds of mucosa or may "stick" to the gastric wall	Tube does not respond to gentle pulling motions	Tube does not respond to gentle pulling motions	Place the patient in a side lying position and flush the tube with 20–50 ml of water. Then pull back gently on the tube. If unsuccessful, repeat flushing of tube with patient in Trendelenburg position (if not contraindicated). If both measures are unsuccessful, the tube should be cut, allowing the lower portion of it to be evacuated per rectum.	

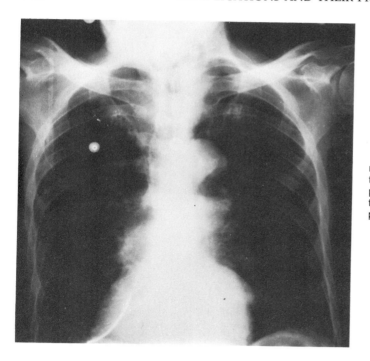

Figure 29–5. Misplacement of a soft nasoenteric tube into the right lung. The patient was asymptomatic following the tube placement. A chest roentgenogram was obtained because of the patient's inability to aspirate gastric contents.

the posterior pharynx. There is limited mobility of both the tube and the anatomic structures of the area. Use of the soft, small-bore tube in patients requiring prolonged feeding should decrease the incidence of this complication.

Esophagitis. Esophagitis in patients with nasoenteric tubes has been reported most frequently in conjunction with other predisposing factors, such as intestinal obstruction, persistent vomiting, and poor nu-

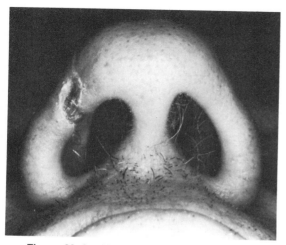

Figure 29–6. Necrosis of the nasal ala secondary to an improperly taped nasoenteric tube. (Courtesy of Michael Meguid, M.D., Ph.D.)

tritional status.[102, 103] Nagler and Spiro reported an increase in gastroesophageal reflux in patients with nasogastric tubes that were placed when the patient was in the supine position.[104] They suggest that in the supine position, there is no gravitational force to help propel the acid from the distal esophagus back into the stomach. This mechanism is enhanced by the obstruction of the esophageal lumen by the tube. Symptoms of esophagitis include heartburn, sour stomach, and substernal and epigastric burning sensations with pain referred to the head, neck, and arms. Careful evaluation of the severity of these symptoms should be taken into account, and caution used in the selection of a nasoenteric tube as the method for delivery of enteral feeding. Personnel caring for the patient should be alert for the development of the above symptoms after placement of a nasoenteric tube.

Esophageal Ulceration and Stenosis. Excessive pressure against the esophageal wall may result in ulceration with stenosis.[105, 106] This is most likely to occur in the patient with prior esophagitis from reflux of juices from the stomach. Vomiting, regurgitation, poor nutritional status, and dehydration contribute to the development of esophageal ulceration and stenosis. Esophageal dilatation and/or surgical repair may be required to correct stenosis. Peripheral parenteral nutrition may be appropriate in patients who require only short-term nutritional support. Gastrostomy, jejunostomy, or placement of a gastrojejunal tube may prevent or reduce the symptoms of esophagitis. Soft, small-bore tubes may exert less pressure against the esophageal wall and therefore decrease the likelihood of this complication.

Tracheoesophageal Fistula. This complication generally occurs in the patient with a large-bore tube and a concurrent nasotracheal or tracheostomy tube in place. Therapy is symptomatic. The fistula occurs as a result of severe pressure necrosis, with erosion occurring through the posterior wall of the tracheostomy and anterior wall of the esophagus. The use of soft, small-bore tubes may minimize this complication. Patients who require long-term ventilatory support may benefit from a gastrostomy, jejunal, or gastrojejunal tube.

Rupture of Esophageal Varices. Irritation or excessive pressure from stiff, large-bore tubes can result in rupture of esophageal varices with resultant hemorrhage.[107] Soft, small-bore nasoenteric tubes may decrease the possibility of rupture of esophageal varices. However, the risk of irritation and subsequent fatal hemorrhage still exists.

Patients with esophageal varices without ascites may be more appropriate candidates for gastrostomy, jejunostomy, or gastrojejunal tube. Central venous nutrition may be indicated if the patient is not expected to tolerate oral intake for more than a month. These patients' nutritional needs generally are too high to be met with peripheral parenteral nutrition.

Gaseous Distention of Intestinal Balloons. Use of nasoenteric feeding tubes with a mercury-filled finger cot can produce small bowel obstruction.[108, 109] In unvented "balloons" the intestinal gases diffuse across the rubber membrane producing an obstructing bolus in the intestinal tract (Fig. 29–7). The patient will exhibit symptoms of intestinal obstruction: nausea, distention, vomiting, and abdominal cramping. Surgical intervention may be necessary. This complication can be avoided by placing a small needle hole in the finger cot or "balloon," or more appropriately by using commercially prepared mercury-weighted nasoenteric catheters.

Knotting of the Tube. Hyperactive peristalsis has been postulated as the cause of knotting of nasoenteric tubes. This complication should be suspected when one is able to remove the majority of the tube prior to feeling resistance. The tube may be removed by cutting it and allowing the lower portion to be evacuated per rectum. If the majority of the tube can be removed prior to feeling resistance, a McGill forceps can be used to grasp the portion of the tube in the back of the throat. The tube should then be cut, and the remainder of the tube may be pulled through the mouth. An emesis bag and tissues should be on hand, as this procedure may result in gagging or emesis. An alternative method is to try to remove the knot with the aid of the interventional radiologist (see Chapter 14).

Inability to Withdraw the Tube. Removal of the tube may not be possible if it has become lodged within folds of the intestinal mucosa (Fig. 29–8). The nasoenteric tube may "stick" to the gastric wall. This has occurred most frequently when gastric suction has been used, but it can occur in tubes without suction. This complication should be considered when the tube does not respond to gentle pulling motions. Place the patient on his or her side and flush the tube with 20 to 50 ml of water, and then pull

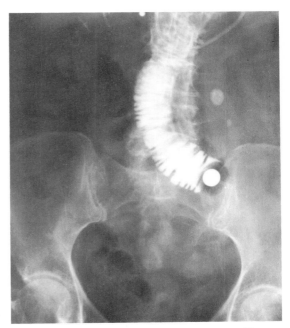

Figure 29–7. Abdominal roentgenogram, with contrast material injected, demonstrating an obstruction of the small intestine secondary to intestinal gases dilating the balloon of a nasoenteric feeding tube.

back gently on the tube. This may result in removal. If this is unsuccessful, flush the tube with the patient in the Trendelenburg position. If both of these measures are unsuccessful, the tube should be cut, allowing the lower portion of the tube to be evacuated per rectum

Duodenal and Intestinal Perforations. Mechanical complications associated with transpyloric nasoenteric tubes, as well as gastric tubes, include intestinal perforation, renal penetrations, and intussusception.[94, 110–114] These complications, associated with the use of polyvinyl chloride and polypropylene tubes, can be minimized by checking the position of the feeding tube radiologically. The hazard of a perforation appears to be greatest when the tube tip is in the proximal duodenum, at its superior flexure.[115] In addition, avoiding manipulation of the tube once in place will minimize the likelihood of intestinal perforation. A decreased incidence of complications has been reported with the use of the silicone tubes, though they still are occasionally reported.

Complications of Gastrostomy. The complications associated with feeding by a gastrostomy tube are relatively few. The rate of many of these complications is dependent upon the surgeon's experience with the procedure (see Chapter 17 on Tube Enterostomy).

Early Postoperative Complications. Hemorrhage and leakage of gastric contents, with associated peritonitis, can occur. There may also be premature or delayed closure of the stoma, wound dehiscence, hernia, or gastric prolapse.[117, 118] These complications usually occur relatively soon after surgery.

Late Tube-Related Complications. With long-term use of a feeding gastrostomy, most complications are related to the catheter itself. These include local irritation, bleeding, and clogging of the tube. Gastric obstruction by the balloon catheter can occur, particularly in the pediatric age group.[112, 119] When the gastrostomy tube is not adequately anchored, the entire tube can migrate into the duodenum as a result of peristalsis,[120] leading to partial or complete outlet obstruction.

Complications of Jejunostomy. Complications from jejunostomy tubes are similar, whether a subserosal tunnel with a large-bore tube or a fine-bore polyvinyl chloride tube is used.[89, 91, 118, 121, 122] Fistulas and intestinal obstruction may occur less frequently with fine-bore tubing. The most frequent mechanical complications related to jejunostomy feedings are discussed below.

Dislodgement of Tube. This may occur when the bowel has not been sutured to the abdominal wall, allowing extraluminal, intraperitoneal infusion of an elemental diet. Appropriate suturing of the bowel to the peritoneum will minimize this complication. Excessive pulling or pushing on the catheter with irrigation of the tube may also result in

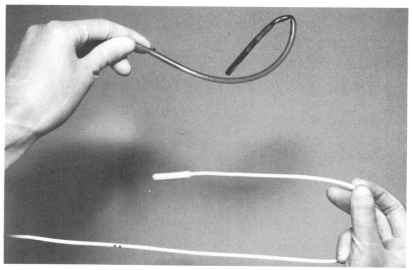

Figure 29–8. Rigid polyethylene feeding tube that was difficult to withdraw following three months of tube placement. Comparison with soft, silicone rubber tube.

dislodgement. Patients will exhibit symptoms of peritonitis. Initial infusion of a sterile 5 per cent dextrose and water solution and confirmation of catheter position by study with meglumine diatrizoate (Gastrografin) is essential.

Hemorrhage. Postoperative hemorrhage can occur and patients should be observed for symptoms.

Intestinal Obstruction. Intestinal obstruction may occur from formation of adhesions at the enterostomy site. If a feeding catheter such as a Foley with a balloon is used, obstruction from gaseous distention of the balloon can occur. Symptoms include abdominal pain, cramping, constipation, nausea, and vomiting. Surgical correction may be necessary. This complication has been reported less frequently with the needle catheter jejunostomy.[91]

Irritation and Excoriation of Skin. These complications may occur with drainage of digestive juices from the stoma site. Keeping the area dry and clean is essential. Use of karaya and stoma adhesive may protect the skin. Problems inducing drainage should be identified and treated.

Cervical Esophagostomy Tubes for Feeding. Cervical esophagostomy has often been used for prolonged tube feeding in patients with head and neck cancer. Mechanical complications of cervical esophagostomy feeding tubes include injury with stricture of the distal esophagus, irritation of skin and soft tissue, tubal obstruction, and accidental extubation. These complications occur most frequently with the use of the hard, rubber tubes and have been minimized or eliminated with the use of the short, wide-lumen silicone tube.[123]

MECHANICAL COMPLICATIONS OF TUBE FEEDING IN PEDIATRIC PATIENTS

Mechanical complications described in the section on adults can occur in the pediatric population. Mechanical complications that are specific to, or occur more frequently in, the pediatric population include the following.

Upper Gastrointestinal Trauma. Esophageal perforation and induction of pharyngeal and cervical esophageal pseudodiverticula are among the mechanical complications seen with gavage feeding in the infant.[124–126] These are potentially fatal complications in the small, premature baby. Caution must be used in inserting the nasoenteric tube. Perforation has been reported to occur more frequently with polyvinylchloride than with Silastic nasoenteric tubes.

Respiratory Alterations. Transient respiratory alterations have been reported with intermittent bolus feedings, particularly in the small, premature infant.[127–131] The infants experience bradycardia, a decrease in functional residual capacity, increased respiratory rate and minute ventilation, and a decrease in arterial PO_2. The reduction in functional residual capacity after bolus feeding is associated with an elevated transpulmonary pressure, which causes airway closure to a greater extent than before feeding. Gastric distention with upward displacement of the diaphragm may also be a contributing factor. Smaller bolus feedings or continuous feeding can decrease or eliminate this complication.

Formation of Lactobezoar. Formation of lactobezoar has increased with the use of low birth weight formula in the premature infant.[132–134] No specific reason for the increase is known. A number of factors must be considered: techniques of feeding, age at onset of feedings, gastric emptying in the premature infant, gastric acidity in the preterm infant, and composition of the formula in relation to protein concentration (casein : lactalbumin ratio) and amount and type of fat. The most common clinical symptoms are abdominal distention, an abdominal mass on palpation, gastric retention, regurgitation, and diarrhea. Gastric perforation requiring surgical intervention has been reported as a result of the lactobezoar formation. Therapy in infants without gastric perforation includes withholding feeding for 24 hours, followed by a change of formula.

SUMMARY

Further reports are needed to provide accurate identification of the metabolic, infectious, psychological, and mechanical complications related to the delivery of enteral nutrition by tube. These potential complications can be lessened and ameliorated by applying specific preventive measures and by thorough monitoring.

REFERENCES

1. Heymsfield, S. B., Bethel, R. A., Ansley, J. D., Nixon, D. W., and Rudman, D.: Enteral hyperalimentation: An alternative to central venous hyperalimentation. Ann. Intern. Med., 90:63–71, 1979.

2. Koretz, R. L., and Meyer, J. H.: Elemental diets—Facts and fantasies. Gastroenterology, 78:393–410, 1980.

3. Bury, K. D., and Jambunathan, G.: Effects of elemental diets on gastric emptying and gastric secretion in man. Am. J. Surg., 127:59–64, 1974.

4. Heitkemper, M. E., Martin, D. L., Hansen, B. C., Hanson, R., and Vanderburg, V.: Rate and volume of intermittent enteral feeding. J.P.E.N., 5:125–129, 1981.

5. Phillips, S. F., and Giller, J.: The contribution of the colon to electrolyte and water conservation in man. J. Lab Clin. Med., 81:733–746, 1973.

6. Debongnie, J. C., and Phillips, S. F.: Capacity of the human colon to absorb fluid. Gastroenterology, 74:698–703, 1978.

7. Curran, P. F., and Solomon, A. K.: Ion and water fluxes in the ileum of rats. J. Gen. Physiol., 41:143–168, 1957.

8. Kaminski, M. V., Jr.: Enteral hyperalimentation. Surg. Gynecol. Obstet., 143:12–16, 1976.

9. Walike, B. C., and Walike, J. W.: Relative lactose intolerance: A clinical study of tube-fed patients. J.A.M.A., 238:948–951, 1977.

10. Walike, B. C., and Walike, J. W.: Lactose content of tube feeding diets as a cause of diarrhea. Laryngoscope, 83:1109–1115, 1973.

11. Christopher, N. L., and Bayless, T. M.: Role of the small bowel and colon in lactose-induced diarrhea. Gastroenterology, 60:845–852, 1971.

12. Gray, G. M.: Carbohydrate digestion and absorption: Role of the small intestine. N. Engl. J. Med., 292:1225–1230, 1975.

13. Stephenson, L. S., and Latham, M. C.: Lactose intolerance and milk consumption: The relation of tolerance to symptoms. Am. J. Clin. Nutr., 27:296–303, 1974.

14. Platt, B. S., Heard, C. R. C., and Stewart, R. J. C.: The effects of protein-caloric deficiency on the gastrointestinal tract. In Munro, H. N. (ed.): The Role of the Gastrointestinal Tract in Protein Metabolism. Philadelphia, F. A. Davis Co., 1964, pp. 227–238.

15. Chernoff, R.: Enteral feedings. Am. J. Hosp. Pharm., 37:65–74, 1980.

16. Kagawa-Busby, K. S., Heitkemper, M. M., Hansen, B. C., Hanson, R. L., and Vanderburg, V. V.: Effects of diet temperature on tolerance of enteral feedings. Nurs. Res., 29:276–280, 1980.

17. Cobb, L. M., Cartmill, A. M., and Gilsdorf, R. B.: Early postoperative nutritional support using the serosal tunnel jejunostomy. J.P.E.N., 5:397–401, 1981.

18. Steiner, M., Bourges, H. R., Freedman, L. S., and Gray, S. J.: Effect of starvation on the tissue composition of the small intestine in the rat. Am. J. Physiol., 215:75–77, 1968.

19. McManus, J.P.A., and Isselbacher, K. J.: Effect of fasting versus feeding on the rat small intestine: Morphological, biochemical, and functional differences. Gastroenterology, 59:214–221, 1970.

20. Frank, H. A., and Green, L. C.: Successful use of a bulk laxative to control the diarrhea of tube feeding. Scand. J. Plast. Reconstr. Surg., 13:193–194, 1979.

21. Voitk, A. J.: The place of elemental diet in clinical nutrition. Br. J. Clin. Pract., 29:55–62, 1975.

22. Russell, R. I.: Progress report: Elemental diets. Gut, 16:68–79, 1975.

23. Gault, M. H., Dixon, M. E., Doyle, M., and Cohen, W. M.: Hypernatremia, azotemia, and dehydration due to high-protein tube feeding. Ann. Intern. Med., 68:778–791, 1968.

24. Howman-Giles, R. H., and Roy, L. P.: Extreme hypernatraemia in a child receiving gastrostomy feeding. Aust. Paediatr. J., 12:167–170, 1976.

25. Telfer, N., and Persoff, M.: The effect of tube feeding on the hydration of elderly patients. J. Gerontol., 20:536–543, 1965.

26. Walike, J. W.: Tube feeding syndrome in head and neck surgery. Arch. Otolaryngol., 89:533–536, 1969.

27. Isaacson, L. C.: Urinary osmolality in thirsty normal subjects. Lancet, 1:467–469, 1960.

28. Lindeman, R. D., Van Buren, H. C., and Raisz, L. G.: Osmolar renal concentrating ability in healthy young men and hospitalized patients without renal disease. N. Engl. J. Med., 262:1306–1309, 1960.

29. Brenner, W. I., Lansky, Z., Engelman, R. M., and Stahl W. M.: Hyperosmolar coma in surgical patients: An iatrogenic disease of increasing incidence. Ann. Surg., 178:651–654, 1973.

30. Alberti, K. G. M. M., Hockaday, T. D. R., and Turner, R. C.: Small doses of intramuscular insulin in the treatment of diabetic "coma." Lancet, 2:515–522, 1973.

31. Page, M. McB., Alberti, K. G. M. M., Greenwood, R., Gumaa, K. A., Hockaday, T. D. R., Lowy, C., Nabarro, J. D. N., Pyke, D. A., Sönksen, P. H., Watkins, P. J., and West, T. E. T.: Treatment of diabetic coma with continuous low-dose infusion of insulin. Br. Med. J., 2:687–690, 1974.

32. Vanlandingham, S., Simpson, S., Daniel, P., and Newmark, S. R.: Metabolic abnormalities in patients supported with enteral tube feeding. J.P.E.N., 5:322–324, 1981.

33. Morris, L. R., McGee, J. A., and Kitabchi, A. E.: Correlation between plasma and urine glucose in diabetes. Ann. Intern. Med., 94:469–471, 1981.

34. Malone, J. I., Rosenbloom, A. L., Grgic, A., and Weber, F. T.: The role of urine sugar in diabetic management. Am. J. Dis. Child., 130:1324–1327, 1976.

35. Primrose, J. N., Carr, K. W., Sim, A. J. W., and Shenkin, A.: Hyperkalemia in patients on enteral feeding. J.P.E.N., 5:130–131, 1981.

36. Zarchy, T. M., Lipman, T. O., and Finkelstein, J. D.: Elevated transaminases associated with an elemental diet. Ann. Intern. Med., 89:221–222, 1978.

37. Sherman, J. O., Hamley, C., and Khachadurian, A. K.: Use of an oral elemental diet in infants with severe intractable diarrhea. J. Pediatr., 86:518–523, 1975.

38. Grant, J. P., Cox, C. E., Kleinman, L. M., Maher, M. M., Pittman, M. A., Tangrea, J. A., Brown, J. H., Gross, E., Beazley, R. M., and Jones, R. S.: Serum hepatic enzyme and bilirubin elevations during parenteral nutrition. Surg. Gynecol. Obstet., 145:573–580, 1977.

39. Freeman, J. B., Egan, M. C., and Millis, B. J.: The elemental diet. Surg. Gynecol. Obstet., *142*:925–932, 1976.

40. Wene, J. D., Connor, W. E., and DenBesten, L.: The development of essential fatty acid deficiency in healthy men fed fat-free diets intravenously and orally. J. Clin. Invest., *56*:127–134, 1975.

41. Abel, R. M., Beck, C. H., Jr., Abbott, W. M., Ryan, J. A., Jr., Barnett, G. O., and Fischer, J. E.: Improved survival from acute renal failure after treatment with intravenous essential L-amino acids and glucose: Results of a prospective, double-blind study. N. Engl. J. Med., *288*:695–699, 1973.

42. Fischer, J. E., Rosen, H. M., Ebeid, A. M., James, J. H., Keane, J. M., and Soeters, P. B.: The effect of normalization of plasma amino acids on hepatic encephalopathy in man. Surgery, *80*:77–91, 1976.

43. Winterbauer, R. H., Durning, R. B., Jr., Barron, E., and McFadden, M. C.: Aspirated nasogastric feeding solution detected by glucose strips. Ann. Intern. Med. *95*:67–68, 1981.

44. Hamelberg, W., and Bosomworth, P. P.: Aspiration pneumonitis: Experimental studies and clinical observations. Anesth. Analg. (Cleve.), *43*:669–677, 1964.

45. Greenfield, L. J., Singleton, R. P., McCaffree, D. R., and Coalson, J. J.: Pulmonary effects of experimental graded aspiration of hydrochloric acid. Ann. Surg., *170*:74–86, 1969.

46. Mendelson, C. L.: The aspiration of stomach contents into the lungs during obstetric anesthesia. Am. J. Obstet. Gynecol., *52*:191–205, 1946.

47. Teabeaut, J. R., II: Aspiration of gastric contents. An experimental study. Am. J. Pathol., *28*:51–68, 1952.

48. Awe, W. C., Fletcher, W. S., and Jacob, S. W.: The pathophysiology of aspiration pneumonitis. Surgery, *60*:232–239, 1966.

49. Bannister, W. K., and Sattilaro, A. J.: Vomiting and aspiration during anesthesia. Anesthesiology, *23*:251–264, 1962.

50. Vandam, L. D.: Aspiration of gastric contents in the operative period. N. Engl. J. Med., *273*:1206–1208, 1965.

51. Schwartz, D. J., Wynne, J. W., Gibbs, C. P., Hood, C. I., and Kuck, E. J.: The pulmonary consequences of aspiration of gastric contents at pH values greater than 2.5. Am. Rev. Respir. Dis., *121*:119–126, 1980.

52. Moran, T. J.: Experimental aspiration pneumonia. IV. Inflammatory and reparative changes produced by intratracheal injections of autologous gastric juice and hydrochloric acid. Arch. Pathol., *60*:122–129, 1955.

53. Moran, T. J.: Experimental food-aspiration pneumonia. Arch. Pathol. *52*:350–354, 1951.

54. Moran, T. J.: Milk-aspiration pneumonia in human and animal subjects. Arch. Pathol., *55*:286–301, 1953.

55. Moran, T. J.: Pulmonary edema produced by intratracheal injection of milk, feeding mixtures, and sugars. Am. J. Dis. Child, *86*:45–50, 1953.

56. Pecora, D. V.: Aspiration pneumonia following gavage feeding [Letter]. Chest, *76*:714, 1979.

57. Magnin F: Interêt de la gastrostomie dans la prévention des inhalations alimentaires. [Value

58. Spray, S. B., Zuidema, G. D., and Carmeron, J. L.: Aspiration pneumonia. Incidence of aspiration with endotracheal tubes. Am. J. Surg., *131*:701–703, 1976.

59. Cameron, J. L., Reynolds, J., and Zuidema, G.: Aspiration in patients with tracheostomies. Surg. Gynecol. Obstet., *136*:68–70, 1973.

60. Cameron, J. L., Sebor, J., Anderson, R. P., and Zuidema, G. D.: Aspiration pneumonia: Results of treatment by positive pressure ventilation in dogs. J. Surg. Res., *8*:447–457, 1968.

61. Broe, P. J., Toung, T. J. K., and Cameron, J. L.: Aspiration pneumonia. Surg. Clin. North Am., *60*:1551–1564, 1980.

62. Bannister, W. K., Sattilaro, A. J., and Otis, R. D.: Therapeutic aspects of aspiration pneumonitis. Anesthesiology, *22*:440–443, 1961.

63. Bosomworth, P. P., and Hamelberg, W.: Etiologic and therapeutic aspects of aspiration pneumonitis. Surg. Forum, *13*:158–159, 1962.

64. Lawson, D. W., Defalco, A. J., Phelps, J. A., Bradley, B. E., and McClenathan, J. E.: Corticosteroids as treatment for aspiration of gastric contents: An experimental study. Surgery, *59*:845–852, 1966.

65. Lewiński, A.: Evaluation of methods employed in the treatment of the chemical pneumonitis of aspiration. Anesthesiology, *26*:37–44, 1965.

66. Toung, T. J. K., Bordos, D., Benson, D. W., Carter, D., Zuidema, G. D., Permutt, S., and Cameron, J. L.: Aspiration pneumonia: Experimental evaluation of albumin and steroid therapy. Ann. Surg., *183*:179–184, 1976.

67. Wynne, J. W., DeMarco, F. J., and Hood, I.: Physiological effects of corticosteroids in foodstuff aspiration. Arch. Surg., *116*:46–49, 1981.

68. Chapman, R. L., Jr., Downs, J. B., Modell, J. H., and Hood, C. I.: The ineffectiveness of steroid therapy in treating aspiration of HCl. Arch. Surg., *108*:858–861, 1974.

69. Downs, J. B., Chapman, R. L., Jr., Modell, J. H., and Hood C. I.: An evaluation of steroid therapy in aspiration pneumonitis. Anesthesiology, *40*:129–135, 1974.

70. Bynum, L. J., and Pierce, A. K.: Pulmonary aspiration of gastric contents. Am. Rev. Respir. Dis., *114*:1129–1136, 1976.

71. Wolfe, J. E., Bone, R. C., and Ruth, W. E.: The effects of corticosteroids in the treatment of patients with gastric aspiration. Am. J. Med., *63*:719–722, 1977.

72. Bartlett, J. G., and Gorbach, S. L.: Treatment of aspiration pneumonia and primary lung diseases: Penicillin G versus clindamycin. J.A.M.A, *234*:935–937, 1975.

73. Bartlett, J. G., and Finegold, S. M.: Anaerobic infections of the lung and pleural space. Am. Rev. Respir. Dis., *110*:56–77, 1974.

74. Lorber, B., and Swenson, R. M.: Bacteriology of aspiration pneumonia: A prospective study of community- and hospital-acquired cases. Ann. Intern. Med., *81*:329–331, 1974.

75. Gutman, L. T., Idriss, Z. H., Gehlbach, S., and Blackmon, L.: Neonatal staphylococcal enterocolitis: Association with indwelling feeding catheters and *S. aureus* colonization. J. Pediatr., *88*:836–839, 1976.

of gastrostomy in the prevention of food inhalation.] Poumon Coeur, *33*:383–385, 1977.

76. Cook, J., Elliott, C., Elliot-Smith, A., Frisby, B. R., and Gardner, A. M. N.: Staphylococcal diarrhoea: With an account of two outbreaks in the same hospital. Br. Med. J., 1:542–547, 1957.

77. De Vries, E. G. E., Mulder, N. H., Houwen, B., and De Vries-Hospers, H. G.: Enteral nutrition in adult patients treated with intensive chemotherapy for acute leukemia. Am. J. Clin. Nutr., 35:1490, 1982.

78. Hostetler, C., Lipman, T. O., Geraghty, M., and Parker, R.: Bacterial safety of reconstituted continuous drip tube feeding. J.P.E.N., 6:232–235, 1982.

79. Schreiner, R. L., Eitzen, H., Gfell, M. A., Kress, S., Gresham, E. L., French, M., and Moye, L.: Environmental contamination of continuous drip feedings. Pediatrics, 63:232–237, 1979.

80. White, W. T., III, Acuff, T. E., Jr., Sykes, T. R., and Dobbie, R. P.: Bacterial contamination of enteral nutrient solution: A preliminary report. J.P.E.N., 3:459–461, 1979.

81. Casewell, M. W., Cooper, J. E., and Webster, M.: Enteral feeds contaminated with *Enterobacter cloacae* as a cause of septicemia. Br. Med. J., 282:973, 1981.

82. Andrassy, R. J., Page, C. P., Feldtman, R. W., Haff, R. C., Ryan, J. A., Jr., and Ratner, I. A.: Continual catheter administration of an elemental diet in infants and children. Surgery, 82:205–210, 1977.

83. Mitty, W. F., Jr., Nealon, T. F., Jr., and Grossi, C.: Use of elemental diets in surgical cases. Am. J. Gastroenterol., 65:297–304, 1976.

84. Bury, K. D., Stephens, R. V., and Randall, H. T.: Use of a chemically defined, liquid, elemental diet for nutritional management of fistulas of the alimentary tract. Am. J. Surg., 121:174–183, 1971.

85. Stephens, R. V., Bury, K. D., DeLuca, F. G., and Randall, H. T.: Use of an elemental diet in the nutritional management of catabolic disease in infants. Am. J. Surg., 123:374–379, 1972.

86. Levy, E., Charles, J. F., Malafosse, M., Huguet, C. I., and Loygue, J.: Continuous low rate enteral feeding. J. Med., 7:113–122, 1976.

87. Dobbie, R. P., and Hoffmeister, J. A.: Continuous pump-tube enteric hyperalimentation. Surg. Gynecol. Obstet., 143:273–276, 1976.

88. Voitk, A. J., Echave, V., Brown, R. A., and Gurd, F. N.: Use of elemental diet during the adaptive stage of short gut syndrome. Gastroenterology, 65:419–426, 1973.

89. Moore, E. E., Dunn, E. L., and Jones, T. N.: Immediate jejunostomy feeding. Arch. Surg., 116:681–684, 1981.

90. Cheek, J. A., Jr., and Staub, G. F.: Nasojejunal alimentation for premature and full-term newborn infants. J. Pediatr., 82:955–962, 1973.

91. Delany, H. M., Carnevale, N., Garvey, J. W., and Moss, C. M.: Postoperative nutritional support using needle catheter feeding jejunostomy. Ann. Surg., 186:165–170, 1977.

92. Roy, F. N., Pollnitz, R. P., Hamilton, J. R., and Chance, G. W.: Impaired assimilation of nasojejunal feeds in healthy low-birth-weight newborn infants. J. Pediatr., 90:431–434, 1977.

93. Loo, S. W. H., Gross, I., and Warshaw, J. B.: Improved method of nasojejunal feeding in low-birth-weight infants. J. Pediatr., 85:104–106, 1974.

94. Chen, J. W., and Wong, P. W. K.: Intestinal complications of nasojejunal feeding in low-birth-weight infants. J. Pediatr., 85:109–110, 1974.

95. Padilla, G. V., Grant, M., Wong, H., Hansen, B. W., Hanson, R. L., Bergstrom, N., and Kubo, W. R.: Subjective distresses of nasogastric tube feeding. J.P.E.N., 3:53–57, 1979.

96. Peteet, J. R., Medeiros, C., Slavin, L., and Walsh-Burke, K.: Psychological aspects of artificial feeding in cancer patients. J.P.E.N., 5:138–140, 1981.

97. Fallis, L. S., and Barron, J.: Gastric and jejunal alimentation with fine polyethylene tubes. Arch. Surg., 65:373–381, 1952.

98. Hayhurst, E. G., and Wyman, M.: Morbidity associated with prolonged use of polyvinyl feeding tubes. Am. J. Dis. Child., 129:72–74, 1975.

99. Hafner, C. D., Wylie, J. H., Jr., Brush, B. E.: Complications of gastrointestinal intubation. Arch. Surg., 83:147–160, 1961.

100. Seebacher, J., Nozik, D., and Mathieu A: Inadvertent intracranial introduction of a nasogastric tube, a complication of severe maxillofacial trauma. Anesthesia, 42:100–102, 1975.

101. Wyler, A. R., and Reynolds, A. F.: An intracranial complication of nasogastric intubation: Case report. J. Neurosurg., 47:297–298, 1977.

102. Mason, L. B., and Ausband, J. R.: Benign stenosing esophagitis associated with vomiting and intubation. Surgery, 32:10–16, 1952.

103. Graham, J., Barnes, N., and Rubenstein, A. S.: The nasogastric tube as a cause of esophagitis and stricture. Am. J. Surg., 98:116–119, 1959.

104. Nagler, R., and Spiro, S. M.: Persistent gastroesophageal reflux induced during prolonged gastric intubation. N. Engl. J. Med., 269:495–500, 1963.

105. Douglas, W. K.: Oesophageal strictures associated with gastroduodenal intubation. Br. J. Surg., 43:404–409, 1955.

106. McCredie, J. A., and McDowell, R. F. C.: Oesophageal stricture following intubation in a case of hiatus hernia. Br. J. Surg., 46:260–261, 1958.

107. Dobbie, R. P., and Butterick, O. D.: Continuous pump/tube enteric hyperalimentation—use in esophageal disease. J.P.E.N., 1:100–104, 1977.

108. Fricke, F. J., and Niewodowski, M. A.: Hazardous gaseous distention of intestinal balloons. J.A.M.A., 235:2611–2613, 1976.

109. Iyer, S. K., Chandrasekhara, K. L., Narayanaswamy, T. S.: Small bowel obstruction due to gaseous distention of an intestinal balloon. J. Natl. Med. Assoc., 72:371–373, 1980.

110. Sun, S. C., Samuels, S., Lee, J., and Marquis, J. R.: Duodenal perforation; a rare complication of neonatal nasojejunal tube feeding. Pediatrics, 55:371–375, 1975.

111. Siegle, R. L., Rabinowitz, J. G., and Sarasohn C: Intestinal perforation secondary to nasojejunal feeding tubes. Am. J. Roentgenol., 126:1229–1232, 1976.

112. Fonkalsrud, E. W.: Intestinal obstruction from gastrostomy tube in infants. J. Pediatr., 69:809–811, 1966.

113. Boros, S. J., and Reynolds, J. W.: Duodenal perforation: A complication of neonatal nasojejunal feeding. J. Pediatr., 85:107–108, 1974.

114. Haws, E. B., Sieber, W. K., and Kiesewetter, W. B.: Complications of tube gastrostomy in infants and children: 15-Year review of 240 cases. Ann. Surg., 164:284–290, 1966.

115. Merten, D. F., Mumford, L., Filston, H. C., Brumley, G. W., Jr., Effmann, E. L., and Grossman, H.: Radiological observations during transpyloric tube feeding in infants of low birth weight. Radiology, *136*:67–75, 1980.

116. Pérez-Rodrígues, J., Quero, J., Frías, E. G., and Omeñaca, F.: Duodenal perforation in a neonate by a tube of silicone rubber during transpyloric feeding. J. Pediatr., *92*:113–114, 1978.

117. Engel, S.: Gastrostomy. Surg. Clin. North Am., *49*:1289–1295, 1969.

118. Torosian, M., and Rombeau, J. L.: Feeding by tube enterostomy. Surg. Gynecol. Obstet., *150*:918–927, 1980.

119. Goodman, L. R., Wittenberg, J., and Messner, R.: Duodenal obstruction—an unusual complication of a gastrostomy feeding catheter. Br. J. Radiol., *44*:883–884, 1971.

120. Sherman, M. L., Cosgrove, M. J., and Dennis, J. M.: Gastrostomy tube migration. Am. Surg., *39*:122–123, 1973.

121. Boles, T., Jr., and Zollinger, R. M.: Critical evaluation of jejunostomy. Arch. Surg., *65*:358–366, 1952.

122. Delaney, H. N., Carnevale, N. J., and Garvey, J. W.: Jejunostomy by a needle catheter technique. Surgery, *73*:786–790, 1973.

123. Balkany, T. J., Jafek, B. W., and Wong, M. L.: Complications of feeding esophagotomy: Advantages of a new esophagotomy tube. Arch. Otolaryngol., *106*(2):122–123, 1980.

124. Eklöf, O., Löhr, G., and Okmian, L.: Submucosal perforation of the esophagus in the neonate. Acta Radiol. [Diagn.] (Stockh.), *8*:187–192, 1969.

125. Girdany, B. R., Sieber, W. K., and Osman, M. Z.: Traumatic pseudodiverticulums of the pharynx in newborn infants. N. Engl. J. Med., *280*:237–240, 1969.

126. Kassner, G. E., Baumstark, A., Balsam, D., and Haller, J. O.: Passage of feeding catheters into the pleural space: A radiographic sign of trauma to the pharynx and esophagus in the newborn. Am. J. Roentgenol., *128*:19–22, 1977.

127. Pitcher-Wilmott, R., Shutack, J. G., and Fox, W. W.: Decreased lung volume after nasogastric feeding of neonates recovering from respiratory disease. J. Pediatr., *95*:119–121, 1979.

128. Hasselmeyer, E. G., and Hon, E. H.: Effects of gavage feeding of premature infants upon cardiorespiratory patterns. Milit. Med., *136*:252–257, 1971.

129. Russell, G., and Feather, E. A.: Effects of feeding on respiratory mechanics of healthy newborn infants. Arch. Dis. Child., *45*:325–327, 1970.

130. Yu, V. Y. H., and Rolfe, P.: Effects of feeding on ventilation and respiratory mechanics of healthy newborn infants. Arch. Dis. Child., *51*:310–313, 1976.

131. Yu, V. Y. H.: Cardiorespiratory response to feeding in newborn infants. Arch. Dis. Child., *51*:305–309, 1976.

132. Duritz, G., and Oltorf, C.: Lactobezoar formation associated with high-density caloric formula. Pediatrics, *63*:647–649, 1979.

133. Erenberg, A.: Lactobezoar, in Feeding the Neonate Weighing Less that 1500 Grams—Nutrition and Beyond—Report of the Seventy-Ninth Ross Conference in Pediatric Research, Columbus, Ohio, Ross Laboratories.

134. O'Malley, J. M., Ferrucci, J. T., Jr., and Goodgame, J. T., Jr.: Medication bezoar: Intestinal obstruction by an Isocal bezoar—case report and review of the literature. Gastrointest. Radiol., *6*:141–144, 1981.

CHAPTER 30

Animal Models for Enteral Feeding of Defined Formula Diets

ELEANOR A. YOUNG
ELLIOT WESER

Animal models have recently been acclaimed as the best single key to the biologic functioning of man.[1] This is true, notwithstanding the modern technologic advances in alternate models such as mathematical and computer systems. These adjunctive models can provide useful information, but cannot eliminate the need for animal models in biomedical research. The use of animal models is directed primarily at the understanding of and attempted elimination of human disease.[1] In this pursuit almost all important advances stem from research performed with animal models.[2]

Ethical and economic considerations, and the limitations of time and study design, curtail the use of human subjects for nutrition experiments, and for studies in other biologic areas of investigation.[3] Currently there remain numerous problems in nutrition for which we do not yet have reliable answers. Nevertheless, studies carried out using animal models provide an approach to learning about the energy requirements of man as related to body composition. In the use of experimental animals, the genetic and environmental conditions that may alter nutritional requirements can be controlled. The discovery of essential nutrients as well as the assessment of toxic ranges of nutrients indicate the important role of experimental animals. Without their use, the discovery, isolation, and synthesis of the essential vitamins required by man would in all probability never have happened. This knowledge alone has almost completely wiped out all of the classic vitamin deficiency diseases (scurvy, beriberi, pellagra) that were epidemic in the United States during the early years of this century. Animal studies have also served as essential steps in establishing the requirements of amino acids, linoleic acid, zinc, and other trace elements. With this knowledge we can now formulate a synthetic mixture containing all of the known nutritional requirements of man and can utilize this formula to sustain a patient with total nutrition for extended periods of time. This scientific advancement has been acclaimed as one of the most important advances in modern medicine. Currently numerous basic animal studies are exploring the contribution of nutrition to the "killer diseases" of modern society, such as coronary heart disease, diabetes, hypertension, and obesity. Basic animal research has been the major contributor to human metabolic studies as well as to clinical trials.

In 1966 Dudrick, Vars, and Rhoads[4] reported for the first time in any animal species that long-term total intravenous feeding could support normal growth and development in beagle puppies. The animal model used by these investigators is shown in Fig. 30–1. Key to the success of this study was not only the availability of complete synthetic nutrient formulation, but also the development of intravenous technology.[5, 6] Subsequently, numerous other investigators developed techniques of parenteral feeding in animal models.[7–13] Some animal models used in these studies are illustrated in Figures 30–2 to 30–8. These studies played an impor-

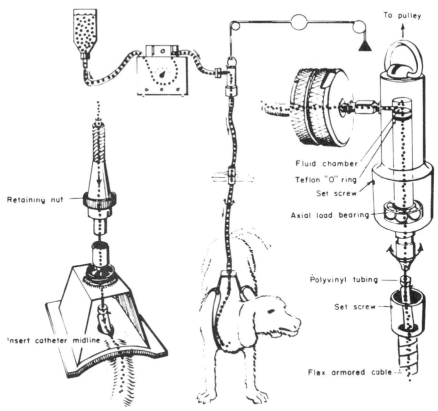

Figure 30–1. Solution is pumped through the membrane filter, swivel assembly (inset on right), and vinyl tubing (protected by the flexible armored cable) to the indwelling catheter secured to the animal's back by the stainless steel support assembly and canvas harness. The animal can be disconnected from the delivery apparatus as desired. (*From* Dudrick, S. J., et al.: Continuous long-term intravenous infusion in unrestrained animals. Lab. Anim. Care, 20:521–529, 1970, with permission.)

tant role in the rapid and dramatic development in assessing the requirements for and benefits of total intravenous nutritional support in surgical and medical patients.

From 1957 to 1967, intense investigations led to the development of water-soluble, chemically defined enteral diets that were successfully used in animal models.[14-24] These diets were designed with specific characteristics: (1) essential and non-essential nitrogen provided in the form of highly purified L-amino acids; (2) high nutritive efficacy in ultra-compact form; (3) complete water solubility; (4) no dietary fiber or bulk; (5) flexibility of formulation; (6) completely digestible; and (7) excellent storage stability. These studies of defined formula diets (DFD) were designed to permit the large-scale preparation of optically pure amino acids for the synthesis of peptides to be used as sub-

strates in in vitro studies of peptidase specificity, and to provide the amino acid components for a completely synthetic diet that would be suitable for long-term nutritional studies with experimental animals and appropriate for administration to human beings.

Couch et al.[25] were the first to take advantage of the knowledge gained from these basic animal studies and to make clinical application of DFD. Clinical trials using these formulas for hospitalized patients indicated that they were practical, safe, and biologically effective.[25] These diets were then evaluated for their adequacy and potential for long-term sustenance for man-in-space.[26-28] Since this time, enteral DFD have been used extensively for a wide variety of clinical conditions.[29-34]

A historical perspective demonstrates the importance of basic animal studies in the

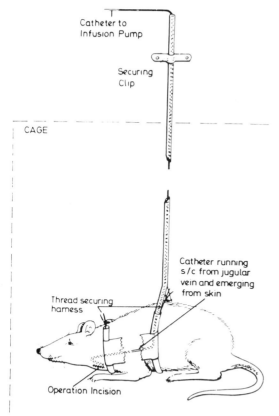

Figure 30–2. Diagram of rat model for parenteral feeding. (*From* Dalton, R. G., et al.: A simple technique for continuous intravenous infusion in rats. J. Lab. Clin. Med., *74*:813–815, 1969, with permission.)

development of enteral liquid DFD and their clinical applicaton. The commercialization of a wide variety of DFD[35–38] and their clinical use[29–34] suggest that the medical use of these diets has been extensive, and that basic ani-

mal studies have not kept pace with clinical investigations using DFD. Koretz and Meyer have recently suggested the need for additional basic studies to gain a greater understanding of the efficacy of these diets.[39]

SELECTED ANIMAL MODELS

INTACT ANIMAL MODELS

Importance of the "Starvation" Models

The influence of enteral feeding on the gastrointestinal tract has perhaps been most dramatically demonstrated by a total lack of nutrients (starvation) and by a lack of luminal nutrients while the animal is maintained on total parenteral nutrition (TPN). Starvation models have consistently verified the significant influence of the absence of nutrients on the structure and function of the gastrointestinal tract of a number of animal species.[40–48] Reduced rate of cell division and cell migration, reduced synthesis of DNA, atrophy of intestinal villi, decreased mucosal protein and water, diminished total intestinal cell population, reduced intestinal enzymes, reduced transport of nutrients through the mucosal cell, and decreased serum and antral gastrin concentrations have been reported.[40–48] Not only are starvation models of importance to demonstrate physiologic response to a lack of nutrients, but these studies also provide important clues as to the specific role of nutrients in maintain-

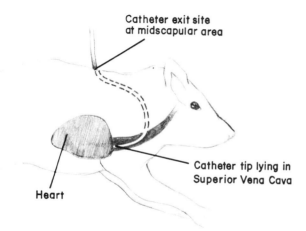

Figure 30–3. Sterile silicone rubber catheter is passed down jugular vein and into superior vena cava or right atrium. Right atrium in the rat is at the level of the axilla. (*From* Steiger, E., et al.: A technique for long-term intravenous feeding in unrestrained rats. Arch. Surg., *104*:330–332, 1972, with permission. Copyright 1972, American Medical Association.)

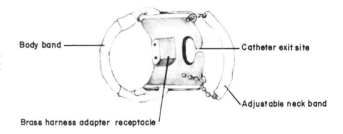

Figure 30–4. Metal rat harness is padded on its undersurface and is securely fastened to rat's back. Neck band is adjustable body band that fits snugly around lower thorax behind front legs. (*From* Steiger, E., et al.: A technique for long-term intravenous feeding in unrestrained rats. Arch. Surg., *104*:330–332, 1972, with permission. Copyright 1972, American Medical Association.)

ing normal structure and function of the gastrointestinal tract in the presence of adequate nutrition.

The Influence of Enteral DFD on Body Growth

It is well known that the specific nutritional composition of the diet can significantly influence body growth. The DFD were designed to provide a balanced ratio of all essential nutrients required for normal growth.[49, 50] Reviewing the wide variation of nutrient composition of commercially available liquid formula diets,[35-38] it is not surprising that animal models maintained on DFD demonstrate significant differences in body growth. Not only does the formula composition influence body growth, but the route of administration of the formula into the gastrointestinal tract may also modify body

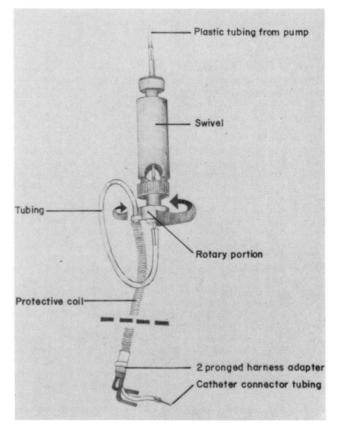

Figure 30–5. Fluid infusion swivel with attached polyvinyl tubing and protective coil of tightly wound stainless steel. Apparatus is preassembled and sterilized as a unit. (*From* Steiger, E., et al.: A technique for long-term intravenous feeding in unrestrained rats. Arch. Surg., *104*:330–332, 1972, with permission. Copyright 1972, American Medical Association.)

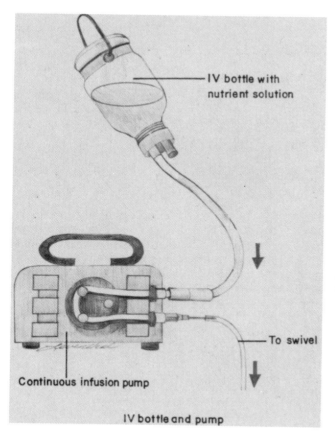

IV bottle with nutrient solution

Continuous infusion pump

To swivel

IV bottle and pump

Figure 30–6. Sterile nutrient solution is pumped through a silicone rubber pump chamber with a nylon Luer adapter to accept intravenous tubing at one end and blunt 22-gauge needle at the other. Short segment of polyvinyl tubing delivers solution to swivel. Copper-containing metallic Luer fittings have caused severe hemolysis in this rat model and should be avoided. (*From* Steiger, E., et al.: A technique for long-term intravenous feeding in unrestrained rats. Arch. Surg., *104*:330–332, 1972, with permission. Copyright 1972, American Medical Association.)

growth. The length of time animals are maintained on a specific feeding regimen, and other conditions of the experimental design, make it difficult to compare growth rates of animal models sustained on DFD.

In the development of chemically defined diets, Greenstein et al.[14] demonstrated that rats maintained on various liquid formulas for periods of up to 90 days were able to grow normally, breed, lactate, and rear their young. Figure 30–9 illustrates the growth curves of rats on diets containing various mixtures of amino acids. Growth rates varied according to the nutritional composition of the diet. Young weanling mice and rats maintained ad libitum on DFD were less

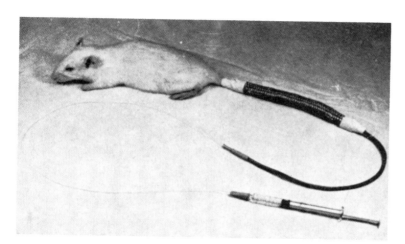

Figure 30–7. The electrical shielding has been secured and the rat is now ready for infusion. (*From* Born, C. T., and Moller, M. L.: A simple procedure for long-term intravenous infusion in the rat. Lab. Anim. Sci., *24*:355–358, 1974, with permission.)

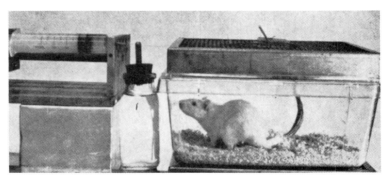

Figure 30–8. A rat in a flat-topped cage connected to the infusion assembly. (*From* Born, C. T., and Moller, M. L.: A simple procedure for long-term intravenous infusion in the rat. Lab. Anim. Sci., *24*:355–358, 1974, with permission.)

than normal size compared to chow-fed controls (Fig. 30–10).[19] Growth rates in a mouse model were either similar to those observed in chow-fed control mice (diet 26) or less than those observed in controls (diet 3). It was also observed that newborn mice did not grow at optimal rates when lactating

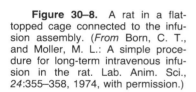

Figure 30–9. Growth curves of male weanling rats on diets containing various mixtures of nonessential amino acids. These are averaged gain values of six animals on each diet. (*From* Greenstein, J. P., et al.: Quantitative nutritional studies with water-soluble, chemically defined diets. I. Growth, reproduction and lactation in rats. Arch. Biochem. Biophys., *72*:396–416, 1957, with permission.)

from mothers on the liquid diets, and when weaned on to the same diet grew at rates distinctly less than those of their parents at the same stage of development and the same liquid diet, but who had been born to and lactated by mothers on a chow diet.[14] Growth rates were also influenced by modification of the amino acid[16] and carbohydrate[17] composition of the formulas.

Young et al.[51] demonstrated reduced body growth in young weanling rats fed isocaloric amounts of DFD by continuous intragastric drip when compared to reference animals eating regular chow orally (Fig. 30–11). The continuous intragastric drip model was modified from the parenteral model of Steiger et al.[11] to allow for intragastric feeding. This model provided for the suture of a Silastic catheter in the rumen portion of the stomach (Fig. 30–12). The proximal end of the catheter was threaded around the animal subcutaneously and exited dorsally between the scapular blades. The animals were harnessed to prevent access to the catheter, and maintained unrestrained in individual metabolic cages. The catheter was threaded up a steel spring and through a swivel at the top of the cage, thus allowing free movement of the animal. The catheter was then threaded through an infusion pump up to the formula bottle. While all animals received isocaloric amounts of liquid formula or rat chow, it was clear that formula-fed animals did not achieve the same growth as chow-fed animals. The authors speculated on several possible contributing factors: (1) the nitrogen : caloric ratio (chow, 1:83; Vivonex HN, 1:150; Ensure, 1:179; Flexical, 1:286; Vivonex, 1:302) may be more conducive to growth in some formulas;[49, 50] (2) nutrients delivered intragastrically may not be digested or absorbed as efficiently or in the same manner

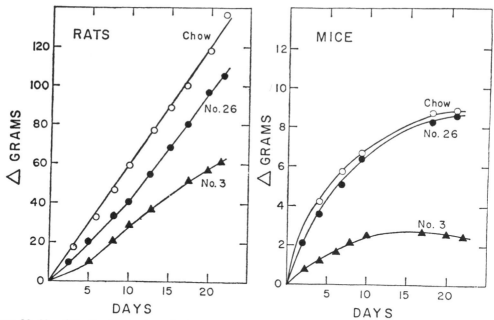

Figure 30–10. Growth rate of rats and mice maintained on regular chow or on liquid formula diet No. 26 or No. 3. (*From* Birnbaum, S. M., et al.: Quantitative nutritional studies with water-soluble, chemically defined diets. VI. Growth studies on mice. Arch. Biochem. Biophys., *78*:245–247, 1958, with permission.)

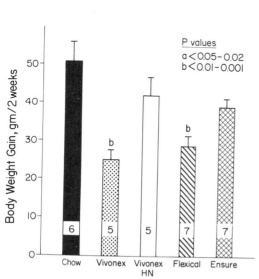

Figure 30–11. Mean ± SE body weight gain of chow reference and DFD groups. Numbers in bars correspond to number of animals in each group. (*From* Young, E. A., et al.: Comparative study of nutritional adaptation to defined formula diets in rats. Am. J. Clin. Nutr., *33*:2106–2118, 1980, with permission.)

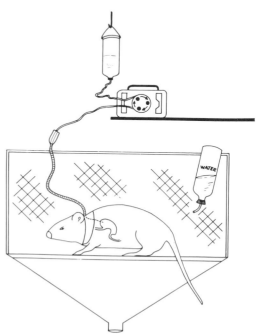

Figure 30–12. Diagrammatic animal model for continuous intragastric feeding. (*From* Young, E. A., et al.: Comparative study of nutritional adaptation to defined formula diets in rats. Am. J. Clin. Nutr., *33*:2106–2118, 1980, with permission.)

as when the same diets are consumed orally; (3) bypassing the cephalic phase of digestion by utilizing a continuous intragastric drip model may alter stimulation of gastrointestinal hormones, as well as the quantity or quality of digestive secretions, thereby modifying growth; or (4) differences in gastric acid output as well as gastric emptying may influence digestion and absorption.[51] Johnson et al.,[52] Ecknauer et al.,[53] and Morin et al[54] have also demonstrated lower body weight gains in rats maintained on DFD compared to isocaloric chow-fed controls. In other studies, body growth rate in rats fed isocaloric regular chow or DFD were virtually identical.[55] When DFD or chow is allowed ad libitum, growth rate has been shown to be similar[56, 57] or greater in DFD-fed rats.[58] Although a similar model was used in these studies, experimental circumstances were not similar.

When the same liquid DFD are isocalorically administered orally or gastrically over a two-week period, body weight gain has been shown to be altered by the specific DFD used and by the route of delivery.[59] As illustrated in Fig. 30–13, Young et al.[59] have demonstrated differences in body weight gain in oral-fed *(A)* and gastric-fed *(B)* animals receiving C (control rat liquid diet), V (Vivonex), VHN (Vivonex High Nitrogen), F (Flexical), or Vit (Vital). In the composite section *(C)* of this figure, body weight gain over a two-week period was less in all gastric-fed animals but was significantly different only for the C, V, and F formulas.[59]

Influence of Enteral DFD on the Gastrointestinal Tract

DFD Versus Fiber-Containing Diets

Esophagus.   Several animal models have been used to develop liquid feeding techniques that would be suitable for patients with esophageal stricture, necrosis of the larynx, head or neck cancer, or physical injury. Feeding pharyngostomies and esophagostomies have been studied in the horse,[60] dog,[61] and pony.[62] These models permit the administration of fiber-free, liquid DFD, and can sustain the nutritional status of the animal.

Stomach.   Utilizing an animal model to study the effects of DFD on gastric acid se-

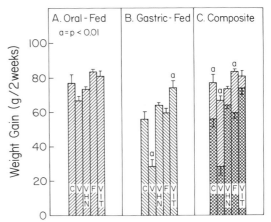

Effect of DFD on Body Weight Gain

Figure 30–13.   Body weight gain in grams per two weeks in animals maintained on the control rat liquid formula or one of several DFD orally *(A)* or gastrically *(B)*. Statistical analysis compare weight gain for each DFD group with the control group. The composite panel (C) compares body weight gain in oral-fed versus gastric-fed animals maintained on the control or DFD formulas. Bars are mean values ± standard error of the mean. Diets are C = Control; V = Vivonex; VHN = Vivonex High Nitrogen; F = Flexical; Vit = Vital. (*From* Young, E. A., et al.: Gastrointestinal response to oral versus gastric feeding of defined formula diets. Am. J. Clin. Nutr., *35:*715–726, 1982, with permission.)

cretion, Rivilis et al.[63] demonstrated approximately an eightfold decrease in gastric acid output with Flexical compared with regular laboratory chow in dogs with Pavlov pouches. The dog food evoked about five times the volume of gastric output compared to the DFD. The use of this animal model subsequently led to several studies in humans. Malagelada et al.[64] compared gastric acid output after an eaten meal versus a gastric infusion of a homogenate of a similar meal. A significantly greater acid output after the eaten meal was thought to reflect a more intense cephalic drive than the liquid meal. Bury and Jambunathan[65] compared acid secretion after blenderized food for each of two elemental diets given intragastrically. They concluded that greater acid secretion resulted from the homogenized meal. These studies suggest that fiber-free liquid DFD are less stimulating to gastric acid and total volume output compared to that stimulated by whole or blenderized food.

Small Intestine.   In the developmental stages of DFD, Greenstein et al.[14] noted at sacrifice that the gastrointestinal tract of rats maintained on one of a variety of DFD contained virtually no measurable contents compared to that found in chow-fed animals. The entire length of the gastrointestinal tract was reported to be free of pathologic lesions, gross or microscopic.[14]

Young et al.[51] have demonstrated that intestinal mucosal weight and concentrations of protein and DNA are significantly decreased in rats maintained on DFD instilled intragastrically when compared to control animals receiving chow isocalorically. A normal proximal to distal gradient was noted for all small intestinal parameters studied (Fig. 30–14); however, the high-fiber chow results in greater mucosal mass despite isocaloric feeding of the two-week period. The high-fiber chow used in the control group of this experimental design may

exert different effects on digestion and absorption of nutrients compared to nonresidue DFD. It has been reported that dietary fiber increases gastrointestinal bulk,[66–68] alters gut transit time,[66–69] may change the gut microflora,[70–72] alters bile acids,[73–74] and may decrease the absorption of the nutrients zinc, iron, calcium, nitrogen, and fat.[75, 76] Reduced small intestinal mass may also be a reflection of reduced body weight gain in the DFD-fed animals.

The gastrointestinal response in rats nourished by continuous intragastric infusion of one of a variety of DFD was compared with response observed in animals consuming the same diets orally.[59] In this study a fiber-free liquid rat diet served as the control diet in both the oral-fed and gastric-fed groups. In the proximal segments of the small intestine of both the oral-fed and

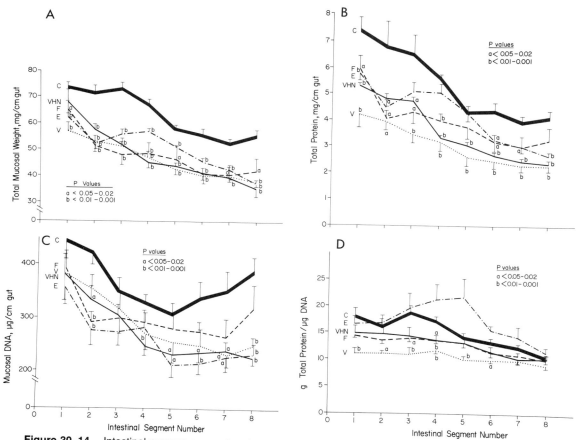

Figure 30–14. Intestinal mucosa parameters (mean ± SE) for chow reference and DFD groups: A, total mucosal weight, mg/cm gut; B, total protein, mg/cm gut; C, mucosal DNA, μg/cm gut; and D, total protein, g; DNA, μg. (*From* Young, E. A., et al.: Comparative study of nutritional adaptation to defined formula diets in rats. Am. J. Clin. Nutr., 33:2106–2118, 1980, with permission.)

gastric-fed groups the segment weight, mucosal weight, protein, and DNA of animals nourished by DFD were significantly lower than those observed in animals consuming the C formula. These parameters were similar in the distal segments. The trend toward greater weights and concentrations of proximal intestinal parameters in the oral-fed animals on C, V, and F diets, and in the gastric-fed animals on VHN and Vital, suggests that the contributions of these diets to intestinal mass are modified to a lesser degree by the route of administration than by the specific diets used.

Morin et al.[54] demonstrated similar findings in a rat model comparing small intestinal changes in animals given a continuous intragastric (IG) infusion of Vivonex, and intravenous (IV) liquid diet of Travasol, or regular rat chow (CH). The caloric intake of all groups was similar. Mucosal DNA and protein of the small intestine was lowest in the IV animals, highest in the CH animals, with the IG animals falling midway between the other two groups (Fig. 30–15). The DFD-fed animals were able to maintain an intestinal mass greater than that of the IV animals, but not as great as that of the CH animals.

Lorenz-Meyer et al.[77] studied the morphology of the intestinal mucosa of rats maintained on elemental diet and pair-fed to control rats on regular chow. Morphometric analysis of the DFD-fed animals showed a decrease of the base and tips of the villi, while the length of the villi increased slightly. The surface of the villi and the depth of the crypts were significantly reduced. When the experimental and control diets were adjusted with similar protein content, no significant differences in the intestinal parameters were noted.[77] These results suggest that the protein content of the diet rather than the presence of fiber was a more important factor in maintaining intestinal mass.

Ecknauer et al.[53] devised a rat model to determine whether or not the physical form of the diet contributes to mucosal growth. In this model, rats were placed on one of three different isocaloric diets: regular chow, an elemental diet, Vivonex High Nitrogen (VHN), or VHN plus bulk added in the form of alpha-cellulose. All dimensions of the

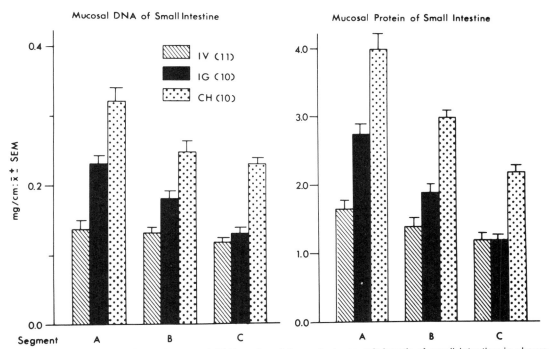

Figure 30–15. Comparison of mucosal DNA and protein content per unit length of small intestine is shown in three segments (A, B, C) of the small intestine fed intravenously (IV), a chemically defined diet (IG), or with rat chow (CH). Figures in parentheses indicate the number of animals. (*From* Morin, C. L., et al.: Small intestinal and colonic changes induced by a chemically defined diet. Dig. Dis. Sci., 25:123–128, 1980, with permission.)

small intestinal villi studied except thickness were greatest in chow-fed rats. Although there were some differences noted in the VHN and the VHN plus bulk groups, it was clear that the addition of dietary bulk did not prevent the reduction in size of the villus compared to the chow-fed groups.[53]

Nelson et al.[57, 58] have used an ad libitum feeding rat model to compare small intestinal changes induced by the elemental diets Vivonex and Flexical compared to regular chow. These investigators have reported a significant reduction in the ratio of crypt height to villus height in the DFD-fed rats compared to the controls, suggesting an improved survival of the mature enterocyte population. In these studies it is important to note the ad libitum feeding of all animals. No information was provided to indicate total caloric intake, a factor of importance in assessing changes in the intestinal mucosa in response to dietary manipulation.

The rat model of Nelson et al.[57] was also used to assess small intestinal function. Segments of jejunum or ileum were perfused in vivo and water absorption was studied. No significant differences in water absorption

were reported between control chow rats and rats on diet 1 (Vivonex), but there was reduced water absorption in rats on diet 2 (Flexical) (Fig. 30–16). These results suggested that small intestinal absorptive function is influenced by the composition of the specific DFD used. Differences in total intake of DFD or chow may also account for some of the observations noted in this study.[57]

Using a mouse model, Lehnert[78] has studied changes in growth kinetics of jejunal epithelium in mice maintained on an elemental diet or mouse chow. The DFD-fed animals show an increase in the number of cells per column in the villus as compared to chow-fed controls. It was speculated that this may be the result of reduced friction from dietary bulk and reduced attrition of cells from the villi tip. Total caloric intake was not assessed, which places a limitation on the interpretation of this study.

Adaptation of intestinal enzymes has been demonstrated in response to dietary sugars,[79] iron deficiency,[80] and protein.[80–84] Moreover, oral intake of food is of major importance in maintaining gut mass and di-

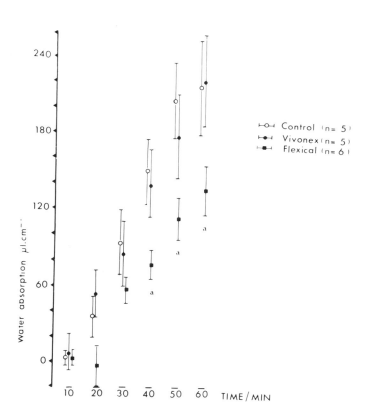

Figure 30–16. Effect of elemental diets 1 and 2 on water absorption by rat jejunum (a, p <0.05 control versus diet 2). (*From* Nelson, L. M., et al.: Elemental diet composition and the structure and function of rat small intestine: comparison of the effects of two diets on morphology and in vivo absorption of water. JPEN, 5:204–206, 1981, with permission. Copyright 1981 by The American Society of Parenteral and Enteral Nutrition.)

saccharidase activity.[85, 86] Thus it is not surprising that variations in the composition of DFD as well as their mode of delivery may impact on intestinal mucosal enzyme activity.

Studies of intestinal mucosal disaccharidases in a rat model comparing intragastrically fed DFD rats with oral chow-fed control animals[51] demonstrated significant differences resulting from the specific formulation of the diet. The maltase activity *(A)* and specific maltase activity *(B)* were similar in the distal intestinal segments (Fig. 30–17). Maltase activity of DFD-fed animals was higher in the proximal segments when compared to the chow-fed controls, likely reflecting the nutrient composition of the various diets.[51] Morin et al.[54] have reported sucrase activity in intravenously and intragastrically fed DFD, and oral chow (CH) rat models. The intestinal sucrase activity of the three isocalorically fed groups showed a proximal to distal gradient (Fig. 30–18). Sucrase activity was greater in IG and CH animals compared to IV animals. The IG and CH animals had similar sucrase activity in proximal segments, but in more distal segments the sucrase activity was greater in CH animals.

Pancreas. Pancreatic response to liquid DFD may depend on how the formula is administered (orally, intragastrically, or intraduodenally)[87–91] or on the various nutrient constituents of the formulas.[92–96] The effect of DFD on pancreatic secretion is unclear. Some studies indicate that DFD do not stimulate pancreatic secretion as well as does regular food[87–89] after duodenal or jejunal instillation, whereas other studies[90, 91] have demonstrated that instillation of DFD into the duodenum evoked a high rate of protein secretion from the pancreas. Koretz et al.[39] have recently reviewed studies of the effect of DFD on the pancreatic secretion and conclude that pancreatic response to DFD is as yet poorly characterized. While a dog model has been used for most of the studies exploring the effect of DFD on pancreatic secretion,[87–91] Buonous et al.[97] have used a mouse model to study the effect of DFD on pancreatic proteases, and have shown that the more elemental diet provided less stimulation of pancreatic secretion than did a polymeric formula. Using a rat model, Young et al.[51] have studied pancreatic response to several DFD given intragastrically compared to oral rat chow given isocalorically. Pancreas total weight (gm) and per cent of body weight, as well as serum and pancreatic amylase are shown in Fig. 30–19. The weight of the pancreas as well as serum and/or pancreatic amylases were significantly lower in response to DFD compared to the response to the control chow diet. In other studies comparing pancreatic amylase response to oral versus gastric isocaloric feeding of a variety of DFD, gastric feeding was shown to stimulate greater pancreatic specific activity than oral feeding when rats were maintained on control liquid rat diet, Vivonex High Nitrogen (VHN), Flexical, or Vital.[59] No other animal models could be found describing the pancreatic amylase response of oral versus gastric isocaloric feeding of DFD. This study also demonstrated variation in pancreatic secretion in response to the specific nutritional composition of the formulas used. Green et al.[98] have developed a rat model in which the bile and pancreatic se-

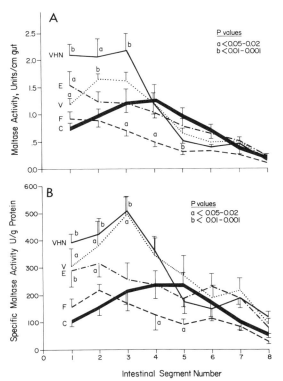

Figure 30–17. Mucosal maltase activity (mean ± SE) mucosal maltase activity of chow reference and DFD groups: A, maltase activity, units/cm gut; and B, specific maltase activity, units/g protein. (*From* Young, E. A., et al.: Comparative study of nutritional adaptation to defined formula diets in rats. Am. J. Clin. Nutr., *33*:2106–2118, 1980, with permission.)

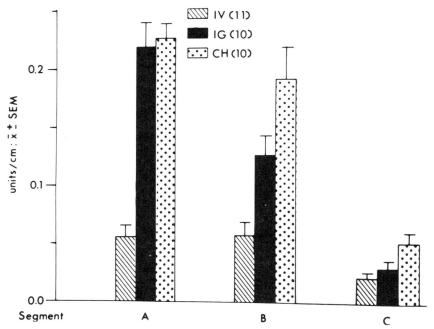

Figure 30–18.   Sucrase activity per unit length of small intestine is shown in the three segments (A, B, C) of the small intestine of rats fed intravenously (IV), a chemically defined diet (IG), or with rat chow (CH). Figures in parentheses indicate the number of animals. (*From* Morin, C. L., et al.: Small intestinal and colonic changes induced by a chemically defined diet. Dig. Dis. Sci., *25*:123–128, 1980, with permission.)

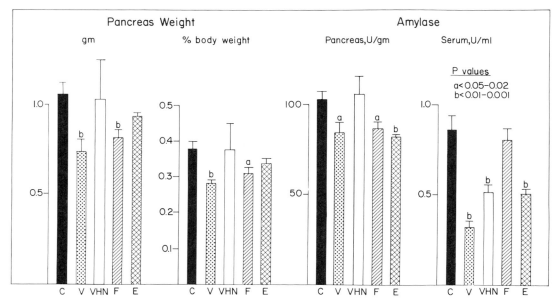

Figure 30–19.   Pancreas weight and pancreatic and serum amylase (mean ± SE) of chow reference and DFD groups. Diets are C = chow; V = Vivonex; VHN = Vivonex High Nitrogen; F = Flexical; E = Ensure. (*From* Young, E. A., et al.: Comparative study of nutritional adaptation to defined formula diets in rats. Am. J. Clin. Nutr., *33*:2106–2118, 1980, with permission.)

cretion can be collected and continuously returned to the intestine. This elegant model lends itself to a manipulation of the diet composition and a more direct assessment of the effect of DFD (Fig. 30–20). In this model pancreatic juice and bile can be collected separately or together, and can be returned mechanically by a peristaltic pump servo-system. This system is simple and has been proved reliable. Pancreatic juice and bile can also be redirected to the intestine (see Fig. 30–20).

Liver. It is well known that variations in the nutrient composition can significantly influence the accumulation of lipid of the livers of rodents.[99–101] As early as in the developmental stages of chemically DFD, Greenstein et al.[14] reported liver toxicity in rats maintained on some of the experimental liquid diets. Ferguson et al.[102] showed that mice reared on an elemental diet during the first 10 weeks after weaning had extensive fatty infiltration of the liver. Campbell et al.[103] reported fatty liver in rats maintained on an elemental diet; however, this was thought to result from a deficiency of choline. Young et al.[51] reported an accumulation of liver lipid in a rat model fed one of several DFD. In this study comparing the liver response to a variety of DFD given intragastrically to regular rat chow, the liver lipid

as percentage of body weight was greater in animals fed Vivonex and Vivonex HN. This finding was also demonstrated when these same diets were lapped up orally (Fig. 30–21),[104] or when these diets were isocalorically oral-fed or gastric-fed (Fig. 30–22).[59] In the latter study, no statistically significant differences were found as a result of the route of administration (see Fig. 30–22C). In these studies all animals were in positive nitrogen balance; however, nitrogen retention was less in animals on Vivonex and Flexical, reflecting a low nitrogen intake compared to the other formulas used. In addition, Vivonex and Vivonex HN have a very low fat content (1.3 per cent) and a very high glucose content (90 per cent). It has been suggested that increasing the proportion of either glucose or fat from a ratio of 75:25 glucose to fat calories could result in hepatic fatty infiltration in parenteral feeding.[105] The underlying mechanism leading to fatty liver in rats maintained on some DFD is not known.

Colon. There are few studies investigating changes in colonic mucosa associated with nutrient intake. Janne et al.[56] studied the influence of a liquid DFD (Vivonex) on weight, crypt cell number, and proliferative parameters in the colon of rats. In this model, DFD-fed rats were compared to a

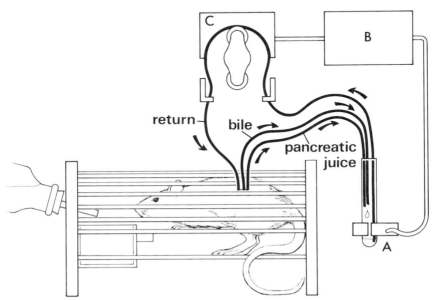

Figure 30–20. Diagram of rat model for selective collection of pancreatic and/or bile secretions. (*From* Green, G. M., et al.: Protein as a regulator of pancreatic enzyme secretion in the rat. Proc. Soc. Exptl. Biol. Med., *142*:1162–1167, 1973, with permission.)

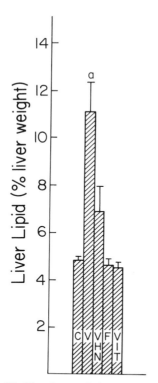

Figure 30–21. Accumulation of liver lipid as % of liver weight. Bars are mean value ± standard error for control and DFD groups (V = Vivonex; VHN = Vivonex High Nitrogen; F = Flexical; Vit = Vital). (*From* Young, E. A., et al.: Gastrointestinal response to nutrient variation of defined formula diets. J.P.E.N., 5:478–484, 1981, with permission. Copyright 1982 by The American Society of Parenteral and Enteral Nutrition.)

control group of rats eating regular rat chow ad libitum. After four weeks the weight of the colon was 43.7 per cent of control values. The crypt column length was decreased 49 per cent, crypt column count in the colonic mucosa 45.5 per cent, and the total cell population per crypt was decreased at 75.8 per cent of control values. It was suggested that the colonic mucosal and muscle atrophy observed in the DFD-fed rats may be caused by reduction in the residue bulk passing through the colon, deprivation of essential nutrients that normally reach the colon from the intestinal lumen, alteration of the bacterial flora of the colon, or modification of bile salts.[56]

Ryan et al.[55] compared the parenteral and enteral feeding of a DFD with the same DFD plus bulk (alpha-cellulose) or rat chow in a rat model. The animals fed parenterally

and enterally showed a 25 per cent loss of colonic weight as well as a decrease in mucosal DNA compared to chow-fed animals (Fig. 30–23). The addition of unabsorbable bulk to the DFD stimulated colonic DNA and growth without elevating serum or antral gastrin. The authors suggested that the gastrointestinal hormone gastrin and the physical effects of luminal contents were independently capable of stimulating colonic growth in rats.[55]

In a similar study[54] three groups of rats were fed a DFD intragastrically, an equivalent diet parenterally, and solid chow. All diets were given isocalorically over an eight day period. Colonic weight, DNA, and protein were significantly lower in animals receiving the liquid diets as compared to the chow (Fig. 30–24). The atrophied colon was similar to that observed in parenterally fed animals. These investigators also speculated

Effect of DFD on Accumulation of Liver Lipid

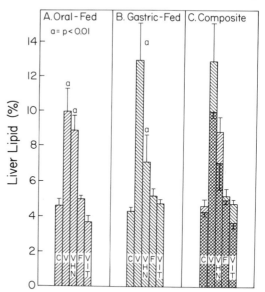

Figure 30–22. Accumulation of liver lipid as % of liver weight in animals maintained on the control or one of several DFD orally (A) or gastrically (B). Statistical analyses compare liver lipid for each DFD group with the control group. The composite panel (C) compares % liver lipid in oral-fed versus gastric-fed animals maintained on control or DFD formulas (V = Vivonex; VHN = Vivonex High Nitrogen; F = Flexical; Vit = Vital). Bars are mean values ± standard error of the mean. (*From* Young, E. A., et al.: Gastrointestinal response to oral versus gastric feeding of defined formula diets. Am. J. Clin. Nutr., 35:715–726, 1982, with permission.)

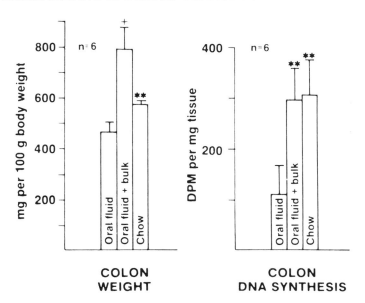

Figure 30–23. Colonic weight and DNA synthesis in oral fluid, oral fluid plus bulk, and chow groups. $^+$P <0.01; **P <0.05 compared with oral fluid group. (*From* Ryan, G. P., et al.: Effect of various diets on colonic growth in rats. Gastroenterology, 77:658–663, 1979, with permission. Copyright 1979 by The American Gastroenterological Association.)

that distal intestinal atrophy may simply result from lack of stimulation in that region.

Enteral Nutrients Versus Intravenous Nutrients

While the starvation model demonstrates small intestinal atrophy and hypoplasia,[40–48] this model does not distinguish between the negative nitrogen balance of fasting and the lack of enteral intake as the cause for the changes observed. These observations led some investigators to develop an animal model that would receive complete nutrient requirements intravenously to maintain positive nitrogen balance while receiving no oral nutrients. These animals

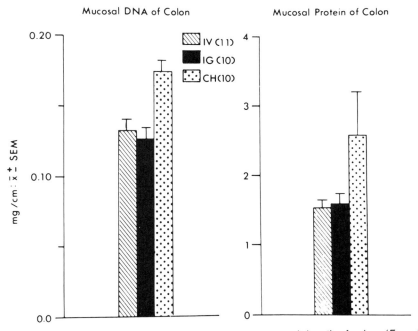

Figure 30–24. Comparison of mucosal DNA and protein content per unit length of colon. (*From* Morin, C. L., et al.: Small intestinal and colonic changes induced by a chemically defined diet. Dig. Dis. Sci., 25:123–128, 1980, with permission.)

could then be compared to a control group receiving the same diet enterally. Using this model with rats, Levine et al.[85] showed that the body weight gain of intravenously fed (IV) and gastrically fed (IG) rats had similar body weight gains over a seven-day infusion. Using a similar model, Lanza-Jacoby et al.[106] showed that the weight gain over a 14-day period was 13 ± 6 gm for rats fed IG and 16 ± 4 gm for rats fed IV.

In the parenteral versus enteral model of Levine et al.,[85] gut length was similar; however, whole small intestinal weight was 22 per cent less in the parenterally fed animals. The gut weight per centimeter of eight proximal to distal segments was significantly lower in the IV animals. Intestinal mucosal weight, protein, and DNA were lower than in orally fed animals by 28, 35, and 25 per cent, respectively. Similarly, parenterally fed animals showed a 46 per cent lower maltase, a 62 per cent lower sucrase, and a 44 per cent lower lactase activity compared to the orally fed animals. Using this enteral versus parenteral model, Levine et al.[85] conclusively demonstrated the importance of oral intake in the maintenance of gut mass and disaccharidase activity. The mechanism(s) by which these effects occur are not yet fully characterized. Possible processes relating to the digestion, secretion, and absorption of dietary intake that contribute to maintenance of gut mass include the following: the luminal presence of nutrients;[107, 108] factors present in biliary and/or pancreatic secretions;[109, 110] trophic properties of the gastrointestinal hormones;[47, 52] neural factors;[111, 112] and blood flow.[113]

Spector et al.[114, 115] have developed an elegant animal model designed to examine the effects of selective individual nutrients of elemental diets on the small intestine while the animals were supported by TPN. (Fig. 30–25). Rats were maintained on intravenous alimentation for one week while simultaneously receiving 30 per cent dextrose, 5 per cent dextrose, 5 per cent amino acids, and 30 per cent mannitol or saline by intragastric or ileal infusion. Proximal infusion of 30 per cent dextrose or amino acids had a direct effect on the proximal gut mass. Ileal infusion of 30 per cent dextrose and amino acids led to local hyperplasia of the site of infusion, and the dextrose infusion also produced hyperplasia of the proximal gut. These investigators concluded that intralum-

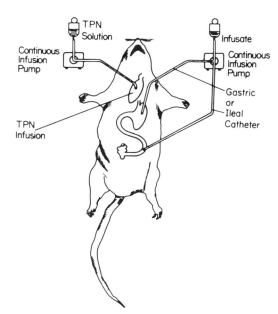

Figure 30–25. Gastric and ileal infusion system in parenterally nourished (TPN) rats. (*From* Spector, M. H., et al.: Stimulation of mucosal growth by gastric and ileal infusion of single amino acids in parenterally nourished rats. Digestion, *21*:33–40, 1981, with permission.)

inal dextrose and amino acids exert direct effects in maintaining gut mass, and speculated that the remote effect in the proximal gut observed after ileal infusion of 30 per cent dextrose may be elicited by hormonal, neural, or vascular responses that secondarily promote an increment in gut mass.[114]

In further studies utilizing this same model, Spector et al.[115] studied the effect on the intestinal mucosa of continuous infusion of single amino acids (glycine, valine, histidine) into the stomach and ileum of rats fed by parenteral nutrition. The mucosal growth responses noted in this study clearly demonstrated differences related to the gut region of infusion as well as the specific amino acid infused. Histidine infusion increased mucosa in the proximal bowel equal to a nutritionally complete amino acid mixture. After ileal infusion of all single amino acids, increased mucosal mass occurred at the site of infusion. In addition, ileal infusion of valine and histidine increased mucosal mass in the remote proximal small intestine. The mechanism(s) responsible for this remote effect of ileal perfusion of single amino acids has not yet been determined. This unique model permits the selective assessment of single nutrient intestinal infusions on intestinal mucosal growth.

Studies comparing liver response to parenteral versus enteral feeding of DFD have not yet been reported. As previously discussed, the enteral feeding of select DFD have demonstrated frank fatty liver.[51, 59, 104] The mechanisms leading to accumulation of lipid in the liver of animals maintained on enteral DFD have not been determined. Nevertheless, this finding is not surprising considering the several reports of fatty liver in animal models[116–121] and human patients[122–129] sustained on high carbohydrate parenteral feeding. This is a particular problem in infants, occurring in as many as 42 per cent of neonates receiving TPN.[122, 127, 128] Several studies of liver toxicity in human infants being nourished on oral elemental diets[130, 131] emphasize the importance that should be given to this aspect of enteral feeding. Various factors have been suggested as possible contributors to abnormal accumulation of liver lipid during parenteral feeding: (1) increasing the proportion of calories : fat from a 75:25 glucose : fat ratio;[105, 118] (2) depression of albumin synthesis and low plasma protein concentrations resulting in a shortage of protein needed to transport fat out of the liver;[125, 129, 132] (3) the synthesis of certain proteins may have a higher priority than some of the liver secretory proteins;[129] (4) the appetite regulatory mechanism is bypassed by force feeding, and fatty acids accumulate as the input of calories may be in excess of the liver's metabolic capability;[121, 129, 133] (5) a high carbohydrate, no-fat formulation could lead to essential fatty acid deficiency with consequent impairment of release of lipid;[134] (6) a continuous excess intake may lead to chronic hepatomegaly.[121, 129] Any single one or combination of these factors could also occur in continuous force feeding of an enteral formulation. Additional studies with animal models to elucidate the underlying mechanisms of fatty liver and abnormal liver function observed in both parenteral and enteral feeding are needed.

Pancreatic secretions have been shown to be decreased as a result of TPN.[91, 135–138] As previously noted, the effect of enteral feeding on pancreatic secretion is not well characterized,[39] but has been shown to be modified by the specific nutrient composition of DFD and also by the route of formula administration.[87–92] Animal models have been extensively used to study the pancreatic response to both parenteral and enteral feeding of DFD, and will continue to be used to further characterize pancreatic response to DFD.

While several reports have demonstrated atrophy in the proximal gastrointestinal tract of animals maintained on parenteral nutrition, little emphasis has been given to possible adaptive changes in the colon. As previously discussed,[54, 55, 114] the colonic mucosa and muscle are reduced in animals maintained on DFD compared to those on chow containing fiber. When colonic changes of DFD-fed animals are compared to those of parenterally fed animals (see Figs. 30–23 and 30–24), atrophy of the colon is similar.[54, 55] Mucosal weight, DNA, and protein are significantly and similarly reduced in both the parenteral and enteral DFD groups compared to fiber-containing chow or DFD plus added bulk.[54, 55]

Diversion of Pancreaticobiliary Secretion

The effect of diverting bile and pancreatic secretions into the ileum on small bowel mucosa has been studied in rats fed a DFD. The duodenal papilla containing the biliary and pancreatic ducts was transplanted by Altmann[109] into the ileum (Fig. 30–26), and rats were fed either a semisynthetic diet (10 per cent casein, 20 per cent lactalbumin hydrolysate, 42 per cent dextrose, 10 per cent sucrose, 9 per cent mixture of vitamins, salt, and yeast, 2 per cent corn oil, and 7 per cent cellulose residue; and weekly 10 per cent ethyl linoleate) or Purina Chow. In both instances villus size doubled in the ileal segment nearest to the transplanted duodenal papilla. This effect of relocating the duodenal papilla into the ileum was noted even in a "blind" or isolated loop of ileum not in continuity with the nutrient stream, suggesting that pancreaticobiliary secretions stimulated by ingested nutrients were responsible for the increase in villus size. Similar studies transplanting only the bile duct into the ileum revealed much less change in villus size indicating that pancreatic secretions or the combination of pancreatic secretions and bile were the potent factor(s) for villus growth.

More recent studies in rats have also

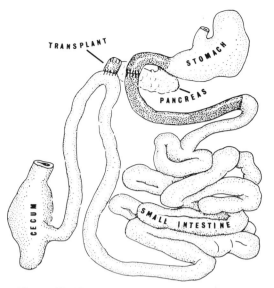

Figure 30–26. Transplantation of the duodenal papilla to the functional ileum. The duodenum is blackened. The pancreas is shown schematically; it is more diffuse in reality. (*From* Altmann, G. G.: Influence of bile and pancreatic secretion on the size of the intestinal villi in the rat. Am. J. Anat., *132*:167–177, 1971, with permission.)

shown that pancreaticobiliary diversion into ileum produces ileal mucosal hyperplasia in rats orally fed a DFD or given the same diet intravenously.[110, 139, 140] Not only does pancreaticobiliary diversion stimulate adaptive mucosal hyperplasia in the pancreaticobiliary secretion enriched ileum, but surprisingly, also in the pancreaticobiliary secretion deprived jejunum. Actually, the absence of these secretions from the jejunum prevented the hypoplasia typically seen in animals maintained on total intravenous feeding.[140] Thus the adaptive responses to bile and pancreatic secretions differ between jejunum and ileum.

In similar studies performed on rats maintained on a DFD after 50 per cent resection of the proximal small intestine, pancreaticobiliary diversion into ileum enhanced the mucosal hyperplasia usually seen in the ileal remnant.[110, 141] However, no changes were observed in the jejunum of these rats in the absence of pancreatic and biliary secretions.[141] In rats fed a DFD, neither bile nor pancreatic juice alone affected ileal mucosa when separately diverted into the ileum. However, pancreatic juice draining into the duodenum while bile was diverted into ileum induced hypoplastic changes in the duodenojeju-

num, again suggesting different regulatory mechanisms of mucosal growth by bile and pancreatic secretions in different parts of the small intestine.

Hormonal Effects of DFD

Dramatic changes in the small intestinal structure and function occur as a result of starvation[40-48] and parenteral feeding.[85] Since gastrointestinal hormones may play a significant role in these changes, recent investigations of possible hormonal response to starvation,[47, 142] parenteral feeding,[51, 55, 56] and to liquid DFD[56, 142, 143] have been carried out. Chemically, DFD given orally to rats can maintain gastrin levels and gastrointestinal structure and growth more effectively than when the diet is given parenterally[52, 85] but not as well as an oral chow diet.[52, 55, 56, 142] In studying the effect of various diets on colonic growth, Ryan et al.[55] demonstrated that neither intravenous nor oral liquid formulas maintained serum duodenal or antral gastrin as well as regular chow (Figs. 30–27 and 30–28). The addition of nonabsorbable bulk to the diet did not stimulate gastrin levels. Similarly, Sircar et al.[143] demonstrated that rats fed on a variety of DFD or pelleted diets can maintain the animals in positive

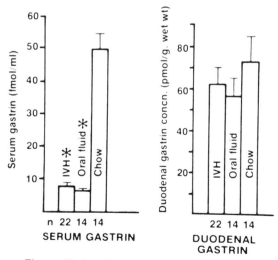

Figure 30–27. Serum and duodenal gastrin concentrations in intravenously hyperalimentated (IVH), oral fluid, and chow groups. *P <0.001 compared with chow-fed controls. (*From* Ryan, G. P., et al.: Effect of various diets on colonic growth in rats. Gastroenterology, 77:658–663, 1979, with permission. Copyright 1979 by The Gastroenterological Association.)

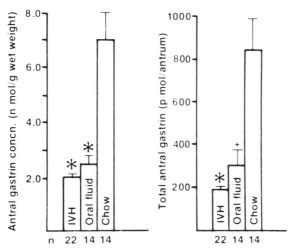

Figure 30–28. Antral gastrin levels in intravenously hyperalimentated (IVH), oral fluid, and chow groups. Results are expressed both as gastrin concentration (n mol/g wet weight) and as total antral gastrin (p mol/antrum). *P = 0.001; +P <0.001 compared with chow fed controls. (*From* Ryan, G. P., et al.: Effect of various diets on colonic growth in rats. Gastroenterology, 77:658–663, 1979, with permission. Copyright 1979 by The American Gastroenterological Association.)

pared to rats on fiber-containing chow (Figs. 30–29 and 30–30). These changes did not appear to be related to the protein, fat, or bulk present in the diets, or to antral acidification by the diets constituents. While gastrin has been identified as an important trophic gastrointestinal hormone, it has been proposed that the inability of synthetic diets to maintain normal gastrin levels may have important clinical significance.[142] Further studies are needed to sort out the relationships between gastrin and the use of liquid DFD.

In studies of rats infused enterally or parenterally with chemically formulated nutritionally complete diets, the enterally fed animals showed greater weight gain,[144] and elicited greater serum immunoreactive insulin, immunoreactive pancreatic glucagon, and enteroglucagon than in parenteral feeding. These hormones are possible candidates for mediation of more effective disposal of enteral nutrients than when these same nutrients are given parenterally.[144]

nitrogen balance with adequate weight gain. However, serum gastrin and antral gastrin were reduced 20 to 30 per cent and 40 to 50 per cent, respectively, in animals maintained on a variety of synthetic DFD com-

DFD and Cancer Models

Demographic reviews of the prevalence of human intestinal cancer[145–147] and studies of metabolic epidemiology[148, 149] have suggested that dietary factors are likely to have

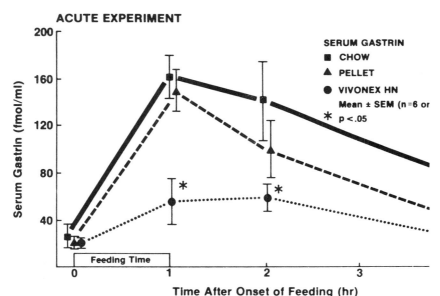

Figure 30–29. Postprandial rise in serum gastrin levels of rats fed chow, Vivonex HN, or ICN pelleted diet. Serum gastrin levels were measured after rats consumed respective diets in I-h test meal. Each point represents means of 6 or 7 rats ± SE. (*From* Sircar, B., et al.: Effect of chemically defined diets on antrol and serum gastrin levels in rats. Am. J. Physiol., *238* (Gastrointest. Liver. Physiol. 1):G376–G383. 1980, with permission.)

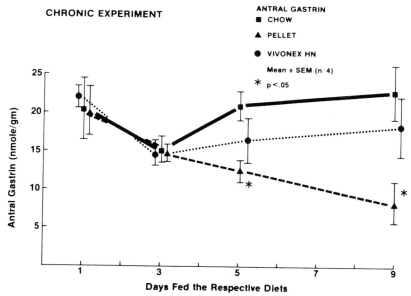

Figure 30–30. Antral gastrin levels of rats fed chow, Vivonex HN, or ICN pelleted diet for 1, 3, 5, and 9 days. (*From* Sircar, B., et al.: Effect of chemically defined diets on antrol and serum gastrin levels in rats. Am. J. Physiol., *238* (Gastrointest Liver Physiol. 1):G376–G383, 1980, with permission.)

an important role in the etiology of intestinal cancer. Castleden[150] has evaluated the influence of a chemically defined diet on intestinal tumor induction using a rat model. After treatment with 1,2-dimethylhydrazine (DMH), experimental animals received DFD (Vivonex) as the sole source of nutrition for a period of 24 weeks. A control nontreated group of rats were similarly nourished. It was apparent from the results of this study that the elemental diet protected the animals from DMH toxicity and significantly reduced the incidence of tumors of the small and large bowel.[150] Further investigation is needed to explore the possible protective effect of DFD in carcinogenesis.

The role of DFD in protecting the intestinal epithelium against ischemic necrosis[151] and lesions produced by 5-fluorouracil (5-FU)[152–155] have been reported. Bounous et al.[152, 153] carried out a series of experiments to determine the effects of an elemental diet upon changes produced by 5-FU in the intestinal mucosa of the rat. Their results indicated that there was a protective effect on the intestine of those animals receiving the DFD, although there was no improvement in survival time. Subsequent studies using this model suggested that the protective effect was due to the substitution of whole

protein by protein hydrolysate. With about 66 per cent of the nitrogen being in the form of free amino acids, it was suggested that the elemental diet would be more suitable for absorption than a formula containing a greater percentage of oligopeptides.[153] In contrast Gardner and Heading[154] were unable to demonstrate a protective effect of an elemental diet in rats after treatment with 5-FU. More recent studies reported by Stanford et al.[155] indicated that elemental diets enhanced the toxicity of 5-FU and suggested that this was related directly to the degree of protein hydrolysis of the specific elemental diet used. Differences in the results of these studies may, at least in part, be the result of differences in achieving consistent formula intake. These studies indicate that this model could be effectively used to elucidate the efficacy versus adversity of DFD in 5-FU treatment as well as treatment with other drugs. The potential contribution of this model to clinical medicine merits further investigation.

Castro et al.[156] have used a rat model to study the effect of enteral versus parenteral feeding on malabsorption in intestinal parasitism. After infection with *Trichinella spiralis*, rats were fed either a stock chow, or an elemental formula orally, intraduodenally, or intravenously. A control group of uninfected animals were similarly fed. The animals receiving DFD by continuous infusion intraduodenally or intravenously were able to maintain body weight and did not demonstrate deficiencies in membrane digestion induced by parasitism as did the rats fed orally. The investigators suggested that metabolic changes leading to weight loss in hosts on the stock diet during trichinosis resulted from a decreased food intake rather than from other metabolic effects caused by the parasites.[156] In other studies Ferguson et al.[102] used a mouse model to study the effects of parasite infection on the intestinal mucosa. Mice infected with *Mippostrongylus brasiliensis* or *Giardia muris* showed increased mucosal damage when sustained on DFD (Vivonex) as compared to parasitized mice maintained on regular mouse chow. The use of DFD was associated with enhanced mucosal damage, enhanced malabsorption, and a prolonged course of infection. These parasitized animal models used to study the effect of DFD on malabsorption and intestinal mucosal changes provide another model with important clinical potential.

The possibility that the gut may act as an important organ of drug metabolism has only recently been considered. Knodell et al.[157] assessed the contribution of intestinal pentobarbital metabolism to overall in vivo pentobarbital pharmacokinetics in a rat model maintained enterally (intragastrically) or parenterally on a DFD. These studies demonstrated a reduced systemic availability of the drug after oral administration as compared to portal vein administration in both the enterally and parenterally nourished group. This suggested that significant intestinal metabolism of the drug occurred. This study did not define the mechanism(s) involved; however, they suggested that the differences in pentobarbital pharmacokinetics may be attributed to effects on hepatic metabolism of the drug, differences in gut hormone release, or to differences in pancreatic secretion in response to the two different routes of alimentation.[157] Because of the increasing use of enteral and parenteral alimentation in clinical medicine, studies to determine the influence of route of feeding on drug metabolism are needed.

Using a mouse model, Hugon et al.[158] and Hugon[159] have demonstrated a positive effect of an elemental diet on the survival, weight recovery and the intestinal mitotic index of γ-irradiation. After prolonged administration of the DFD and several weeks after repeated irradiation doses, comparison was made with a control group receiving regular chow or a whole casein formula. These investigators reported no morphologic abnormalities in the intestinal mucosa during prolonged administration of the DFD. It was suggested that the synthetic DFD provides a balance of amino acids and dipeptides that may be beneficial for mucosal recovery.

Moore et al.[160] have utilized a dog model to quantitatively evaluate the effect of an elemental DFD on the patterns of motility of the small intestine. This study was prompted by suggestions that elemental diets "rest" the small bowel by decreasing motility and secretions because the nutrient substrates are all absorbed in the proximal gut. Slow wave and spike potentials were recorded from 14 electrode sites that were fixed equidistant along the serosal surface of the entire small intestine. These studies demonstrated that the myoelectrical activity of the small intestine of the dog is significantly greater after ingestion of DFD compared to during fasting, but significantly less than when regular dog food was eaten. Since it has been shown that the myoelectrical activity of the dog's small bowel during parenteral alimentation is unchanged from the prefasted pattern,[161] the investigators concluded that for optimal bowel "rest" in the dog, parenteral nutrition is the preferable form of nutritional therapy.

Circadian rhythms in liver and blood parameters in a rat model adapted to a nutrient formula by oral, parenteral, and discontinuous parenteral feeding have been recently reported by Sitren et al.[162] While a continuous drip of DFD has been advocated for optimal clinical efficacy, a constant input of nutrients into the body is not consistent with the normal pattern of food intake in humans or in most animals. Thus the results of this study of circadian rhythms when oral, parenteral, or discontinuous parenteral feeding methods are used indicate distinct differences in liver glycogen and protein, intestinal protein concentrations and disaccharidase activity, and circulating glucose and insulin concentrations. These findings have clear implications for enteral and parenteral administration of DFD under various clinical circumstances.

ANIMAL MODELS WITH A SURGICALLY MODIFIED GASTROINTESTINAL TRACT

Gut Segment Transposition Models

The rat has been used to study the effects of transpositions of small bowel segments on villus size. In a classic paper, Altmann and Leblond[163] transposed jejunal segments into ileum and ileal segments into jejunum (Fig. 30–31). Initially these rats were maintained on a semisynthetic diet containing 31 per cent protein hydrolysate, 63 per cent dextrose, and 6 per cent salt and vitamin mixture; after one week they were completely converted to Purina Chow ad libitum. After two months, in ileal segments inserted into the jejunum, villi enlarged to the size of local jejunal villi. In jejunal segments inserted into ileum, villi decreased almost to the size of local ileal villi. Thus villus size was influenced by the environment, most probably by different composition of chyme in jejunum and ileum. Similar findings have been reported by other investigators.[164]

Short-Gut Models

Chemically defined diets have been used in animal models of small bowel resection to study the effects of resection, type of diet, and route of feeding on structure and function of the remaining gastrointestinal tract. No studies have been reported comparing the effects of small bowel resection on the gastric mucosa in animals fed complex diets as compared to DFD. In chow-fed rats however, the gastric glandular mucosa undergoes hyperplasia after extensive small bowel resection compared with sham-surgery controls.[165, 166] Animals maintained on total intravenous nutrition after small bowel resection were shown to increase gastric mucosal mass if intravenous pentagastrin was administered for eight days.[167] In this study, no measurements were made in paired animals fed isocalorically with DFD by intragastric tube.

It has been well established that intestinal adaptation after small bowel resection occurs in both dogs and rats fed enterally with a DFD but is absent when isocaloric amounts of the same diet are given intravenously.[168-170] These studies established that

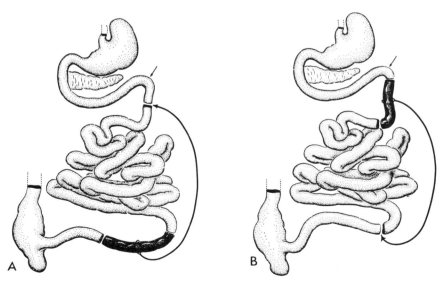

Figure 30–31. *A*, Transplantation of an ileal segment (darkened) to the jejunum. *B*, Transplantation of a jejunal segment (darkened) to the ileum. (*From* Altmann, G. G., and Leblond, C. P.: Factors influencing villus size in the small intestine of adult rats as revealed by transposition of intestinal segments. Am. J. Anat., *127*:15–30, 1970, with permission.)

enteral nutrients were a necessary stimulus for small intestinal hyperplasia after resection. In comparing the degree of intestinal adaptation with various types of enteral nutrition in rats, Buts et al.[171] showed that macromolecular diets were superior to chemically defined diets, which in turn led to greater adaptation than 30 per cent glucose. All these diets were given in isocaloric amounts and contrasted with intravenous administration of equal calories. Other workers have found similar results.[110] More recently, the influence of lipid on intestinal adaptation after resection was specifically studied. Long-chain triglycerides (corn oil) were found to stimulate significantly greater adaptation than protein, polysaccharides, or medium-chain triglycerides.[172] It is not clear whether this effect is primarily related to direct luminal mechanisms or is mediated by the release and circulation of enteric hormones. Recent studies in rats maintained on TPN for 7 or 14 days after small bowel resection have shown that octapeptide-cholecystokinin and secretin may stimulate intestinal adaptation in the remaining small bowel.[173] While the degree of adaptation was less than in rats given the DFD diet intragastrically, it was suggested that continued infusion of the hormones might produce adaptation equal to that of the enterally fed group. In addition to cholecystokinin and secretin, gastrin may also produce mucosal hyperplasia in some parts of the gastrointestinal tract. However, the intravenous infusion of pentagastrin for eight days in rats maintained on TPN after small bowel resection produced mucosal hyperplasia only in the proximal intestine and not in the typical distal small bowel as noted in control rats fed a chemically defined diet.[167] Therefore it is unlikely that circulating gastrin plays a role in small intestinal adaptation after small bowel resection.

CONCLUSIONS

The technologic capability of providing all essential nutrients in a bulk-free, liquid, defined formula diet is a major milestone in medicine. A variety of animal models have been used to determine the nutritional adequacy of DFD. The effect of variation in formulation of DFD and of the route of administration on the growth rate and on functional and structural aspects of the gastrointestinal tract have been reported. Both intact animal models as well as surgically modified models have been used, thus increasing our understanding of adaptation to dietary manipulation under a broader spectrum of experimental circumstances. Animal models have been used to explore the effect of various DFD on hormonal response; intestinal tumor induction; the protective effect on the intestinal epithelium against ischemic necrosis and lesions produced by 5-fluorouracil; the protective effect on malabsorption in intestinal parasitism; the importance of the gut as a drug-metabolizing organ; the protective effect of DFD on the survival, weight recovery and intestinal mitotic index following irradiation; the myoelectrical activity of the intestines; and the circadian rhythms in liver glycogen and proteins, intestinal protein and disaccharidase activities, and circulating glucose and insulin concentrations.

The results of these animal model studies suggest numerous clinical implications. Since nutrient intake plays such an essential role in metabolism and in structural and functional aspects of the gastrointestinal tract, the use of animal models in which the nutrient intake is precisely controlled can be effectively utilized in future research in a variety of medically related areas.

REFERENCES

1. Wood, E. H.: Testimony given before the U.S. House Subcommittee on Science, Research and Technology, October 13, 1981. FASEB Newsletter, 14:2–4, 1981.
2. Raub, W.: Testimony given before the U.S. House Subcommittee on Science, Research and Technology, October 13, 1981. Fed. Proc., 40:17a, 1981.
3. Hegarty, P. V.: Use of experimental animals in human nutrition research—some justifications and precautions. Contemp. Nutr., 6:1–2, 1981.
4. Dudrick, S. J., Vars, H. M., and Rhoads, J. E.: Growth of puppies receiving all nutritional requirements by vein. Fortschr. Parenteral Ernahrung, 2:16–18, 1966.
5. Epstein, A. N., and Teitelbaum, P.: A watertight swivel joint permitting chronic injection into moving animals. J. Appl. Physiol., 17:171–172, 1962.
6. Weeks, J. R., and David, J. D.: Chronic intravenous cannulas for rats. J. Appl. Physiol., 19:540–541, 1964.

7. Dalton, R. G., Touraine, J. L., and Wilson, T. R.: A simple technique for continuous intravenous infusion in rats. J. Lab. Clin. Med., 74:813–815, 1969.

8. Dudrick, S. J., Steiger, E., Wilmore, D. W., and Vars, H. M.: Continuous long-term intravenous infusion in unrestrained animals. Lab. Anim. Care, 20:521–529, 1970.

9. Edmonds, C. J., and Thompson, B. D.: A method allowing intravenous infusion of unrestrained rats for several weeks. J. Physiol. (Lond.), 207:41P–42P, 1970.

10. Edmonds, C. J., and Thompson, B. D.: Further development of a method for prolonged infusion of unrestrained rats. J. Physiol. (Lond.), 232:10P–12P, 1973.

11. Steiger, E., Vars, H. M., and Dudrick, S. J.: A technique for long-term intravenous feeding in unrestrained rats. Arch. Surg., 104:330–332, 1972.

12. Nicolaidis, S., Rowland, N., Meile, M.-J., Marfaing-Jallat, P., and Pesez, A.: A flexible technique for long-term infusions in unrestrained rats. Pharmacol. Biochem. Behav., 2:131–136, 1974.

13. Born, C. T., and Moller, M. L.: A simple procedure for long-term intravenous infusion in the rat. Lab. Anim. Sci., 24:355–358, 1974.

14. Greenstein, J. P., Birnbaum, S. M., Winitz, M., and Otey, M. C.: Quantitative nutritional studies with water-soluble, chemically defined diets. I. Growth, reproduction and lactation in rats. Arch. Biochem. Biophys., 72:396–416, 1957.

15. Birnbaum, S. M., Greenstein, J. P., and Winitz, M.: Quantitative nutritional studies with water-soluble, chemically defined diets. II. Nitrogen balance and metabolism. Arch. Biochem. Biophys., 72:417–427, 1957.

16. Birnbaum, S. M., Winitz, M., and Greenstein, J. P.: Quantitative nutritional studies with water-soluble, chemically defined diets. III. Individual amino acids as sources of "non-essential" nitrogen. Arch. Biochem. Biophys., 72:428–436, 1957.

17. Winitz, M., Birnbaum, S. M., and Greenstein, J. P.: Quantitative nutritional studies with water-soluble chemically defined diets. IV. Influence of various carbohydrates on growth, with special reference to D-glucosamine. Arch. Biochem. Biophys., 72:437–447, 1957.

18. Winitz, M., Greenstein, J. P., and Birnbaum, S. M.: Quantitative nutritional studies with water-soluble, chemically defined diets. V. Role of the isomeric arginines in growth. Arch. Biochem. Biophys., 72:448–456, 1957.

19. Birnbaum, S. M., Greenstein, M. E., Winitz, M., and Greenstein, J. P.: Quantitative nutritional studies with water-soluble, chemically defined diets. VI. Growth studies on mice. Arch. Biochem. Biophys., 78:245–247, 1958.

20. Sugimura, T., Birnbaum, S. M., Winitz, M., and Greenstein, J. P.: Quantitative nutritional studies with water-soluble, chemically defined diets. VII. Nitrogen balance in normal and tumor-bearing rats following forced feeding. Arch. Biochem. Biophys., 81:439–447, 1959.

21. Sugimura, T., Birnbaum, S. M., Winitz, M., and Greenstein, J. P.: Quantitative nutritional studies with water-soluble, chemically defined diets. VIII. The forced feeding of diets each lacking in one essential amino acid. Arch. Biochem. Biophys., 81:448–455, 1959.

22. Sugimura, T., Birnbaum, S. M., Winitz, M., and Greenstein, J. P.: Quantitative nutritional studies with water-soluble chemically defined diets. IX. Further studies on D-glucosamine-containing diets. Arch. Biochem. Biophys., 83:521–527, 1959.

23. Greenstein, J. P., Otey, M. C., Birnbaum, S. M., and Winitz, M.: Quantitative nutritional studies with water-soluble, chemically defined diets. X. Formulation of a nutritionally complete diet. J. Nat. Can. Instit., 24:211–219, 1960.

24. Winitz, M., Birnbaum, S. M., Sugimura, T., and Otey, M. C.: Quantitative nutritional and in vivo metabolic studies with water-soluble, chemically defined diets. In Edsall, J. T. (ed.): Amino Acids, Proteins and Cancer Biochemistry. Jesse P. Greenstein Memorial Symposium. New York, Academic Press, 1960, pp. 1–21.

25. Couch, R. B., Watkin, D. M., Smith, R. R., et al.: Clinical trials of water-soluble chemically defined diets [Abstract]. Fed. Proc., 19:13, 1960.

26. Winitz, M., Graff, J., Gallagher, N., et al.: Evaluation of chemical diets as nutrition for man-in-space. Nature, 205:741–743, 1965.

27. Winitz, M., Seedman, D. A., and Graff, J.: Studies in metabolic nutrition employing chemically defined diets. I. Extended feeding of normal human adult males. Am. J. Clin. Nutr., 23:525–545, 1970.

28. Winitz, M., Adams, R. F., Seedman, D. A., et al.: Studies in metabolic nutrition employing chemically defined diets. II. Effects on gut microflora populations. Am. J. Clin. Nutr., 23:546–559, 1970.

29. Heymsfield, S. B., Bethel, R. A., Ansley, J. D., et al.: Enteral hyperalimentation: An alternative to central venous hyperalimentation. Ann. Intern. Med., 90:63–71, 1979.

30. Shils, M. E.: Enteral nutrition by tube. Can. Res., 37:2432–2439, 1977.

31. Kaminski, M. V.: Enteral hyperalimentation. Surg. Gynecol. Obstet., 143:12–16, 1976.

32. Heymsfield, S. B., Horowitz, J., and Lawson, D. H.: Enteral hyperalimentation. In Burke, E. (ed.): Developments in Digestive Diseases. Vol. 3. Philadelphia, Lea and Febiger, 1980, Chapter 4.

33. Goode, A., Feggetter, J. G. W., Hawkins, T., and Johnston, I. D. A.: Use of an elemental diet for longterm nutritional support in Crohn's disease. Lancet, 1:122–124, 1976.

34. Torosian, M. H., and Rombeau, J. L.: Feeding by tube enterostomy. Surg. Gynecol. Obstet., 150:918–927, 1980.

35. Young, E. A., Heuler, N., Russell, P., and Weser, E.: Comparative nutritional analysis of chemically defined diets. Gastroenterology, 69:1338–1345, 1975.

36. Wilmore, D. W., McDougal, W. S., and Peterson, J. P.: Newer products and formulas for alimentation. Am. J. Clin. Nutr., 30:1498–1505, 1977.

37. Chawla, K. K., and Wright, J.: A primer on liquid formula diets. Pract. Gastroenterol., 11:9–15, 1978.

38. Shills, M. E., Bloch, A. S., and Chernoff, R.: Liquid Formulas for Oral and Tube Feeding. New York, Memorial Sloan-Kettering Cancer Center, 1979.

39. Koretz, R. L., and Meyer, J. H.: Elemental diets—facts and fantasies. Gastroenterology, 78:393–410, 1980.

40. Brown, H. O., Levine, M. L., and Lipkin, M.: In-

hibition of intestinal epithelial cell renewal and migration induced by starvation. Am. J. Physiol., 205:868–872, 1963.

41. Steiner, M., Bourges, H. R., Freedman, L. S., and Gray, S. J.: Effect of starvation on the tissue composition of the small intestine in the rat. Am. J. Physiol., 215:75–77, 1968.

42. Hooper, C. S., and Blair, M.: The effect of starvation on epithelial renewal in the rat duodenum. Exp. Cell Res., 14:175–181, 1958.

43. Imondi, A. R., Bales, M. E., and Lipkin, M.: Nucleic acid metabolism in the gastrointestinal tract of the mouse during fasting and restraint-stress. Exp. Mol. Pathol., 9:339–348, 1968.

44. McManus, J. P. A., and Isselbacher, K. J.: Effect of fasting versus feeding on the rat small intestine. Gastroenterology, 59:214–221, 1970.

45. Altman, G. G.: Influence of starvation and refeeding on mucosal size and epithelial renewal in the rat small intestine. Am. J. Anat., 133:391–400, 1972.

46. Clarke, R. M.: The effect of growth and of fasting on the number of villi and crypts of the small intestine of the albino rat. Am. J. Anat., 112:27–33, 1972.

47. Lichtenberger, L., Welsh, J. D., and Johnson, L. R.: Relationship between the changes in gastrin levels and intestinal properties in the starved rat. Am. J. Dig. Dis., 21:33–38, 1976.

48. Ecknauer, R., and Raffler, H.: Effect of starvation on small intestinal enzyme activity in germ-free rats. Digestion, 18:45–55, 1978.

49. Joint FAO/WHO: Ad Hoc Expert Committee. Report on energy and protein requirements. Geneva, World Health Organ. Tech. Rept. Ser. No. 522, 1973. Rome, FAO Nutrition Meetings Rept. Ser. No. 52, 1973.

50. National Academy of Science, National Research Council: Nutrient requirements of the laboratory rat. In Nutrient Requirements of Laboratory Animals. Washington, D.C., NAS-NRC, 1972, pp. 56–93.

51. Young, E. A., Cioletti, L. A., Winborn, W. B., Traylor, J. B., and Weser, E.: Comparative study of nutritional adaptation to defined formula diets in rats. Am. J. Clin. Nutr., 33:2106–2118, 1980.

52. Johnson, L. R., Copeland, E. M., Dudrick, S. J., Lichtenberger, L. M., and Castro, G. A.: Structural and hormonal alterations in the gastrointestinal tract of parenterally fed rats. Gastroenterology, 68:1177–1183, 1975.

53. Ecknauer, R., Sircar, B., and Johnson, L. R.: Effect of dietary bulk on small intestinal morphology and cell renewal in the rat. Gastroenterology, 81:781–786, 1981.

54. Morin, C. L., Ling, V., Bourassa, D.: Small intestinal and colonic changes induced by a chemically defined diet. Dig. Dis. Sci., 25:123–128, 1980.

55. Ryan, G. P., Dudrick, S. J., Copeland, E. M., and Johnson, L. R.: Effect of various diets on colonic growth in rats. Gastroenterology, 77:658–663, 1979.

56. Janne, P., Carpentier, Y., and Willems, G.: Colonic mucosal atrophy induced by a liquid elemental diet in rats. Am. J. Dig. Dis., 22:808–812, 1977.

57. Nelson, L. M., Russell, R. I., and Lee, F. D.: Elemental diet composition and the structure and function of rat small intestine: Comparison of the effects of two diets on morphology and in

vivo absorption of water. J.P.E.N., 5:204–206, 1981.

58. Nelson, L. M., Carmichael, H. A., Russell, R. I., and Lee, F. D.: Small intestinal changes induced by an elemental diet (Vivonex) in normal rats. Clin. Sci. Mol. Med., 55:509–511, 1978.

59. Young, E. A., Cioletti, L. A., Traylor, J. B., and Balderas, V.: Gastrointestinal response to oral versus gastric feeding of defined formula diets. Am. J. Clin. Nutr., 35:715–726, 1982.

60. Freeman, D. E., and Naylor, J. M.: Cervical esophagostomy to permit extraoral feeding of the horse. J. Am. Vet. Med. Assoc., 172:314–320, 1978.

61. Balkany, T. J., Baker, B. B., Bloustein, P. A., and Jafek, B. W.: Cervical esophagostomy in dogs. Endoscopic, radiographic and histopathologic evaluation of esophagitis induced by feeding tubes. Ann. Otol., 86:588–593, 1977.

62. Stick, J. A., Derksen, F. J., and Scott, E. A.: Equine cervical esophagostomy: Complications associated with duration and location of feeding tubes. Am. J. Vet. Res., 42:727–732, 1981.

63. Rivilis, J., McArdle, H., Wlodek, G. K., and Gurd, F. N.: The effects of an elemental diet on gastric secretion. Ann. Surg., 179:226–229, 1974.

64. Malagelada, J. R., Go, V. L. W., and Summerskill, W. H.: Different gastric, pancreatic and biliary responses to solid-liquid or homogenized meals. Dig. Dis. Sci., 24:101–110, 1979.

65. Bury, K. D., and Jambunathan, G.: Effects of elemental diets on gastric emptying and gastric secretion in man. Am. J. Surg., 127:59–64, 1974.

66. Bond, J. H., and Levitt, M. D.: Effect of dietary fibers on intestinal gas production and small bowel transit time in man. Am. J. Clin. Nutr., 31:S169–S174, 1978.

67. Eastwood, M. A.: Fiber in the gastrointestinal tract. Am. J. Clin. Nutr., 31:S30–S32, 1978.

68. Devroede, G.: Dietary fiber, bowel habits and colonic function. Am. J. Clin. Nutr., 31:S157–S160, 1978.

69. Floch, M. H., and Fuchs, H.-M.: Modification of stool content by increased bran intake. Am. J. Clin. Nutr., 31:S185–S189, 1978.

70. Finegold, S. M., and Sutter, V. L.: Fecal flora in different populations: With special reference to diet. Am. J. Clin. Nutr., 31:S116–S122, 1978.

71. Bornside, G. H.: Stability of human fecal flora. Am. J. Clin. Nutr., 31:S141–S144, 1978.

72. Drasar, B. S., and Jenkins, D. J. A.: Bacteria, diet and large bowel cancer. Am. J. Clin. Nutr., 29:1410–1416, 1976.

73. Kern, F., Jr., Birkner, H. J., and Ostrower, V. S.: Binding of bile acids by dietary fibers. Am. J. Clin. Nutr., 31:S175–S179, 1978.

74. Story, J. A., and Kritchevsky, D.: Bile acid metabolism and fiber. Am. J. Clin. Nutr., 31:S199–S202, 1978.

75. Sandstead, H. H., Muñoz, J. M., Jacob, R. A., et al.: Influence of dietary fiber on trace element balance. Am. J. Clin. Nutr., 31:S180–S184, 1978.

76. Cummings, J. H.: Nutritional implications of dietary fiber. Am. J. Clin. Nutr., 31:S21–S29, 1978.

77. Lorenz-Meyer, H., Fimmel, C., and Teutenberg, M.: The effect of the elemental diet on the morphology and function of the intestinal mucosa after long-term exposure. Aktuel. Ernahrungsmedizin, 5:74–80, 1980.

78. Lehnert, S.: Changes in growth kinetics of jejunal

epithelium in mice mantained on an elemental diet. Cell Tissue Kinet., *12*:239–248, 1979.

79. Rosensweig, N. S.: Dietary sugars and intestinal enzymes. J. Am. Diet. Assoc., *60*:483–486, 1972.

80. Sriratanaban, A., and Thayer, W. R.: Small intestinal disaccharidase activities in experimental iron and protein deficiency. Am. J. Clin. Nutr., *24*:411–415, 1971.

81. McCarthy, D. M., Nicholson, J. A., and Kim, Y. S.: Intestinal enzyme adaptation to normal diets of different composition. Am. J. Physiol., *239* (6):G445–G451, 1980.

82. Bowie, M. D., Barbezat, G. O., and Hansen, J. D. L.: Carbohydrate absorption in malnourished children. Am. J. Clin. Nutr., *20*:89–97, 1967.

83. Solimano, G., Burgess, E. A., and Levin, B.: Protein-calorie malnutrition: Effect of deficient diets on enzyme levels of jejunal mucosa of rats. Br. J. Nutr., *21*:55–68, 1967.

84. Prosper, J., Murray, R. L., and Kern, F., Jr.: Protein starvation and the small intestine. II. Disaccharidase activities. Gastroenterology, *55*:223–228, 1968.

85. Levine, G. M., Deren, J. J., Steiger, E., and Zinno, R.: Role of oral intake in maintenance of gut mass and disaccharidase activity. Gastroenterology, *67*:975–982, 1974.

86. Dworkin, L. D., Levine, G. M., Farber, N. J., and Spector, M. H.: Small intestinal mass of the rat is partially determined by indirect effects of intraluminal nutrition. Gastroenterology, *71*:626–630, 1976.

87. Neviackas, J. A., and Kerstein, M. D.: Pancreatic enzyme response with an elemental diet. Surg. Gynecol. Obstet., *142*:71–74, 1976.

88. Ragins, H., Levenson, S. M., Signer, R., et al.: Intrajejunal administration of an elemental diet at neutral pH avoids pancreatic stimulation. Am. J. Surg., *126*:606–614, 1973.

89. Cassim, M. M., and Allardyce, D. B.: Pancreatic secretion in response to jejunal feeding of elemental diet. Ann. Surg., *180*:228–231, 1974.

90. Wolfe, B. M., Keltner, R. M., Kaminski, D. L.: The effect of an intraduodenal elemental diet on pancreatic secretion. Surg. Gynecol. Obstet., *140*:241–245, 1975.

91. Kelly, G. A., and Nahrwold, D. L.: Pancreatic secretion in response to an elemental diet and intravenous hyperalimentation. Surg. Gynecol. Obstet., *143*:87–92, 1976.

92. Desnuelle, P., Reboud, J. P., and Abdeljid, A. B.: Influence of the composition of the diet on the enzyme content of rat pancreas. *In* deReuck, A. V. S., and Cameron, M. (eds.). The Exocrine Pancreas. Ciba Foundation Symposium on the Exocrine Pancreas. Boston, Little, Brown and Co., 1961, pp. 90–114.

93. Snook, J. T., and Meyer, J. H.: Response of digestive enzymes to dietary protein. J. Nutr., *82*:409–414, 1964.

94. Snook, J. T., and Meyer, J. H.: Effect of diet and digestive processes on proteolytic enzymes. J. Nutr., *83*:94–102, 1964.

95. Howard, F., and Yudkin, J.: Effect of dietary change upon the amylase and trypsin activities of the rat pancreas. Br. J. Nutr., *17*:281–292, 1963.

96. Snook, J. T.: Dietary regulation of pancreatic en-

zymes in the rat with emphasis on carbohydrate. Am. J. Physiol., *221*:1383–1387, 1971.

97. Bounous, G., Devroede, G., Hugon, J. S., and Charuel, C.: Effects of an elemental diet on the pancreatic proteases in the intestine of the mouse. Gastroenterology, *64*:577–582, 1973.

98. Green, G. M., Olds, B. A., Matthews, G., and Lyman, R. L.: Protein as a regulator of pancreatic enzyme secretion in the rat. Proc. Soc. Exp. Biol. Med., *142*:1162–1167, 1973.

99. MacDonald, R. A.: Pathogenesis of nutritional cirrhosis. Arch. Intern. Med., *110*:424–434, 1962.

100. Zaki, F. G., Hoffbauer, F. W., and Grande, F.: Fatty cirrhosis in the rat. Arch. Pathol., *80*:323–331, 1965.

101. Harper, A. E.: Nutritional fatty liver in rats. Am. J. Clin. Nutr., *6*:242–253, 1958.

102. Ferguson, A., Logan, R. F. A., and MacDonald, T. T.: Increased mucosal damage during parasite infection in mice fed an elemental diet. Gut, *21*:37–43, 1980.

103. Campbell, A. H., Sewell, W. R., Chudkowski, M., et al.: The effects of feeding an elemental chemical diet to mature rats: Toxicologic and pathologic studies. Toxicol. Appl. Pharmacol., *26*:63–71, 1973.

104. Young, E. A., Cioletti, L. A., Traylor, J. B., and Balderas, V.: Gastrointestinal response to nutrient variation of defined formula diets. J.P.E.N., *5*:478–484, 1981.

105. Buzby, G. P., Mullen, J. L., Stein, T. P., et al.: Optimal TPN calorie substrate for correction of protein malnutrition of the liver. Surg. Forum, *30*:64–67, 1979.

106. Lanza-Jacoby, S., Sitren, H. S., Stevenson, N. R., et al.: Comparative adaptation to intragastric and intravenous feeding with a hypertonic alimentation diet. Surg. Forum, *31*:101–103, 1980.

107. Dowling, R. H.: Compensatory changes in intestinal absorption. Br. Med. Bull., *23*:275–278, 1967.

108. Gleeson, M. H., Cullen, J., Dowling, R. H.: Intestinal structure and function after small bowel bypass in the rat. Clin. Sci., *43*:731–742, 1972.

109. Altmann, G. G.: Influence of bile and pancreatic secretion on the size of the intestinal villi in the rat. Am. J. Anat., *132*:167–177, 1971.

110. Weser, E., Heller, R., and Tawil, T.: Stimulation of mucosal growth in the rat ileum by bile and pancreatic secretions after jejunal resection. Gastroenterology, *73*:524–529, 1977.

111. Dupont, J. R., Biggers, D. C., and Sprinz, H.: Intestinal renewal and immunosympathectomy. Arch. Pathol., *80*:357–362, 1965.

112. Silen, W., Peloso, O., and Jaffe, B. F.: Kinetics of intestinal epithelial proliferation: Effect of vagotomy. Surgery, *60*:127–135, 1966.

113. Touloukian, R. J., and Spencer, R. P.: Illeal blood flow preceding compensatory intestinal hypertrophy. Ann. Surg., *175*:320–325, 1972.

114. Spector, M. H., Levine, G. M., and Deren, J. J.: Direct and indirect effects of dextrose and amino acids on gut mass. Gastroenterology, *72*:706–710, 1977.

115. Spector, M. H., Traylor, S., Young, E. A., and Weser, E.: Stimulation of mucosal growth by gastric and ileal infusion of single amino acids in parenterally nourished rats. Digestion, *21*:33–40, 1981.

116. Steiger, E., et al.: Postoperative intravenous nutrition: Effects on body weight, protein regeneration, wound healing and liver morphology. Surgery, 73:686–691, 1973.

117. Daly, J. M., Steiger, E., Vars, H. M., and Dudrick, S. J.: Postoperative oral and intravenous nutrition. Ann. Surg., 180:709–715, 1974.

118. Chang, S., and Silvis, S. E.: Fatty liver produced by hyperalimentation of rats [Abstract]. Gastroenterology, 64:178, 1973.

119. Machytka, B., Hoos, I., and Förster, H.: Fatty liver in rats following parenteral hyperalimentation with glucose or glucose substitutes. Nutr. Metab., 21 (Suppl. 1):110–112, 1977.

120. Mashima, Y.: Effect of calorie overload on puppy livers during parenteral nutrition. J.P.E.N., 3:139–145, 1979.

121. Buzby, G. P., Mullen, J. L., Stein, T. P., Rosato, E. F.: Manipulation of TPN caloric substrate and fatty infiltration of the liver. J. Surg. Res., 31:46–54, 1981.

122. Bernstein, J., Chang, C.-H., Brough, A. J., and Heidelberger, K. P.: Conjugated hyperbilirubinemia in infancy associated with parenteral alimentation. J. Pediatr., 90:361–367, 1977.

123. Broviac, J. W., and Schribner, C. H.: The artificial gut: Two years' experience with total parenteral nutrition in the home [Abstract]. Gastroenterology, 62:727, 1972.

124. Peden, V. H., Witzleben, C. L., and Skelton, M. A.: Total parenteral nutrition. J. Pediatr., 78:180–181, 1971.

125. Sheldon, G. F., Scott, R. P., and Sanders, R.: Hepatic dysfunction during hyperalimentation. Arch. Surg., 113:504–508, 1978.

126. Touloukian, R. J., and Downing, S. E.: Cholestasis associated with long-term parenteral hyperalimentation. Arch. Surg., 106:58–62, 1973.

127. Touloukian, R. J., and Seashore, J. H.: Hepatic secretory obstruction with total parenteral nutrition in the infant. J. Pediatr. Surg., 10:353–360, 1975.

128. Hirai, Y., Sanada, Y., Fujiwara, T., et al.: High calorie infusion-induced hepatic impairments in infants. J.P.E.N., 3:146–150, 1979.

129. Stein, T. P., Buzby, G. P., Gertner, M. H., et al.: Effect of parenteral nutrition on protein synthesis and liver fat metabolism in man. Am. J. Physiol., 239:G280–287, 1980.

130. Sherman, J. O., Hamly, C. A., and Khachadurian, A. K.: Use of an oral elemental diet in infants with severe intractable diarrhea. J. Pediatr., 86:518–523, 1975.

131. Hirai, Y., Sanada, Y., and Nakagawa, T.: An enteral elemental diet for infants and children with surgical disorders. J.P.E.N., 4:460–463, 1980.

132. Flores, H., Sierralta, W., and Monckeberg, F.: Triglyceride transport in protein-depleted rats. J. Nutr., 100:375–379, 1970.

133. Burke, J. F., Wolfe, B. B., Mullany, C. J., et al.: Glucose requirements following burn injury. Ann. Surg., 190:274–285, 1979.

134. Fukazawa, T., Privett, O. S., and Takahashi, Y.: Effect of EFA deficiency on lipid transport from liver. Lipids, 6:386–393, 1971.

135. Hughes, C. A., Bates, T., and Dowling, H.: Cholecystokinin and secretin prevent the intestinal mucosal hypoplasia of total parenteral nutrition in the dog. Gastroenterology, 75:34–41, 1978.

136. Hamilton, R. E., et al.: Effects of parenteral hyperalimentation on upper gastrointestinal tract secretions. Arch. Surg., 102:348–352, 1971.

137. Towne, J. B., Hamilton, R. E., and Stephenson, D. V., Jr.: Mechanism of hyperalimentation in the suppression of upper gastrointestinal secretions. Am. J. Surg., 126:714–716, 1973.

138. Kotler, D. P., Levine, G. M.: Reversible gastric and pancreatic hyposecretion after long-term total parenteral nutrition. N. Engl. J. Med., 300:241–242, 1979.

139. Weser, E., Drummond, A., and Tawil, T.: Effect of diverting bile and pancreatic secretions into ileum on small bowel mucosa in rats fed a liquid formula diet. J.P.E.N., 6:39–42, 1982.

140. Miazza, B. M., Levan, H., Vaja, S., and Dowling, R. H.: Effect of pancreatico-biliary diversion on jejunal and ileal structure and function in the rat. In Intestinal Adaptation 2. Proceedings of International Conference, Titisee/Black Forest, West Germany, May 24–31, 1981. Lancaster, England, MTP Press, 1982, pp. 467–479.

141. Gélinas, M. D., and Morin, C. L.: Effects of bile and pancreatic secretions on intestinal mucosa after proximal small bowel resection in rats. Can. J. Physiol. Pharmacol., 58:1117–1123, 1980.

142. Lichtenberger, L. M., Lechago, J., and Johnson, L. R.: Depression of antral and serum gastrin concentration by food deprivation in the rat. Gastroenterology, 68:1473–1479, 1975.

143. Sircar, B., Johnson, L. R., and Lichtenberger, L. M.: Effect of chemically defined diets on antral and serum gastrin levels in rats. Am. J. Physiol., 238 (4):G376–G383, 1980.

144. Lickley, H. L. A., Track, N. S., Vranic, M., and Bury, K. D.: Metabolic responses to enteral and parenteral nutrition. Am. J. Surg., 135:172–176, 1978.

145. Doll, R.: The geographical distribution of cancer. Br. J. Cancer, 23:1–8, 1969.

146. Wynder, E. L.: The epidemiology of large bowel cancer. Cancer Res., 35:3388–3394, 1975.

147. Bjelke, E.: Epidemiologic studies of cancer of the stomach, colon and rectum; with special emphasis on the role of diet. Scand. J. Gastroenterol., 9(Suppl. 31):1–235, 1974.

148. Hill, M. J.: Metabolic epidemiology of dietary factors in large bowel cancer. Cancer Res., 35:3398–3402, 1975.

149. Reddy, B. S., and Wynder, E. L.: Large bowel carcinogenesis: Fecal constituents of populations with diverse incidence rates of colon cancer. J. Natl. Can. Inst., 50:1437–1442, 1973.

150. Castleden, W. M.: Prolonged survival and decrease in intestinal tumours in dimethylhydrazine-treated rats fed a chemically defined diet. Br. J. Cancer, 35:491–495, 1977.

151. Bounous, G., Sutherland, N. G., McArdle, A. H., and Gurd, F. N.: Prophylactic use of an "elemental" diet in experimental hemorrhagic shock and intestinal ischemia. Ann. Surg., 166:312–343, 1967.

152. Bounous, G., Hugon, J., and Gentile, J. M.: Elemental diets in the management of the intestinal lesion produced by 5-fluorouracil in the rat. Can. J. Surg., 14:298–311, 1971.

153. Bounous, G., and Maestracci, D.: Use of an elemental diet in animals during treatment with 5-fluorouracil (NSC-19893). Cancer Treat. Rep.,

60:17–22, 1976.

154. Gardner, M. L. G., and Heading, R. C.: Effects of elemental diets on absorptive and enzymic activities and on 5-fluorouracil toxicity in rat small intestine. Clin. Sci., 56:243–249, 1979.

155. Stanford, J. R., Carey, L. C., King, D. R., and Anderson, G. W.: Adverse effects of elemental diets on tolerance for fluorouracil (5-FU) toxicity in rats. Surg. Forum, 27:42–43, 1976.

156. Castro, G. A., Copeland, E. M., Dudrick, S. J., and Ramaswamy, K.: Enteral and parenteral feeding to evaluate malabsorption in intestinal parasitism. Am. J. Trop. Med. Hyg., 28:500–507, 1979.

157. Knodell, R. G., Spector, M. H., Brooks, D. A., et al.: Alterations in pentobarbital pharmacokinetics in response to parenteral and enteral alimentation in the rat. Gastroenterology, 79:1211–1216, 1980.

158. Hugon, J. S., and Bounous, G.: Protective effect of an elemental diet on radiation enteropathy in the mouse. Strahlentherapie, 146:701–712, 1973.

159. Hugon, J. S.: Intestinal ultrastructure after prolonged use of an elemental diet. Strahlentherapie, 151:541–548, 1976.

160. Moore, E. P., Copeland, E. M., Dudrick, S. J., and Weisbrodt, N. W.: Effect of an elemental diet on the electrical activity of the small intestine in dogs. J. Surg. Res., 20:533–537, 1976.

161. Weisbrodt, N. W., Copeland, E. M., Thor, P. J., and Dudrick, S. J.: Small bowel motility during intravenous hyperalimentation in the dog [Abstract 154]. Gastroenterology, 68:1011, 1975.

162. Sitren, H. S., and Stevenson, N. R.: Circadian fluctuations in liver and blood parameters in rats adapted to a nutrient solution by oral, intravenous and discontinuous intravenous feeding. J. Nutr., 110:558–566, 1980.

163. Altmann, G. G., and Leblond, C. P.: Factors influencing villus size in the small intestine of adult rats as revealed by transposition of intestinal segments. Am. J. Anat., 127:15–30, 1970.

164. Grönqvist, B., Engström, B., and Grimelius, L.: Morphological studies of the rat small intestine after jejuno-ileal transposition. Acta Chir. Scand., 141:208–217, 1975.

165. Winborn, W. B., Seelig, L. L., Jr., Nakayama, H., and Weser, E.: Hyperplasia of the gastric glands after small bowel resection in the rat. Gastroenterology, 66:384–395, 1974.

166. Seelig, L. L., Jr., Winborn, W. B., and Weser, E.: The effect of small bowel resection on the gastric mucosa in the rat. Gastroenterology, 72:421–428, 1977.

167. Morin, C. L., and Ling, V.: Effect of pentagastrin on the rat small intestine after resection. Gastroenterology, 75:224–229, 1978.

168. Feldman, E. J., Dowling, R. H., McNaughton, J., and Peters, T. J.: Effects of oral versus intravenous nutrition on intestinal adaptation after small bowel resection in the dog. Gastroenterology, 70:712–719, 1976.

169. Levine, G. M., Deren, J. J., and Yezdimir, E.: Small bowel resection. Oral intake is the stimulus for hyperplasia. Am. J. Dig. Dis., 21:542–546, 1976.

170. Morin, C. L., Long, V., Van Caillie, M.: Role of oral intake on intestinal adaptation after small bowel resection in growing rats. Pediatr. Res., 12:268–271, 1978.

171. Buts, J., Morin, C. L., and Ling, V.: Influence of dietary components on intestinal adaptation after small bowel resection in rats. Clin. Invest. Med., 2:59–66, 1979.

172. Morin, C. L., Grey, V. L.: Influence of lipid on intestinal adaptation after resection. In Intestinal Adaptation 2. Proceedings of an International Conference, Titisee/Black Forest, West Germany, May 24–31, 1981. Lancaster, England, MTP Press, 1982, pp. 175–185.

173. Weser, E., Bell, D., and Tawil, T.: Effects of octapeptide-cholecystokinin, secretin, and glucagon on intestinal mucosal growth in parenterally nourished rats. Dig. Dis. Sci., 26:409–416, 1981.

174. Weser, E., Tawil, T., and Fletcher, J. T.: Stimulation of small bowel mucosal growth by gastric infusion of different sugars in rats maintained on total parenteral nutrition. In Robinson, J. W. L., Dowling, R. H., and Riecken, E. O. (eds.): Mechanisms of Intestinal Adaptation: Proceedings of the Second International Conference on Intestinal Adaptation (Falk Symposium 30), 1981. Lancaster, England, MTP Press Ltd., 1982, pp. 141–152.

Index

Note: Page numbers in italics refer to illustrations; those followed by t refer to tables.